Cardiac Surgery

Perioperative Patient Care

Cardiac
Surgery
Perioperative Patient Care

Patricia C. Seifert, RN, MSN, CRNFA, FAAN

Coordinator, Cardiovascular Service Line
Virginia Hospital Center–Arlington
Arlington, Virginia

With 665 Illustrations

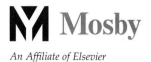 Mosby

An Affiliate of Elsevier

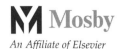
Mosby
An Affiliate of Elsevier

Vice-President, Nursing Editorial Director: Sally Schrefer
Senior Editor: Michael S. Ledbetter
Senior Developmental Editor: Lisa P. Newton
Publishing Services Manager: Deborah L. Vogel
Project Manager: Ann E. Rogers
Design Manager: Bill Drone
Cover Designer: Christine Fullgraf

NOTICE

Pharmacology is an ever-changing field. Standard safety precautions must be followed, but as new research and clinical experience broaden our knowledge, changes in treatment and drug therapy may become necessary or appropriate. Readers are advised to check the most current product information provided by the manufacturer of each drug to be administered to verify the recommended dose, the method and duration of administration, and contraindications. It is the responsibility of the treating physician, relying on experience and knowledge of the patient, to determine dosages and the best treatment for each individual patient. Neither the publisher nor the editor assumes any liability for any injury and/or damage to persons or property arising from this publication.

Mosby, Inc.
An Affiliate of Elsevier
11830 Westline Industrial Drive
St. Louis, Missouri 63146

Printed in the United States of America

Library of Congress Cataloging in Publication Data
Seifert, Patricia C.
  Cardiac surgery: perioperative patient care/Patricia C. Seifert.
    p.; cm.
  Includes bibliographical references and index.
  ISBN 0-323-01426-7
  1. Heart—Surgery. 2. Heart—Surgery—Nursing. 3. Operating room nursing. I. Title.
  [DNLM: 1. Cardiac Surgical Procedures—nursing. 2. Operating Room
  Nursing—methods. WY 162 S4592c 2002]
  RD598 .S3862 2002
  617.4'12—dc21

                                                    2002019265

04 05 06 GW/MVY 9 8 7 6 5 4 3 2

To my husband, Gary

Contributors

Patricia E. Chapek, RN, BA, CNOR
Chapter 16
Staff Nurse, Cardiothoracic O.R.
Cleveland Clinic Foundation
Cleveland, Ohio

Vicki J. Fox, MSN, RN, ACNP-CS
Chapter 19
Acute Care Nurse Practitioner
Trauma Service–Trinity Mother Frances Health System
Tyler, Texas

Tonya Kraus, RN, MSN
Chapter 15
Assist Device and Heart Transplant Coordinator
Inova Transplant Center
Fairfax Hospital
Falls Church, Virginia

Jane C. Rothrock, DNSc, RN, CNOR, FAAN
Chapter 5
Professor and Director, Perioperative Programs
Delaware County Community College
Media, Pennsylvania

Reviewers

Bea Colburn, RN, BS, CNOR
Nurse Clinician, Cardiothoracic, Vascular Services
Mt. Diablo Medical Center
Concord, California

Reneé Lynn Dodge, RN, MSN, CNOR, RNFA
Cardiovascular Specialty Service Coordinator
Sutter Memorial Hospital
Sacramento, California

Christine C. Espersen, RN, CNOR, CRNFA
CRNFA Cardiac Surgery
Buffalo General Hospital
Buffalo, New York

Rebecca Freda, RN, RNFA, CNOR
Assistant Coordinator CVOR
Virginia Hospital Center–Arlington
Arlington, Virginia

John R. Garrett, MD, FACS
Chief of Cardiac Surgery
Chief of Non-Cardiac, Thoracic, and Vascular Surgery
Virginia Hospital Center–Arlington
Arlington, Virginia

Michael H. Goldman, MD, FACC
Consultative Cardiologist for Congenital Heart Disease
Inova Fairfax Hospital
Consultative Cardiologist
Virginia Hospital Center–Arlington
Arlington, Virginia

Lauren Holwager, CST
Staff member, CVOR Team
Virginia Hospital Center–Arlington
Arlington, Virginia

Edward A. Lefrak, MD
Chief, Cardiac Surgery
Inova Fairfax Hospital and the Inova Heart Institute
Annandale, Virginia

Shawn W. Palmiter, BS, RCIS
Quality Improvement Outcomes Database Analyst
Virginia Hospital Center–Arlington
Arlington, Virginia

Rebecca Rose, RN, BSN, CCRN
Patient Care Director
Virginia Hospital Center–Arlington
Arlington, Virginia

Leslie A. Wyatt, RN, CRNFA
Patient Care Director CVOR
Virginia Hospital Center–Arlington
Arlington, Virginia

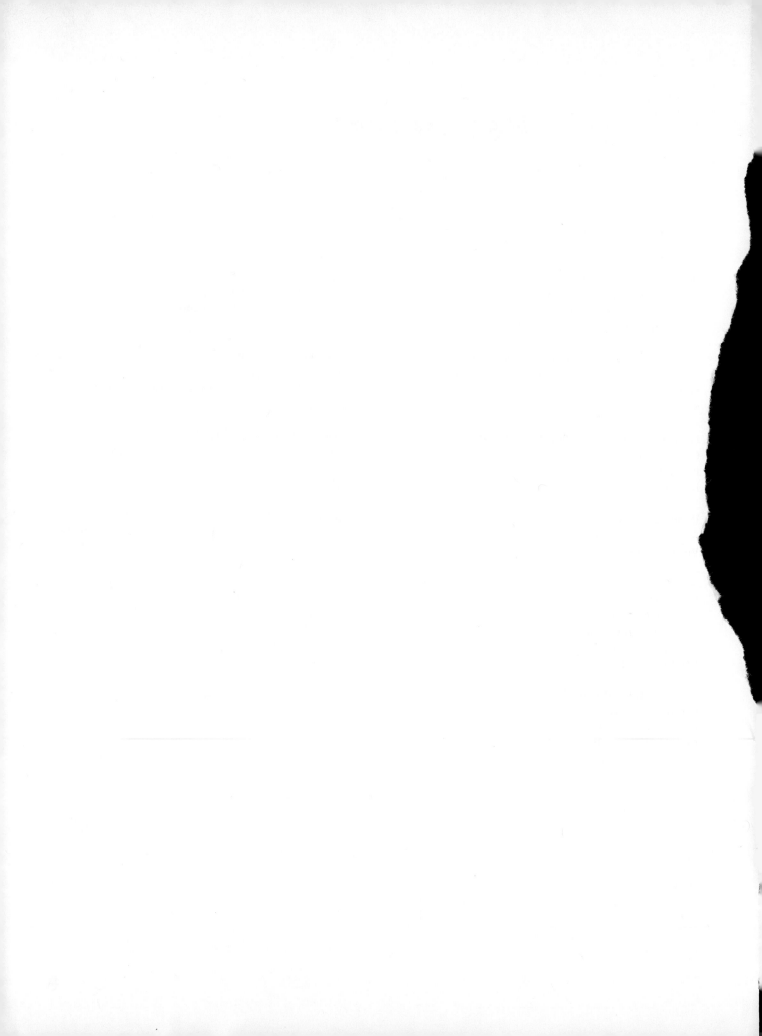

Preface

When *Mosby's Perioperative Nursing Series: Cardiac Surgery* was published in 1994, minimal access procedures and minimally invasive techniques for cardiac surgery were just being introduced into clinical practice. Xenotransplantation, decoding of the human genome, mechanical ventricular assistance as end-destination therapy, robotic manipulation, and a wide array of percutaneous coronary interventions were largely in the investigational stage. Since 1994, these research activities and technologies have entered the clinical realm to expand the array of treatment options for patients and are represented in this updated *Cardiac Surgery*. Learning about these advances enables the nurse to meet evolving patient needs, whether these needs are related to safety, education, or rehabilitation. This knowledge is also needed by the nurse to make informed, competent decisions about patient care. The purpose of this book is to serve as a resource for perioperative nurses to meet patient needs and to facilitate effective clinical problem solving.

Consumer and payer demands for cost-effective and efficient care have been no less important to professional practice than clinical advances. In demanding greater value for their health care dollar, consumers have also played an important role in stimulating the growth of evidence-based practice, promoting more effective error-reduction strategies, and effecting greater accountability from all team members. These trends have led to safer, more effective care not only in cardiac surgery, but in all surgical specialties.

The growing number of cardiac surgical programs nationwide makes this text especially useful to clinicians and managers involved in developing or expanding these programs. *Cardiac Surgery* contains perioperative nursing competencies, a course outline, problem-solving exercises, a pretest and posttest, and nursing standards to guide novices as well as more experienced nurses. In addition, rationales and alternative techniques are included throughout the section on surgical interventions to assist nurses in adapting to changing circumstances.

Part One of *Cardiac Surgery* includes a historical review of the individuals (including nurses) and the technological advances that have made cardiac surgery possible (Chapter 1); characteristics of the cardiac nurse and the cardiac team, nursing competencies, error-reduction and stress-management strategies, and a cardiac surgery course outline (Chapter 2); structural components of cardiac surgery including instruments and supplies for traditional and minimally invasive procedures, and updated diagnostic related group (DRG) codes (Chapter 3); nursing process elements of assessment, diagnosis, outcome identification, planning, implementation, and evaluation (Chapters 4 through 7); and surgical anatomy and physiology (Chapter 8).

Part Two includes surgical procedures such as basic cardiac procedures for surgical exposure, cardiopulmonary bypass, and myocardial protection (Chapter 9); surgery for coronary artery disease, including newer percutaneous and off-pump procedures (Chapter 10); valvular heart disease (Chapters 11 through 13); thoracic aneurysms and dissections (Chapter 14); mechanical and biological circulatory assistance (Chapter 15); transplantation of the heart and lungs (Chapter 16); surgical procedures for dysrhythmias (Chapter 17); adult congenital heart disease (Chapter 18); trauma and emergency procedures (Chapter 19); and miscellaneous procedures such as pericardiectomy (Chapter 20).

Acknowledgments

The individuals listed in the Preface from the original textbook continue to demonstrate their generosity, and I thank them once again. I am especially grateful to the contributors and reviewers of the present textbook, and also to Drs. Warren Levy, Michael Mack, and Frederick Schwab; and to Dr. Nathan Belkin, Judy Blanchard, Brian J. Kilgore, Bill Manganaro, Andy Reding, Dick Reid, Steve Rowe, Brigid Scanlon, Lyn Thompson, Amy Wiggins, and Sarah Wright. A special "thank you" goes to my perioperative nursing colleagues for their persistence in requesting an updated textbook.

Editors are a writer's guardian angels, and I thank Lisa Newton, Michael Ledbetter, and Ann Rogers at Mosby and Keith Roberts at Graphic World Publishing Services for their guidance and recommendations. My family, and in particular my husband, have been very patient and supportive. Everyone is pleased that we can use the dining room table once again.

Patricia C. Seifert
2002

Preface from the Original Textbook, Part of Mosby's Perioperative Nursing Series

Cardiac surgery places the patient in a uniquely vulnerable situation, and the perioperative nurse plays a vital role as patient advocate within the continuum of care. Among the numerous texts written by nurses, physicians, and perfusionists addressing the needs of patients undergoing cardiac surgery, none has been devoted to perioperative nursing care. *Cardiac Surgery* is intended to close a gap in the cardiac literature.

The purpose of this book is twofold: (1) to identify the needs of adult patients during surgery and (2) to demonstrate the perioperative nursing considerations and interventions that form the basis for professional practice in the cardiac operating room. Although adult congenital lesions (and infant patent ductus arteriosus) are included, pediatric cardiac surgery is not discussed in detail; the special needs of this patient population warrant a book devoted solely to the subject. Medical/surgical nursing care, critical care, and rehabilitation have been thoroughly discussed elsewhere and thus are only briefly mentioned in this book.

Part One of *Cardiac Surgery* addresses the foundations of cardiac surgical nursing, including a historical perspective (Chapter 1); attributes of perioperative cardiac nurses and the cardiac team (Chapters 2 and 3); surgical anatomy and physiology (Chapter 4); environment, instrumentation, and equipment, including structural standards (Chapter 5); and elements of the nursing process, including process and outcome standards (Chapters 6 through 10).

Part Two describes surgical interventions that focus on generic procedures (Chapter 11); surgery for coronary artery disease (Chapter 12), valvular heart disease (Chapters 13 through 15), and thoracic aortic aneurysms and dissections (Chapter 16); ventricular assist devices for the failing heart (Chapter 17); transplantation of the heart and lungs (Chapter 18); surgery for conduction disturbances (Chapter 19), adult congenital heart disease (Chapter 20), and trauma and emergencies (Chapter 21); and miscellaneous procedures (Chapter 22).

The procedures discussed include those commonly done for frequently encountered disorders, as well as those performed for rarer disorders. No single method of repair is universally suited to a particular problem, and each operation will be influenced by the training and experience of team members. However, there are basic principles that can be applied to many situations. The appropriate operation depends on the lesion, anatomic features, patient factors, and available resources. Moreover, surgical procedures are constantly evolving. When the underlying rationale for familiar techniques is understood, the nurse should be able to modify current practices and adapt to new ones in light of this rationale.

Some of the special features of *Cardiac Surgery* are:
- Comments and reminiscences about the history of cardiac surgery from perioperative nurses who participated in the formation of cardiac surgery programs
- Competency statements for perioperative nurses based on AORN's Standards and Recommended Practices and the American Nurses Association and American Heart Association's Council on Cardiovascular Nursing Standards of Cardiovascular Nursing Practice
- Characteristics of cardiac perioperative nurses based on the Benner/Dreyfus model for progressing from novice to expert
- A cardiac surgery course outline and pretests and posttests for nurses learning the perioperative cardiac role

- Anatomic drawings illustrating a surgical perspective
- Nursing standards of care for cardiac procedures
- Step-by-step procedures with rationales and possible alternative maneuvers
- RN first assistant considerations related to cardiac surgery
- "Pearls" by nurses and surgeons who are experts in their fields, and by others, that provide special insights into the subject under discussion

In performing the perioperative role, the nurse focuses on issues related to patient safety, protection from hazards, comfort, prevention of infection, emotional support, and educational needs regarding the surgery and its impact on the patient's functional status postoperatively. Although these issues have global significance, within the context of surgery they take on a distinctive character requiring special interventions. Alterations in myocardial oxygen supply and demand, temperature, and blood flow to major organs are only a few of the stressors affecting patients during surgery. Perioperative nurses must understand the underlying pathoanatomy, monitor hemodynamic status, anticipate patient needs, and intervene appropriately and quickly. Responding effectively requires knowledge, skill, compassion, and clinical judgment.

Of special concern to all cardiac team members are the temporal constraints imposed by the need for induced cardiac arrest. "Time is muscle," and the difference between reversible and irreversible ischemic myocardial injury is difficult to determine with precision. That cardiac surgery is considered "stressful" is due in large part to the tyranny of the clock. This consideration places great importance on mental and manual skill, efficiency, and, above all, teamwork.

The public and professional esteem enjoyed by cardiac surgeons has been greatly influenced by their manual skill, as well as their mental acumen. Such skill and acumen are equally important in the perioperative nurse. The patient's safety and welfare depend both on the nurse's critical thinking skills and on the safe and appropriate use of the myriad instruments, equipment, prosthetics, and other items within the cardiac technologic armamentarium.

The concept of the "team" is essential to a cardiac service. The team is the primary unit and one that exemplifies the principle that the whole is greater than the sum of its parts. Nurses and surgeons alike consistently emphasize the necessity of teamwork. Team members may have special roles and responsibilities, but these are interdependent and necessitate flexibility and an appreciation of one another's duties and functions if successful outcomes are to be achieved. The strong bonds that often develop among team members are evidence of the mutual support and respect that characterize the group.

Although, out of necessity, proportionately more time is devoted to the physiologic needs of patients who are anesthetized, meeting psychosocial needs is also a critical component of the perioperative nurse's role. Comfort measures and anxiety-reducing interventions preoperatively are integral components of perioperative nursing practice. They reflect not only a compassionate attitude, but also a means of reducing endogenous catecholamine release and myocardial oxygen consumption. Communicating with the family of a critically ill patient requires the ability to provide a realistic appraisal of the situation without taking away all sense of hope for a successful outcome. When patients die in the operating room, it is the perioperative nurse who routinely prepares the body and is there to support the family and loved ones when they make their final farewells.

Cardiac surgery has a profound physiologic and emotional impact on the patient, the family, and friends. Probably no other organ carries with it such deep psychologic and spiritual significance. As it was centuries ago, the heart is still believed to be the seat of the soul and the wellspring of emotion. An awareness of what the patient experiences during surgery and the appropriate nursing care that is provided in collaboration with surgeons, anesthesiologists, perfusionists, and other members of the surgical team enhances continuity of care and facilitates recovery, recuperation, and rehabilitation. *Cardiac Surgery* has been written as a testament to the outstanding contributions of perioperative nurses and to the art and science that are reflected in their practice.

Acknowledgments

The decision to write *Cardiac Surgery* on my own was based on the desire to achieve consistency throughout the book and to reflect certain beliefs about the demands of cardiac disease, surgery, and the clinicians who participate in surgical procedures. It has been my good fortune throughout my professional life to have a diverse and flexible job description that allowed me to engage in a variety of practice roles: staff nurse, RN first assistant, educator, clinical coordinator, and administrator. These experiences have given me valuable insights into the needs of patients and families, as well as professional associates. They also inspired me to write about the special needs of surgical patients and the vital role played by perioperative cardiac surgical nurses. I am especially indebted to my present and former colleagues at The Arlington Hospital, the Fairfax Hospital, and the Washington Hospital Center.

However, this book could not have been written without the help of many persons. Few have the knowledge and experience to treat as complex a subject as cardiac surgery completely without relying on those with expertise in the field; I am no exception. I am most grateful to the consultants listed in the front of this book who have reviewed the manuscript and offered valuable suggestions and comments.

I would like to thank my nursing colleagues for their unstinting support and encouragement in the development of this book. Their compassion and competence have made them exemplary role models: Nancy Abou-Awdi, Ursula Anderson, Sonia Astle, Gwyn Baumgarten, Alice Cannon, Nancy Davis, Jodee Desilets, Diane Fecteau, Dr. Cathie Guzzetta, Chris Esperson, Peggy Hartin, Kim Hill, Nancy Holloway, Dena Houchin, Edwinia Ion, Gail Kaempf, Cecil King, Linda Lewis-Sims, Brad Manuel, Dr. Rosemary McCarthy, Jill Montgomery, Cheryl Nygren, Pat Palmer, Dottie Platt, Leanna Revell, Pat Rogers, Dr. Jean Reeder, Dr. Jane Rothrock, Bridget Schall, Anne Weiland, Chizuko Williams, and the nursing colleagues with whom I have had the privilege of working.

I am deeply grateful to the surgeons for whom I have been a first assistant. Their patience and their faith in me during thousands of operations have provided me with learning opportunities afforded to few. They have demonstrated the art and the science of surgery elegantly and skillfully: Drs. David C. Cleveland, John R. Garrett, Cleland Landolt, Edward A. Lefrak, Quentin Macmanus, and Alan M. Speir. I also wish to express my great appreciation to the many surgeons, anesthesiologists, cardiologists, and other physicians who responded to my requests and who generously shared with me their knowledge and experiences: in particular, Drs. W. Gerald Austen, Richard Bjierke, Peter Conrad, Denton A. Cooley, Paul Corso, Willard Daggett, Richard DeWall, Paul A. Ebert, Rene Favaloro, O.H. Frazier, Ted Friehling, Jorge Garcia, Nevin M. Katz, C. Walton Lillehei, Robert S. Litwak, Kenneth L. Mattox, Luis Mispretta, Albert Pacifico, William S. Pierce, John D. Randolph, Bruce A. Reitz, William C. Roberts, Emil Roushdy, Sandy Schaps, Mohammed Shakoor, John A. Walhausen, and Scott Walsh.

The assistance of perfusionists has been invaluable, and I am especially thankful to Aaron Hill, Bob Groom, John O'Connell, and William Yorde.

The contributions of artists Peter Stone, M. LaWaun Hance, SA, Dan Beisel, and Edna Hill, and photographers Howard Kaye, Kip Seymour, and Doug Yarnold, CRNA, have been vital to the book.

To Leo Rosenbaum, a special thank you.

No book can be written without the assistance of librarians. I am indebted to Cecelia Durkin, Donna Giampa, Susan Osborn, Sue Polucci, Nell E. Powell, Alice Sheridan, and Norma Stavetski.

Supporters within the business community have provided valuable information and generously shared resources: Steve Aichele, Barry Hopper, Bertie Janney, William Merz, Alan Mock, William Pilling, Dick Reid, and Charles Riall.

I am most grateful to the individuals at Mosby who worked on this project. Their attention to detail and guidance in no small way helped to make this book a reality; thank you, Nancy Coon, Beverly Copland, Suzie Epstein, Michael Ledbetter, Teri Merchant, Judi Bange, Donna Walls, Gayle Morris, and Susan Lane.

Finally, to my husband and children, thank you for your patience and love.

Patricia C. Seifert

Contents

PART ONE
Foundations of Cardiac Surgical Nursing

1 History of Cardiac Surgery, 1

Early Crucial Developments, 2
Surgical Procedures, 11
Valvular Heart Surgery, 12
Development of Cardiac Surgical Nursing:
    The Perioperative Role, 16
Conclusion, 19

2 The Perioperative Nurse and the Cardiac Team, 22

Development of the Team, 22
Staffing Issues, 23
Collaboration, 24
Nursing Roles, 26
Team Roles, 32
Stress and Stress Reduction Within the Cardiac
    Service, 33
Error Detection, Recovery, and Prevention, 37
Conclusion, 40
Appendix 2A: Pretest/Posttest, 41
Appendix 2B: Competency Statements in Perioperative
    Cardiac Nursing, 43
Appendix 2C: "What If?" Simulations and Decision-
    Making Exercises, 49

3 Structural Elements of Cardiac Surgery, 51

Financial Considerations, 52
Regulatory Considerations, 53
The Cardiac Suite, 53
Furniture, 56
Equipment, 56
Instruments, 69
Suture, 78
Supplies, 81
Prosthetic Implants, 83
Conclusion, 93

4 Preoperative Assessment, 95

Background Information, 95
Diagnostic Procedures, 98
Laboratory Tests, 112
Preoperative Patient Interview, 117
Conclusion, 127

5 Nursing Diagnoses, Outcomes, and Plans for Patient Care, 129

Perioperative Nursing Data Set, 129
Human Response Patterns and Associated
    Diagnoses, 132
Planning Patient Care, 135
Generic Care Plans, 135
Conclusion, 144

6 Implementation of Perioperative Nursing Care, 146

Admission to the Cardiac Service, 146
Preoperative Patient Teaching, 146
Advance Directives, 151
Room Preparation, 151
Entry into the Operating Room, 151
Intraoperative Medications, 155
Positioning and Skin Preparation, 155
Draping, 158
Infection Control Measures, 159
Transfusion Therapy and Blood Conservation, 160
Defibrillation, 161
Temporary Epicardial Pacing, 163
Hemostasis, 165
Chest Tube Insertion, 166
Completion of the Procedure, 168
Fast-Track Cardiac Surgery, 169
Postoperative Management, 170

7 Evaluating Outcome Achievement, 173

Research, 174
Patient Care Management, 175
Human Resource Management, 183

Evaluation of Fiscal and Material Resources, 184
Additional Methods of Evaluation, 185
Conclusion, 185

8 Anatomy and Physiology, 187

Introduction, 187
Location of the Heart, 187
Size and Position of the Heart, 189
External Features of the Heart, 191
Cardiac Chambers, 191
Cardiac Valves, 194
Coronary Arteries, 196
Cardiac Veins, 199
Conduction System, 199
Innervation of the Heart, 200
Excitation-Contraction of the Cardiac Cell, 202
Cardiac Cycle, 204
Cardiac Output, 205
Myocardial Oxygen Consumption, 207
Circulatory System, 207

PART TWO
Surgical Interventions

9 Basic Cardiac Procedures, 213

Thoracic Incisions, 213
Other Thoracic Incisions, 226
Cardiopulmonary Bypass, 230
Myocardial Protection, 250

10 Surgery for Coronary Artery Disease, 258

Coronary Artery Disease, 258
Thrombolytic/Antiplatelet Therapy, 263
Percutaneous Coronary Intervention, 264
PCI and CABG, 266
Surgery for Coronary Artery Disease, 267
Completion of Procedures, 303
Postoperative Considerations and
    Complications, 304
Reoperation for Coronary Artery Disease, 304

11 Mitral Valve Surgery, 309

Atrioventricular Valves, 309
Mitral Valve Apparatus, 309
Mitral Valve Disease, 310
Diagnostic Evaluation of Mitral Valve Disease, 315
Surgery for Mitral Valve Disease, 315
Completion of the Procedure, 339
Postoperative Considerations, 340

12 Aortic Valve Surgery, 343

Anatomy and Physiology of the Aortic Valve, 343
Aortic Valve Disease, 344
Diagnostic Evaluation of Aortic Valve Disease, 350
Surgery for Aortic Valve Disease, 351
Completion of the Procedure, 371
Postoperative Complications, 371

13 Tricuspid and Pulmonary Valve Procedures, 375

Tricuspid Valve Procedures, 375
Tricuspid Apparatus, 375
Tricuspid Valve Disease, 375
Diagnostic Evaluation of Tricuspid Valve
    Disease, 378
Postoperative Considerations, 390
Pulmonary Valve Procedures, 391
Pulmonary Valve Disease, 391

14 Surgery on the Thoracic Aorta, 395

The Aorta, 395
The Aortic Wall, 395
Aortic Aneurysms and Aortic Dissections, 396
Classification of Aortic Aneurysms and Aortic
    Dissections, 397
Diagnostic Evaluation of Thoracic Aortic
    Disease, 401
Surgery on the Thoracic Aorta, 403
Surgery on the Aortic Arch, 414
Surgery on the Descending Thoracic Aorta, 419
Completion of the Procedure, 425
Postoperative Complications, 425

15 Mechanical and Biologic Circulatory Assistance, 430

Heart Failure, 431
Compensatory Mechanisms in Heart Failure, 432
Initial Medical Management, 434
Circulatory Assist Devices, 435
Hemopump, 438
Ventricular Assist Devices, 438
Pulsatile Devices, 441
Implantable Systems, 448
Total Artificial Heart, 451
HeartSaver VAD, 451
Implantable Axial Flow Systems, 452
General Considerations to Prepare for Mechanical
    Circulatory Support Implants, 452
Complications of Mechanical Circulatory
    Systems, 454

Other Surgical Interventions for Heart Failure, 457
Pericardial Devices, 459
Future Challenges, 459

16 Transplantation for Heart and Lung Disease, 463

General Considerations, 463
Emotional Aspects of Transplantation, 464
Organ Recovery, 465
Recipient Preparation, 466
Heart Transplantation, 467
Heart-Lung Transplantation, 483
Lung Transplantation, 487
Conclusion, 492

17 Surgery for Cardiac Dysrhythmias, 495

Conduction System, 495
Conduction of Electrical Impulses, 497
Categorizing Dysrhythmias, 501
Diagnostic Evaluation of Dysrhythmias, 503
Supraventricular Dysrhythmias, 508
Ventricular Dysrhythmias, 521

18 Surgery for Adult Congenital Heart Disease, 527

Intrauterine Circulation, 529
Postnatal Circulatory Changes, 530

Congenital Malformations, 530
Diagnostic Evaluation of Congenital Heart Disease, 531
Patent Ductus Arteriosus, 532
Atrial Septal Defect, 536
Coarctation of the Aorta, 542
Conclusion, 546

19 Cardiac Trauma and Emergency Surgery, 547

Trauma, 547
Mechanism of Injury, 548
Nursing Considerations, 549
Blunt Thoracic Injuries, 550
Penetrating Thoracic Injuries, 552
Perioperative Nursing Considerations, 557
Inadvertent Hypothermia, 557
Pulmonary Embolus, 559
Postoperative Complications of Cardiac Surgery, 561

20 Miscellaneous Procedures, 565

Cardiac Tumors, 565
Pericardial Disease, 568

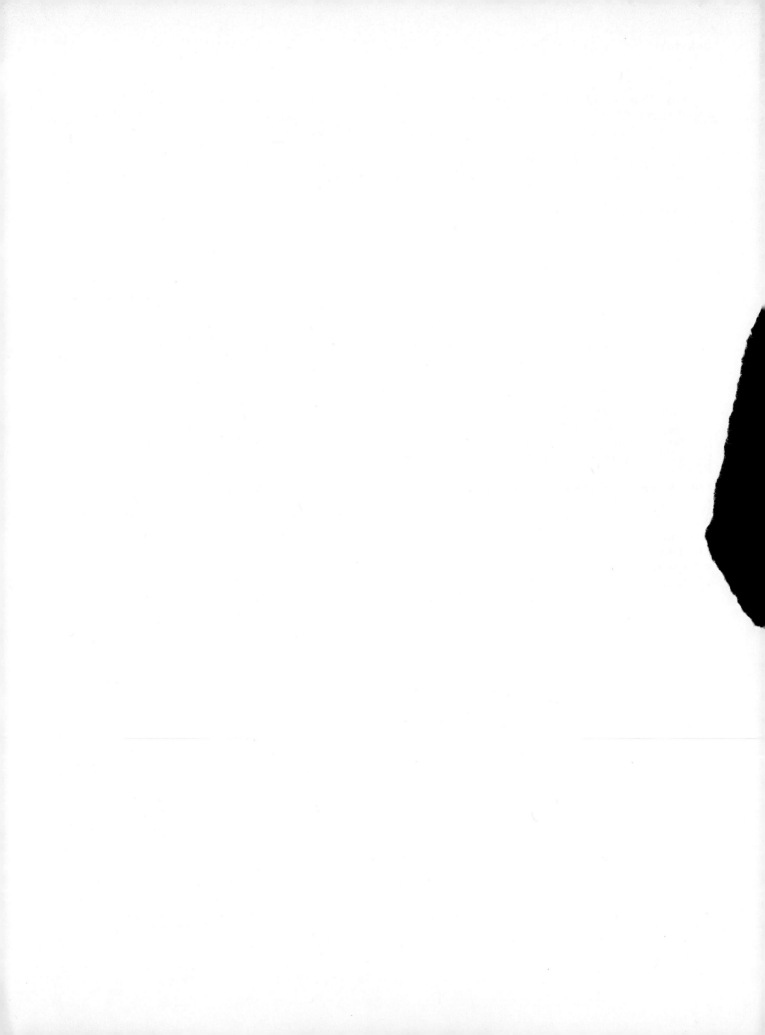

1

History of Cardiac Surgery

I may have made the progress reported sound easy, effortless, and unobstructed. That most certainly was not the case. There were innumerable failures, disappointments, frustrations, and obstacles—nature's as well as man's. The only solution was a mixture of persistence and stubbornness.

C. Walton Lillehei, MD, 1986 (p. 21)

Many of the innovations came from surgeons themselves and their helpers.

Harris B. Shumacker, MD, 1992 (p. 366)

Probably no other achievement focused the public's attention on the world of cardiac surgery as did the first human heart transplant, performed by Christiaan Barnard (1967) on December 3, 1967, in Cape Town, South Africa (Fig. 1-1). Not only was this hailed as a technologic miracle, it also had a profound emotional impact because the object of attention was no less than what was considered the seat of the soul.

For centuries curiosity about the structure and function of the heart had been tempered by injunctions against touching it and by reverence for it as the principal and most noble organ of the body (Shumacker, 1992). Although William Harvey studied the hearts of animals, his deduction that dual pumps—the right and left sides of the heart—propelled the blood to the body in a continuous cycle through the interconnecting pulmonary and systemic circulations was the result of human experiments on the valves of veins and not on the heart itself (Comroe, 1983).

As late as 1896 surgeons were hesitant to perform cardiac procedures and risk the wrath or ridicule of their peers (Nissen, 1963). Theodor Billroth, the noted abdominal surgeon, is reported to have said in a lecture circa 1875 that "a surgeon who would attempt the suture of a heart should lose the respect of his colleagues because the operation is not compatible with a surgeon's responsibility" (Westaby, 1997, p. 15). As if that were not enough to chill the enthusiasm of surgeons, Sir Stephen Paget predicted in that same year that "surgery of the heart has probably reached the limits set by Nature to all surgery; no new method, and no new discovery can overcome the natural difficulties that attend a wound of the heart" (Paget, 1896, p. 121).

These statements were not without some foundation, given the obstacles to open chest surgery during that era—infection, hemorrhage, and the difficulty of avoiding the lethal cardiopulmonary consequences of pneumothorax (Brieger, 1991). Ironically, the beginning of heart surgery is often considered to have been in 1896, when a German, Ludwig Rehn, successfully sutured a stab wound to the right ventricle of a young man. In doing this, Rehn demonstrated that touching the heart would not necessarily cause a lethal dysrhythmia and that the myocardium could hold sutures (Rashkind, 1982). The first cardiac surgical procedure in the United States occurred in 1902 and was also the closure of a stab wound.

In a world rarely free from fighting and war, it is not surprising that early attempts at cardiac repair often focused on battle injuries. One of the most famous wartime accomplishments was Dwight Harkin's World War II series of 134 operations to remove retained missiles from the heart and great vessels: There were no deaths, and all patients were discharged from the chest surgery hospital (Johnson, 1970).

These and other achievements—from Rehn's 1986 myocardial suture repair to Barnard's 1967 cardiac transplantation to Denton Cooley's 1969 and William DeVries' 1982 (DeVries, 1988) implantation of a total artificial heart, and to the introduction of port-access, robotically assisted minimally invasive techniques—are singular examples of the progress made in cardiac surgery, which, as Lillehei (1986) has noted, sounds "easy, effortless, and unobstructed" (p. 21). Such was

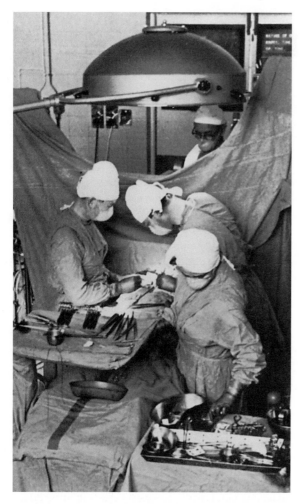

FIGURE 1-1   Dr. Christiaan N. Barnard performing world's first heart transplant in Cape Town, South Africa, on December 3, 1967. (Courtesy Berchtold Corp., Charleston, SC.)

not the case, however, as these pioneers would surely agree. The history of cardiac surgery is the result of many investigations that paved the way for momentous achievements. It is meticulous research and serendipitous discoveries. It is numerous trials and errors by physicians and technicians in experimental laboratories and imaginative solutions to seemingly insurmountable problems by surgeons, nurses, and others involved in surgery. Whether they were elucidating anatomy and physiology, enhancing diagnostic capabilities, developing surgical techniques, creating prosthetic replacements, or designing instruments and sutures, many persons were responsible for transforming ideas into clinical reality.

When Rene Favaloro (1992) wrote, "It is very dangerous to say 'I was first'; there is almost always a precedent" (p. 111), he captured the relationship between the reassessment of earlier insights and the application of current knowledge to forge new advances. There are

many precedents in the development of cardiac surgery, and they attest to the creativity and persistence of many individuals.

Early Crucial Developments

A number of developments laid the groundwork for cardiac surgery as we know it today. From the electrocardiogram to vascular clamps that would not traumatize blood vessels, numerous inventions and discoveries paved the way for the successful treatment of congenital and acquired heart disease (Comroe and Dripps, 1977; Table 1-1).

ELECTROCARDIOGRAPHY, CHEST RADIOGRAPHS, AND SELECTIVE CORONARY ARTERIOGRAPHY

The invention of the stethoscope by Laennec in 1819 brought medicine into the age of physical examination. Physicians could begin to understand *what* was happening, but the *why* and *how* of cardiac disease required new methods of detection.

Electrocardiography
Investigations in the 1850s uncovered the electrical current that accompanied cardiac contraction. By the 1870s scientists were familiar with the electrical activity of the heart. Measurement of these electrical currents was first achieved by recording the activity of the exposed hearts of experimental animals. In 1887 Augustus Waller made a surface recording, which he called an *electrogram* or *cardiogram* (Johnson, 1970, p. 17). It was not until Willem Einthoven's work in the late 1890s, however, that normal and abnormal waveforms and deflections of the electrocardiogram were described. Studies of the cardiac dysrhythmias were greatly expanded by Sir Thomas Lewis in a 1912 monograph titled *Clinical Disorders of the Heart Beat,* and by 1920 the electrocardiogram was an established component of the cardiac examination.

Chest radiographs
The diagnosis and treatment of heart disease was greatly simplified by Wilhelm Roentgen's discovery of x rays in 1895. Within a short time x-ray films were used to evaluate cardiomegaly, aneurysms, pericardial and pleural fluid, and pulmonary edema (Johnson, 1970).

Selective coronary arteriography
Radiographic opacification of the vascular system allowed diagnosticians to analyze a problem affecting the systemic circulation and plan appropriate treatment. Probably the most significant advancement affecting the treatment of

TABLE 1-1

Clinical Advances in Cardiovascular Surgery: Surgical Instruments, Supplies, and Prostheses

DATE	SCIENTIST	EVENT (AND CITATION)
1902-1912	Carrel	Used arteries, veins, metal tubes, rubber tubes, and gold-plated aluminum tubes as vascular grafts in animals; developed atraumatic needles and clamps, petrolatum-coated sutures (*Lyon Med* 98:859, 1902; *Surg Gynecol Obstet* 2:266, 1906; with Guthrie: *Bull J Hopkins Hosp* 18:18, 1907; *J Exp Med* 16:17, 1912; *Surg Gynecol Obstet* 15:245, 1912)
1910	Stewart	Devised clamp to permit blood flow to continue through one channel of a large artery while remainder was closed and available for surgical procedures (partial occlusion clamp); rediscovered in 1946 by Potts (*JAMA* 55:647, 1910)
1937	Demikhov	First to design a mechanical pump as a cardiac replacement (*Biull Eskp Biol Med* 32:22, 1951; Russian)
1946	Potts, Smith, and Gibson	Used Stewart clamp (see above) for anastomosis of aorta to pulmonary artery (*JAMA* 132:627, 1946)
1947	Hufnagel	Used rigid tubes of methyl methacrylate for permanent intubation of thoracic aorta (*Arch Surg* 54:382, 1947)
1948	Potts	Designed clamp to permit surgical division of ductus arteriosus (*Q Bull Northwestern U Med School* 22:321, 1948)
1949	Donovan and Zimmerman	Used polyethylene as an artificial surface to replace arteries (*Blood* 4:1310, 1949; *Ann Surg* 130:1024, 1949)
1949	LaVeen and Barberio	Studied tissue reaction to plastics used in vascular surgery (*Ann Surg* 129:74, 1949)
1950	Dubost and others	Used preserved human aortas to replace narrowed arteries; first blood vessel bank (*Semin Hop Paris* 26:4497, 1950)
1951	Grindlay and Waugh	Used Ivalon plastic sponge as framework (*Arch Surg* 63:288, 1950)
1951	Hufnagel	Inserted plastic (methyl methacrylate) valve in descending aorta of dogs (*Bull Georgetown U Med Center* 4:128, 1951)
1952-1954	Vorhees, Jaretzki, and Blakemore; Blakemore and Voorhees	Used Vinyan "N" cloth in dogs to bridge arterial gap; fashioned first synthetic artery from a woven material (fibroblasts grew over cloth to form "new" intima); used clinically; used woven material to replace metal or plastic (*Ann Surg* 135:332, 1952; 140:324, 1954)
1955	Deterling and Bhonslay	Made first objective evaluation of nylon and 15 other fabrics being used or proposed as prosthetic materials (*Surgery* 38:71, 1955)
1955	Hufnagel	Introduced flexible, seamless vascular prosthesis to replace an arterial bifurcation (*Surgery* 37:165, 1955)
1955	Edwards and Tapp	Used crimped accordian nylon tubing to provide flexibility without kinking (crimped graft) (*Surgery* 38:61, 1955)
1955-1960	Ethicon, Inc.	Developed miniaturization of sutures; used monofilaments in small diameters (*The Ethicon contribution to cardiac, vascular, and pulmonary surgery during the last 25 years,* Somerville, NJ, 1972, Ethicon)

Modified from Comroe JH, Dripps RD: *The top ten clinical advances in cardiovascular-pulmonary medicine and surgery between 1945 and 1975: how they came about*—final report, Bethesda, Md, Jan 31, 1977, National Heart and Lung Institute. An article describing this information was also published by the authors: Scientific basis for the support of biomedical science, *Science* 192:105, 1976.

Continued

heart disease was F. Mason Sones' (1962) development of selective coronary arteriography in 1958. As with many discoveries, this one was quite unexpected, but Sones and his colleagues were quick to recognize the tremendous potential of this technique. Not only did it improve the diagnosis of coronary artery disease and other cardiac pathologic conditions, but most important, according to Effler (1970), "it defined the needs of the individual patient" (p. xi). Thus clinicians could tailor surgical therapy (e.g., number and location of bypass grafts) and individualize patient teaching needs (e.g., lifestyle/risk factor modification and genetic counseling).

CARDIAC RESUSCITATION AND THORACIC ANESTHESIA

Cardiac resuscitation

Cardiac arrests during the administration of chloroform or ether for general anesthesia had been documented from the mid-1800s, but the cause of these arrests was not determined until 1911, when ventricular fibrillation (which was already familiar to scientists) was implicated. Early attempts at resuscitation were largely unsuccessful until Morris Schiff described a method of open cardiac massage. The first successful attempt at cardiac massage was made in the early 1900s by a surgeon who performed

TABLE 1-1
Clinical Advances in Cardiovascular Surgery: Surgical Instruments, Supplies, and Prostheses—cont'd

DATE	SCIENTIST	EVENT (AND CITATION)
1956	Wesolowski and Sauvage	Studied mesh versus solid materials for prostheses (*Ann Surg* 143:65, 1956)
1956	Murray	Used homografts for mitral and aortic valves (*Angiology* 7:466, 1956)
1960s	Various instrument companies	Manufactured microforceps, clamps, scissors, and apparatus for tying knots for microsurgery
1960	Harken and others	Devised prosthesis for replacing regurgitant aortic valve (*J Thorac Cardiovasc Surg* 40:744, 1960)
1960	Starr and Edwards	Devised caged ball valve to replace stenotic mitral valve (*Ann Surg* 154:726, 1961)
1962	Usher and others	Used polypropylene monofilament suture to close wounds (*JAMA* 179:780, 1962)
1962	Ross	Developed homograft replacement of aortic valve (*Lancet* 2:487, 1962)
1963	Gott, Whiffen, and Dutton	Used heparin bonding on colloidal graphite surfaces (*Science* 142:1297, 1963)
1964	Barratt-Boyes	Used homografts of aortic valves to replace stenotic or regurgitant valves (*Thorax* 19:131, 1964)
1965	Simmons and others	Used Teflon terry cloth to encourage growth of neointima (*Surg Forum* 16:128, 1965)
1965	Binet and others	Used preserved aortic valves from pig to replace human valves (*Acad Sci Paris* 261:5733, 1965)
1966	Liotta and others	Used Dacron prostheses (woven, knitted, velour, flocked) to encourage growth of a "new" intima (*Cardiovasc Res Center Bull* 4:69, 1966)
1968	Carpentier and others	Performed mitral valve replacement with frame-mounted aortic heterograft (*J Thorac Cardiovasc Surg* 56:388, 1968)
1969	Carpentier and others	Denatured proteins in porcine valves by treating with glutaraldehyde to prevent antigenic reactions (*J Thorac Cardiovasc Surg* 58:467, 1969)
1970	Björk	Created Björk-Shiley valve, a tilting disk mitral valve prosthesis (*J Thorac Cardiovasc Surg* 60:355, 1970)
1970	Gonzalez-Lavin and others	Used autologous pulmonary valve to replace diseased aortic valve (*Circulation* 42:781, 1970)
1980	Mirowski and others	Reported first use of implantable cardioverter defibrillator (*Am Heart J* 100:1089)
1996	St. Goar and others	Early clinical use of port-access, endovascular cardiopulmonary bypass (*Circulation* 94 [suppl 1]:52)
1998	Hansen and others	First reported clinical use of a suction-based mechanical coronary stabilizing system ("octopus") for off-pump coronary bypass surgery (*J Thorac Cardiovasc Surg* 116:60)
1998	Mohr and others	First reported clinical use of a computer-assisted robot for coronary artery surgery (*J Thorac Cardiovasc Surg* 117:1212)

an emergency thoracotomy to gain access to the heart. The intracardiac injection of epinephrine was first attempted a few years later, and drug treatment for cardiac arrest with epinephrine and calcium chloride eventually gained popularity. It seems strange that closed cardiac massage should be introduced years after open chest resuscitation, but the closed method (with artificial respiration) was not known until 1960, when it was introduced by William Kouwenhoven, James Jude, and Guy Knickerbocker (1960).

Defibrillation

Research on induced ventricular defibrillation with alternating current, as well as termination of the dysrhythmia with a larger amount of the same type of current, was published in 1900. This work was largely ignored until the 1930s, when Kouwenhoven, Donald Hooker, O.R. Langworthy, and colleagues from Johns Hopkins Hospital in Baltimore started experiments on ventricular fibrillation in open and closed chests of animals. Although there was little initial success in electrically terminating the dysrhythmia, they did learn about the damaging effects of hypoxia on cardioversion. Work by Carl Wiggers in the 1930s showed that combining cardiac massage (to perfuse the heart) with electrical shock resulted in the revival of fibrillating animal hearts. Claude Beck first applied these findings to the clinical arena, but it was not until 1947 that he succeeded in performing the first successful operative defibrillation in a human (Johnson, 1970). The direct-current defibrillator used today was introduced a few years later. Direct current was much less traumatic and more efficient than alternating current (Harkin, 1989). Theo Raber (1992), a nurse working at Hahnemann Hospital in Philadelphia in the 1950s, recalls the frequent shocks received by surgeons using defibrillators that were plugged into ordinary wall (alternating-current) outlets.

The problem of sudden cardiac death (SCD) resulting from lethal ventricular dysrhythmias was studied by Michel Mirowski and his associates, who in 1980 published their work on the use of an internal defibrillator. Their introduction of the automatic implantable cardioverter defibrillator has led to the creation of antidefibrillation technology that has resulted in the prevention of SCD in thousands of patients.

Thoracic anesthesia

Before thoracic anesthesia became available, operations on the chest wall were limited by the constraints imposed by an open thorax and the body's need for a constant supply of oxygenated blood. At the time chest surgery consisted mainly of incision and drainage for empyema or pleural effusion. The problem of opening the pleura and exposing the lungs to atmospheric pressure, which would cause the lungs to collapse, was solved in two ways in the early 1900s. Ferdinand Sauerbruch designed a complex subatmospheric pressure chamber in which the thorax could be opened without the lungs collapsing and causing asphyxia. The apparatus enclosed all of the patient's body except the head; surgeons would operate by placing their hands in gloves that allowed entry into the chamber without loss of negative pressure. The introduction of closed, positive-pressure endotracheal anesthesia in the early 1900s provided a preferable alternative to the cumbersome and impractical Sauerbruch apparatus and eventually became the accepted standard for thoracic surgery anesthesia (Frost, 1985). The impact of these two types of anesthetic management is evident in the 1921 *Textbook of Surgical Nursing,* written by Ralph Colp and Manela Wylie Keller, former chief operating room nurse at St. Luke's Hospital in New York. In describing operations for pulmonary lobectomy, the authors refer to both negative-pressure chambers and positive-pressure endotracheal inflation of the lungs, adding in an understated manner that the latter "is successful, and does not require as much time or preparation as the negative-pressure variety of operations" (p. 129).

BLOOD VESSEL SURGERY

Developments in vascular surgery had a major impact on cardiac surgery. Early attempts to anastomose blood vessels had failed mainly because of thrombosis and infection. In the early 1900s Alexis Carrel, often in collaboration with Charles Guthrie, devised techniques of end-to-end anastomoses that resulted in a

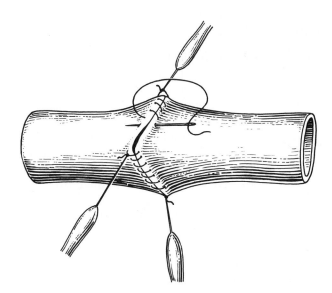

FIGURE 1-2 Alexis Carrell's technique of "triangulation" (see text). (Modified from Comroe JH: Who was Alexis who? Cardiovascular disease, *Bull Tex Heart Inst* 6[3]:251, 1979; based on Carrell A: La technique operatoire des anastomoses vasculaires et la transplantation des visceres, *Lyon Med* 98:859, 1902.)

smooth intraluminal lining that did not contain excess tissue that could become the focus for clot formation. The suture method (Fig. 1-2), still used today, consisted of triangulating the rounded openings of blood vessels by inserting three equidistant retraction sutures close to the open end of the vessel. By gently retracting the stay sutures, a triangle was formed, allowing Carrel to sew along straight lines rather than in a circle. He would sew one side of the triangle, then the second side, and then complete the third side of the anastomosis. Another improvement was to include all three layers of the vessel wall in the anastomosis. Carrel's success is often attributed to his dexterity, gentle handling of tissue, and strict asepsis in an era before antibiotics were available. He also designed special instruments and sutures, which he coated with petrolatum to facilitate their sliding through blood vessels. One of his few innovations that has not been widely adopted was his preference for black surgical attire to reduce the glare from operating lights and enhance visibility (Comroe, 1979).

The desire for easier, quicker, and less-damaging methods of creating vascular anastomoses has prompted the development of stapling and coupling devices and the investigation of glues and lasers to attach blood vessels (Werker and Kon, 1997). The growth of minimally invasive techniques has stimulated the development of a fast, reliable, and reproducible facilitated anastomotic technique.

BLOOD, BLOOD TRANSFUSIONS, AND HEPARIN

Blood typing and transfusions

Blood transfusions have been attempted for centuries, with little success because of transfusion reactions and blood clotting. Although by the end of the nineteenth century scientists had learned about the mechanism of such reactions and had begun to use citrate experimentally to prevent clotting, blood transfusions were still dangerous and rarely performed. Delays in finding a solution to the problem were partly due to the introduction in 1875 of intravenous saline infusion to treat hemorrhage. Progress was made when George Crile, using Carrel's vascular anastomotic techniques, connected donor arteries to recipient veins. The resulting smooth inner lining of the conjoined blood vessels prevented clotting, but the method was time consuming and impractical. Also, the problem of transfusion reaction remained. It was Karl Landsteiner who first discovered, in 1900, three of the four blood groups (which he called A, B, and C); the fourth blood group, O, was discovered in 1902 by Alfred von Decastello and Adriano Strurli. The discovery of blood groups was largely unappreciated by all except a few until 1911, when cross-agglutination testing before blood infusions demonstrated significant reductions in transfusion reactions (Johnson, 1970).

Blood preservation was first developed during World War I, and the first blood bank was created in 1937 at Cook County Hospital in Chicago. During World War II whole-blood transfusions to treat shock gained widespread use, and methods were devised to prolong the storage life of blood.

The search for a red blood cell substitute that can both deliver oxygen to the body's tissues and avoid the risk of blood-borne pathogens has led to the introduction of blood substitutes. One is a bovine-derived, noncellular oxygen-carrying hemoglobin that is ultrapurified and capable of circulating in human plasma. This product is compatible with all blood types and can be stored at room temperature for 2 years (IR@biopure.com, 2001). A genetically engineered hemoglobin is being investigated for possible use as an artificial blood replacement product (Ho, 2000).

Heparin and protamine

Both blood banking and the discovery of heparin by Jay McLean in 1915 were crucial to the development of cardiac surgery. Early use of McLean's discovery provided a means of anticoagulating postoperative patients, whose recovery was often complicated by thromboembolism. Later use of this knowledge enabled cardiopulmonary bypass circuits to remain free of blood clots. The discovery in 1937 by Erwin Chargoff and Kenneth Olson that protamine sulfate neutralized the effects of heparin was another milestone that allowed animal ex-

perimentation on the heart and enabled the development of John Gibbon's heart-lung machine.

CARDIOPULMONARY BYPASS

Early investigations

Although thoracic anesthesia gave investigators surgical access to the lungs, it could do little more than provide clear visualization of the surface of the beating heart. Stopping the heart with cessation of blood flow to the coronary and systemic circulations created a risk for ventricular fibrillation and anoxia of the brain and other organs. In the absence of a method to perfuse the body without having to rely on cardiac contraction, surgeons were limited to "closed" procedures that could be performed without stopping or opening the heart. Surgery for acquired diseases was mainly limited to closed mitral commissurotomy for mitral stenosis, pericardiectomy for constrictive pericarditis, and drainage of pericardial effusion. Procedures for intracardiac congenital lesions (e.g., tetralogy of Fallot) were generally limited to extracardiac palliative operations. Only those congenital defects outside the heart, such as patent ductus arteriosus and coarctation of the aorta, could be repaired directly.

Techniques to repair atrial septal defects were developed that reduced the possibility of air embolus during surgery, but these were "blind" procedures that were technically difficult. The poor results associated with these and other procedures to repair intracardiac defects made investigators continue to look for a method of performing "open" procedures. Surgeons needed a quiet, dry operating field (Johnson, 1970).

Two techniques had the potential to make this a reality. One was occlusion of venous return, introduced into clinical practice in the late 1940s; the venae cavae were clamped, and the repair was performed. This method could be used for pulmonary valve stenosis and other right-sided lesions wherein air embolus was less of a danger than it was on the left side of the heart. However, the danger of anoxia still limited safe operating time. The other technique was the institution of total-body hypothermia, which had been shown to reduce myocardial oxygen demand and thereby prolong the "safe" anoxic period. Studies by W.G. Bigelow and his associates in Toronto around the same time had demonstrated the feasibility of this technique. Interest became widespread, and researchers attempted to develop methods to avert the ventricular fibrillation and air embolism that plagued the method (Litwak, 1970).

A workable technique was finally devised by the early 1950s. Patients were anesthetized, intubated, and immersed in an ice-water bath. When the desired temperature was reached, the patients were removed from the ice-water bath and placed on the operating table, where the surgery was performed. Although the introduction of cardiopulmonary bypass a few years later superceded the use of hypothermia as the principal method of performing open heart surgery, the concept of reducing myocardial (and systemic organ) oxygen consumption by using hypothermia eventually became an important addition to bypass technology for protecting the myocardium (as well as the brain and other organs) during surgery.

Extracorporeal circulation

Research by physiologists and others had shown that the idea of extracorporeal circulation was feasible. (Alexis Carrel and Charles Lindbergh had collaborated in the 1930s on an early heart-lung apparatus.) The "azygos (low) flow principle" had shown that when the venae cavae were occluded, enough blood returned to the heart via the azygous vein (which empties into the superior vena cava) to provide a sufficient (albeit greatly reduced) cardiac output to sustain life. The significance of this was appreciated by those wondering whether reduced bypass flows would produce irreversible injury. A number of investigators were interested in devising a mechanical means of removing carbon dioxide and adding oxygen to the blood. Different methods of gas exchange had been tried, but none seemed to be workable in humans until John Gibbon (1954) introduced his heart-lung machine in Philadelphia on May 6, 1953, to close an atrial septal defect in an 18-year-old woman. Venous blood drained into the pump from the superior vena cava and was returned, freshly oxygenated, to the body through the femoral artery. Gibbon and his wife, Maly, had worked for nearly two decades on the project; what seems simple today was exceedingly difficult then. According to Shumacker (1992), who described one of the last talks Gibbon gave before his death, Gibbon received almost no encouragement from his colleagues; heparin had recently become available, but not its antagonist, protamine; there was no plastic, so the system was mainly rubber and glass; circuit components were purchased from secondhand shops!

It seems incredible today, but few surgeons initially understood or accepted the significance of this achievement, perhaps partly because Gibbon's original paper was published in a regional journal (rather than one with a national circulation) and because few surgeons had the knowledge or resources to use the device (Dobell, 1990; Shumacker, 1992). The popularity of the machine increased in a few years, however, when John Kirklin and his colleagues at the Mayo Clinic in Rochester, Minnesota, built a similar machine, which they used in a series of successful operations. Richard DeWall, with the encouragement of C. Walton Lillehei of the University of Minnesota, simplified the device by creating a bubble oxygenator that was nontoxic, inexpensive, and disposable. This modification enabled many surgeons to use extracorporeal techniques (Litwak, 1970).

However, obstacles persisted, one of the greatest being the need for large amounts of blood to "prime" the pump. Denton Cooley (1989) had described having to draw blood from seven or eight donors on the morning of surgery in the 1950s. Cooley himself made an important contribution when he started to prime the pump with intravenous solutions rather than blood. This was not only safer and more efficient, but it also enabled him to operate on Jehovah's Witnesses. Membrane oxygenators, which produce less adverse physiologic alterations than the bubble method, were introduced in the late 1950s and early 1960s. Continuous-flow, roller-type pump heads, widely used today for blood propulsion, were popularized by Michael DeBakey, who at the time was at Tulane University (but later went to The Methodist Hospital in Houston) (Shumacker, 1992).

There is some irony in the fact that John Kirklin, who played such a vital role in popularizing the use of cardiopulmonary bypass (CPB), was also one of the first to elucidate its damaging sequelae. Describing the effects of complement activation on the immune system, James Kirklin (the son and fellow author of John Kirklin) and his colleagues (1983) described the inflammatory response that occurs when blood contacts the foreign surfaces of the CPB circuit. As the deleterious effects of CPB became increasingly evident, a number of investigators were motivated to develop "off-bypass" cardiac surgical procedures to prevent the untoward effects of CPB.

Cross-circulation

One cannot discuss the subject of extracorporeal circulation without mentioning the cross-circulation studies of Lillehei and others at the University of Minnesota. The idea of using a human donor as a biologic oxygenator was conceived in the early 1950s. In April 1954 the first successful operation using this technique was performed on a 1-year-old boy, with his father as the donor. The first total correction of tetralogy of Fallot was accomplished with this technique. Although the heart-lung machine became the standard for extracorporeal circulation, Lillehei's group, using the cross-circulation technique, showed what could be achieved with a dry, quiet operative field. They made remarkable advancements in the surgical correction of a number of congenital defects and malformations that previously had been considered "uncorrectable" (Miller, 2000).

SURGICAL INSTRUMENTS, SUPPLIES, AND PROSTHESES

Instruments

Many surgical techniques could not be perfected until appropriate instruments and supplies became available that would allow the surgeon to perform new, more complex procedures. Early failures often were due partly to clamps that slipped or tore delicate tissue. Because atraumatic jaws did not exist before the 1940s, surgeons in that era used rubber boots ("rubber-shods") over the jaws of clamps to reduce their crushing effects. These difficulties led to many working relationships between instrument makers and surgeons and nurses looking for a particular clamp or retractor.

Willis Potts enabled patent ductus ligations to be performed with less risk of massive hemorrhage with a clamp he designed in 1944 that could grasp the tissue firmly. Potts also introduced the partial-occlusion clamp for shunt palliation of congenital defects such as tetralogy of Fallot. The clamp isolates the portion of the blood vessel to be repaired or anastomosed, while allowing blood flow through the unclamped portion of the vessel.

Many nurses were also involved in these endeavors. Instruments were frequently borrowed from other specialty services. The Himmelstein retractor, used by some as a sternal retractor, was originally designed for neurosurgery. Sternal retractors evolved from thoracotomy rib spreaders, which are still used for minithoracotomy approaches to the heart (Hagopian and others, 2000).

Theo Raber (1992) from Hahnemann Hospital recalls "inventing" many instruments in collaboration with surgeons and instrument manufacturers. Alice Cannon (1992) (Fig. 1-3), a nurse working with Albert Starr at the University of Oregon Hospital in Portland, devel-

oped, in collaboration with two of the surgical residents, a pediatric retractor, as well as arterial catheters and the use of orthopedic stockinette as sternal wound towels for cardiac surgery. Gwyn Baumgarten (1992) (Fig. 1-4) was a nurse at St. Luke's Hospital working with Denton Cooley when she designed numerous instruments, including the aorta clamp that bears her name (Fig. 1-5) and a wire twister needleholder, first made by Hoenig Instruments and presently manufactured by the V. Mueller Company and the Pilling Company. These and many other nurses were frequently called on to design and develop clamps, retractors, and other instruments that would enhance the operative procedure. Master craftsmen such as William Merz from the V. Mueller Company and William Pilling from the Pilling Company, along with numerous engineers working in hospitals, made important contributions. The number of cardiovascular instruments that bear the surname of Cooley, Potts, DeBakey, or Baumgarten—to name a

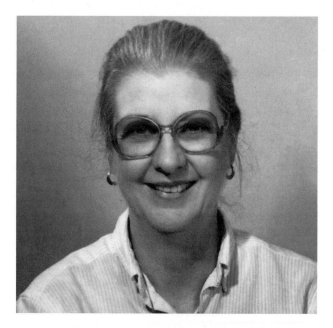

FIGURE 1-4 Gwyn Baumgarten, RN.

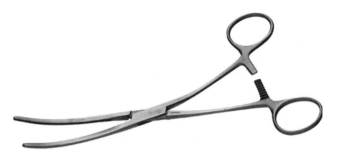

FIGURE 1-5 Cooley-Baumgarten aorta clamp. (Courtesy Baxter Health Care Corp., V. Mueller Div., Chicago, Ill.).

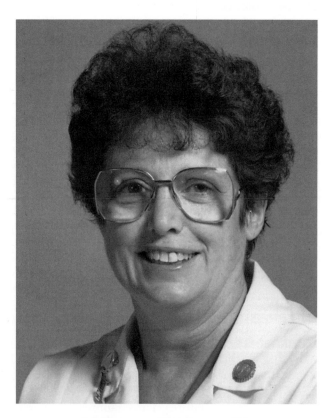

FIGURE 1-3 Alice Cannon, RN.

few—also attest to the mutually rewarding efforts between clinicians and manufacturers.

Suture

Early sutures consisted mainly of catgut and silk. These materials and the free needles that were used often traumatized blood vessels and fostered thrombosis at the anastomotic site. Operating room nurses were also called on to consult with suture companies to devise less-traumatic needles and suture materials (Raber, 1992). With the introduction of monofilaments (e.g., polypropylene) and multifilaments of braided Dacron, as well as swedged-on needles (which reduced the size mismatch between suture and needle), vascular anastomoses could be performed that were not only less traumatic, but also stronger, less irritating to surrounding tissue, less likely to become infected, and longer lasting.

In a 1951 article titled "Surgery of the Heart and Great Vessels," Lisbeth Brandt, head nurse of the operating room at The Presbyterian Hospital in Chicago, described existing cardiac procedures, and outlined the supplies and instruments required. The only types of suture listed were silk and catgut.

Supplies and equipment

Interestingly, most of the items listed by Brandt (1951) are still familiar to contemporary perioperative nurses; what is remarkable is what is omitted by Brandt: synthetic sutures, sternal retractors (rib spreaders are included), pacemaker wires, disposable drapes, prosthetic implants, cautery, and a defibrillator. Pacemaker wires in the early 1950s and 1960s consisted of bare wire attached to the heart and pulled through the chest wall. Raber (1992) has described insulating these early leads with polyethylene tubing so that patients (or staff) would not be inadvertently shocked. In addition to these items, the creation of plastics and synthetic fibers, as well as improvements in existing materials, broadened the array of surgical supplies and led to refinements that made surgery more efficient and effective. Reusable equipment and supplies, common during the early period of heart surgery, were eventually replaced by disposable items (Cooley, 1989; Box 1-1).

Nancy Davis (1992) (Fig. 1-6), a nurse practitioner who worked with Albert Starr at St. Vincent's Hospital in Portland, Oregon, in the mid-1960s and later started a cardiac surgery service in Boise, Idaho, recalls the numerous, complex supplies needed for operative procedures. To make the process more efficient, especially as it related to turnover time, the nurses designed special packs for various types of supplies: bypass tubing packs,

---

BOX 1-1
Five Periods in the Development of Cardiac Surgery

Period 1 (1956 to 1962)
- Homologous blood bypass pump prime
- Reusable equipment
- Surgery for congenital heart disease

Period 2 (1963 to 1969)
- Nonblood pump prime
- Disposable equipment
- Surgery for acquired valvular heart disease

Period 3 (1970 to 1979)
- Moderate hypothermia for myocardial protection
- Surgery for coronary atherosclerotic heart disease
- Cardiac transplantation and mechanical circulatory assistance

Period 4 (1980 to 1989)
- Cardioplegia
- Impact of interventional cardiology (percutaneous transluminal coronary angioplasty [PTCA], balloon valvuloplasty)
- Refinement of surgical techniques
- Surgery for atrial and ventricular dysrhythmias

Period 5 (1990 to Present)
- Minimally invasive approaches
- Percutaneous catheter endovascular technology
- Surgery without cardiopulmonary bypass
- Hybrid surgical/cardiologic procedures (e.g., bypass grafting with concomitant stent insertion)
- Genetic identification and treatment of cardiovascular disease

Modified from Cooley DA: Recollections of early development and later trends in cardiac surgery, *J Thorac Cardiovasc Surg* 98(5 pt 2):817, 1989.

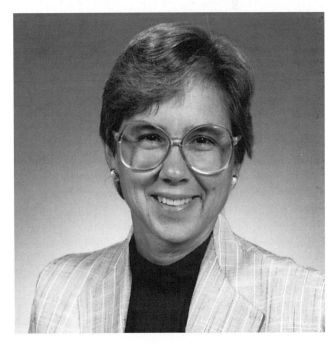

FIGURE 1-6 Nancy Davis, RN, NP.

drape packs, sponge and gown packs, and suture packs. This change streamlined the process for preparing the operating room, and it has been widely implemented in cardiac operating rooms (see Chapter 3).

Minimally invasive (e.g., smaller incisions, port access) and off-bypass surgery techniques have spawned the creation of many new devices: retractors with attached components that can illuminate the confined operative site, suction fluid, and stabilize portions of the (beating) myocardium. Double-action instruments allow surgeons to insert clamps through narrow incisions between the ribs to cut and suture, retract, and clamp tissue with the working end of the instrument. Voice-controlled, computer-assisted robotic technology has provided greater precision in closed-chest and open-chest procedures (Reichenspurner and others, 1999).

Prosthetic implants

The development of vascular substitutes was important for the fields of both vascular and cardiac surgery. Early tube grafts to replace portions of diseased aortas and peripheral blood vessels were made from Vinyon "N," a fine, porous nylon derivative. These grafts were introduced by Arthur Voorhees, Alfred Jaretzki, and Arthur Blakemore in a 1952 report. Although aortic homografts had been used for bridging arterial defects, their supply was scarce and their insertion technically challenging. Voorhees' contribution was significant because he was one of the first to find an arterial substitute that would act like a native vessel and not cause thrombosis or anastomotic breakdown (Voorhees, 1988).

Nylon, Orlon, and Ivalon (a styrofoam-like material) proved disappointing because prolonged exposure to body fluids caused them to lose tensile strength and degenerate; Dacron and polyester (Teflon) were more successful and are now the most widely used synthetic materials for vascular conduits. Patch grafts to repair intracardiac defects were also made from Dacron and Teflon, but many early procedures used Ivalon to patch atrial and ventricular septal defects.

Further refinements included crimping to prevent kinking of the graft, different porosities to either allow rapid tissue ingrowth or to prevent interstitial hemorrhage (depending on the degree of heparinization), collagen and albumin impregnation of the graft to eliminate the need for preclotting the graft, and improved sterilization techniques (Cooley, 1986). Cooley and DeBakey both made many contributions to the development of these prosthetic materials, and tube and patch grafts of woven, knitted, and velour material are now widely used for arterial repair (Brieger, 1991).

Nurses contributed to these developments in a number of ways. Baumgarten (1992), who recalls late nights in the hospital kitchen slicing graft material to make ar-

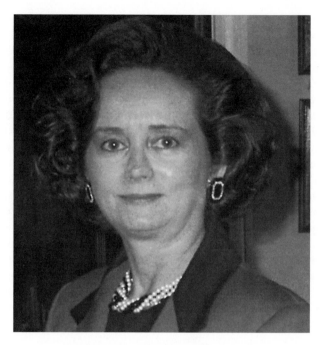

FIGURE 1-7 Edwinia James Ion, RN.

terial conduits, instituted a system of tracking the names and serial numbers of prosthetic implants in the 1960s—a standard practice today.

In 1976 Edwinia James Ion (Fig. 1-7) designed and received a patent for a set of graduated graft sizers made of stainless steel. Before this time grafts were delivered to the operating room unsterilized. The surgeon would have to compare the diseased vessel with the available grafts, and then the appropriate graft would be sterilized; this delay prolonged cross-clamp time and led to the practice of an array of grafts in various sizes being sterilized first and placed on the field; as a result, many blood-soiled but unused grafts were wasted or had to be soaked in peroxide and resterilized for future use (Cardiovascular nurse, 1976; Ion, 1992). Use of the sizers enhanced patient safety by reducing cross-clamp time, eliminating the guesswork in the selection of grafts, and reducing the risk of infection posed by resterilized grafts; also, they saved money.

Cardiac valve prostheses. Because the introduction of the heart-lung machine in the 1950s enabled surgeons to expose the inside of the heart, interest in a substitute heart valve grew. Reparative procedures were insufficient for valves that were too calcified or immobile. Early substitutes to replace individual cusps were made of pericardium, Teflon, and Dacron. Even artificial chordae tendineae from silk suture were devised. Most of these attempts failed because of thrombosis, dehiscence, or loss of leaflet mobility (Lefrak and Starr, 1979).

Hufnagel implanted a ball valve in the descending thoracic aorta of a patient with aortic insufficiency (see

Chapter 12), but it only partly corrected the physiologic problem. A substitute that could be implanted in the native position (e.g., the aortic root or the mitral annulus) was needed. Dwight Harkin solved the problem for aortic valve disease by implanting a ball-cage valve (see Chapter 12) in the subcoronary position in 1960. Around the same time, Albert Starr implanted a mitral ball-cage valve (see Chapter 11). Over the next few years, Starr's aortic and mitral (Starr-Edwards) prostheses were implanted throughout the United States and abroad.

Davis (1992) (see Fig. 1-6), working with Cannon (see Fig. 1-3) and Starr, remembers the excitement as visitors from all over the world came to Portland to observe the new valve procedure and learn about the use of these prostheses.

The work of Starr, Harkin, and other researchers confirmed that valvular problems, rather than intrinsic myocardial disease, were the cause of disability and that valve replacement instead of drugs alone could improve morbidity and mortality (Lefrak and Starr, 1979). This idea provided incentive to Donald Ross and Brian Barratt-Boyes to use aortic homografts in the mid-1960s to replace stenotic or regurgitant valves. Within a few years Carpentier and his colleagues in Paris introduced the porcine valve and made valve replacement a reality for patients who could not undergo the chronic anticoagulation required with mechanical valves (see Table 1-1).

Surgical Procedures

CONGENITAL HEART DISEASE

Patent ductus arteriosus

Before Robert Gross and John Hubbard of Boston performed the first successful suture ligation of a patent ductus in 1938, many physicians were knowledgeable about the effects of this persistent connection between the aorta and the pulmonary artery after birth. The function of the ductus was understood in the first century AD; the "machinelike" murmur had been described in 1898; and a ligating procedure had been suggested in 1907. According to Rashkind (1982), one of the factors that enabled Gross to attempt the procedure was the collaborative relationship that had been established with pediatricians and cardiologists; this was to help others perform daring surgical procedures in the future. Also contributing to the success of these procedures were the ductus clamps that had been designed by Potts (see earlier discussion).

Coarctation of the aorta

Like the patent ductus, coarctation of the aorta was known to physicians, but its consequences were unappreciated until Maude Abbott classified these disorders

in her *Atlas of Congenital Heart Disease* in 1936. Both Gross and Alfred Blalock at Johns Hopkins had considered operations that would either bypass the narrowed segment of the descending aorta or resect it and reconnect the cut ends. Resection was a problem because no one had cross-clamped (totally occluded) an aorta for fear of causing vascular injury or lower-extremity paralysis. Clarence Crafoord of Stockholm discovered that the aorta could be clamped temporarily without the development of these complications and in 1944 used the technique to resect the coarctation and reanastomose the aorta with Carrel's suture techniques (Johnson, 1970; Shumacker, 1992). Crafoord's techniques had a tremendous impact on vascular surgery for aortic and other blood vessel diseases.

Tetralogy of Fallot

In 1888 Étienne-Louis Arthur Fallot described the cardinal manifestations of the "blue malady": stenosis of the pulmonary artery, ventricular septal defect, right ventricular hypertrophy, and dextroposition of the aorta. The idea for a surgical intervention came from Helen Taussig, a physician at Johns Hopkins Hospital. Realizing that the degree of cyanosis was inversely proportional to the amount of pulmonary blood flow, she thought that if there were a way to connect a systemic artery and the pulmonary artery to increase blood flow to the lungs, the severity of the disorder could be reduced. She proposed her idea of creating a systemic artery–pulmonary artery anastomosis to Blalock. With the assistance of Vivian Thomas, Blalock's laboratory technician, Blalock performed the first shunt procedure in 1944. With modification of the procedure—anastomosing the innominate artery, and later the subclavian artery, to the pulmonary artery—results improved, and the Blalock-Taussig palliative shunt became firmly established. Potts' side-to-side descending aortic–left pulmonary artery anastomosis (with the partial occlusion clamp he designed) and other procedures followed (Johnson, 1970; Shumacker, 1992).

Credit to Blalock and Taussig for devising the procedure did not appear right away in nursing texts. It was described, but not named, by Stafford and Diller in 1947 as a "brilliant recent advance [that] has been made in extending the benefits of surgery to 'blue babies'" (p. 167); it was again described, but not attributed to Blalock and Taussig, in West, Keller, and Harmon's 1950 text.

Atrial septal defects

Various operations to repair atrial septal defects were attempted, but the risk of air traveling to the left side and embolizing to the systemic circulation hampered these efforts. One of the most intriguing procedures, developed in the early 1950s by Robert Gross in Boston, was described in the 1962 book *Cardiovascular Surgical Nursing,* by Mary E. Fordham. A "well," a funnel-shaped receptacle, was sewn to a right atriotomy, and blood was allowed to fill the container. Surgeons could insert their fingers through the blood-filled well and attempt to repair the defect using this "underwater" technique. The method was complicated, and the results were difficult for other surgeons to duplicate. The use of caval occlusion and hypothermia finally allowed John Lewis and Richard Varco from the University of Minnesota to repair the defect under direct vision in 1952 (Johnson, 1970).

Palliation for other defects

Excessive pulmonary blood flow, as well as restricted pulmonary flow, could be a problem, and the artificial creation of pulmonary stenosis by banding the artery was introduced in 1952. Creation of an atrial septal defect to increase mixed pulmonary-systemic blood flow in babies with transposition of the great arteries was introduced in 1950.

Correction of defects became possible with the introduction of CPB and with Lillehei's cross-circulation techniques. Often bypass was used in conjunction with surface cooling. Jill Gorman Montgomery (1992) (Fig. 1-8), a nurse working with Robert Gross and Aldo Castenada, has described surface cooling techniques used in Boston during the early 1970s. Infants were placed in a large green plastic bag—with endotracheal tube and intravascular lines in place—and immersed in a bathtub of ice slush. When the infants were cooled to the desired temperature (or when they fibrillated), they were taken out of the bag and placed on the operating table. The chest was opened, CPB was instituted, and the operation was performed. Postoperative neurologic sequelae were rare, even 20 years later.

Improved operative results permitted the development of corrective procedures for ventricular septal defects (VSDs), tetralogy of Fallot, transposition of the great arteries (TGA), and many other intracardiac disorders. In her 1962 book Fordham describes the palliative procedures (shunts) that had been developed and lists corrective operations for VSD, TGA, tetralogy of Fallot, partial and total anomalous pulmonary venous return, and partial and complete atrioventricular canal. (Fordham had been head nurse of the intensive care unit for cardiovascular patients at St. Mary's Hospital in Rochester, Minnesota; supervisor at the Chest Hospital in London, England; and supervisor of the Brooklyn Chest Hospital in Cape Town, South Africa.)

Valvular Heart Surgery

EARLY PROCEDURES

The surgical treatment of valvular heart disease was first directed toward the problems created by rheumatic valvulitis, which produced mitral stenosis.

Mitral valve surgery

Early attempts to treat mitral valve stenosis were encouraged by Rehn's successful suturing of a heart wound. A number of researchers had considered the possibility of relieving the obstruction to blood flow caused by mitral stenosis by excising portions of the deformed valve. Surgeons began to use finger dilatation, valvotomy, or partial valvectomy on aortic, pulmonary, and mitral valves. Elliott Cutler, Claude Beck, and Samuel Levine built a device called a *cardiovalvulotome,* which was inserted through the left ventricle to excise a portion of a stenotic mitral valve. In 1923 they used the device on an 11-year-old girl with severe mitral stenosis. She survived the operation but succumbed 4½ years later from progression of her disease. Other instruments were developed, and expectations were high that surgical correction of mitral stenosis had finally become a reality (Johnson, 1970).

In 1929 Cutler and Beck published their summary of the results of 12 operations for chronic valvular heart disease performed between 1913 and 1928. The dismal results (only three patients were alive after 1 week, and most died within a few hours after surgery) caused a furor, and attempts to relieve mitral stenosis were halted for the next 15 years (Shumacker, 1992).

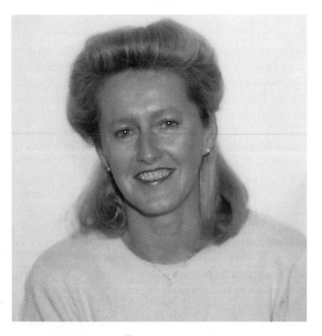

FIGURE 1-8　Jill Gorman Montgomery, RN.

The modern era of mitral valve surgery was initiated by Charles Bailey in the 1940s. While at the Hahnemann Medical School in Philadelphia, Bailey realized that a left atrial approach to the mitral valve would avoid damage to the left ventricle. Ventricular dysfunction was of concern because patients were almost always severely debilitated, and defibrillation, safe thoracic anesthesia, blood transfusion, antidysrhythmic drugs, and other advancements taken for granted today were unavailable or in the early stages of development.

After working on dogs to refine techniques for enlarging the mitral valve orifice without creating severe mitral regurgitation, Bailey performed his first procedure in 1945 on a 37-year-old man. The operation was a failure, in large part because of the lack of vascular clamps that would not tear friable cardiac tissue (Johnson, 1970). The next three patients also died, but his fifth patient, a 24-year-old woman, survived. The procedure, called a *commissurotomy*, was significant because it involved splitting the valve commissures, rather than removing a portion of the leaflet or digitally enlarging the valve orifice, which often led to severe regurgitation. Around the same time, similar successful attempts by Dwight Harken in Boston and Lord Brock in London confirmed the feasibility of surgery for mitral stenosis, and closed mitral commissurotomy became an established procedure (Lefrak and Starr, 1979).

Aortic valve surgery

Surgical correction for aortic stenosis was first attempted in humans by Theodore Tuffier, a French surgeon, in 1912. When he opened the chest of a young man and palpated the aorta, it felt soft rather than firmly calcified as expected, and Tuffier decided to invaginate the aortic wall into the aortic valve to dilate it. (Alexis Carrel was present at the operation.) After he had done this, Tuffier noticed an appreciable reduction in the intensity of the vibratory "thrill" that is caused by blood squirting through a stenotic valve and hitting the wall of the aorta. The patient survived and recovered. However, it was not until the 1950s that Charles Bailey, spurred on by the death of a colleague with aortic stenosis, performed the first successful aortic valve commissurotomy (Johnson, 1970; Shumacker, 1992).

Correction of aortic insufficiency was attempted by Charles Hufnagel at the Georgetown University Hospital in Washington, D.C. Although his prosthesis (see earlier discussion and Chapter 12) provided only partial relief, it did set the stage for Harkin's and Starr's accomplishments. The development of prostheses that could perform the function of their natural counterparts enabled clinicians to treat severe valvular heart disease.

Coronary artery disease

Angina pectoris and its symptoms were named and described by Herberden in 1768, and coronary thrombosis was diagnosed 100 years later.

Indirect methods. Cervical and upper dorsal sympathectomy was an early attempt to alleviate anginal pain. This method of pain relief for angina pectoris was described in 1947 by surgeon Edward S. Stafford and nurse Doris Diller in *A Textbook of Surgery for Nurses:* The sensory nerve fibers were interrupted by alcohol injection of the upper thoracic sympathetic ganglia. The book also refers to "surgical methods to improve the circulation of the heart following coronary occlusion [that] are now under trial. . . . Perhaps the future will bring success" (p. 168).

Another indirect method was to excise the thyroid gland to lower the body's metabolic requirements. Sympathectomy and alcohol injection for pain relief and thyroidectomy for decreasing metabolic activity (and myocardial oxygen demand) were listed as surgical options by surgeon Walter Modell in his 1952 *Handbook of Cardiology for Nurses,* but the author noted that these attempts had not been very successful. The author also included the Beck procedure but noted that it had been unsuccessful for the problem of "deficient coronary circulation" (p. 210).

Direct myocardial revascularization for atherosclerotic coronary artery disease had to await the development of extracorporeal techniques and selective coronary arteriography to provide a motionless field and to identify the precise location of the coronary lesions, respectively. Since the 1930s Claude Beck had been aware of the vascular interconnections between the coronary arteries and extracardiac portions at the base of the heart, and within adhesions between the heart and the pericardium. He theorized that grafting adjacent tissues to the myocardium would provide a new blood supply to the heart (Beck, 1935). Beck would roughen the surface of the heart with a burr or bone rasp to remove the visceral pericardium and then graft parietal pericardium, pericardial fat, or pectoral muscle directly onto the exposed myocardium.

A similar technique was tried in the 1930s by Laurence O'Shaughnessy in England. He pulled omentum up through the diaphragm and sutured it to the myocardial surface ("cardio-omentopexy"). O'Shaughnessy and others stimulated the formation of adhesions with powdered bone, talc, and other abrasive substances. Results of these operations were generally poor, but the work was a stimulus to others to find more direct methods to increase the coronary blood supply.

A brief allusion to the Beck procedure is made by surgeon John West, nurse Manelva Keller (who had coauthored the 1921 text with Colp), and nurse Elizabeth

Harmon in their 1950 book *Nursing Care of the Surgical Patient:*

> Attempts have been made to establish a collateral blood supply in such cases [e.g., narrowing or occlusion of a coronary artery] by placing muscle or other well vascularized tissues in contact with the heart, but the results have not been very satisfactory. The *chief surgical interest in the disease* is related to the danger of carrying out operative procedures upon patients with damaged coronary arteries. The increased risk in such cases is considerable but by no means prohibitive (pp. 191-192).

Although the authors could not envision a bright future for the surgical repair of hearts afflicted with coronary artery disease, they did reflect a growing awareness of the increased morbidity and mortality resulting from preexisting ischemic heart disease in patients undergoing surgery on other body systems.

Arthur Vineberg from McGill University in Montreal devised a different approach to coronary artery disease. He speculated that tunneling the internal mammary artery (IMA) into the myocardium would stimulate the development of new blood vessels between the artery and the myocardium. He first performed the operation clinically in 1950, and by 1964 he reported impressive results. Others attempted similar procedures using a variety of arterial sources such as the IMA and the gastroepiploic artery; surgeons even experimented with autogenous vein grafts attached to the aorta at one end and implanted into a myocardial tunnel at the other end. Beck interposed a segment of autogenous systemic artery between the descending thoracic aorta and the coronary sinus to increase myocardial blood flow retrogradely. Although these indirect procedures were never consistently effective, they did increase the knowledge and skill of surgeons. Information about coronary sinus retrograde perfusion, flow characteristics of arterial grafts (IMA and the gastroepiploic), intraoperative rhythm disturbances, anatomic variations, and other findings eventually enhanced methods of direct revascularization and myocardial protection (Favaloro, 1992; Shumacker, 1992).

Although Fordham's 1962 book has an extensive section on surgical repair of congenital heart disease, the section on acquired disorders is limited to valvular heart disease and aortic aneurysms; there is no discussion of coronary artery disease. In the 1969 publication by Maryann Powers and Frances Storlie (both nurses in Portland, Oregon) titled *The Cardiac Surgical Patient,* three "revascularization procedures for coronary artery disease" (p. 74) are included: (1) the Vinebery procedure (using IMA and gastroepiploic pedicle grafts), as well as "more direct attack[s] on coronary occlusion" (p. 76); (2) coronary endarterectomy; and (3) incision and patch enlargement of an obstructed coronary artery. Direct anastomoses are not mentioned.

Direct methods. Direct revascularization techniques came under investigation in the 1950s. Once again, Carrel's studies in the early 1900s provided a foundation for future techniques. He had performed aortocoronary bypass grafting in dogs, with carotid artery grafts attached proximally to the descending aorta and distally to the left coronary artery. Other early attempts were aimed at replacing diseased portions of a coronary artery with venous or arterial grafts. Some tried embolectomy or Carrel's carotid-coronary anastomoses. Direct IMA–coronary artery anastomosis had been performed in the early 1960s by Vasily Kolessov (1967) in Leningrad and Robert Goetz (Favaloro, 1992) in New York City. They worked on beating hearts and were guided largely by electrocardiograms and chest x-ray films. Sones' (Sones and Shirey, 1962) introduction of cineangiography enabled surgeons to target the coronary anastomotic sites with precision; CPB technology provided a motionless field on which to sew.

As early as 1958, William Longmire and John Cannon from the University of California at Los Angeles described an IMA–coronary bypass. Shumacker (1992) has attributed the first successful aortocoronary bypass with autogenous saphenous vein to Michael DeBakey of The Methodist Hospital (Houston) in 1964; Austen (1992) has attributed this feat to Edward Garrett (a colleague of DeBakey's). Publication of Garrett and DeBakey's results did not occur until 1973 (Garrett, Dennis, and DeBakey, 1973). Others—George Green, Rene Favaloro, Dudley Johnson—followed quickly, and with the heart-lung machine and the creation of microsurgical instruments, saphenous vein bypass grafting spread rapidly. Favaloro's report (1968) of his operation in 1967 at The Cleveland Clinic is often considered the beginning of the coronary bypass era (Austen, 1992). Direct anastomoses with the IMA were slower to take hold, but their use became widespread when their long-term patency was demonstrated by Loop and others (1986).

Although the early investigators' off-pump techniques have been described as nontransferable to coronary artery bypass grafting on arrested hearts (Shumacker, 1992), the current popularity of off-pump surgery is a testament to the creative application of these earlier techniques by Benetti and his colleagues (1991) and others.

Transplantation

Carrel and Guthrie had performed cardiac transplantation in animals early in the twentieth century. Solid organ transplantation in human started with kidney transplants in 1954, but problems with rejection limited the procedure to identical twins, who were least likely to reject each other's organs. With the introduction of azathioprine (Imuran) and steroid immunosuppression in

1962, survival rates improved in patients receiving organs from donors who were not identical twins, and interest in heart transplantation began to grow. Tissue typing and studies on the histocompatibility of antigens were shown to affect outcomes positively, but finding and matching donors to recipients remained difficult. Norman Shumway from Stanford University recalled his early experiences with transplantation in dogs (starting in 1958) and the uncertainty of immune responses. Shumway stated, "At the outset we thought the dog would be wise enough not to reject something as important to his survival as an orthotopically transplanted heart, [but] the usual laws of immunology . . . prevailed" (Shumway, 1992).

Because of rejection problems, efforts were increased to develop more nonspecific immunosuppressive agents (Austen, 1992). The discovery of antilymphocyte serum in the 1960s resulted in a third immunosuppressive agent that, when added to the other two drugs, enabled surgeons to attempt other organ transplants. Barnard (1967) performed his historic human transplantation in 1967, and there was tremendous interest in the procedure.

One of the first nursing texts to include transplantation of the human heart, titled *Cardiovascular Nursing: Rationale for Theory and Nursing Approach,* was published in 1970 and written by Jeanette Kernicki, Barbara Bullock, and Joan Matthews (all nurses at The Methodist Hospital in Houston). The authors provided a detailed description with drawings of the transplant operation that no doubt was helpful to operating room nurses familiarizing themselves with the steps of the procedure. Kernicki, Bullock, and Matthews were also among the first to discuss the legal ramifications of "brain death," ethical questions surrounding the procedure, and the emotional stress felt by families and the nurses and physicians caring for the recipient and the donor. The operative setup and preparation was also described in 1972 by Virginia Higgins (a nurse at Barnes Hospital in St. Louis) in her chapter on cardiothoracic operations in the fifth edition of *Alexander's Care of the Patient in Surgery* (Higgins, 1972).

However, problems of rejection quickly reduced the global fervor for cardiac transplantation. Shumway, Richard Lower (who later continued his transplant investigations at the Medical College of Virginia in Richmond), and colleagues from Stanford continued to study the problem and improved the 1-year survival rate from 22% in 1968 to almost 70% in 1978 (Jamieson, Stinson, and Shumway, 1979). They were among the few during this period, however, who continued to study transplantation techniques.

By 1975 and the publication of Ouida King's *Care of the Cardiac Surgical Patient* (King had been a critical care nurse at the Texas Heart Institute), the poor results of transplantation were reflected in the one-paragraph discussion of the subject. Tissue rejection and limited donor availability were cited, and mention was made of the search for a mechanical heart as an alternative cardiac pump. This trend was echoed in Rita Chow's 1976 book *Cardiosurgical Nursing Care,* which also briefly referred to heart transplantation and the possibility of total mechanical heart replacement for end-stage heart disease.

The introduction of cyclosporine and monoclonal antibody immunosuppression in the late 1970s had a significant effect on survival rates, and transplantation moved from experimental status to clinical reality. In 1981 Bruce Reitz and his colleagues at Stanford University Hospital performed the first successful long-term heart-lung transplant (Reitz, Pennock, and Shumway, 1981). Cooley had performed a heart-lung transplant in the late 1960s on a young child, but rejection developed not long afterward, according to Ion (1992), who was the scrub nurse during the procedure. Joel Cooper and his associates in Toronto achieved the first successful long-term lung transplant in 1983 (Toronto Lung Transplant Group, 1988).

The excitement of these early transplant procedures is still vivid for Baumgarten and Ion, who worked with Cooley in Houston. According to Ion, one of the operating rooms was converted into a "sterile" room for recuperating transplant patients (Baumgarten, 1992; Ion, 1992).

Peggy Hartin (Fig. 1-9), who was at Stanford during the early transplant era, also remembers the excitement. In 1968 at the Association of periOperative Registered Nurses' (AORN) Boston Congress, Hartin, along with Ludmilla Davis, Operating Room Director of

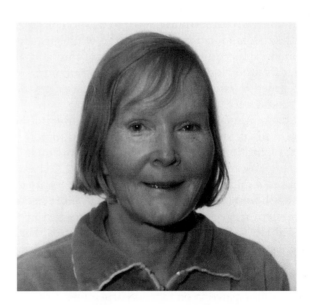

FIGURE 1-9 Peggy Hartin, RN.

Stanford University Hospital, participated in a panel on "The Role of the Nurse in Heart Transplant." Nationwide press coverage, including coverage in *Life* and *Time* magazines, was given to this conference, largely because of the enthusiasm surrounding the recent heart transplantation that had been performed by Shumway at Stanford (Driscoll, 1990).

Hartin had come to Stanford University Hospital in 1959 and had joined the cardiac team in 1964. One of her most memorable experiences concerning that cardiac transplant procedure (the first at Stanford and the third in the world) was keeping away from the operating room and the intensive care unit the newspaper reporters who had resorted to climbing the walls of the hospital and dressing as central service attendants. In contrast, when Shumway and Reitz performed the first heart-lung transplant, the news media and curiosity seekers were conspicuously absent (Hartin, 1992).

Development of Cardiac Surgical Nursing: The Perioperative Role

EARLY OPERATING ROOM NURSING

The history of perioperative cardiac nursing is as brief as the specialty of cardiac surgery itself. Its origins can be found in the development of surgery that "specializes in the treatment of physical disorders through mechanical measures" (West, Keller, and Harmon, 1950, p. 5).

The era of modern surgery—and consequently perioperative nursing—began with the introduction of anesthesia and antisepsis, and the subsequent development of surgical techniques that were made possible by these advancements. Operative procedures had been performed for centuries before the mid-1900s, but usually as a last resort, because pain, hemorrhage, and infection exacted a high toll. Early surgery was limited to excision of superficial lesions, amputation, and drainage of infected fluid. Operative procedures on the heart were rare and, like Rehn's suture closure of a myocardial laceration, were performed in emergent situations. Surgical gloves, hats, and masks were unknown.

Change came with Louis Pasteur's discovery of bacteria as the causative agent of infection and Joseph Lister's application of this knowledge to the treatment of wounds (West, Keller, and Harmon, 1950). The introduction of antisepsis "made it absolutely necessary that nurses should be of such an intellectual calibre and development as would permit them to be trained in the prevention of infection through absolute cleanliness" (Metzger, 1976; Walsh, 1929, p. 125).

Operating room nursing education began in 1876 at Massachusetts General Hospital in Boston, when student nurses participated in an extensive operating room rotation. Operating room nursing as a specialty, and the concept of an operative "team" consisting of surgeons, nurses, and assistants, originated at Johns Hopkins Hospital in Baltimore (Lee, 1976). During this initial period nurses accompanied patients from their units to the operating room to assist surgeons with the technical tasks of surgery. After the operation, these same nurses followed the patient back to the surgical ward and provided care until the patient was discharged. A few nurses might be permanently assigned to the surgical suite to supervise the visiting nurses and manage the operational details of the suite (Kneedler, 1987).

EARLY TEXTBOOKS

Surgical textbooks before the midtwentieth century reflected this continuum and discussed the patient's entire surgical experience from admission to postoperative recuperation and discharge. Intraoperative duties were described in detail, from organization of the operating room to sterilization procedures (steam sterilizers), antisepsis and asepsis, instrument passing, and dressing of wounds. These early texts even addressed preparation and management of surgery in the home, including "improvised operative positions" (Colp and Keller, 1921, table of contents). In addition to the content addressing surgical nursing, Colp and Weller's (1921) table of contents listed common operations on the following body systems: alimentary, glandular, nervous, osseous, reproductive, respiratory, skin and appendages, and urinary. Omission of the cardiovascular system reflected the relative lack of knowledge about surgery on the heart and blood vessels. This omission was gradually rectified as scientists learned more about the cardiovascular system and surgical techniques were devised to treat a growing number of congenital and acquired disorders.

Surgical nursing textbooks published in 1947 by Stafford and Diller and in 1950 by West, Keller, and Harmon continued to reflect the relative lack of cardiac surgical experience. Although these books did include chapters on surgery for heart disease, the sections were brief and amounted to three and four pages, respectively. However, by this time diseases and malformations of the heart were being widely investigated, and the clinical application to surgery—spurred on by the introduction of extracorporeal circulation—soon became evident. This in turn fostered the development of the specialty of cardiovascular nursing.

DEVELOPMENT OF CARDIOVASCULAR NURSING

With the progress made in understanding cardiovascular disorders came the need to meet the educational demands of nurses caring for this patient population. By the end of the 1940s, cardiovascular disease had become a national concern, stimulating the creation of the American Heart Association (AHA). In January 1950 the "First National Conference on Cardiovascular Diseases" was held by the AHA in Washington, D.C. The purpose of the meeting was to summarize existing knowledge, find ways to use that knowledge more effectively, and define areas where research was most needed to answer basic questions (AHA, 1950). In keeping with the goals of the conference, the planners stressed the preparation of nurses to participate effectively in prevention, "assistance to the physician in diagnosis and treatment" (p. 247), nursing care, administration, rehabilitation, and research. "Each one of these areas of service involves special relationships and specialized knowledge" (p. 247), and a listing of essential abilities emphasized specialization and teamwork. Among these were

> carrying out technical and social procedures for prevention, cure, or rehabilitation, and managing the nurse's role in the teamwork process for the care of the family and patient, and for program planning in the cardiovascular field (p. 248).

The abilities required to care for cardiovascular patients promoted by the AHA were applicable to the operating room nurse, but formal educational programs for nurses were starting to delete the operating room component from their curricula. This trend was reflected in general surgical nursing textbooks. Whereas Keller's earlier text (Colp and Keller, 1921) had included an extensive section on the operating room nurse's duties, her 1950 text (West, Keller, and Harmon, 1950) reflected this change. In their preface to the fifth edition, the authors wrote, "The section on the operating room has been omitted since it was felt that such a highly specialized field of nursing could be more effectively presented in a separate text." The 1943 publication of Edythe Louise Alexander's *Operating Room Technique* (known in later editions as *Alexander's Care of the Patient in Surgery*) provided a reference text devoted to the operative care of surgical patients. Neither the first (1943) nor the second (1949) edition of Alexander's book included cardiac procedures ("heart" was not listed in the index of either edition). In these editions chapters titled "Chest Operations" discussed breast surgery and a few thoracotomy procedures. In the first edition Carrel's anastomotic techniques (with credit to Carrel) appeared in the chapter on "Vascular Operations" under the section discussing open embolectomy procedures (p. 377). Extracardiac repairs for patent ductus arteriosus and coarctation of the aorta appeared in the second edition, as did pericardiectomy.

The third (1958) edition of Alexander's book was the first to include a chapter on "Cardiovascular Operations," but it did not refer to extracorporeal circulation or the heart-lung machine. The focus was mainly on surgery for congenital heart disease, performed without CPB.

Publication of the fourth edition (1967), which was coauthored with Wanda Burley, Dorothy Ellison, and Rosalind Vallari, greatly expanded the number and complexity of cardiovascular operations and included extracorporeal technology. In addition to the congenital malformations, acquired diseases and their treatment were described. However, revascularization of the coronary arteries was limited to descriptions of the Beck procedure, endarterectomy, and myocardial implantation of the IMA. The section on valvular heart disease included an extensive array of valve prostheses that were being used at the time.

FORMATION OF AORN

Meeting the special educational needs of perioperative nurses and transmitting the knowledge required to provide operative care was a major motivating force in the development of the AORN, which held its first national Congress in 1954. In one effort to accomplish the goal of providing continuing education for operating room nurses, AORN's Audiovisual Committee, in collaboration with the Davis and Geck Company, premiered its first film in 1959 at the sixth annual AORN Congress in Houston (Driscoll, 1990). Titled *Cardiac Surgery and the OR Nurse,* it featured Denton Cooley; Marie Ellison, Operating Room Supervisor at St. Luke's Episcopal–Texas Children's Hospitals in Houston; and Mary Schwendeman, editor of *OR Supervisor.* The film depicted the operating room nurse's role as a member of the cardiac surgery team and emphasized operating room nursing involvement before and during surgery (Nineteen years of AORN films, 1978). The *AORN Journal* and other perioperative nursing journals continue to publish articles pertinent to the cardiac nurse, and AORN has a Specialty Assembly to meet the needs of cardiovascular perioperative nurses (Riese, 2000; www.aorn.org).

CARDIOVASCULAR NURSING LITERATURE

Other than the educational opportunities provided by AORN, book chapters, and published articles, there were few resources devoted exclusively to the special needs of perioperative cardiac nurses. There were, however, a number of excellent nursing texts and papers devoted to the preoperative and postoperative care of these patients. Most had no perioperative component, but these books were valuable resources in expanding the knowledge base of operating room nurses interested in cardiac surgery.

Fordham's 1962 text *Cardiovascular Surgical Nursing,* reflecting the impact of Gibbon's heart-lung machine, is probably one of the earliest dealing with this subject. Fordham related the advancements of the heart-lung machine, the use of hypothermia, and the development of "adequate" cardiovascular prostheses to the evolution of a "more specialized and intensive type of [nursing] care. . . . Modern cardiovascular care can be provided only by the highly skilled and trained nursing attendant" (p. v).

Articles started to appear in journals. Edwinia Ion (see Fig. 1-7), under her maiden name of Edwinia E. James, contributed to furthering cardiovascular knowledge by writing "The Nursing Care of the Open Heart Patient" in the *Nursing Clinics of North America* in 1967 as a result of her experiences as a private-duty cardiovascular nurse.

The demand for knowledge, skill, physical strength, and emotional stability were stressed by Powers and Storlie (1969) as necessary qualities for cardiac intensive care nurses. It was also becoming increasingly evident that there was a shift from "training" nurses to perform duties to "educating" them to solve problems. Powers and Storlie emphasized the importance of questioning: *why* is a drug used, *what* is the mechanism of a particular dysrhythmia, *how* does a surgical procedure affect the heart? Such questions were not viewed as encroaching on the "traditional province of the physician" (p. 111), but as a means of making effective observations that, when correlated with basic knowledge, enabled the nurse to form (in the authors' words) a "nursing diagnosis" (p. 110).

This philosophy was reiterated in the 1970 publication of *Cardiovascular Nursing* by Kernicki, Bullock, and Matthews, which emphasized the "rationale for therapy and nursing approach"—the book's subtitle. In the book's preface, the authors noted a change from the primary role of executing physician's orders to a more collaborative role in the care of patients. This role required active participation rather than passive observation.

Mary Jo Aspinall's 1973 book *Nursing the Open-Heart Surgery Patient* also focused attention on the nurse's need for theoretical knowledge and the ability to use it in making clinical decisions. According to Aspinall, "[The nurse] must understand the operation of the machines . . . , recognize critical physiological changes, make interpretive judgments, and take necessary action" (preface).

Ouida M. King wrote in the preface of *Care of the Cardiac Surgical Patient*, which was also published in 1973, that her book was "designed to present a discussion of the principles involved in cardiac disease, thereby providing a background on which skill in caring for the cardiac surgical patient may be developed" (p. ix).

The need for skilled and informed nurses was echoed by their surgeon colleagues. Albert Starr and Denton Cooley each wrote a foreword in Powers and Storlie's book and in King's book, respectively, attesting to the importance of the cardiovascular nurse's professional role. In their surgical text *Coronary Artery Surgery,* John Ochsner and Noel Mills (1978) highlighted the role of the cardiovascular nurse specialist and referenced research from the nursing literature (Elsberry, 1972) in their chapter on patient education for coronary artery bypass surgery.

PERIOPERATIVE CARDIAC NURSE

Although the role of the perioperative nurse appeared in few cardiovascular-specific nursing texts of the period, there were exceptions. One was Chow's 1976 book *Cardiosurgical Nursing Care,* which included a short paragraph on preoperative visits by operating room nurses. Chow wrote:

> It is encouraging that some operating room nurses visit patients who are scheduled for major surgical procedures. This practice helps to alleviate the patient's anxieties, and helps the nurse to make observations about the mental and physical status of the patient and to anticipate his needs in personalized care (p. 319).

Chizuko Williams (Fig. 1-10), former operating room supervisor at Deborah Heart and Lung Center in Brown Mills, New Jersey, recognized the importance of the preoperative visit early in her 25-year tenure at the center. Her staff visited "each surgical patient preoperatively to perform a nursing assessment and [develop] a nursing care plan. This enabled them to provide

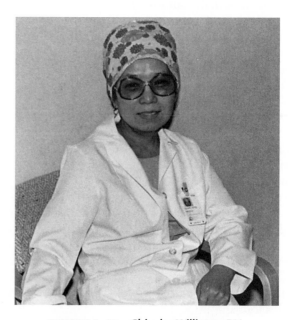

FIGURE 1-10   Chizuko Williams, RN.

highly individualized care to their patients intraoperatively" (Williams, 1992). Her philosophy was described in an article in 1985 (Williams, Czapinski, and Graf, 1985) and in an accompanying interview (Conversation with the author, 1985).

Awareness of the profound physiologic effects of cardiac surgery, as well as the emotional effects of fear and anxiety, prompted other nurses (including those represented in this chapter) participating in the development of cardiac surgery programs to promote patient and family interactions. This trend was reflected in the perioperative nursing literature, which stressed the need to incorporate a psychosocial component in preoperative patient assessments.

In addition to relying on available nursing and surgical literature to expand their knowledge, perioperative cardiac nurses worked closely with the surgeon to increase their skill and experience within the surgical setting. These interactions with surgeons, perfusionists (not mentioned in this chapter, but deserving much credit), and other members of the cardiac team were important in achieving successful patient outcomes. Surgeons were among the first to support the development of a professional perioperative nursing role that would foster a calm, competent, and efficient operative environment. Shumacker (1992) reflected the need for knowledge, as well as skill, when he wrote that "especially trained nurses, assistants, and technicians superseded willing but untutored ones" (p. 366).

Perioperative cardiac nurses were highlighted in a book describing the history of the Texas Heart Institute (THI) (THI Foundation, 1989), one of the most well-known cardiac centers in the world. Susan J. Kadow, at the time an assistant nurse manager of cardiovascular surgery at THI, was one of the many nurses depicted and quoted in the book. Her emphasis on the importance of close working relationships with the surgeon and the ability to anticipate needs represents some of the critical attributes of perioperative cardiac nurses.

These attributes and the importance of consistency in the performance of operations were factors that led to expanded perioperative nursing roles. The RN First Assistant (RNFA) is one such role that has been widely adopted by perioperative cardiac nurses. The efforts of Nancy Davis (see Fig. 1-6) have been crucial to the development of the role and its widespread acceptance throughout the Untied States. The establishment of a college-level educational program for the RNFA by Jane Rothrock (1993) has enabled numerous perioperative nurses to engage in first-assisting duties that are based on a sound theoretical foundation, as well as extensive clinical practice. RNFA Christine Espersen (1993) describes the range of responsibilities of the RNFA during the preoperative, intraoperative, and postoperative periods and illustrates the positive impact that the RNFA has on patient care.

In 1994 Patricia Seifert published the first comprehensive textbook devoted to the perioperative nursing care of cardiac patients. This book integrated the nursing process; RNFA considerations; descriptions of cardiac surgical procedures; standards of care; and "pearls" from physicians, nurses, patients, and manufacturers.

Conclusion

The history of cardiac surgery and the role of the perioperative nurse have been largely associated with technical achievements. However, these achievements, important as they are, do not reflect the essence of what cardiac surgery is or what cardiac surgery team members do. A truer representation can be found in the personal characteristics of its participants: curiosity, flexibility, compassion, and persistence. These qualities have enabled surgeons and nurses to perform the technical feats for which they are justifiably esteemed. Such qualities have motivated persons to go beyond what was expected and to extend their responsibilities above what was considered allowable. These are the significant achievements that represent cardiac surgery. Perioperative cardiac nurses need to be aware of their heritage so that they can appreciate how important their contributions have been and how necessary it is for them to continue to contribute to the welfare of patients with cardiac disease.

References

Abbott M: *Atlas of congenital heart disease*, New York, 1936, American Heart Association.

Alexander EL: *Operating room technique*, St Louis, 1943, Mosby.

Alexander EL: *Operating room technique*, ed 2, St Louis, 1949, Mosby.

Alexander EL: *The care of the patient in surgery including techniques*, ed 3, St Louis, 1958, Mosby.

Alexander EL and others: *Care of the patient in surgery including techniques*, ed 4, St Louis, 1967, Mosby.

American Heart Association: *Proceedings of the first national conference on cardiovascular diseases*, New York, 1950, AHA.

AORN Online (The Association of PeriOperative Registered Nurses). www.aorn.org, accessed 11/5/01

Aspinall MJ: *Nursing the open-heart surgery patient*, New York, 1973, McGraw-Hill.

Austin WG: Presidential address: surgery is a great career, *Am Coll Surg Bull* 77(12):6, 1992.

Barnard CN: The operation. A human cardiac transplant: an interim report of a successful operation performed at Groote Schuur Hospital, Cape Town, *S Afr Med J* 41(48):1271, 1967.

Baumgarten G: Personal communication, 1992.

Beck CS: The development of a new blood supply to the heart by operation, *Ann Surg* 102:801, 1935.

Benetti FJ and others: Direct myocardial revascularization with extracorporeal circulation, *Chest* 100(2):312, 1991.

Brandt L: Surgery of the heart and great vessels, *OR Supervisor*, Dec 1951.

Brieger GH: The development of surgery. In Sabiston DC Jr, editor: *Textbook of surgery*, ed 14, Philadelphia, 1991, WB Saunders.

Cannon A: Personal communication, 1992.

Cardiovascular nurse designs graft sizers, *Methodist J*, April 9, 1976.

Chow RK: *Cardiosurgical nursing care: understandings, concepts, and principles for practice*, New York, 1976, Springer.

Colp R, Keller MW: *Textbook of surgical nursing*, New York, 1921, Macmillan.

Comroe JH Jr: Who was Alexis who? Cardiovascular diseases, *Bull Tex Heart Inst* 6(3):251, 1979.

Comroe JH Jr: Doctor, you have six minutes, *Science*, Jan/Feb:64, 1983.

Comroe JH Jr, Dripps RD: *The top ten clinical advances in cardiovascular-pulmonary medicine and surgery between 1945 and 1975: how they came about*—final report, Bethesda, Md, Jan 31, 1977, National Heart and Lung Institute.

Conversation with the author (Chizuko Williams, R.N.), *Cardiothorac Nurse* 3(1):5, 1985.

Cooley DA: *Surgical treatment of thoracic aneurysms*, Philadelphia, 1986, WB Saunders.

Cooley DA: Recollections of early development and later trends in cardiac surgery, *J Thorac Cardiovasc Surg* 98:817, 1989.

Cooley DA and others: Organ transplantation for advanced cardiopulmonary disease, *Ann Thorac Surg* 8(1):30, 1969.

Cutler E, Beck C: The present status of the surgical procedures in chronic valvular disease of the heart, *Arch Surg* 18:403, 1929.

Davis N: Personal communication, 1992.

DeVries WC: The permanent artificial heart: four case reports, *JAMA* 259(6):849, 1988.

Dobell ARC: Surgery in the era of technology, *Am Coll Surg Bull* 75(4):8, 1990.

Driscoll J: *Preserving the legacy: AORN 1949-1989*, Denver, 1990, Association of Operating Room Nurses.

Effler DB: Introduction. In Favaloro RG: *Surgical treatment of coronary arteriosclerosis*, Baltimore, 1970, Williams & Wilkins.

Elsberry NL: Psychological responses to open heart surgery: a review, *Nurs Res* 21(3):220, 1972.

Espersen CC: The RN first assistant in cardiac surgery. In Rothrock JC: *The RN first assistant: an expanded perioperative nursing role*, ed 2, Philadelphia, 1993, JB Lippincott.

Favaloro R: Saphenous vein autograft replacement of severe segmental coronary artery occlusion operative technique, *Ann Thorac Surg* 5(4):334, 1968.

Favaloro RG: *The challenging dream of heart surgery: from the Pampas to Cleveland*, Cleveland, 1992, The Cleveland Clinic Foundation.

Fordham ME: *Cardiovascular surgical nursing*, New York, 1962, Macmillan.

Frost EAM: *Essays on the history of anesthesia*, Georgetown, Conn, 1985, McMahon.

Garrett HE, Dennis EW, DeBakey ME: Aortocoronary bypass with saphenous vein grafts: seven-year follow-up, *JAMA* 223(7):792, 1973.

Gibbon J: Application of a mechanical heart and lung apparatus to cardiac surgery, *Minn Med* 37:171, 1954.

Hagopian EJ and others: The history of thoracic surgical instruments and instrumentation, *Chest Surg Clin N Am* 10(1):9, 2000.

Harkin DE: The emergence of cardiac surgery, *J Thorac Cardiovasc Surg* 98(5, pt 2):805, 1989.

Hartin P: Personal communication, 1992.

Higgins V: Cardiothoracic operations. In Ballinger WF, Treybal JC, Vose AB: *Alexander's care of the patient in surgery*, ed 5, St Louis, 1972, Mosby.

Ho C and others: Genetically engineered hemoglobin, *Biochemistry* 39:13719, 2000.

Ion E: Personal communication, 1992.

IR@biopure.com: World's first oxygen therapeutic for human use approved in South Africa to Treat Anemia in surgery patients, electronic mail communication, 2001.

James EE: The nursing care of the open heart patient, *Nurs Clin North Am* 2(3):543, 1967.

Jamieson SW, Stinson EB, Shumway NE: Cardiac transplantation in 150 patients at Stanford University, *Br Med J* 1(6156):93, 1979.

Johnson SL: *The history of cardiac surgery: 1896-1955*, Baltimore, 1970, Johns Hopkins University Press.

Kernicki J, Bullock BL, Matthews J: *Cardiovascular nursing: rationale for therapy and nursing approach*, New York, 1970, GP Putnam's Sons.

King OM: *Care of the cardiac surgical patient*, St Louis, 1975, Mosby.

Kirklin JK and others: Complement and the damaging effects of cardiopulmonary bypass, *J Thorac Cardiovasc Surg* 86:845, 1983.

Kneedler JA: Origins of operating room nursing. In Kneedler JA, Dodge GH: *Perioperative patient care: the nursing perspective*, ed 2, Boston, 1987, Blackwell Scientific.

Kolessov VI: Mammary artery-coronary artery anastomosis as method of treatment for angina pectoris, *J Thorac Cardiovasc Surg* 54:535, 1967.

Kouwenhoven WB, Jude JR, Knickerbocker GG: Landmark article July 9, 1960: Closed-chest cardiac massage, *JAMA* 251(23):3133, 1984.

Lee RM: Early operating room nursing, *AORN J* 24(1):124, 1976.

Lefrak EA, Starr A: *Cardiac valve prostheses*, New York, 1979, Appleton-Century-Crofts.

Lillehei CW: Discussion of Lillehei CW and others: The first open-heart repairs of ventricular septal defects, atrioventricular communis, and tetralogy of Fallot using extracorporeal circulation by cross-circulation: a 30-year follow-up, *Ann Thorac Surg* 41(1):4, 1986.

Litwak RS: The growth of cardiac surgery: historical notes, *Cardiovasc Clin* 3(2):5, 1971.

Loop FD and others: Influence of the internal-mammary-artery graft on 10-year survival and other cardiac events, *N Engl J Med* 314(1):1, 1986.

Metzger RS: The beginnings of OR nursing education, *AORN J* 24(1):73, 1976.

Miller GW: *King of hearts*, New York, 2000, Random House.

Modell W: *Handbook of cardiology for nurses*, New York, 1952, Springer.

Montgomery JG: Personal communication, 1992.

Nineteen years of AORN films, *AORN J* 27(3):511, 1978.

Nissen R: *Billroth and cardiac surgery,* Lancet 2:25, 1963.

Ochsner JL, Mills NL: *Coronary artery surgery,* Philadelphia, 1978, Lea & Febiger.

Paget S: *Surgery of the chest,* London, 1896, John Wright.

Powers M, Storlie F: *The cardiac surgical patient,* London, 1969, Macmillan.

Raber T: Personal communication, 1992.

Rashkind WJ: Historical aspects of surgery for congenital heart disease, *J Thorac Cardiovasc Surg* 84(4):619, 1982.

Reichenspurner H and others: Use of the voice-controlled and computer-assisted surgical system ZEUS for endoscopic coronary artery bypass grafting, *J Thorac Cardiovasc Surg* 118:11, 1999.

Reitz BA, Pennock JL, Shumway NE: Simplified operative method of heart and lung transplantation, *J Surg Res* 31(1):1, 1981.

Riese S: A historical review of the AORN Journal, *AORN J* 71(3):606, 2000.

Rothrock JC: *The RN first assistant: an expanded perioperative nursing role,* ed 2, Philadelphia, 1993, JB Lippincott.

Seifert PC: *Cardiac surgery,* St Louis, 1994, Mosby.

Shumacker HB: *The evolution of cardiac surgery,* Bloomington, 1992, Indiana University Press.

Shumway NE: *Transplantation of the heart and heart-lung.* Paper presented at Cardiac Surgery: 1993 "State of the Art," The Academy of Medicine of New Jersey, Division of Cardiothoracic Surgery, School of Cardiovascular Perfusion, Department of Nursing Education and Quality Assurance, Cooper Hospital/University Medical Center, St Thomas, Virgin Islands, Nov 14, 1992.

Sones FM, Shirey EK: Cine coronary arteriography, *Mod Concepts Cardiovasc Dis* 31(7):735, 1962.

Stafford ES, Diller D: *A textbook of surgery for nurses,* Philadelphia, 1947, WB Saunders.

Texas Heart Institute Foundation: *Twenty-five years of excellence: a history of the Texas Heart Institute,* Houston, 1989, THI Foundation.

Toronto Lung Transplant Group: Experience with single lung transplantation for pulmonary fibrosis, *JAMA* 259:2558, 1988.

Voorhees AB: The origin of the permeable arterial prosthesis: a personal recollection, *Surg Rounds* Feb:79, 1988.

Voorhees AB Jr, Jaretzki A 3rd, Blakemore AH: The use of tubes constructed from Vinyon "N" cloth in bridging arterial defects, *Ann Surg* 135(3):332, 1952.

Walsh JJ: *History of nursing,* New York, 1929, PJ Kennedy.

Werker PM, Kon M: Review of facilitated approaches to vascular anastomosis surgery, *Ann Thorac Surg* 63:S122, 1997.

West JP, Keller MW, Harmon E: *Nursing care of the surgical patient,* ed 5, New York, 1950, Macmillan.

Westaby S: *Landmarks in cardiac surgery,* Oxford, 1997, Isis Medical Media.

Williams C: Personal communication, 1992.

Williams C, Czapinski N, Graf D: Perioperative nursing: implications for open-heart surgery, *Cardiothorac Nurs* 3(1):1, 1985.

2

The Perioperative Nurse and the Cardiac Team

Perioperative patient care is a complex and comprehensive physiologic and psychologic undertaking; it is at times precise and scientific, and at times fluid, intuitive, and subjective.

Jane C. Rothrock, RN, 1990

It is now widely accepted that error tolerance, error detection, and error recovery are as important as error prevention.

Marc R. de Leval, MD, and colleagues, 2000

The team concept is a fundamental principle of cardiac surgery. Complex technologic resources, distinctive patient populations, and, frequently, sudden and life-threatening physiologic alterations require that individual efforts be integrated efficiently and effectively into a unified effort. Achieving this high level of coordination requires collaboration to create the team, an understanding of tam members' roles, stress management strategies, competence, ongoing skill development, continuing knowledge acquisition, and a systematic plan for error reduction. Perioperative nursing considerations are the main focus of this chapter, but other team members are included to illustrate the multidisciplinary nature of an effective cardiac service.

Development of the Team

A team is more than a collection of people. It is a cohesive group of individuals whose personal and professional goals are congruent with the objectives of the service: to achieve optimal outcomes by providing knowledgeable, skilled, and cost-effective care in a safe and therapeutic environment to patients with cardiovascular disease. Among individual team members, personal goals may include meeting the challenges presented by these patients, being rewarded for performance, learning new skills, and receiving recognition for contributions to patient care.

The qualities that are sought in prospective members reflect the values of the service and the organization. The ability to function within the group depends not only on knowledge and skill but also on qualities such as flexibility, dedication, a sense of humor, and the ability to reset or modify priorities. A positive attitude, an appreciation for quality and excellence, and respect for loyalty are additional attributes desired in new and experienced staff. Because the tempo of the operating room (OR) is fast and demanding, a solid work ethic is imperative (Houchin, 1994). In recruiting new team members, specific cardiac-related knowledge is less important than a "can-do" attitude and a desire to be the best; individuals with these traits tend to be enthusiastic learners who can acquire the technical and cognitive knowledge required to function as a cardiac team member.

Integrating individual and team goals is achieved through a process that fosters camaraderie among group members. It is influenced by frequent interaction, interesting work, effective communication, a history of success, high performance standards, team members' knowledge and experience, and support and encouragement from group leaders. Box 2-1 describes a study by Pisano, Bohmer, and Edmundson (2001) that confirms the value of effective teamwork in implementing new technologies into a cardiac service.

As a result of the ego strength derived from clinical competence, team members are often highly motivated and possess strong characters. Such personal qualities lend themselves to environments in which independent thinking is encouraged. A structured environment is suitable during the formative stages of a cardiac program, but decentralized units provide a more appropriate forum for the problem solving and decision making required in an established cardiac surgical service. Communication must be open and information shared freely if team

---

BOX 2-1
Organizational Learning Factors

Pisano, Bohmer, and Edmondson studied how organizations learn and implement new highly technical services to determine whether, in addition to the level of experience possessed by individual team members, there are organizational factors that contribute to a collective learning process. Sixteen hospitals were selected for study; they all had similar state-of-the-art operating rooms, all were using essentially the same Food and Drug Administration-approved devices, and all members of the surgical teams participated in the same training course. The authors found that there were different rates of learning (i.e., learning curves) among the institutions.

Four factors characterized the fastest-learning institutions.

1. The team members selected to attend the initial, manufacturer-sponsored 3-day training program were picked on the basis of the individual team members' prior experience working together and working well together (team members were not selected randomly or on the basis of seniority).

2. Considerable cross-department communication and cooperation was evident even before the first operation. After returning from the training, the surgeon organized a series of meetings with other departments that might be affected by the new technology. Cardiologists, perfusionists, nurses, and anesthesia care providers learned about the indications for the use of the new technology, agreed on standard ter-

minology, and met on a regular basis to discuss the procedure. The surgeon regularly met with cardiologists to discuss upcoming cases.

3. The first 30 procedures were carefully managed by the surgeon. Both the makeup of the team and the performance of the procedure remained stable; the same team performed the first 15 cases. When new team members were added, they were required (regardless of rank) to observe 4 cases and be preceptored on 2 cases before they were allowed to join the team. Before each of the first 10 cases, the entire surgical team met to discuss the planned procedure. The team also met again after the first 20 cases to debrief. Team members collected and analyzed outcome data, and presented their findings to local and national audiences.

4. The surgeon engendered a high degree of cooperation among the team members, and actively became a partner with the rest of the team. The surgeon encouraged input and feedback from other team members. A trusting relationship was developed among the team members.

The authors concluded that learning from experience is not automatic; some organizations capitalize on their experience more effectively than others. Opportunities for learning should be exploited.

Modified from Pisano GP, Bohmer RMJ, Edmondson AC: Organizational differences in rates of learning: evidence from the adoption of minimally invasive cardiac surgery, *Management Science* 47(6):752, 2001.

---

members are to be able to make appropriate decisions and resolve problems both individually and collectively.

Staffing Issues

Considerable interest has been focused on staffing shortages, diversity issues, generational differences, and the impact of an aging workforce.

STAFFING SHORTAGES

Staffing shortages affect nursing and other professions. One strategy to expand the pool of cardiac nurses is to cross-train staff from the general OR to the cardiac OR. This can be effective when the trainee receives a comprehensive orientation to the service, works with a preceptor who is committed to the trainee's success, and functions within a team that welcomes and encourages new members. Cross-training fails if the new staff member is not provided sufficient clinical and psychologic support. Similarly, a supportive environment is necessary for retaining staff; recruitment is more difficult when retention is a problem.

Another strategy is to hire cardiac staff from a different unit, such the intensive care unit (ICU) or the cardiac catheterization laboratory. These individuals usually have excellent knowledge of patient assessment, cardiac

pathophysiology, hemodynamic monitoring, and pharmacology. A structured perioperative nursing course provides the foundation for functioning in the OR.

Cardiac perioperative nurses also can work with schools of nursing to provide clinical study sites for their students or can participate in perioperative nursing programs. The Association of periOperative Registered Nurses (AORN) is committed to addressing the shortage of perioperative nurses; additional information can be found at www.aorn.org.

DIVERSITY ISSUES

Cultural diversity among patients, nurses, physicians, and other staff members provides both enriching and occasionally frustrating experiences. Differing languages, diets, health beliefs, religions, and values may test the team's ability to function as a unit, but managers and staff need to effect policies and behaviors that promote cultural understanding. Diversity can also apply to generational differences.

GENERATIONAL DIFFERENCES

The various characteristics of different generations have been studied, and differentiating between the rhetoric and the reality can be a challenge (Cufaude,

TABLE 2-1
Generational Categories

CATEGORY	BORN	GROUP SIZE (APPROXIMATE)	KEY VALUES
Mature	1909-1945	62 million	Teamwork, commitment, sacrifice, discipline
Baby Boomers	1946-1964	77 million	Idealism, individualism, self-improvement, high expectations
Generation X	1965-1978	52 million	Pragmatism, diversity, quality of life, savvyness, entrepreneurial spirit
Generation Y, Millenialists, or Echo Boomers	born after 1979	78 million	Optimism, technologic adeptness, ritual, multiculturalism, compartmentalized work and leisure

Modified from Cufaude JB: Cultivating new leadership, *Assoc Manage* (January):73-78, 2000.

2000). Individuals in one generational category (Table 2-1) may attribute stereotypical characteristics to those in another (older or younger) category. This perception or conclusion may be the result of a failure to understand the motivating factors and social contexts that affect the behaviors or values of a particular generation. Rather than stereotype the "Boomers" or the "X-ers," individuals should look at the special strengths and skills that staff members bring to a cardiac service (or any other work setting). The technologic adeptness often attributed to one age group can be a valuable skill in the current environment of outcomes databases and Web-based information systems. The high expectations and idealism associated with another group may be helpful in creating a meaningful link between long hours and positive patient outcomes. The important point is that although there are generational characteristics, people should not be automatically pigeonholed. There are technologically savvy 80 year olds and dedicated 20 year olds. Both managers and staff should look for the strengths that individuals bring to the group.

AGING WORKFORCE

Another related issue is the aging workforce and its impact in the workplace. Creative strategies to redesign the work environment to make it "older worker–friendly" can have real benefit in an era of staffing shortages. Experienced nurses can be invaluable preceptors and mentors to younger, less-experienced staff. In a cardiac service there is a complex, sophisticated experiential and cognitive body of knowledge, and the knowledge based on the expertise of mature nurses must be transferred to the newer members of the team.

The question of when a surgeon should retire (Greenfield and Procter, 1999) also has been addressed. Visual, cognitive, and psychomotor changes associated with aging can affect surgical risk and patient outcomes. Objective measures to test sensory and cognitive impairment are needed not only so that patients are protected but also so that clinicians (physicians, nurses, and others) are not subject to discrimination.

Collaboration

Collaboration among caregivers (e.g., nurses, physicians, anesthesia care providers, perfusionists, and others) fosters consumer well-being in the clinical setting (Pew Health Professions Commission, 1995; Lassen and others, 1997; Knaus and others, 1986; Seifert, 1999; Institute of Medicine, 1999). Examples specific to cardiac surgery have been published (Carthey, de Leval, and Reason, 2001; de Leval and others, 2000) that demonstrate the value of collaboration and positive professional relationships.

COLLABORATION IN THE CLASSROOM

Developing a culture of professional collaboration starts in the classroom. Students of medicine, nursing, perfusion, and other professions can build a strong foundation for future teamwork by sharing not only classes on subjects such as anatomy and physiology but also through nonclass activities such as breakfast and luncheon meetings, journal clubs, and other gatherings. One program described by Zarbock (1999) included topics such as the use and abuse of power, deaf culture, and cultural disparities in the delivery of health care. In cultures with a hierarchical model of interprofessional relationships (whether within another country or within the United States), changing role stratification requires both the presence of role models of collaboration to serve as champions of the culture change and the implementation of interprofessional education to enhance understanding of the complementary roles of physicians and nurses (Hojat and others, 2001).

Partnering with schools of nursing (and medicine) to incorporate knowledge and practice skills related to infection control (e.g., aseptic practices), injury prevention (e.g., positioning, laser safety, skin preparation), and systems improvement (e.g., structure, process and outcome standards) are ways of enhancing safety (Seifert, 2000).

Additional opportunities for joint education and training of physicians and nurses have arisen with the rapid growth of new cardiac surgical techniques. Minimally invasive interventions, video-assisted technologies, and computerized robotic surgery have produced a demand for nontraditional training programs (Satava and Jones, 2000). In describing minimally invasive surgical training solutions for the twenty-first century, Rosser, Murayama, and Gabriel (2000) stress the need for a perioperative nursing component that parallels the medical portion of training programs. Additionally, the authors strongly suggest that nurses be exposed to the same lecture series as the surgeons. These recommendations reflect the interactive nature of many newer interventions that require a high level of coordination among all members of the surgical team.

Historically, skill development in new technologies has been provided by industry, professional meetings (often supported by industry), visits by surgeons and team members to other institutions, and informal communication (Lytle, 2001). Although Ricci and colleagues (2000) found that 88% of physicians in cardiac surgical residency programs wanted to perform off-pump surgery after completion of their training, less than 12% of residents had performed more than 20 off-pump surgeries. Professional cardiac surgical organizations, notably the Society of Thoracic Surgeons (STS) and the American Association for Thoracic Surgery (AATS), have offered conceptual continuing education but little detailed technical training. In order to minimize the learning curve and accelerate the acquisition of expertise for technologic advances, the STS (see www.sts.org) and the AATS (see www.aats.org) have jointly developed a demonstration project for beating heart surgery, including didactic sessions, live animal and cadaver training, observational visits to institutions experienced in the new techniques, and visits by mentoring surgeons to the surgeons in training (Lytle, 2001). These educational programs (and others) also may employ three-dimensional visualization, telepresence and distant learning components, video conferencing, and access to the Internet. Virtual reality (VR) technology is especially valuable for the education and training of physicians and nurses. VR enables the user to become immersed in and interact with the artificial environment. The ability to simulate the senses of sight, sound, and touch have been developed to a fairly high degree in VR technology; the simulation of smell and taste is in the early experimental stages (Meier, Rawn, and Krummel, 2001).

CLINICAL COLLABORATION

Practicing clinicians also have many opportunities to promote collaboration and teamwork. A simple but effective method is for department managers to incorporate field trips by members of their department to another department or to include time in another unit as part of a staff member's orientation. Perioperative nurses, cardiac catheterization laboratory technologists, and critical care nurses (to name a few examples) can benefit from spending time in other units. Although staff time must be allowed for this, the positive effects are well worth the challenges faced by managers in scheduling such visits. Not only do these visits educate and inform staff about patient needs on other units (thereby fostering a more global view of the patient's movement through the hospital stay), but they also allow individuals from one department to meet their respective colleagues on another unit. Communication is enhanced, and when emergencies arise, established personal relationships promote the sharing of pertinent information and foster seamless care.

The value of such interaction is exemplified by two scenarios. The first relates to the patient brought to the catheterization laboratory for an acute coronary intervention that results in emergency surgery, and the second scenario concerns a postoperative patient hemorrhaging in the surgical intensive care unit (SICU) who requires reoperation to control the bleeding. Perioperative nurses who have established good communication channels with their colleagues in these departments can anticipate patient needs sooner and intervene more expeditiously.

Partnerships are not always easy to achieve. Greenfield (1999) addressed a troubled partnership between doctors and nurses. He surveyed physicians and nurses and found areas of polarity between the two groups. For example, one survey question stating that "the major responsibility of the nurse is to serve as the patient's advocate" (p. 284) elicited strong support from nurses but opposition from physicians. The current environment tends to promote competition rather than cooperation between the professions. This is a source of concern for many nurses and physicians who see the conflict as interfering with patient care. Suggestions offered by Greenfield (1999) for improving the partnership include the following:

- Joint clinical training of nursing and medical students
- Daily communication between nurses and physicians to improve the coordination of care
- Incentives that reward collegial behavior and discourage dictatorial behavior
- Promotion of a clinical curricula that provides patients the very best that both disciplines have to offer

Numerous additional learning opportunities are available from representatives in radiology, pharmacy, blood bank, laboratory, other institutional departments, and manufacturer's representatives. For example, partnering with industry to design ergonomically sound devices that consider human factors, such as fine motor skills, visual cues, and energy expenditure, has been a fruitful collaboration for many years and has become

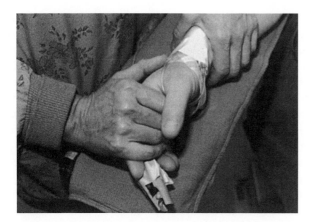

FIGURE 2-1 The patient is wearing a pulse oximetry finger cot. Perioperative cardiac nursing combines sophisticated technology and compassionate care. (Courtesy Howard Kaye.)

> **BOX 2-2**
> ## *Tips for Patients*
>
> - Make sure that you, your surgeon, and other members of the health care team all agree and are clear on exactly what will be done.
> - Speak up if you have questions or concerns.
> - Make sure that one person (such as your personal physician) is in overall charge of your care.
> - Make sure that all health care professionals involved in your care have the necessary health information about you.
> - Ask a family member or friend to be with you and serve as your advocate to speak up for you and get things done.
> - If you have a test, know why it is being done. Don't assume that no news is good news; ask about the results.
> - Learn about your condition and treatments by asking your physician and nurses and by using other reliable sources.

Modified from Agency for Healthcare Research and Quality: 20 tips to help prevent medical errors. Patient fact sheet, AHRQ Pub no 00-P038, February 2000, http://www.ahrq.gov/consumer/20tips.htm (accessed July 13, 2001).

increasingly important with the explosion of minimally invasive and other high-technology devices, tools, and practices. Perioperative cardiac nurses and surgeons have a long history of mutually beneficial partnerships with industry.

PATIENT PARTNERSHIPS

Information exchanges between perioperative nurses and patients are especially important. Patient-provider partnerships can be fostered by working together to achieve the same goals. It is helpful to recognize and validate patient's feelings through verbal and nonverbal skills, provide understanding and clarification of the patient's situation (Fig. 2-1), and encourage patient participation in the selection of treatment options (Zarbock, 2000). Even within the fairly structured universe of surgery, patients do have choices, as witnessed by patients who select their physician, institution, or intervention based on a thorough Internet search. For example, the rapid growth of off-pump and minimal-incision surgery has been caused in no small part by consumer demand for these minimally invasive techniques.

Although there are managed care and payor-imposed restrictions, patients often can identify their preference for a caregiver and a procedure. By providing information about various therapeutic options, clinicians can empower patients with knowledge about available treatments and promote informed acceptance and cooperation. According to the Agency for Healthcare Research and Quality's "Patient Fact Sheet," the single most important way for a patient to prevent medical errors is to be an active member of the health care team by taking part in every decision regarding one's health care (AHRQ, 2000).

Patients have an important role in reducing medical errors. Mishaps can be caused by the complexity of the health care system itself, but communication problems between patients and their caregivers also can foster errors. An involved and informed patient is more likely to become an active member of the health care team. Patients should be encouraged to ask questions that provide a basis for informed decision making and participation. Box 2-2 lists tips, which are recommended by AHRQ (2000), for patients anticipating surgery.

Nursing Roles

The core of a cardiac service consists of nurses, surgeons, surgical assistants, anesthesia care providers, cardiopulmonary technologists, perfusionists, and patients. Surgical technologists and support staff, such as aides and orderlies, perform many vital functions and should be considered cardiac team members.

Nursing roles have been influenced by collaborative practice models and the multidisciplinary integration of resources. This is especially evident in the cardiac operating room, where patient outcomes are dependent on shared decision making and responsibility for judging the appropriateness of interventions. This emphasis on clinical nursing judgment implies that nurses demonstrate the knowledge and skills required to function as partners in collaborative efforts. The nurse must have knowledge of an extensive array of cardiovascular disorders and their treatments, be able to manipulate complex equipment, and interact effectively with patients and families coping with illnesses that have a profound physiologic and emotional impact on their lives. These skills are acquired gradually while performing the traditional roles of circulator and scrub nurse; they

---

BOX 2-3
Five Stages of Proficiency

Novice: The nurse has no experience with cardiac surgery and bases performance on rules and instructions from the preceptor. The novice is unable to place patient situations into context.

Advanced beginner: The nurse has had limited experience with cardiac surgery and is able to identify critical activities but is unable to discern subtle cues or to prioritize actions.

Competent nurse: The nurse has sufficient experience to formulate an efficient and organized plan of care but still lacks flexibility and speed in unusual situations.

Proficient nurse: The nurse is capable of placing actions in context and sees situations holistically rather than as a series of steps. The proficient nurse works interdependently with other members of the cardiac team.

Expert: The nurse has a wealth of experience and responds automatically to familiar situations rather than depending on analysis and rules. Performance is fluid and flexible. The expert works interdependently with professionals within and outside the cardiac operating room.

Modified from Benner P: *From novice to expert*, Menlo Park, Calif, 1984, Addison-Wesley.

---

also form the basis for more expanded clinical nursing practice, represented by the registered nurse first assistant (RNFA) role, and advanced nursing practice, represented by clinical specialists and practitioners.

DEVELOPMENT OF CLINICAL SKILL

Clinical skill develops as one learns to integrate theoretical knowledge and experience in the perioperative arena. Nurses specializing in cardiac surgery progress from a beginner level to an advanced level of practice as they apply these "head and hand" skills to patient situations. Benner (1984) identified five stages of proficiency to describe this progression: novice, advanced beginner, competent, proficient, and expert (Box 2-3). The model has been applied to numerous clinical settings, including the operating room (Benner, Hooper-Kyriakidis, and Stannard, 1999).

These designations are situational. A perioperative nurse, proficient in general surgery, enters a cardiac surgery service as a novice or advanced beginner because the patient population, the operative procedures, and the cardiac team are unfamiliar. The nurse with past open heart surgery experience is likely to adapt more quickly to the new setting but still functions as a beginner. Specific attributes of the environment and the team need to be learned. Among these are the structure of the unit, the location of supplies, surgeon preferences, and the personalities of individual team members.

The RNFA novice has demonstrated proficiency as a scrub nurse and circulator, but as a beginning cardiac RNFA the novice needs to develop new skills specific to the practice of cardiac surgical first assisting.

Other characteristics of developing proficiency include (1) a shift from relying on abstract principles to using past concrete experiences, (2) viewing the situation more as a whole rather than a compilation of parts, and (3) moving from detached observation to involved performance (Benner, 1984).

NOVICE

Novice nurses orienting to cardiac surgery have no previous open heart experience on which to base their performance. Because of the complexity of patients' problems, most beginning cardiac nurses come to a cardiac service with some perioperative nursing experience. At this stage they rely on a structured educational process that focuses on checklists and textbook rules, such as instrument and supply lists, or on patient vital signs and allergies. Novices may have minimal theoretical knowledge of cardiac disease, diagnostic studies, or surgical techniques; the course outline in Box 2-4 lists knowledge basic to cardiac nursing. A pretest and posttest (Appendix 2A) can be used to identify specific learning needs. Often novices are not aware of their knowledge or skills because they are too unfamiliar with the situation to ask questions; they may be unaware of what they don't know.

A preceptor assists the novice to begin the process of transforming abstract knowledge into clinical skill by applying theory to patient situations. For example, novice nurses may know that the purpose of coronary bypass surgery is to improve blood flow to the myocardium, but they may not know how this is achieved with bypass grafts. In planning preoperative teaching for the patient, the novice needs to understand the goal of the planned surgery, how that goal is met, and what the patient's responses to the intervention may be.

Psychomotor skills are enhanced by frequent hands-on practice and return demonstration with instruments and equipment such as vascular clamps, bypass lines, sternal saws, and defibrillators. Over time the nurse develops habits that enhance the efficient use of these devices.

Psychosocial skills can be developed by role playing and interacting with patients under the guidance of the preceptor. The preceptor can adapt the novice's previous experience and level of understanding to the situation, making it a learning experience for both patient and nurse.

Often the best preceptors for novices and advanced beginners are those at the competent and proficient levels because they can relate better than experts to the structured learning needs of beginners. They are able to assimilate the novice into the unit culture by interpreting new experiences in light of what the novice knows and what needs to be learned. The preceptor provides a

---

BOX 2-4
Cardiac Surgery Course Outline

Unit I

Introduction to the cardiac service
Anatomy and physiology
Perioperative nursing roles
Competency skills checklist
Standards of clinical practice
Standards of professional performance
Patient safety and error reduction
Policies, procedures
Inventory
Supplies (packs, carts)
Equipment (e.g., saws, defibrillators, endoscopic setup, video monitors)
Prostheses
   Grafts
   Valves and allografts
   Obturators
Room setup
Basic instrumentation
   Traditional
   Minimally invasive
Table setups

Unit II

Cardiovascular disease/pathology
   Congenital
      Normal fetal circulation
      Circulation after birth
      Increased pulmonary blood flow
      Decreased pulmonary blood flow
      Malformations, anomalies, defects
   Acquired
      Coronary artery disease
      Valvular heart disease
      Thoracic aneurysms, dissections
      Conduction disturbances, pacemakers, ICDs
      Emergencies
      Miscellaneous
Diagnostic studies
   Noninvasive (e.g., ECG, echocardiogram, nuclear studies, CT scan, MRI)
   Invasive (cardiac catheterization)

Interventional cardiology
   Percutaneous coronary intervention (PTCA, stent insertion, atherectomy)
   Valve balloon repair
   Occlusive devices for congenital defects
Laboratory tests
Blood bank
Cardiovascular drugs
Infection control
Perioperative care
Cardiac anesthesia
Hemodynamic monitoring
Ventricular function monitoring
Basic cardiac procedure (incision, bypass, closing)
Extracorporeal circulation, cardiopulmonary bypass
Circulatory arrest
Myocardial protection (cardioplegia: antegrade, retrograde)
Cerebral protection (cerebroplegia)

Unit III

History of cardiac surgery
Contributions of perioperative cardiac nurses
Procedures for congenital heart disease
   Special patient/family needs
   Special equipment and supplies
   Special instrumentation
Procedures for acquired heart disease
   Special patient/family needs
   Special equipment and supplies
   Special instrumentation
On-pump/off-pump considerations
Emergency procedures
   Trauma
   Postoperative hemorrhage
   Conversion from off-pump to on-pump
Pacemakers, ICDs
Patient/family teaching
Discharge planning and rehabilitation
The Mended Hearts (support group)
Research
Ethical issues

CT, Computed tomography; *ECG*, electrocardiogram; *ICD*, internal cardiovertor defibrillator; *MRI*, magnetic resonance imaging; *PTCA*, percutaneous transluminal coronary angioplasty.

---

balanced perspective and assists the novice to make the transition from detached observer to involved performer.

Novice circulating nurses may fear that they will be left alone in an emergency situation (such as a patient in cardiac arrest) or that they will be incapable of learning their new cardiac role sufficiently to function independently. The novice observes the situation but may not feel capable of becoming an active participant. Thoughts are disjointed and do not reflect a focus on achieving a goal. The novices' anxiety level is increased by a lack of practice in using the equipment and supplies common to cardiac surgery and by the fear that they will be expected to do something for

which they have no preparation. They are not yet aware that patient care requires both individual actions and mutually shared responsibilities. Commonly there is a feeling of sensory overload, which can be overwhelming without the guidance and support of the preceptor and other members of the team. Preceptors need to reassure nurses while at the same time monitoring their progress.

ADVANCED BEGINNER

The advanced beginner still follows preset rules but is starting to perceive patterns, set priorities, and anticipate needs based on patient cues during routine procedures. Both the novice and the advanced beginner learn basic skills by focusing on tasks. The competencies outlined in Appendix 2B reflect the knowledge, skills, and behaviors associated with the clinical practice and professional performance of the cardiac nurse. Not all the elements listed may require assessment; the selection of which elements are necessary is driven by each patient's individual situation.

The nurse at the advanced beginner level may be able to perform the skills but is not able to make associations between them. For instance, the proficient or expert nurse continuously assesses the hemodynamic status of the patient by comparing the information displayed on the monitor with the directly observable beating heart. (The expert may not even be conscious of doing this unless questioned.) Correlating subtle, progressive alterations in pressures (decreasing systemic pressure, increasing pulmonary pressure after the termination of cardiopulmonary bypass [CPB]) to a distended, sluggish heart alerts the expert to anticipate the reinstituting of pharmacologic support, cardiopulmonary bypass, intraaortic balloon counterpulsation, or other measures to rest the heart and conserve its energy resources. Alternatively, a patient undergoing off-pump surgery who suddenly demonstrates hemodynamic collapse may require the institution of CBP and conversion to an on-pump procedure. This transition is relatively seamless for the expert. The expert prepares for these procedures before being specifically requested to do so by the surgeon. The advanced beginner may be aware of these clinical signs but is unable to recognize the significance of them or identify available options and interventions appropriate to the clinical situation.

Preceptors assist beginning nurses to identify recurring aspects of situations. The advanced beginner starts to differentiate between what is normal and abnormal and what is significant and what is not, but he or she is still learning to judge the relative importance of these different aspects.

A circulating nurse at this level may express confusion or uncertainty about the appropriate timing of activities, such as counting instruments and remaining with the patient during anesthesia induction or determining when to use cold solutions versus warm solutions. In these cases the advanced beginner knows that the principles of patient safety and temperature control are important but cannot integrate them efficiently.

Another difficulty encountered by the advanced beginner is the formulation of a procedural timetable for completing tasks sequentially and in order of priority. The scrub nurse at this level may not be able to load the sternal wires, perform the counts, prepare the dressings, connect the chest tubes, and clean up the back table in an appropriate sequence. The preceptor helps the nurse to prioritize and do the most important things first and to identify what is important.

The scrub nurse is attempting to complete these tasks without identifying what has to be done first and what can wait. Whereas it may be obvious to the proficient nurse that the sternal wires need to go in before the dressing is applied or that cleaning up the table can be done after the case is completed, that kind of common sense is the result of participating in enough cases that the nurse is able to view the situation as a whole and not as a set of separate and unrelated activities.

It is not uncommon for the advanced beginner to forget certain basic activities or go through a transient dip in the learning curve. The scrub nurse may omit a step during the cannulation procedure (e.g., giving the surgeon a heavy suture to tie the cannula to the tourniquet); the circulator may neglect to apply the dispersive pad; the RNFA may forget when to use the cardiotomy suction in preference to the discard suction. One reason for this is that the nurse at this stage is trying to focus on both the particular and the general. He or she is trying to remember numerous details while at the same time attempting to plan ahead, perceive the situation on a more global scale, and group individual activities into sets (e.g., cannulation, opening or closing the chest, inserting temporary pacing wires). These lapses are disconcerting to the nurse, and it is helpful to review basic steps with emphasis on why actions are performed. When previously learned rules are explained in the context of situations experienced, nurses arrive at a deeper and more meaningful understanding of their performance.

COMPETENT

The competent nurse is able to place aspects of the situation into perspective and formulate a deliberate plan that is efficient and organized. Tasks are incorporated into the plan and are no longer the center of attention. Although lacking in speed and flexibility, the nurse has sufficient knowledge and skill to organize care, as illustrated by the ability to prepare a patient from the cardiac catheterization laboratory for emergency surgery. The competent nurse ensures that blood has been ordered and that lines are in place; the nurse has called the OR front desk to page the perfusionist and the anesthesia staff, opened the packs while the scrub nurse performed a hand scrub, and assisted with the transfer of the patient to the OR bed. After the patient is anesthetized, dispersive pads are applied and the patient placed in the supine position. The skin preparation is completed by the time the surgeon enters the OR to perform surgery.

Emergency cases like the one just described are typical, and a nurse who has been with a cardiac service for 2 or 3 years will have encountered a number of such cases.

These experiences allow nurses to develop a perspective and to put actions into terms of goals. In the situation described, the goal is to minimize the patient's myocardial damage and improve blood flow to the heart. This commonly is achieved by putting the patient on bypass and revascularizing the myocardium as expeditiously as possible. Nursing interventions of the circulator are aimed at facilitating this process by focusing on activities pertinent to the goal, such as comfort, safety, and anxiety-reducing measures, and monitoring and prepping procedures. The scrub nurse focuses on preparing instruments and supplies for incision, cardiopulmonary bypass, and coronary anastomoses. Activities not directly related to the goal (dressings, chest tubes, pacing wires) can be deferred. The nurse is capable of judging what is and what is not critical for preparation of an emergency case.

At this level of skill nurses benefit from simulations and decision-making exercises (Appendix 2C). Various imagined scenarios enable the nurse to detect the problem and define it, collect and analyze information, select options, identify available resources, develop plans, and evaluate the relative effectiveness of these plans. By placing the problem within a context (e.g., a particular surgeon's preferences, unit-specific characteristics, team members' designated responsibilities), nurses can avoid actions that are not pertinent. They can focus on plans that are congruent with the structure of the unit and the performance of its team members.

These simulations can be practiced with a proficient or expert preceptor, or they can be done alone. The value of these exercises is that the nurse can think through a problem without the attendant stress of real-life situations and reduce the margin for error by narrowing the selection to only the most appropriate options.

Such "what if" exercises are helpful not only to the competent nurse but also to the novice and advanced beginner who are often being precepted by the nurse at the competent level. Deliberate, conscious planning enables the competent nurse to verbalize to the novice step by step the rationale for actions and to put those actions into context. Compared with the expert, the competent nurse still relies on a linear analysis of performance, which can be broken down into discrete parts. The competent nurse is not yet fully capable of seeing the situation as a seamless whole.

PROFICIENT

Proficient nurses have learned from experience what to expect in a given situation and how to make modifications in response to changes in the patient's status. They know what the usual course of events is and plan appropriately without obvious effort. They are not deterred by unusual circumstances or untoward events. Unlike the competent nurse, the proficient nurse has advanced beyond a checklist mentality and has an overall picture of the situation. This holistic view is a hallmark of the proficient nurse.

The proficient nurse considers fewer options in deciding how to proceed, even in complex situations. In the case of a patient presenting with a thoracic aortic aneurysm, the proficient nurse wants to determine the location of the aneurysm because many nursing actions are dictated by this. For instance, if the patient has a descending thoracic aneurysm, the nurse knows that the patient will be placed laterally and that the surgeon will require thoracotomy instruments and equipment to achieve a lateral thoracotomy procedure.

Perfusion of the kidneys and other organs distal to the aneurysm may require extracorporeal techniques while the aorta is cross-clamped. The nurse does not dwell on gathering instruments and supplies for a median sternotomy and induced cardiac arrest, because in this situation the aneurysm is approached from the left lateral thoracotomy incision, and the heart does not need to be stopped.

Conversely the nurse awaiting a patient with an ascending aortic aneurysm knows that the position will be supine, that sternotomy instruments will be used, and that cardiopulmonary bypass will be used to perfuse the body's organs while the heart is arrested. The size and the location of the aneurysm will dictate cannulation techniques, which in turn will affect skin preparation, surgical exposure, and instrumentation. If the aneurysm has dilated the aortic annulus to the point of valvular incompetence (as seen on echocardiogram of the left ventricle), aortic valve replacement may be indicated, necessitating valve instruments. If the aortic root and ascending aorta must be resected, thereby obliterating the entrance to the coronary arteries, aortocoronary continuity must be reestablished by either coronary ostial reimplantation or bypass grafts (if coronary artery disease is documented). This would necessitate coronary bypass instruments and exposure of the saphenous vein if bypass grafts are required.

The description of these activities is linear, but the thought processes of the nurse do not proceed in such a step-by-step manner. The proficient nurse focuses on the salient features (ascending or descending) and considers the multiple options available almost simultaneously. In considering the important aspects of a case, proficient nurses talk to each other in a way that may not be easily understood by less-experienced clinicians. In discussing plans for an ascending aortic aneurysm, the scrub nurse, circulator, and RNFA might talk in disjointed lingo, referring to the "root," "opening the groin before the chest," "ostial reimplantation," and "clean coronaries."

In this scenario the RNFA is stating that because of the location and extent of the aneurysm, the ascending aorta and the aortic valve (located in the root of the aorta) will be replaced. Because there is a danger of lacerating this aneurysm during sternotomy and because placing a cannula in the aneurysmal aorta would risk rupture, the surgeon will first cannulate the femoral vein and femoral artery to initiate cardiopulmonary bypass. To reestablish blood flow to the coronary arteries (necessitated by excision of the aortic root, which contains the right and left coronary ostia that are the entrance to the coronary system) the ostia of the coronary arteries will be anastomosed to the prosthetic graft. Coronary bypass grafts are not indicated because the patient has no evidence of significant coronary artery disease (the coronary arteries are "clean").

In addition, the circulating nurse knows that the patient will probably require a prosthesis (and appropriate sizers) that combines a prosthetic graft and a manufactured valve. The circulator also will have available separate grafts and valves in the event that these are indicated. The nurse is familiar with similar cases and knows to cleanse the groin for exposure of the femoral artery and vein for cannulation. Patients with ascending aneurysms frequently present on an emergency basis, so family members' anxiety levels tend to be high during this high-risk procedure. The nurse is aware of this and can talk to the family once the procedure is under way.

Proficient nurses anticipate what can be expected and what modifications may be required. At this stage nurses demonstrate the following characteristics: basing performance on experience, viewing the situation as a whole, and becoming actively involved. With extensive knowledge and experience, proficient nurses are flexible enough to develop contingencies when operations do not proceed as planned, but novices may not understand why and how such modifications were chosen. Only when the nurse has attained a competent level of skill can she or he grasp the holistic nature of the proficient or expert nurse's performance. Case studies enable nurses to decipher the decision-making process in selecting interventions to meet specific patient needs, and they test nurses' ability to compare the expected with what actually occurs. Additionally, case studies highlight the most important aspects of a situation so that nurses can focus on them.

EXPERT

Experts have attained a level of skill that is difficult to describe because of the many contextual nuances associated with their clinical interventions. They respond automatically to situations and rarely analyze their decisions. Only when nurses have had little or no previous experience with a situation do experts need to reduce a situation to its component parts. Through repeated practice, experts have acquired habits that are ingrained in their performance.

The grace and rhythm of many experts and their seeming ability to read minds are the result not only of extensive experience with patient situations but also of working closely with team members. Excellence in the health care setting is often the result of collaborative relationships, as well as individual efforts. This is especially evident in the cardiac service, where mutual trust and respect, based on clinical competence, are themselves factors that promote positive patient outcomes.

RNFAs who have worked with a surgeon make few unnecessary motions and facilitate the performance of highly exacting surgical techniques such as anastomoses and cannulation. The expert scrub nurse displays a graceful familiarity with the stages of an operation and is unlikely to be directed by the surgeon in any but those situations in which the surgeon has not yet decided how to proceed. The expert circulator is known by the controlled calm created in the operating room and the efficient progression of the surgery.

Unlike less-skilled nurses, experts and proficient nurses approach a situation with the self-assurance that comes from knowing what is happening and what can (or cannot) be done about it. For example, if a patient who has just undergone a mitral valve replacement suddenly loses a large amount of blood in the SICU, the expert is capable of immediate intervention in the unit. This person will open the SICU's emergency chest set and supplies on an available surface, put on a gown and gloves, drape the patient, and assist the surgeon to open the chest in order to control the bleeding. If the hemorrhage cannot be controlled because of severity of the injury (e.g., a lacerated ventricular wall), more aggressive intervention is planned and implemented (such as replacing the valve). The nurse and the surgeon must quickly assess the options and select the one most likely to save the patient's life. This may mean that valve replacement needs to be performed in the unit because transport to the OR is not possible for a patient who is extremely unstable as a result of uncontrollable hemorrhage.

In viewing such a situation a novice might be appalled at the perceived lack of attention to the "basics" (e.g., performing a valve replacement outside the sterile confines of the OR), but in fact the basic consideration was to fix the ventricular tear and stop the bleeding so that the patient could survive. Deliberating over appropriate sterile technique or optimum surgical environments would have hindered the eventual successful outcome for this patient. What is significant in this instance is the shared responsibility and the collaborative plan that was implemented for the patient. Had there not been both competence and good working relationships, the outcome might not have been as positive.

It is the anticipation of problems and the selection of appropriate interventions that characterize the expert. But outlining the mental progression from problem identification to implementation of clinical strategies is difficult for experts to explain. Much of their practice is based on well-formed habits and intimate knowledge of co-workers' problem-solving processes, as well as extensive clinical experience. For this reason the use of case studies and simulations (see Appendix 2C) relating to actual events are recommended for maintaining the expert's competence. Experts may have to describe their experiences to proficient nurses, who in turn can interpret the expert's performance in a way that is understandable to nurses with less contextual experience. The expert identifies clinical situations in which his or her actions made a difference. The proficient or competent nurse can reduce those actions into quantifiable sets of activities that can be more easily comprehended by the novice or advanced beginner.

The development of expertise in perioperative cardiac surgical nursing is quantitative and qualitative. It is knowing anatomy, pathophysiology, and technique and using the knowledge to provide care. It is understanding the needs of the patient and fellow team members, as well as the requirements of the surgical procedure. It is a continuing process that depends not only on self-reliance but also on the support and encouragement of those who know the environment. A fellowship requires understanding the roles of the other team members.

Team Roles

Cardiac surgery team members include the surgical staff, anesthesia care providers, nurses, perfusionists, and others; supporting staff members from other departments (e.g., laboratory, environmental services) are also valuable contributors to the cardiac service. The following are brief descriptions of cardiac team members; more extensive information can be found in textbooks and articles devoted to individual team member performance.

SURGEON

The surgical staff is represented by the attending surgeon, who has received extensive education and training in cardiac procedures. Cardiac training programs often have a uniquely characteristic philosophy and methodology that is transmitted to the surgeon-in-training. Familiarity with that training offers useful insights into preferences for instruments and supplies, perceptions about roles and functions of team members, and procedural considerations such as cannulation for bypass and anastomotic techniques. Discussing aspects of the service with the surgeon and contacting a colleague from the surgeon's alma mater can be helpful to nurses who are establishing a new service or preparing for the arrival of an additional member of the surgical staff.

FIRST ASSISTANT

The first assistant helps the surgeon to perform an optimal repair. Whether retracting, suctioning, sewing, or performing any of the other duties required to ensure a smooth-flowing operation, the assistant is also the patient's advocate by constantly monitoring the surgical site and the overall physiologic status of the patient. Additional classroom study and guided clinical experience are required for the role; a firm foundation in perioperative patient care (e.g., asepsis, safety, basic instrumentation) are mandatory (Vaiden, Fox, and Rothrock, 2000; Rothrock, 1999).

Depending on the nature of the institution, another surgeon may perform first assistant duties. Fellows, residents, and medical students are often involved in university-based training programs; individuals with less direct operative experience often function in the role of second assistant (e.g., retractor holder). In some hospitals surgical (physician) assistants, surgical technologist first assistants, or RNFAs, employed by the surgeon or the hospital or self-employed, provide assistance before, during, and after the procedure.

ANESTHESIA PROVIDER

Physician anesthesiologists and certified registered nurse anesthetists (CRNAs) provide relief from pain, monitor patient functions, and create safe operative conditions for the patient. Cardiovascular anesthesiologists have specialized knowledge of the circulatory dynamics of the patient with cardiac disease and frequently are the physicians who employ echocardiography to monitor the patient's left ventricular function. They may serve as teachers for students of anesthesia, nursing, and medicine.

PERFUSION TECHNOLOGISTS

Perfusionists are specially trained in the use of extracorporeal circulation and myocardial protection. Special cerebral protection techniques are employed when circulatory arrest is used (and the brain is not perfused by the bypass circuit). Perfusionists run the CPB machine (the pump), which oxygenates returning venous blood and pumps it back into the arterial system.

Although perfusionists are not required during off-pump procedures, their immediate availability is necessary should the surgeon wish to convert from an off-pump procedure to one requiring CPB. Partial ventricular assistance (e.g., right-sided heart bypass) may be used during some off-pump cases, and perfusionists are generally responsible for using these devices. They also may have additional responsibilities related to the intraaortic balloon pump and other left or right ventricular assist devices.

CARDIOPULMONARY TECHNOLOGISTS

These individuals assist the perfusionist and the anesthesia care provider by performing intraoperative laboratory analyses of blood gas levels, electrolyte levels, bleeding and coagulation times, and heparin concentration levels. They also may aid with hemodynamic monitoring by preparing systems for intravascular venous and arterial pressure monitoring; anesthesia technicians may perform these functions in some institutions.

SUPPORTIVE STAFF

Within the immediate surgical environment, supportive staff may have tasks delegated to them by anesthesia or nursing personnel for the preparation, maintenance, and cleaning of equipment, instruments, and supplies. Surgical technologists perform scrub role duties and, with additional education and training, may serve as the surgeon's assistant.

Environmental service employees help with the rapid room turnovers required for emergency cases and routine cleaning duties; it is important to recognize the valuable functions that these individuals perform and actively recognize them as members of the team.

Because many cardiac services operate under a separate budget, supply coordinators enhance inventory control by keeping track of the numerous (often expensive) items used during surgery. When such a position is unavailable, responsibility for these items may be divided among nursing team members.

OTHER TEAM MEMBERS

The cardiac team also can be thought of on a more global scale. In addition to the surgical team are the staff of the nursing units caring for cardiac patients before and after surgery, cardiologists and other referring physicians, and members of other departments, such as the pathology laboratory, the blood bank, the cardiac catheterization and electrophysiology laboratories, the noninvasive diagnostic and imaging laboratories, the pharmacy, and the respiratory, radiology, and cardiac rehabilitation departments.

With the constant introduction of new devices and technologies (and the widespread reduction of staff educators), representatives from industry (including industry clinical educators) should be considered members of the team. These individuals provide valuable information about the appropriate and safe use of devices and supplies, present inservices and continuing education programs, offer troubleshooting recommendations, and help to minimize expensive misuse of items, thereby reducing repair costs.

Members of administration, finance, quality improvement, infection control, and utilization review departments and managed care (and other) payors are all interested in the performance of the cardiac service and its outcomes relating to clinical criteria, revenue generation, and patient satisfaction. The perioperative cardiac nurse can learn from these individuals and apply the knowledge to improving the service. Cardiac surgery places demands on practically every department within a health care institution. Political sensitivity and group process skills facilitate productive interdepartmental and interdisciplinary relationships.

Stress and Stress Reduction Within the Cardiac Service

A cardiac service is stressful, and for many this provides an opportunity to excel. There are times, however, when stressful challenges become burdens. Team members usually cannot routinely engage in formal stress reduction activities; however, there are some stress reduction strategies that can be employed during the work day (Box 2-5) (Scott, 1999). Cardiac procedures routinely last longer than 3 hours and may be especially prolonged

---

BOX 2-5
Stress Reduction on the Job

Work schedules rarely allow time for a long physical workout or a long mental break during a given shift. The following can be performed by most individuals daily.

- Avoid negative self-talk ("I'm no good at this," "I'll never learn this"); switch to more positive statements ("I've been chosen to learn this because my boss knows I'm capable of succeeding").
- Count to 10; count to 20 or 30, if necessary.
- Perform deep abdominal breathing; combine with imagery.
- Perform simple exercises such as shoulder crunches, head rolls, and arm and leg stretches (often these can be done during surgery).
- Mentally picture a pleasant or humorous situation (e.g., a favorite funny movie).
- Remain curious; learn new techniques or skills.
- Share your knowledge and expertise with less-expert colleagues and students (this includes experienced nurses sharing clinical problem-solving knowledge with medical students, nursing students, and others).
- Ask a more expert colleague to teach you something new.
- Eat healthful foods, even if only snack food such as peanut butter crackers; minimize caffeinated beverages.
- When offered a break, take it! Offer a break to a colleague.
- Take a brisk 15-minute walk.
- Put up pictures of family, friends, or pets on your locker door or bulletin board.
- Visit a patient . . . any patient.

Modified from Scott A: More tips for eliminating stress. In Siomko AJ: Stress and the mind–body connection, *Advance Nurses* 4:22, 1999.

in complex cases. Given the prolonged time frames and the close working relationships, it should not be surprising that disharmony occurs occasionally.

A growing body of literature is devoted to the causes of stress and its effects in the workplace (Gaba, Howard, and Jump, 1994). Stress factors pertaining to cardiac surgery in particular are related to the work environment, equipment and material resources (including ergonomic factors), patient factors, ethical concerns, and staff dynamics (and other human factors). These factors also play a major role in error management (see p. 37).

WORK ENVIRONMENT

Early research by Weinger and Englund (1990), who studied anesthesia performance, described a number of stressful factors affecting surgical team members that remain applicable to a cardiac service. Among the most stressful were noise level, temperature and humidity, ambient lighting, and the arrangement of equipment and furniture.

Noise levels tend to be prolonged and loud, given the combined sounds of the bypass machine, electrosurgical units, physiologic monitors, light sources, suction equipment, sternal saws, airflow systems, and background music. Performing off-bypass surgery only removes a few of these noise-producing devices. In settings with similar noise levels, short-term memory losses and distractions during critical periods were noted (Weinger and Englund, 1990).

Adjustments to ambient temperature levels are common. It is not unusual to set the thermostat to 55° F (12° C) for most adult and pediatric procedures to conserve energy resources. During rewarming of the patient, room temperatures are routinely increased. When off-pump procedures are performed, active measures are taken to avoid the drifting down of the patient's internal temperature. This may mean that the room temperature is uncomfortably high for the gowned members of the surgical team. Extremes in temperature can produce an increase in errors, and when possible, room temperatures should be adjusted to achieve a more comfortable environment. Low humidity also can be a problem, leading to dehydration when the staff's access to fluids is limited.

Illumination of the surgical field, requiring up to 20,000 lux, can produce uncomfortable glare (Weinger and Englund, 1990). Excess lighting (from no-longer-required ceiling surgical lights and headlight and endoscopic light sources) should be turned off to avoid unnecessary discomfort.

The arrangement of equipment and furniture may be a problem, especially in small operating rooms. The large array of machines, supply carts, and other big pieces of equipment pose challenges not only for effi-

cient movement within the OR but also for infection control. Ceiling-mounted outlets for electricity, suction, and medical gases can reduce floor clutter; wall- or ceiling-mounted display screens for hemodynamic monitoring and video-assisted endoscopic surgery can replace some of the bulky carts formerly required.

Storage space is often inadequate, necessitating creativity in the arrangement of supplies. Throughout a given procedure the circulating nurse is responsible for using and repositioning many of these items; this can be a source of frustration in a confined work area and may increase the risk of surgical site infections. Storage problems can be improved with the use of exchange carts, which obviate the need for maintaining the entire inventory in the cardiac suite. Custom packs (see Chapter 3) save shelf space and reduce the need for excess inventory; they also save time that would be needed for opening numerous individual supplies (this is especially beneficial during emergencies), and they reduce the number of lost charges by consolidating multiple items. These custom packs can be as simple as a few basic sterile supplies or as comprehensive as an oil drum–size container of drapes, supplies, and fluids.

EQUIPMENT AND MATERIAL RESOURCES

Nonfunctioning equipment, lost or unavailable instruments and supplies, and dirty equipment are major stressors for perioperative nurses (and others). Thorough cleaning and careful checking of instruments before surgery, along with a regular maintenance program for equipment, will eliminate many problems, but unexpected events may still occur. Backup instruments sets, equipment, and supplies that are critical (e.g., cannulation instruments, sternal saw, anastomotic suture) should be available.

Adequate room preparation (with no missing supplies or instruments) is a team responsibility and an individual responsibility. Because emergencies are not uncommon, it is helpful at the conclusion of procedures to have the room cleaned and stocked with sterile items that are ready to be opened. After a long and strenuous day when staff have worked beyond their scheduled shift time, it is understandable that they would want to leave. However, when called for an emergency, the staff will appreciate having the OR clean and ready for another case with suction setup, sterile instruments, supplies, and other items available. The patient should not have to wait unnecessarily for a room to be cleaned and prepared.

New cardiac surgical programs with small caseloads cannot afford to rely on a single sternal saw or defibrillator. The same defibrillator model may be available on another nursing unit; receiving prior permission from the unit's department head will help facilitate borrowing the machine if the need arises. A list of similar defibrillator models throughout the hospital can be helpful, but the perioperative nurse *must* confirm that the defibrillator is compatible with the *internal paddles* used in the cardiac OR. Internal paddles are model specific; internal paddles from one defibrillator model will not function in another, dissimilar defibrillator.

Borrowing critical items such as a valve or graft prosthesis may be necessary when the supply of a particular-size prosthesis has been depleted unexpectedly. Establishing a collaborative network with nurses in other institutions can form the basis for a mutually beneficial system of borrowing (and loaning) needed items for emergencies. This does not mean that nurse managers should not be held accountable for maintaining an adequate inventory, but there are occasions when, for example in this author's experience, three patients within one 24-hour period all required a 21-mm aortic valve prosthesis. The current competitive environment should never preclude helping the patient of a colleague at another institution.

Poorly designed devices also produce stress and can increase the chance of accidents and errors. Basic considerations such as the color of a machine, the shape of a handle, and the location of knobs can affect the probability of error in the use of equipment and supplies (Berguer, 1999). The impact of design factors (ergonomics) in the delivery of safe care can be seen in the results of a Food and Drug Administration study that links the poor design of medical instruments with half of the 1.3 million unintentional patient injuries occurring in hospitals each year (Burlington, 1996). Cardiac nurses are a valuable resource to designers and manufacturers of medical equipment that will function effectively with reduced risk of error.

PATIENT FACTORS

Patient factors may be among the most stressful: patients die. Cardiac surgery patients are at greater risk for complications because of the underlying severity of most heart conditions requiring surgery. Patient variables such as age at operation, sex, weight, anatomic cardiac and noncardiac anomalies, and comorbidities affect surgical outcomes (de Leval and others, 2000).

The nurse and other team members on occasion must deal with feelings of powerlessness or loss when patient outcomes are not as expected, and it is normal to reflect on one's performance and its effect (if any) on the final outcome. These feelings of powerlessness were evident during the September 11, 2001 attack on the World Trade Center buildings in New York City when nurses and other health care providers, who were mentally and operationally prepared for numerous casualties, cared for only the relatively small number of individuals who survived the tragedy.

Caring for dying patients and their families requires balancing obligations to others with obligations to oneself. Clarifying these obligations with a counselor and turning to a compassionate listener or other support system may assist the nurse in dealing with these situations.

Other patient-related factors include the potential for transmission of blood-borne diseases, such as various forms of hepatitis and human immunodeficiency virus (HIV). Strict adherence to standard precautions and other guidelines recommended by AORN (2001) and other professional organizations and regulatory agencies helps to minimize the risk to both patients and health care workers. Suggestions to decrease occupational exposure include greater use of disposable scalpels and electrosurgical units for incising and dissecting tissue, disposable containers for sharp items in all ORs, impervious gowns, stronger gloves, modifications in the design of surgical instruments, and more self-defensive surgical techniques.

Federal and state laws and regulations exist to ensure that patients are informed of their right to consent or refuse treatment and to make their wishes known and respected concerning what course of treatment they would desire if they become incapacitated or incompetent or their condition becomes terminal. Do-not-resuscitate orders and other end-of-life decisions must be respected even when the health care providers are in disagreement. Organ and tissue donation requires careful consideration by the potential donor, the family, and the members of the health care team.

ETHICAL CONSIDERATIONS

Many patient-related issues can produce ethical dilemmas concerning patients' rights and staff rights, just and equitable distribution of technologic resources and organs for transplantation, interventions that benefit or potentially harm the patient, and advanced directives. Patients have a right to have their wishes respected, and caregivers have a duty to respect those wishes.

Perioperative nurses can refer to a number of documents to guide their deliberation of ethical issues. AORN's (1993) explication of the American Nurses' Association's (ANA) Code for Nurses (1985) for perioperative nurses represents one of the first attempts by a specialty nursing organization to identify the unique relationship between patients and families and the members of a specialty practice. The American Nurses' Association's newly revised Code of Ethics for Nurses (2001) reaffirms the nurse's primary commitment to the patient in providing ethical care (Fowler, 2001).

The Tavistock Group's "Shared Statement of Ethical Principles for Everyone in Health Care" (Smith, Hiatt, and Berwick, 1999; Davidoff, 2000; Hanlon, 2001) was developed in response to the conviction that the existence of separate moral frameworks designed by physicians, nurses, hospital executives, and others does not reflect the interdependencies of all health care workers. The principles enumerated emphasize cooperation among professionals, safety, openness, and the ongoing responsibility for improving health care.

STAFF DYNAMICS

There can be problems associated with interdisciplinary collaboration. Teams composed of highly diverse, skilled professionals may be hindered in accomplishing their functions by goal conflicts, role conflicts, problems with decision making, and difficulties with interpersonal communication.

Goals

Although the main goal of a cardiac team is to provide quality care to patients, individual and group goals contribute to this. Among these goals are task and maintenance goals, short- and long-term goals, and client, professional, and organizational goals. Conflict can arise when goals are not clearly specified or when team members' perceptions of the goals and their achievement are incongruent. Often these differences are related to dissimilar philosophic, religious, or professional values.

Clear identification of goals, assessment of individuals' perceptions about desired goals, consensus regarding which goals are most important, and unity on actions to be taken are some of the things that can foster a less-divisive environment (Tiffany and Lutjens, 1998).

Roles

Disagreement about role performance can exist among nurses, physicians, and other team members and also among nurses themselves. In the cardiac arena this may be compounded by the presence of physician assistants (PAs) and perfusionists—all highly trained professionals. Often there is an overlapping of roles. For example, first assistant duties may be performed by other surgeons, by PAs, by surgical technologists, or by RNFAs. The scrub role may be fulfilled by a surgical technologist or a registered nurse (RN). Differing expectations of persons performing within the same role can produce ambiguity, frustration, and distrust. This may be aggravated by inequalities in reward systems (monetary or nonmonetary), recognition of performance, little opportunity for career growth, and varying degrees of autonomy, responsibility, and accountability.

Methods to reduce role conflicts focus on clarifying role perceptions and expectations, identifying members' professional competencies, exploring overlapping responsibilities, and possibly renegotiating role assignments. Position descriptions and competency-based evaluations can help reduce role ambiguity and provide objectivity. Persons responsible for assigning their respective staffs, such as nurses or PAs, should jointly discuss staffing needs on a case-by-case basis or through a mutually agreed-on schedule. Flexibility and cooperation promote collaborative working relationships that enhance professional harmony and improve team function (Seifert, 1999).

Emergencies are often good examples of flexibility: PAs, perfusionists, or anesthesia personnel can assist the circulating nurse or the RNFA in preparing the patient for surgery or in elevating the legs of a patient requiring vein harvest for a coronary artery bypass procedure. Nurses can assist in procuring medications or assisting with endotracheal intubation.

It is evident from research on collaborative practice models that a solid knowledge base in one's discipline and an appreciation of the knowledge and skills required in others' disciplines offer a strong foundation for effective interdisciplinary working relationships. In a cardiac service, as in other specialized services, there is a large overlapping knowledge base from which all members can draw. The depth and scope of that knowledge may vary, and its application to practice may distinguish one discipline from another, but the concepts are mutually understood. Consider the concept of balancing myocardial oxygen supply and demand and how implementing that goal is interpreted by different disciplines. Anesthesia staff engage in the pharmacologic manipulation of intravascular pressures and resistances; perfusionists prepare and infuse cardioplegia solutions that preserve and protect myocardial function; nurses employ anxiety-reducing measures that diminish endogenous catecholamine release; surgeons use techniques that minimize cross-clamp time. These interventions all aim at optimizing the balance between oxygen supply and demand.

Decision making

Achieving successful outcomes is hampered if problems are not clearly identified or if team members' roles in the decision-making process are poorly defined. Consensus is achieved not by unanimity but by providing an opportunity for all members to participate, based on sufficient and relevant data, discussion of alternatives, commitment to action, and mutual respect for all members' contributions.

Such a process may not be appropriate during an emergency situation; but neither can the resolution of emergencies be entirely satisfactory if consensus building has not already been established as a team value. A patient with a life-threatening problem is more likely to have a successful outcome when team members are sure of their roles, individual strengths are promoted, their knowledge base is secure, and appropriate interventions are implemented.

The cultural norms of the group promote or hinder joint problem solving. In teams in which nursing managers and staff freely discuss problems and possible solutions, a favorable climate is likely to exist.

A culture in which mistakes or lapses can be admitted without fear of retribution is more likely to use these incidents as opportunities to learn from the mistake and improve the overall system. Nurses in such an atmosphere are more comfortable discussing treatment alternatives with physician colleagues. One's understanding of the rationales for treatment can be enhanced by attending cardiac catheterization conferences, surgical grand rounds, or critical care meetings. Insight into why a surgeon makes a certain patient care decision is invaluable in preparing for an operative procedure. One is better able to anticipate the needs of both the surgeon and the patient if one is aware of the options a surgeon is likely to consider. What are the individual surgeon's indications for selecting a particular valve prosthesis? For returning a patient to the OR for mediastinal exploration? For inserting a ventricular assist device? By better understanding the surgeon's decision-making process, the nurse becomes more capable of anticipating the most likely options and preparing for them. Similarly, nurses can plan and jointly implement care with anesthesia personnel based on a knowledge of preferred vasoactive medications, the sequence of inserting central pressure lines and endotracheal tubes, and the transportation of patients to postoperative care units.

Surgeons, anesthesiologists, and other team members can be made aware of issues of importance to nurses and the need to coordinate and integrate the elements of the service. For example, nurses who include a psychosocial assessment of the patient often obtain information crucial to the successful outcome of the procedure. They may discover that for a particular patient the optimum placement of a pacemaker generator is the abdomen rather than the chest wall or that geographic location may preclude insertion of a valve prosthesis requiring follow-up laboratory testing for anticoagulation-related bleeding times. This process also enables patients to participate in the decision-making process affecting their care.

Communication

Communication between the clinical staff fosters continuity of patient care. It is also the vehicle for reassessing and redefining how the team functions. It is necessary for the reappraisal process, which includes improving knowledge and skill, engaging in frank self-evaluation, and offering constructive and issue-oriented criticism.

Team members communicate by speaking and listening, negotiating, and expressing opinions and feelings without recrimination (IOM, 1999, 2000).

Forums for communication may be formal or informal. Committees may be organized to discuss problems on a regular basis. Informal meetings between two or more people can be held as the need arises. Interpersonal problems are best handled by those involved. Managers should intervene only when a resolution cannot be found and the ongoing antagonism affects team function and patient care. Managers should not attempt to force mutual admiration, but they do have a duty to ensure fair treatment of staff, to communicate acceptable levels of performance to team members, to offer unit orientations and continuing education, and to provide the resources necessary for the nurse to practice effectively and efficiently.

Error Detection, Recovery, and Prevention

Physicians, nurses, pharmacists, and other caregivers alone cannot prevent all errors, nor should they attempt to do so. Mishaps will continue to occur, if only because there are always unforeseen circumstances. These circumstances may be related to unknown (and undetectable) patients factors, environmental variables, time constraints, or some other phenomenon (Gaba, Howard, and Jump, 1994). Emphasis must be on preventing the adverse consequences of unavoidable human error and minimizing the factors that foster errors. Effective clinical error management requires a team approach (Bodenheimer, 1999).

A steady trend has been seen in journal articles and reports that focus on human errors causing patient harm in the health care setting. The National Patient Safety Foundation (see www.npsf.org), first conceived by the American Medical Association in 1996 (Hatlie and Wagner, 1999), was created to explore the problem of patient injury and potential solutions. National concern over the impact of avoidable and unavoidable medical errors received widespread media attention with the publication of the Institute of Medicine's *To Err is Human: Building a Safer Health System* (IOM, 1999) and *Crossing the Quality Chasm: a New Health System for the 21st Century* (IOM, 2000). Among the problems identified by the IOM that contribute to adverse outcomes are illegible handwriting, wrong diagnoses as a result of mislabeled specimen containers, drug miscalculations, and lack of continuity in care as patients are passed from one provider to another. Not only are patient morbidity and mortality rates increased, but there are also substantial costs in the form of dollars, reduced satisfaction, and loss of trust in the system by patients and health care professionals.

One study of surgery-related errors cited by the IOM concluded that more than 50% of the adverse events described could have been prevented (Gawande and others, 1999). Improving the quality of health care by reducing errors not only promotes positive patient outcomes but also can reduce the costs associated with the misuse of services (Chassin and Galvin, 1998; Bodenheimer, 1999). Quality initiatives to reduce errors reflect a professional duty to the patient and professional colleagues.

TYPES OF ERROR

Error is defined by the IOM as "the failure of a planned action to be completed as intended or the use of a wrong plan to achieve an aim" (IOM, 1999, p. 3). Different forms of human error can be classified (Spencer, 2000; Leape, 1994). A *knowledge error* (a *mistake*) may result when an individual has inadequate or incorrect information. An example might be the novice cardiac nurse who does not know that heparin needs to be given before instituting cardiopulmonary bypass. (If heparin is not given, blood throughout the pump circuit will clot.)

A *rule-based error* (a *lapse*) refers to a situation in which the information is correct, but it is incorrectly applied. The novice nurse may know that heparin prevents clotting of the bypass circuit but (incorrectly) assumes that the heparin can be given by the perfusionist once CPB has been initiated.

A *skill-based error* (a *slip*) involves faulty performance, often because of distraction or inattention. The tired nurse may not notice sudden hemorrhage and delays giving the surgeon a suture ligature.

Accidents are another form of adverse event. Accidents may occur after multiple small errors combine unpredictably to produce a disaster. The introduction of root cause analysis techniques often can uncover multiple *root causes* rather than one single precipitating factor. Often there are active and latent failures (Table 2-2) that contribute to errors and accidents. *Active* failures are errors committed by people at the service delivery end of the system (e.g., surgeons, RNFAs, circulating nurses, and other members of the OR team) and have an immediate impact on patient safety. *Latent* failures usually are the result of flawed administrative decisions by executives in hospitals, regulatory agencies industry, and so on. Latent failures weaken the organization's defenses and increase the likelihood that when active failures occur, the combination of latent and active failures will produce a disaster (Fig. 2-2) (Carthey, de Leval, and Reason, 2001). An example might be a situation in which policies and procedures for obtaining blood for surgical patients are not in place or are not strictly en-

TABLE 2-2 *Examples of Latent and Active Failures in Health Care*	
LEVEL	EXAMPLES OF LATENT AND ACTIVE FAILURES
Health care organizations	Lack of investment in health care at government and state levels
	Poor working conditions for nursing staff
	No continuity in health care management initiatives
Hospital management	Nursing shortages lead to overreliance on agency nurses
	Lack of investment in high technology equipment
	Poor organizational communication networks
Cardiac surgery department	Poor organization of staff roles and responsibilities
	Failure to invest in staff training
	Absence of, or inadequate, policies and protocols for treatment
	Poor intradepartmental communication
Preoperative decision making	Incorrect diagnosis of the patient's condition
	Communication failures between teams
	Conflicts between clinical, research, and management goals
	Poor scheduling of cases
Intraoperative problems	Major errors: accidental injury of a coronary artery, pincushioning during catheter insertion leading to a serious cardiac event
	Minor errors: tension and positioning errors by surgical assistants, instrument handing errors by the scrub nurse, communication failures between the operating room team

From Carthey and others: The human factor in cardiac surgery, *Ann Thorac Surg* 72:300, 2001.

forced. Over time there may be a number of instances when a close check of names and blood types was not done but did not result in injury. When two patients with the same name but very different blood types are both scheduled for surgery on the same day (this happens!), the wrong blood is given and severe anaphylactic shock ensues.

IOM RECOMMENDATIONS

Safety is defined by the IOM as "freedom from accidental injury" (IOM, 1999, p. 3). In order to improve the nation's safety record and minimize the risk of er-

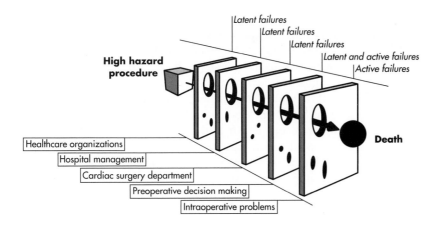

High hazard procedure

Latent failures
Latent failures
Latent failures
Latent and active failures
Active failures

Death

Healthcare organizations
Hospital management
Cardiac surgery department
Preoperative decision making
Intraoperative problems

FIGURE 2-2 A generic organizational accident model applied to health care systems in general and to a cardiac service in particular. Multiple, cumulative latent failures related to the organization, management policies, the cardiac surgery department, and preoperative decision-making processes eventually can result in preoperative and intraoperative active failures that lead to death. (Modified from Carthey and others: The human factor in cardiac surgery, *Ann Thorac Surg* 72:300, 2001.)

rors and accidents, a comprehensive approach is needed that makes safety and the prevention of error an integral part of the health care culture. Currently there are legal and cultural barriers that make it difficult to analyze errors, learn from them, and implement practice changes that could prevent future errors. Shifting the focus from blaming individuals for past errors to designing systems that focus on the prevention of future errors is one of the key recommendations. The IOM refers to other high-risk industries (e.g., aviation) that have successfully implemented safety initiatives and calls for a four-tiered approach to reduce medical errors:

1. Establish a national focus to create leadership, research tools, and protocols to enhance the knowledge base about safety.
2. Identify and learn from errors through immediate and strong mandatory reporting efforts.
3. Raise standards and expectations for improvements in safety through the actions of oversight organizations, group purchasers, and professional groups.
4. Create safety systems inside health care organizations through the implementation of safe practices at the delivery level.

Creating safe systems at the clinical level is the ultimate target of the IOM's recommendations. The institute's focus on the role of professional groups and the need for change at the clinical interface is especially pertinent because perioperative nurses have a long tradition of partnering with others to develop standards, recommended practices, guidelines, competencies, and position statements that promote safe practice and illustrate their role as patient advocates (AORN, 2001). The IOM's promotion of an interdisciplinary approach to enhance patient safety is especially relevant for cardiac nurses. The growing complexity of care suggests that even greater collaboration is necessary for achieving safe systems.

CARDIAC NURSE'S ROLE IN ERROR REDUCTION

The cardiac nurse's responsibility for safety can be demonstrated in the structural and process elements of practice that affect the outcomes of care. New equipment and complex instrumentation require hands-on practice before use on a patient. Partnering with the manufacturer to learn how to use a new device is one important step toward error reduction. Given the time constraints in today's work environment, it is often difficult to gather the entire staff for inservice training. One nurse can be the designated "learner/teacher"; this nurse can then educate other staff members (including physicians) about the new item.

Processes affecting interdepartmental communication and interaction are also critical. If a vital instrument (e.g., the chest wire cutter in the emergency chest set) is missing, it is potentially dangerous to the patient whose chest needs to be opened quickly in the SICU. If this situation occurs, it is important to (1) get a wire cutter immediately so that the procedure can be performed promptly; (2) train the staff responsible for putting up the set and help them understand why the instrument is vital (a field trip to the OR or a slide show in the staff's department is invaluable); (3) develop a system to minimize the chance of an instrument's being missing; and (4) promote a system of accountability in partnership with colleagues to fix the system. Unfortunately, the first response is often blame, and blame rarely produces positive change. What the IOM recommends—systems improvement rather than blame—is notable because improving a system to achieve better results implicitly and

---

BOX **2-6**
Lessons on Patient Safety

1. The problem is not errors; the problem is *harm*.
2. Rules don't create safety; rules and breaking the rules create safety.
3. Telling stories to gain knowledge is more important than reporting that tracks problems and progress.
4. Conversation, not technology, is the foundation of safety.
5. Health care is not the same as other high-hazard industries.
6. What happens after the injury is as important as what happens before the injury.

Modified from Berwick DM: Patient safety: lessons from a novice, *Focus on Patient Safety* (Newsletter from the National Patient Safety Foundation) 4(3):3, 2001.

---

explicitly links processes and outcomes. Processes from the basis for good outcomes. The IOM's and others' recommendations reinforce this by addressing the need for system improvements using a team approach (process) to reduce errors (outcomes) (Seifert, 2000).

Berwick (2001) describes lessons learned about patient safety (Box 2-6). The lessons seem to go against conventional wisdom (e.g., "Rules and breaking the rules create safety"), but careful consideration of Berwick's points reflect his clinical experience. The idea that errors are inevitable reflects the reality of the clinical realm. The emphasis should be on avoiding harm to the patients by developing processes and systems that minimize injury and harm. One example could be to ensure that the defibrillator is *not* routinely kept in the synchronous mode because if the patient does fibrillate—and the defibrillator is set to the synchronous mode, which requires sensing and synchronizing to an R wave—the device will not discharge because ventricular fibrillation produces no R wave.

The second lesson refers to rules and knowing when to break them. Berwick compares this activity to driving a car: the driver must constantly adapt to the changes in the road. A clinical example could be the "rule" that a thorough skin preparation should be performed before the incision is made. If a patient arrests suddenly on induction, a full body preparation may delay exposing the heart for manual compression. In this scenario the risk of death outweighs the risk of infection.

The third lesson emphasizes the importance of clarification rather than focusing solely on enumerating quantifiable factors. Telling stories that clarify what happened (or what can happen) can give a deeper meaning to the numbers. For example, if an extra sternal saw is unavailable because one has been used and the other is out for repair, it may be helpful to justify the purchase of a new saw by telling a story that incorporates both patient safety factors (including institutional liability) and financial arguments for increasing inventory.

The fourth lesson refers to the role of technology. It is easy to rely on patient monitors, for example, but the accuracy of such devices should be constantly confirmed by the clinician's senses: sight, sound, feel, and smell.

The fifth lesson reminds clinicians that health care is not like other industries because a health care worker's goal is to postpone death, not prevent it. Clinicians must accept death and assist patients and families to live or die with dignity.

The final lesson reflects the reality that injuries will occur. Saying "I'm sorry" to the patient or a colleague demonstrates the principle of truth telling and reaffirms the bond that forms the foundation of professional relationships.

Conclusion

Cardiac surgery is a team process that reflects a comprehensive approach to patient care. Communication remains one of the most important methods for maintaining an integrated and cohesive team, for minimizing injury, and for enhancing group processes that lead to quality outcomes. Understanding the needs of both patients and fellow team members contributes to the success of the individual, the service, and the institution.

References

Agency for Healthcare Research and Quality (AHRQ): Patient fact sheet: 20 tips to help prevent medical errors. In *Patient fact sheet* [on-line], AHRQ Pub No 00-PO38, February 2000. Available: http://www.ahrq.gov/consumer/20tips.htm (accessed July 13, 2001).

American Nurses' Association (ANA): *The code of ethics for nurses,* Washington, DC, 2001, ANA.

American Nurses' Association (ANA): *ANA code for nurses with interpretive statements,* St Louis, 1985.

Association of periOperative Registered Nurses: The ANA code for nurses with interpretive statements—explications for perioperative nursing. In AORN: *Standards and recommended practices,* Denver, 1993, AORN.

Association of periOperative Registered Nurses (AORN): *Standards, recommended practices & guidelines,* Denver, 2001, AORN.

Benner P: *From novice to expert: excellence and power in clinical nursing practice,* Menlo Park, Calif, 1984, Addison-Wesley.

Benner P, Hooper-Kyriakidis P, Stannard D: *Clinical wisdom and interventions in critical care: a thinking-in-action approach,* Philadelphia, 1999, WB Saunders.

Berguer R: Surgery and ergonomics, *Arch Surg* 134(9):1011, 1999.

Berwick DM: Patient safety: lessons from a novice, *Focus on Patient Safety* (Newsletter from the National Patient Safety Foundation) 4(3):3, 2001.

Bodenheimer T: The American health care system—the movement for improved quality in health care (Health Policy Report), *N Engl J Med* 340(6):488, 1999.

Burlington DB: Human factors and the FDA's goals: improved medical device design, *Biomed Instrum Technol* 30(2):107, 1996.

Carthey J, de Leval MR, Reason JT: The human factor in cardiac surgery: errors and near misses in a high technology medical domain, *Ann Thorac Surg* 72(1):300, 2001.

Chassin MR, Galvin RW: The urgent need to improve health care quality. Institute of Medicine, National Roundtable on Health Care Quality, *JAMA* 280(11):1000, 1998.

Cufaude JB: Cultivating new leadership, *Assoc Manag* (January):73, 2000.

Davidoff F: Changing the subject: ethical principles for everyone in health care, *Ann Int Med* 133(5):386, 2000.

de Leval MR and others: Human factors and cardiac surgery: a multicenter study, *J Thorac Cardiovasc Surg* 119(4 Part 1):661, 2000.

Fowler MD: Implementing the new code of ethics for nurses: an interview with Marsha Fowler, *Am J Crit Care* 10(6):434, 2001.

Gaba DM, Howard SK, Jump B: Production pressure in the work environment. California anesthesiologists' attitudes and experiences, *Anesthesiology* 81(2):48, 1994.

Gawande AA and others: The incidence and nature of surgical events in Colorado and Utah in 1992, *Surgery* 126(1):66, 1999.

Greenfield LJ: Doctors and nurses: a troubled partnership, *Ann Surg* 230(3):279, 1999.

Greenfield LJ, Procter MC: When should a surgeon retire? *Adv Surg* 32:385, 1999.

Hanlon CR: Ethical principles for everyone in health care, *J Am Coll Surg* 192(1):72, 2001.

Hatlie MJ, Wagner SM: The National Patient Safety Foundation: creating a culture of safety, *Surg Serv Manage* 5(7):35, 1999.

Hojat M and others: Attitudes toward physician-nurse collaboration: a cross-cultural study of male and female physicians and nurses in the United States and Mexico, *Nurs Res* 50(2):123, 2001.

Houchin D: Comments about the members of a cardiac team. In Seifert PC: *Cardiac surgery*, St Louis, 1994, Mosby.

Institute of Medicine: *Crossing the quality chasm: a new health system for the 21st century*, Washington, DC, 2000, National Academy Press.

Institute of Medicine (IOM): *To err is human: building a safer health system*, Washington, DC, 1999, National Academy Press.

Knaus WA and others: An evaluation of outcome from intensive care in major medical centers, *Ann Intern Med* 104(3):410, 1986.

Lassen AA and others: Nurse/physician collaborative practice: improving health care quality while decreasing cost, *Nurs Econ* 15(2):87, 1997.

Leape LL: Error in medicine, *JAMA* 272(23):1851, 1994.

Lytle BW: Evolving technology: recognition and opportunity, *Ann Thorac Surg* 71(5):1409, 2001.

Meier AH, Rawn CL, Krummel TM: Virtual reality: surgical application—challenge for the new millennium, *J Am Coll Surg* 192(3):372, 2001.

Pew Health Professions Commission: *Reforming health care workforce regulation: policy considerations for the 21st century*, San Francisco, 1995, Center for Health Professions, University of California.

Pisano GP, Bohmer RMJ, Edmondson AC: Organizational differences in rates of learning: evidence from the adoption of minimally invasive cardiac surgery, *Management Science* 47(6):752, 2001.

Ricci M and others: Survey of resident training in beating heart operations, *Ann Thorac Surg* 70(2):479, 2000.

Rosser JC Jr, Murayama M, Gabriel NH: Minimally invasive surgical training solutions for the twenty-first century, *Surg Clin North Am* 80(5):1607, 2000.

Rothrock JC: The RN first assistant: an expanded perioperative nursing role, ed 3, Philadelphia, 1999, JB Lippincott.

Rothrock JC: *Perioperative nursing care planning*, St Louis, 1990, Mosby.

Satava RM, Jones SB: Preparing surgeons for the 21st century, *Surg Clin North Am* 80(4):1353, 2000.

Scott A: More tips for eliminating stress. In Siomko AJ: Stress and the mind–body connection, *Advance Nurses* 4:22, 1999.

Seifert PC: Partnering for quality, *AORN J* 71(3):466, 2000.

Seifert PC: The RN first assistant and collaborative practice. In Rothrock JC: T*he RN first assistant: an expanded perioperative nursing role*, ed 3, Philadelphia, 1999, JB Lippincott.

Smith R, Hiatt H, Berwick D: A shared statement of ethical principles for those who shape and give health care: a working draft from the Tavistock group, *Ann Intern Med* 130(2):143, 1999.

Spencer FC: Human error in hospitals and industrial accidents: current concepts, *J Am Coll Surg* 191(4):410, 2000.

Tiffany CR, Lutjens LR: *Planned change theories for nursing*, London, 1998, Sage Publications.

Vaiden RE, Fox VJ, Rothrock JC, editors: *Core curriculum for the RN first assistant*, ed 3, Denver, 2000, AORN.

Weinger MB, Englund CE: Ergonomic and human factors affecting anesthetic vigilance and monitoring performance in the operating room environment, *Anesthesiology* 73(5):995, 1990.

Zarbock SF: How to create successful patient-provider partnerships, *Clin News* (February):29, 2000.

Zarbock SF: Health care students get a head start on interdisciplinary teamwork, *Clin News* (May):30, 1999.

Appendix 2A

Pretest/Posttest

Use the following terms to answer questions 1 through 14.

Left ventricular aneurysm	Mechanical valve prosthesis
Supine	Tricuspid valve
Superior vena cava	Lesser saphenous vein
Lateral	Dopamine
Right atrium	Inferior vena cava
Left atrium	Aortic valve
Mediastinum	Aorta
Cephalic vein	Right ventricle
Radial artery	Ventricular septal rupture
Mitral valve	Left ventricle
Air	Right ventricle
Gastroepiploic artery	Calcium chloride
Lungs	Mitral regurgitation
Blood	Greater saphenous vein
Internal mammary artery	Pulmonary veins
Dobutamine	Biologic valve prosthesis
Inferior epigastric artery	Anterior thoracotomy

1. Which valves are in the right side of the heart?

   _____

   _____

2. Describe the movement of blood through the heart and lungs from the inferior and superior vena cavae to the ascending aorta.

   _____

   _____

3. Which valves are in the left side of the heart?

   _____

   _____

4. What type of valve prosthesis generally requires chronic postoperative anticoagulation?

   _____

   _____

5. Which valve(s) is (are) most likely to become diseased in the adult?

   _____

   _____

6. Complications of myocardial infarction include the following (list three):

   _____

   _____

7. The patient position for off-pump coronary artery bypass (OPCAB) is:

   _____

   _____

8. The patient position for minimally invasive direct coronary artery bypass (MIDCAB) is:

   _____

   _____

9. Which *vein* is most likely to be used as a graft/conduit in coronary artery bypass grafting?

   _____

   _____

10. Which coronary bypass graft/conduit displays the greatest long-term patency?

    _____

11. List at least three autologous arterial conduits:

    _____

    _____

12. The patient position for a descending aortic thoracic aneurysm is:

    _____

    _____

13. During typical cardiopulmonary bypass, blood is diverted from the _____ and _____, oxygenated, and pumped into the _____.

14. The *main* reason for inserting chest tubes into the cardiac surgical patient is to remove _____ from the _____.

15. Of the following the most *likely* setting (in joules) for internal defibrillation in the adult is (circle the best answer):
    a. 10   b. 30   c. 60   d. 250   e. 400

16. Only patients with a single lesion of the left anterior descending coronary artery are suitable candidates for off-pump coronary bypass surgery.
    a. True   b. False

ANSWER KEY

1. Tricuspid, pulmonary
2. Right atrium→tricuspid valve→right ventricle→pulmonary valve→pulmonary artery→lungs→pulmonary veins→left atrium→mitral valve→left ventricle→aortic valve
3. Mitral, aortic
4. Mechanical valve prosthesis
5. Mitral, aortic
6. Ventricular septal rupture, left ventricular aneurysm, mitral regurgitation
7. Supine
8. Anterior thoracotomy
9. Saphenous vein
10. Internal mammary artery
11. Internal mammary artery, radial artery, gastroepiploic artery, inferior epigastric artery
12. Lateral
13. Superior vena cava and inferior vena cava, aorta
14. Blood, mediastinum
15. a
16. b

Appendix 2B

Competency Statements in Perioperative Cardiac Nursing

Assessment

1. Competency to assess the physical health status and physiologic response of the patient

  1.1. Assesses physical cardiovascular risk factors
      Age
      Obesity
      Hypertension
      Smoking
      Alcohol intake
      Drug abuse (e.g., cocaine)
      Hypercholesterolemia
      Diabetes

  1.2. Identifies current medical diagnosis and therapy

  1.3. Identifies other congenital and acquired conditions

  1.4. Assesses previous health state
      Past medical history (angina, MI, CHF, vascular disease, syncope, TIA, stroke)
      Hospitalizations
      Surgery (sternotomy, thoracotomy, vein stripping, transurethral resection)
      Injuries
      Chronic illnesses: lupus, arthritis, multiple sclerosis, myasthenia gravis, pulmonary disease, thyroid disorders
      Infectious diseases (rheumatic fever, endocarditis)

  1.5. Identifies presence of prostheses/implants
      Pacemaker, internal defibrillator
      Prosthetic heart valve
      Joint prostheses (hip, knee)

  1.6. Assesses medication history
      Antiplatelets
      Aprotinin (especially during previous bypass surgery)
      Aspirin
      Dipyridamole
      Anticoagulants
      Nitrates
      ACE inhibitors
      Digitalis
      Diuretics
      Antidysrhythmics
      Beta blockers
      Calcium channel blockers
      Inotropes
      Antihypertensives
      Immunosuppressants
      Statins, lipid-lowering drugs
      Steroids, antiinflammatories

  1.7. Notes diagnostic studies
      Electrocardiogram
      Exercise stress test
      Echocardiogram
      Cardiac catheterization
      Nuclear studies
      CT scans
      MRI
      Arteriograms
      Pulmonary function studies
      Roentgenograms

  1.8. Reports deviation of laboratory studies
      Complete blood count
      Blood glucose
      Coagulation profile (prothrombin time, partial thromboplastin time, platelets)
      Urinalysis
      BUN, creatinine
      Liver function studies
      Serum enzymes
      Serum lipid levels
      Serum electrolytes
      Arterial blood gases, pulse oximetry
      Reports blood type (units available, cold antibodies, donor-directed units)

  1.9. Verifies allergies (medications, chemical, food, contact)

  1.10. Assesses cardiovascular status
      Blood pressure(s) (legs and arms, bilaterally)
      Pulse (legs and arms, bilaterally)
      Dysrhythmias
      Presence of monitoring lines
      Edema
      Pain in the chest, arms, shoulders, back, neck, jaw, stomach
      Murmurs
      Fatigue
      Claudication
      Bruits
      Cyanosis
      Left ventricular function

  1.11. Assesses respiratory status
      Respiratory rate
      Intercostal retractions, bulging
      Use of accessory respiratory muscles
      Breath sounds

Modified from AORN: Competency statements in perioperative nursing. In AORN: *standards, recommended practices, and guidelines for perioperative nursing*, Denver, 2001, AORN.

Chest tubes
Shortness of breath, dyspnea, cough
Prolonged expiration
Increased anterior/posterior diameter

1.12. Assesses skin condition
Previous incisions
Rashes, bruises
Skin turgor
Diaphoresis
Petechiae
Temperature
Skin color
Nail beds
Clubbing
Invasive lines

1.13. Assesses urinary/renal status
History of benign prostatic hypertrophy, prostate surgery
Intake and output
Serum creatinine and BUN

1.14. Assesses neuropsychiatric status
Syncope, dizziness
Level of consciousness
Confusion, restlessness
Numbness, tingling
Anger
Anxiety, fear
Tension, depression

1.15. Notes weight and height

1.16. Notes sensory impairments (hearing, vision, tactile)

1.17. Assesses nutritional status
Weight
NPO status

1.18. Determines mobility of body parts
Presence of indwelling catheters
History and physical
Medication

1.19. Communicates/documents physical health status

2. Competency to assess the psychosocial health status and psychophysiologic response of the patient/family

2.1. Assesses psychosocial cardiovascular risk factors
Family history
Stressful life events
Sedentary living

2.2. Assesses personal and social factors
Meals, caffeine intake
Sleep patterns
Occupation, activities, hobbies
Economic status, insurance
Living arrangements

Geographic location
Cultural/spiritual beliefs
Education
Basic language

2.3. Identifies coping mechanisms
Denial, withdrawal, anger
Information seeking

2.4. Identifies support systems
Family, significant others
Nurse liaison (preoperative, intraoperative, and postoperative)
Support groups (The Mended Hearts)
Counseling/pastoral services

2.5. Assist significant others with postmortem care
Prepare body for viewing
Provide private viewing area
Respect refusal to see deceased
Allow mothers/fathers to hold babies/children
Accompany to chapel or other suitable area
Refer to appropriate personnel for support/assistance

2.6. Assesses ability to comply with prescribed therapy

2.7. Elicits perception of surgery (e.g., on/off bypass)

2.8. Elicits expectation of care and verifies consent

2.9. Determines knowledge level of patient/family
Diagnosis
Therapy, surgery
Postoperative care
Rehabilitation

2.10. Communicates/documents psychosocial health status

3. Competency to analyze and interpret health status data in determining nursing diagnoses

3.1. Analyzes and interprets assessment data
Selects pertinent data
Sets priorities for data based on acuity
Emergent
Semiemergent
No acute distress

3.2. Identifies nursing diagnoses/patient problems consistent
With clinical manifestations
With human responses to cardiovascular problems

3.3. Validates diagnoses with patient, significant others, and cardiac team members, when possible

3.4. Supports nursing diagnoses with evidence-based, scientific knowledge
Nursing

> Medical
> Physical sciences
> Social sciences

3.5. Communicates/documents nursing diagnoses to health care team in a manner that facilitates the determination of outcomes and plan of care

Planning

4. Competency to identify expected outcomes unique to the patient

    4.1. Develops outcome statements based on nursing diagnoses and related to needs of cardiac surgery patients in collaboration with patient, significant others, and cardiac team members, when possible

    4.2. Identifies outcomes that are consistent with patient's cardiovascular history and therapeutic interventions

    4.3. Formulates outcomes that are measurable

    4.4. Develops outcomes that provide direction for continuity of care

    4.5. Sets priorities for outcome achievement based on
    > Clinical signs
    > Laboratory data
    > Patient preference, physical capabilities, and behavior patterns
    > Human and material resources available to patient

    4.6. Directs interventions to correct, alter, or maintain the nursing diagnoses

    4.7. Communicates and documents outcomes to appropriate persons in retrievable form

5. Competency to develop a plan of care that prescribes nursing actions to achieve patient outcomes

    5.1. Coordinates planned activities with patient, significant others, and cardiac team members

    5.2. Identifies nursing actions in a logical sequence specific to type of surgery
    > Coronary bypass grafting
    > Valve surgery
    > Thoracic aneurysms
    > Congenital defects
    > Conduction disturbances
    > Trauma/emergencies
    > Other cardiac conditions

    5.3. Identifies nursing actions to achieve patient outcomes based on best practices

    5.4. Identifies patient teaching needs to achieve expected outcomes

    5.5. Maintains availability of appropriate sterile equipment, instruments, and supplies

    5.6. Maintains equipment in functional order

    5.7. Coordinates scheduling of elective and emergency cases

    5.8. Notifies control desk and team members of possible cases/unstable patients

    5.9. Organizes instruments, equipment, and supplies to facilitate rapid and efficient room preparation

    5.10. Controls environment to meet patient needs
    > Temperature/humidity
    > Traffic patterns
    > Noise level

    5.11. Prepares for potential emergencies
    > Certified in CPR
    > Follows assigned call schedule
    > Maintains backup instruments, supplies, equipment

    5.12. Assigns activities to personnel based on
    > Qualifications
    > Demonstrated competency
    > Patient needs
    > Availability of personnel

    5.13. Communicates/documents patient's plan of care to appropriate personnel in retrievable form

Implementation

6. Competency to implement nursing actions in transferring the patient to the OR according to the prescribed plan

    6.1. Confirms identity of patient

    6.2. Selects personnel for transport depending on need
    > Sufficient number
    > Patient acuity

    6.3. Determines appropriate and safe method according to need
    > Nitroglycerin available
    > Transport personnel CPR certified
    > Use of monitoring devices as indicated

    6.4. Provides for emotional needs during transfer
    > Allows significant others to accompany patient to entrance of cardiac suite
    > Used comfort measures and touch
    > Greets patient by name and introduces self

    6.5. Communicates/ documents patient's transfer

7. Competency to participate in patient and family teaching

    7.1. Identifies teaching/learning needs of cardiac surgical patient and family related to
    > Expected sequence of events
    > Surgical procedure
    > Immediate postoperative events

Prevention of complications

Discharge planning

7.2. Assesses readiness to learn

Anxiety level

Acuity level

Level of consciousness

7.3. Provides instructions based on identified needs, readiness to learn, desires of patient and significant others, and reading level

7.4. Determines teaching effectiveness

7.5. Respects patient's use of therapeutic coping strategies

7.6. Communicates/documents patient/family teaching to provide for continuity of care

8. Competency to create and maintain a sterile field

8.1. Maintains sterility of bypass lines

8.2. Confines and contains instruments used in groin

8.3. Maintains sterility while supplying sterile items for procedure

Heart valves

Grafts

Donor organs

Solutions and supplies

Other items as needed

8.4. Uses aseptic technique to prepare grafts

8.5. Changes gown and gloves after contamination from

Team member's back

Groin procedures

OR bed elevated or lowered

8.6. Maintains sterility of setup until patient exits OR

8.7. Follows procedure for culturing tissue or solutions per institutional protocol

8.8. Follows procedure for rinsing glutaraldehyde-preserved tissue or valve prostheses per institutional protocol

8.9. Keeps instruments clean of blood and particulate matter during procedure

8.10. Communicates/documents maintenance of sterile field

9. Competency to provide equipment and supplies based on patient needs

9.1. Ensures equipment is functioning properly before use

Defibrillator, cords, and paddles

Fibrillator

Sternal saw and power source

Overhead lights

Headlight and light source

Autotransfusion system

Discard suction system

Electrosurgical equipment

External pacemaker generator

OR bed

Hypothermia/hyperthermia unit

Refrigerator (for cold solutions)

Cooling unit (for iced solutions)

Blood refrigerator

Blanket warmer

Positioning equipment

Other items as requested

9.2. Operates and maintains equipment (above) according to manufacturer's instructions

9.3. Selects instruments appropriate to procedure and size of patient in organized and timely manner

Basic sternotomy

Coronary artery bypass

Valve surgery

Thoracic aneurysm

Congenital defects

Conduction disturbances

Trauma/emergencies

9.4. Ensures instruments are functioning properly before use

Vascular clamps

Retractors

Forceps

Scissors and needle holders

9.5. Anticipates the need for equipment and supplies

Suture

Prostheses and sizers

Patch material (synthetic and biologic)

Medications

Special items per protocol

9.6. Documents lot and serial numbers of all prosthetic implants

9.7. Completes implant documentation forms for patient identification

9.8. Uses supplies judiciously and cost-effectively

As indicated from discussion with surgeon

According to surgeon preference

According to surgical technique

9.9. Ensures emergency equipment and supplies are available at all times

Items checked daily

Replacements/backups available

Replacements ordered promptly

9.10. Follows policy for reporting unsafe medical devices

9.11. Communicates/documents provision of equipment and supplies

10. Competency to account for sponges, "sharps," instruments, and other items as indicated per protocol

10.1. Accounts for sponges, "sharps," instruments

10.2. Accounts for specialty items per protocol

Bulldog clamps

Hypodermic needles
Umbilical tapes
Vessel loops, coronary snares
Rubbershods
Cannulas
Stopcocks
Prosthetic sizers/handles
Coronary stabilizers
Other items per policy and procedure

10.3. Communicates/documents results of counts according to institutional protocol

11. Competency to administer drugs and solutions as prescribed

11.1. Identifies drugs and solutions used
Heparin solution
Heparin bolus
Protamine
Papaverine
Calcium chloride
Epinephrine
Antibiotic solution
Cardioplegia solution
Topical cold solutions (normal saline, lactated Ringer's)
Topical hemostatic agents
Antidysrhythmic medications

11.2. Provides medications and solutions at proper temperature per protocol
Cold during induced arrest
Warm before or after induced arrest/when danger of producing fibrillation with cold solutions

11.3. Avoids ice chips in slush or liquid cold topical solutions

11.4. Communicates/documents administration of drugs and solutions

12. Competency to monitor the patient physiologically during surgery

12.1. Monitors physiologic status of patient
Skin color
Temperature (skin, esophageal, rectal, urinary, septal, within bypass lines)
Systemic blood pressure
Mean arterial pressure
Pulmonary artery systolic/diastolic/mean pressures
Pulmonary artery wedge pressure
Central venous pressure
Intracardiac pressure (left atrial, coronary sinus)
Oxygen saturation of arterial hemoglobin
Cardiac output, cardiac index
Electrocardiogram

12.2. Identifies lethal dysrhythmias
Ventricular fibrillation

Ventricular tachycardia
Asystole

12.3. Calculates intake and output
Blood loss, blood salvaged/reinfused
Urinary output
Pericardial effusion
Irrigating solutions

12.4. Assists/monitors behavioral changes preoperatively and during induction of anesthesia
Restlessness
Anxiety
Tenseness

12.5. Initiates nursing actions based on interpretation of physiologic changes
Anxiety-reduction measures
Comfort measures
CPR
Defibrillation
Notification of surgeon, anesthesiologist, perfusionist, and other team members as indicated

12.6. Operates monitoring equipment according to manufacturers' instructions

12.7. Communicates/documents physiologic responses

13. Competency to monitor and control the environment

13.1. Regulates room temperature as indicated
Cool during cardiopulmonary bypass
Warmer before and after bypass (as indicated)

13.2. Communicates with engineering department as necessary to maintain room temperature/humidity

13.3. Regulates hypothermia/hyperthermia unit as indicated

13.4. Implements OR sanitation policies

13.5. Confines and contains contaminated items (e.g., those used in the groin, lung biopsies)

13.6. Properly disposes of waste materials
"Sharps"
Bloody or body fluid–soiled items
Infected material

13.7. Maintains traffic patterns that
Avoid contamination
Provide sufficient space for operative preparation
Facilitate smooth transport of patient to and from OR

13.8. Avoids pressure on body parts from heavy instruments or leaning on patient

13.9. Follows policy for observers in OR (or in a special viewing area): number, purpose, etc.

13.10. Communicates/documents environmental controls

14. Competency to implement nursing actions in transferring the patient to the SICU according to the prescribed plan.
    14.1. Reports patient status to SICU prior to patient's leaving OR; includes
        Patient's name
        Procedure (bypass grafts, valves, grafts, etc)
        Difficulties associated with operative procedure (poor-quality saphenous vein, small aortic root, etc.)
        Weight, height
        Allergies
        Location of central and peripheral lines
        Intraoperative problems
            Excessive blood loss
            Dysrhythmias
            Blood pressure
            Difficulty cardioverting/defibrillating
            Bypass problems
        Blood/blood products (given and available)
        Urinary output
        Medications: used and required, dosage, route
            Vasoactive drugs
            Dysrhythmic drugs
            Coagulation/anticoagulation drugs
            Additional medications
        Tubes, drains, catheters
        Temporary pacing leads
            Atrial
            Ventricular
        Most recent electrolyte levels
            Calcium
            Magnesium
            Potassium
            Sodium
        Patient problems/concerns
        Notification of family members of patient's status
        Pertinent past medical history
        Pertinent past psychosocial history
    14.2. Selects personnel for transport based on patient acuity and staff needs
    14.3. Transports remaining blood/blood products to SICU (or blood bank) as indicated by hospital policy
    14.4. Ensures patient safety, privacy, and dignity during transport
    14.5. Verifies SICU bed is ready for transport
        Properly made
        Warming blanket applied
        X-ray cassette applied (if requested)
        Sufficient oxygen in portable tank

        Transport monitor
        Defibrillator
    14.6. Covers patient with warm blankets
    14.7. Accompanies patient to SICU with anesthesia and surgical staff (per protocol)
    14.8. Communicates physiologic and psychosocial data relevant to discharge planning to SICU staff and documents in perioperative records
    14.9. Assesses patient's physiologic stability prior to departing for SICU
15. Competency to respect the patient's rights
    15.1. Demonstrates consideration of patient's rights
        Association of periOperative Registered Nurses: *ANA Code for Nurses with Interpretive Statements—Explications for Perioperative Nursing*
        American Nurses' Association: *The Code of Ethics for Nurses* (2001)
        American Hospital Association: *A Patient's Bill of Rights*
    15.2. Provides privacy through confidentiality and physical protection
    15.3. Identifies cultural and spiritual beliefs
        Attitudes toward blood transfusions
        Heart as "seat of the soul"
        Family support
        Expressions of fear/anxiety
        Desire for religious counseling
    15.4. Communicates/documents respect for patient's rights

Evaluation

16. Competency to perform nursing actions that demonstrate professional accountability
    16.1. Completes an orientation based on individualized learning needs
    16.2. Remains current with newer trends in
        Cardiovascular technology
        Nursing/medical research
        Patient care practices
    16.3. Demonstrates flexibility and adaptability to changes in patient's status
    16.4. Demonstrates tact and understanding when dealing with the public, patients, and staff
    16.5. Communicates appropriate information to team members and representatives of other departments
    16.6. Seeks new learning opportunities for personal and professional development
    16.7. Promotes nursing research and incorporates research findings in practice
    16.8. Bases judgments and decisions on knowledge, skill, and experience

16.9. Fosters professional growth of team members, peers, colleagues, and others

16.10. Practices within ethical and legal guidelines

16.11. Participates in self-evaluation and peer review

16.12. Seeks and provides constructive feedback

16.13. Demonstrates accountability for maintaining competency as a cardiac team member

16.14. Seeks assistance when needed

16.15. Fosters collaborative working relationships in delivery of patient care

16.16. Considers factors related to efficient and effective use of human and material resources

16.17. Communicates/documents nursing accountability

17. Competency to evaluate patient outcomes

17.1. Develops criteria for outcome measurement

17.2. Measures outcome achievement in collaboration with patient, significant others, and cardiac team members

17.3. Evaluates patient responses to nursing interventions

17.4. Communicates/documents degree of goal achievement as appropriate to promote continuity of care

18. Competency to measure effectiveness of nursing care

18.1. Establishes criteria to measure quality of nursing care through a systematic quality assessment/improvement process

18.2. Evaluates practice in context of standards of clinical practice and professional performance, and relevant statutes and regulations, including but not limited to

AORN: *Standards, Recommended Practices, and Guidelines for Perioperative Nursing*

American Nurses' Association and American Heart Association Council on Cardiovascular Nursing: *Standards of Cardiovascular Nursing Practice* (in revision)

JCAHO standards

Other standards relevant to care of patients undergoing cardiac surgery

18.3. Assesses patient postoperatively

18.4. Evaluates effectiveness of nursing actions in relation to desired patient outcomes

18.5. Communicates/documents results of nursing care

19. Competency to reassess continuously all components of patient care based on new data

19.1. Reassess physiologic and psychosocial health status

19.2. Revises nursing diagnoses based on changes in health status

19.3. Reestablishes outcomes based on changes in signs and symptoms/laboratory data/patient preferences

19.4. Revises plan of care to reflect changes in priorities

19.5. Implements revised plan of care

19.6. Reevaluates patient outcomes and outcome criteria

19.7. Communicates/documents process of reassessment

Abbreviations

ACE (inhibitor)   Angiotensin-converting enzyme

AORN   Association of periOperative Registered Nurses

BUN   Blood urea nitrogen

CHF   Congestive heart failure

CPR   Cardiopulmonary resuscitation

CT   Computed tomography

JCAHO   Joint Commission on Accreditation of Healthcare Organizations

MI   Myocardial infarction

MRI   Magnetic resonance imaging

NPO   Nothing by mouth

OR   Operating room

SICU   Surgical intensive care unit

TIA   Transient ischemic attack

Appendix 2C

"What If?" Simulations and Decision-Making Exercises

SITUATION 1

You are planning to use the left radial artery as a bypass conduit; the surgeon asks you if there is adequate collateral circulation.

Questions to ask

How do you determine if there will be sufficient perfusion to the arm/hand after removal of the radial artery?

What is Allen's test? How is it performed? If the results of Allen's test are equivocal, what are your options?

How might a Doppler be used to test perfusion by the ulnar artery?

SITUATION 2

The surgeon is about to split the sternum, and the saw does not work.

Questions to ask

Is the saw power source connected?

Is the saw put together correctly?

Is there a procedure for testing the saw before use?

Is there a sterile backup saw available? If not, how can you ensure that there will be a sterile backup in the future?

What other resources are available in the operating room (e.g., Lebsche knife, orthopedic saws)?

SITUATION 3

You are preparing for a repair of a tricuspid valve. You notice that the anesthesia provider is getting ready to insert a pulmonary artery catheter.

Questions to ask

Where will the surgical site be located in the heart?

Why might a pulmonary artery catheter *not* be inserted in a patient with a right-sided lesion?

What technical difficulties would be associated with the presence of the catheter?

Why might a pulmonary artery catheter be indicated?

Could the placement of the catheter be adjusted?

Could the catheter be inserted postoperatively?

SITUATION 4

The patient, recently transported to the surgical intensive care unit (SICU), has suddenly started to bleed copiously through the chest tube.

Questions to ask

What are the responsibilities of the cardiac OR staff? Of the SICU staff?

What supplies and instruments are available in the SICU?

How would you access the heart if the original incision was a sternotomy? A lateral thoracotomy?

What supplies and instruments need to be brought from the OR?

How are nursing roles and responsibilities differentiated?

What information should be communicated to the OR? To the blood bank? To the sterile processing/supply department?

SITUATION 5

During an off-pump procedure performed through a median sternotomy, the patient's heart is retracted to expose the target coronary artery. Suddenly the patient's blood pressure drops to 30 mm Hg, and the heart starts to produce a series of premature ventricular contractions.

Questions to ask

Is the heart undergoing a temporary, reversible hemodynamic alteration? How do you know?

If the surgeon determines that cardiopulmonary bypass must be instituted, what do you do first?

Is the perfusionist immediately available? Is the bypass pump set up? Are the cannulas opened and ready?

Is heparin drawn up? How will the heparin be given? Directly into the right atrium? Through a central line?

SITUATION 6

You are talking with a patient preoperatively, and the family starts to ask you questions about the surgery (including how long it will last, whether the patient will be okay, why the procedure is being performed, and if the surgeon is competent).

Questions to ask

What is it that the patient and family want to know?

Are you qualified (legally and professionally) to answer every question?

What should you do if you are unable to answer their questions? Whom do you contact?

What can you do to reduce their level of anxiety?

3

Structural Elements of Cardiac Surgery

Why should a cardiac surgical unit be organized or developed? Where should such units be organized? When should they be organized? With what resources should they be developed? Finally, how does one go about it and what does it take to make it go?

Arthur E. Baue, MD, Alexander S. Geha, MD, and Hugh O'Kane, MD, 1974 (p. 31)

The technology is here, the potential is enormous, and the path is minimal.

Michael Mack, MD, 2001 (p. 572)

Questions asked more than a quarter of a century ago about organizing a cardiac surgical unit remain pertinent today because of the intense demands that such a service places on an institution's human, material, and fiscal resources. At the same time, advances in minimally invasive procedures—supported by new devices and equipment that integrate many operating room (OR) functions—are transforming surgical suites (Popolow, 1999). This transformation has not occurred without a price. As medical costs escalate and reimbursement decreases, the appropriateness and expense of diagnosing and treating cardiovascular disease continue to be intensely scrutinized.

One consequence of this is the public's demand for greater accountability and safety from health care professionals. The Institute of Medicine (IOM, 1999; 2001) has issued two reports that question whether consumers receive care that meets their needs and is based on the best scientific knowledge. The IOM's concerns about patient safety prompted the Joint Commission on the Accreditation of Healthcare Organizations (JCAHO, 2001) to revise its standards to incorporate error-reduction mechanisms, in addition to their requirements for specific evidence of acceptable standards of clinical practice and patient outcomes.

The Society of Thoracic Surgeons (STS, www.sts.org) and the American College of Cardiology (ACC, www.acc.org) both maintain a national database to track morbidity and mortality data on patients undergoing cardiac surgery and percutaneous coronary interventions, respectively. Hospitals participating in the ACC and STS databases can compare their patient outcomes with regional and na-

tional benchmarks and target areas for their own improvement. Patient satisfaction scores are tracked by a number of groups, such as the Gallup organization; an institution's scores enable its care team members to enhance the quality of the services they provide. Other activities by nursing and medical organizations promote continuous quality improvement, including patient satisfaction.

Standards that promote safe and effective nursing practice are published by the American Nurses Association (ANA, www.nursingworld.org) and the Association of peri-Operative Registered Nurses (AORN, 2001; www.aorn.org). The American Heart Association (AHA, www.americanheart.org), often in association with both nursing and medical groups, develops standards and guidelines related to heart disease. Both the ACC and the AHA jointly have developed guidelines for coronary artery bypass graft (CABG) surgery (Eagle and others, 1999) that identify conditions for which CABG is useful and effective. The American College of Surgeons (ACS, www.facs.org) has expanded earlier guidelines for cardiac surgery by adding sections that address structural elements, minimum procedure volume, patient follow-up, and professional performance.

This emphasis on the process and outcome of care is reflected in standards that, respectively, guide the manner in which care is provided and monitor the results that are achieved. In addition to *Process* and *Outcome Standards* identified by AORN in the Standards, Recommended Practices, & Guidelines (AORN, 2001), *Structural Standards*—the "Standards of Perioperative Administrative Practice" (AORN, 2001)—exist that relate to the professional, ethical, financial, regulatory, and material aspects of the OR and other interventional suites.

In addition to Structural Standards, AORN develops Recommended Practices. AORN's document—*Recommended Practices for Safety through Identification of Potential Hazards in the Perioperative Environment* (AORN, 2001)—provides guidance in identifying and avoiding those potential hazards associated with patient transport, patient temperature, chemicals in the OR, and electrical equipment. These hazards should be addressed in policies and procedures (Box 3-1), and safe practices should be instituted to protect patients.

Professional and ethical standards are addressed in Chapter 2, The Perioperative Nurse and the Cardiac Team. This chapter describes those structural aspects of the cardiac OR that the perioperative nurse manages in order to maintain a safe environment and to employ available resources efficiently, effectively, and cost consciously. Included are financial and regulatory considerations and the material resources of a cardiac OR: the cardiac suite, equipment, instrumentation, supplies, and prosthetic implants.

Financial Considerations

Increasingly, perioperative nurses (Ward, 1999) and surgeons (Canales, Macario, and Krummel, 2001) are expected to understand the financial aspects of the care they provide and the resources that they use. Being familiar with key accounting principles promotes effective dialogue with clinical colleagues, hospital administrators, payers, and regulatory agencies. Knowledge of the prospective payment system and diagnosis-related groups (DRGs) enables the nurse to be a more active participant and a key decision maker in the cardiac service.

For example, Medicare and Medicaid reimbursement schedules for cardiovascular (and other) cases are regulated by the Center for Medicare and Medicaid Services (CMS, formerly known as the Health Care Financing Administration [HCFA]). Cases (e.g., procedures) are classified into DRGs (Box 3-2) for payment under the prospective payment system based on the principal diagnosis, up to eight additional diagnoses, and up to six procedures performed during the hospital stay, as well as age, sex, and discharge status of the patient. The diagnosis and procedure information is reported by the hospital using codes from the International Classification of Diseases, ninth revision, Clinical Modification (ICD-9-CM). Cases are assigned to one of 503 DRGs in 25 major diagnostic categories (MDCs). Most MDCs are based on a particular organ system of the body; MDC-5 includes diseases and disorders of the circulatory system. Within most MDCs, cases are then divided into surgical DRGs and medical DRGs. Some surgical and medical DRGs are further differentiated based on the presence or absence of complications or comorbidities (HCFA, 2001).

BOX 3-1

Policies and Procedures Related to Cardiac Surgery

Policies and procedures specific to cardiac surgery are listed below. When policies and procedures are already available in the main operating room (such as those related to counts, electrosurgical safety, and positioning), they can be used by the cardiac service and need not be reformulated.

Autotransfusion system
Blood refrigerator
Hypothermia/hyperthermia unit
Preparation of iced saline/"slush"
Rinsing and preparation of glutaraldehyde-preserved valve prostheses
Policy for compliance with *The Safe Medical Devices Act of 1990*
Borrowing and lending of cardiac supplies and equipment
Availability/maintenance of sterile cardiac instrument sets during steam shutdown
Use of emergency generators during power failure
Use of internal/external defibrillator
Posting of cardiac procedures: scheduled, emergent
Position descriptions for cardiac staff (circulating and scrub nurses, RN first assistants)
Orientation program to the cardiac service
Staffing of the cardiac suites
Catheter Interventions, percutaneous coronary interventions (PCI)
Emergency sternotomy outside the cardiac operating room (e.g., intensive care unit, emergency room)
Use of cardiac personnel in noncardiac operating rooms
On-call policy for cardiac personnel
Notification of on-call personnel in emergency situations
Visitor policy for the cardiac operating room
Death procedure/procedure for family viewing of the deceased
Preoperative patient assessment
Patient/family teaching of the cardiac surgery patient
Postoperative report to the surgical intensive care unit
Postoperative patient assessment
Sterilization methods, recommendations for cardiac instruments/supplies/equipment
Policy for compliance with the *Anatomical Gift Act*
Policies related to organ transplantation/retrieval of donor organs
Cardiac quality improvement
Policy on *Patient Self-Determination Act*
Cardiac new product selection
Indication for/use of robot
Insertion/removal of ventricular assist device
Cardiac operating room setup for furniture, equipment, supplies, packs, and instrument sets
Policy on reprocessing of cardiac supplies/devices
Staffing coverage for PCI (e.g., percutaneous transluminal coronary angioplasty, stent insertion)
Cardiac laser policy

With declining reimbursements, practices within the cardiac suite are under constant review. Cost analyses of cardiothoracic procedures may focus on resource use, activity-based accounting, standardization of practices

> ### BOX 3-2
> ### Common Cardiac Diagnosis-Related Group Codes
>
> | | |
> |---|---|
> | DRG 103 | Heart transplantation |
> | DRG 104 | Cardiac valve procedure and other major cardiothoracic procedures with cardiac catheterization; formerly included ICDs (see DRG 514) |
> | DRG 105 | Cardiac valve procedure and other major cardiothoracic procedure without cardiac catheterization; formerly included ICDs (see DRG 515) |
> | DRG 106 | Coronary bypass with PTCA |
> | DRG 107 | Coronary bypass with cardiac catheterization |
> | DRG 108 | Other cardiothoracic procedures |
> | DRG 109 | Coronary bypass without cardiac catheterization |
> | DRG 112 | Formerly *percutaneous cardiovascular procedures;* has been *removed* from the DRG listing; new DRG numbers have been given a variety of percutaneous coronary interventions, such as stent insertion, PTCA, and intravascular brachytherapy (e.g., use of radioactive elements in coronary arteries) |
> | DRG 116 | Other cardiac pacemaker implantation; formerly titled *other permanent cardiac pacemaker implantation or PTCA, with coronary artery stent implant* |
> | DRG 495 | Lung transplant |
> | DRG 514 | Cardiac defibrillator implant with cardiac catheterization |
> | DRG 515 | Cardiac defibrillator implant without cardiac catheterization |

Modified from Health Care Financing Administration: *Proposed changes to DRG classifications and relative weights,* http://www.hcfa/gov/regs/hcfa1158p/pp021_111.doc (accessed Nov 28, 2001).
ICD, Internal cardioverter defibrillator; *PTCA,* percutaneous transluminal coronary angioplasty.

and inventory, and other areas that can improve tracking and controlling the cost of each patient treated (Mishra and others, 2001; Chiang, 2001; Kirshner, 2000). Nurses with knowledge of and experience in the financial aspects of running a cardiac suite are best qualified to identify waste and enhance efficiency without compromising the quality of care. These nurses can play an important advocacy role for their patients.

Regulatory Considerations

Structure standards also include compliance with regulatory and legislative mandates. The *Safe Medical Devices Act of 1990* (Public Law 101-629) reflects the public's concern about the development and use of current and future technologies and makes users of these devices accountable for their actions. The Food and Drug Administration (FDA, www.fda.gov) develops many performance standards on a range of devices and processes, from monitoring devices to reprocessing surgical supplies. Consideration of patients' rights legislation also illustrates society's interest in ensuring the well-being of patients within the health care delivery system.

The Cardiac Suite

Minimum requirements for performing cardiac procedures continue to be debated, but standards for construction of a cardiac suite have remained fairly constant, albeit with modifications reflecting new technology (such as video-assisted, port-access surgery and other minimally invasive procedures). Guidelines by the Inter-Society Commission for Heart Disease Resources (Judkins and others, 1976; Optimal resources, 1975) and the American College of Surgeons (1997) reflect not only the intensive demand for clinical competence but also the need for sufficient space that allows adequate monitoring, electrical safety, protected power supplies, availability of hot and cold water, infection control mechanisms, and other resources that support an optimum cardiac surgical environment (Fig. 3-1; Box 3-3).

Diagnosis and treatment facilities should be closely linked both geographically and operationally to promote the flow of information and the continuity of care. Interdisciplinary cooperation and communication promote efficient and effective care among the OR and units such as the emergency department, intensive care units (ICUs, surgical and nonsurgical), neonatal ICU, laboratory, cardiac catheterization laboratory, and imaging suite. Newer delivery models, such as the use of a mobile cardiac catheterization laboratory (Hubbard, 1999), also require close communication and planning for contingencies, even though the units are not physically connected.

ORs under construction or expansion may include diagnostic imaging devices such as fluoroscopy machines, magnetic resonance imagers, and computerized and digitized tomographic scans that can be integrated with traditional surgical resources (*Surgical Services Management,* 2001; entire issue devoted to construction/renovation). One example is the use of OR-based fluoroscopy to both identify coronary lesions and perform angioplasty or stent insertion in conjunction with traditional CABG surgery (so-called hybrid procedures). Future ORs will be technologically savvy and capable of providing both traditional surgery and computer-enhanced robotic interventions.

Traffic patterns are of special concern within the operating room, as well as to and from other departments. Transport routes should be preplanned to avoid delays. For instance, the fastest routes from the cardiac catheterization laboratory and the surgical intensive care unit to the cardiac OR should be identified, because patients requiring emergency surgery often come from these areas. (Mock runs can be practiced to test

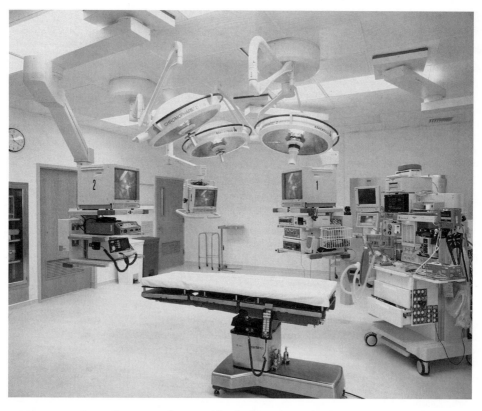

FIGURE 3-1 Operating room that provides both open and minimally invasive surgery capabilities. (Courtesy Community Medical Center, Scranton, Pa; and Berchtold Corp., Charleston, SC.)

BOX 3-3
Recommended Resources for Cardiac Surgery

Cardiac Operating Room

600 to 800 square feet
Large enough to accommodate 8 to 12 (or more) staff members
Large enough to maneuver without contamination of sterile areas

Storage Space

Sufficient for cardiac instrument, supplies, and equipment
Easily accessible to cardiac staff

Pump Room

Adequate for storage of pump oxygenators and assist devices
Located within surgical suite
Accessible from inside and outside suite

Plumbing

Installation of plumbing to provide hot, cold, and waste water
 for pump oxygenator

Suction

3 to 4 separate and independent sources of suction
1 dedicated suction source for anesthesia

Anesthesia Utility Pedestal

Ceiling-mounted units for gases, oxygen, suction, electrical outlets, and
Floor-mounted multipurpose pedestals

Blood Gas Core Laboratory

Capable of performing analyses of blood gases, pH, and electrolytes
Located adjacent to or near operating suite
Capable of providing blood gas results within 5 to 10 minutes
 during cardiopulmonary bypass

Modified from Optimal resources for cardiac surgery: guidelines for program planning and evaluation, *Am J Cardiol* 36:836, 1975; Judkins and others: Report of the Inter-Society Commission for Heart Disease Resources. Optimal resources for examination of the chest and cardiovascular system, *Circulation* 53(2): A1, 1976; American College of Surgeons: Guidelines for standards in cardiac surgery, *Bull Am Coll Surg* 82(2): 27-29, 1997.

BOX 3-3

Recommended Resources for Cardiac Surgery—cont'd

Infection Control

Installation of air-handling equipment capable of at least 25 operating room air changes per hour

Maintenance of temperature between 20° and 24° C (68° and 75° F), with capability of attaining 15.5° C (60° F)

Maintenance of humidity between 50% and 55%

Installation of high-efficiency particulate air filtering of incoming air (state codes may vary)

Unobstructed exhaust vents

Higher air pressure in operating room than outside operating room

Compliance with dress codes

Appropriate sterilization techniques

Electrical Hazard Control

Sufficient electrical outlets for equipment

90 to 120 amperes for peak load electrical current

Availability of alternative sources of power in case of power failure

Compliance with national electric codes

Electrical Interference and Shielding

Avoidance of monitoring signal distortion

Operating Room Illumination

Capability of lighting two operating fields simultaneously

200 to 250 foot candles for ambient light in operating room

2500 to 4000 foot candles for operative site

Instruments and Prostheses

Preventive maintenance and repair program

Appropriate storage and sterilization

Monitoring

Capability to monitor cardiorespiratory systems, blood gases, pH, electrolytes, temperature, renal function, and coagulation abnormalities

Data Handling

Capability to input and retrieve patient data via computer and digitized format, as well as hard copy

Pump Oxygenator

Availability of backup pump oxygenator

Preventive maintenance program

Record system for each pump oxygenator

Radiology

Capability of flexibility and maintenance of sterility of surgical field

Availability of a rapid processing unit in close proximity to operating room

Preventive Maintenance Program

Availability of policies and procedures for preventive maintenance of equipment and plant of operating room

Regular surveillance of medical devices for safety and efficacy

Availability of policies and procedures for emergency repairs and replacement of equipment

Qualifications of Professional Team

Orientation of new personnel

Sufficient number of assignments in cardiac OR to maintain proficiency

Need for special training for surgeons, first assistants, anesthesia care providers, nurses (OR and ICU), technologists, and perfusionists

Quality Improvement

Peer review to maintain adequate standard of practice

Participation in a registry for the recording of cardiac surgical results

Educational programs to maintain competence

Patient follow-up system

Surgical Volume Standards

Individual surgeon's volume greater than 200 cases per year, per hospital

Diagnostic and Laboratory Facilities

Cardiac catheterization laboratory available 24 hours a day

Laboratory, including blood bank, available 24 hours a day

Communication

Emergency alarm system

Capability for direct audio communication with blood bank and OR control desk

Telephone with inside and outside calling capability

---

the system.) If an elevator must be used, it should be called to the floor and held so that the patient can be moved into it without delay. It should be of sufficient size to accommodate the patient, the staff, and equipment such as monitors and ventricular support devices. In some hospitals freight elevators may provide the only adequately sized lifts.

Occasionally, cardiovascular procedures are performed outside the OR suite because patients are too critically ill to be transported. Such cases include emergency sternotomies for postoperative cardiac tamponade in the surgical intensive care unit, portable cardiopulmonary bypass for failed angioplasty patients in circulatory collapse, and patent ductus arteriosus ligations in the neonatal intensive care unit. In planning procedures to be performed outside the OR, perioperative nurses must consider (1) how sterility is to be maintained; (2) how to supply all necessary equipment, instruments, and other items; and (3) how to work within the confines of an unfamiliar environment (Box 3-4).

Maintenance of Sterility

Control traffic
Isolate the room (close doors, place screens)
Limit personnel in room
Provide inservices to unit personnel on asepsis, sterile technique
Bring disposable supplies as needed
   Hats, masks, gowns, shoe covers
   Scrub brushes, skin preparation solution
Assist unit with developing inventory for surgical procedures
Create sterile field on overbed table or bed
Use large disposable laparotomy sheet to cover bed

Availability of Supplies

Have portable carts with instruments and supplies
Have internal defibrillator paddles (ensure that they fit into unit's defibrillator)
Develop emergency sets with minimum but sufficient instrumentation
Have a runner to obtain additional items from operating room
Bring headlight, electrosurgical unit as requested

Working in a New Environment

Practice mock runs, simulations
Have joint meetings with unit staff
Discuss roles/responsibilities
   Monitoring
   Attaching suction
   Giving medications
   Obtaining blood
   Obtaining supplies
   Availability of perioperative staff
   Cleaning, reprocessing of unit instruments
Orient perioperative staff to unit
Have unit orientees observe surgery

Furniture

Standard furnishings found in the cardiac OR include the OR bed and accessories, small and standard-size tables, kick buckets, ring stands, Mayo stands, linen and waste hampers, intravenous (IV) poles, suction, sitting and standing stools, patient monitors, and anesthesia machines. Additional tables and stands may be needed for extra basins, instrument containers, and drapes. They also may be needed to provide surfaces for setting up a sterile field to insert intravascular lines by anesthesia personnel or for rinsing biologic valve prostheses, thawing cryopreserved homografts, or arranging components of ventricular assist devices. Portable carts may be used to store sutures, prosthetic implants, or other supplies.

The OR bed may be modified to enable it to be raised higher than usual for exposure of the internal mammary arteries (located on either side of the retrosternal borders). Surgery on neonates and infants may require a special, smaller bed constructed to reflect and maintain body temperature.

Typically, cardiac ORs are dedicated to open heart procedures. Furniture is selected and arranged according to the preference and needs of the staff and often is consistent with an established plan. Some ORs use one or more Mayo stands and a back table; others may use an overbed table without a Mayo stand. The staff can determine what works best for them.

Whatever the plan, it should be diagrammed for environmental service employees to assist them in returning items to their proper location after cleaning. This diagram should include instructions about reconnecting electrical cords that have been unplugged during cleaning. A diagram is also useful for OR personnel who are not familiar with the routine arrangement and must begin the initial room preparation for an emergency procedure. This may occur on the evening or night shifts when cardiac staff are not yet in-house. Orientation to the cardiac OR enables those unfamiliar with the cardiac routine to help during emergencies. Of special importance is the location of supplies, instruments, and medications and the identification of what items to open. Wasted supplies can be minimized if only those items that need to be opened are set around the room when the cardiac staff leaves for the day.

Equipment

POSITIONING EQUIPMENT

The patient position for most cardiac procedures is supine because it affords the best exposure of the heart and great vessels. However, some minimally invasive procedures (i.e., employing smaller incisions) and those performed without cardiopulmonary bypass may employ a semilateral or full thoracotomy position. Positioning devices and supplies should be kept near the cardiac OR. Padding for the head, hands, elbows, and feet can be kept near the OR bed. If the lower extremities do not need to be exposed, an anesthesia screen placed at the foot of the bed will keep heavy drapes off the feet. In obese patients padded sleds may be needed to keep the arms tucked next to the body. Armboards attached to the bed can provide extra width for very large patients. Very tall patients may require a footboard to extend the length of the bed.

An anesthesia screen or IV poles keep drapes off the face and provide access to the airway and intravascular lines. Some services use an overbed frame that is placed over the patient's head. These frames may have a shelf that, after being draped, can be used by the surgeon and assistant to place instruments. Splints may be used

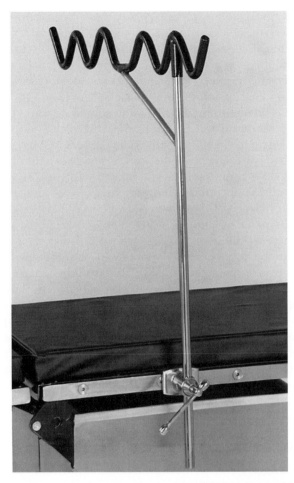

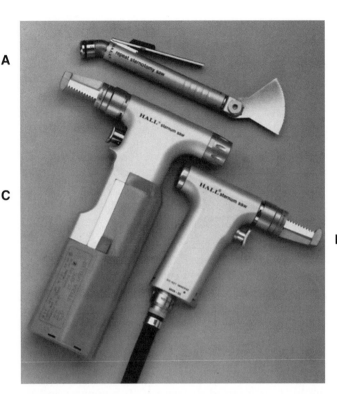

FIGURE 3-3 **A,** Air-driven, hand-controlled sternal saw powered by nitrogen from a portable tank; **B,** battery-powered (reciprocating) sternal saw (especially convenient for sternal splitting during distal procurement of donor hearts for transplantation); **C,** oscillating saw (may be used for repeat sternotomy). (Courtesy Zimmer, Hall Surgical Div., Carpinteria, Calif.)

FIGURE 3-2 "Picket fence" used to elevate one or both legs for circumferential skin preparation. Other models may have two legs that attach to the OR bed. (Courtesy OSI, Orthopedic Systems, Inc., Hayward, Calif.)

to maintain the position of the wrist in which a radial arterial monitoring line has been inserted.

When saphenous leg vein must be excised for coronary bypass grafting, leg holders can be used to elevate the legs for circumferential skin preparation (Fig. 3-2). Elevating or flexing the legs may be contraindicated when a femoral artery sheath is in place, so the nurse should first confer with the surgeon about which skin preparation and positioning technique to use. Foam rubber leg supports that elevate and externally rotate the legs are available for intraoperative use to provide optimal exposure for harvesting saphenous leg veins (see Chapter 10).

Cardiovascular lesions such as those involving the descending thoracic aorta are best approached through a left lateral thoracotomy incision. Lateral positioning equipment and supplies include overarm boards (or Mayo stands), axillary rolls, and pillows to support the legs and feet. A vacuum pillow on the bed that hardens

into the desired shape when suction is applied is useful for lateral positioning. For some minimally invasive procedures an anterolateral position can be achieved with a small roll, sandbag, or IV bag placed under the operative side, thereby slightly tilting the chest to provide the necessary exposure.

HEADLIGHT, LOUPES

A fiberoptic headlight and light source offer supplemental lighting, which is usually necessary for illuminating deep chest cavities. In addition to the surgeon, the assistant also may require a headlight. Loupes with $2\frac{1}{2} \times$ to $3\frac{1}{2} \times$ magnification are commonly used and may be stored in the cardiac suite.

STERNAL SAW

When a sternotomy incision is used to expose the mediastinum, the sternum is divided (or partially divided for mini-sternotomy) from the xiphoid process to the sternal notch with a saw that is air driven (Fig. 3-3, *A*), battery powered (Fig. 3-3, *B*), or electrically powered

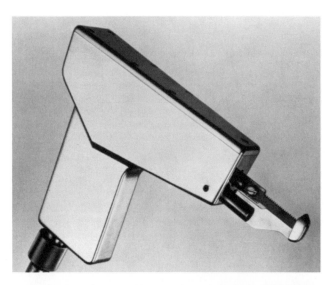

FIGURE 3-4 Electric (reciprocating) sternal saw with a foot pedal. (Courtesy Sarns 3M Health Care, Ann Arbor, Mich.)

(Fig. 3-4). The blade is inserted with the teeth facing up. Some surgeons prefer to saw from the sternal notch to the xiphoid process; in this case the toothed edge of the blade is inserted downward. (In neonates and infants, heavy scissors can be used to transect the cartilaginous sternum.)

An oscillating saw with sagittal saw blades (Fig. 3-3, *C*) may be used for repeat sternotomies, where the presence of adhesions from a previous sternotomy increases the risk of injuring underlying structures adhering to the sternum. The action of the saw allows the bone to be divided from the anterior table of the sternum to the posterior table. Saw blades may be wide or narrow depending on surgeon preference. Some surgeons prefer to use the reciprocating saw (see Fig. 3-4) for repeat sternotomies.

When a saw is unavailable, a Lebsche knife and mallet may be the only available means of splitting the sternum to expose the heart in acute settings such as an emergency room (see Chapter 21). Thoracotomy incisions are made with a knife.

When a portion of rib is to be removed, rib shears are used.

HYPOTHERMIA/HYPERTHERMIA UNITS

The ability to control the temperature of both the patient and the environment is critical to the success of cardiac surgery, even when a procedure is performed under normothermia. When hypothermia is employed, the patient must be both cooled and rewarmed during the same operation. External patient cooling and warming is achieved with mobile hypothermia/hyperthermia units. Some units have only a warming function. A disposable

or nondisposable thermia blanket is placed under a sheet (or other padding) on the OR table and connected to hoses running to the unit. The desired temperature is selected, and water within the machine's reservoir is pumped through the hoses into the channels within the blanket. The unit must be kept filled with water to function properly. The unit should be turned on early so that it will be warm when the patient is positioned on it. (In addition, the filling process will be completed more quickly if the unit is activated before the blanket is compressed by the patient's weight.) Recommended temperature settings are between 38° and 40° C (100.4° and 104° [Maldonado and Nygren, 1999]). In addition to monitoring water temperature, some machines also monitor the patient's temperature via a rectal probe that is inserted before the patient is draped.

Hypodermic needles, towel clips, or other sharp objects stuck into a water-filled blanket will cause the circulating water to leak out of the thermia pad and may pose an electrosurgical hazard. Thermal burns are a potential danger, although most hyperthermia units do not exceed the safe setting of 41° to 42° C. A more probable cause of injury from these units is pressure necrosis. Recommendations for preventing such injuries include placing additional padding between the patient and the blanket, confirming the proper position of the temperature probe, and maintaining electrical safety practices when electrosurgical instruments are used.

RADIANT HEATERS

Radiant heaters may be employed as an additional heat source for maintaining body temperature. These are often used in pediatric procedures. Precautions are necessary to avoid burns or insensible water loss from prolonged use.

SALINE ICE UNITS

During induced hypothermia, cold topical solutions may be used to enhance cooling of the myocardium. Various methods of cooling normal saline (or lactated Ringer's solution) are available, such as refrigerator or freezer storage of bags or bottles or using dry ice or isopropyl alcohol as the cooling agent. Specially designed units that have a depression in the top (occasionally called *bird baths*) into which a sterile transfer basin (or a cold- or heat-resistant drape) is placed can be used to either cool or warm solutions, depending on the temperature desired.

Cold topical solutions are also available in dispenser bags (Fig. 3-5), making them especially useful for transplant organ preservation during the procurement period. The bags can be cooled, transported to the procurement site, and opened to expose a sterile, wrapped

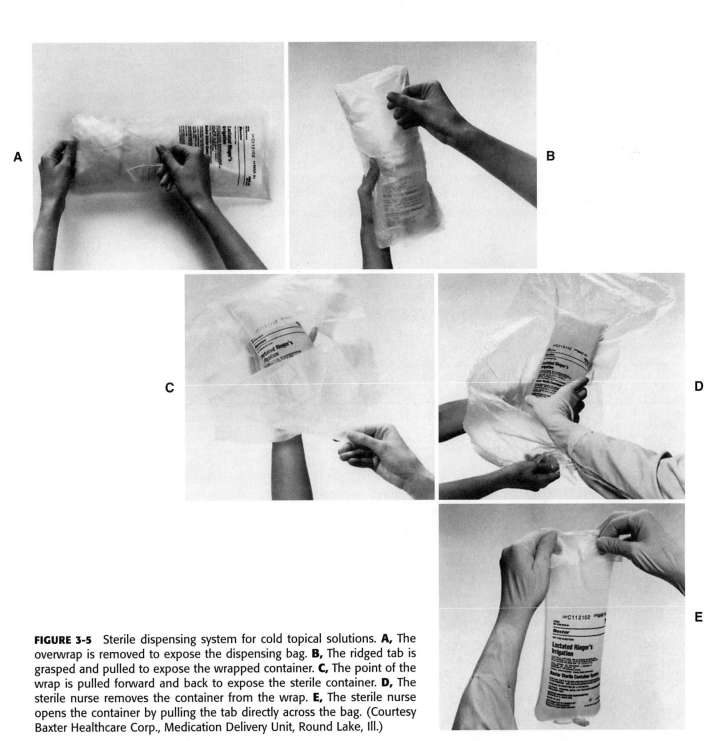

FIGURE 3-5 Sterile dispensing system for cold topical solutions. **A,** The overwrap is removed to expose the dispensing bag. **B,** The ridged tab is grasped and pulled to expose the wrapped container. **C,** The point of the wrap is pulled forward and back to expose the sterile container. **D,** The sterile nurse removes the container from the wrap. **E,** The sterile nurse opens the container by pulling the tab directly across the bag. (Courtesy Baxter Healthcare Corp., Medication Delivery Unit, Round Lake, Ill.)

solution container. The wrapping is removed, and the contents are poured or squeezed into a basin.

DEFIBRILLATOR

Defibrillation by the external or internal application of a direct-current (DC) electrical shock to the myocardium is instituted when the heart fibrillates. It is the only reliable therapy for persistent ventricular tachycardia and ventricular fibrillation. The amount of current selected varies depending on the size of the patient and on whether internal or external defibrillation is being performed (Table 3-1). It should be noted that defibrillation will not convert a heart that is asystolic; the heart must be fibrillating. (A pacemaker would be needed for the heart to start beating.)

Defibrillators (Fig. 3-6) should be tested before use. The unit may not function if the power cord has been disconnected and there is insufficient battery power. The unit should be inspected routinely to ensure that it is connected to line power when it is not in use.

Both external and internal paddle tips come in an assortment of sizes (Fig. 3-7). Disposable defibrillator electrodes (Fig. 3-8, *E*) can be applied securely to the chest. Some manufacturers make pediatric adaptors that slip over the standard external paddles (Fig. 3-8, *B*). Internal paddles (Fig. 3-8, *D*) are screwed into handles attached to cords that are connected to the defibrillator (or the adapters [Fig. 3-8, *A*] that inserts into the defibrillator).

Internal handles, cords, and tips can all be sterilized with low-temperature hydrogen peroxide gas plasma

TABLE **3-1**	
External and Internal Defibrillator Settings for Children and Adults	
PATIENT AGE GROUP	SETTING
External Defibrillator	
Neonates	2 joule (J)/kg (1 J/lb)
Children	2 J/kg (1 J/lb)
Adults	200 J First shock
	300 J Second shock
	360–400 J Subsequent shocks
Internal Defibrillator	
Neonates and children	Lowest possible setting, starting at 3 J for neonates and 5 J for children, increasing the energy in small increments; no definitive data are available for defibrillation energy requirements in neonates and children
Adults	10–20 J Lower energy levels may be effective; higher levels or repeated shocks may cause myocardial necrosis

Modified from Myerburg RJ, Castellanos A: Cardiac arrest and sudden cardiac death. In Braunnold E, Zipes DP, Libby P, editors: *Heart disease,* ed 6, Philadelphia, 2001, WB Saunders. Emergency Cardiac Care Committee and Subcommittees, American Heart Association: Guidelines for cardiopulmonary resuscitation and emergency cardiac care, *JAMA* 268(16):2172, 1992; Kerber RE and others: Open chest defibrillation during cardiac surgery: energy and current requirement, *Am J Cardiol* 46(3):393-396, 1980; Pugsley WB and others: Low energy level internal defibrillation during cardiopulmonary bypass, *Eur J Cardiothorac Surg* 3(3):273-275, 1988; Bossert L, Koster R: Defibrillation: methods and strategies, Resuscitation 24(3):211-223, 1992.

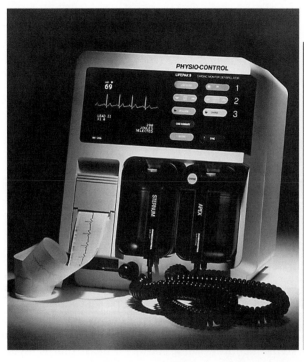

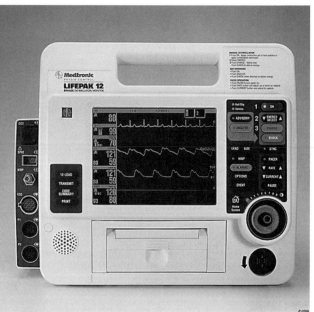

A   B

FIGURE 3-6   Defibrillator. **A,** The unit provides internal and external defibrillation or cardioversion. **B,** LIFEPAK 12. This defibrillator can be used to treat dysrhythmias encountered during surgery and as an automatic external defibrillator. (Courtesy Medtronic, Inc.)

(75-minute cycle time) or with ethylene oxide (EO) gas (minimum 12-hour cycle time). Steam sterilization (approximately 1-hour cycle time) can be used for the metal defibrillator tips but not on the nonmetal handles and cords (Medtronic Physio-Control, 1997).

Hydrogen peroxide sterilization has a number of advantages over EO and steam sterilization. EO is toxic and has a relatively long cycle time; the prolonged turnaround time to process internal defibrillator components requires a larger inventory of these items in order to have

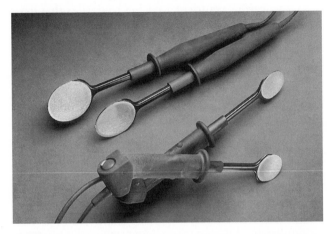

FIGURE 3-7 Internal defibrillator paddle tips come in an array of sizes. Smaller tips are used for infants and children. A large tip placed under the patient's back (with padding) and a standard adult tip placed directly on the heart provide external-internal defibrillation. Paddles will function only in defibrillator units for which they were designed. (From Meeker MH, Rothrock JC: *Alexander's care of the patient in surgery,* ed 11, St Louis, 1999, Mosby; courtesy Hewlett-Packard Co., Andover, Mass.)

sterile paddles readily available. Steam sterilization can only be used for the metal paddle tips; when different sterilization methods are used, there is a danger of misplacing one part of the required internal defibrillation system components. With hydrogen peroxide sterilization, components can be quickly sterilized/resterilized and kept together in one package; both time and money can be saved.

Sterilizable (with hydrogen peroxide or EO) external paddles are available, but most often disposable sterile adhesive electrode patches are used. Sterile external defibrillation capability may be required when a recently draped patient's heart fibrillates (and the sternum is not yet opened) or when incisions are too small to allow the use of internal paddles.

For defibrillation, direct electrical current must traverse the myocardium. To achieve this, internal paddles are commonly placed laterally on the right and left ventricles. They do not need to be moistened with conductive paste because the heart is already lubricated with blood and pericardial fluid. Personnel should stand away from the table to avoid being shocked. In the presence of pericardial adhesions from prior sternotomy, sterile external paddles (or patches) can be used. Another method is to perform anteroposterior defibrillation with a large, flat external paddle placed against the patient's back and an internal paddle placed on top of the heart (see Fig. 3-7). Precautions should be taken to pad the handle of the external paddle so as not to cause pressure injury to the patient's back. If the patient fibrillates during dissection of the adhesions, anteroposterior defibrillation with internal-external paddles can be performed. Alternatively the pleura can be opened and the internal paddles placed on the pleural surface and pressed against the heart.

A

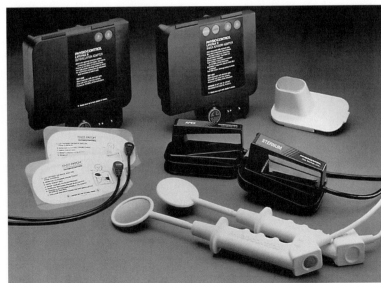

FIGURE 3-8 Accessories for LIFEPAK 9 defibrillator. **A,** Defibrillator adapter cassettes (required for internal paddles); **B,** pediatric clip-on external paddle, which slides over adult paddles; **C,** sterilizable external paddles (hydrogen peroxide or ethylene oxide recommended for sterilization); **D,** internal defibrillator handles and tips with remote discharge control; **E,** disposable defibrillator/electrocardiogram electrodes for external defibrillation (commonly used for repeat sternotomy and minimally invasive procedures). (Courtesy Medtronic, Inc.)

The defibrillator also can be used for cardioversion. The difference between defibrillation and cardioversion is that the former delivers an unsynchronized shock to the heart. A patient requiring cardioversion has a pulse (e.g., the ventricle is not fibrillating), and the shock is synchronized with the R wave of the QRS complex. In the OR the procedure is most commonly indicated to convert recent-onset atrial fibrillation to normal sinus rhythm. When cardioversion is to be performed, the patient is attached by electrocardiogram (ECG) cables to the defibrillator, which has been set to the "synchronous" mode. This is done to synchronize the delivery of electrical current to the R wave of the QRS complex (ventricular systole). If the shock is not synchronized to the R wave, it can produce ventricular fibrillation if it is discharged during the vulnerable period (the T wave of the ECG).

The unit is then charged and activated. Successful cardioversion depolarizes all excitable myocardium, interrupts abnormal electrical circuits, and establishes electrical homogeneity, which fosters normal sinus rhythm. When no QRS complex exists (e.g., in ventricular fibrillation), the defibrillator will not discharge if it is in the synchronous mode because there is no regular waveform that the machine can "read" and synchronize to. If the patient fibrillates, valuable time may be lost trying to change settings to "asynchronous"; therefore it is recommended that the defibrillator routinely be kept in the asynchronous mode unless cardioversion specifically is requested.

Automatic External Defibrillator

Because early defibrillation improves survival, it is the standard for both in-hospital and out-of-hospital cardiac arrest (Myerburg and Castellanos, 2001). Automatic external defibrillators (AEDs) (Fig. 3-6) are devices that may be used in a variety of settings (e.g., airports, business offices) by persons without formal training in cardiac rhythm recognition and manual defibrillation (see Chapter 17). The AED is attached to the patient via adhesive electrode patches (sternum-apex placement). A computerized detection system analyzes the cardiac rhythm, identifies rhythms that require a shock, and delivers the appropriate defibrillation energy. AEDs should not be used on children under 8 years of age.

AEDs are beneficial not only in public places but also on general nursing floors, where early defibrillation can be performed before the code team arrives. Defibrillators are currently available that can be used either as an AED or as the main intraoperative defibrillator.

FIBRILLATOR

Although some cardiac procedures are intentionally performed on a beating heart with the use of CPB, there are situations when ventricular contractions make precise suturing difficult (even with the use of coronary stabilizers

and blood pressure–reducing drugs). In addition, when extensive bleeding occurs after the discontinuation of CPB, repair may be technically difficult and may put the patient at risk of further injury. The beating heart produces a systolic force and a pulse wave that can disrupt sutures as they are being inserted or tied. A cardiac fibrillator (approximately the size of a 2-inch × 3-inch × 5-inch box) capable of delivering 25 to 50 volts of alternating current (AC) produces a fine fibrillation, enabling the surgeon to repair the injury on a quiet field.

To perform this technique, the surgeon uses the temporary epicardial ventricular pacing lead wires that have been attached before termination of cardiopulmonary bypass. The distal ends of the leads are passed off the field and attached to the fibrillator. The fibrillator is activated, producing fine fibrillation. Once the repair is accomplished and the bleeding controlled, cardiac massage followed by defibrillation with DC countershock (with internal paddles) will cause cardiac action to resume. (The pacing leads may then be removed from the fibrillator and attached to an external pacemaker for pacing if indicated.)

Nurses must understand the different indications for fibrillation and defibrillation if serious accidents are to be avoided. Fibrillation is used to produce a relatively motionless field so that tissue being repaired is not torn; defibrillation is used to reverse fibrillation and initiate cardiac contractions. To reduce confusion between the fibrillator and the defibrillator, some have suggested painting the fibrillator red or another bright color.

ELECTROSURGICAL UNIT

Electrosurgical units use high-frequency electrical current to cut tissue and cauterize bleeding vessels. The development of solid-state generators has significantly decreased the potential for burns and electrical shocks that were associated with spark-gap units.

Two electrosurgical units may be used when more than one surgical site is exposed. This may occur during coronary artery bypass procedures in which the saphenous vein is being excised simultaneously with opening of the chest and preparation for cannulation. When two units are in use, each unit must be connected to its own dispersive pad, which has been applied to the patient. Commonly, dispersive pads are applied bilaterally to the patient's buttocks. When two units are in use, caution must be taken to ensure that changes in current settings are made only to the unit being used by the surgeon making the request and that the unused electrosurgical pencil is not discharged inadvertently by leaning on the control button. The amount of current needed will vary during the operation depending on the type of tissue being cauterized. Often the surgeon will request a lower setting when cauterizing close to vascular structures such as the aorta or internal mammary artery.

Precautions are warranted in patients with permanent pacemakers or internal cardioverter defibrillators. Problems encountered with the use of electrocautery include damage or alterations to pulse generator functions, electrical and thermal burns at the myocardial insertion site of the electrode, and ventricular fibrillation. Some authors have suggested the use of bipolar cautery to reduce the amount of electricity transmitted to surrounding tissue. When monopolar probes are used, precautions include placing the dispersive pads as far as possible from the pulse generator, using short bursts of electrocautery, monitoring pacer function frequently, and having ready access to a pulse-generator programmer. If possible, the type of pacemaker or ID and the manufacturer should be identified in the event that reprogramming or other alterations have to be made.

ULTRASONIC SCALPEL

Another form of energy that is not based on heat generation (used for cautery) is *ultrasonic energy,* which is especially useful during dissection of the internal mammary artery (IMA) to minimize thermal injury to the vessel and surrounding structures. The ultrasonic scalpel consists of an energy generator, a hand piece with cable, an assortment of blades, and a foot pedal. The device denatures tissue protein into a coagulum that seals blood vessels and bleeding tissue. The scalpel's cutting action is produced by longitudinal vibration of the blade tip at 55,500 times per second. The protein coagulum is formed as the mechanical energy from the blade combines with the tissue protein (Higami and others, 2000). Because there is reduced damage to surrounding tissue, the ultrasonic scalpel is also beneficial during minimally invasive procedures, where there is a restricted surgical field (Lamm and others, 2000).

AUTOTRANSFUSION SYSTEM

Autotransfusion systems (Fig. 3-9) that salvage, process, and return blood back to the patient have several advantages, including avoidance of incompatible bank blood, decreased risk of infection, and less danger of donor-related disease. Contraindications to the use of autologous blood transfusions include sepsis, severe coagulopathy, renal failure, bowel perforation, and cancer (Reger and Roditski, 2001).

Blood is collected by suction, filtered, and anticoagulated with a heparin solution or citrated phosphate dextrose. A cell processor separates and packs the red blood cells, which have been washed to remove the anticoagulant and reinfused as indicated (Fig. 3-10). Precautions should be taken to avoid suctioning topical

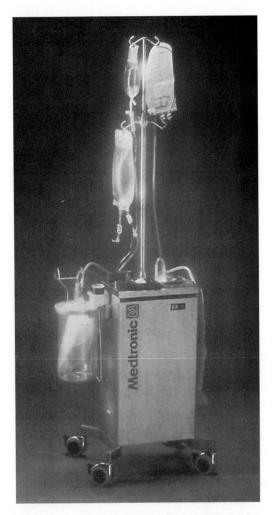

FIGURE 3-9 Autotransfusion system; used when excessive bleeding is anticipated or encountered. (Courtesy Medtronic, Inc.)

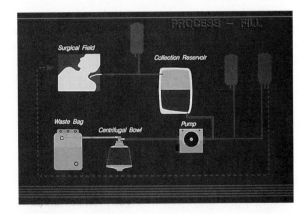

FIGURE 3-10 Diagram of autotransfusion system. (Courtesy Haemonetics Corp., Braintree, Mass.)

hemostatic agents such as thrombin, fibrin glue, or microfibrillar collagen compounds into the reservoir because they can trigger clotting mechanisms. The aspiration of topical antibiotics should be avoided as well.

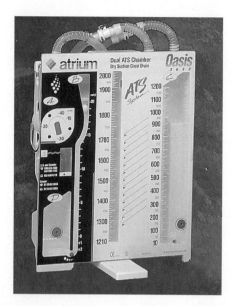

FIGURE 3-11 Chest drainage system that also can be used to reinfuse shed mediastinal blood when significant drainage is anticipated. (Courtesy Atrium Medical Corporation, Hudson, NH.)

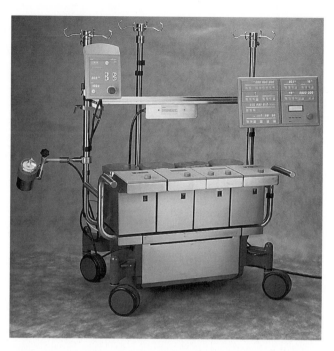

FIGURE 3-12 Cardiopulmonary bypass pump: Stöckert S III modular HLM with integrated centrifugal pump driver. (Courtesy Stöckert Instrumente, Gmbh, Munich; photo courtesy of US distributor: COBE CV, division of Sorin Biomedica, Arvada, CO.)

Because there is a variable amount of trauma to blood cells that can impair the patient's clotting function, autotransfusion systems are indicated mainly in situations in which there is extensive blood loss (e.g., more than one unit of packed red blood cells). The cost of a setup pack also can be saved when the device is used mainly for significant bleeding. When patients are at risk for hemorrhage (or are actively hemorrhaging), the autotransfusion system should be used.

Autotransfusion can be used postoperatively to salvage mediastinal shed blood. Chest tube drainage is collected, filtered, and reinfused within a 1- to 2-hour period. The collecting chamber (Fig. 3-11) may be a unit designed solely for chest tube drainage, or it may be the venous reservoir used during the bypass procedure and modified for autotransfusion. Collection systems should be labeled with the patient's name. Small amounts of chest tube drainage are not reinfused.

PUMP OXYGENATOR

Although there is a trend toward performing cardiac procedures (mainly coronary artery bypass) without the use of CPB, extracorporeal circulation is still required for many procedures (e.g., valve replacement, ascending aortic and arch aneurysms). Because there is the potential for profound hemodynamic instability even in the most healthy surgical candidates with normal left ventricular function, perioperative cardiac nurses should *always* be prepared to institute CPB on a patient when needed. This necessitates that supplies and equipment be immediately available and that performance competencies be maintained.

Extracorporeal circulation can be achieved with a variety of devices. These include the standard bypass system (Fig. 3-12) or an endovascular system (Fig. 3-13) that employs a series of percutaneous multilumen catheters, which can be used to institute femoral venous–femoral arterial bypass, infuse solutions, vent air, measure intravascular pressures, and occlude the aorta via inflation of an endoaortic balloon. Smaller, more portable (percutaneous) systems are also available that can be used to support patients in the cardiac catheterization laboratory and the intensive care unit (see Chapter 9).

The pump oxygenator (Fig. 3-12), also called the *heart-lung machine, bypass pump,* or *pump,* supports the patient's cardiorespiratory function during cardiac surgery. It does this by draining or siphoning venous blood, removing waste gases, oxygenating and filtering the blood, and pumping it back into the patient's arterial system. The unit incorporates an oxygenator, a heat exchanger to warm or cool the blood, a device to propel the blood into the arterial system, and monitoring and safety devices.

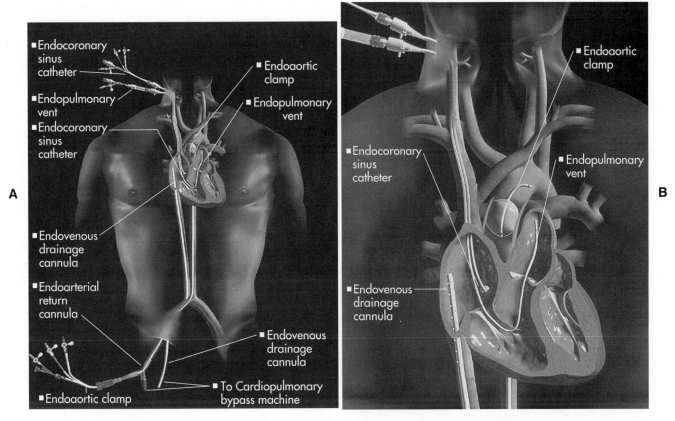

FIGURE 3-13 A, Endovascular cardiopulmonary bypass and myocardial protection system (see text). **B,** Intracardiac placement of catheters. (Courtesy CARDIOVATIONS, a division of ETHICON, Inc.)

Returning blood is diverted from the right atrium via one or two cannulas attached to tubing that leads to the pump. A single, two-stage cannula (Fig. 3-14) is used in many procedures in which the right atrium is not opened. The cannula is inserted through the right atrium, with the fenestrated distal end placed in the inferior vena cava to collect returning blood from the lower body. The portion of the cannula sitting in the right atrium also has openings, which collect blood from the superior vena cava and coronary sinus. The cannula is attached to tubing that goes to the pump.

The inferior and superior venae cavae may be cannulated separately, with the cannulas "Y'd" to the venous returning tubing. This is necessary when the right atrium is the surgical site and must remain free of excess blood. Venous blood also may be returned via the femoral vein for percutaneous procedures or when the right atrium cannot be cannulated safely (e.g., in the presence of a very large ascending aortic aneurysm).

Various kinds of cannulas are available depending on the size of the patient, the exposure required, and the

flow rates needed. Because inflow with oxygenated blood is dependent on the amount of venous outflow, the surgeon optimizes returning blood flow by inserting as large a catheter as possible into the venous system. (Larger catheters also produce less shear forces and are less traumatic to the formed elements in the blood.)

Arterial catheters (Fig. 3-15) to return oxygenated blood commonly are inserted into the ascending aorta. When entry into the thorax of a patient who has previously undergone a sternotomy poses a risk of injuring the heart or aorta, the surgeon may cannulate the femoral artery. Arterial cannulas (femoral or aortic) are secured to the drapes or the patient's skin to aid in preventing the accidental removal of the catheter. Both venous and arterial cannulas may be reinforced with wire to avoid kinking.

Two methods of blood oxygenation have evolved to remove carbon dioxide and restore oxygen: the bubble method and the membrane method (Fig. 3-16). The bubble method works by pumping oxygen directly through a column of venous blood. This creates a foam of air bubbles, necessitating the use of a chemical

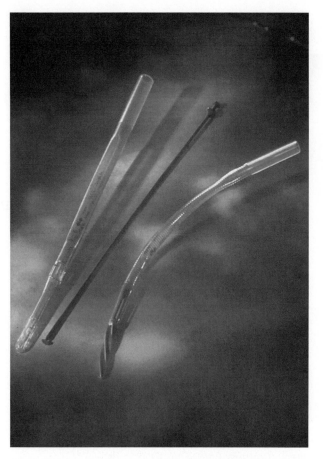

FIGURE 3-14 Venous cannulas. (Courtesy Medtronic, Inc.)

surfactant to defoam the blood and filters to remove the bubbles. Membrane oxygenators use a gas-permeable membrane through which oxygen diffuses into and carbon dioxide diffuses out of the desaturated blood. Advocates of the membrane method stress that because of the absence of a direct blood-gas interface, there is a reduced risk of air emboli, as well as less trauma to the cellular components of the blood, resulting in improved renal function and less use of bank blood. Membrane technology also facilitates control of oxygen (PaO_2 and carbon dioxide ($PaCO_2$) levels in the blood during hypothermia. These are among the major reasons why membrane oxygenators are more commonly used.

A heat exchanger is routinely incorporated into the oxygenator. This is used to alternatively cool and rewarm the blood within the bypass circuit. Hoses connected at one end to a water supply built into the operating room are attached to the heat exchanger at the other end. The temperature is controlled by the regulation of warm or cold water circulating around the tubing encasing the blood.

In most extracorporeal circuits the roller pump is used to propel oxygenated blood through polyvinyl chloride (PVC) tubing. Blood inside the tubing is displaced by the compression of the rotating pump head. Although some damage occurs to the blood, relatively atraumatic blood flow can be achieved with careful calibration and judicious use. Cellular trauma is also attributed to prolonged pump runs and overuse or misuse of suctioning devices.

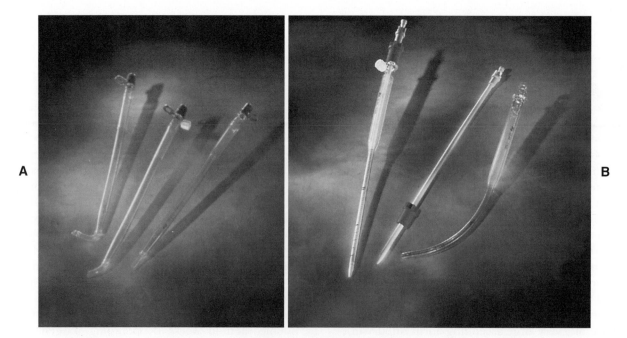

FIGURE 3-15 Arterial cannulas. **A,** Standard aortic cannulas. **B,** Elongated arterial cannulas that can be inserted transfemorally. (Courtesy Medtronic, Inc.)

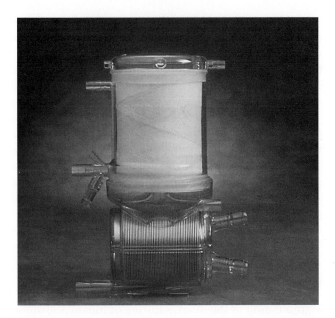

FIGURE 3-16 Membrane oxygenator. (Courtesy Medtronic, Inc.)

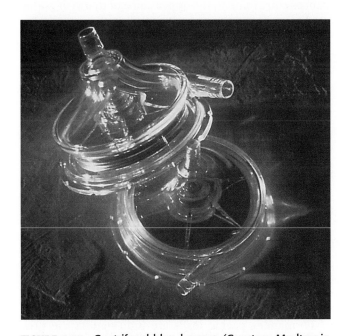

FIGURE 3-17 Centrifugal blood pump (Courtesy Medtronic, Inc.)

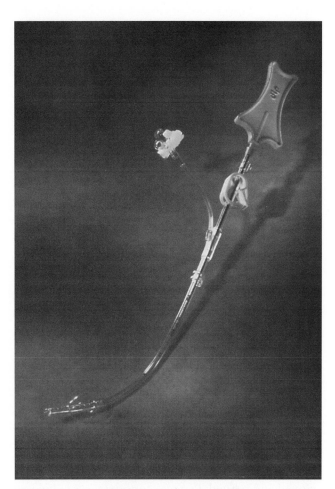

FIGURE 3-18 Retrograde cardioplegia infusion catheter. The distal tip is inserted through an incision in the right atrial wall and into the orifice of the coronary sinus. The balloon at the distal tip autoinflates to occlude the sinus. (Courtesy Medtronic, Inc.)

In many cases a centrifugal pump (Fig. 3-17), rather than a roller head, is used for maintaining blood flow. Centrifugal pumps use kinetic energy that transfers high volumes of flow at low pressure. Rotating cones within the pump create centrifugal force, which provides the energy to drive the blood. Safety features such as the prevention of excessive pressures in the arterial line have resulted in widespread use of this pumping device (Kirklin and Barratt-Boyes, 1993).

Although blood normally flows in pulsatile waves with systolic and diastolic phases (seen on the arterial waveform), blood flow with roller heads or centrifugal pumps is usually nonpulsatile (no phasic waveform is seen). This is manifested by a "mean" arterial waveform on the oscilloscope during total cardiopulmonary bypass. Pulsatile flow can be produced in some models.

Additional components of the bypass system include blood filters and bubble traps, which are incorporated into the circuit to trap gaseous and particulate matter that could produce emboli. Cardioplegia infusion devices are added to the system as well. Catheters are available for antegrade (aortic root infusion) and retrograde (coronary sinus infusion) cardioplegia delivery (Fig. 3-18). Monitoring devices are used to measure blood gases, pH, temperature, and intravascular pressures. Suction lines return shed blood to the cardiotomy filter and then to the oxygenator for reinfusion. Other suction lines can be used to vent air and blood from the heart. These lines serve both to decompress the ventricle and to reduce the possibility of air emboli escaping into the aorta and traveling to the brain.

Percutaneous systems for femoral vein–femoral artery bypass (see Fig. 3-13) may be employed for minimally invasive procedures and for emergencies in which the environment is not conducive to traditional CPB techniques. The system uses a thin-walled, wire-reinforced catheter inserted into the femoral artery and another similar (but longer) catheter placed in the femoral vein. The venous catheter uses assisted (e.g., vacuum) drainage to siphon venous blood into a portable bypass circuit. (Assisted drainage is required because the longer, smaller-bore venous cannula does not allow adequate venous return through simple passive drainage, unlike a shorter and larger bore [e.g., 36 French, two-stage] cannulas used in the right atrium.) These systems also can employ multilumen arterial and venous catheters to infuse solutions and measure pressures, and the arterial catheter can be used as an endovascular clamp with inflation of the balloon contained in its distal tip.

Another form of percutaneous CPB used for minimally invasive procedures employs cannulas that are first inserted through stab wounds in the chest and then placed into the right atrium for venous drainage and into the aorta for arterial inflow. Other techniques for inserting devices for CPB without taking up additional space in confined areas are constantly being developed and refined. Percutaneous systems can be used in the cardiac catheterization laboratory, the intensive care unit, the emergency department, and any other area where a patient may benefit from temporary, emergency extracorporeal circulation.

CIRCULATORY ASSIST DEVICES

The extracorporeal heart-lung machine is the prototype of assisted circulation. It takes over the functions of oxygenating and pumping blood, and by diverting venous return to the pump, it also decompresses the heart. This decreases the work normally performed by the volume- and pressure-loaded ventricles.

In cases where prolonged support of the myocardium is indicated, however, the pump oxygenator is not an optimum choice because of the trauma to the blood and the need for systemic heparinization (even with heparin-coated cannulas). Thus in the presence of low cardiac output caused by myocardial dysfunction, a number of other assist devices are used to reduce the workload of the heart and to improve organ perfusion. These range from systems that offer temporary relief to the myocardium to devices that support a heart that has suffered irreversible damage and is awaiting transplantation.

The intraaortic balloon pump (IABP) is a device used to support patients with postoperative left ventricular failure who have not responded to fluid or pharmacologic therapy. It works on the principle of volume displacement to propel blood into the systemic and coronary circulations (see Chapter 15).

Ventricular assist devices (VADs) may be used when the IABP fails to produce improvement. VADs are extravascular, volume-capturing devices that augment the existing circulation. The devices may use a centrifugal pump, a pneumatic pump, battery-powered pump, or an electric pump to propel the blood. The centrifugal pump maintains unidirectional blood flow; the other devices require prosthetic valves to achieve one-way flow (see Chapter 15).

PACEMAKERS

Manipulation of the heart, suturing of the myocardium, hypothermia, electrolyte imbalances, trauma to conduction tissue, and underlying conduction disturbances contribute to the appearance of dysrhythmias in cardiac surgery patients. Bradydysrhythmias are frequent in patients undergoing myocardial revascularization. Atrial dysrhythmias are often seen in patients with valvular heart disease, and temporary or permanent heart block can occur during surgery involving the atrial or ventricular septum.

Temporary pacing leads are inserted routinely to optimize cardiac output by preventing bradydysrhythmias or maintaining normal sinus rhythm (see Chapter 17). Epicardial leads are attached to the atrium when atrioventricular (AV) conduction is unimpaired. Ventricular leads are used in the presence of heart block when atrial beats are not conducted to the ventricle consistently. When AV conduction is delayed, both atrial and ventricular leads may be attached. The distal ends of the leads are inserted into a temporary pacemaker generator, and the patient is paced at a rate of 90 to 100 beats per minute to optimize cardiac output.

Permanent pacing leads are indicated in the presence of impulse formation or conduction disorders leading to complete heart block, bradydysrhythmias, and tachydysrhythmias. Various screw-in or stab leads are available (but infrequently used) for epicardial attachment to the atrium, ventricle, or both. Pulse generators are attached to the leads, programmed, and tested before being inserted into a subcutaneous pocket. Newer pacemakers offer antitachydysrhythmia functions and rate-responsive modes to change the heart rate as needed to meet demands for increased cardiac output (see Chapter 17). Most pacemakers are inserted transvenously.

IMPLANTABLE CARDIOVERTER DEFIBRILLATORS

Unlike pacemaker electrodes, which sense asystole or slow heart rates, the internal cardioverter defibrillator senses malignant ventricular dysrhythmias such as ventricular fibrillation and ventricular tachycardia. When these conditions are not amenable to pharmacologic or surgically ablative therapy, the internal defibrillator is implanted transvenously for the purpose of defibrillating the patient. These devices have pacing capabilities (see Chapter 17).

ADDITIONAL EQUIPMENT

Lasers (often used in other specialty areas) are also found in the cardiac OR. These may be used for transmyocardial revascularization (TMR), a procedure whereby a series of small laser-generated tunnels are made in the myocardium in order to stimulate neovascular growth. Laser safety guidelines and policies should be strictly enforced.

Monitoring devices are found in all cardiac ORs to provide a continuous flow of information about the patient's hemodynamic status. Doppler devices may be available to assess blood flow where palpation is difficult or does not provide sufficient information about blood flow. Video monitors are used for endoscopic procedures.

Additional equipment found in the cardiac suite includes "blood refrigerators" for storing packed red blood cells or whole blood. These refrigerators are specially designed to maintain the blood at the proper temperature and to trigger an alarm if the temperature becomes too warm or too cold. Blood refrigerators must have a system to identify which blood belongs to the patient; blood for one patient should be separated from that for another patient.

Also commonly available are standard refrigerators for solutions and medications requiring cold storage, as well as ice machines to provide ice for chilling cardioplegia solutions and blood gas samples.

Blanket warmers keep blankets at a comfortable temperature and can be used to warm saline or water. Occasionally these warmers are used to store medications that would crystallize at room temperature. Devices are also available to warm and maintain the desired temperature of saline for irrigation; these devices can be incorporated into some cooling units.

Blood test results may be transmitted to the OR from the laboratory via computer or over a fax machine if there is no facility adjacent to the operating room for analyzing blood samples. Computer terminals may be located in the room where patient lab results, charges, documentation of care, and other information may be put into or received from the system. One or two (or more) telephone lines are a valuable resource for contacting personnel, giving reports, and receiving information about the patient; extra-long extension cords enable the circulating nurse to remain close to the operating field.

A machine for reviewing coronary cineangiograms before surgery also may be available within the suite; digitalized transmission is increasingly available.

Instruments

ROBOTS

Automation, miniaturization, computerization, and increasingly complex procedures in combination with endoscopic, minimally invasive approaches have prompted the development of new techniques and new technology (Table 3-2). For example, the precise, steady retraction required during endoscopic procedures can be achieved with robotic assistance (Fig. 3-19). Video cameras held by robots are more effectively manipulated and controlled than those held by their human counterparts (Kavoussi and others, 1995; Eckberg, 1998). Robots can be voice controlled, provide microdexterity without tremor, and be manipulated remotely (Mack, 2001; Popolow, 1999). Voice-activated robots for CABG are in use in a number of centers (Damiano, Reichenspurner, and Ducko, 2000). Port-access (e.g., "keyhole"), thoracotomy, or sternal incisions can be employed with the robot holding retractors and a camera (two-dimensional or three-dimensional) for video-assisted exposure.

Specially designed instrument tips attached to robotic arms are manipulated from a computerized surgeon interface device that digitizes the surgeon's motions and relays the information in real time to the computer-driven robotic arms. Robotic instrumentation, unlike conventional instrumentation, offers two to six (or more) *degrees of freedom* that mimics the "wrist" joint to produce a more natural, handlike movement. Thus motions made by the operator can be reproduced precisely at the tip of the instrument. The motions can be *scaled* down by the computer, thereby enabling the surgeon to operate on extremely small structures. Robotic systems also provide *haptic* feedback (e.g., the sense of touch) (Damiano, Reichenspurner, and Ducko, 2000).

Instruments used in cardiac surgery are designed for specific purposes and selected according to the weight of the patient, anatomic requirements, and surgeon preference. They must be capable of securely grasping and holding blood vessels, cardiac structures, and other tissue without injury. In addition, they must be available in an array of sizes and shapes to meet the needs of a range of patients, from a 2-kg neonate to a 90-kg adult.

TABLE 3-2
Technology Development and Forecast: Robotics and Computer Assistance in Surgery

TASK	FUNCTION	FORECAST
Surgical assistant	Voice-activated endoscopic holder positioner	Becoming routine

Dexterity enhancement
   Motion scaling
   Tremor filtration
   Force feedback
	Facilitate precision endoscopic procedures	Of 1000 procedures now performed, 50% are cardiac and 50% are laparoscopic

Operating room systems networking	Surgeon control of or via voice activation, touch screen	Rapid integration of operating room systems in near future
Telepresence surgery Remote surgery	Surgeon at remote site from patient using broadband transmission or internet	No clear path to clinical application
Telementoring	Proctoring from a remote site	Demonstrated to have potential for new educational paradigm

Information enhancement
   3-dimensional modeling and reconstruction
   Image referencing guidance
	Real-time data acquisition and nonvisual imaging	3-dimensional reconstruction of computed tomography, magnetic resonance imaging, and ultrasonography with surgical overlays to facilitate percutaneous therapy

Virtual stillness (motion stabilization)	"Gate" time visualization and surgical instruments to heart motion to create illusion of stillness	Facilitate endoscopic "beating heart" surgery
Virtual simulators	Flight simulators for surgery	About to become realistic and affordable
Information enhancement sensory feedback	Action in response to nonvisual feedback	Potential for integrated "smart" local delivery of drug/energy based on tissue-level feedback
Microelectronic mechanical systems	Miniature autonomous robots	Remote diagnosis and delivery via body lumina

From Mack M: Minimally invasive and robotic surgery, *JAMA* 285(5):568-572, 2001.

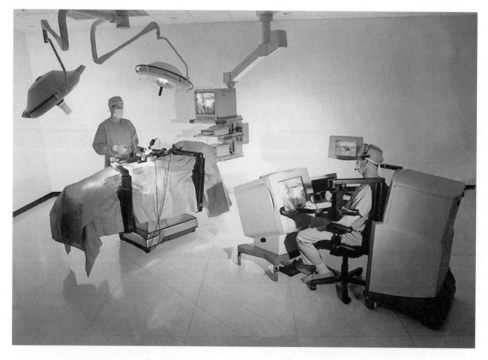

FIGURE 3-19 Robot. (Courtesy Computer Motion, Santa Barbara, Calif.)

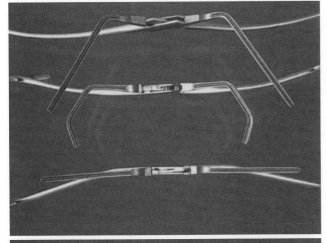

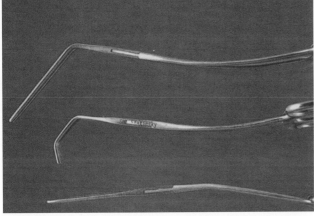

FIGURE 3-20 Vascular clamps for occluding blood vessels. **A,** *Top to bottom:* DeBakey multipurpose vascular clamp tip (total occluding); Beck aorta clamp tip (partial occluding); Glover patent ductus clamp tip (total occluding). **B,** *Top to bottom:* DeBakey multipurpose vascular clamp, 60-degree obtuse angle; Beck aorta clamp; Glover patent ductus clamp, straight. (From Brooks-Tighe SM: *Instrumentation for the operating room: a photographic manual,* ed 3, St Louis, 1989, Mosby.)

Sturdy instruments are required for procedures such as reapproximating sternal bone, and fine instruments must be available for sewing arteries that may be 2 mm or less in diameter and often are the consistency of cooked spaghetti. Of particular interest are the vascular clamps (Fig. 3-20). Their atraumatic jaw serrations are specially designed for occluding or partially occluding blood vessels without damaging their walls. The master instrument maker William Merz collaborated with me and with many other perioperative nurses and surgeons to craft instruments for cardiac surgery that were functional, atraumatic, and aesthetically pleasing. Although many new instruments have been manufactured for minimally invasive procedures, Merz' comments published in 1994

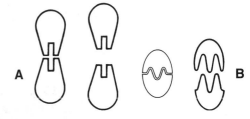

FIGURE 3-21 Types of jaws in vascular clamps. **A,** Cooley jaws have two opposing rows of serrated teeth, closed and open. **B,** DeBakey jaws have a single row of serrated teeth opposing a double row of teeth, closed and open. (Courtesy Pilling-Weck Co, Fort Washington, Pa.)

(Seifert, 1994) remain as pertinent today as when they were first written (Box 3-5). Figure 3-21 illustrates two common jaw patterns used for forceps and occluding clamps. Clamps are constructed with multiple rachets that allow the surgeon to adjust the clamp according to the blood pressure inside the blood vessel. Rachets also enable the surgeon to release the clamp gradually, thereby avoiding a sudden increase or decrease in vascular volume.

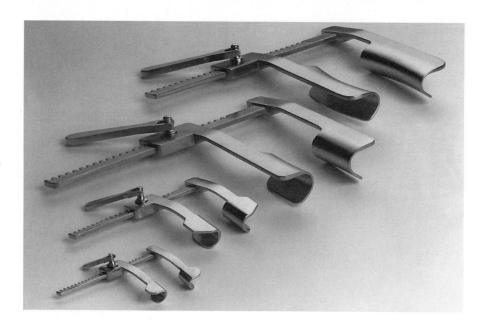

FIGURE 3-22 Cooley sternal retractors in various sizes. (Courtesy Pilling-Weck, Fort Washington, Pa.)

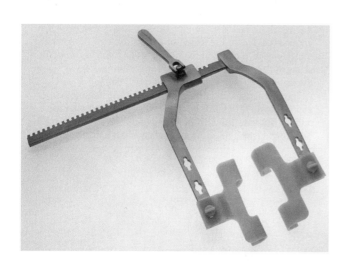

FIGURE 3-23 Collins sternal retractor with disposable, radiopaque blades. (Courtesy Codman & Shurtleff, Inc, a Johnson & Johnson company, Randolph, Mass.)

FIGURE 3-24 Himmelstein sternal retractor *(left)* and Ankeney sternal retractor *(right)*. (From Brooks-Tighe SM: *Instrumentation for the operating room: a photographic manual*, ed 5, St Louis, 1999, Mosby.)

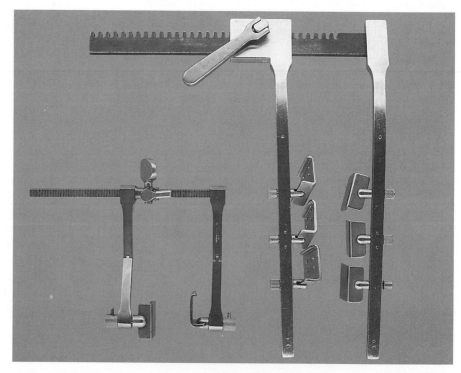

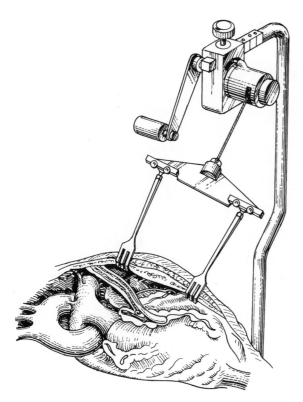

FIGURE 3-25 Retractor used to elevate the sternal border for exposure of the internal mammary artery. (Courtesy Rultract, Inc., Cleveland, Ohio.)

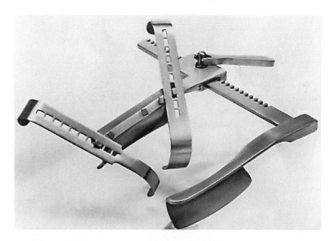

FIGURE 3-26 Sternal self-retaining retractor with attachments for left atrial retraction during mitral valve replacement. (Courtesy Pilling-Weck Co., Fort Washington, Pa.)

Standard self-retaining retractors for exposing the mediastinum are shown in Figures 3-22 through 3-24. Some are constructed to meet different needs (Figs. 3-25 through 3-27). Cardiac valves also can be exposed with handheld retractors.

A variety of scissors and needle holders should be available. Potts-type scissors (Fig. 3-28) are frequently used to incise blood vessels. Castroviejo needle holders (Fig. 3-29) are popular for delicate anastomoses. Instrument kits for pediatric procedures and internal mammary artery procedures (Fig. 3-30) can be added to complement basic sets.

Vascular instruments can be made of tungsten carbide, stainless steel, or titanium. Titanium is stronger yet lighter than stainless steel, and these properties make it popular for some microsurgical instruments.

BEATING HEART SURGERY

Beating heart surgery for coronary artery bypass grafting has been greatly facilitated by the introduction of stabilizing devices that isolate the section of myocardium undergoing coronary anastomosis. Before the introduction of stabilizers, the technical difficulty of

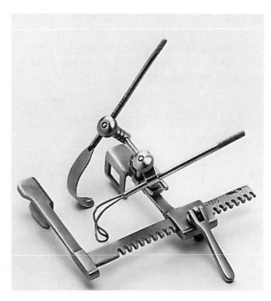

FIGURE 3-27 Pediatric cardiac self-retaining retractor with detachable blades. The retractor can be used for midline sternotomy or lateral thoracotomy. The blades are similar to those used for mitral valve exposure in adult-size retractors. (Courtesy Pilling-Weck, Fort Washington, Pa.)

sewing on a contracting heart (even when the force of contraction was reduced with blood pressure–lowering drugs) increased the risk of producing technically imperfect anastomoses or conversion to CPB and induced cardiac arrest.

Some stabilizers (Fig. 3-31) function by compressing a portion of the myocardium between the prongs of the instrument. Other devices use suction to bring

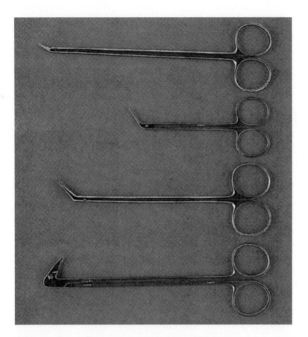

FIGURE 3-28 Dietrich and Potts-Smith scissors in an array of forward and backward cutting angles (frequently used to incise coronary arteries). (From Brooks-Tighe SM: *Instrumentation for the operating room: a photographic manual,* ed 3, St Louis, 1989, Mosby.)

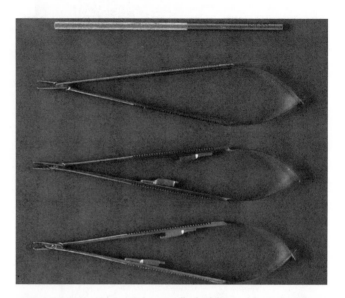

FIGURE 3-29 Castroviejo needle holders with and without locks are used for delicate anastomoses. Some surgeons prefer fine standard needle holders with ratchet locking mechanisms for performing anastomoses. (From Brooks-Tighe SM: *Instrumentation for the operating room: a photographic manual,* ed 3, St Louis, 1989, Mosby.)

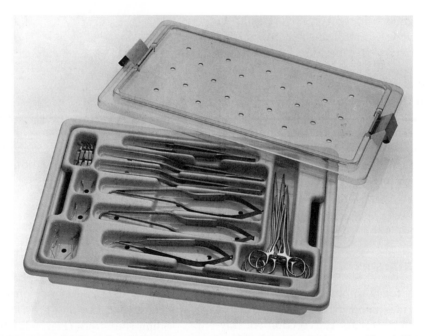

FIGURE 3-30 Codman internal mammary artery kit. Courtesy Codman & Shurtleff, Inc., a Johnson & Johnson company, Randolph, Mass.)

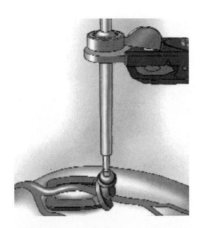

FIGURE 3-31 The AXIS 360-degree coronary stabilizer gently compresses tissue around the arteriotomy to immobilize the anastomotic site. This allows the surgeon to perform a more technically facile anastomosis. (Courtesy CARDIOVATIONS, a division of ETHICON, Inc.)

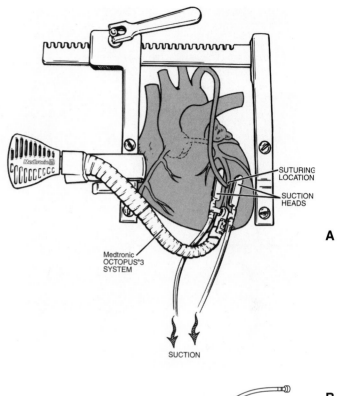

A

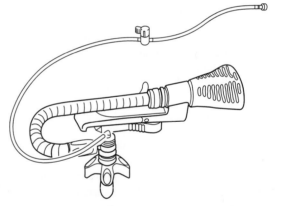

B

FIGURE 3-32 A, The Octopus 3 coronary stabilizer attaches to the sternal retractor proximally and immobilizes the coronary artery. The device uses suction pads to minimize tissue motion at the anastomotic site. **B,** The Starfish left ventricular suction device holds the left ventricular apex and allows it to be retracted for access to lateral and posterior coronary arteries. (Courtesy Medtronic, Inc.)

the tissue snugly up against the stabilizing device (Fig. 3-32, *A*). Stabilizers may be part of a system that includes a retractor and additional attachments such as a suction catheter, a light source, and the stabilizer itself. A blower-mister and a small shunt (Fig. 3-33) can keep the anastomotic site clear of blood. Silicone vessel loops with a blunt needle may be used to encircle and gently occlude the coronary artery during anastomosis (Fig. 3-34).

Elevating the left ventricular apex to access the posterior and lateral coronary arteries can be a challenge off pump, especially when torsion of the heart causes a reduction in venous return (e.g., preload), producing hypotension. Devices to elevate the heart can be positioned under the apex and gently inflated. These items may be "homemade" (e.g., a sterile glove partially filled with warm saline) or manufactured (e.g., an inflatable/deflectable balloon with an attached tube containing a one-way valve for infusion/removal of air or saline. Box 3-6 lists special considerations for beating heart surgery.

MINIMAL ACCESS SURGERY

Surgery may be performed through small incisions (i.e., *minimal access, minimally invasive surgery*) in the sternum or the lateral chest wall. These procedures may be performed off pump (e.g., "beating heart") or on pump with endovascular CPB systems (see Fig. 3-13) not requiring a sternotomy for cannulation.

Instrumentation for minimally invasive surgeries has been modified to reflect the smaller incisions often seen in these procedures. For example, clamps need a longer shaft (Fig. 3-35) with the box lock closer to the handles (or a double-action mechanism) to allow the handle (and lock box) to be positioned outside of the incision, so that it can be opened as widely as necessary. Endoscopic instrumentation is also available, although some basic laparoscopic dissecting instruments (e.g.,

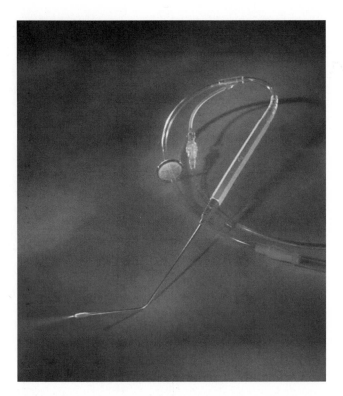

FIGURE 3-33 Blower-mister uses CO_2 to keep blood out of the coronary anastomotic site; mister keeps the heart moist and prevents drying of the endothelium. Small shunts may be inserted into the proximal and distal coronary arteriotomy to provide distal blood flow and create a clear anastomotic site. (Courtesy Medtronic, Inc.)

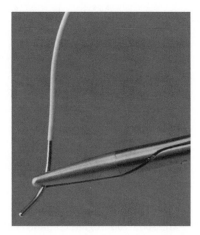

FIGURE 3-34 A Silastic vessel loop with a blunt needle is used as a tourniquet around the proximal and distal portion of the coronary artery during beating heart anastomoses; the loop can also be used for retraction. (Courtesy Scanlon International, St Paul, Minn.)

scissors, forceps, cautery devices) can be used for cardiac procedures.

Appropriate use, careful handling, and proper cleaning will prolong the life of instruments and minimize costly repairs and replacements. Most instrument damage is caused by misuse and abuse. Scissors constructed to incise coronary arteries should not be used to cut heavy suture; delicate needle holders and forceps should not be used to remove knife blades. Instruments should not be dropped, stacked, or forced into sterilizing pans; care should be taken to avoid placing heavy pans on top of delicate instruments.

Before surgery, check instrument jaws for burrs by running them over a sponge. Vascular clamps, especially the cross-clamp, which is likely to be used, should be checked for proper alignment and a secure grip. If they are damaged or not working properly, the instruments should be removed from the setup immediately and replacements obtained. During and after the procedure, keep instruments clean of blood and debris; this will help to prevent damage from hardening of the material in the jaws and box locks and re-

duce the possibility of introducing dried blood into blood vessels.

At the end of an operation the instruments should be thoroughly cleaned and decontaminated. A nonmetallic brush should be used to clean them. A soft-bristled toothbrush or scrub brush is good for cleaning micro-size instruments and those with serrated vascular jaws. Instruments should be inspected for cracked, chipped, broken, worn, or otherwise damaged parts. In particular, vascular forceps and clamps should be inspected for bent tips, burrs, or misaligned jaws that could damage vascular structures. Damaged instruments should be sent out for repair immediately. Instruments should be arranged so that the heavier ones are not placed on more delicate ones. Fine instruments can be placed in separate containers for their protection. Placing instruments in instrument milk will help to keep the jaws and box locks working properly. A regular schedule for sharpening scissors is recommended.

Basic sternotomy sets that are too heavy to place in one pan can be divided into two separate parts. One method is to arrange those instruments needed to open the chest and cannulate on a Mayo tray and to place the remaining instruments in a back pan. The advantage of such a system is apparent in an emergency when the Mayo tray can be opened to provide its own sterile field, with the instruments made available for rapid institution of cardiopulmonary bypass. The Mayo tray should contain knife handles, wire cutters, a chest retractor, dissecting instruments, tubing clamps, needle holders, and vascular clamps needed for putting a patient on

BOX 3-6
Beating Heart Surgery Considerations

Safety

Use disposable adhesive defibrillator pads on all patients
Have internal (pediatric and adult) defibrillator paddles opened

Maintenance of Normothermia

Warm fluids for topical irrigation and coronary misting
Provide warming blanket
Maintain warm ambient OR temperature

Coronary Stabilization

Avoid placing stabilizer over infarcted or aneurysmal tissue
Suction devices (e.g., Octopus) require separate suction at −400 mm Hg (regulator is required)
Compression devices should employ only enough pressure to stop bleeding from coronary artery

Surgical Site Exposure

Discard suction setup × 2
Have available:

Retractors for sternotomy, mini-sternotomy, or thoracotomy with attachments for illumination, suction, stabilization, apical retraction (to expose posterior surface of heart)
Left ventricular apical elevator
Coronary vessel occluder/tourniquet (silastic loop)
Blower device (usually CO_2) to keep anastomotic site clear of blood; CO_2 tank (have O_2 as backup)
Mister device (usually saline, warmed) to keep anastomotic site clear of blood and heart moist (CO_2 can cause drying of epithelium)
Coronary shunts for distal perfusion
Coronary occluders
Suction retractor to elevate apex of heart
Video monitors and endoscopic setup may be requested

Conversion to Cardiopulmonary Bypass

Have ready supplies and instruments (including sternal saw if chest not yet opened)
Have CPB supplies and equipment (and perfusionist) immediately available

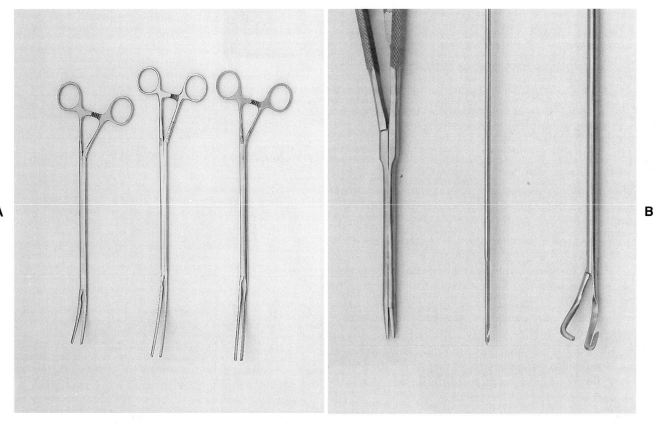

A

B

FIGURE 3-35 A, Transthoracic DeBakey vascular clamps are designed to pass through the chest wall via smaller incisions for minimally invasive procedures. **B,** Closeup view of minimally invasive needle holder, trocar/suture puller, and knot slider. (From Meeker MH, Rothrock JC: *Alexander's care of the patient in surgery,* ed 11, 1999, St Louis, Mosby; courtesy Scanlon International, St Paul, Minn.)

bypass. Additional instruments should be placed in the second pan.

Special sets can be developed for valve surgery, coronary bypass, and thoracic aneurysms. The list in Box 3-7 outlines a variety of instruments (including those used for minimally invasive procedures) that can be selected to create these sets. Included are cutting, retracting, holding, clamping, suturing, and miscellaneous instruments. Because personal preference and training are so critical in the selection of needle holders, forceps, clamps, and other items, nurses should first confer with the surgeon (or the surgeon's former perioperative nursing colleagues) to determine which instruments to purchase. This will help to avoid the unnecessary expense of buying instruments that will not be used.

The sterility of the instruments should be maintained until the patient has left the operating room; then they can be used to reopen the sternum if chest tube drainage is excessive, to insert an additional chest tube, or to secure an intravascular line.

Suture

Various types and sizes of cardiovascular sutures and needles are used on the heart, surrounding tissue, and blood vessels. Box 3-8 lists sutures commonly used for a number of procedures.

In performing vascular anastomoses, surgeons are concerned with creating a patent and leakproof vessel lumen. The development of inert synthetic suture materials such as nylon, polyester, and polypropylene has reduced the incidence of tissue reaction and thrombus formation, which in the past were frequently the cause of failed anastomoses.

Sutures may be constructed as a multifilament or a monofilament. Multifilament polyester sutures allow clotting to occur within the interstices and thereby reduce leaking from the suture line. This factor, as well as the tensile strength of the material, makes these sutures popular for the fixation of vascular grafts and heart valves. They also are used frequently for pursestring stitches used with tourniquets to anchor bypass cannulas or venting catheters. Monofilament sutures may be more desirable than multifilament sutures in the presence of sepsis or trauma because there are no interstices in the suture to harbor bacteria.

The use of swaged needles with tapered tips also has minimized vessel trauma. Cardiovascular suture often is made with needles at each end of the filament. Double-ended stitches allow the surgeon to perform half an anastomosis with one end of the

stitch and then use the other end to complete the anastomosis (Fig. 3-36).

Vessel anastomoses are commonly performed using a continuous suturing technique with polypropylene, a monofilament material. Tension around the circumference of the suture line is distributed evenly with this method and helps to avoid constricting the lumen. When tying polypropylene, surgeons will find the process easier if their hands are first moistened with saline.

When sewing on friable tissue or tissue that does not hold sutures well (such as the myocardium), felt pledgets can be used to buttress the sutures and avoid tearing or cutting of tissue (Fig. 3-37). Pledgets are available precut, or they can be made by cutting a larger piece of felt material. Strips of felt are used to buttress the myocardium for resection of left ventricular aneurysms; these can be prepared at the field by cutting a patch of felt into strips.

Suture is available in single packs or multipacks. Multipacks of polypropylene suture are helpful during coronary artery bypass procedures in which several anastomoses are anticipated. Alternately colored polyester suture within multipacks (green/white or blue/white) are helpful for avoiding confusion in procedures such as valve replacements, which require numerous interrupted stitches to be placed and tied.

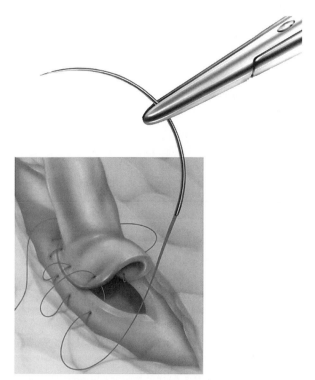

FIGURE 3-36 End-to-side vascular anastomosis with double-ended (also called *double-armed*) suture. (Courtesy USSDG, Division of Tyco Healthcare, Norwalk, Conn.)

BOX **3-7**
Cardiac Instrumentation (Partial Listing)

Basic Sternotomy Instruments
CUTTING INSTRUMENTS

No. 3 Bard-Parker knife handles: No. 10 blade
No. 4 Bard-Parker knife handles: No. 20 blade
No. 7 Bard-Parker knife handles: No. 15 blade, No. 15c blade,
   No. 11 blade
Beaver handles and blades
Sternal wire cutter
Temporary epicardial pacing wire cutter
Lebsche knife and mallet
Cooley "My" scissors: $7\frac{1}{4}$-inch
Bladder scissors
Metzenbaum scissors: 7-inch (and longer)
Straight Mayo scissors: $6\frac{3}{4}$-inch
Curved Mayo scissors: $6\frac{3}{4}$-inch
Potts forward-cutting scissors
Potts backward-cutting scissors
Tenotomy scissors: 7-inch
Bandage/tube–cutting scissors

RETRACTORS

Cooley sternotomy retractor
Ankeney retractor
Himmelstein retractor
Codman retractor
Weitlaner retractors
Gelpi retractors
Richardson retractors, assorted sizes
Army-Navy retractors
Rake retractors
Semb retractors
Vein retractors
Ribbon retractors

HOLDING INSTRUMENTS

Regular towel clips: blunt and sharp
Baby towel clips
Kocher clamps with teeth: $7\frac{1}{4}$-inch
Cooley vascular forceps: $7\frac{3}{4}$-inch, $9\frac{1}{2}$-inch
DeBakey vascular forceps: $7\frac{3}{4}$-inch, $9\frac{1}{2}$-inch
Russian forceps: 10-inch
Adson forceps with teeth
English Bonney forceps
Cooley "gold" forceps: $7\frac{3}{4}$-inch
Dressing forceps: $9\frac{1}{2}$-inch
Geralt forceps: 7-inch, $9\frac{1}{4}$-inch
Sponge stick forceps
Allis clamps

CLAMPING INSTRUMENTS

Hemostats, straight and curved
Criles, curved
Mosquito clamps, straight and curved
Right-angle clamps, assorted lengths
Mixter clamps
Tonsil clamps
Kelly (Pean) clamps, assorted lengths
Tube-occluding clamps

VASCULAR CLAMPS

Total-occluding clamps
   Fogarty cross-clamp, straight and angled
   Femoral artery clamps
   Cooley aortic aneurysm clamp
   Crafoord coarctation clamp
   Iliac clamp
   Bulldog clamps
   Patent ductus clamps
   DeBakey multipurpose clamps
Partial-occluding clamps
   Glover clamp
   Derra clamps
   Kay aorta clamp
   Kay-Lambert clamps
   Weck-Beck clamps
   Statinsky clamps
   Beck aorta clamps
   Cooley aorta clamps
   Cooley curved and angled clamps
   Auricular appendage clamp
   DeBakey tangential occlusion clamps

SUTURING INSTRUMENTS

Sarot needle holders
Mayo-Hegar needle holders
Wire needle holders
Vascular needle holders, assorted sizes
Castroviejo needle holders

ACCESSORY ITEMS

Cooley vena caval occlusion clamps
Suction tips, assorted sizes
Rumel tourniquet stylets
Ligating clips and appliers
Nerve hook
Freer elevator
Bypass tubing holder
Banding gun (to tighten cannulas to tubing connectors)
Fogarty clamp inserts
Instrument stringers
Rubbershods

Coronary Artery Bypass Instrument Extras
CUTTING INSTRUMENTS

Castroviejo micro scissors, forward- and backward-cutting
Dietrich scissors
Potts micro scissors, forward- and backward-cutting
Aortic punch

RETRACTORS

Favalaro internal mammary artery retractor
Rultract internal mammary artery retractor
Parsonnett epicardial retractor
Balfour retractor (for exposure of gastroepiploic artery)
Lighted retractor for endoscopic vein harvest

HOLDING INSTRUMENTS

Delicate vascular forceps

Continued

BOX **3-7**
Cardiac Instrumentation (Partial Listing)—cont'd

VASCULAR CLAMPS

Micro bulldog clamps

SUTURING INSTRUMENTS

Castroviejo micro needle holders
Ryder needle holders
Microvascular needle holders

ACCESSORY ITEMS

Fine suction tips
Coronary dilators: 0.5 to 5.0 mm
Small clip appliers and clips
Radiopaque graft markers
Endarterectomy spatulas
Blunt internal mammary artery infusion needle
Vein irrigation cannulas

BEATING HEART CORONARY EXTRAS

Stabilizer
Suction regulator to achieve −400 mm Hg
CO_2 blower/mister/suction devices
Retractors with coronary retraction accessories
Left ventricular apical retractors/positioners

Valve Instrument Extras
CUTTING INSTRUMENTS

Curved mitral scissors
Long Bard-Parker No. 3 knife handles: No. 10 blade, No. 15 blade

RETRACTORS

Handheld right and left atrial retractors
Handheld aortic root retractors
Self-retaining sternal retractors with atrial retraction accessories (for traditional or minimally invasive surgery)

HOLDING INSTRUMENTS

Curved Allis clamp
Long smooth forceps

CLAMPING INSTRUMENTS

Baby tubing clamps
Carmalt clamps with rubbershods
Long right-angle clamp

SUTURING INSTRUMENTS

Long needle holders
Suture holder

ACCESSORY ITEMS

French-eye needles
No. 3 dental mirror
Culture tubes
Mitral hook
Sizing obturators and handles
Prosthesis handles
Handheld coronary perfusion tips
Tubbs dilator
Hegar dilators, assorted sizes

Pituitary rongeurs: up, down, straight
Debridement suction tip

Thoracotomy Instrument Extras
CUTTING INSTRUMENTS

Rib cutters
Nelson scissors, curved: 10-inch
Periosteal elevators

RETRACTORS

Finochietto rib spreader
Burford retractor
T malleable lung retractors
Scapular retractor
Bailey rib approximators

HOLDING INSTRUMENTS

Duval lung clamps
Rumel thoracic clamps

CLAMPING INSTRUMENTS

Bronchus clamps
Right-angle clamps

VASCULAR CLAMPS

Crafoord coarctation clamps
Patent ductus clamps, angled and straight

SUTURING INSTRUMENTS

Long hemaclip appliers, assorted sizes
Bronchus, vascular staplers
Long needle holders
Port-access endoscopic instruments
  Camera
  Clamps
  Needle holders
  Suction
  Cautery

Pediatric Instrumentation

Most of the instrumentation listed above is also used for pediatric procedures. The size of the child and the patient's position determine which instruments are most appropriate. The working end of the instrument may be finer, but often it is of standard length to allow the surgeon's and assistants' hands to remain outside the relatively confined surgical field. The following also may be used:

RETRACTORS

Finochietto rib retractor, infant/child sizes
Cooley sternal retractor, infant/child sizes
"T" malleable lung retractors, assorted sizes
Silicone-coated brain retractors

VASCULAR CLAMPS

Downsized and proportionally balanced for smaller vessels
Cooley pediatric clamps
Castaneda pediatric clamps

BOX 3-8
Sutures for Selected Procedures*

Pericardial retraction: 2-0 braided polyester, nylon, or silk
Cannulation for cardiopulmonary bypass:
 Aortic pursestring: 2-0 braided polyester (with or without pledget)
 Right atrial pursestring: 2-0 braided polyester or nylon
Cardioplegia infusion
 Aortic vent/antegrade cardioplegia infusion pursestring: 4-0 polypropylene (with or without pledget)
 Right atrial retrograde cardioplegia infusion pursestring: 3-0 polyester
Temporary epicardial pacemaker leads: lead wire attached with 5-0 silk
Chest tubes: 0, 2-0 silk
Sternum: 5 chest wire; polyester (children)
Linea alba: 0, 2-0 polyester
Fascia, subcutaneous tissue: 2-0 absorbable suture
Skin: 3-0, 4-0 absorbable suture or polypropylene, nylon; skin staples (legs)
Coronary anastomoses
 Distal anastomosis:
  Saphenous vein: 6-0, 7-0 polypropylene

 Internal mammary artery: 7-0, 8-0 polypropylene
Proximal anastomosis
  Saphenous vein to aorta: 5-0, 6-0 polypropylene
Valve replacement or repair
 Aortic: 2-0 polyester, alternately colored (blue or green and white)
  Closure of aorta: 4-0 polypropylene
 Mitral: 2-0 polyester, alternately colored
  Closure of left atrium: 3-0 polypropylene
 Tricuspid: 3-0 polyester or polypropylene
  Closure of right atrium: 4-0 polypropylene
Closure of left ventricular aneurysm: 0, 2-0 polyester (with felt strips)
Closure of atrial septal defect: Patch/primary repair: 4-0 polypropylene
Coarctation of aorta (child): Primary repair: 5-0, 6-0 absorbable suture
Thoracic aortic aneurysms
 Ascending aorta: 2-0, 3-0 polyester, polypropylene
 Descending aorta: 3-0, 4-0 polyester, polypropylene

*The sutures listed vary depending on the patient's size and surgeon's preference.

Made-to-order suture packs (Fig. 3-38) contain a variety of sutures arranged in a predetermined order to meet the requirements of a particular surgeon or a specific procedure. Packs may be developed for opening and cannulation procedures, coronary artery bypass grafting, and valve procedures. Because 80 or more needles may be used, much time can be saved by opening one or two packs versus numerous individual packs. Inventory space is reduced, and there is less waste. If cost savings are to be realized, however, the packs should contain only those sutures that will be used routinely. When additional sutures are needed, individual packs should be provided to the scrub nurse. If premade suture packs are not available, it is helpful to have the individual sutures already collected and placed in a bag so that if an emergency arises, the sutures need not first be retrieved from the storage area.

Suturing during endoscopic procedures has been performed extensively in laparoscopic surgery (Ball, 1999) and can be expected to be applied increasingly to cardiac surgery. Automated devices that perform interrupted suture anastomoses have been laboratory tested, and clinical studies are in progress in some centers (Shennib and others, 2000; Solem and others, 2000). These devices can be expected to facilitate minimally invasive, endoscopic cardiac procedures.

Supplies

Numerous supplies are used during cardiac surgery, and among the most common are those listed in Box 3-9. Specific items depend on surgeon preference, as well as on purchasing agreements that many hospitals have with distributors and vendors.

Because of the large number of items that must be opened for surgery, many cardiac services work with vendors to develop custom trays or case carts. These may include items used for basic sternotomy procedures (such as rubbershods [Fig. 3-39]) or specialty trays for valve or coronary artery bypass surgery (such as coronary graft markers [Fig. 3-40], bulldog clamps [Fig. 3-41], or aortic punches [Fig. 3-42]). The user determines what items to include. Like the suture packs discussed earlier, custom products are cost-effective when they include only those items that will be used on all procedures for which the pack is intended. Standardization of pack contents is an important cost-saving strategy (Kirshner, 2000).

Prosthetic Implants

In addition to the items listed in Box 3-9, numerous materials are used to replace or repair cardiovascular structures. These prosthetic materials may be synthetic

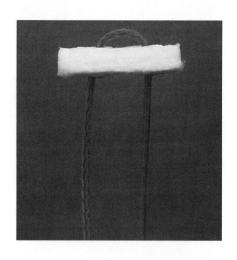

FIGURE 3-37 Pledgeted suture. The suture loop should be placed in the central part of the pledget. (Courtesy Ethicon, Inc., a Johnson & Johnson company, Somerville, NJ.)

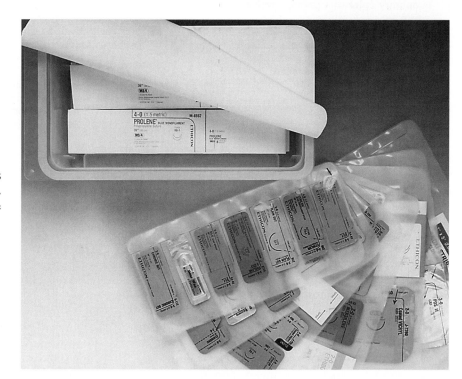

FIGURE 3-38 Customized suture packs save turnover time and setup time. (Courtesy Ethicon, Inc., a Johnson & Johnson company, Somerville, NJ.)

BOX 3-9
Supplies Commonly Used in a Cardiac Service

Adaptors, connectors, stopcocks
Aortic punches
Autotransfusion supplies
Bulb syringes
Cannulas and catheters for cardiopulmonary bypass
Chest tubes, chest drainage system
Coronary graft markers
Coronary occluders (Silastic loop or clips)
Cotton gloves (for retracting the heart)
Disposable drapes, gowns, gloves
Disposable towels
Disposable vascular (bulldog) clamps
Dressing supplies
Electrosurgical pencils: foot-control and hand-control
Graduated pitchers, cups, emesis basins, rinsing bowls
Guidewires
Hypodermic and venting needles

Knife blades
Marking pens
Needle counters
Polyvinylchloride or Silastic tubing in various sizes
Pressure tubing
Rubbershods
Solutions, medications
Shunts (coronary)
Sponges (lap tapes, peanuts, radiopaque 4 × 4s)
Suction tips, tubing
Syringes and needles for injections, infusions, and blood samples
Tourniquet catheters
Trash bags
Ultrasonic scalpel
Urinary drainage system (catheters, urine meters, lubricant)
Vascular clamp inserts

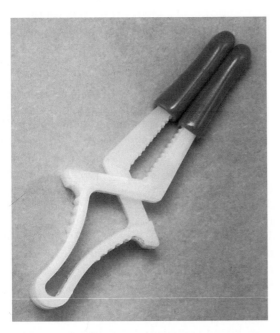

FIGURE 3-39 Rubbershods applied to the tips of a bulldog clamp. (Courtesy Scanlon International, St Paul, Minn.)

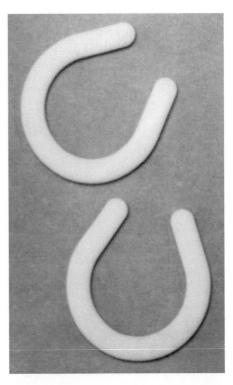

FIGURE 3-40 Radiopaque coronary graft markers enable the clinician to identify the site of proximal anastomoses postoperatively. (Courtesy Scanlon International, St Paul, Minn.)

or biologic (Table 3-3) and include intracardiac patches, tube grafts, and heart valves. They should be stored in a clean, dry, protected environment. Care in handling helps to prevent damage or contamination of the implant.

SYNTHETIC GRAFTS

Synthetic prostheses are available in a variety of meshes, fabrics, felts, tapes, and sutures (Fig. 3-43). Many synthetic materials can be resterilized by steam autoclaving or by using ethylene oxide with adequate aeration unless otherwise advised by the manufacturer (follow manufacturer's instructions). However, numerous resterilization cycles (e.g., more than three or four times) can jeopardize the integrity of the fibers, so a record should be kept of the number of times a graft has been resterilized. Unused grafts that have been in contact with blood or tissue should be discarded.

Synthetic tube and patch grafts made of Dacron are either woven or knitted; tube grafts may be straight or bifurcated (Fig. 3-44). (Knitted materials can be compared to the construction of a sweater, whereas woven grafts are more comparable to the tighter weave of a shirt.) The decision to use a woven or a knitted graft is based primarily on whether heparin has been adminis-

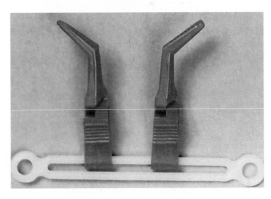

FIGURE 3-41 Disposable bulldog clamps. These come in a variety of sizes, colors, and angles. (Courtesy Scanlon International, St Paul, Minn.)

tered to the patient (such as required for cardiopulmonary bypass) and the speed of tissue ingrowth.

Woven grafts are less porous than knitted grafts because their fibers are closer together. They are indicated when the patient is being given heparin because there is less bleeding through the interstices of the fabric. Many fabrics are treated with collagen impregnation by the manufacturer to minimize interstitial bleeding.

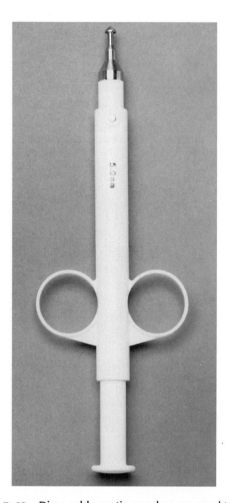

FIGURE 3-42 Disposable aortic punches are used to create the aortotomy for proximal coronary anastomoses. A smaller punch can be used to create an opening in a vein graft for a side-to-side anastomosis. (Courtesy Scanlon International, St Paul, Minn.)

Tube grafts are used to resect a portion of a blood vessel, bypass obstructions, or create an alternative route for blood flow. Woven patch material can be used to repair a portion of a blood vessel, replace the wall of a cardiac chamber, or close a ventricular septal defect. When flat patch material is unavailable, a patch can be cut from a piece of tube graft.

Knitted grafts have a higher porosity and thus allow more bleeding between the fibers. Tissue ingrowth is more rapid when the fibers are farther apart, which facilitates the creation of a new endothelial lining. This process can be enhanced with a textured surface made of filamentous loops ("velour"), which attract and provide a structure for cells that form the neointima. Knitted prostheses are also available as straight or bifurcated tubes or patch grafts.

Knitted grafts may be preclotted with unheparinized autologous venous blood, or they may be precoated by the manufacturer with albumin or collagen to retard bleeding. When preclotting the graft with blood, the surgeon will aspirate enough blood to moisten the graft (approximately 5 to 10 ml). This blood must be withdrawn before the patient receives heparin.

Advantages of knitted grafts are their ease of handling and less fraying at the cut edges as compared with woven grafts. They are used predominantly in the abdominal aorta, in visceral and peripheral arteries, and for patch repairs of endarterectomized carotid arteries. In cardiac repairs knitted patches are used to close atrial septal defects because they are easier to handle, fray less when cut, and endothelialize once heparin is reversed. Temporary residual bleeding through the graft from one atrial chamber to the other causes little problem. The use of unaltered knitted materials outside the heart in patients receiving heparin, however, is avoided because there would be ex-

TABLE **3-3**		
Sources of Graft Materials for Repair or Reconstruction		
TYPE	DEFINITION	EXAMPLES
Synthetic	Made from artificial sources	
Teflon	Fluorocarbon fiber	Felt pledgets for suture
Dacron	Polyester fiber	Straight or bifurcated tube grafts
PTFE	Polytetrafluoroethylene	Patch material
Biologic	Made from living or previously living tissue	Tube or patch grafts
Autograft	Tissue from one part of a person's body placed in another part	Saphenous vein graft
		Pulmonary artery autograft to replace aorta
Heterograft/xenograft	Tissue from another species placed in a person's body	Porcine valve
		Bovine pericardial patch
Allograft/homograft	Tissue from one person's body placed in another person	Transplant donor heart
		Cadaver aortic valve
		Human umbilical vein

From Carthey and others: The human factor in cardiac surgery, *Ann Thorac Surg* 72:300, 2001.

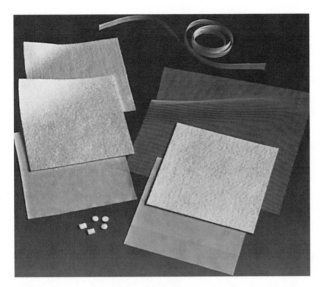

FIGURE 3-43 Assorted prosthetic materials to repair intracardiac and extracardiac defects: tapes, Teflon and Dacron patches, and felt pledgets. (From Meeker MH, Rothrock JC: *Alexander's care of the patient in surgery,* ed 11, 1999, St Louis, Mosby; courtesy Boston Scientific, Natick, Mass.)

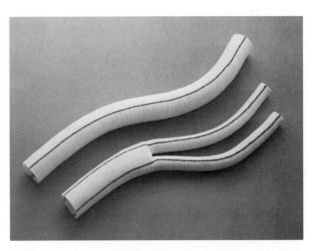

FIGURE 3-44 Straight and bifurcated arterial tube grafts. Most currently available grafts are treated with collagen to minimize interstitial bleeding. (From Meeker MH, Rothrock JC: *Alexander's care of the patient in surgery,* ed 11, St Louis, 1999, Mosby; courtesy Boston Scientific, Natick, Mass.)

cessive bleeding into the pericardium, causing tamponade. However, some knitted and woven grafts that are impregnated with collagen to prevent interstitial bleeding can be used in these situations.

Most tube grafts are crimped to reduce the possibility of compression. Some grafts are externally supported with plastic rings. Grafts made of polytetrafluoroethylene (PTFE) are not crimped but also may be reinforced with external plastic coils. Such grafts can be used to replace a segment of thoracic aorta or vena cava or to provide a conduit for blood flow from one vessel or cardiac chamber to another (such as the creation of a shunt from a systemic artery to a pulmonary artery in pediatric patients who have inadequate pulmonary blood flow). The appropriate-size tube graft diameter may be determined with the use of graft sizers. Sizing of PTFE grafts to the appropriate length, as well as diameter, is critical because these grafts do not stretch as crimped grafts do.

Occasionally a small-diameter straight-tube graft will be needed. If one is unavailable, the nurse can scan the bifurcated graft inventory for an appropriately sized "leg." This can be cut from the bifurcated graft and implanted.

Intraluminal tube grafts—reinforced at one or both ends with metal rings—were originally designed for rapid insertion into an aneurysmal aorta. The devices were anchored with tapes around the rings (or secured with stitches sewn into the rings and the aortic tissue). Problems with migration of the prosthesis and reduced time savings when conventional anastomoses were performed diminished the enthusiasm for these devices. However, the concept of a rapidly inserted graft has continued to evolve with the development of percutaneously inserted endoluminal stent grafts (see Chapter 14). This minimally invasive technology has significant potential for aneurysm repair of the descending thoracic and abdominal aorta (Diethrich, 2001).

BIOLOGIC GRAFTS

Biologic prostheses can be derived from human tissue or the tissue of another species (see Table 3-3). Human tissue grafts may be one of two types: autografts (the patient's own tissue) or allografts, also called homografts (tissue from another human). Autografts include the saphenous vein segments used during coronary artery bypass surgery and pericardium, a portion of which may be excised and used for patch repairs (it may be first immersed in glutaraldehyde to toughen it, then rinsed in saline and implanted). Heterografts are obtained from other species and include bovine pericardium and porcine heart valves. Heterografts are stored in sterile solutions and placed in sealed containers. Before implantation the storage solution is removed by rinsing with normal saline.

PROSTHETIC HEART VALVES

The era of prosthetic valve replacement began over three decades ago. Various designs and materials have been used as substitutes for native cardiac valves, but the ideal valve prosthesis has yet to be created (Box 3-10) (Autschbach and others, 2000).

Cardiac valve prostheses are of two types: mechanical and biologic. Each has advantages and disadvantages (see Chapter 11). The major advantage of mechanical valves is their durability. However, mechanical valves are thrombogenic, requiring patients to undergo chronic anticoagulation postoperatively. This is the major disadvantage of these prostheses.

Biologic valves (Figs. 3-45 through 3-50) have the advantage of not being inherently thrombogenic, thus obviating the need for chronic anticoagulation in the absence of other thromboembolic risk factors, such as atrial fibrillation or a history of transient ischemic attacks. Their disadvantage is that they are less durable than their me-

chanical counterparts and may need to be replaced, with the attendant risks associated with reoperations.

Other selection criteria include anatomic factors (such as the size of the aortic root or the left ventricle), blood flow and residual pressure gradients, ease of insertion, intensity of valve noise, patient preference, and (in the case of homografts) ease of procurement.

Obturators specific to each kind of prosthesis are available for determining the appropriate-size valve. Valve holders facilitate suturing and placement (seating) of the prosthesis.

Some manufacturers make aortic prostheses that can be inserted into the annulus itself or in the supraannular position. Because the area above the aortic annulus is generally larger than the annular area, supraannular valves allow a larger prosthesis to be inserted. This is advantageous in a person with a small aortic annulus (e.g., 19 mm). Before inserting this type of valve, the surgeon will confirm that the supraannular prosthesis does not occlude the coronary orifices. The appropriate obturators should be used for sizing.

Currently available mechanical prostheses use a ball-and-cage (Figs. 3-51 through 3-53) or tilting disk design (Figs. 3-54 through 3-57) and are made of a variety of materials. These include Silastic for ball-and-cage poppets; pyrolytic carbon for disks; titanium, Stellite alloy, or pyrolytic carbon for orifice rings; and Dacron or Teflon fabric for sewing cuffs. The valves allow closure with slight regurgitation to prevent stasis of blood. Care should be taken to avoid scratching or injuring the prosthesis.

Valve insertion during minimally invasive procedures (e.g., through a small thoracotomy in the right side of the chest) can be achieved with a valve holder/rotator system

---

BOX 3-10
The Ideal Prosthetic Heart Valve

Good blood flow
Durable
Nonthrombogenic
Atraumatic to blood
Biocompatible/nonreactive
Easy to insert
Silent
Acceptable to the patient

Modified from Autschbach and others: Prospectively randomized comparison of different mechanical aortic valves, *Circulation* 102(19 Suppl 3): III 1-4, 2000.

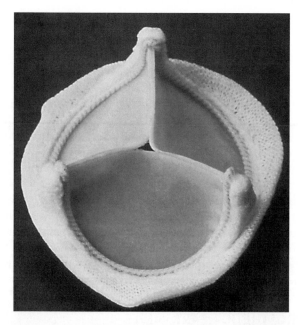

FIGURE 3-45 Carpentier-Edwards Perimount bovine pericardial valve prosthesis. (From Meeker MH, Rothrock JC: *Alexander's care of the patient in surgery,* ed 11, St Louis, 1999; courtesy Edwards Lifesciences, Irvine, Calif.)

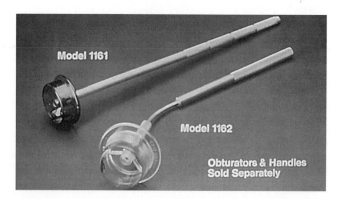

FIGURE 3-46 Sizing obturators and handles for Carpentier-Edwards aortic *(top)* and mitral *(bottom)* porcine and bovine pericardial valves. The malleable mitral handle facilitates insertion into the mitral annulus of the left atrium. (From Meeker MH, Rothrock JC: *Alexander's care of the patient in surgery,* ed 11, St Louis, 1999, Mosby; courtesy Edwards Lifesciences, Irvine, Calif.)

designed to introduce the prosthesis through a small incision and then seat the valve in its proper position.

Biologic valves approved for sale are made from porcine aortic valves or bovine pericardium cut into leaflets and sutured to Dacron or Teflon cloth-covered stents. They are treated and preserved in a glutaraldehyde solution, which must be rinsed off for 2 minutes in each of three separate baths of normal saline (for a

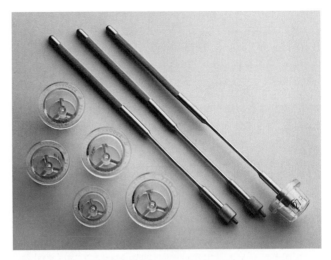

FIGURE 3-49 Sizing obturators and handles for Medtronic mitral porcine valve. (Courtesy Medtronic, Inc.)

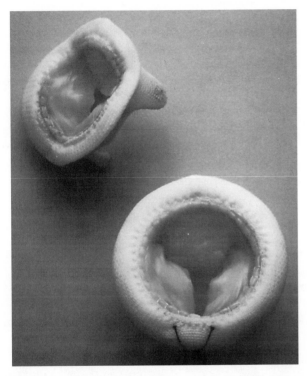

FIGURE 3-47 Medtronic Mosaic aortic porcine bioprosthesis *(top)* and Medtronic Mosaic porcine mitral bioprosthesis *(bottom)*. (Courtesy Medtronic, Inc.)

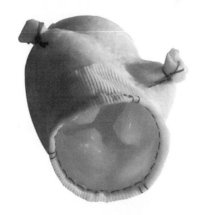

FIGURE 3-50 Medtronic Freestyle aortic root bioprosthesis. The absence of a stent and a sewing ring allow a greater orifice area through which blood can flow. (Courtesy Medtronic, Inc.)

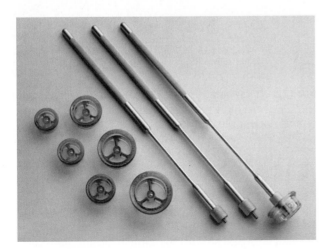

FIGURE 3-48 Sizing obturators and handles for Medtronic aortic porcine valve. (Courtesy Medtronic, Inc.)

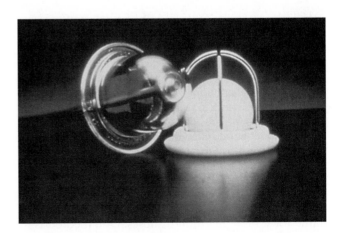

FIGURE 3-51 Starr-Edwards mitral sizing obturator and ball-and-cage valve prosthesis. (Courtesy Edwards Lifesciences, Irvine, Calif.)

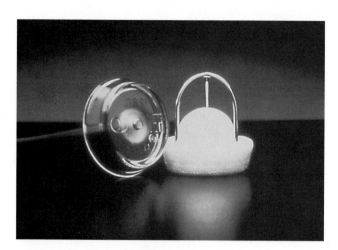

FIGURE 3-52 Starr-Edwards aortic and ball-and-cage valve prosthesis. (Courtesy Edwards Lifesciences, Irvine, Calif.)

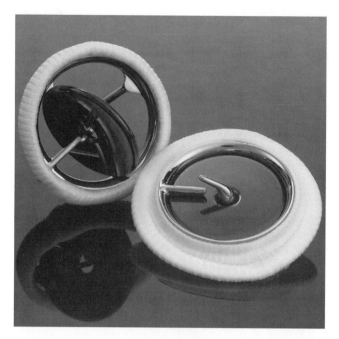

FIGURE 3-54 Medtronic Hall aortic *(left)* and mitral *(right)* tilting disk valve prostheses. (Courtesy Medtronic, Inc.)

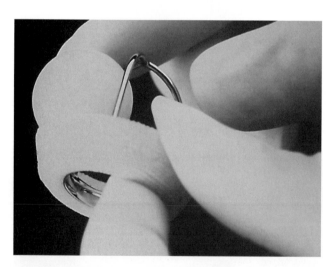

FIGURE 3-53 The poppet from the Starr-Edwards aortic valve can be removed to facilitate sewing the suture ring. It is inserted once the prosthesis is seated and the stitches are tied. (The poppet from the mitral valve prosthesis is not removable.) (Courtesy Edwards Lifesciences, Irvine, Calif.)

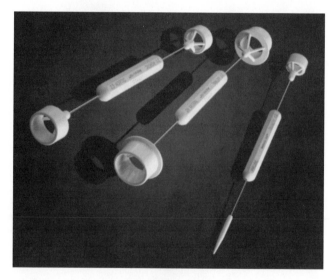

FIGURE 3-55 Medtronic Hall double-ended sizing obturators *(left, center)* and probe *(right)* used to test leaflet movement. (Courtesy Medtronic, Inc.)

total of 6 minutes [Fig. 3-58]). This required preparation time may influence the surgeon's suture technique for implanting bioprostheses. One method is to place stitches into the native valve annulus while the prosthesis is being rinsed. When the valve is ready, sutures are then placed in the prosthetic sewing ring.

Porcine *stentless* aortic bioprostheses (Fig. 3-50) are available for the small aortic root. The absence of a stent and sewing cuff give this prosthesis a larger internal orifice than a prosthesis with the same external dimension; thus a larger prosthesis (with greater flow) can be implanted. With a stentless valve it is possible to implant a

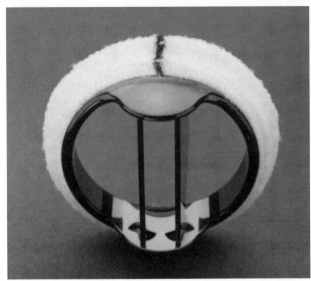

FIGURE 3-56 St. Jude Medical bileaflet tilting disk valve prosthesis. (Courtesy St. Jude Medical, Inc., St Paul, Minn.)

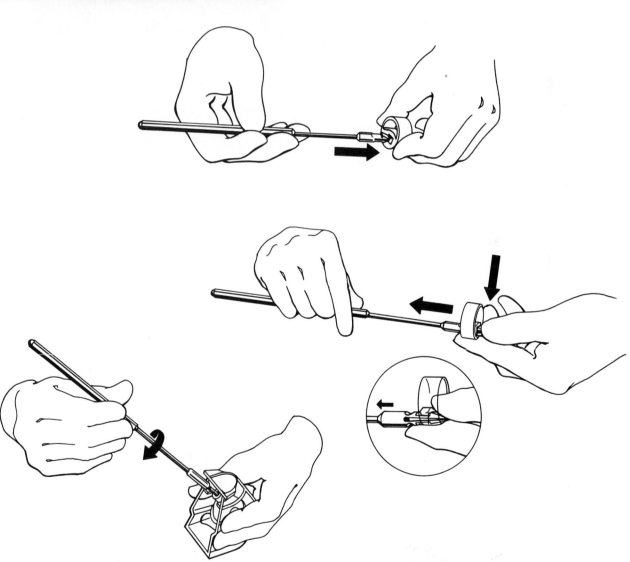

FIGURE 3-57 St. Jude Medical handles for obturators and prostheses. Procedure for attaching the St. Jude Medical obturator handle to the obturator/sizer *(top)*. Prosthesis handle is screwed into valve holder containing the prosthesis *(bottom)*. Note that the prosthesis is still inside its storage container; the handle and attached prosthesis are removed from the container after the handle has been screwed in. (Courtesy St. Jude Medical, Inc., St Paul, Minn.)

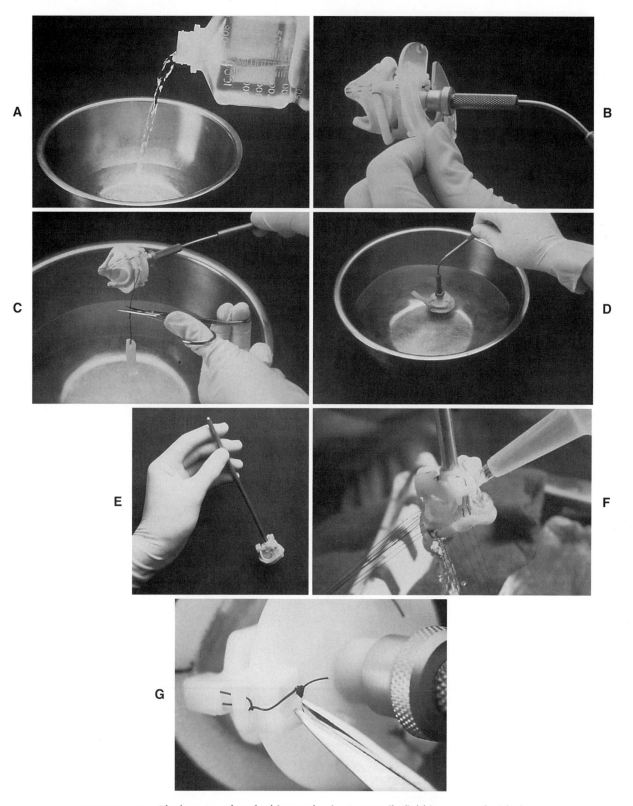

FIGURE 3-58 Rinsing procedure for bioprosthesis. **A,** A sterile field is prepared with three basins of normal saline. **B,** After the circulating nurse opens the valve container, the sterile nurse screws the prosthesis handle into the valve holder, which is attached to the prosthesis, and removes the valve. **C,** The circulating nurses and the sterile nurse check the size, type, and serial number on the tag, which the sterile nurse then cuts and removes before rinsing the prosthesis. **D,** The prosthesis is placed in the first basin of saline and gently agitated for a minimum of 2 minutes. The procedure is repeated in the second and third basins of saline. **E,** The valve with the holder and handle still attached is ready for insertion. It should not be allowed to dry out. **F,** The prosthesis is kept moist with frequent saline irrigation using a bulb syringe. **G,** The valve holder is removed by cutting the fixation stitch and pulling away the holder. (Courtesy Edwards Lifesciences, Irvine, Calif.)

prosthesis one or two sizes larger than a stented (e.g., Fig. 3-45) valve. Insertion is more technically difficult than with a conventional valve replacement.

In addition, the prosthesis shown in Figure 3-50 is manufactured with an anticalcification treatment to retard valve cusp calcification and degeneration. This is advantageous in prolonging the time before reoperation may be required. Obturators specific to the prosthesis should be used for correct sizing.

When the use of a biologic valve is anticipated, a sterile team member should be available to function as a valve rinser before the valve size is determined. It is recommended that even when the surgeon intends to use a mechanical prosthesis, a person should be ready to rinse a bioprosthesis in the event that circumstances favor its use. Delays in preparing the valve should be avoided in order to minimize cross-clamp time. During insertion the prosthesis should be kept moist with saline to avoid drying of the tissue.

AORTIC AND PULMONARY ALLOGRAFTS (HOMOGRAFTS)

Aortic and pulmonary allografts from cadaver donors (see Chapter 12) are used frequently for acquired and congenital lesions. A number of advantages have fostered their increasing popularity: little or no risk of thromboembolism, optimal hemodynamic function, no need for anticoagulant medications, and minimal risk of sudden catastrophic failure. They also demonstrate a lower incidence of infective endocarditis than do mechanical or biologic valves, and their long-term durability is superior to that of bioprostheses. Allografts may be fresh, but more frequently they are cryopreserved (frozen) and must be thawed according to strict protocol before implantation. Aortic allografts include the entire ascending aorta or the valve alone (Fig. 3-59). The graft is trimmed, and the valve alone or the valve and attached aortic wall are implanted.

Pulmonary allografts are also popular for use in children as conduits or patches for right ventricular outflow tract reconstruction, coarctation of the aorta, and hypoplastic left heart syndrome.

AORTIC GRAFT VALVE PROSTHESES

Conduits consisting of mechanical (Fig. 3-60) or biologic (Fig. 3-61) valves attached to a tube graft are used in procedures that require replacement of the native aortic valve and ascending aorta. If vein grafts must be inserted into the conduit during concomitant coronary artery bypass surgery or if a direct coronary ostial anastomosis is required, an eye cautery can be used to make the opening into the graft. In neonates conduits with

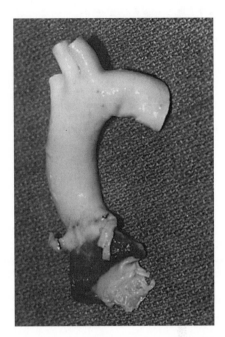

FIGURE 3-59 Aortic allograft (homograft) with the aortic valve and arch vessels attached. (From Meeker MH, Rothrock JC: *Alexander's care of the patient in surgery,* ed 11, St Louis, 1999, Mosby; courtesy CryoLife, Inc., Kennesaw, Ga.)

valves interposed between tube graft material can be used to reconstruct right ventricle–pulmonary artery continuity if, for example, there is an absent pulmonary valve. Pulmonary allograft valves have been used for these procedures as well.

When sizing graft valve conduits, one needs to remember that in the manufacturing process, the addition of the graft to the valve prosthesis adds 2 mm to the size of the valve sewing ring. For instance, a 25-mm valve sewing ring would contain a 23-mm valve prosthesis. When using the sizers specific for the valve incorporated into the conduit, the sizer with the best fit determines the size of the aortic graft valve prosthesis (e.g., the sewing ring annulus), not the size of the valve within the conduit (which would be 2 mm smaller). Thus if a 27-mm St. Jude Medical sizer fit best into the native annulus, a 27-mm conduit (containing a 25-mm valve) would be selected and implanted.

ANNULOPLASTY RINGS

The complications associated with replacement of the mitral and tricuspid valves in particular have fostered widespread use of reparative techniques with or without prosthetic devices. Moreover, the use of intraoperative echocardiography to assess valve function has taken much of the guesswork out of evaluating mitral and tricuspid repairs. The prosthetic devices include

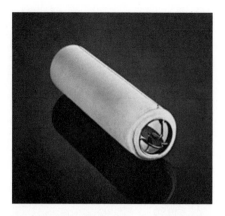

FIGURE 3-60 Aortic rotatable conduit containing a Medtronic-Hall disk valve prosthesis. (From Meeker MH, Rothrock JC: *Alexander's care of the patient in surgery,* ed 11, St Louis, 1999, Mosby; courtesy Medtronic, Inc.)

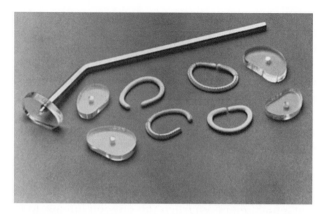

FIGURE 3-62 Carpentier-Edwards tricuspid and mitral annuloplasty rings and sizing obturators and holder. Note the gap in the tricuspid rings *(left)* that correlates to the area in the heart containing bundle of His conduction tissue; this helps the surgeon to avoid placing sutures in the area. Carpentier-Edwards rings are available in two models: the Classic ring *(shown)* has a semirigid shape; the Physio ring is similar in gross appearance but is more flexible. (Courtesy Edwards Lifesciences, Irvine, Calif.)

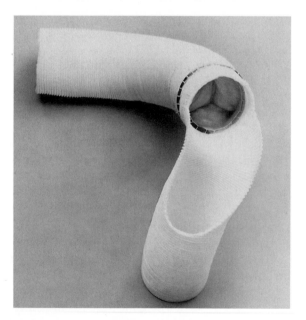

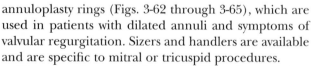

FIGURE 3-61 Conduit with a porcine valve within the tube graft. (Courtesy Medtronic, Inc.)

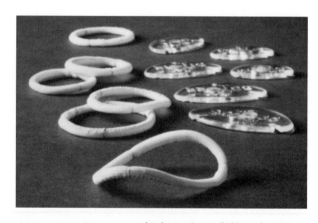

FIGURE 3-63 Duran annuloplasty rings *(left)* and sizing obturators *(right).* (Courtesy Medtronic, Inc.)

annuloplasty rings (Figs. 3-62 through 3-65), which are used in patients with dilated annuli and symptoms of valvular regurgitation. Sizers and handlers are available and are specific to mitral or tricuspid procedures.

Rings may be semirigid or flexible. The semirigid rings are used to *remodel* the annulus into its normal (beanlike) shape; the flexible rings enhance the physiologic function (e.g., annular contraction at the end of *atrial systole*) of the native valve. Another type of ring is shaped like the letter C lying on its side. This ring is

used to reduce annular dilation that occurs predominantly in the posterior leaflet of the mitral valve (see Chapter 11). Surgeon preference guides the selection of the most appropriate ring for the patient.

Patch repairs of valve leaflets can be performed with the patient's own pericardium or with commercially available tissue. Autologous tissue may be treated by soaking it for a few minutes in glutaraldehyde, but the glutaraldehyde must be rinsed off before the treated tissue is implanted.

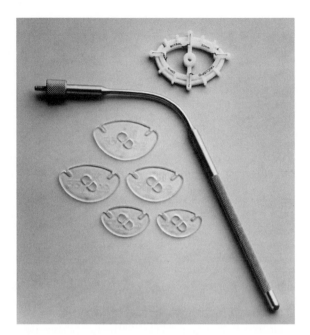

FIGURE 3-64 Accessories for Duran annuloplasty rings: ring holder *(top)*, handle for prosthetic ring holder *(center)*, and sizing obturators *(bottom)*. A handle can be made for the sizing obturator by grasping the central portion of the sizer with a tonsil or Kelly clamp. (Courtesy Medtronic, Inc.)

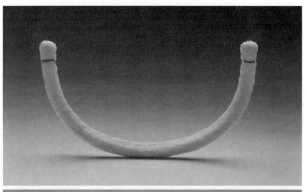

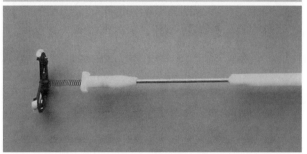

FIGURE 3-65 **A,** Cosgrove annuloplasty ring. **B,** Ring attached to ring holder and handle. (Courtesy Edwards Lifesciences, Irvine, Calif.)

Conclusion

Structural standards guide the perioperative nurse in organizing and administering the cardiac OR. Consideration must be given to the array of equipment and supplies, the complexity of patient care, and the demands placed on a hospital's human, fiscal, and material resources.

References

Advisory Council for Cardiothoracic Surgery, American College of Surgeons: Guidelines for standards in cardiac surgery, *Bull Am Coll Surg* 82(2):27, 1997.

Association of periOperative Registered Nurses (AORN): *Standards, recommended practices & guidelines,* Denver, 2001, AORN.

Autschbach R and others: Prospectively randomized comparison of different mechanical aortic valves, *Circulation* 102 (19 Suppl 3): III 1, 2000.

Ball KA: Surgical modalities. In Meeker MH, Rothrock JC, *Alexander's care of the patient in surgery,* ed 11, St Louis, 1999, Mosby.

Baue AE, Geha AS, O'Kane H: Organization of a cardiac surgical unit, *Angiology* 25(1):45, 1974.

Bossert L, Koster R: Defibrillation: methods and strategies, *Resuscitation* 24:(3)211, 1992.

Canales MG, Macario A, Krummell T: The surgical suite meets the new health economy, *J Am Coll Surg* 192(6):768, 2001.

Chiang B: Activity-based benchmarking in cardiac surgery, *Surg Serv Manage* 7(1):30, 2001.

Diethrich EB: AAA stent grafts: current developments, *J Invasive Cardiol* 13(5):383, 2001.

Damiano RJ, Reichenspurner H, Ducko CT: Robotically assisted endoscopic coronary artery bypass grafting: current state of the art, *Adv Card Surg* 12:37, 2000.

Eagle KA and others: ACC/AHA Guidelines for coronary artery bypass graft surgery *J Am Coll Cardiol* 34(4):1262, 1999.

Eckberg E: The future of robotics can be ours, *AORN J* 67(5):1018, 1998.

Emergency Cardiac Care Committee and Subcommittees, American Heart Association. Guidelines for cardiopulmonary resuscitation and emergency cardiac care, *JAMA* 268(16):2171, 1992.

Health Care Financing Administration (HCFA): *Proposed changes to DRG classifications and relative weights,* http://www.hcfa.gov/regs/hefal158p/pp021_111.doc (accessed Aug 3, 2001).

Higami T and others: Histologic and physiologic evaluation of skeletonized internal thoracic artery harvesting with an ultrasonic scalpel, *J Thorac Cardiovasc Surg* 120(6):1142, 2000.

Hubbard W: Mobile cardiac cath: a revolutionary tool, *Surg Serv Manage* 5(6):8, 1999.

Institute of Medicine (IOM): *Crossing the quality chasm: a new health system for the 21st century,* Washington, DC, 2001, National Academy Press.

Institute of Medicine (IOM): *To err is human: building a safer health system,* Washington, DC, 1999, National Academy Press.

Joint Commission on the Accreditation of Healthcare Organizations: (2001) *Revisions to Joint Commission standards in support of patient safety and medical/health error (1) reduction,* http://www.jcaho.org/standard/fr_ptsafety.html (accessed Feb 14, 2001).

Judkins and others: Report of the Inter-Society Commission for Heart Disease Resources. Optimal resources for examination of the chest and cardiovascular system, *Circulation* 53(2):A1, 1976.

Kavoussi LR and others: Comparison of robotic versus human laparoscopic camera control, *J Urol* 154(6)2134, 1995.

Kerber RE and others: Open chest defibrillation during cardiac surgery: energy and current requirement, *Am J Cardiol* 46:(3)393, 1980.

Kirklin JW, Barratt-Boyes BG: *Cardiac surgery,* ed 2, New York, 1993, Churchill Livingstone.

Kirshner E: Standardization is key to streamlining cardiac surgery, *Surg Serv Manage* 6(9):18, 2000.

Lamm P and others: The harmonic scalpel: optimizing the quality of mammary artery bypass grafts, *Ann Thorac Surg* 69(6):1833, 2000.

Mack M: Minimally invasive and robotic surgery, *JAMA* 285(5):568, 2001.

Maldonado SS, Nygren C: Pediatric surgery. In Meeker MH, Rothrock JC: *Alexander's care of the patient in surgery,* ed 11, 1999, St Louis, Mosby.

Medtronic Physio-Control: *Defibrillation: what you should know* (manufacturer's instructions), Redmond, Wash, 1997, Physio-Control.

Mishra V and others: Cost analysis of cardiothoracic procedures, *Surg Serv Manage* 7(3):44, 2001.

Myerburg RJ, Castellanos A: Cardiac arrest and sudden cardiac death. In Braunwald E, Zipes DP, Libby P, editors: *Heart disease,* ed 6, Philadelphia, 2001, WB Saunders.

Optimal resources for cardiac surgery: guidelines for program planning and evaluation, *Am J Cardiol* 36:(6)836, 1975.

Popolow G: How robotics is transforming the OR, *Surg Serv Manage* 5(12):35, 1999.

Pugsley WB and others: Low energy level internal defibrillation during cardiopulmonary bypass, *Eur J Cardiothorac Surg* 3(3):273, 1988.

Reger TB, Roditski D: Bloodless medicine and surgery for patients having cardiac surgery, *Crit Care Nurse* 21(4):35, 2001.

Seifert PC: *Cardiac surgery,* St Louis, 1994, Mosby.

Shennib H and others: An automated interrupted suturing device for coronary artery bypass grafting: automated coronary anastomosis, *Ann Thorac Surg* 70(3):1046, 2000.

Solem JO and others: Evaluation of a new device for quick sutureless coronary artery anastomosis in surviving sheep, *Eur J Cardiothorac Surg* 17(3):312, 2000.

Surgical Services Management 7(4), 2001. [Entire issue devoted to construction and renovation.]

Ward SF: Financial management: an important millennium skill, *Surg Serv Manage* 5(9):6, 1999.

4

Preoperative Assessment

Nurses today . . . are assuming a more collaborative role in the care of their patients. They are, therefore, interested in knowing why certain manifestations of disease appear and why a specific therapeutic regimen is chosen rather than simply observing these events passively.

Jeannette Kernicki, RN, Barbara L. Bullock, RN, and Joan Matthews Register, RN, 1970

The preoperative consultation should be performed with at least as much care as the technical operation.

Daniel James Waters, DO, 1995

The preoperative assessment is performed to identify patient problems and diagnoses. Perioperative nurses are guided by the process and outcome standards developed by the Association of periOperative Registered Nurses (AORN, 2001) that assist clinicians in formulating clinical judgments. (The *Standards of Cardiovascular Nursing Practice,* jointly developed by the American Nurses' Association and the American Heart Association Council on Cardiovascular Nursing, published in 1981, are currently undergoing revision.)

Another important resource for perioperative nurses is the *Perioperative Nursing Data Set* (Beyea, 2000), which describes, defines, and establishes a data set that incorporates perioperative nursing diagnoses, nursing interventions, and patient outcomes. The identification of appropriate patient outcomes (more fully discussed in Chapter 5) is based on assessing patients to identify risk factors, pathophysiology, abnormal diagnostic testing results, and the effects of cardiac disease on each patient. Based on the patient's history, physical examination, and tests and studies, diagnostic judgments are formed and provide the foundation for planning, implementation, and outcome achievement (Seifert, 1999).

Information required for patient care can be obtained from the hospital record, the preoperative interview, and other sources such as professional colleagues and the patient's family and friends. In many instances, before the perioperative nurse conducts the preoperative interview, the patient will have undergone diagnostic studies to identify the clinical problem and laboratory tests to measure various physiologic parameters pertinent to the surgical management. Based on the results of these tests and the find-ings from prior assessment interviews (conducted by the patient's primary and consulting physicians and by admitting nurses), the perioperative nurse communicates with the patient to formulate a plan of care that promotes physiologic and psychologic well-being. Intraoperatively the nurse continues to assess the patient by monitoring the clinical status and comparing it with preoperative baseline data; interventions can be adjusted or modified depending on the patient's response to surgery. During the postoperative evaluation the perioperative nurse can apply significant findings to future patient care.

This chapter describes diagnostic and laboratory procedures commonly performed before surgery. Many of these preoperative diagnostic tests (e.g., echocardiography, electrocardiography, radiography, blood testing) also are employed during the perioperative period, and familiarity with these modalities will assist the perioperative nurse in monitoring patients more effectively. A format for a preoperative interview of the patient based on functional health patterns also is presented (Carpenito, 1999).

Background Information

In arriving at a diagnosis, clinicians consider etiology, anatomy, and physiology (Box 4-1); these factors are often interrelated. For example, in a patient with myocardial ischemia, the underlying causes may be related to obstructive coronary artery disease (CAD) or to left ventricular hypertrophy (LVH) secondary to aortic stenosis. The anatomic changes associated with CAD and LVH (narrowed coronaries arteries and increased myocardial wall thickness, respectively) can themselves produce myocardial ischemia. Physiologically, ischemia

---

BOX 4-1
Examples of Etiologic, Anatomic, and Physiologic Factors Contributing to Heart Disease

Etiology
Congenital: genetic, gestational, environmental
Infection: viral, bacterial, fungal
Hypertension: essential hypertension, arteriosclerosis
Ischemia: coronary atherosclerosis, left ventricular hypertrophy

Anatomy
Cardiac chambers: hypertrophy, dilation, combination
Valves: stenosis, regurgitation, combination
Myocardium: infarction
Pericardium: effusion, thickening
Great vessels: calcification, dissection, aneurysm

Physiology
Dysrhythmias: reentry, tachydysrhythmias, fibrillation
Heart failure: cardiomyopathy, ischemia
Myocardial ischemia: coronary artery disease, coronary vasospasm

Modified from Braunwald E: Approach to the patient with heart disease. In Braunwald E and others, *Harrison's principles of internal medicine,* ed 15, New York, 2001a, McGraw-Hill.

BOX 4-2
New York Heart Association Functional and Cardiac Status Classification System

Class I: Patients with cardiac disease do not display symptoms of syncope, fatigue, dyspnea, palpitation, or anginal pain with ordinary physical activity; cardiac status is uncompromised.
Class II: Patients with cardiac disease are comfortable at rest but display symptoms during ordinary physical activity; cardiac status is slightly compromised.
Class III: Patients with cardiac disease, although comfortable at rest, are markedly limited functionally and display symptoms with less than ordinary exercise; cardiac status is moderately compromised.
Class IV: Patients with cardiac disease are unable to engage in any physical activity without discomfort and may have symptoms of cardiac insufficiency even at rest; cardiac status is severely compromised.

Modified from Criteria Committee of the New York Heart Association: *Nomenclature and criteria for diagnosis,* ed 9, Boston, 1994, Little, Brown; Braunwald E: The history. In Braunwald E. Zipes DP, Libby P, editors: *Heart disease,* ed 6, Philadelphia, 2001, WB Saunders.

BOX 4-3
Canadian Cardiovascular Society Classification System for Angina Pectoris

Class 0: No angina.
Class I: Walking, climbing stairs, and other ordinary physical activity does not produce angina; angina may occur with strenuous, prolonged, or rapid exertion.
Class II: Ordinary activity may be slightly limited; angina may occur with moderate activity such as walking rapidly, walking uphill, or walking after meals or in cold weather.
Class III: Ordinary activity is markedly limited; angina may occur after walking one or two blocks on level ground or climbing one flight of stairs at a normal pace.
Class IV: Angina may be present at rest; any physical activity produces discomfort.

Modified from Campeau L: *Circulation* 54:522, 1975; Braunwald E: The history. In Braunwald E, Zipes DP, Libby P, editors: *Heart disease,* ed 6, Philadelphia, 2001, WB Saunders.

(from whatever cause) can lead to heart failure. An initial review of the hospital record (i.e., the patient's chart) provides valuable historical and diagnostic information about these three elements.

Braunwald (2001a) has suggested that the impact of the cardiovascular disorder on the functional status of the patient also should be considered in addition to etiology, anatomy, and physiology. The New York Heart Association (NYHA) classification system has been used widely to relate functional activity to the ability to participate in normal activity. The NYHA system has been broadened to include cardiac status (Box 4-2) (Criteria Committee, 1994). Another classification scale is that of the Canadian Cardiovascular Society (CCS); it specifically grades the amount of activity that produces angina pectoris (Box 4-3) (Campeau, 1975).

The underlying causes, anatomic changes, and physiologic disturbances may be described in the progress notes from primary and referring physicians, reported in laboratory tests, and documented by clinicians in their admission assessments. Commonly the patient's internist or cardiologist records the events and the symptoms that initially prompted the patient to seek treatment. These entries provide valuable information to the perioperative nurse in preparation for the preoperative interview.

Frequently a patient with heart disease complains about symptoms such as dyspnea, chest pain or discomfort, syncope, palpitation, edema, cough, and excessive fatigue (Box 4-4) (Braunwald, 2001b). The clinician determines whether these symptoms are caused by heart disease by eliciting the patient's history and performing a physical examination. Because there is a subjective

BOX **4-4**
Cardinal Symptoms of Heart Disease

Dyspnea

- Characterized by uncomfortable awareness of breathing
- Cardiac dyspnea commonly associated with pulmonary congestion
- Associated with diseases of heart and lungs, chest wall, and respiratory muscles
- Sudden onset suggestive of pulmonary embolism, acute pulmonary edema, airway obstruction
- Chronic dyspnea suggestive of left ventricular failure, pulmonary vascular disease, chronic obstructive pulmonary disease
- Noncardiac causes include anxiety, obesity, anemia

Chest Pain or Discomfort

- Cardiac causes include myocardial ischemia, myocardial infarction (MI), pericarditis, aortic dissection, pulmonary embolus
- Anginal "pain" secondary to myocardial ischemia is sensed commonly as tightening around chest or pressure on chest; may radiate to neck, jaw, epigastrium, and arm or shoulder (commonly on left side)
- Women may experience "atypical" chest pain: sharp or fleeting pain, unrelated to exercise, relieved by antacids; palpitations without chest pain, especially at rest, during sleep, or during mental stress
- MI pain often substernal and may radiate to neck, jaw, arm, or shoulder
- Pericarditis pain may begin over sternum or cardiac apex; may radiate, but less than MI
- Aortic dissection pain may begin in anterior chest and radiate to back; commonly characterized as ripping, knifelike pain
- Pulmonary embolism may produce substernal pain, but chest pain often not felt

Cyanosis

- Both a physical sign and a symptom; bluish discoloration of the skin commonly caused by reduced hemoglobin in blood
- Key feature in patients with congenital heart disease
- Central cyanosis characterized by decreased arterial oxygen saturation caused by left-to-right shunting of blood (e.g., desaturated blood mixing with oxygen-saturated blood)
- Peripheral cyanosis commonly secondary to cutaneous vasoconstriction caused by low cardiac output (or exposure to cold air or water)

Syncope

- Characterized by loss of consciousness from reduced perfusion to brain
- May result from cardiac dysrhythmias (e.g., heart block), seizures
- Syncope in aortic stenosis usually precipitated by effort

Collapse

- Characterized by cardiogenic shock, inadequate cardiac output, severe hypotension, life-threatening cellular dysfunction
- May result from extensive MI, anaphylaxis, excessive blood loss, infection, uncontrolled diabetes

Palpitation

- Characterized by unpleasant awareness of forceful or rapid beating of the heart, described as pounding, jumping, racing, flip-flopping
- May be caused by heart block, tachydysrhythmias, other heart rate or rhythm disturbances

Edema

- Characterized by abnormal accumulation of fluid in interstitial spaces
- May be caused by heart failure from left or right ventricular dysfunction, mitral stenosis, fluid overload, constrictive pericarditis
- Visible edema of both lower extremities usually preceded by weight gain (3-5 kg)

Cough

- Frequent symptom of heart disease; frothy, pink sputum associated with pulmonary edema; bloody sputum associated with carcinoma of the lung, tuberculosis, pulmonary infarction
- May be caused by infection, allergy, pulmonary disease, mitral valve disease, or compression of tracheobronchial tree secondary to aortic aneurysm

Hemoptysis

- Characterized by expectoration of blood or bloody sputum
- May result from escape of red blood cells or rupture of bronchial or pulmonary vessels secondary to pulmonary edema or infarction, lung carcinoma, or aortic aneurysm
- Associated shortness of breath may indicate mitral stenosis

Fatigue

- Common symptom; very nonspecific
- May be related to depressed cardiac output, drugs (e.g., beta blockers or diuretics)
- Extreme fatigue sometimes precedes or accompanies MI

Other Symptoms

- **Fever and chills** are common in infective endocarditis
- **Nocturia** may be an early complaint in patients with congestive heart failure
- **Cachexia** (malnutrition and emaciation) is symptomatic of advanced heart failure
- **Hoarseness** may be caused by compression on recurrent laryngeal nerve by aortic aneurysm, enlarged pulmonary artery, or greatly enlarged left atrium

Modified from Braunwald E: The history. In Braunwald E, Zipes DP, Libby P, editors: *Heart disease: a textbook of cardiovascular medicine,* ed 6, Philadelphia, 2001b, WB Saunders.

component to any evaluation of a patient, direct contact between physician and patient or nurse and patient enables the clinician to arrive at a more complete and accurate assessment.

Previous illnesses are an important part of the history. Episodes of rheumatic fever or tonsillitis as a child are significant because the sequelae of rheumatic fever and streptococcal infections can lead to damage of the cardiac valves. Other significant diseases include thyroid disease, recent dental disease requiring manipulation or extraction, and immunologic disorders.

Congenital malformations may be present and may be the result of genetic factors (e.g., certain forms of atrial septal defect can be inherited). If genetic factors and chromosomal defects have been eliminated as the cause, congenital heart disease likely is triggered by gestational and environmental factors (Milewicz, 2000). The clinician inquires about the prenatal history of the infants, including family history, maternal viral illnesses (such as rubella), and alcohol and drug use during the pregnancy. Maternal diabetes mellitus and parental congenital heart disease are associated with a higher incidence of congenital heart disease in children (Friedman and Silverman, 2001). Some congenital malformations may not require surgery until adulthood (e.g., atrial septal defect and bicuspid aortic valve) (Milewicz, 2000).

Once the history is completed, a review of the patient's systems is performed to determine cardiovascular involvement and other systemic illnesses that may affect the heart. Among these are muscular dystrophies than can cause cardiomyopathies, metabolic disorders that can produce heart failure and conduction disturbances, and inherited connective tissue disorders associated with aortic dissection and mitral valve prolapse (Friedman and Silverman, 2001). A systems review is described under the "Exchanging" pattern in the section on the preoperative patient interview later in this chapter.

Based on the findings from the history and physical examination, a preliminary diagnosis is formulated. To confirm the medical diagnosis and guide treatment, the physician orders specific diagnostic tests. Although the clinical examination can establish a diagnosis for a number of disorders (e.g., hypertension, aortic stenosis, mitral valve prolapse, and cardiac tamponade), supplemental tests are used to arrive at a complete cardiac diagnosis (Braunwald, 2001a).

Diagnostic Procedures

In addition to confirming the diagnosis, specific tests are selected to evaluate the degree of injury or extent of the disorder and select the most appropriate interventions. There are four categories of tests: (1) electrocardiogram, (2) chest roentgenogram, (3) noninvasive

graphic tests (e.g., echocardiogram, radionuclide and imaging techniques), and (4) invasive examinations (e.g., cardiac catheterization, angiocardiography, and coronary angiography). Some common diagnostic procedures are described in this chapter.

Not all the following tests are performed on every patient; generally only those needed to confirm the diagnosis or to provide additional data for the selection of the appropriate therapy are ordered. One consideration is the current emphasis on quality improvement, cost containment, and professional peer review. Physicians select tests on the basis not only of the clinical indication but also on whether the data provided by particular procedures are worth the cost, inconvenience, and risk to the patient. The economic scrutiny of tests also focuses on whether the information gained will actually be used to guide treatment and enhance clinical outcomes (i.e., provide clinical and economic value) (Hlatky and Mark, 2001; Beller, 2001).

Increasingly, gender differences are also taken into account in the selection of tests because certain studies (e.g., exercise electrocardiography, radionuclide perfusion imaging) are less accurate in women than in men (Lee and Boucher, 2001; Miller, 2000). In part this is because of certain difficulties in diagnosing heart disease (especially CAD) in women (Table 4-1). For example, the presence of estrogens may create an abnormal electrocardiogram (ECG) finding when in fact there is no abnormality (i.e., a *false positive* test result). In other instances there may be a normal result when in fact there is underlying disease (i.e., a *false negative* test result). The value of different diagnostic tools for CAD in women is illustrated in Table 4-2.

Diagnostic studies requiring arterial (or central venous) puncture are characterized as invasive; noninvasive studies do not require vascular access. Occasionally the technique may be semiinvasive, such as radiographs with the intravascular injection of dye. Noninvasive studies include the ECG, stress testing, radiography, echocardiography, cardiac Doppler studies, and nuclear imaging (Goldstein and Hendel, 1996). Invasive tests, such as electrophysiology studies, cardiac catheterization, and endomyocardial biopsy, require the insertion of intravascular catheters, electrodes, or bioptomes. Test results are usually in the patient record and should be reviewed by the perioperative nurse.

Patients electively scheduled for surgery may have had cardiac catheterization, echocardiography, and other tests performed during a previous admission (or outpatient visit). The old chart should be available so that these test results can be reviewed preoperatively by the surgical team. Hospitalized patients requiring urgent or emergent surgery undergo diagnostic procedures and tests as needed to prepare for operation.

TABLE 4-1
Difficulties Diagnosing Coronary Artery Disease in Women

DIAGNOSTIC TOOL	R OR R/S	COMPARED WITH MEN, WOMEN SHOW:
History of chest discomfort	R/S	More false (+)
ECG–ST	R/S	More false (+) because of unknown factors (estrogens?)
SPECT MPI ± LV function	R/S	More false (+) because of soft tissue attenuation Radiation risk if pregnant
LV function (RNA)	R/S	More false (+) because of different hemodynamic responses in women: less increase in LVEF and more increase in LVED volume, less increase in systolic BP Radiation risk if pregnant Gender-related differences in attenuation make little difference
LV function (Echo)	R/S	Same as above (but no radiation) Often difficult to acquire images of all walls of left ventricle caused by more limited "window" in women
PET MPI ± LV function	R/S	Best current test because gender-related differences in attenuation are corrected Radiation risk if pregnant but less radiation with ^{82}Rb versus with other radionuclide methods
MRI: LV function and MPI	R/S	Promising, but more validation is needed
MRA	R	Gender differences in attenuation do not alter cardiovascular images
UFCT: LV function and MPI	R/S	Promising, but more validation is needed
Angiography (contrast)	R	Radiation risk if pregnant Gender differences in attenuation have little effect on cardiovascular images
UFCT: Coronary calcification in arterial walls	R	Very promising; preliminary data for gender differences at various ages show less CA^{++} in women Radiation risk if pregnant Gender differences in attenuation have little effect on cardiovascular images
Cardiac catheterization with contrast coronary angiography	R	More arterial access complications caused by smaller size arteries in women Radiation risk if pregnant Gender differences in attenuation have little effect on cardiovascular images

(+), Positive; *ECG–ST*, electrocardiographic ST segments; *SPECT*, single photon emission computed tomography with thallium-201 or technetium-99m-sestamibi; *MPI*, myocardial perfusion imaging; *LV*, left ventricular; *Echo*, echocardiography; *LVED*, LV and end-diastolic; *PET*, positron emission tomography; *MRA*, MR angiography; *R*, rest only; *RNA*, radionuclide angiocardiography; *LVEF*, LV ejection fraction; *BP*, blood pressure; *MRI*, magnetic resonance imaging; *UFCT*, ultrafast computed tomography; *R/S*, rest and stress.
Modified from Julian DG, Wenger NK: *Women & heart disease,* St Louis, 1997, Mosby.

TABLE 4-2
Value of Diagnostic Tools for Coronary Artery Disease in Women (0 to ++++)

	R OR R/S	FALSE (+)	FALSE (−)	NONDIAGNOSTIC	VALIDATION	RISK	COST
History	R	+++	++	++++	++	0	+
ECG	R/S	+++	++	+++	+++	++	++
SPECT MPI	R/S	++	+	++	+++	++	+++
RNA	R/S	++	+	++	+++	++	+++
Echo	R/S	++	+	++	++	++	+++
PET–MPI	R/S	+	+	+	++	++	++++
MRI LV function/perfusion	R/S	++	+	++	+	++	++++
MRA	R	++	+	++	+	0	++++
UFCT: LV function/perfusion	R/S	+	+	+	+	+	++++
UFCT: Rest angiography	R	+	+	++	+	+	++++
UFCT:							
Calcification	R	++	+	+	++	0	++
Coronary angiography	R	0	0	0	++++	++++	++++

(+), Positive; *ECG–ST*, electrocardiographic ST segments; *SPECT*, single photon emission computed tomography with thallium-201 or technetium-99m-sestamibi; *MPI*, myocardial perfusion imaging; *LV*, left ventricular; *Echo*, echocardiography; *LVED*, LV and end-diastolic; *PET*, positron emission tomography; *MRA*, MR angiography; *R*, rest only; *RNA*, radionuclide angiocardiography; *LVEF*, LV ejection fraction; *BP*, blood pressure; *MRI*, magnetic resonance imaging; *UFCT*, ultrafast computed tomography; *R/S*, rest and stress.
Modified from Julian DG, Wenger NK: *Women & heart disease,* St Louis, 1997, Mosby.

ELECTROCARDIOGRAM

A resting 12-lead ECG, the most commonly used diagnostic test in cardiology, provides baseline information about the electrical activity of the heart (see Chapter 17 on dysrhythmias). Although the ECG rarely points to a specific diagnosis, it can detect abnormal cardiac rhythms, conduction disturbances, and signs of ischemia (ST segment changes) or infarction (Q waves), and it can provide information about the position of the heart and the size and wall thickness of the cardiac chambers (Figs. 4-1 and 4-2). QRS complex, ST segment, T wave, and P wave changes may be the results of cardiac factors or noncardiac causes such as age, the effects of drugs, or electrolyte imbalances. Results of the ECG are correlated to clinical data obtained from the history and physical examination

ECG results may be normal with the patient at rest, even in the presence of CAD; abnormal changes may become apparent only with exercise. These patients may be referred for an exercise ECG (stress test); they also may undergo continuous electrocardiography testing with a Holter monitor. This is worn by the patient for 24 to 48 hours, after which the recorded ECG is scanned for abnormalities. Patients with periodic "spells" may be attached to event recorders that are activated when the patients feel dysrhythmias or symptoms such as syncope, palpitations, or chest pain.

EXERCISE ELECTROCARDIOGRAPHY (STRESS TEST)

Exercise ECG, stress echocardiogram, and myocardial perfusion imaging are the three most commonly used noninvasive tests to determine myocardial ischemia. Guidelines from the American College of Cardiology, American Heart Association, American College of Physicians, and American Society of Internal Medicine (Gibbons and others, 1999) recommend exercise electrocardiography as the appropriate first test for patients with suspected chronic stable angina.

The exercise ECG is used to uncover myocardial dysfunction and other signs of ischemia that become apparent only with the increased metabolic demands created by exertion (or strong emotion). An exercise treadmill (or stationary bicycle) is used to stress the heart of patients who may be asymptomatic at rest or who have atypical chest pain. An exercise ECG may have little diagnostic value in patients with ECG abnormalities at rest. Whenever possible, drugs such as beta-adrenergic blocking agents, vasodilators, and other antihypertensive medications that alter hemodynamic responses should be stopped for approximately 2 days. If withdrawal of these drugs is not feasible, an alternative test may be required. Stress ECG is contraindicated in patients with unstable angina, aortic valve stenosis, or

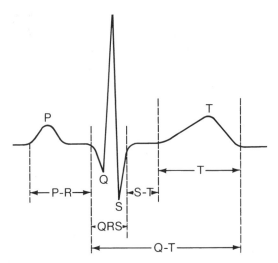

FIGURE 4-1 ECG waveform components. P wave: electrical activity associated with sinoatrial (SA) node impulse and depolarization of the atria (absent with atrial fibrillation or flutter). PR interval: the time the impulse takes to travel through the atria to the atrioventricular (AV) node, the His-Purkinje system, and the ventricles; interval between the onset of the P wave and the onset of the QRS complex (normal duration: 0.12 to 0.20 second). QRS complex: electrical depolarization and contraction of the ventricles (normal duration: 0.04 to 0.12 second). QT interval: from the onset of the QRS complex to the end of the T wave. ST segment: period between completion of depolarization and the beginning of depolarization of the ventricles; interval between the end of the QRS complex and the beginning of the T wave. Displacement of 0.5 mm or more (up or down) is generally indicative of inadequate myocardial perfusion. T wave: recovery or repolarization phase of the ventricles. (From Canobbio MM: *Cardiovascular disorders,* St Louis, 1990, Mosby).

other forms of left ventricular outflow tract obstruction that can increase the risk of ventricular fibrillation and cardiac arrest (Lee and Boucher, 2001).

Patients exercise on the treadmill or bicycle until they reach a target heart rate or demonstrate symptoms of hypotension, ventricular dysrhythmias, ST segment changes, or chest pain. The degree of ST segment changes and the level of exercise at which they occur, and the patient's symptoms and hemodynamic changes (e.g., blood pressure, heart rate), all are considered in determining the severity of CAD and the patient's functional status (see Boxes 4-2 and 4-3). A positive stress test may warrant cardiac catheterization with coronary arteriography. Complications of exercise testing include syncope, hypotension, dysrhythmia, and death.

Exercise ECGs tend to be less reliable in predicting CAD in women because there are differences in the response of men and women to exercise (Julian and Wenger, 1997). For example, both men and women demonstrate an increased left ventricular stroke volume (SV), but women tend to achieve increased SV by increasing

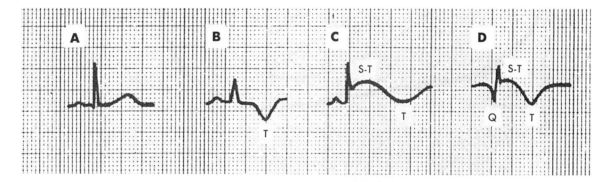

FIGURE 4-2 ECG wave changes indicative of ischemia, injury, and necrosis of the myocardium. **A,** Normal left ventricular wave pattern. **B,** Ischemia indicated by inversion of the T wave. **C,** Ischemia and current of injury indicated by T wave inversion and ST segment elevation. The ST segment may be elevated above or depressed below the baseline, depending on whether the tracing is from a lead facing toward or away from the infarcted area and depending on whether epicardial or endocardial injury occurs. Epicardial injury causes ST segment elevation in leads facing the epicardium. Intraoperatively ST segment changes may indicate temporary or permanent ischemic injury resulting from the presence of air in the coronary arteries, a vascular clamp placed too close to a coronary ostium, or incomplete surgical revascularization. **D,** Ischemia, injury, and myocardial necrosis. The Q wave indicates necrosis of the myocardium. (From Andreoli KG and others: *Comprehensive cardiac care,* ed 6, St Louis, 1987, Mosby.)

left ventricular end-diastolic volume, with little change in the left ventricular ejection fraction (the percentage of blood within the left ventricle expelled with each contraction). Men are more likely to increase SV by increasing their ejection fraction (Table 4-3). Current guidelines do not recommend replacing the stress test with nuclear imaging as the first evaluation method in women (Lee and Boucher, 2001; Gibbons and others, 1999)

Patients unable to perform physical exercise may be pharmacologically "stressed" through the administration of vasodilators such as dipyridamole and adenosine, which unmask coronary narrowing by promoting increased blood flow in nondiseased coronary arteries. Another agent is dobutamine, a positive inotropic agent that provokes ischemia by increasing myocardial work. Administration of these drugs increases perfusion to myocardium supplied by coronary arteries without significant stenosis but does not increase the blood supply to areas supplied by an obstructed coronary artery. After administration of the drug, the heart is assessed.

RADIOGRAPHY

Posteroanterior (PA), anteroposterior (AP), and lateral chest radiographs provide information about the size, shape, and positioning of the heart, the ribs, and the great vessels, such as the aorta, the pulmonary vessels, and the vena cavae (Malarkey and McMorrow, 2000). Chest films can detect the presence of calcium (on valves, in the aorta, or in coronary arteries), implants, wires, and catheters (Table 4-4). In patients with coarctation of the

TABLE 4-3
Gender Difference in Hemodynamic Responses to Exercise

VARIABLE	WOMEN	MEN
Systolic blood pressure	+++	++++
Left ventricular end-diastolic volume	+ (most)	0 (most)
	0 (some)	− (some)
Left ventricular end-systolic volume	0 (most)	−
	− (some)	
Left ventricular ejection fraction	0 (many)	++
	+ (some)	

From Julian DG, Wenger NK: *Women & heart disease,* St Louis, 1997, Mosby.

TABLE 4-4
X-ray Image Densities of Intrathoracic Structures

METAL OR BONE (WHITE)	STRUCTURES OR FLUID (GRAY)	AIR (BLACK)
Ribs, clavicle, sternum, spine	Blood	Lung
Calcium deposits	Heart	
Surgical wires or clips	Veins	
Prosthetic valves	Arteries	
Pacemaker, ICD	Edema	
Pacemaker wires		

ICD, Internal cardioverter defibrillator.
Modified from Thelan LA and others: *Critical care nursing: diagnosis and management,* ed 2, St Louis, 1994, Mosby.

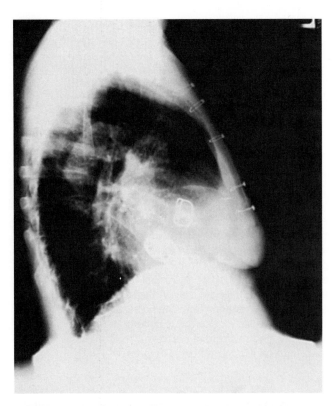

FIGURE 4-3 Lateral chest x-ray film. (From Meeker MH, Rothrock JC: *Alexander's care of the patient in surgery,* ed 11, St Louis, 1999, Mosby.)

aorta, rib notching may be evident on the left side of the thorax because of the tortuous path of hypertrophied intercostal arteries.

Because blood, myocardium, and other cardiac tissues have similar radiodensities, the normal heart provides a homogenous shadow with little internal detail. Detection of cardiac (or pulmonary) disease depends mainly on changes in the silhouette of the heart and great vessels. Dilation of one or more chambers may be caused by myocardial weakening or volume overloading, and a characteristic bulging can be seen on the radiograph. Ventricular hypertrophy shows little change on the chest film because as the myocardial wall thickens, it tends to extend inward and encroach on the chamber lumen; occasionally blunting or rounding of the cardiac apex can be seen (Baron, 2000). A recognizable change in the cardiac outline becomes apparent only after the hypertrophied wall starts to dilate.

Cardiac size is assessed by calculating the cardiothoracic ratio, which is the relationship between the transverse cardiac diameter and the widest diameter of the chest. Generally the cardiac diameter is approximately 50% of the thoracic diameter on inhalation. Traditionally a ratio of heart size to chest size greater than 50% was considered evidence of cardiac "enlargement." However,

some authors (Baron, 2000) have recommended that a 60% ratio be employed as the top normal value because body builds vary widely and some radiographic techniques (e.g., portable and supine radiographs) tend to magnify the image of the heart.

Assessing the pulmonary portion of the chest film provides information about the lungs, such as the presence of chronic obstructive pulmonary disease (COPD), effusion, or malignant lesions, which may contraindicate or change the timing of surgery. Tumors or other mediastinal masses may be apparent and if present also should be investigated before the planned cardiac procedure is performed.

The most recent, as well as previously taken, chest x-ray films should be available for review at the time of surgery (as a hard copy of the film or in electronically retrievable format). In patients with prior sternal operations, lateral chest x-ray films can demonstrate chest wires, the proximity of the heart to the sternum, and the extent of pericardial adhesions (Fig. 4-3).

ECHOCARDIOGRAPHY

Echocardiography (echo) is one of the most widely used diagnostic cardiovascular imaging techniques. It is often considered the initial imaging procedure of choice for assessing cardiac chamber and great vessel morphology, and two-dimensional echocardiography is the "gold standard" for the diagnosis of mitral stenosis (Nishimura, Gibbons, and Tajik, 2001). For assessing left ventricular function, echocardiography displays the most versatility, offers considerable additional information, and has the lowest cost compared with most other imaging studies (Beller, 2001).

High-frequency sound waves are transmitted from a probe (the transducer) to the heart and surrounding structures. These ultrasound waves bounce off the internal organ, echo back to the transducer, and are electronically converted into waveforms or images that are displayed on a monitor or videotape (Doty, 2000). The transducer may be positioned over the sternum (transthoracic), inside the esophagus behind the heart (transesophageal), or over the exposed heart during surgery (epicardial). When positioned directly on the heart, the transducer is placed in a sterile plastic sheath and kept on the operative field.

Because echocardiography is portable, noninvasive, provides immediate (real-time) information, and does not require the use of ionizing radiation, it is especially attractive for the assessment of many conditions in both children and adults. Studies can be videotaped for future study, but direct digital acquisition capability has improved storage and retrieval of images. The family of echocardiographic tests in-

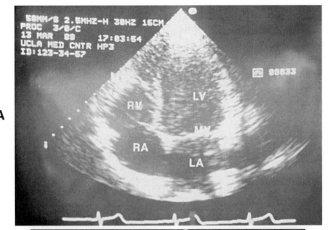

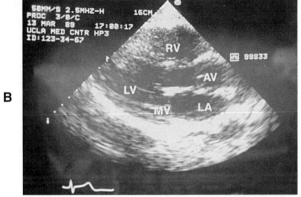

FIGURE 4-4 Two-dimensional echocardiography. Labels have been added to identify the structures. **A,** Short-axis view. **B,** Long-axis view. *RA,* Right atrium; *RV,* right ventricle; *LA,* left atrium; *LV,* left ventricle; *MV,* mitral valve. (From Canobbio MM: *Cardiovascular disorders,* St Louis, 1990, Mosby.)

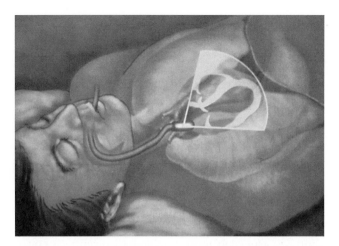

FIGURE 4-5 Transesophageal echocardiography is performed with the probe positioned in the esophagus; this allows a view of the cardiac chambers that is unobstructed by the sternal bone. (Courtesy Hewlett-Packard Co., Palo Alto, Calif.)

cludes M-mode, two-dimensional (2-D), Doppler, color flow, and stress echocardiography. Three-dimensional (3-D) imaging and intravascular ultrasound are also available.

M-mode recordings display one-dimensional time-motion (*M* for motion) views of the heart. The earliest form of cardiac ultrasound, M-mode is used to identify the timing of events during the cardiac cycle (Barasch, 2000). M-mode echocardiography can provide a limited, quantitative measurement of the systolic and diastolic dimensions of the ventricles (an "ice pick" view [Doty, 2000]). The M-mode technique now is used mainly for very precise timing measurements when 2-D imaging cannot provide the necessary temporal resolution; examples include the timing of a regurgitant valve and the rate of blood flow into the left ventricle. Color can be superimposed on M-mode techniques (Armstrong and Feigenbaum, 2001).

Two-dimensional echocardiograms visualize more of the heart and provide cross-sectional images along numerous planes (Fig. 4-4), most commonly the precordial

sagittal plane (long-axis view of the heart and great vessels) and the transverse plane (short-axis view of the heart and great vessels). Spatial anatomic relationships between cardiac chambers, wall motion abnormalities, valvular movement, anatomic alterations, and the dynamic geometry of cardiac contractions can be visualized, and 2-D echocardiograms are ideal for assessing left ventricular size and function. *Transthoracic* echocardiographic (TTE) imaging is obtained with a handheld transducer placed directly on the chest wall. In patients with thick chest walls, large breasts, or severe lung disease, it is difficult to obtain high-quality images with TTE. *Transesophageal* echocardiography (TEE) offers a better "window" through which to view the heart because there is less excess tissue or bone between the transducer and the heart; thus it provides a relatively unimpeded view of the posterior cardiac structures (Fig. 4-5).

TEE has become an important adjunct during surgery and is routinely employed to establish a baseline for ventricular function, assess the need for repair versus replacement of cardiac valves, and evaluate the effectiveness of a valve repair. TEE also can be used to detect the presence of residual intracardiac air (seen as bright white specks); additional venting maneuvers then can be performed by the surgeon to remove remaining air bubbles that could otherwise embolize to the brain (Shively, 2000).

With the addition of *Doppler* ultrasound, sound waves echo back from moving red blood cells at different velocities, allowing blood flow to be heard and visualized. Information is provided on pulmonary and intracardiac blood pressures, transvalvular gradients, septal shunts, valve areas, and valvular stenosis and regurgitation. The addition of *color* illustrates the direction, velocity, and flow patterns of the blood. Flow moving toward the transducer is seen in shades of red; flow away from the transducer is seen as blue; greater intensity or hue of the color parallels the flow velocity (Armstrong and Feigenbaum, 2001). Turbulent flow may be yellow or green. Color Doppler is especially useful for diagnosing acquired and congenital abnormalities of cardiac structures and hemodynamic function.

Three-dimensional echocardiography (through either a TTE or TEE window) incorporates different reference views to achieve a 3-D picture. Although the time required to process the 3-D image and the lack of clear resolution currently limit widespread use, 3-D has advantages, especially in unusually shaped ventricles or in complex congenital lesions.

Stress echocardiography enables the clinician to compare myocardial function at rest and after physical exercise (or after pharmacologic stress with dobutamine or dipyridamole). Transthoracic baseline images are obtained while the patient is at rest and during or immediately (1 to 2 minutes) after exercise. A test is considered positive if abnormalities develop with stress in a previously normal image or if there is worsening in an abnormal baseline image. Stress echocardiography is indicated mainly to confirm the presence of coronary artery disease and to estimate its severity, although it may provide additional information in patients with valvular heart disease (Nishimura, Gibbons, and Tajik, 2001). The test may be especially useful in high-risk patients, such as those who have marked myocardial ischemia at low exercise levels. Low-risk patients (no angina, minimum or no ischemia with exercise) may receive no additional benefit from exercise echocardiography versus stress ECG (Lee and Boucher, 2001).

Intravascular ultrasonography (IVUS) is used mainly in the cardiac catheterization laboratory during coronary angiography. A very small transducer is incorporated into the tip of an intracardiac catheter. Angiographic IVUS catheters are small enough to be introduced into the epicardial coronary arteries, where the operator can visualize the shape and character of the coronary lumen. Some of the uses for IVUS include assessment of coronary calcification and atherosclerosis, determination of the position of the plaque within the coronary lumen (e.g., concentric or eccentric), confirmation (or refutation) of the angiographic estimation of the degree of stenosis, and postinsertion evaluations of intracoronary stentings (Popma and Bittl, 2001).

Technologic advances in echocardiography have improved access to images and enhanced the quality of those images. *Digital conversion* of images makes storage, retrieval, and playback easier. *Harmonic imaging* improves visualization of the myocardium by increasing

the range of ultrasound frequencies. *Contrast echocardiography* uses a contrast agent (saline is the simplest agent), which is agitated to form *microbubbles;* the bubbles increase the reflection of the ultrasound waves, thereby improving the clarity of the image.

CARDIAC NUCLEAR IMAGING

Nuclear studies are used to test myocardial perfusion, function, and metabolism and are widely applied to assess ischemic heart disease. When an ECG stress test (or stress echocardiography) cannot be performed because the patient is unable to undergo physical or pharmacologic stress or when an ECG or echo stress test is contraindicated because of potentially lethal conduction disturbances, nuclear imaging with pharmacologic stress is considered an appropriate initial test for CAD (Nishimura, Gibbons, and Tajik, 2001).

All nuclear cardiology studies depend on injecting the patient intravenously with an isotope that emits photons as the isotope decays into progressively lower energy levels. A special camera images the photons that are emitted from the isotope. The two most commonly used isotopes are technetium-99 (Tc-99) (which has a half-life of 6 hours), and thallium-201 (T-201) (which has a half-life of 73 hours). The advantages of thallium imaging include lower cost and more widespread experience using the isotope for imaging. However, because of its shorter half-life, higher energy level (which reduces scatter and absorption of photons), better imaging quality (especially in women), and shorter imaging time, technetium is often a more desirable imaging agent for assessing ventricular function.

Technetium angiography is performed by labeling the red blood cells with the isotope, which enters damaged myocardial cells, creating "hot spots." The technetium is combined with tracer agents (most commonly sestamibi) that allow the isotope to cross cell membranes by diffusion and enter functioning mitochondria. Measuring the initial distribution of these tracers within the cardiac cells correlates to myocardial blood flow and provides an assessment of myocardial viability. Images obtained 3 to 4 hours later assess cellular viability (and are unrelated to blood flow). A defect observed in the initial scan that resolves in the later image indicates viable myocardium (Fig. 4-6). Defects that persist in the subsequent scan suggest myocardial injury or death (Lee and Boucher, 2001).

Computer-assisted technetium scanning of the ventricle in motion is performed with multiple-uptake gated acquisition (MUGA) studies. Sequential photographs are taken during systole and diastole and are synchronized to the ECG. By "gating" the images, cardiac motion (which would produce an unclear picture)

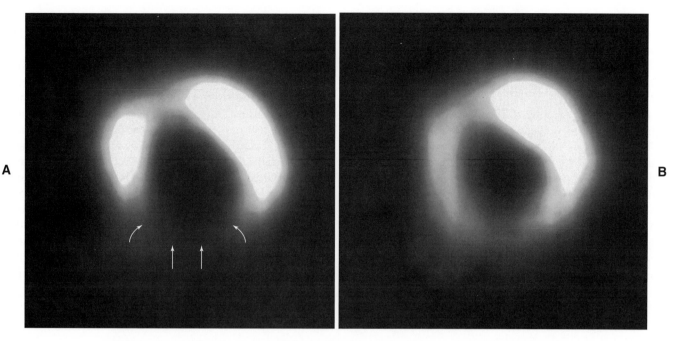

FIGURE 4-6 Technetium-sestamibi single photon emission computed tomography (SPECT) images of the heart after stress and at rest. **A,** During stress (exercise), the ventricular inferior wall demonstrates reduced uptake of isotope *(arrows)*. **B,** Normal distribution of isotope is seen in the resting image. (Courtesy Frederick J. Schwab, MD.)

is minimized. The ejection fraction can be calculated with this technique; regional and global ventricular wall motion and regurgitant valve lesions can be evaluated by comparing sequential images.

Myocardial perfusion imaging at rest and during stress (exercise or pharmacologic stress with dobutamine, adenosine, or dipyridamole) can be achieved with both thallium and technetium. Thallium enters the cell like its analogue, potassium, and is distributed throughout the myocardium, reflecting regional blood flow. Thallium is injected into the bloodstream after vigorous exercise, which is continued to stress the heart and circulate the thallium. The heart is scanned for perfusion defects ("cold spots"), indicating the absence of blood flow. If there are no defects, the test is negative. If a defect is present, the patient is scanned again within a few hours. If at that time the defect has taken up the thallium, the area is considered to be ischemic; if the defect persists, infarction is thought to have occurred. In patients with a persistent defect but without a known prior infarction or electrocardiographic evidence of infarction, delayed thallium scanning may be performed 24 hours later to differentiate between stunned and scarred myocardium. Because it may not be feasible to perform another test a day or more later, thallium may be reinjected just after redistribution imaging is performed. The purpose is to differentiate between viable but jeopardized myocardium. The dis-

tinction is important for determining the appropriateness of myocardial revascularization because coronary artery bypassing is effective for ischemic but not infarcted myocardium.

Ejection fraction and regional wall motion also can be assessed with gating of single photon emission computed tomographic (SPECT) myocardial perfusion images using thallium or technetium-sestamibi. Anatomic slices are reconstructed by computer, and both color and monochrome images can be created (Goldin, Ratib, and Aberle, 2000). In addition to simultaneously evaluating global left ventricular function, myocardial perfusion, and regional wall thickening, gated SPECT imaging also has enhanced the detection of coronary artery disease in patients with chest pain (Beller, 2001).

Positron emission tomography (PET) measures myocardial blood flow and metabolism with the introduction of very high energy photons. These photons are recorded by a series of detectors placed in a ring around the patient. Metabolic activity and myocardial viability are detected by measuring the hypoperfused myocardium's preferential use of glucose (rather than fatty acid or lactate—the heart's normal metabolic substrate). PET can differentiate ischemic or hibernating myocardium from infarcted tissue and is regarded as the gold standard for assessing myocardial viability. PET cameras are more expensive than conventional nuclear imaging devices, and the very short half-life of the radionuclides restricts use of PET imaging to specific situations where it is most beneficial (Goldin, Ratib, and Aberle, 2000).

COMPUTED TOMOGRAPHY

Computed tomography (CT) is a method of scanning the density of tissue with multiple narrow x-ray beams. These beams are blocked by the tissue in proportion to the density of the tissue. A three-dimensional image is formed by computer analysis and transferred to x-ray film or digital format (Fig. 4-7). Contrast material often is added to enhance the clarity of the images. Scans are taken at multiple levels to provide "slices" of tissue during multiple phases of the cardiac cycle. CT scanning, with or without the injection of radioactive substances, can be used to identify cardiac, thoracic, abdominal, and distal aortic aneurysms, intracardiac tumors, and calcium; it also can be used to assess the patency of coronary arterial bypass grafts. This imaging technique

is one of the best methods for determining cardiac chamber and great vessel morphology (Higgins, 2001).

Electron beam computed tomography (EBCT) is an ultrafast technique that provides enhanced imaging of global and regional myocardial mass and wall thickness. It also can be used to detect and quantify coronary artery calcium. This very rapid (e.g., in 50 *milliseconds*) imaging technique eliminates cardiac motion artifact (and removes the need for ECG gating). The CT image is then scored to arrive at a predictive value for coronary atherosclerosis. Limitations of EBCT (e.g., variability, inconsistent reproducibility) and lack of consensus regarding the predictive value of EBCT scores for correlating coronary calcification to subsequent atherosclerotic coronary events have produced some debate about the appropriate use of EBCT (Goldin, Ratib, and Aberle, 2000; Higgins, 2001, Halberl and others, 2001). Lending support to the use of EBCT is a study of 1764 patients by Halberl and colleagues (2001), which found that the negative predictive value of EBCT was

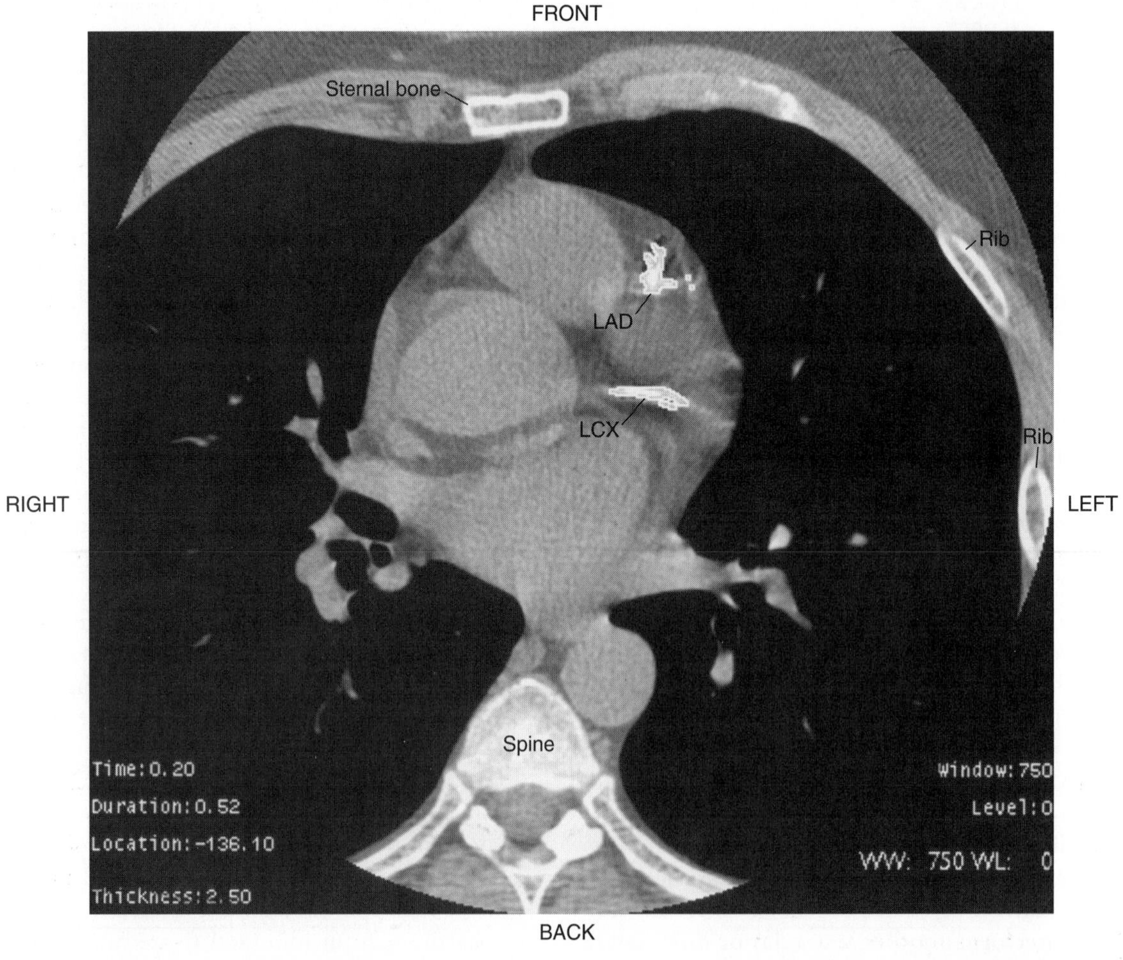

FIGURE 4-7 High-resolution cross-sectional CT scan of the heart showing dense calcification in the area of the left anterior descending (LAD) coronary artery and left circumflex (LCX) coronary artery. (Courtesy Frederick J. Schwab, MD.)

extremely good (i.e., individuals with very low or zero scores did not have significant coronary artery disease).

MAGNETIC RESONANCE IMAGING

Magnetic resonance imaging (MRI) acts on the magnetic field created by spinning atomic particles within the body. A powerful external magnetic field is applied, which aligns these particles. The patient is placed within a cylindrical scanner (the MRI tube) containing the magnet. When the magnetic field is removed, the particles return to their former position. MRI measures these changes and thereby provides details about anatomy and function. The technique is used to evaluate the heart and great vessels and the abdominal aorta in patients with acquired and congenital cardiovascular disease. Wall motion abnormalities and myocardial ischemia and infarction can be imaged. Image-guided surgery with MRI has been performed for neurosurgical patients (Leblanc, Aubry, and Gervin, 1999), and the ability to use MRI technology to measure blood vessel density, vessel permeability, and blood flow is likely to be applied to cardiovascular interventions (Tempany and McNeil, 2001).

An advantage of MRI is that neither contrast media nor ionizing radiation is needed (although the former can be added—see the following). Disadvantages include the claustrophobic environment and the need to remain very still during the procedure, which may be difficult in highly anxious or very young patients. Sedation may be required. As a result of powerful magnetic forces exerted during the procedure, the presence of metallic implants (e.g., pacemakers, cerebral aneurysm clips) in a patient are generally a contraindication for MRI, although most prosthetic valves and vascular stents that have been in place for at least 6 weeks are acceptable (Lee, 2001).

Contrast-enhanced, three-dimensional images make MR imaging especially valuable for diagnosing thoracic aortic diseases such as aneurysm and coarctation, as well as congenital heart disease. Magnetic resonance angiographic (MRA) techniques—using intravenous contrast agents, multiple detectors, and faster acquisition speeds—to image coronary vessels and congenital anomalies will enhance the ability to make accurate diagnoses (Fig. 4-8). Improvements in techniques are likely to promote greater use of MR imaging for the noninvasive assessment of coronary artery disease (Goldin, Ratib, and Aberle, 2000).

CARDIAC CATHETERIZATION

Although some intracardiac pressures and coronary artery anatomy can be evaluated with noninvasive techniques such as MRI and echocardiography, diagnostic cardiac catheterization remains the gold standard for defining the presence or severity of obstructive coronary artery disease. Cardiac catheterization in patients with discrete valvular or congenital heart disease may be performed only after an initial full echocardiographic evaluation; however, many clinicians continue to rely on cardiac catheterization as a beneficial adjunctive diagnostic technique in patients with valvular heart disease. For patients with congenital lesions, gross cardiac anatomy can be defined well with MRI and echocardiography, but catheterization may be required for calculating hemodynamic information (Table 4-5) such as shunt size, pulmonary vascular resistance, and intracardiac blood flow and pressures (Davidson and Bonow, 2001).

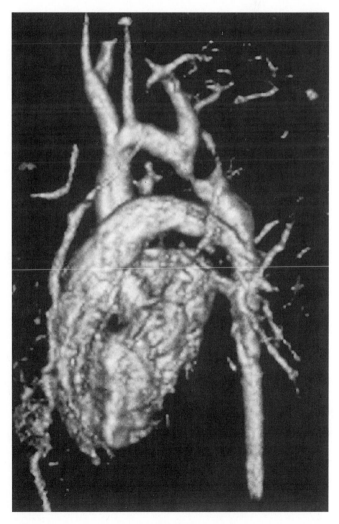

FIGURE 4-8 Three-dimensional MR angiogram of the heart and great vessels. (From Braunwald E, Zipes DP, Libby P, editors: *Heart disease,* ed 6, Philadelphia, 2001, WB Saunders.)

TABLE 4-5
Cardiac Catheterization Data

HEMODYNAMIC DATA	NORMAL VALUES

Flow

Cardiac output (CO)	4.0–8.0 L/min
Cardiac index (CI)	2.5-4.0 L/min/m²
Ejection fraction (EF)	60%–70%
Left ventricular end-diastolic volume (LVEDV)	90–180 ml
Stroke volume (SV)	60–130 ml/beat
Stroke volume index (SVI)	35–70 ml/beat/m²

	SYSTOLIC	DIASTOLIC	MEAN
Resistances			
Systemic vascular resistance (SVR)	<20 Wood units		
Total pulmonary resistance	<3.5 Wood units		
Pulmonary vascular resistance (PVR)	<2.0 Wood units		

Shunts (Q_P/Q_S)

Pulmonary flow/systemic flow		1:1

Oxygen Saturations

Venae cavae	70%
Right atrium	70%
Right ventricle	70%
Pulmonary artery	70%
Pulmonary veins	97%
Left atrium	97%
Left ventricle	97%
Aorta	97%

Valve Orifices (Adult)

Aortic	2–4 cm²
Mitral	4–6 cm²
Tricuspid	10 cm²

Pressures (mm Hg)

	SYSTOLIC	DIASTOLIC	MEAN
Venae cavae			0–5
Right atrium (RA)			2–6
Right ventricle (RV)	20–30	0–5	
Pulmonary artery (PA)	20–30	10–20	10–15
Pulmonary artery wedge pressure (PAWP)			4–12
Left atrium (LA)			4–12
Left ventricle (LV)	120	0–5	
Left ventricular end-diastolic pressure (LVEDP)			5–12
Aorta	120–140	60–80	70–90
Brachial artery	120	70	
Femoral artery	125	75	

Angiographic Data	FINDINGS
Coronary arteries	Anatomy/function coronary vascular bed; distal coronary flow; AV fistula; atherosclerosis; anomalous origin of coronary arteries
Ventriculography	Anatomy/function of ventricles and associated structures; LV aneurysm; congenital abnormalities; valvular stenosis/regurgitation; shunts
Valvular angiography	Intact mitral/tricuspid complex; valvular incompetence/stenosis/regurgitation
Pulmonary angiography	Pulmonary embolism; congenital abnormalities
Aortography	Patency of aortic branches; normal mobility, competence, and anatomy of aortic valve; aneurysms: saccular, fusiform; origin of aortic dissection; shunts or anomalous connections; congenital defect or obstructions

From Meeker MH, Rothrock JC: *Alexander's care of the patient in surgery,* ed 11, St Louis, 1999, Mosby.

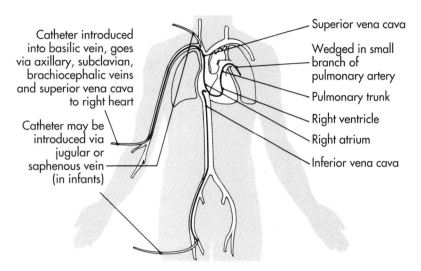

Catheter introduced into basilic vein, goes via axillary, subclavian, brachiocephalic veins and superior vena cava to right heart

Catheter may be introduced via jugular or saphenous vein (in infants)

Superior vena cava

Wedged in small branch of pulmonary artery

Pulmonary trunk

Right ventricle

Right atrium

Inferior vena cava

FIGURE 4-9   Right-sided heart catheterization. The heart is approached from the basilic vein (Sones technique) or the femoral vein (Judkins technique). (From Kern MJ: *The cardiac catheterization handbook,* St Louis, 1991, Mosby.)

Because the indications for cardiac catheterization are changing with improvements in other imaging modalities, guidelines for diagnostic coronary angiography have been developed to identify which diseases and conditions are more (or less) appropriate for cardiac catheterization (Scanlon and others, 1999). In general, patients with known or suspected CAD (including myocardial infarction) and those with coronary anomalies are considered candidates, especially if surgical or nonsurgical interventions for coronary, valvular, or congenital conditions are planned. Studies also may be performed to assess coronary artery spasm or thrombosis, left ventricular (LV) dysfunction, ischemic valvular disorders, LV aneurysm, or cardiomyopathy.

In addition to diagnostic assessment, interventional catheterization procedures (e.g., angioplasty, stent insertion, coronary atherectomy) are performed for patients with CAD. Other procedures include balloon dilation of stenotic valves or blood vessels and umbrella or coil occlusion of atrial or ventricular septal defects, patent ductus arteriosus, or coarctation of the aorta.

Catheterization is performed by inserting catheters into arteries or veins and threading them to the heart to obtain x-ray movies (cineangiograms) of cardiac chambers and coronary arteries and to measure intracardiac and intravascular pressures. Various insertion sites may be used depending on the age of the patient, the anatomy, and the information required. Among these are the femoral artery or vein in the groin (Judkins technique); the median basilic vein and brachial artery in the antecubital fossa (Sones technique); the

subclavian, saphenous, or jugular vein; and, in neonates, the umbilical artery and vein (Kern, 1999). The femoral artery is generally the preferred entry site because of the ease of insertion and relatively few complications, but aortoiliac disease or other lower-extremity vascular problems may necessitate the use of arm veins.

Right-sided heart catheterization (Fig. 4-9) is indicated for patients with intracardiac shunts, pulmonary disease, a history of dyspnea, or right-sided cardiac valve disorders. The catheter is inserted percutaneously (or via cutdown when necessary) into the femoral or basilic vein, threaded to the respective vena cava, and passed into the right atrium. Contrast media may be injected to opacify defects or shunts, and pressures are recorded. Blood samples from the venae cavae and right atrium may be taken to measure oxygen saturations when atrial septal defects, anomalous pulmonary venous return, or other shunts are suspected. The catheter is advanced into the right ventricle and the outflow tract and then through the pulmonary valve to the proximal and distal pulmonary arteries. Anatomic information and hemodynamic data, including blood pressures, blood oximetry, and cardiac output, are recorded.

Left-sided heart catheterization (Fig. 4-10) is performed to study CAD, cardiomyopathy, pericardial constriction, left-sided valvular lesions, and congenital abnormalities. The catheter is inserted into the femoral or brachial artery and threaded in retrograde fashion to the ascending aorta. Coronary arteriograms and left ventriculograms then can be performed.

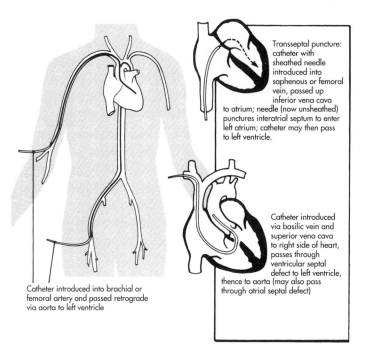

Transseptal puncture: catheter with sheathed needle introduced into saphenous or femoral vein, passed up inferior vena cava to atrium; needle (now unsheathed) punctures interatrial septum to enter left atrium; catheter may then pass to left ventricle.

Catheter introduced via basilic vein and superior vena cava to right side of heart, passes through ventricular septal defect to left ventricle, thence to aorta (may also pass through atrial septal defect)

Catheter introduced into brachial or femoral artery and passed retrograde via aorta to left ventricle

FIGURE 4-10 Left-sided heart catheterization. The heart is approached from the brachial (Sones technique) or femoral (Judkins technique) artery. The left side of the heart also can be approached via the right side with a catheter passed through an atrial or ventricular septal defect. (From Kern MJ: *The cardiac catheterization handbook,* St. Louis, 1991, Mosby.)

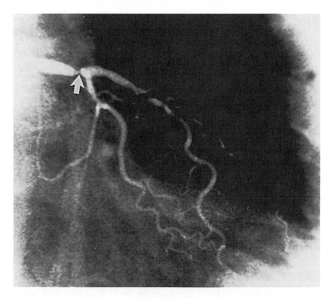

FIGURE 4-11 Cineangiographic (moving picture) frame showing left main coronary artery stenosis *(arrow)* in the RAO projection. (From Kern MJ: *The cardiac catheterization handbook,* St Louis, 1991, Mosby.)

Coronary arteriography is performed by selectively injecting dye into the right and left coronary ostia. Obstructions, flow, and distal perfusion ("run-off") are evaluated. To maximize clarity, each vessel is viewed from several angles and recorded so that arteries overlapping one another in one position may be visualized clearly from a different angle. The right anterior oblique (RAO) projection provides good visualization of the left main coronary artery (Fig. 4-11). This projection at 30 degrees also offers a clear view of the left anterior descending (LAD) coronary artery, LAD septal perforators, and the circumflex system. A 45-degree RAO demonstrates the right coronary artery and posterior descending (interventricular) coronary artery (Fig. 4-12). The left anterior oblique (LAO) projection at 55 to 60 degrees is used to study the mid and distal LAD coronary artery, as well as the diagonal branches of the LAD. Depending on the lesion, cranial and caudal projections also may be recorded.

Intravascular ultrasound can provide detailed information about the coronary vessel wall, including plaque histology and stability. This can be especially useful in selecting the appropriate-size angioplasty balloon or coronary stent for small vessels and long coronary lesions.

Coronary anomalies may be identified, such as the left main coronary artery arising from the right sinus of Valsalva (instead of its normal take-off from the left sinus), the right coronary artery arising from the left sinus of Valsalva, or the presence of only one main coronary artery arising from the aorta. Such anomalies are significant for a variety of reasons, among them that

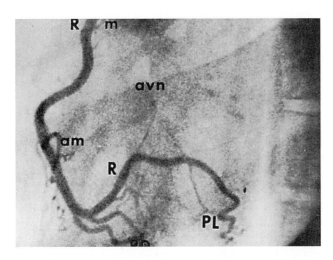

FIGURE 4-12 Coronary angiogram of a normal right coronary artery in the RAO position. *R (top)*, Proximal right coronary artery; *m*, main right artery; *am*, acute marginal coronary artery; *avn*, atrioventricular nodal artery; *R (bottom)*, distal right coronary artery; *PL*, posterior lateral coronary artery. (From Canobbio MM: *Cardiovascular disorders*, St Louis, 1990, Mosby.)

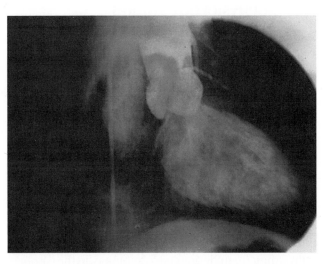

FIG. 4-13 Left ventriculogram in the RAO position. Note opacification of the aortic valve and the sinuses of Valsalva. (From Kern MJ: *The cardiac catheterization handbook*, St Louis, 1991, Mosby.)

patients with proximal obstructions of a single large coronary artery are at increased risk of myocardial infarction, and pediatric patients being considered for arterial switch procedures to repair transposition of the great arteries may need to undergo an alternative operation.

Left ventriculography is performed by passing a catheter through the aortic valve into the left ventricle. Rarely the left ventricle also may be approached through a transseptal puncture from the right atrium. When congenital atrial or ventricular septal defects are present, the physician may use these openings to enter the left side of the heart from the right side.

Blood sampling and pressure measurements are performed. Ventricular wall motion is studied by injecting dye into the ventricular chamber (Fig. 4-13); this demonstrates regional and global wall motion and displays areas that may be hypokinetic (weakly contractile), akinetic (not contractile), or dyskinetic (paradoxic motion such as that seen with left ventricular aneurysms). Shunts and regurgitating blood are revealed. The cardiac output and ejection fraction are estimated.

Cardiac valves (most commonly the aortic and mitral) are studied to determine their structure and function. The cardiologist can assess valvular orifice size, impedence to flow (stenosis), and reflux (regurgitation), as well as the structural integrity of the valvular components. Valves that have become stenotic often demonstrate some degree of regurgitation as well.

Differences in pressure behind and in front of primarily stenotic valves (the pressure gradient) can be calculated for aortic valve stenosis by simultaneously measuring the systolic blood pressure in the ascending aorta and the left ventricle. The difference in pressure (which is normally equal when the aortic valve is open) provides an indication of the severity of the stenosis. When cardiac failure is present, however, the ventricle may be too weak to generate a high intraventricular pressure and the gradient may be considerably diminished. This may be apparent on the left ventriculogram as hypokinesis of the ventricular wall. Occasionally stenosis of the aortic valve may be too severe to allow transvalvular passage of the catheter from the aorta into the left ventricle; a transseptal approach from the right side may then be used, or the test may be deferred. Stenotic mitral valve gradients can be similarly computed.

Endomyocardial biopsy requires cardiac catheterization and is employed most commonly to monitor cardiac transplant rejection and to test for cardiotoxicity; occasionally it is used to diagnose cardiomyopathy or myocarditis. Bioptomes are inserted, using fluoroscopic or echocardiographic guidance, through the internal jugular vein or the femoral vein and advanced to the right atrium, threaded through the tricuspid valve, and inserted into the right ventricle. Left ventricular samples may be taken; the LV is commonly approached via femoral artery cannulation. Four to six specimens of endocardium are obtained and tested (Kern, 1999).

ELECTROPHYSIOLOGY STUDIES

Electrophysiology studies involve procedures similar to cardiac catheterization and are performed to study cardiac rhythms. Of particular concern are recurrent ventricular tachydysrhythmias and ventricular fibrillation. These often are associated with coronary artery disease, but other etiologic factors include cardiomyopathy, ventricular dysplasia, and congenital abnormalities.

The goal of the studies is to confirm the dysrhythmia, locate its origin and path of conduction, define the mechanism, and assess treatment modalities (e.g., pharmacologic, cryothermic or electrical ablation, or surgical excision or implantation of a device) (Kern, 1999).

The procedure is similar to right-sided heart catheterization. Multiple electrode catheters are placed high in the right atrium (to study sinus node impulses), in the coronary sinus (to study the bundle of His and bundle branches), and in the right ventricle (to study the Purkinje system). Occasionally catheters are placed in the left side of the heart. Ventricular tachydysrhythmias are induced by electrical stimulation of different areas of the heart that have been "mapped," and dysfunctional areas are identified. Patients considered suitable for ablative treatment or insertion of antidysrhythmia devices are referred as necessary. Direct mapping and stimulation of the epicardium and the endocardium may be performed as part of a surgical procedure.

Laboratory Tests

The referring physician who first evaluated the patient will have ordered a number of blood and urine studies in association with the initial history and physical examination (H & P). The laboratory tests described in this section are those commonly ordered on admission (or a few days before admission) in preparation for surgery. Some of these tests (e.g., coagulation studies, blood gases, electrolyte levels, and complete blood cell counts) are performed at regular intervals during surgery to monitor physiologic function (Table 4-6). Laboratory values commonly vary from institution to institution; nurses should familiarize themselves with their laboratory's normal and abnormal values.

A complete blood cell count is performed to determine the number, percentage, and oxygen-carrying capacity of red blood cells (RBCs) and to count the total number and percentage of each type of white blood cell (WBC). This provides baseline data for comparison intraoperatively and postoperatively. A low hematocrit preoperatively (normal: 42% to 52% for males, 35% to 47% for females) may require infusion of packed RBCs. Intraoperatively and immediately postoperatively, a hematocrit of 25% (or less) in adults may be well tolerated and not require infusion if intravascular volume is adequate for perfusion. A hematocrit of 60% or higher

(polycythemia) may be seen in patients with chronic hypoxia (e.g., tetralogy of Fallot), who compensate by increasing the percentage of oxygen-carrying RBCs. These patients may undergo preoperative phlebotomy to lower the hematocrit, thereby reducing blood viscosity and the risk of thromboembolism.

Blood is tested for viral contamination, including the human immunodeficiency virus (HIV) and hepatitis. Increasingly patients are donating their own blood preoperatively ("autologous predonation") to avoid the risks of homologous blood transfusions. Blood also is tested for the presence of cold antibodies, which could cause agglutination of the patient's blood when the patient is cooled intraoperatively to hypothermic temperatures.

Hematologic tests provide a detailed coagulation profile to uncover bleeding tendencies or disorders that could affect the operative course. This information creates a baseline for future comparison and enables the clinician to treat the disorder appropriately. In addition, the medication history should be reviewed because certain drugs prolong the clotting time or interfere with coagulation function (Table 4-7; Fig. 4-14). Aspirin and dipyridamole block the effectiveness of circulating platelets, thrombolytic agents (streptokinase or tissue plasminogen activator) break down clots, and warfarin (Coumadin) and heparin prolong bleeding time. Effective hemostasis can be hindered further by the destruction of platelets and clotting factors that occurs intraoperatively from the trauma to blood contacting plastic bypass tubing and suctioning devices. A low platelet count is notable and alerts the nurse to anticipate possible replacement of this blood product.

The use of herbal medicines should be investigated explicitly because some of these substances may impair coagulation, increase blood pressure, or interfere with immunosuppression regimens, which would affect organ transplantation recipients (Table 4-8) (Ang-Lee, Moss, and Yuan, 2001; Liu and others, 2000; Brumley, 2000).

Determination of electrolyte levels is important because of their effects on cardiac function. In particular, low potassium (K+) levels may trigger dysrhythmias on induction of anesthesia and throughout the perioperative period. When possible, replacement therapy is initiated before surgery to bring electrolyte levels into the normal range.

Cardiac enzymes are markers of myocardial damage (Siomko, 2000). Patients admitted for symptoms suggesting an acute myocardial infarction (AMI) undergo testing of serum cardiac enzymes to establish or exclude the diagnosis of AMI. When cardiac cells die, intracellular enzymes and other substances released into the bloodstream can be measured to provide an estimation of the rate and extent of myocardial damage. Among these are creatinine kinase (CK), myoglobin, and troponins. Lactic

TABLE **4-6**
Laboratory Data

TEST	CONVENTIONAL VALUES	TEST	CONVENTIONAL VALUES
Arterial blood gases		3–6 months old	$3.1–4.5 \times 10^6/\mu l$
pH 7.38–7.44		2–6 years old	$3.9–5.3 \times 10^6/\mu l$
Po_2 95–100 mm Hg		Adult	
Pco_2 35–40 mm Hg		Male	$4.6–6.2 \times 10^6/\mu l$
Blood chemistry		Female	$4.2–5.4 \times 10^6/\mu l$
Glucose (fasting)	70–110 mg/dl	White blood cells (WBCs)	
Protein (total)	6.8–8.5 g/dl	1 day old	$9.4–34.0 \times 10^3/\mu l$
Blood urea nitrogen		1 month old	$5.0–19.5 \times 10^3/\mu l$
(BUN)	8.0-25 mg/dl	Adult	$4.5–11.0 \times 10^3/\mu l$
Uric acid	3.0–7.0 mg/100 ml	Creatinine (urine, 24-hr)	
Cardiac enzymes		Male	20–26 mg/kg/24 hr
Creatine kinase (CK)	5–75 mU/ml	Female	14–22 mg/kg/24 hr
CK-MB (isoenzyme)	0%	Electrolytes	
Troponin T	$<0.2\ \mu g/L$	Potassium (K)	3.8–5.0 mEq/L
Troponin I	$<0.35\ \mu g/L$	Sodium (Na)	136–142 mEq/L
Coagulation profile		Chloride (Cl)	95–103 mEq/L
Platelet count	$150,000–400,000/\mu l$	Magnesium (Mg)	1.5–2.0 mEq/L
Prothrombin time (PT)	Depends on thromboplastin re-agent used: typically 9.5–12.0 sec	Lipids	
		Cholesterol	<200 mg/dl
Thrombin time	Depends on concentration of thrombin reagent used; typically 20–29 sec	Triglycerides	10–190 mg/dl
		Phospholipids	150–380 mg/dl
		Free fatty acids	9.0–15.0 mM/L
Partial thromboplastin time (PTT)	Depends on phospholipid reagent used; typically 60–85 sec	Liver function	
		Albumin (serum)	3.5–5.0 g/dl
Activated PTT	Depends on activator and phos-pholipid reagents used; typically 20–35 sec	Alkaline phosphatase	20–90 IU/L
		Globulin (serum)	2.3–3.5 g/dl
		Serum bilirubin (total)	0.2–1.4 mg/dl
Fibrinogen	200–400 mg/dl	Pulmonary function	
Fibrinogen split products	10 mg/L	*Normal values vary depending on the patient's age, sex, weight, and race. The following are generally calculated:*	
Complete cell blood count (CBC)		Residual volume (RV)	
Hemoglobin (Hgb)		Tidal volume (TV)	
1–3 days old	14.5–22.5 g/dl	Expiratory reserve volume (ERV)	
2 months old	9.0–14.0 g/dl	Inspiratory reserve volume (IRV)	
6–12 years old	11.5–15.5 g/dl	Total lung capacity (TLC)	
Adult		Vital capacity (VC)	
Male	13.5–18.0 g/dl	Urinalysis	
Female	12.0–16.0 g/dl	Color	Amber, yellow
Hematocrit (Hct)		Clarity	Clear
2 days old	48%–75%	pH	4.6–8.0
2 months old	28%–42%	Specific gravity (SG)	1.002–1.035
Adult		Protein	0.0–8.0 mg/dl
Male	42%–52%	Sugar, ketones, RBCs, WBCs, casts	Negative
Female	35%–47%		
1 week old	$3.9–6.3 \times 10^6/\mu l$		

Modified from Malarkey LM, McMorrow ME: *Laboratory tests and diagnostic procedures,* ed 2, St Louis, 2000, Mosby.

dehydrogenase (LDH), formerly routinely analyzed, is no longer recommended because it has been superceded by newer, more cardiac-specific markers such as the troponins (Antman and Braunwald, 2001).

CK has three isoenzymes, one of which, CK-MB (*MB* refers to myocardial bands), is found primarily in cardiac muscle. Elevations of CK-MB provide a specific marker of myocardial damage. The degree of CK-MB elevation can indicate myocardial injury or infarction. Two CK-MB *isoforms,* CK-MB1 and CK-MB2, have been identified that further increase the diagnostic specificity. Isoform measurements are expressed either as an absolute level or a ratio. A CK-MB2 level of 1 unit per liter of CK-MB1 or a ratio of 2.5 or greater (derived by dividing CK-MB2 by CK-MB1) may indicate infarction (Antman and Braunwald, 2001; Gavaghan, 1999).

TABLE **4-7**
Agents Affecting Coagulation and Thrombosis

AGENT	ACTION	CONSIDERATIONS
Antithrombotic Agents		
Heparin	Interacts with antithrombin III to accelerate heparin's ability to bind to and neutralize thrombin and other clotting factors, thereby inhibiting clotting	Anticoagulant of choice for rapid-acting anticoagulation; reversed by protamine sulfate. Used during cardiopulmonary bypass; requires laboratory monitoring (e.g., heparin concentration)
Low-molecular-weight heparin	Inhibits and neutralizes platelet-bound factor Xa	Less fractionated than heparin; effects on coagulation cascade restricted, thereby causing less bleeding risk. Less effective on platelet function and vascular integrity compared with heparin; does not routinely require laboratory monitoring
Warfarin (Coumadin)	Vitamin K antagonist	Most frequently used oral anticoagulant; requires laboratory monitoring to determine prothrombin time. Commonly used in patients with mechanical heart valves or atrial fibrillation
Antiplatelet Agents		
Aspirin (acetylsalicylic acid)	Blocks platelet aggregation, particularly in the arterial circulation; inhibits cyclooxygenase (COX) enzyme, which promotes platelet aggregation and vasoconstriction	Widely used, effective, relatively safe; platelet function impaired for 4–7 days after a single dose of aspirin, but prolonged bleeding time generally returns to normal within 24–48 hours of aspirin ingestion (because of bone marrow release of new platelets); used to reduce risk of coronary thrombosis
Ticlopidine (Ticlid)	Inhibits adenosine diphosphate pathway of platelet activation	Oral administration, relatively slow onset (full effect occurs in 3–5 days) and persists 4–8 days after discontinuation of the drug. Rarely causes thrombocytopenia purpura
Clopidogrel (Plavix)	Similar to ticlopidine	Similar to ticlopidine
Dipyridamole	Mechanism unclear, but may enhance effect of warfarin	Unlike aspirin, does not prolong bleeding time. May be used with warfarin to prevent prosthetic heart valve embolization
Glycoprotein (Gp) IIb/IIIa Antagonists		
Abciximab (ReoPro)	Binds fibrinogen to Gp IIb/IIIa receptor complex; monoclonal antibody with extended duration of antiplatelet activity	Used to prevent coronary restenosis and thrombus generation after coronary interventions. Administered intravenously; oral forms under development
Eptifibatide (Integrilin)	Peptide antagonist	Similar to abciximab
Thrombolytic (Fibrinolytic) Drugs		
Streptokinase	Isolated from hemolytic streptococci; forms a complex with plasminogen to enzymatically autolyse the plasminogen	Because of its bacterial source, has antigenic properties, especially in patients with previous streptococcal infections. Used for lysis of coronary thrombosis
Urokinase	Made from human fetal kidney cells; activates plasminogen to plasmin, thereby degrading fibrin and fibrinogen	Does not cause allergic reactions. Used for lysis of coronary thrombosis
Tissue-type plasminogen activator (t-Pa)	Naturally occurring molecule released from vascular endothelial cells. Promotes activation of plasminogen to plasmin localized on a fibrin clot; fibrin then becomes substrate for lysis by the plasmin generated on it surface	Used for lysis of coronary thrombosis
Reteplase (r-PA)	Variant of t-PA; has a prolonged half-life	Used for lysis of coronary thrombosis

Modified from Schafer AI, Ali NM, Levine GN: Hemostasis, thrombosis, fibrinolysis, and cardiovascular disease. In Braunwald E, Zipes DP, Libby P, editors: *Heart disease: a textbook of cardiovascular medicine,* ed 6, Philadelphia, 2001, WB Saunders.

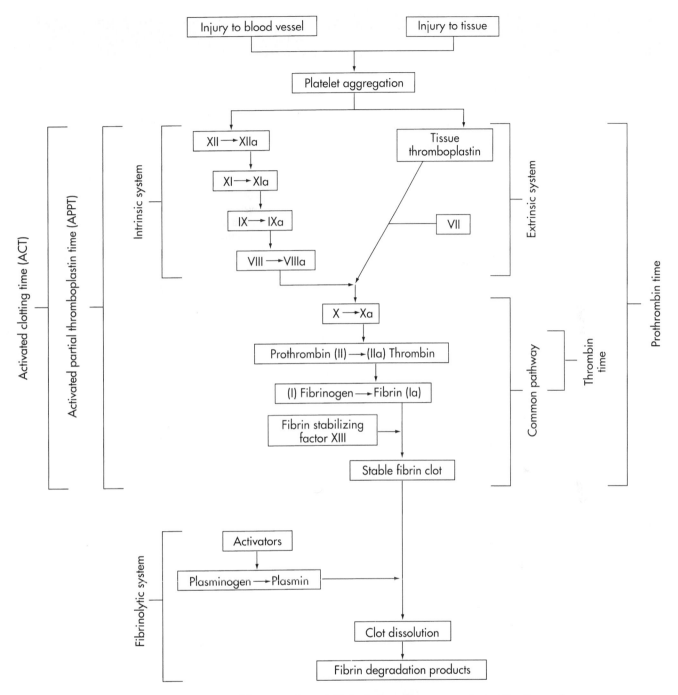

FIGURE 4-14 Process of hemostasis and fibrinolysis, with common tests of anticoagulation. Injury to the blood vessel or the tissue activates, respectively, the intrinsic and extrinsic coagulation pathways, which join to form the common pathway. If the coagulation process is not inhibited, a fibrin clot is formed and then undergoes dissolution by the fibrinolytic system. The activated clotting time is prolonged when factors of the intrinsic or common pathway are severely decreased. Activated partial thromboplastin time is a more sensitive test; it is prolonged when the level of coagulation factors of the intrinsic and common system decreases to 10% to 40% of the normal level. Prothrombin time detects low levels of factors of the extrinsic or common system. Thrombin time is prolonged in the presence of abnormally low fibrinogen. Heparin prolongs the times of all these tests. (Modified from Pagana KD, Pagana TJ: *Mosby's diagnostic and laboratory test reference,* St Louis, 1992, Mosby.)

TABLE **4-8**
Perioperative Effects of Herbal Medicines

AGENT	PHARMACOLOGIC ACTION	CONCERNS AND CONSIDERATIONS
Echinacea (purple cone-flower root)	Activates cell-mediated immunity	Decreases effectiveness of immunosuppressants; should not be taken by organ transplant patients
Ephedra	Increases heart rate and blood pressure through sympathomimetic effects	Increases risk of stroke and myocardial ischemia; may cause intraoperative hemodynamic instability
Garlic	Inhibits platelet aggregation; increases fibrinolysis	Increases risk of bleeding, especially in combination with other platelet inhibitors
Ginkgo	Inhibits platelet activation	Increases risk of bleeding, especially in combination with other platelet inhibitors
Ginseng	Inhibits platelet activation; lowers blood glucose; has many diverse effects	Increases risk of bleeding; has potential to decrease anticoagulation effect of warfarin; may cause hypoglycemia
St John's wort	Inhibits neurotransmitter reuptake	Induces enzymes that affect warfarin and many other drugs; may affect calcium channel blockers and decrease serum digoxin levels

Modified from Ang-Lee MK, Moss J, Yuan CS: Herbal medicines and perioperative care, *JAMA* 286(2):208, 2001; Liu EH and others: Use of alternative medicine by patients undergoing cardiac-surgery, *J Thorac Cardiovasc Surg* 120:335, 2000; Brumley C: Herbs and the perioperative patient, *AORN J* 72(5):785, 2000.

Myoglobin is a low-molecular-weight heme protein that is released into the circulation from injured myocytes. They can be detected within a few hours after infarction; peak levels of serum myoglobin are reached much earlier than peak values of serum CK. Myoglobin is a less specific cardiac marker than troponin.

Three subunits of troponin have been identified that form a troponin complex. These include troponin C(TnC), which binds calcium (important for cardiac contraction); troponin I (TnI), which binds to actin (part of the cardiac contractile mechanism); and troponin T(TnT), which binds to tropomysin (part of the cardiac contractile system). Although both TnI and TnT are present in cardiac and skeletal muscle, they are encoded in different genes and differ in their amino acid sequences. This allows antibodies to be produced and quantified in assays of the markers. As each generation of the assay process undergoes refinement, the results have become increasingly more accurate in detecting myocardial injury. Clinicians should be aware of their own laboratory's range of values. In patients with AMI, TnT and TnI begin to increase above the upper limit within 3 hours of the onset of chest pain. (The majority of TnC released into the bloodstream is combined with TnI.) TnT and TnI may continue to be released for 7 to 14 days. Troponin assays can detect myocardial necrosis before CK-MB levels reach levels indicative of AMI.

Patients who have suffered a myocardial infarction preoperatively may not be able to withstand the stress of surgery; these patients may undergo more conservative treatment (e.g., coronary care monitoring, rest, antidysrhythmia medications).

Some elevation of these enzymes is seen in the postoperative patient as a result of the intraoperative trauma caused by median sternotomy, atrial cannulation, and other maneuvers performed on the heart. The clinician evaluates the degree of elevation of the CK-MB and troponin levels, in addition to other clinical signs, such as new Q waves, to determine whether perioperative myocardial infarction has occurred or whether the elevation is due to surgical trauma.

Liver and kidney function tests results may be abnormal in patients with chronic heart failure, possibly because of congestion related to right-sided failure in the former case and reduced cardiac output in the latter case. Occasionally, kidney function is affected by the injection of contrast media during cardiac catheterization. Surgery may be delayed to allow the kidneys to recover so that the anticipated additional stress from cardiopulmonary bypass does not aggravate the injury; off-pump surgery may be an alternative.

Renal function is assessed by testing blood urea nitrogen and creatinine levels. Renal failure may produce electrolyte imbalances of potassium and calcium, both of which are important for cardiac conduction and contractility. Elevated potassium levels (hyperkalemia) decrease the rate of ventricular depolarization and repolarization and depress atrioventricular conduction. Potassium levels in excess of 10 to 14 mEq per liter can lead to cardiac standstill. The effects of hyperkalemia are evident during surgery when cardiac standstill (evidenced by a flat-line ECG) is purposely induced by the infusion of hyperkalemic cardioplegia solutions.

Low potassium levels (hypokalemia) prolong the period of ventricular repolarization, allowing supraventricular and ventricular dysrhythmias to occur. Low potassium levels are commonly caused by diuretic therapy, which promotes potassium excretion.

Liver disease can affect the synthesis of clotting factors and thereby prolong bleeding times. The liver also produces enzymes, proteins, and other products vital to maintaining homeostasis; detoxifies and breaks down many endogenous and exogenous substances; and metabolizes and stores carbohydrates, proteins, and fats (Malarkey and McMorrow, 2000).

Preoperative Patient Interview

Before the preoperative patient interview, the perioperative nurse can review the admission nursing assessment in the patient's chart for background information about the patient's physical, psychologic, and social status. Because the format of the assessment questionnaire influences the data collected, the admission assessment form should reflect a holistic view of the patient, facilitate identification of nursing diagnoses, and assist the nurse in predicting patient outcomes (Seifert, 1999). The assessment form should reflect a systematic, logical, and ordered process that incorporates observation, interviewing, and physical assessment and communication skills.

Some perioperative nurses may be unaccustomed to performing a holistic evaluation of the patient. In this era of cost containment, when many patients are admitted on the morning of surgery, the perioperative clinician may be the only nurse to see the patient before surgery and to assess the patient's needs. For most patients, emotional and social needs are as important as physical needs. An assessment based on human response patterns (Thelan and others, 1994) can assist the perioperative nurse in identifying all these needs and problems (see Chapter 5). When the perioperative nurse uses a similar format based on these patterns, information is elicited that provides insight not only into the patient's physiologic condition but also into how the illness has affected psychologic and social aspects of the patient's life.

Assessing the physical, mental, and emotional needs of neonates and children should be familiar to perioperative nurses, even if their cardiac programs focus only on adults with acquired lesions (or congenital lesions becoming apparent in adulthood). When a pediatric cardiac program is not available, many heart centers that perform adult surgery may operate on babies requiring ligation of a persistent patent ductus. The procedure does not require cardiopulmonary bypass and can be performed in the operating room (OR) or neonatal intensive care unit (NICU). Although pediatric considerations are not described in detail, some guidelines are offered in this and subsequent chapters that may assist the perioperative nurse in caring for these patients and their significant others.

The order of the following patterns and the guidelines for obtaining information within each may be altered according to the perioperative nurse's judgment about the patient's condition. The initial interview can take place in the OR suite, physician's office, surgical inpatient unit, diagnostic laboratory, or some other location. In urgent or emergent situations, priority sections of the assessment form (e.g., physiologic data within the exchanging pattern) are completed first and other sections are completed at a later time (Seifert, 1996). A patient who is very young or elderly may be unable to verbalize information, and the perioperative nurse may need to depend on significant others for information about the patient's psychosocial status.

COMMUNICATING

The nurse assesses the patient and, whenever possible, the family's ability to communicate verbally and nonverbally. Does the patient understand, speak, read, and write English? If not, and if the patient is alert and oriented, is a translator available? If speech is impaired, it should be determined whether the cause is physiologic or psychologic (e.g., stroke, oral anatomic defect, severe anxiety). With very young children, the parents are interviewed and their ability to communicate is assessed; elderly patients may have children or significant others who can contribute information.

The patient may be intubated, comatose, severely short of breath, or premedicated. Nonverbal communication, such as restlessness, wanting to hold the nurse's hand, or clinging to a religious object, may be the only indicator that the patient is in distress, is anxious, or is fearful.

PERCEIVING

Sensory deficits may result from physical or emotional factors and may be related or unrelated to the illness. Information should be elicited about changes in vision, hearing, movement, smelling, and tasting.

The patient's or significant others' perceptions of the effects of the illness and the proposed surgical intervention should be determined, as well as whether the functional restrictions often imposed by cardiovascular disease influence the individual's self-perception. Self-esteem, body image, and personal identity may be affected. The inability to perform activities of daily living may lead to feelings of hopelessness and powerlessness with the realization that activities once taken for granted can no longer be accomplished. The perceived loss of control may be a source of frustration and anger in patients such as business executives, who are used to making their own decisions.

Elderly patients may be accompanied by family members or other caretakers, who should be included in the preoperative preparations. This also applies to children, who may have separation anxiety and a fear of being abandoned by their parents. Parents and other members of the family may demonstrate feelings of inadequacy or guilt about the child's illness.

FEELING

The human response pattern of feeling relates to both physical and emotional feelings. Patients often have a history of pain. Pain may be chronic (e.g., angina pectoris) or acute and unrelieved (e.g., aortic dissection). Patients with ischemic heart disease may complain of chest pain with or without radiation to the neck, jaws, and arms. Some patients complaining of chest pain typical of myocardial ischemia have angiographically normal coronary arteries, a condition called *syndrome X* (Kaski and Russo, 2000). Patients with the syndrome have normal left ventricular function despite ECG evidence of ischemia and may be subjected to an expensive and extensive array of tests and treatment. Symptomatic management may be effective, but the condition remains a public health concern. The syndrome is associated with estrogen deficiency, and the majority of patients with syndrome X are perimenopausal or postmenopausal women (Kaski and others, 1998; Kaski and Russo, 2000).

Women also tend to have atypical anginal pain: nausea, gastrointestinal discomfort, or pain at rest, during sleep, or with mental stress. The atypical nature of the symptoms in women is probably related to their presenting with symptoms at an older age than men. As a result, women tend to have more comorbid conditions (Julian and Wenger, 1997).

Patients with valvular heart disease may complain of shortness of breath, syncope, fatigue, and anginal or upper abdominal pain. Postoperatively, pain and altered comfort are commonly related to the incisions, positioning, and restrictions imposed by tubes, drains, and monitoring devices.

The nurse asks the patient about pain or discomfort, including the onset, duration, quality, location, radiation, associated symptoms, precipitating factors, and relieving factors of each symptom. Does the patient have palpitations or other cardiac rhythm disturbances? Objective manifestations of pain, such as guarding, and protective behaviors, such as moaning, crying, grimacing, or withdrawal, should be looked for. The patient's muscle tone or nervous system responses, such as changes in blood pressure, respiratory rate, pulse, and pupils, are evaluated. Diaphoresis, if present, is noted. The patient may complain of being cold. Patient complaints about any of these discomforts are significant because pain and the shivering that accompanies chilling elevate the metabolic rate and increase the workload of the heart.

Children may have unique words or expressions that denote pain and discomfort. Some children perceive themselves as feeling well. They should not be told that the surgery will make them feel better, because immediately postoperatively they will feel worse as a result of incisional pain, monitoring lines, and drainage tubes. They can be told that within a few days they will have less discomfort.

Emotional responses should be elicited as well. Fear and anxiety can affect both psychologic and physical well-being. Mental stress has been implicated in the development of myocardial ischemia (Rozanski, Blumenthal, and Kaplan, 1999; Krantz and others, 2000). The nurse elicits the expression of fears and unspecified threats from the patient, answers questions, and communicates reassurance through body language and tone of voice. Specific questions about morbidity or mortality should be directed to surgeons or attending physicians.

Occasionally patients express extreme fear that they will die during surgery. The nurse should not tell the patient that this is an unfounded fear. Rather, the nurse should allow the patient to discuss the concern. The surgeon should be informed in order to discuss the fear with the patient; a consultation with psychiatric or social services may be requested. Although unusual, surgery has been cancelled when such a situation arises.

KNOWING

The nurse may briefly assess what the patient (or family member) knows about the planned surgical intervention. Misconceptions may be uncovered that can be clarified, and expectations can be correlated to the planned interventions and outcomes. Patients are normally anxious, which may interfere with eliciting necessary information. Many patients and family members use the Internet and World Wide Web to learn about their diagnosis and its treatment (Taylor, Alman, and Manchester, 2001). Although there are many excellent Internet Web sites providing accurate information, clinicians should be alert to patients' questions or confusion caused by inaccurate or contradictory sources, inappropriate reading levels, or too much technical jargon (Jadad and Gagliardi, 1998). Reviewing material that has been downloaded or recommending Web sites that supply useful and appropriate information helps patients and significant others to increase their understanding of and their ability to deal with their condition.

Psychologic reactions to stress are often seen in the form of coping mechanisms such as denial or withdrawal. By alleviating fears and providing comfort measures, the nurse may be able to reduce the patient's overall anxiety and obtain a more accurate description of the patient's past experiences (Bednash, 2001).

The level of consciousness and orientation to person, place, and time are assessed to determine the patient's ability to understand instructions and ask questions. Assessment of knowledge and learning needs may be complicated by the patient's unreadiness to learn or the lack of adequate time to complete the evaluation. If an abbreviated assessment must be performed, learning needs should be documented so that they can be met at a later date by another member of the cardiac team. Many hospitals have a nurse who performs preoperative patient teaching; specific details about the OR can be communicated by the perioperative nurse. Communicating with the patient also allows a relationship to develop between the perioperative nurse and the patient. Knowing one of the surgical team members may allay some of the patient's fears about the unknown and fearful OR environment.

The presence of risk factors for coronary artery disease (Table 4-9) and the patient's perception and level of knowledge about these risk factors can influence the long-term results of surgery. What the patient knows and how he or she has responded to illnesses and problems in the past can provide some indication of teaching needs and future adherence to prescribed therapeutic regimens.

Newer risk factors also are being investigated. *Homocysteine* is an amino acid that in certain rare inherited defects can develop into severe hyperhomocystinemia and premature atherosclerosis. The mechanism is not known, but it may be related to endothelial toxicity, impairment of endothelial-derived relaxing factor (a vasodilator), and other arterial vasodilation mechanisms. *High-sensitivity C-reactive protein* (hs-CRP) is a marker for inflammation that plays a role in the pathogenesis of atherosclerosis. Because other inflammatory conditions (e.g., infection, rheumatic conditions) produce CRP, special care should be used in interpreting test results (Ridker, Genest, and Libby, 2001).

Information about recent medications and the patient's response to them may be elicited or reviewed in the chart. Among those of particular interest are cardiotonics, diuretics, myocardial depressants (such as antidysrhythmics, calcium channel blockers, and beta-adrenergic blockers), antibiotics, anticoagulants, immunosuppressants, antihypertensives, corticosteroids, and herbal medicines (see Table 4-8). This information is pertinent during surgery because medications can have many effects. For example, they may alter coagulation, pose an increased risk of infection, signal the potential development of dysrhythmias, influence tissue healing, and produce toxicity, sensitivity, or allergic reaction.

Information pertinent to discharge planning may require an optimum teaching environment, which is difficult to create in the immediate preoperative period. This has become more of a challenge in the era of cost containment, when patients are admitted on the day of surgery. Patient teaching may need to be performed during the preoperative screening that generally occurs a few days before surgery. It may be done via telephone, or in some cases it can take place in the physician's office or in the patient's home. The Mended Hearts, Inc., a support group for patients who have had cardiac surgery, has had to modify its visiting program as a result of these changes, and their suggestions for patient teaching include those just described, as well as establishing day or evening teaching sessions at the hospital and developing a referral system with cardiologists and surgeons. When preoperative teaching cannot be performed, the perioperative nurse can communicate the need for education on lifestyle and risk factor modifications or prescribed postoperative therapeutic regimens to the nurses caring for the patient after surgery.

To prioritize teaching needs, the nurse should determine what the patient knows, what the patient does not know, what the patient needs to know, and what the patient wants to know. Patients are often unaware of the technical details of a procedure, and many do not want vivid descriptions of sternal splitting, saphenous vein excision, or chest wiring. The nurse should respect the patient's desire to remain ignorant of those details. Conversely, some individuals are able to cope by gaining extensive knowledge of a procedure. These patients have done their "homework" and inquire about cardiopulmonary bypass or off-pump techniques and the

TABLE 4-9 **Risk Factors for Coronary Artery Disease**	
NONMODIFIABLE	MODIFIABLE
Age	Elevated serum cholesterol
Sex	Hypertension
Family history	Cigarette smoking
Race	Obesity
Menstrual status (estrogen levels may be modifiable)	Elevated serum lipids
	Diabetes mellitus
	Psychologic stress
	Personality type

Modified from Ridker PM, Genest J, Libby P: Risk factors for atherosclerotic disease. In Braunwald E, Zipes, DP, Libby P, editors: *Heart disease,* ed 6, Philadelphia, 2001, WB Saunders.

long-term patency of saphenous vein grafts versus internal mammary artery conduits. These patients can achieve a greater sense of control with knowledge about their condition and treatment plan.

Preoperatively patients need to have information that facilitates a positive experience. Patients will be less frightened and more cooperative (and release fewer endogenous catecholamines) if they are aware of the sequence of events that will take place immediately before anesthesia induction and surgery. The nurse can describe the transportation to the OR, explain the preinduction area and insertion of intravascular lines, and comment on what the patient will see, hear, and feel in the OR. The patient should be told how many people are in the room and what they do. Many patients are aware that a urinary drainage catheter is inserted, and they may ask when the catheter is inserted, if it hurts, and if they are awake when it is inserted.

Postoperatively family members may be reassured to know that they will be able to see, talk to, and touch the patient, even though the patient may be sedated. They should be aware that the patient may appear pale and feel cool and clammy. They should also be prepared for the array of tubes, lines, and drains that are used to monitor the patient and provide access for medications and blood samples.

In some cases family members or significant others may not want to see the patient in the intensive care unit (ICU). They can be reassured that there is no correct or incorrect protocol for visiting. It may be too stressful for some individuals and will only increase their (and the patient's) anxiety (Seifert, 1996).

Patients appreciate forewarning about being intubated and unable to talk. Recovered patients often mention the frustration of being alert but unable to speak. The nurse can assure the patient that alternative methods of communication will be available in the ICU.

MOVING

Cardiovascular disease can have an impact on the patient's ability to move, perform activities of daily living and self-care, sleep, and play. These alterations are often associated with symptoms of varying severity that affect the patient's functional status (see Boxes 4-1 and 4-2).

The nurse can investigate the presence and the effects of fatigue, pain, and dyspnea on sleep patterns and self-care regarding hygiene, grooming, feeding, and diversional activity. Impaired physical mobility, activity intolerance, and inability to manage a home are not uncommon in patients with a cardiac output that is insufficient to meet exercise-induced demands.

Children with severe congenital anomalies may demonstrate altered growth and development and feeding difficulties. Elderly patients frequently have joint problems that impair mobility. Postoperatively patients will have some impairment of mobility as a result of pain and the effects of positioning and immobility of 3 to 4 hours or more during surgery.

EXCHANGING

The human response pattern of exchanging relates to the patient's physical condition and includes most of the physiologic diagnoses and collaborative problems commonly encountered during surgery. The exchanging pattern also reflects many of AORN's (2001) patient outcome standards pertaining to injury, skin integrity, fluid and electrolyte balance, infection, and physiologic responses to surgery. Data within this category take priority if the patient's condition is unstable and immediate surgical intervention is indicated. Many of the findings associated with the patient's physiologic status can be anticipated by reading the H & P in the chart. On occasion this may be the only way to obtain sufficient information about the patient.

During surgery and the first few hours postoperatively, assessment of the physiologic parameters enables the nurse to anticipate alterations in cardiovascular function and act on those changes to restore physiologic stability. In assessing the patient, the nurse should identify whether the patient's condition and the presenting signs and symptoms are acute or chronic. In addition, the preoperative data should be distinguished from intraoperative and postoperative data so that the clinician can evaluate the significance of any changes or new events. Physiologic differences between the very young and the elderly should be integrated into the assessment when appropriate (Table 4-10).

General appearance

Initial inspection of the patient should focus on the ABCs of basic life support: airway, breathing, and circulation. Is the patient intubated or wearing a nasal cannula for oxygen? Does the patient's facial expression (signs of apprehension and pain) or body posture (sitting upright or leaning forward) indicate dyspnea, shortness of breath, or labored breathing? Are the neck veins distended? Is chest expansion symmetric and rhythmic? Is there nasal flaring or use of accessory respiratory muscles? Is cyanosis present? The bluish discoloration of cyanosis reflects a decreased oxygen saturation of circulating hemoglobin and may be a result of right-to-left intracardiac shunting, impaired pulmonary function, peripheral vasoconstriction from severe heart failure, or hypoxia from any cause. Clubbing of the nail beds (spongy or swollen nail bases with an angle of greater than 180 degrees between the nail and the nail

TABLE 4-10
Physiologic Features of the Very Young and the Very Old (Compared With the Adult)

VERY YOUNG	VERY OLD	VERY YOUNG	VERY OLD
Cardiovascular System		**Respiratory System—cont'd**	
MYOCARDIUM		Higher oxygen consumption	Reduced vital capacity, maximum ventilation volume
Less contractile tissue	Increased subendocardial fat		
Less compliant	Increased heart weight	Short, narrow airway obstructed easily	
Cardiac output increased by faster heart rate	Reduced resting cardiac output		
		Renal System	
VALVES		Glomeruli small and immature	Fewer functional glomeruli
Less tension created by papillary muscle	Fibrous thickening, calcification of leaflets and annulus	Tubular concentration of fluids and electrolytes diminished	Reduced renal blood flow and glomerular filtration rate
CORONARY ARTERIES		Unable to excrete increased electrolytes and hydrogen ions (acids)	Impaired ability to excrete increased amount of water and electrolytes; reduced ability to secrete hydrogen ions
Rarely, anomalies of coronary arteries	Coronary arteriosclerosis, atherosclerosis; tortuous epicardial arteries		
CONDUCTION SYSTEM		**Other**	
Impulse conduction faster	Impulse conduction slower	**TEMPERATURE CONTROL**	
		Immature regulating system: rapid heat loss	Decreased control
BLOOD VOLUME			
Total circulating amount small, volume per kilogram of body weight relatively greater	Reduced plasma volume	**METABOLIC RATE**	
	Reduced blood water content	Higher	Lower
Respiratory System		**STRESS RESPONSE**	
Inadequate cough reflex	Decreased ability to eliminate secretions	Decreased phagocytic capability of leukocytes	Limited capability to retain homeostasis
Increased chest wall compliance, decreased pulmonary compliance	Increased chest wall rigidity, decreased lung compliance	Immature immunoglobulin synthesis	Decreased adrenal activity

From Meeker MH, Rothrock JC: *Alexander's care of the patient in surgery,* ed 11, St Louis, 1999, Mosby.

base) also is associated with cyanosis and is a sign of chronic oxygen deficiency (Thelan and others, 1994).

What is the color of the skin, lips, tongue, nail beds, conjunctiva, and mucous membranes: cyanotic, pale, dusky, or jaundiced? The color may be an indication of hypotension, low cardiac output, or hepatic congestion related to right ventricular heart failure.

Skin integrity
It should be determined whether the patient has any allergies to medications, antimicrobial solutions, dressing tape, or other substances. The presence of rashes, abrasions, lacerations, bruises, petechiae, varicosities, nodules, or other lesions are noted, as well as signs of hydration, edema, elasticity, texture, turgor, mobility, and thickness. Does the skin feel cool or warm? Does the patient have a fever? Fever is significant because of the increased workload that it places on the heart.

Are there percutaneous intravascular lines? Are they patent? Is there swelling, redness, or pain at the inser-

tion site? Are there stomas or drains that should be covered during surgery?

Past surgical incision sites should be identified. Is there a bulge in the abdomen or chest indicating the presence of a pacemaker or internal defibrillator? Is there evidence of greater saphenous vein stripping or removal from previous surgery that will require the use of alternative conduits in the patient scheduled for coronary bypass grafting? Patients who have undergone a previous median sternotomy will have mediastinal adhesions that obscure anatomic landmarks; these adhesions must be cautiously dissected to avoid injury to the right ventricle or major blood vessels. Adhesions are less of a problem in patients with previous lateral thoracotomies who are scheduled for a procedure using a median sternotomy incision. These can include adults who have previously undergone closed mitral commissurotomy via a lateral incision or children who have received palliative shunts through a thoracotomy before median sternotomy for repair of the congenital defect.

The skin over dependent areas of the body, such as the heels, buttocks, sacrum, back, and occipital area of the head, is assessed, and any existing marks, lesions, or areas of breakdown are noted. Elderly or very young patients may be at increased risk for skin breakdown because their skin is less sturdy than the integumentary system of adults. Additional padding may be indicated for surgery that may last 3 or 4 hours or more. The sites where the dispersive pads are to be applied should be checked. Dispersive pads are generally applied to the buttocks, thereby avoiding bony prominences and the sacrum.

Respiratory status

It should be determined whether the patient has had anything to eat before the scheduled surgery; food or fluid in the stomach is an anesthetic risk for aspiration. The patient's respiratory rate, rhythm, and depth, as well as chest wall expansion and symmetry with respiration, are noted. Normally the adult breathes 16 to 20 times per minute; children under 1 year of age may have rates of up to 40 breaths per minute. Is the depth of breathing shallow, moderate, or deep? Neonates are obligatory nose breathers. Children are normally diaphragmatic muscle breathers; anything that compromises air flow or the movement of the diaphragm can be a source of rapid respiratory failure and can lead to cardiac dysrhythmias and arrest.

Does the patient complain of dyspnea, and is it a chronic problem or sudden in onset? Labored breathing accompanies a number of cardiac conditions; it often occurs with exertion and may be affected by position. When it occurs at rest, it is frequently a manifestation of congestive heart failure.

Paroxysmal nocturnal dyspnea occurs at night; the patient awakens with a frightening sense of suffocation. Patients with orthopnea have difficulty breathing when lying flat and may require two or more pillows for sufficient elevation to be able to sleep. These patients may become extremely anxious in the OR if left in the supine position without the head elevated. They should be offered pillows, or the bed can be elevated to facilitate breathing.

If the patient has a cough, is it productive or nonproductive? Is it weak or strong? The color, amount, odor, and consistency of the sputum are noted. Coughing up of blood may be a sign of pulmonary edema or acute pulmonary embolus. A history of tuberculosis also is noted.

The nurse listens to breath sounds and notes if they are diminished or if abnormal sounds such as crackles are heard. Rales occur when air passes through bronchi that contain fluid of any kind, and they may be found in patients who are fluid overloaded, who have mitral stenosis, or who are in left ventricular failure with pulmonary edema.

The patient's arterial blood gases (see Table 4-6) are evaluated for the level of oxygen and carbon dioxide and the acid-base balance of the arterial blood. The method of oxygen delivery (e.g., endotracheal tube or nasal cannula) is noted, as well as the percentage of oxygen delivered and the flow rate or setting. Pulse oximetry monitors may be attached to the foot, finger, earlobe, or nose by a finger clip or an adhesive to measure arterial blood oxygen saturation (SaO_2). Transcutaneous patches may be applied to very young patients to measure oxygen and carbon dioxide levels.

Pulmonary function testing may be ordered for patients at risk for postoperative acute respiratory failure, such as those with mitral or aortic valve disease.

Cardiovascular status

In addition to dyspnea, common symptoms of heart disease are chest pain, palpitations, syncope, and fatigue (see Box 4-4). Their severity will affect the functional capacity of the patient (see Boxes 4-1 and 4-2). In addition to these symptoms, children may demonstrate feeding difficulties, lack of weight gain, frequent respiratory infections, or irritability.

Pain. The most common cause of chest pain in the cardiac surgery patient is myocardial ischemia, which generally is described as an uncomfortable sensation of pressure, tightness, or squeezing. It may be dull or aching rather than sharp or spasmodic. The discomfort associated with myocardial ischemia, angina pectoris, may be triggered by exertion, strong emotion, eating a large meal, or exposure to cold. It usually subsides with the administration of nitroglycerin and cessation of exertional activity. Acute onset of chest pain should be reported immediately to the surgeon or anesthesiologist for treatment.

The pain accompanying myocardial infarction is more severe and prolonged and is unrelieved by rest or medications. Some patients have variant (Prinzmetal's) angina—by definition, pain that occurs at rest—or syndrome X (see p. 118). These patients may have evidence of coronary artery spasm with or without fixed coronary artery obstruction.

Ischemic pain may accompany hypertrophy of either ventricle or aortic valve disease. Pain also may be produced by pulmonary hypertension, pericarditis, myocarditis, and mitral valve prolapse. Aortic dissection produces tearing or stabbing pain of great intensity that often radiates to the back.

Palpitations. Patients may complain of palpitations or an awareness of their heartbeat. This may or may not be hemodynamically significant.

Premature ventricular contractions may be felt as missed beats, and ventricular tachycardia may be sensed as fluttering. Atrial fibrillation is seen often in patients with valvular disease (and postoperatively in patients who have undergone coronary artery bypass surgery). These findings are significant when there is a decline in left ventricular filling and cardiac output that leads to reduced perfusion of the brain. This can produce momentary dizziness, blurring of vision, or loss of consciousness (syncope), especially when the patient is in the upright position. Syncope also may occur in patients with aortic valve stenosis or hypertrophic obstructive cardiomyopathy and is usually exertional or postexertional.

Fatigue. Fatigue is common in patients with cardiovascular disease, but it is nonspecific (Braunwald, 2001). The patient may complain of muscle weakness as a consequence of reduced cardiac output, or the fatigue may be a result of diuresis, excessive blood pressure reduction in hypertensive patients, or the use of beta-adrenergic blocking agents.

Edema. Edema may be present in the lower extremities in ambulatory patients or in the dependent parts of the body (i.e., the back and sacral regions) in patients on bed rest. It is characteristic of bilateral chronic venous insufficiency (which may be significant if the saphenous vein is to be used as a conduit in coronary artery bypass surgery) or heart failure. When edema is cardiac in origin, fluid collection results from elevated right atrial pressure secondary to right ventricular failure, left ventricular failure, or pulmonary hypertension.

Blood pressure. Systemic blood pressures in the arms and legs are checked bilaterally and noted to be equal or unequal and high, normal, or low. Hypertension can produce a chronically increased afterload, which predisposes the patient to left ventricular hypertrophy.

Unequal pressures in the arms may be a contraindication to the use of the internal mammary artery as a bypass graft because the perfusion pressure could be suboptimal. Patients with coarctation of the aorta may demonstrate higher blood pressures in the upper extremity as compared with the lower extremity, and patients with aortic dissections may have unequal bilateral carotid, femoral, brachial, or radial artery blood pressures when the dissection occludes one or more of these vascular branches. The patient may have a radial artery pressure line. Preoperatively the nurse can palpate the carotid pulse for comparison and correlate the readings to the arterial waveform displayed. Intraoperatively the femoral pulse can be palpated to compare central pressures with peripheral (radial) pressures.

Pulses. Carotid, left ventricular apical, femoral, brachial, radial, ulnar, popliteal, dorsalis pedis, and posterior tibial pulses may be palpated preoperatively to determine a baseline for future comparison. This information is especially important to nurses caring for patients in the postoperative period who have had the femoral artery cannulated for cardiopulmonary bypass or have undergone the insertion of an intraaortic balloon.

It should be noted whether the pulses are symmetric, regular or irregular, bounding or thready, and fast or slow. The following values may be assigned:

Absent	0
Thready	1+
Diminished	2+
Normal	3+
Bounding	4+

A weak pulse may be caused by hypovolemia, heart failure, or mitral valve stenosis; a bounding pulse may be associated with increased stroke volume, anxiety, anemia, or fever.

Heart sounds. Heart sounds are auscultated and correlated with other data. The first heart sound (S_1) is associated with changes in flow related to the closing of the mitral and tricuspid valves at the beginning of ventricular systole and is almost simultaneous with the carotid impulse and QRS complex of the ECG. The second heart sound (S_2) reflects changing flow patterns associated with the closure of the aortic and pulmonic valves at the beginning of ventricular diastole. Both S_1 and S_2 are normal sounds.

The presence of a third heart sound (S_3), creating a "gallop" rhythm, is abnormal in adults and is related to the filling of a distended or noncompliant ventricle. A fourth heart sound (S_4) reflects the vibrations of the ventricular wall with the influx of blood from atrial contraction. A distinctly audible S_4 is considered abnormal (O'Rourke and Braunwald, 2001).

Bruits and murmurs. Are there bruits (turbulent blood flow around obstructions) in the carotid or femoral arteries or in the abdominal aorta? Bruits can be a sign of vascular disease. Significant carotid stenosis increases the risk of stroke in patients undergoing cardiac surgery; this increased risk is a result of the brief periods of hypotension that are necessary during cardiac operations (e.g., when flow is momentarily decreased to allow the aortic cross-clamp to be applied without excessive tension on the vessel). Carotid endarterectomy may be performed before or concurrently with the cardiac procedure in patients with significant, symptomatic carotid disease.

Murmurs are sounds produced by turbulent blood flow into a cardiac chamber or through a heart valve. They are classified as systolic, diastolic, or continuous. They are further described according to their location, radiation, intensity, configuration, duration, and quality. Patients with valvular stenosis, regurgitation, or a combination of the two commonly have murmurs, as do patients with some intracardiac shunts. Other sounds that may be heard with a stethoscope include pericardial and pleural friction rugs. These are signs of inflammation and produce characteristic leathery or scratchy sounds, respectively.

Patients also may have thrills, vibratory sensations felt over the location of the ascending aorta in patients with aortic stenosis. The narrowed valve orifice produces a jet of squirting blood against the aortic wall, which can be palpated.

Cardiac rhythm. Assessment of the cardiac rhythm enables the nurse to evaluate the baseline rhythm, obtain information about myocardial oxygen supply and demand, and use the information as an indication of myocardial ischemia, injury, or infarction. Coronary artery disease, ventricular hypertrophy, drug toxicity, and electrolyte imbalances are among the conditions that may produce changes in rhythm, although these conditions are not always reflected on the ECG.

Many of the dysrhythmias have a deleterious effect on the oxygen supply/demand balance because they produce inefficient contractions. For instance, ventricular tachydysrhythmias shorten the diastolic period during which the ventricles fill and most myocardial blood flow occurs; if this rhythm persists, cardiac output and myocardial perfusion are jeopardized and the patient is at increased risk for ventricular fibrillation. In atrial fibrillation, atrial activity is disorganized and ineffective. With the loss of atrial contractions the atrial contribution to diastolic ventricular filling is absent, eventually resulting in a reduction of stroke volume.

Alterations in the heart rate include tachydysrhythmias (100 to 160 beats per minute) and bradydysrhythmias (40 to 60 beats per minute). The origin of the dysrhythmia—the atrium, the atrioventricular junction, or the ventricle—is noted. It is determined whether alterations are new in onset, and the patient's ability to tolerate the dysrhythmia is assessed.

Is there atrioventricular heart block (indicating damage to the conduction tissue from ischemia, infarction, drug effects, or other causes)? Are the ST segments elevated (see Fig. 4-2) or depressed (which can indicate myocardial ischemia)? Other signs and symptoms associated with dysrhythmias include low urinary output, dizziness, transient ischemic attacks, hypotension, weakness, and confusion.

Hemodynamic data. The patient's systemic blood pressure and cardiac output (normal for adults is 5 liters per minute) are noted. Large patients may have higher outputs. To determine if the cardiac output is appropriate for the body size, the cardiac index is noted; this is derived by dividing the cardiac output by the body surface area (normal for adults ranges from 2.5 to 4 liters per minute per m^2).

The central venous pressure and the pulmonary artery systolic, diastolic, and capillary pressures are assessed (see Table 4-5). These values provide information about right and left ventricular function and volume status and can alert the nurse to changes in cardiac status before clinical signs of failure become apparent.

Peripheral vascular status

It should be determined whether previous vein harvests, vein stripping, or varicosities will preclude the use of saphenous vein as a bypass conduit. Atherosclerotic aortoiliac disease may create problems if femoral access is required for blood pressure monitoring or insertion of an intraaortic balloon. It also should be noted if abdominal aortic or lower-extremity arterial bypass graft surgery has been performed because this also could preclude the insertion of invasive catheters. When blood pressure monitoring lines are inserted into the radial artery, the nurse should be aware that ulnar artery patency is necessary to prevent ischemic injury to the hand. This can be ascertained by performing Allen's test (Box 4-5).

Cerebrovascular disease, especially significant carotid artery stenosis, should be noted and may require carotid endarterectomy either before or at the same time as the cardiac procedure. Carotid artery disease (identified from a history of transient ischemic attacks or stroke or documented diagnostic findings) impairs cerebral perfusion and increases morbidity and mortality in the cardiac surgery patient. Inducing hypotension during surgery (e.g., lowering bypass flow rates to reduce bleeding at coronary anastomotic sites) is especially risky in patients with obstructions within one or both carotid arteries.

The nurse also should review the record for preoperative echocardiographic (with or without Doppler) eval-

---

BOX 4-5
Allen's Test

Allen's test is performed to determine the adequacy of collateral (ulnar) blood flow to the hand when the radial artery is cannulated for blood pressure monitoring.
1. Elevate the patient's arm above the heart.
2. Press one thumb on the patient's radial artery and the other thumb on the ulnar artery while the patient clenches the fist (this squeezes the blood from the palm and fingers).
3. Release pressure on the ulnar artery while maintaining pressure on the radial artery.
4. If the blood returns rapidly (within 3 to 5 seconds) to the palm and fingers when the patient opens the hand, ulnar patency is present.
5. To determine the patency of the radial artery, repeat the test and release the radial artery.

Modified from Daily EK: Hemodynamic monitoring. In Guzzetta CE, Dossey BM: *Cardiovascular nursing: holistic practice*, St Louis, 1992, Mosby.

uation of the heart, aorta, and peripheral vascular system to detect potential sources of embolization (e.g., intraluminal calcium and atherosclotic plaque) that could cause neurologic injury. A preoperative assessment also provides a baseline for comparison after surgery.

Neurologic status

The patient's level of consciousness and orientation to person, place, and time are assessed. Papillary size, shape, and equality are noted. Is the reaction to light brisk or sluggish, or is the patient nonreactive? The patient is assessed preoperatively for signs of confusion, restlessness, slurred speech, weakness, numbness, or paralysis that could signal impaired perfusion, abnormal blood glucose concentrations in diabetic patients, or the effects of preoperative medications. The perioperative nurse should report changes in neurologic function to the surgical intensive care nurses, who will want to compare preoperative and postoperative findings.

Urinary/renal status

Has the patient had problems urinating that may suggest a urinary tract infection or some form of obstruction? In male patients with a history of benign prostatic hypertrophy or prostate surgery, residual scar tissue could make urinary catheterization difficult and require the use of urethral sounds to dilate the urethra. In both males and females, if urethral narrowing is severe, insertion of a suprapubic catheter may be necessary.

The kidneys are acutely sensitive to cardiac output. The results of urine studies, including the amount, color, clarity, and odor, are noted, and laboratory data are reviewed for creatinine level, blood urea nitrogen (BUN), and specific gravity to assess kidney function (see Table 4-6). During surgery, urinary output is monitored continuously and calculated at least every 30 minutes. Urinary output measurements before, during, and after cardiopulmonary bypass are documented for comparison and to reflect kidney perfusion and function.

Patients with chronic renal failure who require hemodialysis must be managed perioperatively, with consideration given to their altered excretory function. A dialysis catheter may be inserted in the OR for later use. Cardiac medications, anesthetic agents, and muscle relaxants that are excreted through the kidneys should be avoided when possible or used cautiously and monitored closely. Also, the danger of sepsis is high in patients with renal failure, and additional precautions may be warranted in perioperative management. Renal failure hampers calcium excretion, resulting in increased serum calcium levels; this may be a contraindication to the use of bioprostheses because of the accelerated calcification of the prosthesis in these patients (Oliver, de Castro, and Strickland, 1999).

Acute renal failure may be related to a decrease in circulating blood volume, hypotension, or the effects of cardiopulmonary bypass. In the absence of underlying renal disease, acute renal failure generally is reversible if it is diagnosed and treated quickly.

Nutritional status

The patient's nutritional status is assessed to determine increased risk for skin breakdown, infection, or poor healing. Patients who are obese or very thin may be at risk. Patients with cardiac cachexia have muscle wasting and a marked reduction in tissue mass, as well as a negative nitrogen balance, resulting from heart failure, reduced caloric intake, or increased caloric expenditure (Kotler, 2000).

Ears, eyes, nose, mouth, and throat

It should be determined whether the patient has difficulty hearing, seeing, smelling, tasting, or swallowing. Tracheobronchial problems may make intubation difficult. Patients may require the use of their eyeglasses or hearing aids in the immediate preoperative period, but these and other removable prostheses (such as dentures) should be removed and given to a family member or placed in a safe location before surgery.

Patients with colds, as well as those with loose or carious teeth, have a higher risk of infection. Surgery may be cancelled and rescheduled at a later date once these problems are corrected.

Gastrointestinal system

Laboratory results from liver function tests, if performed, are noted, as well as serum albumin levels; reduced serum albumin levels may indicate a protein deficit that can affect wound healing and the maintenance of vascular oncotic pressure. Low gamma globulin levels also may pose an increased risk of infection for the patient.

It should be determined whether there is a history of stomach or duodenal ulcers, gastrointestinal bleeding, or other bleeding tendencies, which could be a concern perioperatively. A bleeding history is usually a contraindication to mechanical heart valves that require chronic anticoagulation postoperatively.

Bowel preparation may or may not be ordered before surgery. If stool is present, rectal temperature probes will not accurately reflect core body temperature. Esophageal and bladder temperature probes can obviate this problem.

Endocrine system

The endocrine system affects the chemical and energy activities associated with metabolism. The function of the thyroid, pancreatic, adrenal, pituitary, and other hormone-producing glands affects aerobic and anaerobic energy production, which is vital to cardiac function. If these disorders are present, the most recent laboratory results are checked and abnormal findings reported.

Diabetes mellitus accelerates the development of atherosclerosis and is a major risk factor for complications. Individuals with diabetes are also more likely to have a "silent" (without angina) MI. The absence of pain is related to autonomic neuropathy in patients with long-standing diabetes (Weintraub and others, 1998).

Cardiopulmonary bypass induces hyperglycemia, which in diabetic patients requires adjusting the insulin dosages. Neutral protamine Hagedorn (NPH) insulin–dependent patients also may demonstrate a reaction to the protamine sulfate infusion for reversal of heparin and should be monitored closely for swelling, redness, hives or blisters, and other skin changes that may signal anaphylaxis.

Estrogen may serve a protective function against the development of atherosclerosis. Postmenopausal women, who have reduced estrogen levels (unless estrogen supplements are taken) have the same risk as men for heart disease and MI, and heart disease is the leading cause of death in both men and women. Whether hormone replacement therapy actually prevents atherosclerosis is being widely investigated (Penckofer and Schwertz, 2001).

RELATING

The relating pattern is assessed to determine how the patient relates to others in terms of role performance and sexual and social relationships. The marital status of the patient is determined, as well as the presence of a spouse, children, extended family, and friends. If these individuals will be present for the surgery, it should be noted where they will be waiting, and information should be provided about the time frame for surgery and plans for perioperative communication. If surgery has been delayed, family members will appreciate being told so that they can anticipate a longer wait (and not automatically assume that the delay is the result of intraoperative problems).

Also included in this pattern is the establishment and maintenance of bonds that are frequently affected by heart disease and the profound physical and psychologic effect it has. The heart is associated with love and other emotions; the physical consequences of cardiovascular disease affect the patient's ability to maintain personal, professional, and societal roles. Pain and fatigue, two common symptoms, make interpersonal relationships and the performance of familial roles more difficult. Sexual dysfunction also may be attributed to discomfort, fatigue, or the fear of recurring anginal attacks, or it may be the result of poor perfusion.

VALUING

When companionship is denied or compromised by debilitating symptoms, patients may be in spiritual distress. Their religious preference should be determined, as well as whether they desire to have access to a spiritual counselor. Not infrequently, patients have a heightened fear of death before surgery, and prayer, religious services, or religious articles may provide comfort. An attempt should be made to elicit whether any treatments are prohibited by the religion. Jehovah's Witnesses' refusal of blood transfusions should be communicated to the surgeon, anesthesiologist, and other appropriate personnel. The nurse needs to check that the necessary documentation forms are available and signed.

The valuing category also refers to cultural orientation. The nurse identifies the patient's cultural background or heritage and practices, including how the culture defines responses to pain, enactment of the sick role, and the behavior of the family with regard to the illness.

Also included in this category are complementary therapies that can be used as adjuncts or supplements to the perioperative experience. In particular, preoperative interventions such as imagery, massage, Reiki, music, biofeedback, touch, and meditation may enhance relaxation and reduce anxiety (Norred, 2000; Alspach, 1998).

CHOOSING

Choosing relates to the patient's coping abilities, judgment, participation, and wellness behavior. Both the patient's and the family's ability to cope with and adjust to the health problem are assessed. Difficulties may be experienced by both patients and families as the disease progresses and its impact is increasingly felt. Responses such as denial, disbelief, anger, regression, lack of cooperation, or acceptance may be evident.

The assessment should include an evaluation of the patient's willingness to comply with past and proposed future therapeutic regimens, which may necessitate lifestyle changes. Is the patient aware of the implications of the insertion of a mechanical heart valve (which requires chronic anticoagulation)? Will the family understand and support lifestyle changes related to diet, medication, exercise, and follow-up laboratory tests? Patients demonstrating a willingness to make lifestyle changes can be expected to have a successful recuperative and rehabilitative course and to be open to teaching by clinicians. Difficulty in following prescribed behaviors may point to a diagnosis of noncompliance, but the nurse should investigate whether failure to adhere to recommendations is purposeful or a result of inadequate knowledge and support.

Ideally preparation for home care begins on the patient's admission. The perioperative nurse can reinforce, review, clarify, and add to information and instructions the patient and significant others need in order to plan for discharge. Misconceptions should be clarified and questions answered.

Conclusion

The extensive array of diagnostic and laboratory tests enables the clinician to identify anatomic and functional disorders of the heart with greater precision. Interviews with patients and professional colleagues produce additional data, and ongoing monitoring systems provide a continuous source of information that must be interpreted and integrated into the clinical picture.

The perioperative nurse must be selective in assessing this information during the perioperative period and focus on the most pertinent actual or potential problems that exist. When there are changes in the patient's status, whether gradual or sudden and life threatening, priorities are adjusted, diagnoses modified, and plans altered accordingly.

References

Alspach G: Alternative and complementary therapies: treading tentatively out of the mainstream, *Crit Care Nurse* 18(5):13, 1998.

American Nurses' Association (ANA) and American Heart Association Council on Cardiovascular Nursing: *Standards of cardiovascular nursing practice,* Kansas City, Mo, 1981, ANA.

Ang-Lee MK, Moss J, Yuan CS: Herbal medicines and perioperative care, *JAMA* 286(2):208, 2001.

Antman EM, Braunwald E: Acute myocardial infarction. In Braunwald E, Zipes DP, Libby P, editors: *Heart disease: a textbook of cardiovascular medicine,* ed 6, Philadelphia, 2001, WB Saunders.

Association of periOperative Registered Nurses (AORN): *Standards, recommended practices, and guidelines,* Denver, 2001, AORN.

Barasch E: Echocardiography. In Willerson JT, Cohn JN, editors: *Cardiovascular medicine,* ed 2, New York, 2000, Churchill Livingstone.

Baron MG: The cardiac silhouette, *J Thorac Imaging* 15(4):230, 2000.

Bednash G, editor *Ask a nurse: from home remedies to hospital care,* New York, 2001, Simon & Schuster.

Beller GA: Relative merits of cardiovascular diagnostic techniques. In Braunwald E, Zipes DP, Libby P, editors: *Heart disease,* ed 6, Philadelphia, 2001, WB Saunders.

Beyea SC, editor *Perioperative nursing data set: the perioperative nursing vocabulary,* Denver, 2000, AORN.

Braunwald E: Approach to the patient with heart disease. In Braunwald E and others, *Harrison's principles of internal medicine,* ed 15, New York, 2001a, McGraw-Hill.

Braunwald E: The history. In Braunwald E, Zipes DP, Libby P, editors: *Heart disease: a textbook of cardiovascular-medicine,* ed 6, Philadelphia, 2001b, WB Saunders.

Brumley C: Herbs and the perioperative patient, *AORN J* 72(5):785, 2000.

Campeau L: Letter: grading of angina pectoris, *Circulation* 54(3):522, 1976.

Carpenito LJ: *Nursing care plans and documentation: nursing diagnoses and collaborative problems,* ed 3, Philadelphia, 1999, JB Lippincott.

Criteria Committee of the New York Heart Association: *Nomenclature and criteria for diagnosis of diseases of the heart and great vessels,* ed 9, Boston, 1994, Little Brown.

Daily EK: Hemodynamic monitoring. In Guzzetta CE, Dossey BM: *Cardiovascular nursing: holistic practice,* St Louis, 1992, Mosby.

Davidson CJ, Bonow RO: Cardiac catheterization. In Braunwald E, Zipes DP, Libby P, editors: *Heart disease,* ed 6, Philadelphia, 2001, WB Saunders.

Doty JR: Echocardiography. In *Cardiothoracic Surgery Network online curriculum,* http://www.ctsnet.org/doc/4274 (accessed Nov 27, 2000).

Friedman WF, Silverman N: Congenital heart disease in infancy and childhood. In Braunwald E, Zipes DP, Libby P, editors: *Heart disease,* ed 6, Philadelphia, 2001, WB Saunders.

Gavaghan M: Biochemical markers in myocardial injury. *AORN J* 70(5):840, 1999.

Gibbons RJ and others: ACC/AHA/ACP-ASIM [American College of Cardiology/American Heart Association/American College of Physicians—American Society of Internal Medicine] guidelines for the management of patients with chronic stable angina: a report of the American College of Cardiology/American Heart Association Task Force on Practice Guidelines, *J Am Coll Cardiol* 33:2092, 1999. [Erratum, *J Am Coll Cardiol* 34:314, 1999.]

Goldin JG, Ratib O, Aberle DR: Contemporary cardiac imaging: an overview. *J Thorac Imaging* 15(4):218, 2000.

Goldstein SI, Hendel RC: Interpreting noninvasive cardiac tests. In Alpert JS, editor: *Cardiology for the primary care physician,* St Louis, 1996, Mosby.

Haberl R and others: Correlation of coronary calcification and angiographically documented stenoses in patients with suspected coronary artery disease: results of 1,764 patients, *J Am Coll Cardiol* 37(2):451, 2001.

Higgins CB: Newer cardiac imaging modalities: magnetic resonance imaging and computed tomography. In Braunwald E, Zipes DP, Libby P, editors: *Heart disease,* ed 6, Philadelphia, 2001, WB Saunders.

Hlatky MA, Mark DB: Economics and cardiovascular disease. In Braunwald E, Zipes DP, Libby P, editors: *Heart disease,* ed 6, Philadelphia, 2001, WB Saunders.

Jadad AR, Gagliardi A: Rating health information of the Internet: navigating to knowledge or to Babel? *JAMA* 279(8):611, 1998.

Julian DG, Wenger NK: *Women and heart disease,* London, 1997, Martin Dunitz.

Kaski JC and others: Differential plasma endothelin levels in subgroups of patients with angina and angiographically normal coronary arteries, Coronary Artery Disease Research Group, *Am Heart J* 136(3):412, 1998.

Kaski JC, Russo G: Cardiac syndrome X: an overview, *Hosp Pract* 35(2):75, 2000.

Kern MJ: *The cardiac catheterization handbook,* ed 3, St Louis, 1999, Mosby.

Kernicki J, Bullock BL, Matthews J: Preface. In *Cardiovascular nursing: rationale for therapy and nursing approach,* New York, 1970, Putnam.

Kotler DP: Cachexia, *Ann Intern Med* 133(8):622, 2000.

Krantz DS and others: Effects of mental stress in patients with coronary artery disease: evidence and clinical implications, *JAMA* 283(14):1800, 2000.

Leblanc PA, Aubry B, Gervin M: Moveable intraoperative magnetic resonance imaging systems in the OR, *AORN J* 70(2):254, 1999.

Lee TH, Boucher CA: Clinical practice. Noninvasive tests in patients with stable coronary artery disease, *N Engl J Med* 344(24):1840, 2001.

Lee V: Cardiac imaging with Ct & MRI: an update. In *Medscape Surgery update,* http://surgery.medscape.com/Medscape/CNO/2001/SCVIR/SCVIR-01.html (accessed April 17, 2001).

Liu EH and others: Use of alternative medicine by patients undergoing cardiac surgery, *J Thorac Cardiovasc Surg* 120(2):335, 2000.

Malarkey LM, McMorrow ME: *Nurse's manual of laboratory tests and diagnostic procedures,* ed 2, Philadelphia, 2000, Saunders.

Meeker MH, Rothrock JC: Alexander's care of the patient in surgery, ed 11, St Louis, 1999, Mosby.

Milewicz D: Genetic aspects of congenital heart disease. In Willerson JT, Cohn JN: *Cardiovascular medicine,* ed 2, New York, 2000, Churchill Livingstone.

Miller CL: Cue sensitivity in women with cardiac disease, *Prog Cardiovasc Nurs* 15:82, 2000.

Nishimura RA, Gibbons RJ, Tajik AJ: Noninvasive cardiac imaging: echocardiography and nuclear cardiology. In Braunwald E and others: *Harrison's principles of internal medicine,* ed 15, New York, 2001, McGraw-Hill.

Norred CL: Minimizing preoperative anxiety with alternative caring-healing therapies, *AORN J* 72(5):838, 2000.

Oliver WC, de Castro MA, Strickland RA: Uncommon diseases and cardiac anesthesia. In Kaplan JA, editor: *Cardiac anesthesia,* ed 4, Philadelphia, 1999, WB Saunders.

O'Rourke RA, Braunwald E: Physical examination of the cardiovascular system. In Braunwald E and others: *Harrison's principles of internal medicine,* ed 15, New York, 2001, McGraw-Hill.

Penckofer S, Schwertz D: Hormone replacement therapy: primary and secondary prevention, *J Cardiovasc Nurs* 15(3):1, 2001.

Popma JJ, Bittl J: Coronary angiography and intravascular sonography. In Braunwald E, Zipes DP, Libby P, editors: *Heart disease,* ed 6, Philadelphia, 2001, WB Saunders.

Ridker PM, Genest J, Libby P: Risk factors for atherosclerotic disease. In Braunwald E, Zipes DP, Libby P, editors: *Heart disease,* ed 6, Philadelphia, 2001, WB Saunders.

Rozanski A, Blumenthal JA, Kaplan J: Impact of psychological factors on the pathogenesis of cardiovascular disease and implications for therapy, *Circulation* 99(16):2192, 1999.

Scanlon PJ and others: American College of Cardiology/American Heart Association ACC/AHA guidelines for coronary angiography: a report of the Task Force on Practice Guidelines, *J Am Coll Cardiol* 33(6):1756, 1999.

Schafer AI, Ali NM, Levine GN: Hemostasis, thrombosis, fibrinolysis, and cardiovascular disease. In Braunwald E, Zipes DP, Libby P, editors: *Heart disease: a textbook of cardiovascular medicine,* ed 6, Philadelphia, 2001, WB Saunders.

Seifert PC: Cardiac surgery. In Meeker MH, Rothrock JC, editors: *Alexander's care of the patient in surgery,* ed 11, St Louis, 1999, Mosby.

Seifert PC: Cardiac surgery. In Rothrock JC: *Perioperative nursing care planning,* ed 2, St Louis, 1996, Mosby.

Shively BK: The ten most commonly asked questions about echocardiography, *Cardiol Rev* 8(5):252, 2000.

Siomko AJ: Demystifying cardiac markers, *Am J Nurs* 100(1):36, 2000.

Taylor MR, Alman A, Manchester DK: Use of the Internet by patients and their families to obtain genetics-related information, *Mayo Clin Proc* 76(8):772, 2001.

Tempany CMC, McNeil BJ: Advances in biomedical imaging, *JAMA* 285(5):562, 2001.

Thelan LA and others: *Critical care nursing: diagnosis and management,* ed 2, St Louis, 1994, Mosby.

Waters DJ: Instruction #5. In *A heart surgeon's little instruction book,* St Louis, 1995, Quality Medical Publishing.

Weintraub WS and others: Outcome of coronary bypass surgery versus coronary angioplasty in diabetic patients with multivessel coronary artery disease, *J Am Coll Cardiol* 31(1):10, 1998.

5

Nursing Diagnoses, Outcomes, and Plans for Patient Care

The idea of nursing diagnosis broke the link between information collection and care planning. Clinical judgment was inserted as a recognized responsibility.

Marjorie Gordon, RN, 1982 (p. 1)

The ideal way to manage complications is to avoid them, which is best accomplished with a carefully conducted care plan.

Robert S. Litwak, MD, and Simon Dack, MD, 1982 (p. 22)

Review and analysis of the assessment data results in the identification of patient problems, needs, and health status. Many of these problems are related to medical diagnoses, necessitating physician-prescribed orders and collaborative interventions (Carpenito, 1999; Seifert, 1999b). Collaborative problems (potential complications), as well as nursing diagnoses, require judgment and critical thinking by the nurse. Nursing considerations can be found in subsequent chapters that discuss specific cardiac disorders.

Nursing diagnoses (Box 5-1) reflect judgments about the patient's responses to health problems that are amenable to nursing intervention. The use of nursing diagnoses facilitates a common language among nurses; this in turn facilitates choosing nursing interventions and evaluating their effectiveness (Beyea, Killen, and Watson, 1999; Doenges and Moorhouse, 2000). A nursing diagnosis may be categorized as *actual* when the nurse validates its presence by verifying major defining characteristics. For example, perioperative patients often demonstrate some anxiety, which can be modified or reduced through nursing interventions. On the other hand, the perioperative nurse may recognize that an individual patient or group of patients is more vulnerable to developing a problem than others. In this instance, the nursing diagnosis is categorized as a *risk for* the problem to develop. For example, most patients undergoing cardiac surgery do not have an infection as their presenting problem (which commonly would be a contraindication to surgery), but because of the risk of

infection from both exogenous and endogenous sources, the diagnosis of "risk for infection" is often made. Multiple perioperative nursing interventions are aimed at reducing this risk and are integrated into a plan of care for the cardiac surgery patient.

Problems must be resolved and undesirable outcomes avoided. This is achieved by identifying expected outcomes that reflect the unique physical and psychosocial needs of patients. When possible, outcomes should be formulated with the patients as recommended in the Association of periOperative Registered Nurses' (AORN) Patient Outcome Standard 4.1: Patients participate in decisions affecting their perioperative plans of care (AORN, 2001). This and other AORN Outcome Standards (Box 5-2) are nationally recognized standards of patient care.

Perioperative Nursing Data Set

AORN's outcome standards became the basis for further work undertaken by AORN to describe, define, and develop *data elements* of perioperative nursing practice that impact and affect patient outcomes (Beyea, 2000; Research Highlight 5-1). Each of the outcome statements was further refined and defined with interpretive statements, outcome criteria, and related nursing interventions. In 2000 this work was developed into a model for perioperative nursing practice (Fig. 5-1). The model places the patient and family (defined by the patient's perceived meaning of "family") as the central and most

BOX 5-1

Nursing Diagnoses for the Cardiac Surgery Patient: Classification by Human Response Patterns

Exchanging: A Human Response Pattern Involving Mutual Giving and Receiving

Airway clearance, ineffective
Aspiration, risk for
Body temperature, altered, risk for
Breathing pattern, ineffective
Cardiac output, decreased
Fluid volume deficit
Fluid volume deficit, risk for
Fluid volume excess
Gas exchange, impaired
Hyperthermia
Hypothermia
Infection, risk for
Injury, risk for (specify) (electrical, physical, chemical hazards, retained foreign objects)
Nutrition, imbalanced: less than body requirements
Nutrition, imbalanced: more than body requirements
Oral mucous membrane, altered
Peripheral neurovascular dysfunction
Skin integrity, impaired
Skin integrity, impaired, risk for
Tissue integrity, impaired
Tissue perfusion, ineffective (specify) (renal, cerebral, cardiopulmonary, gastrointestinal, peripheral)

Communicating: A Human Response Pattern Involving the Sending of Messages

Communication, impaired verbal

Relating: A Human Response Pattern Involving the Establishing of Bonds

Family processes, altered
Parental role conflict
Parenting, altered
Parenting, altered, risk for
Role performance, ineffective
Sexual dysfunction
Social interaction, impaired
Social isolation

Valuing: A Human Response Pattern Involving the Assigning of Relative Worth

Spiritual distress (distress of the human spirit)

Choosing: A Human Response Pattern Involving the Selection of Alternatives

Adjustment, impaired
Coping, ineffective family: compromised

Coping, ineffective family: disabling
Coping, ineffective individual
Decisional conflict (specify)
Health-seeking behaviors (specify)
Noncompliance (specify)

Moving: A Human Response Pattern Involving Activity

Activity intolerance
Activity intolerance, risk for
Diversional activity deficit
Fatigue
Growth and development, altered
Home maintenance management, impaired
Mobility, impaired physical
Perioperative positioning injury, risk for
Self-care deficit (specify) (bathing/hygiene, dressing/grooming, feeding, toileting)
Sleep pattern disturbance
Swallowing, impaired

Perceiving: A Human Response Pattern Involving the Reception of Information

Body image disturbance
Hopelessness
Personal identity disturbance
Powerlessness
Self-esteem, chronic low
Self-esteem, disturbance
Self-esteem, situational low
Sensory/perceptual disturbances: visual, auditory, kinesthetic, gustatory, tactile, olfactory

Knowing: A Human Response Pattern Involving the Meaning Associated with Information

Knowledge deficit (specify)
Thought processes, altered

Feeling: A Human Response Pattern Involving the Subjective Awareness of Information

Anxiety
Fear
Pain, acute
Pain, chronic

Modified from Rothrock JC: *Perioperative nursing care planning*, ed 2, St Louis, 1996, Mosby.

important aspect of perioperative nursing. Three of the four domains represented in the model reflect important characteristics and critical areas for any patient undergoing a surgical intervention. These three do-

mains are safety, physiologic responses, and the behavioral responses of the individual patient and family. Following the domain, the first focus is on outcomes. As described by Rothrock and Smith (2000), perioperative

---

BOX 5-2
AORN Patient Outcome Standards

Standard 1: The patient is free from signs and symptoms of
- Physical injury
- Injury due to extraneous objects
- Chemical injury
- Electrical injury
- Injury related to positioning
- Laser injury
- Radiation injury
- Injury related to transfer/transport
- The patient receives appropriate prescribed medications, safely administered, during the perioperative period.

Standard 2: The patient
- Is free from signs and symptoms of infection
- Has wound/tissue perfusion consistent with or improved from baseline levels established preoperatively
- Is at or returning to normothermia at the conclusion of the immediate postoperative period
- Has fluid, electrolyte, and acid-base balance consistent with or improved from baseline levels established preoperatively
- Has pulmonary function consistent with or improved from baseline levels established preoperatively
- Has cardiac function consistent with or improved from baseline levels established preoperatively

Standard 3: The patient demonstrates knowledge of
- Physiologic responses to the operative or other invasive procedure
- Psychologic responses to the operative or other invasive procedure
- Nutritional requirements related to the operative or other invasive procedure
- Medication management
- Pain management
- Wound healing
- The patient participates in the rehabilitation process.

Standard 4: The patient
- Participates in decisions affecting his or her perioperative plan of care
- Receives care consistent with the perioperative plan of care
- Is the recipient of competent and ethical care within legal standards of practice
- Receives consistent and comparable levels of care from all caregivers, regardless of the setting
- The patient's right to privacy is maintained.
- The patient's value system, lifestyle, ethnicity, and culture are considered, respected, and incorporated in the perioperative plan of care as appropriate, and the plan of care reflects the patient's level of function and ability during the perioperative period.

Standard 5: The patient demonstrates or reports adequate pain control throughout the perioperative period.

Modified from AORN: patient outcomes: standards of perioperative care. In *Standards, recommended practices, and guidelines,* Denver, 2000, p. 181.

RESEARCH HIGHLIGHT 5-1

Development of the Perioperative Nursing Data Set (PNDS)

In 1993 AORN appointed a Task Force on Perioperative Data Elements to define, describe, and develop the "elements" that described perioperative nursing practice. The 14 expert perioperative nurses on this original task force examined a number of nursing "languages" (ways of describing nursing practice) and determined that none of them thoroughly or comprehensively included the many facets of perioperative nursing patient care. Thus in 1995 four subcommittees were created to examine, define, and validate perioperative nursing diagnoses, interventions, outcomes, and the structural elements necessary to support the nurse in his or her work of providing patient care that resulted in the identified patient outcomes. Over the course of the next 4 years, numerous experts, consultants, and researchers were involved in the validation of each of the four elements. During this process, they were each modified and refined based on the results of research conducted. The end result is a clinically relevant and standardized language of perioperative nursing that can be used during any time frame of the perioperative patient's care and in any perioperative practice setting. Kleinbeck and others (2000) have already begun to test the use of these data elements for patient documentation; their work resulted in a written record tested in clinical settings in California, Kansas, and Missouri. Perioperative nurses in cardiac surgery and other cardiac invasive settings are encouraged to conduct similar clinical validation and testing of the PNDS to further refine and develop it.

Modified from Beyea SC, editor: *Perioperative nursing data set,* Denver, 2000, AORN.

---

from nursing diagnoses, the perioperative nurse selects interventions to achieve the outcomes. The fourth domain in the model represents the structural elements that must be in place in practice areas to enable perioperative patient care that is safe, and marked by quality and excellence. Structural considerations for cardiac surgery are discussed in Chapter 3.

Even with a body of tested data elements and their corresponding outcomes and interventions, it is important whenever possible to validate with the patient the diagnoses selected and the outcomes desired to provide information in planning patient care and facilitating a positive surgical experience. Congruent patient and nurse goals are more likely to be achieved. Congruence also establishes realistic expectations for treatment. Outcomes management further delineates "patient-based factors" (the severity of illness), "practitioner-based factors" (professional competence), and "organization-based factors" (the structural elements of the model and their subsequent allocation of necessary resources) as areas of consideration. Distinguishing among these factors promotes monitoring and more

nurses have in their unique knowledge base a set of outcomes that apply to all patients receiving their care. Such a philosophy is similar to the "risk" diagnoses for certain patient populations. From these outcomes, nursing diagnoses are selected based on patient assessment;

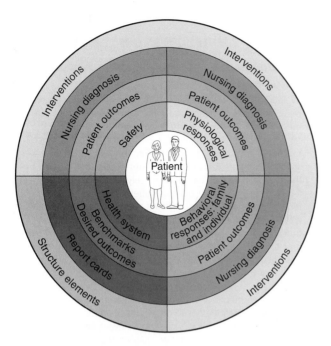

FIGURE 5-1 AORN perioperative patient-focused model. (From AORN: Patient outcomes: standards of perioperative care. In *Standards, recommended practices, and guidelines,* Denver, 2001, AORN.)

precise measurement of performance assessment and improvement efforts. It also highlights the interdependent and collaborative nature of many patient care activities.

Human Response Patterns and Associated Diagnoses

The profound impact of cardiovascular disease on the physical and emotional integrity of the patient suggests a number of nursing diagnoses (Seifert, 1999a). Identification of problems is facilitated by a holistic assessment based on the human response patterns developed by the North American Nursing Diagnosis Association (Rantz and LeMone, 1999). When assessing the patient, the nurse clusters the signs and symptoms to determine whether the diagnosis within that pattern is applicable.

COMMUNICATING

The communicating pattern of human responses includes *impaired verbal communications* and may be related to the inability to speak or understand the dominant language. The cause may also be cardiovascular insufficiency, sedation, dyspnea, reduced level of consciousness, or physical barriers such as endotracheal (ET) tubes.

Postoperatively, intubated patients may be distressed that they cannot talk. The perioperative nurse should prepare patients for this situation, reassuring them that the ET tube will be removed as soon as possible and that a writing tablet or other means of nonverbal communication will be available.

PERCEIVING

Impaired functional status often affects how individuals perceive themselves. *Disturbances in body image* and self-concept are related to the functional restrictions imposed by disease. *Self-esteem* and *personal identity* may be similarly disturbed, and feelings of *hopelessness* and *powerlessness* may become apparent with the realization that activities once taken for granted can no longer be accomplished. As the disease progresses in severity, *disturbed sensory perceptions* may be evident that affect vision, hearing, movement, smell, and taste.

An example of powerlessness may be seen in patients with devices such as a pacemaker or a ventricular assist device that places patients in a situation over which they have no sense of control. These feelings should be explored and factual information given that minimizes specific fears about the function and purpose of the device.

FEELING

Anxiety is a common diagnosis in the cardiac surgical patient population and may be accompanied by the *fear* of more specific threats to the patient. Although these feelings are specific to the individual patient, they may be related to events such as changes in health status, threats to self-concept, or even fear of death (Lenz and Perkins, 2000). Fear and anxiety may aggravate physical discomfort, sympathetic stimulation, increased tension, apprehension, or *pain*. Chronic or acute pain may be produced by the disease or as a result of the surgical intervention, including uncomfortable procedures or positions during the perioperative period.

Pain has become an increasingly important factor in caring for patients, especially those who undergo thoracotomy procedures for certain minimally invasive coronary artery bypass procedures. Patients should be told about anticipated pain, and reassured that pain-reducing medications and other interventions are available (and encouraged).

KNOWING

Although *deficient knowledge* is not uncommon among patients with heart disease, many individuals actively seek more information about their condition in publications and on the Internet. Nurses play a vital role in helping patients to distinguish between correct information and misleading or false information. Nurses can encourage patients to verbalize their understanding of what they have read and share online resources for additional study. Box 5-3 lists some available Internet sites.

Patients may purposely avoid learning more about their disorder because of the perceived threat to their physical and emotional well-being. Coping mechanisms such as denial often play a role. The nurse must assess the patient's ability and readiness to learn, and must distinguish among what the patient knows and wants to know, what the patient chooses not to know, and what the patient needs to know to maximize the benefits of the recommended or prescribed therapy. The underlying disease or the surgical treatment may produce temporary *disturbed thought processes* or *situational low self-esteem*.

MOVING

Functional status not only affects self-concept but also impairs *physical mobility* and the performance of activities of daily living. The *risk for perioperative positioning injury* is related to the immobility associated with surgery, which can last 3 to 6 hours (or more) and also aggravate preexisting musculoskeletal problems. Problems with mobility after surgery are often related to healing of the sternal incision. Patients who have had a median sternotomy incision need to understand that sternal bone healing requires 2 to 3 months. However, early (before hospital discharge) and frequent walking is strongly recommended to promote cardiovascular wellness and optimum healing. Patients should be encouraged to work with cardiac rehabilitation professionals to formulate an exercise plan.

Fatigue itself may be a problem; when fatigue is associated with pain and dyspnea, it can produce *activity intolerance* and restrict *diversional activities* and *home maintenance*. *Self-care deficits* related to hygiene, grooming, feeding, and toileting are not uncommon in cardiac patients. *Sleep patterns* may be disturbed, particularly in patients with paroxysmal nocturnal dyspnea or orthopnea.

EXCHANGING

The exchanging pattern includes most of the physiologic diagnoses that are commonly encountered during the perioperative period. It also reflects many of AORN's Outcome Standards (AORN, 2001) that pertain to injury, skin integrity, fluid and electrolytes, infection, and the physiologic response to surgery.

The circulatory system is the focal point for cardiac surgery patients, and the most common nursing diagnoses related to the exchanging pattern are *decreased cardiac output* and *ineffective tissue perfusion*. Patients with impaired cardiac function have or are at risk for a reduction in the amount of blood pumped out of the heart, which in turn jeopardizes adequate perfusion of organ systems. Alterations in cardiac output may be related to electrical factors (conduction disturbances), mechanical factors (preload, afterload, contractility), or structural factors (valve deformities, aneurysms, congenital anomalies) (Doenges, Moorhouse, and Geissler, 2000).

During procedures performed "off pump" (e.g., without the use of cardiopulmonary bypass [CPB]), the heart is neither cooled nor arrested for protection. During these cases the heart remains normothermic, which increases the risk for injury if there are delays that prolong the period of ischemia. The perioperative nurse can minimize this risk of injury by having equipment and supplies readily available and by closely monitoring the patient for signs of potential myocardial injury.

Diagnoses related to oxygenation and breathing include *ineffective airway clearance, risk for aspiration, ineffective breathing pattern,* and *impaired gas exchange*. These diagnoses often reflect the duration of surgery, the patient's

BOX 5-3
Internet Sites of Interest to Cardiac Patients

American Association for Thoracic Surgery
http://aats.org
American Heart Association
http://www.americanheart.org
Annals of Thoracic Surgery
http://ats.ctsnetjournals.org
AORN Surgical Knowledge Base (ASK)
http://www.aorn.org
Cardiac-Related Breaking News
http://www.theheart.org
Cardiology Compass
http://cardiologycompass.com
Cardiothoracic Digest
http://www.ctdigest.com
Cardiothoracic Surgery Network
http://ctsnet.org
Centers for Disease Control and Prevention
http://www.cdc.gov
Congenital Heart Disease Information and Resources
http://chin.org
Heart Information Network
http://heartinfo.org
Heart Surgery Forum
http://www.hsforum.com
National Institutes of Health
http://www.nih.gov
National Marfan Foundation
http://www.marfan.org
New England Journal of Medicine
http://nejm.org
Society of Thoracic Surgeons
http://www.sts.org

immobility and subsequent retention of secretions, the respiratory effects of anesthesia, and underlying cardiac and pulmonary pathologic conditions.

Regulation of the patient's temperature is common during surgery, and cooling the heart is one method of myocardial protection. *Hypothermia* may become a problem when it occurs inadvertently in the preoperative or postoperative period. In the preoperative period the shivering that accompanies chilling should be avoided because of the increased metabolic demands on the heart that accompany shivering. Actions are implemented to keep the patient warm before the induction of anesthesia and the use of neuromuscular blocking agents that reduce shivering.

Postoperatively some residual hypothermia is often encountered, and rewarming of the patient is performed gradually so that the body is able to adjust to the shifting of blood from central organs to the periphery as rewarming and vasodilation occur. Hypothermia has received considerable attention since the publication of a study by Kurz and colleagues (1996) showing a correlation between prolonged postoperative hypothermia and increased surgical site infection rates, prolonged hospital stays, risk for increased surgical bleeding, and increased risk for cardiac events. Perioperative nurses should be vigilant in monitoring the patient's temperature and implementing warming interventions (Hudson and others, 1999; Fecteau, 1999).

Other diagnoses in the exchanging pattern include risks for *injury, impaired skin integrity, impaired tissue integrity,* and *peripheral neurovascular dysfunction.* Patients with compromised cardiac function require special precautions to avoid skin and tissue injury, especially those who are obese *(imbalanced nutrition, more than body requirements)* or cachectic *(imbalanced nutrition, less than body requirements).* These dangers may be potentiated by the use of equipment such as electrosurgical units, defibrillators, powered equipment, and chemical agents. An important role of the perioperative nurse is protecting patients who are unable to protect themselves from internal or external threats during surgery.

The *risk for infection* is ever present, and this diagnosis is routinely applied to cardiac surgery patients. *Excess fluid volume, deficient fluid volume,* and *imbalanced fluid volume* are related to factors such as blood loss, fluid and electrolyte shifts, dehydration or overhydration, extensive use of banked blood, immobility, and inability to maintain appropriate fluid status as a result of heart failure or renal failure.

RELATING

Establishing and maintaining bonds may be affected by heart disease. The functional restrictions imposed by heart disease often affect the patient's ability to engage in personal, professional, and societal roles. *Social interaction* may be impaired, *role performance* may be ineffective, and *family processes* may be interrupted when pain, fatigue, dyspnea, and other symptoms are present. *Sexual dysfunction* may also accompany these problems.

Cardiac patients come from many different cultures, and the perioperative nurse should be sensitive to specific beliefs that impact the perception of illness, pain, and the role of family members during the perioperative period. If language is a barrier to supporting a patient's wishes, the nurse should use the institution's translation services or have an English-speaking family member communicate with the nurse to ensure that special needs are met.

VALUING

When companionship is denied or restricted by debilitating symptoms, patients may be in *spiritual distress.* They may be unable to participate in religious ceremonies or benefit from the spiritual support of religious counselors. Religious beliefs may affect certain interventions, such as the refusal of Jehovah's Witnesses to receive blood transfusions. Religious and emotional aspects of the heart (the "seat of the soul") combined with the fear of death or disfigurement should be assessed by the nurse.

The importance of religion and spiritual beliefs cannot be underestimated for their impact on the mental well-being of the patient. Patients' requests to visit with a spiritual counselor before surgery should be respected, even if it means a short delay in starting the surgical procedure.

CHOOSING

Problems of *adjustment* and *coping* are not unusual in patients and families as the disease progresses and its impact becomes more and more apparent. Conflicts between patients and health care professionals or between patients and significant others may arise. Adaptive behaviors may be developed, or denial, anger, disbelief, regression, and lack of cooperation may become evident.

Consideration must be given to the ability or desire of the patient to engage in *health-seeking behaviors* and to follow prescribed therapeutic regimens. The potential diagnosis of *noncompliance* requires initial investigation. The nurse should distinguish between a patient's refusal to comply with recommendations and the inability to follow orders because of insufficient information and emotional support (Butcher, 1999). These considerations are significant for patients who are expected to make lifestyle changes such as risk factor modification, adherence to a precise medication schedule, or long-term laboratory follow-up testing. The perioperative nurse can serve as a consultant or as a source for referrals to ensure that emotional support and information are available to the patient and family (Fox, 1999).

Planning Patient Care

The purpose of planning is to identify and implement actions necessary to achieve the desired patient outcomes. Planning is also critical to avoid or lessen the incidence of complications that pose a high risk to the patient during the perioperative period. Safety considerations have long been the focus of perioperative nursing practice and have received additional attention with the publication of the Institute of Medicine's (IOM, 1999) report "To Err is Human: Building a Safer Health System." One study of surgery-related errors cited by the IOM concluded that more than 50% of the adverse events described could have been prevented (Gawande and others, 1999). Among the strongest recommendations made by the IOM were to increase knowledge about safety, design systems that prevent future errors (rather than blame individuals), identify and learn from errors, and implement safe practices. Cardiac perioperative nurses have many opportunities to promote safety, whether by working with central supply personnel to ensure that wire cutters *must* be placed in the emergency chest sets or by communicating with the postoperative critical care nurses to ensure a smooth patient transfer after surgery.

In addition to nursing-related diagnoses, other problems exist that are clearly medical diagnoses: ventricular fibrillation, hemorrhage, infarction, cerebral vascular accident, and anaphylactic reactions. Whether diagnoses are nursing or medical, the nurse must be aware of the various potential problems and complications and the expected patient response, anticipate their occurrence, observe for the expected patient response, and be prepared to act quickly in a collaborative manner should problems or complications arise. Thus the nurse must constantly reassess which needs have the greatest priority and rearrange or modify interventions accordingly. These considerations should be reflected in the plan of care, whether it is written or unwritten. When they are documented, care plans can serve as written evidence of the nurse's knowledge, judgment, and critical thinking.

In some institutions clinical pathways are used; these are abbreviated plans of care (or care maps) that are event-related, providing outcome-based guidelines for goal achievement within a designated length of stay.

Generic Care Plans

Active and skillful analysis, synthesis, and evaluation of information gathered from or generated by experience, observation, research, and reflective reasoning lead to modifications and adaptations of generic care plans. Care plans based on the diagnoses and patient outcomes identified are outlined in the rest of this chapter. Patient outcomes with an asterisk (*) are based on the AORN (2001) Patient Outcome Standards (see Box 5-2). Interventions listed are generic to the cardiac surgery patient and are not intended to be all-inclusive. The perioperative nurse must incorporate the unique physical and psychosocial needs of each patient and place them in order of priority to appropriately implement care regimens. Perioperative considerations related to specific surgical procedures are listed in subsequent chapters.

1. NURSING DIAGNOSIS

Deficient knowledge related to the physiologic effects of the cardiac disorder, proposed surgical procedure, and immediate postoperative events.

PATIENT OUTCOME*

The patient demonstrates knowledge of the physiologic responses to the cardiac disorder (at his or her level of understanding), the proposed surgical treatment, and immediate postoperative events as evidenced by verbalization of disease state, purpose of surgery, sequence of events, anticipated outcomes, and recovery process.

INTERVENTIONS

Assess current physiologic status such as vital signs, fluid/electrolyte balance, heart sounds (see Box 5-4), and level of consciousness.

Confirm patient identity.

Confirm that consent for surgery has been granted.

Assess patient's understanding of cardiac disease.

Assess effects of cardiac disorder on physiologic and functional status.

Assess effects of cardiac medications on patient's thought processes.

Determine patient's knowledge of current medication regimen.

Determine whether patient is taking any herbs or complementary/alternative medicines (some of these can inhibit coagulation, affect blood pressure, cause sedation, have cardiac effects, or alter electrolytes [Norred, Zamudio, and Palmer, 2000]).

Elicit patient's understanding of surgical procedure, possible alternative procedures (e.g., saphenous vein or internal mammary artery).

Respect normal level of denial.

Answer patient's and family's questions.

Elicit understanding of prior cardiac procedures; if patient has questions or misunderstandings, provide

---

BOX 5-4
Auscultating Heart Sounds

How and Where to Listen for Heart Sounds
The table below provides tips on how to position the patient, what part of the stethoscope to use, and where to listen for specific heart sounds

HEART SOUND	PATIENT POSITION	STETHOSCOPE PART	WHERE TO LISTEN
S_1 (first heart sound)	Any position	Diaphragm	• Entire precordium • Heard best at apex
S_2 (second heart sound)	Sitting or supine	Diaphragm	• Aortic area at second right intercostal space (ICS) to the right of the sternum • Pulmonic area at second left ICS to the left of the sternum
S_3 (third heart sound)	Supine or left lateral recumbent	Bell	• Apex
S_4 (fourth heart sound)	Supine or left semilateral	Bell	• Apex
Murmur	High Fowler's and leaning slightly forward	Diaphragm and bell to differentiate between high-pitched and low-pitched sounds	• Entire precordium • Heard best over affected valve's auscultation site
Rub	Any position	Diaphragm	• Entire precordium • Heard best at third ICS, left sternal border

NORMAL FINDINGS	
• S_1 and S_2 sounds producing the *lubb-dubb* associated with normal valve closing • Ventricular rate between 60 bpm and 100 bpm in a resting adult	• Ventricular rate less than 60 bpm (bradycardia) in some young adults, athletes, or patients taking heart-slowing medications, such as beta-blockers • Rhythm consistent and regular, without extra beats • Systolic murmur in a young child • Valve click in a patient who has had a valve replacement

From *Expert 10-minute physical examinations*, St Louis, 1998, Mosby.

---

information or refer to appropriate health care professional as indicated (Butcher, 1999).

Note presence of sternotomy scars; reoperations require longer surgical time and may be accompanied by increased bleeding. Inform patient and family of possible prolonged operative time.

Assess patient's and family's understanding of possible complications: perioperative myocardial infarction, stroke, hemorrhage, renal failure, infection, dysrhythmias, death.

Ascertain where family or significant other will be waiting during surgery; provide communication per institutional protocol.

Describe/explain the following events (use models, diagrams, fact sheets, and so forth):

Preoperative

Nothing by mouth (NPO status)

Premedication

Time and mode of transport to operating room (OR)

Preinduction (holding) area

Interview by circulating nurse

Insertion of peripheral intravascular lines

Transport to OR, transfer to OR bed

OR environment—what patient will see, hear, feel, smell (e.g., numerous staff, what they are wearing, equipment, sound of people moving, cool temperature, uncomfortable procedures)

Induction of anesthesia

Insertion of nasogastric tube, central vascular lines, urinary catheter

Skin preparation

Intraoperative

Anticipated length of surgery

Surgical procedure, intraoperative events, equipment as requested

Postoperative

Surgical intensive care unit (SICU) environment—noises, equipment, protocols

Condition of patient on arrival to the SICU—tubes, lines, catheters, patient cool and pale; medicated/anesthetized; unable to talk while intubated; if normothermic off-pump procedure has been performed, patient may be extubated and have a normal body temperature

Alternative methods of communication

Visiting hours, anticipated length of stay (Reassure family/significant other that it is not necessary to visit patient in SICU if the experience is too frightening; staff can keep family informed and communicate information about patient's progress)

Special Pediatric Considerations (Maldonado and Nygren, 1999; Nygren and Rothrock, 1996)

Determine if the patient and family have participated in the hospital surgical tour.

Orient the patient and family to the nursing unit, playroom, and hospital room.

Be honest about painful procedures (e.g., injections, blood tests).

Encourage the child to bring a special toy for security.

Show the patient and family the surgical staff's clothing, particularly face masks; allow child to play with apparel.

Stress to the patient that surgery is performed only on the part of the body that has been discussed and specified.

Use age-appropriate terminology for all teaching.

Encourage expression of fears.

Special geriatric considerations (Meckes, 1999; Kee and Miller, 1999; Hersey, 1996)

Assess patient's ability to see and hear, and ascertain patient's experience with previous surgery (if any).

Modify teaching plan in accordance with sensory/perceptual alterations; minimize use of audiovisual materials if they create too much confusion for the patient.

Allow sufficient time to answer questions.

Include family members and significant others involved in patient care outside the hospital.

Reduce extraneous noise or music as appropriate; employ a one-on-one approach.

Request that information be repeated; have patient explain planned intervention in his or her own words; use frequent reminders.

Direct speech toward patient's "good" ear; speak face-to-face with patient in a normal tone but clearly and slowly; avoid increased pitch of voice.

Remove surgical mask to speak whenever possible.

Use teaching materials with large print and high-contrast colors.

2. NURSING DIAGNOSIS

Deficient knowledge related to the psychologic responses to the cardiac disorder, the proposed surgical treatment, and/or immediate postoperative events.

PATIENT OUTCOME*

The patient demonstrates knowledge of the psychologic responses to the cardiac disorder (at his or her level of understanding), the proposed surgical treatment, and immediate postoperative events as evidenced by verbalization of perception of cardiac disorder, surgery, and postoperative events; identification of concerns and fears; communication of data relevant to planning; and participation in decisions affecting perioperative plan of care.

INTERVENTIONS

Elicit patient's feelings about the impact of the disease on activities of daily living.

Encourage verbalization of fears, "silly questions," concerns, and perceived threats.

Determine religious, spiritual, cultural, and ethnic beliefs that may affect surgical procedure (e.g., Jehovah's Witnesses' attitude toward blood transfusion).

Identify and reinforce current effective coping strategies.

3. NURSING DIAGNOSIS

Anxiety related to apprehension about surgery and/or perioperative events.

PATIENT OUTCOME

The patient's anxiety is reduced to a manageable level; manifestations of anxiety (increased heart rate, elevated blood pressure, increased respiratory rate, diaphoresis, restlessness, agitation, crying, poor eye contact) are reduced or absent.

INTERVENTIONS

Assess anxiety level and physiologic response, such as increased blood pressure and heart rate (in children, one may also see crying, clinging to parent, restlessness, and trembling).

Assess patient's knowledge of cardiac disease and planned surgery.

Implement perioperative teaching.

Encourage verbalization of concerns, perceived threats, and fears.

Orient patient to OR environment; note if patient has taken preoperative tour.

Explain perioperative events as they occur, describe what patient will see, hear, and feel.

Answer requests for information with simple, concise explanations.

Control external stimuli.

Provide comfort measures, such as warm blankets or religious articles.

In children note developmental stage and plan interventions accordingly.

4. NURSING DIAGNOSIS

Risk for injury related to surgical position.

PATIENT OUTCOME*

The patient is free from signs and symptoms of injury related to surgical position as evidenced by absence of acquired neuromuscular impairment and tissue necrosis.

INTERVENTIONS

Assess airway; confirm effective breathing pattern.

Have extra personnel to position patient.

Use patient transfer roller if patient is unable to move.

Avoid shearing forces and friction during patient positioning and transfer; lift patient rather than pulling or sliding.

Identify patient risk factors (age, body weight, nutritional status, medications, chronic disease status, existing pressure ulcers) (McEwen, 1996).

Anticipate movement of extraneous lines and tubes during transfer; secure or guide them into position.

Secure patient on OR bed, explaining necessity for restraint.

Check pulses in extremities.

Assess range of motion/mobility before positioning; note physical limitations.

Pad pressure points.

Have available necessary positioning supplies.

Maintain accessibility to groin (e.g., femoral artery).

Assess bony prominences and dependent pressure sites at the end of surgery.

Select positioning devices in accordance with skin condition, tissue integrity, and weight.

Protect eyes and ears.

In pediatric patients, one may need to use body restraints.

In elderly patients be especially cautious positioning joints, notably the hips, knees, and ankles (Meckes, 1999).

> *Supine*
> Maintain proper body alignment.
> In patients with reduced range of motion or back problems, place in functional position.
> Use extra padding as necessary on arms, hands, feet, back, sacrum, and back of head.
> Maintain airway; avoid decreased chin-to-chest angle, especially in children and obese patients; assess respiratory rate and rhythm, chest expansion, and oxygenation; monitor pulse oximetry.
> Observe for decrease in blood pressure, heart rate, and peripheral resistance, especially during induction of anesthesia; monitor blood pressure and electrocardiogram (ECG) (Biddle and Cannady, 1990).

> *Lateral*
> If patient is placed on the right side, vena cava may be compressed (especially in obese patients with subsequent reduction in preload; monitor systemic, pulmonary pressures).
> Monitor respiratory rate and rhythm, oxygenation, and ECG; note compromised respiratory function.
> Use axillary rolls, and pillows between legs; provide padding for arms, elbows, feet, and head.
> Attach arm boards and over-arm boards; use stabilizing pillows, sandbags, or other devices anteriorly and posteriorly.
> Place adhesive tape across buttocks (if it does not interfere with access to surgical site or groin).

> *Anterolateral*
> If left side should be slightly elevated for minimally invasive direct coronary artery bypass, use a small roll under left side.
> Ensure access to mediastinum (or groin) for possible cardiopulmonary bypass cannulation.

5. NURSING DIAGNOSIS

Risk for injury related to retained extraneous objects.

PATIENT OUTCOME*

The patient is free from signs and symptoms of physical injury related to retained extraneous objects as evidenced by correct counts or unremarkable x-ray films when necessitated by incorrect counts.

INTERVENTIONS

Account for suture and hypodermic needles, knife blades, umbilical tapes, rubbershods, pledgets, vessel loops, bulldogs, cannulas, pill sponges, guidewires, stopcocks, connectors for tubing, prosthetic materials, instruments, surgical sponges, and other items per institutional protocol.

Remove tissue debris from instruments, such as calcium particles, plaque, thrombus, and vegetations (Seifert, 1996).

Remove suture particles from surgical site.

Complete necessary documentation; follow policy for incorrect counts per institutional protocol.

6. NURSING DIAGNOSIS

Risk for injury related to chemical hazards.

PATIENT OUTCOME*

The patient is free from signs and symptoms of chemical injury as evidenced by the absence of allergic reactions or tissue necrosis to solutions and medications.

INTERVENTIONS

Note allergies (especially to latex, skin preparation solutions, depilatories, and dressing materials).

Identify fluids, solutions, irrigations, injectates, and medications: heparin injectate, heparin solution, topical "slush," cardioplegia solution, papaverine, epinephrine, thrombin, antibiotic solution, "glue" components, normal saline, lactated Ringer's solution, and other fluids on field (Seifert, 1999a).

Follow hospital protocol for allergic/anaphylactic blood reactions.

Inject blood vessels (e.g., saphenous vein) and other tissue with physiologic solutions or prescribed fluids only.

Remove glove powder from outside of gloves after gloving and before handling tissue per manufacturer's instructions.

Remove toxic storage solution (e.g., glutaraldehyde) from grafts/prosthetic material with saline before use per protocol.

7. NURSING DIAGNOSIS

Risk for injury related to physical hazards.

PATIENT OUTCOME*

The patient is free from signs and symptoms of physical injury as evidenced by the availability and proper functioning of appropriate instruments, equipment, and supplies.

INTERVENTIONS

Inspect vascular clamps, forceps, needle holders, and other instruments for malalignment, missing teeth, burrs, and malfunctions; replace as necessary.

Avoid overstretching of sternal (or internal mammary artery [IMA]) retractor; remove IMA posts after IMA dissection if post is impinging on patient's arm.

Use a minimum amount of nonirritating adhesive tape on skin, especially in patients with frail skin (e.g., very young or old patients).

Moisten surgeon's or assistant's hands when tying fine suture to prevent snagging per request.

Visually examine entire length of suture before handing to surgeon; discard suture with knots.

Prevent snagging of suture; avoid clamping suture with unprotected metal jaws (use rubbershods or special suture clamps).

Have available chest x-ray films, cardiac catheterization cineangiograms, arteriograms, angiograms, computed tomography (CT) scans, and so forth as requested.

If performing reoperation, display lateral and antero-posterior chest x-ray films (to note adherence of mediastinal structures to sternum, to count chest wires, to note the presence of prostheses, and so forth); have special supplies and equipment as requested by surgeon (e.g., oscillating saw, topical hemostatic agents).

If doing an off-pump procedure, have backup cardiopulmonary bypass supplies available.

Have backup supplies or alternative source of supplies available (e.g., grafts, valves, pledgets, special suture; list lot and serial number of all implants.

Have additional sterile instruments, equipment, and supplies (e.g., case carts) available in anticipation of emergency procedures.

When OR is not in use, keep room prepared for cardiac procedures: sterile instrument sets in place, sternal saw power source ready for use, light source available, electrosurgical units (ESUs) in working order (attachments available), OR table parts attached to bed, defibrillator plugged in, temporary atrioventricular pacemaker available, and inventory (e.g., supplies, solutions) stocked.

8. NURSING DIAGNOSIS

Risk for injury related to electrical hazards.

PATIENT OUTCOME*

The patient is free from signs and symptoms of electrical injury as evidenced by the absence of redness or blistering of skin at the conclusion of the surgical procedure.

INTERVENTIONS

Ensure appropriate location of ESU dispersive pad site; place pad on clean, dry skin over muscular area; avoid bony prominences and scarred or excessively hairy areas; place pad as far from ECG electrodes as possible.

In patients with pacemakers or internal defibrillators, place dispersive pad away from generator sites; minimize use of electrosurgery (may require a device programmer).

Check that defibrillator (and fibrillator) and external pacemaker are in proper working order; schedule regular maintenance checks with biomedical engineering; report malfunctioning equipment and devices per institutional protocol.

Ensure that the appropriate connector for the anteroposterior paddles/patches is available (some patients scheduled for internal defibrillator insertion may arrive in the OR with disposable external defibrillator patches incompatible with the OR defibrillator).

Insulate proximal tip of electrosurgery pencil when using in deep cavities or in retrosternum (e.g., during IMA dissection); verify with surgeon.

Visually inspect each instrument and use an insulation testing device to check insulation of endoscopic instruments (Dennis, 2001).

Check epicardial pacing leads and wires for kinks or cracks; if pacing wires are not in use postoperatively, place insulating covers over distal tips of each wire; have external pacemaker generator available (unifocal and bifocal).

Verify defibrillator settings with surgeon.

Have surgeon verbalize when defibrillator is to be discharged.

Have appropriate size internal defibrillator paddles; ensure that they fit into OR defibrillator.

For reoperation, have internal and external paddles or adhesive external defibrillator patches available; verify setting with surgeon before discharging.

Apply sufficient electrode paste to external paddles before placing paddles on patient's chest.

9. NURSING DIAGNOSIS

Risk for injury related to thermal hazards.

PATIENT OUTCOME*

The patient is free from signs and symptoms of thermal injury as evidenced by absence of tissue damage secondary to hyperthermia or hypothermia.

INTERVENTIONS

Check setting of thermia unit; maintain temperature per protocol.

Turn warming unit off when patient is being cooled; turn unit on when patient is being rewarmed.

Cover thermia blanket with sheet or thin blanket; avoid direct contact with skin.

Ensure integrity of thermia blanket; avoid puncture injury to blanket from needles or other sharp objects.

In neonates use radiant heater (per protocol), head covering, plastic blankets or wrappers, or warming bed with heaters; avoid excess heat.

Expose only skin area required for operation; both the very young and the elderly are more susceptible to temperature changes.

Ensure that temperature of topical solutions is appropriate for use (cold during induced arrest, warm before or after induced arrest).

Have cardiac insulating pads (if surgeon requests), cold lap tapes, and so forth available to retain hypothermic temperature during cardiac repair; have sufficient cold topical irrigating solution.

When normothermia is used (e.g., off-pump procedure), avoid excessive cooling of ambient temperature.

When profound hypothermia is used, protect ears, nose, and other prominences from frostbite with additional padding.

Avoid direct contact of ice or ice chips with skin or tissue (ice chips in the pericardium may cause phrenic nerve injury).

Maintain cool temperature in room during period of induced arrest; increase temperature during closing of incision; verify with surgeon; have warming blankets on SICU bed per protocol.

Provide warm blankets preoperatively (verify with surgeon) and postoperatively.

Monitor patient's temperatures (rectal, esophageal, bladder, ventricular septal, in-line bypass); verify accuracy of monitoring system; report malfunctions; adjust room temperature as needed.

10. NURSING DIAGNOSIS

Risk for infection at surgical site related to surgical incision, sites of catheters and intravascular lines, and altered cardiac function (CDC, 1999; Fogg, 1999).

PATIENT OUTCOME*

The patient is free from signs and symptoms of infection as evidenced by absence of redness, edema, purulent incisional drainage, or untoward elevation of temperature postoperatively.

INTERVENTIONS

Use depilatories or electric clippers to shave hair; avoid razors if possible.

Assess risk factors for postoperative infection (e.g., previous cardiac operations, duration of surgery, duration of CPB, length of hospitalization [preoperative and in SICU], blood transfusions, postoperative blood loss, diabetes mellitus, results of laboratory studies); review laboratory data; and report abnormal urine or blood values (e.g., elevated white blood cell count) to physician.

Dress all incisions and sites of intravascular lines.

Have prescribed topical antibiotic solution available for irrigation.

Ensure prophylactic antibiotics are given preoperatively.

Use closed urinary drainage system; verify urine flow before draping patient.

Routinely perform skin preparation to knees (or feet if leg vein needed) in anticipation of inserting femoral artery pressure line or intraaortic balloon or instituting femoral vein–femoral artery bypass.

Confine and contain instruments and supplies used in groin or leg; change gown and gloves when they are contaminated.

If the OR bed is elevated or lowered (for some IMA dissections) or turned from side to side (to de-air ventricle), take appropriate measures to retain sterility of field, gowns, gloves, and drapes; take precautions to maintain sterility of bypass lines.

Keep setup sterile until patient leaves OR (in case incision needs to be reopened for exploration).

Document lot and serial numbers of all implants and other information per institutional protocol.

Ensure that hand washing, standard precautions, and appropriate sterilization and decontamination procedures are followed.

11. NURSING DIAGNOSIS

Risk for impaired skin integrity.

PATIENT OUTCOME*

The patient's skin integrity is maintained as evidenced by the absence of bruises, skin breakdown, discoloration, open skin lesions, or excoriation during the perioperative period (Rothrock, 1996).

INTERVENTIONS

Assess skin integrity; note bruises, lesions, discoloration, and other problems; assess skin turgor and elasticity (especially in very young and elderly patients).

Pad hands, elbows, and back of head; pad heels and feet when possible.

Keep drapes off lower extremities and head; use anesthesia screen or special drape holders and equipment.

Ensure that SICU bed is prepared with mattress padding.

Prevent pooling of preparation solutions.

Maintain dry, wrinkle-free linen on OR and SICU bed.

Tape dressings with porous, hypoallergenic tape, using the minimum amount of tape that will secure entire dressing; the length of tape that extends beyond edge of dressing should be approximately one third the width of dressing (Berger and Williams, 1999).

12. NURSING DIAGNOSES

Risk for impaired myocardial, peripheral, and cerebral tissue integrity related to surgery, hypothermia, cardiopulmonary bypass, and/or surgical particulate or air emboli.

PATIENT OUTCOME

The patient's myocardial, peripheral, and cerebral tissue integrity is adequate or improved as evidenced by absence of new electrocardiographic manifestations of infarction, the presence of palpable peripheral pulses, and clear or improving sensorium postoperatively.

INTERVENTIONS

Minimize or limit activities that increase myocardial oxygen demand (e.g., decrease anxiety, decrease environmental stimulation such as noise or direct lighting).

Monitor ECG throughout procedure; note dysrhythmias, ectopic beats for potential cardiac arrest; note bradydysrhythmias and ECG evidence of ischemia (e.g., ST segment changes).

Anticipate need for antidysrhythmic agents if ectopy is noted.

Monitor ECG during induced arrest; if ECG activity noted, prepare to reinfuse cardioplegia solution.

Maintain extra supply of cold topical solution to keep the heart cold.

Keep instruments clean of blood and particulate matter that could become a source of emboli (tissue debris such as fat, bone fragments, suture pieces, excess bone wax); remove particulate matter remaining in the surgical site and notify surgeon.

Check bypass lines before institution of CPB; note presence of air in arterial lines and notify surgeon or perfusionist; ensure that arterial and venous lines are secure.

Use discard suction at site of heart valve excision to remove particulate debris.

Determine whether single or double venous cannulation is to be used (have caval clamps or tapes available for double cannulation per surgeon's preference).

Fill/refill venous lines according to protocol and with designated solutions only; avoid excessive air in venous lines (which can cause airlock).

Be able to readily identify inflow lines from outflow lines; label if necessary.

Verify that vent/suction lines are suctioning (and not infusing).

If femoral vein–femoral artery bypass is to be instituted, have appropriate supplies and instruments to access femoral vessels; have Y-connectors and extra tubing for extending venous line to right atrium (if requested).

Avoid kinks in bypass tubing; avoid pressure on bypass lines; ensure band connections are secure in bypass tubing (especially arterial and other high pressure lines).

When venting catheters and lines are employed, have appropriate connectors, tubing, and so forth.

Have correct heparin dosage if given at field; have additional heparin available if emergency reinstitution of bypass is required after heparin reversal (with protamine sulfate); verify that heparin has been given.

Avoid restrictive leg dressings (when vein is excised).

When intraaortic balloon pump (IABP) or other catheters are used in the femoral artery, avoid bending the patient's legs (resulting in kinking lines or injury to vessel wall).

> *Surgery without cardiopulmonary bypass*
>
> Have immediately available (per protocol): special retractors, coronary stabilizers, coronary artery retraction or occlusion tapes, CO_2 blower/suction device, lighted retractors, and other surgeon-requested items.
>
> Use normothermic or warm irrigation.
>
> Avoid inadvertently touching the heart.
>
> Be prepared to institute cardiopulmonary bypass quickly; have setup supplies readily available.

13. NURSING DIAGNOSIS

Risk for injury related to deficient fluid volume and electrolyte, and/or acid-base imbalance due to blood loss, blood reaction, and/or hyperkalemic cardioplegia solution.

PATIENT OUTCOME*

The patient's fluid, electrolyte, and acid-base balance is consistent with or improved from baseline levels established preoperatively as evidenced by hematocrit within acceptable range, electrolytes, arterial blood gases, urinary output, and blood pressures within normal limits.

INTERVENTIONS

Review patient's record for blood order (type and number of units).

Review laboratory studies: complete blood cell count, coagulation profile, electrolytes, arterial blood gases (ABGs).

Monitor intraoperative blood loss; note sudden or excessive bleeding.

Ensure that suction is available and working properly.

Monitor intraoperative ABGs, electrolytes, blood laboratory values, ECG.

Monitor pulmonary and systemic blood pressures for indication of volume status.

Have packed red blood cells immediately available (in OR or directly adjacent to OR); follow protocol for proper blood storage.

Ensure adequate blood and blood product supply via communication with blood bank; verify with surgeon and anesthesiologist.

Use autotransfusion suction before patient is fully heparinized (and cardiotomy suction is available) to conserve blood.

Use sump (cardiotomy) suction only when heparin has taken full effect; suction with sump suction whenever possible to conserve blood and to return it immediately to the bypass pump; avoid using cardiotomy suction after protamine reversal.

Avoid excessive negative pressure with pump sucker to reduce shear stress on red blood cells.

Use discard suction for irrigation and antibiotic solutions (to reduce amount of irrigation solution and medication returning to bypass pump and causing an undesired drop in hematocrit level).

Use discard suction to remove topical solutions from pleural cavity (if opened) and pericardial cavity.

Ensure that the autotransfusion system is working properly; have available additional supplies (suction tubing, canisters).

Anticipate need for platelets, fresh frozen plasma, or "glue" with reoperations and patients with a history of anticoagulation and antiplatelet therapy; have topical hemostatic agents available.

If patient has been receiving warfarin anticoagulants, note if medication has been discontinued and heparin initiated.

Note if patient discontinued antiplatelet therapy preoperatively.

Monitor intraoperative urine output.

Verify that urine is draining when catheterizing bladder; notify surgeon or anesthesiologist if urine is not visualized; if urethral strictures are present, have available dilators, water-soluble lubricant, large syringe, Coude catheters, and other supplies as requested by surgeon; anticipate possible insertion of suprapubic catheter if other measures fail; have necessary items available.

Have chest tubes available; if pleural cavity is entered, anticipate placement of a tube in the pleural space (during surgery or immediately postoperatively).

Have available additional chest tubes, Y-connectors, and tubing if extra chest tubes are connected; have chest drainage containers or cardiotomy reservoirs to collect drainage.

Monitor chest tube drainage closely; alert surgeon if drainage exceeds acceptable amount (e.g., 150 to 200 ml or more per hour).

Secure tubes and drains (and connections) before leaving OR.

In addition to standard postoperative report, include information on cardiac status, dysrhythmias, difficulties with defibrillation, cardiac medications, baseline pulmonary function, location of pressure monitoring and infusion lines, recent electrolyte levels (especially potassium), and any other information that will facilitate patient care in the SICU.

14. NURSING DIAGNOSIS

Risk for decreased cardiac output related to emotional (e.g., fear), sensory (e.g., pain), or physiologic (electrical, mechanical, or structural) factors.

PATIENT OUTCOME

The patient's cardiac function is consistent with or improved from baseline levels established preoperatively as evidenced by blood pressure within expected range; warm, dry skin; and urine output greater than 30 to 50 ml per hour.

INTERVENTIONS

Institute measures to reduce emotional stress and pain, which can increase myocardial oxygen demand.

Assess pain level; provide nitroglycerine or other pain medication as ordered.

Provide comfort measures before induction (e.g., adjust positioning, apply warm blankets, hold the patient's hand).

Provide requested religious articles.

Monitor pulmonary and systemic pressures; note any drop in systemic pressures or increase in pulmonary pressures, indicating myocardial dysfunction; correlate with distended, sluggish heart.

Monitor cardiac output (CO), cardiac index (CI), pulmonary vascular resistance (PVR), systemic vascular resistance (SVR), and other hemodynamic parameters.

Monitor for fluid volume deficit or excess.

Note reduction in urine output, which may indicate a reduction in cardiac output.

If pulmonary artery pressure line has not been inserted, anticipate insertion of line immediately postoperatively; anticipate possible insertion of left atrial pressure line; have appropriate supplies available.

Observe for reaction during protamine infusion (drop in blood pressure).

Monitor ECG rate and rhythm, especially lethal dysrhythmias (ventricular tachycardia/fibrillation).

Have epicardial temporary pacing wires ready for insertion.

Have defibrillator ready when fibrillation is seen before induced arrest or immediately after removal of cross-clamp; test defibrillator before start of procedure; have backup defibrillator and internal paddles available.

Have appropriate ECG leads and cables available for cardioversion.

Have appropriate ECG leads available for use with IABP; have IABP and supplies available.

15. NURSING DIAGNOSIS

Potential for altered participation (ineffective) in rehabilitation.

PATIENT OUTCOME*

The patient will participate in rehabilitation as evidenced by verbalizing or participating in planning for discharge, identifying knowledge deficits related to potential complications or referral services requiring patient education, and demonstrating ability to perform activities related to postoperative care (Rothrock, 1996). (See Research Highlight 5-2).

RESEARCH **HIGHLIGHT 5-2**

Telephone Follow-Up After Cardiac Surgery

In this study 90 cardiac surgery patients were randomly assigned to one of two groups: the control group, which received routine postoperative care, and the intervention group, which received routine care plus five follow-up phone calls from a cardiovascular nurse research assistant. Eligibility criteria included age over 21; discharge to home 3 to 7 days after surgery; and the ability to read, speak, and understand English. The intervention group's phone calls followed a standardized assessment sheet that included questions related to respiratory, cardiac, and neurologic function; fluid status; pain management; sleep; nutrition; elimination; activity; self-care; psychosocial status; wound management; and patient knowledge. Algorithms and nursing guidelines were developed to ensure consistent intervention and decision making during the phone calls. Analysis of the content of the follow-up phone calls revealed that nurse interventions focused primarily on support and reinforcement, making referrals, and coaching. Questionnaires were sent to both groups 1 month after surgery to measure patient satisfaction, office visits, postoperative complications, and readmission to the hospital. The intervention group demonstrated higher satisfaction, had lower depression scores, and had fewer readmissions and emergency room visits. The researchers concluded that follow-up telephone calls can aid in transition from hospital to home for cardiac surgery patients, providing a means to answer questions, clarify instructions, and reinforce education.

Modified from Weaver LA, Doran KA: Telephone follow-up after cardiac surgery, *Am J Nurs* 101(Suppl 5):2400, 2001.

INTERVENTIONS

Assess patient's ability to deep breathe and cough; teach patient how to use cough pillow and splint.

Assess patient's and family's understanding of procedure performed; clarify misconceptions; and if necessary, refer patient to specialist for additional information.

Assess patient's understanding of prescribed lifestyle modifications, assess feelings of patient and family about these changes, and answer questions or refer to appropriate personnel.

Encourage patient and family to clarify misconceptions and seek additional information and support as needed.

Assess family's ability to assist patient in recuperation and rehabilitation; refer as necessary.

Verify patient's and family's knowledge of reportable signs and symptoms related to specific procedure (e.g., bypass graft closure, valve failure, infection).

Verify patient's and family's knowledge of prescribed medications, including name, dosage, and times, side effects, and signs and symptoms (of allergic reaction, overdose); list medications.

Verify patient's and family's understanding of special considerations related to surgery (e.g., risk factor modification for patients with coronary artery disease, need for laboratory follow-up in patients with prosthetic valves requiring chronic anticoagulation).

Conclusion

Nursing diagnoses and patient outcomes guide the perioperative nurse in selecting the appropriate interventions to achieve the stated goals. Planning enables the nurse to identify interventions that will achieve selected outcomes and avoid complications. These interventions are directed by the nursing diagnoses and collaborative problems that have been formulated to reflect particular patient needs, but they should also incorporate an awareness of the potential hazards common to all cardiac surgery patients. Actions must be continuously reappraised for their appropriateness and effectiveness and the priority given to their implementation.

For cardiac surgery patients, priority nursing interventions include supporting hemodynamic stability and ventilatory function, promoting relief of pain and discomfort, promoting healing, and providing information about perioperative expectations and treatment regimens (Doenges, Moorhouse, and Geissler, 2000). How successfully such interventions are implemented and desired outcomes achieved is determined in part by the nurse's intellectual, interpersonal, and technical abilities. The following chapter provides a broad overview of methodologies for evaluating outcome achievement.

References

Association of periOperative Registered Nurses (AORN): Patient outcomes: standards of perioperative care. In *Standards, recommended practices, and guidelines,* Denver, 2001, The Association.

Berger KJ, Williams MB: *Fundamentals of nursing: collaborating for optimal health,* ed 2, Stamford, Conn, 1999, Appleton & Lange.

Beyea SC, editor: *Perioperative nursing data set: the perioperative nursing vocabulary,* Denver, 2000, AORN.

Beyea SC, Killen AR, Watson D: Perioperative data elements: the contribution of a specialty to nursing language. In Rantz MJ, Lemone P, editors: *Classification of nursing diagnoses: proceedings of the thirteenth conference,* Glendale, Calif, 1999, Cinahl Information Systems.

Biddle C, Cannady MJ: Surgical positions: their effects on cardiovascular, respiratory systems, *AORN J* 52(2):350, 1990.

Butcher L: Teaching: preoperative. In Bulechek GM, McCloskey JC: *Nursing interventions: effective nursing treatments,* ed 3, Philadelphia, 1999, WB Saunders.

Carpenito LJ: *Nursing care plans and documentation: nursing diagnosis and collaborative problems,* ed 3, Philadelphia, 1999, JB Lippincott.

Centers for Disease Control and Prevention (CDC): Guideline for prevention of surgical site infection 1999, *Am J Infect Control* 27:97, 1999.

Dennis V: Implementing active electrode monitoring: a perioperative call, *Surgical Services Management* 7(2):32, 2001.

Doenges ME, Moorhouse MF: *Nurses pocket guide: diagnoses, interventions, and rationales,* ed 7, Philadelphia, 2000, FA Davis.

Doenges ME, Moorhouse NF, Geissler AC: *Nursing care plans: guidelines for individualizing patient care,* ed 5, Philadelphia, 2000, FA Davis.

Fecteau D: Patient and environmental safety. In Meeker MH, Rothrock JC: *Alexander's care of the patient in surgery,* ed 11, St Louis, 1999, Mosby.

Fogg D: Infection control. In Meeker MH, Rothrock JC: *Alexander's care of the patient in surgery,* ed 11, St Louis, 1999, Mosby.

Fox VJ: Patient education and discharge planning. In Meeker MH, Rothrock JC: *Alexander's care of the patient in surgery,* ed 11, St Louis, 1999, Mosby.

Gawande AA and others: The incidence and nature of surgical events in Colorado and Utah in 1992, *Surgery* 126:66, 1999.

Gordon M: *Nursing diagnosis: process and application,* New York, 1982, McGraw-Hill.

Hersey DN: The aging patient. In Rothrock JC: *Perioperative nursing care planning,* ed 2, St Louis, 1996, Mosby.

Hudson G and others: Warming up to better surgical outcomes, *AORN J* 60(1):247, 1999.

Institute of Medicine (IOM): *To err is human: building a safer health care system,* Washington, DC, 1999, National Academy Press.

Kee CC, Miller V: Perioperative care of the older adult with auditory and visual changes, *AORN J* 70(6):1012, 1999.

Kurz A and others: Perioperative normothermia to reduce the incidence of surgical-wound infection and shorten hospitalization, *N Engl J Med* 334(19):1209, 1996.

Lenz ER, Perkins S: Coronary artery bypass graft surgery patients and their family member caregivers: outcomes of a family-focused staged psychoeducational intervention, *Appl Nurs Res* 13(3):142, 2000.

Litwak RS, Dack S: Concepts of patient care. In Litwak RS, Jurado RA: *Care of the cardiac surgical patient,* Norwalk, Conn, 1982, Appleton-Century-Crofts.

Maldonado SS and Nygren C: Pediatric surgery. In Meeker MH, Rothrock JC, *Alexander's care of the patient in surgery,* ed 11, St Louis, 1999, Mosby.

McEwen DR: Intraoperative positioning of surgical patients, *AORN J* 63(6):1059, 1996.

Meckes PF: Geriatric surgery. In Meeker MH, Rothrock JC: *Alexander's care of the patient in surgery,* ed 11, St Louis, 1999, Mosby.

Norred CL, Zamudio S, Palmer SK: Use of complementary and alternative medicines by surgical patients, *AANA J* 68:13, 2000.

Nygren C, Rothrock JC: Pediatric surgery. In Rothrock JC: *Perioperative nursing care planning,* ed 2, St Louis, 1996, Mosby.

Rantz MJ, LeMone P, editors: *Classification of nursing diagnoses: proceedings of the thirteenth conference,* Glendale, Calif, 1999, Cinahl Information Systems.

Rothrock JC: Generic care planning: AORN patient outcome standards. In Rothrock JC: *Perioperative nursing care planning,* ed 2, St Louis, 1996, Mosby.

Rothrock JC, Smith DA: Selecting the perioperative patient focused model, *AORN J* 71:1030, 2000.

Seifert PC: Cardiac surgery. In Rothrock JC: *Perioperative nursing care planning,* ed 2, St Louis, 1996, Mosby.

Seifert PC: Cardiac surgery. In Meeker MH, Rothrock JC: *Alexander's care of the patient in surgery,* ed 11, St Louis, 1999a, Mosby.

Seifert PC: The RN first assistant and collaborative practice. In Rothrock JC: *The RN first assistant: an expanded perioperative nursing role,* ed 3, Philadelphia, 1999b, JB Lippincott.

6

Implementation of Perioperative Nursing Care

We're always ready.

Anonymous

Do whatever it takes.

Anonymous

Although the existence of a well-prepared plan is implied when patients achieve successful outcomes, the actions result in the surgical goal's being met. A plan of care provides guidelines for nursing actions, but there is no one formula that can replace the nurse's judgment and decision-making skill in a given situation. Cardiac surgery patients are complex and do not always respond in a predictable manner. Perioperative nurses in general, and registered nurse first assistants (RNFAs) in particular, must be alert to unexpected changes in the patient's condition and be prepared to intervene appropriately (Box 6-1). The growth of "off-pump" surgery, performed without the use of cardiopulmonary bypass (CPB), is associated with special considerations that are listed in Box 6-2. New information must be assessed, judged for its significance, integrated into the plan of care, and reflected in the actions taken. Priorities may have to be reordered. Interventions may have to be modified or alternative actions followed based on the knowledge, experience, and skill of the nurse.

Nursing actions include not only performing activities to achieve patient outcomes, but also supervising others in carrying out the plan, monitoring the patient's response to interventions, and documenting nursing actions and patient responses. The achievement of patient outcomes provides tangible evidence of the success or failure of the interventions and reflects the nurse's intellectual, interpersonal, and technical ability. A high degree of communication, cooperation, and collaboration among team members is necessary if successful outcomes are to be achieved (Ladden, 1999).

This chapter reviews the activities of a standard cardiac procedure using CPB with myocardial protection; addi-

tionally, off-pump procedures are also addressed. Generic care plan outlines in Chapter 5 are applicable to these activities. Specific operative procedures and related nursing considerations are discussed in the following chapters.

Admission to the Cardiac Service

The admission process varies according to the underlying pathologic condition and the condition of the patient. Patients admitted for symptoms of heart failure may already be in the hospital for a diagnostic workup and cardiac catheterization. Patients who are hemodynamically stable but too debilitated to withstand the stress of immediate surgery may require nutritional support before the operative procedure is done. Emergency admissions (for acute derangements such as postinfarction ventricular septal rupture or aortic dissection) often come to the operating room (OR) directly from the coronary care unit or after emergency admission to the cardiac catheterization laboratory or the radiology imaging suite. Patients undergoing an elective procedure are often admitted the day of surgery. Typical adult admission orders (Box 6-3) are implemented. Same-day admission patients usually have the preoperative laboratory work and consultations performed during the preadmission screening a day or two before they are admitted.

Preoperative Patient Teaching

The preadmission screening period is an especially good time to perform patient teaching because there may be less stress than during the immediate preoperative

---

BOX 6-1
Registered Nurse First Assistant Considerations During Surgery

Patient/Family Interactions*

In addition to meeting specific teaching needs of patients and families, also promote psychologic well-being and a sense of security by alluding to staff nurses' competence and complimenting fellow caregivers. If there are complaints about care, listen to the concerns and investigate the problem or report it to the appropriate persons as warranted.

Always approach families with a positive expression on your face (this does not necessarily mean a broad smile); a frown may cause them to assume that their loved one is in "trouble" and cause unnecessary stress. When talking to families of patients who may die in the OR, be honest about the seriousness of the situation, but always allow the family to retain some hope for improvement (even if survival seems unlikely).

Do not strongly encourage or discourage a family's viewing of a deceased patient. There may be guilt feelings, denial, and other emotions that affect the decision. If the family wishes to view the body, remove excess blood, cover the body with a clean sheet (the head may be left uncovered), and transfer to a quiet room. Accompany the family to the room and provide chairs and tissues. Offer coffee or water. Stay with the family if it seems appropriate, and touch the body (the head, the hands) to show the family that this is "acceptable" behavior.

Peer Relationships

Participate in general perioperative duties: setting up for surgery, patient preparation (washing, positioning, etc.), cleaning up after the case.

Share knowledge gained from assisting duties with staff (including assistive personnel) in the OR, nursing units, and diagnostic laboratories.

Provide rationales for the surgeon's preferences (e.g., suture, instruments); help to differentiate between changes in the surgeon's routine that are exceptions and permanent alterations as a result of new technology, research findings, and so on.

Participate in inservices and staff meetings.

Assist managers with capital and operational budget considerations.

During emergencies, determine whether it is more important for you to scrub in immediately or whether assistance to the circulator (e.g., grounding, positioning, skin preparation) to get the patient ready is of greater priority. This will differ with each emergency and must be decided on an individual basis.

Mentor experienced and inexperienced nurses, participate in orientation activities, and serve as preceptor to nurses new to the unit.

Admit mistakes or errors to team members; notify surgeon of missing items.

Technical Considerations

Develop a "disaster" mentality; anticipate and mentally plan for sudden adverse changes (e.g., acute hemorrhage, ven-

tricular fibrillation) in the patient's hemodynamic status; play "what if?"

Inspect inflow lines for air, especially arterial infusion catheters during cannulation, and cardioplegia infusion lines before each delivery of the solution.

When working on the pericardium, be aware of the location of the phrenic nerve; know the location of the tips of the instruments you are holding to prevent injury to the heart, lungs, and other tissue.

Do not obscure the surgeon's vision with instruments, hands, and so on.

Do not bump the surgeon's arms or hands; if the surgeon is leaning on your arm or hand, don't move without giving advance warning.

Know the location of the entire length of the suture and verify that it is not caught on an instrument or other item.

Use curved scissors to cut the suture; use scissor tips for cutting; point the tips up or down depending on what will pose the least risk of injuring surrounding tissue.

Retract the right pleura to provide more room for the surgeon to insert a right atrial cannulation pursestring and to attach atrial pacing wires (if bypass is terminated and the inflated lungs are in the way).

Stabilize the handle of the cross-clamp with a rolled or folded towel to prevent wobbling (and possible injury to a blood vessel).

If using a long, narrow (e.g., coronary) suction tip, stabilize the midshaft of the sucker on the sternal edge, retractor, or hand for greater control.

Follow the suture so that there is sufficient length between the portion of the suture held in your hand and the needle end of the stitch; then when the surgeon pulls the needle through the tissue, the suture does not tug at your hand and possibly injure tissue.

Avoid holding too much suture between your hand and the needle, which could result in excess suture obscuring the anastomotic site.

When requested to open the jaws of the cross-clamp, do so slowly and smoothly.

Verbalize the patient's systemic blood pressure to the surgeon (especially drops in pressure) when the surgeon is unable to see the monitors during manipulation of the beating heart to inspect anastomoses, potential bleeding sites, and so on.

Suction opened pleural spaces before completion of the procedure.

Look for bleeders in a systematic manner; suction specific areas rather than wide expanses of tissue; suction after cauterizing, applying hemostatic clips, or suture ligating to confirm control of the bleeding site.

Prepare for double cannulation for any surgery on the right side of the heart.

Know the surgeon's indications and technique for converting from an off-pump procedure to a conventional CPB procedure.

---

*Applicable to all perioperative nurses.

---

period. Patient teaching performed before admission can decrease the amount of instruction necessary during the abbreviated and usually tense period immediately be-

fore surgery (Table 6-1). Also, it can ease some of the fear and anxiety caused by the impending surgery, as well as concerns about resumption of functional activities,

BOX **6-2**

Intraoperative Considerations in Beating Heart Coronary Bypass Surgery

Preoperative Assessment

- Similar to that for all revascularization patients
- LV function and exercise tolerance assessed in preparation for short period of ischemia when coronary artery occluded for anastomosis
- Complete revascularization is the surgical goal
- Poor target vessels (small, highly calcified) may favor use of CPB

Premedication

- Cardiac antiischemic drugs (e.g., beta blockers, calcium antagonists, and nitrates) continued
- Diazepam given for sedation
- Low-molecular-weight heparin given subcutaneously for thrombosis prophylaxis

Positioning

- Anterior thoracotomy: semilateral with left side up; a small pillow can be placed under the left side of the chest; left arm may be secured above the head
- Median sternotomy (partial or complete): supine, arms at side
- Legs positioned so that groin can be cannulated for A-line or IABP if necessary

Safety

- CPB equipment and perfusionist should be immediately available
- Instruments, supplies, and equipment for conventional coronary procedures should be available
- Sternal saw immediately available should median sternotomy be required (after nonsternal incision initially made)
- Temporary pacing wires available
- External defibrillator pads applied; internal paddles may be used with larger incisions
- A second assistant useful for keeping field clear of blood
- All team members need to be especially vigilant during anastomoses because hemodynamic changes can occur rapidly (and there is no backup normally provided with CPB)

Monitoring

- Cineangiograms available to assess collateral circulation
- Volume status monitored (reduced preload creates hemodynamic problems)
- TEE often used to monitor LV function
- Temperature monitored and actions implemented to maintain patient at normothermia

Anesthesia

- Thoracic epidural or general anesthesia (Park and others, 1999) used
- Analgesia with bupivacaine and morphine
- General anesthesia with propofol, rocuronium, and sufentanil for rapid induction and emergence from anesthesia (Krucylak, 1999)

- Double-lumen ET tube may be used to selectively deflate lung on affected side during LIMA take-down and left heart anastomosis
- After mobilization of IMAs and before application of coronary stabilizer, heparin given to achieve ACT greater than 250 to 300 seconds; protamine may or may not be given to reverse the heparin

Blood Loss

- Autotransfusion system generally used if more than two bypass grafts are performed; may not be cost effective for fewer grafts (Pfister, 1999)

Preconditioning

- Before anastomosis the coronary artery to be bypassed is temporarily occluded for 5 to 10 minutes and then allowed to reperfuse for 5 to 10 minutes to test ability of heart to withstand ischemia during anastomosis and to precondition the heart for the ischemic period; if heart is unable to tolerate short periods of ischemia, surgery may require use of CPB
- Hearts with coronary lesions greater than 95% usually tolerate vessel occlusion better than hearts with less-stenosed vessels
- Ventricular wall function inspected with TEE before coronary stabilizer application or vessel occlusion

Anastomosis

- Performed after mobilization of left or right IMA
- Local cardiac motion commonly minimized with stabilizer to facilitate technically successful anastomosis; pharmacologic bradycardia may also be induced with esmolol, adenosine, verapamil, or diltiazem
- May use CO_2 blower/mister to keep arteriotomy clear of blood
- Monitor for deteriorating cardiac function when heart is manipulated or elevated to expose lateral or posterior coronary arteries
- LAD coronary artery likely to be first anastomosis of multiple grafts (revascularization of left ventricle enables heart to better tolerate more technically difficult lateral or posterior vessels); in general, order of anastomoses is from site of least cardiac displacement to area requiring most cardiac displacement (normally this would coincide with performing the LAD anastomosis first)
- Calcium channel blocker given intravenously when arterial grafts (e.g., IMA, radial artery) are used

Intraoperative Complications

- Monitor for signs of ischemia, pump failure, dysrhythmias
- Extended episodes of hypotension; may signal a myocardial infarction
- Institute measures to prevent/treat inadvertent hypothermia; check the temperature of topical irrigating solutions before application (cold fluid may cause heart to fibrillate) (see Box 6-4)
- When difficult-to-access target artery or hemodynamic instability occurs, may need to convert to conventional coronary bypass surgery; instruments, supplies, CPB setup need to be immediately available

---

ACT, Activated clotting time; *A-line,* arterial pressure line; *ET,* endotracheal; *IABP,* intraaortic balloon pump; *ICU,* intensive care unit; *IMA,* internal mammary artery; *LAD,* left anterior descending; *LV,* left ventricular; *OR,* operating room; *TEE,* transesophageal echocardiography.
Modified from Nierich AP: In *Minimally invasive cardiac surgery: information for associated professionals,* http://www.medtronic.com/cardiac/mics/phys_associates.html (accessed May 23, 2001); Krucylak PE: *Semin Thorac Cardiovasc Surg* 11(2):116, 1990; Pfister AJ: *Adv Cardiac Surg* 11:35, 1999; Park KW and others. In Kaplan JA: *Cardiac anesthesia,* ed 4, Philadelphia, 1999, WB Saunders.

BOX 6-2
Intraoperative Considerations in Beating Heart Coronary Bypass Surgery—cont'd

Reperfusion

- May see dysrhythmias after release of vessel occluder; lidocaine may be used to reduce dysrhythmias
- May require angiography to confirm graft patency (Krucylak, 1999)

PostoperativeCare

- Patients may be extubated in the OR or within the first few hours in the ICU (depending on the depth of anesthesia and degree of hypothermia)
- Pain aggressively treated to promote ambulation, comfort, and patient satisfaction

- Pain control options include intercostal blocks, patient-controlled analgesia pumps, epidural anesthesia, and nonsteroidal antiinflammatory drugs
- Extubation, chest tube removal, and first time out of bed usually accomplished earlier than conventional post-CPB procedure
- Calcium antagonists continued for approximately 6 weeks postoperatively
- Low-dose aspirin is given to reduce risk of graft thrombosis
- Beta blockers are given to reduce incidence of atrial fibrillation

---

pain, death, absence from home or work, and recuperation (Fox, 1999).

The perioperative nurse's initial contact with the patient may occur during the preadmission screening, on the nursing unit, or in the preinduction area of the OR. The patient can also expect preoperative visits by anesthesia personnel, surgeons and their associates, and others involved in the care of the patient.

Preoperative teaching assignments vary with the institution. Formal patient teaching may be provided by the patient's primary nurse on the unit, a cardiovascular clinical specialist, or the perioperative nurse. Many RNFAs include this function in their role (Espersen, 1999). Whether the perioperative clinician visits the patient during the preadmission period or just before surgery, it is important that the nurse collect sufficient information to plan the most appropriate care. The interaction is also helpful to the patient because it can provide the reassurance of meeting someone who will be directly involved in giving care during the operation.

When teaching is done on the unit, the perioperative nurse can reinforce what has been taught and provide information that is uniquely related to the surgical environment. This may be as simple as the sights and sounds that one can expect on entry into the OR or as complex as the principles involved in extracorporeal circulation. (Whereas some patients use denial to cope with stress, others rely on knowledge as a defense mechanism.) No matter what is discussed, the information should be accurate and meet the patient's identified needs.

The surgeon reviews the operative plan and discusses the benefits and risks of the operation in order to obtain an informed consent from the patient. Patients should also be informed that a planned operation may have to be modified. An example of this is the patient's expectation that surgery is to be performed with a small incision or without the use of CPB; should anatomic or other considerations necessitate reverting to a conventional

---

BOX 6-3
Preoperative Orders: Admission to the Cardiac Service

Diagnosis _____
Allergies _____ Activity _____
Diet _____
Vital signs _____
Height and weight (kg) _____
Chest x-ray examination (PA and lateral) _____
Bilateral carotid ultrasound _____
ECG _____
Blood chemistry,* CBC, PT, PTT, bleeding time

_____
Urinalysis _____
Type and cross-match _____
    4 units packed RBCs _____
    2 units fresh frozen plasma _____
    10 units platelets _____
Test for cold agglutinins (cold screen) _____
ABGs _____
Respiratory consult to teach incentive spirometry_____
Patient teaching by nurse clinician _____
Old chart to floor _____
Night before surgery _____
    Triazolam (Halcion) PO prn hs for sleep _____
    Hibiclens shower at HS _____
    NPO after midnight _____
OR consent for _____
Consent for blood and blood products _____
Medications _____
    Cefuroxime _____
    Vancomycin _____
    Cardiac drips to OR _____

ABGs, Arterial blood gases; *CBC,* complete blood count; *ECG,* electrocardiogram; *hs,* bedtime; *NPO,* nothing by mouth; *OR,* operating room; *PA,* posteroanterior, *PO,* orally; *prn,* as needed; *PT,* prothrombin; *PTT,* partial thromboplastin time; *RBC,* red blood cells.
*Blood chemistry includes the following: glucose, acetone, urea nitrogen, creatinine, CO_2 content, sodium, potassium, chloride, calcium, uric acid, phosphorus, magnesium, alkaline phosphatase, amylase, lipase, total protein, albumin, globulin, bilirubin, cholesterol, and triglycerides.
Courtesy John R. Garrett, MD.

TABLE **6-1**
Patient Teaching Content for Coronary Artery Bypass Graft Surgery and Valve Surgery

TOPIC	CABG SURGERY	VALVE SURGERY
Preoperative Pointers		
Medical diagnosis	Coronary artery occlusive disease	Valve regurgitation, stenosis or mixed
Diagnostic tests	ECG, chest radiograph, nuclear imaging, cardiac catheterization	Same, plus echocardiogram
Routine preoperative tests	CMP, ECG, T&C, pulmonary function, PT, PTT, INR	Same
Incision site	Midsternal or anterior thoracotomy; multiple leg incisions for vein harvest, arm incision for radial artery harvest	Mini- or full sternotomy
Resume eating	2-3 days after removal of ET and NG tubes	Same
Pain control	IM, PO, PCA	Same
Estimated length of procedure	4-6 hours	Same
Estimated length of hospital stay	5-7 days	6-8 days
Long-term effects of surgery	Loss of saphenous vein, possible intermittent lower leg ischemia	Possible chronic anticoagulation; differences between biologic and mechanical prostheses, valve repair
Drains or tubes	2 days: mediastinal chest tube, pleural tube; 2-3 days: leg drains, urinary drainage catheter	2 days: mediastinal and pleural tubes, urinary catheter
Postoperative Pointers/Home Instructions		
Food	Cardiac diet	Same
Wound care	Wounds covered if draining; redress after shower or bath; contact clinician if signs of infection	Same
Bathing	Daily	Same
Driving	4-6 weeks (automatic shift only)	Same
Sex	Restricted by limits of ability to bear weight on upper arms and chest	Same
Return to work	8-12 weeks	Same
Medications	Aspirin anticoagulant, cardiac drugs	Warfarin (Coumadin), cardiac drugs
Follow-up	7-14 days	Same, plus lab tests for determination of bleeding times
Special restrictions	Upper body movement restricted for 6 weeks for sternal healing	Same
Lifestyle changes	Reduction of coronary risk factors; rehabilitation	Risk factor reduction; rehabilitation
Worrisome but normal	Fatigue, swelling in leg; leg discomfort 4-6 weeks; weakness, emotional let down	Fatigue; sound of mechanical valve; weakness; emotional let down

ECG, Electrocardiogram; *ET,* endotracheal; *IM,* intramuscular; *INR,* international normal ratio; *NG,* nasogastric; *PCA,* patient-controlled analgesia; *PO,* by mouth (per os); *PT,* prothrombin time; *PTT,* partial thromboplastin time; *CMP,* comprehensive metabolic panel (includes glucose, blood urea nitrogen, sodium, potassium, chloride, creatinine, albumin, bilirubin, calcium, alkaline phosphatase, total protein); *T&C,* type and cross-match.
Modified from Fox VJ: Patient education and discharge planning. In Meeker MH, Rothrock JC, editors: *Alexander's care of the patient in surgery,* ed 11, St Louis, 1999, Mosby.

sternotomy or instituting CPB, the patient and family should be prepared for this possibility. Preoperative communication between the surgeon, the patient, and the patient's significant others educates the patient and family about associated risks and benefits and provides information to the surgeon and nurse about the patient's expectations, fears, concerns, and coping strategies, all of which are important for perioperative patient management. Ensuring that the patient and family are properly informed and know what to expect before, during, and after surgery can facilitate a smooth postoperative experience.

Any fears of the patient regarding the risks of blood transfusion should be addressed and have prompted some states to enact blood safety laws. These laws require that when blood transfusion may be necessary during

surgery, the patient must be informed preoperatively of all available methods of receiving blood transfusions— autologous and homologous. One of the few exceptions for complying with the law is the need for emergency surgery. Bloodless surgery programs have gained popularity as a result of greater awareness of the potential risks of banked blood transfusions, a decrease in the availability of donor blood, religious objections to blood transfusion, and the costs associated with collecting, testing, storing, and administering blood and blood products (Reger and Roditski, 2001).

Patients can meet the cardiac surgery critical care nurses and visit the postoperative unit to prepare themselves for their postsurgical experience. However, patients and families may not wish to see the intensive care unit

(ICU) if it arouses fear and dread. These wishes should be respected, but family members or close friends planning to see the patient in the immediate postoperative period should be prepared for what they will see in the patient: multiple lines and catheters, pallor, cool skin, some facial edema, and unresponsiveness. Even though the patient may not be able to react, visitors should be encouraged to talk to the patient for their own psychologic welfare, and possibly for the patient's as well.

Advance Directives

Advances in health care technology and the increase in the number of elderly patients undergoing cardiac surgery has created ethical and legal challenges for health care workers. In particular, there is now the capability of extending life beyond the point where patients are capable of making decisions or expressing wishes about future health needs. To avoid uncertainty about a patient's wishes, advance communication among the patient, family, and health care providers can alleviate some of the problems that may arise during a health care crisis. The passage of the 1990 Patient Self-Determination Act enables patients, on admission to the hospital, to provide instructions about their wishes should they become terminally ill or have little hope of being weaned from life support. Advance directives include living wills, durable powers of attorney, and anatomic gifts (Watson, 1999).

Living wills are documents concerning treatment that direct others about the care desired by the patient who is terminally ill and unable to provide further instruction. Generally these documents express a desire not to prolong imminent death; care necessary to maintain comfort and dignity should be provided.

Durable powers of attorney delegate either very broad or specific authority to a proxy, who makes decisions about health care needs. This authority endures if the patient becomes incapable of making his or her own decisions. Often a spouse is the delegated authority. If the patient chooses, the authority can be revoked at any time.

Anatomic donations of body tissue and organs may also be arranged in advance. The Uniform Anatomical Gift Act of 1968, as well as the revisions made to the act in 1987, permits the donor to sign a legally valid document authorizing such gifts without the need for additional permission by family members. In the absence of the patient's documented desire to donate, an anatomic gift may be made by family members in the following order of priority: spouse, adult child, parent, adult brother or sister, or guardian. The Omnibus Reconciliation Act of 1986 was enacted to require hospitals receiving Medicare or Medicaid reimbursement to request organ donation from family members.

Room Preparation

Before the perioperative nurse visits the patient in the immediate preoperative period and transports the patient to the operating room, the nurse should ensure that critical supplies and equipment are available and that certain preparations have been made (Kaempf, 1994). Among these are:

- Banked blood (e.g., packed red blood cells) in the refrigerator
- Atrioventricular pacemaker (with new batteries)
- Backup internal paddles
- Backup sternal saw
- Both single and double venous cannulas available; extra aortic cannula
- Conventional sternal instruments, supplies, and equipment even if plan is to perform minimally invasive procedure
- Prosthetic valve inventory checked at least 24 hours before a scheduled valve procedure, and missing sizes replaced; check again the morning of surgery

If the patient suddenly decompensates hemodynamically, the nurse can focus attention on the patient and not have to worry about supplies or other basic items needed for surgery. This is part of the "disaster" mentality that promotes an alert and ready culture wherein emergencies and other unusual situations can be handled with minimal confusion and disruption.

If a beating heart procedure is planned, special consideration is given to preparing the room to protect the patient from inadvertent hypothermia. Strategies to maintain normal body temperature are listed in Table 6-2.

Entry into the Operating Room

The cardiac surgery patient's risk for sudden decompensation mandates that unpredictability should be expected. Certain assumptions are warranted. Chief among these are the importance of maintaining the balance between myocardial oxygen supply and demand, and the deleterious effects that a disproportionate increase on the demand side (or decrease on the supply side) has on cardiac function. Nursing actions should be implemented with these assumptions in mind.

The preoperative assessment begins as the nurse approaches the patient: Is the patient sitting up and alert to the surroundings? Are there attending critical care nurses, and monitors and other equipment on the transport stretcher, indicating a more unstable status?

The circulating nurse greets the patient by name and checks the identification band. Patients may feel cold and uncomfortable. Offering a warm blanket is not only a comfort measure but also reduces the metabolic impact of shivering. The proposed operation is

TABLE 6-2
Strategies to Prevent and Treat Inadvertent Hypothermia During Off-Pump Cardiac Surgery

STRATEGY/DEVICE	CONSIDERATIONS
Patient Care Management	
Minimize unnecessary exposure to ambient temperature	Keep patient covered before/after surgery; minimize time between skin preparation and and draping
Monitor patient temperature (Normal 37° C; 98.6° F)	Possible sites include esophagus, skin, nasopharynx, urinary bladder, rectum, and pulmonary artery catheter
Drapes/Coverings	
NONSTERILE	
Warm cotton blankets	Lose heat quickly; inexpensive
Reflective coverings (space blanket)	Conserve heat; may not be feasible for covering the large body area that is part of sterile field
Warm air device	Warm air transferred to patient; useful only in limited area; use cautiously in patients with ischemic peripheral vascular limbs
Warm water mattress	Placed on OR bed under patient; avoid puncturing with needles and sharps
Head covering	Towel, hat, stockinette, forced warm air
STERILE	
Surgical draping	Provide maximum coverage without limiting surgical access to chest, groin, and upper legs
Local draping	Cover areas of sterile field not requiring immediate access (e.g., place towels over groin area or site of leg vein excision); can be removed without contaminating the field should access to these sites be required. Replace wet towels as needed
Fluid Warmers	
IV fluid	Warm fluids, blood, and irrigating solutions to reduce heat loss from conduction
Blood	
Topical irrigation/lavage	Check temperature of fluids immediately before use
Anesthetic Gas Warmers	
Heat-moisture exchanger	Reduces heat loss during positive-pressure ventilation
Heated humidifier for gases	
Ambient Room Temperature	
Keep room temperature between 20°-24° C (68°-77° F)	Fairly effective warming strategy; staff discomfort; may foster growth of microorganisms
Infrared lamp directed at patient's body	Not generally recommended because of risk of burns

IV, intravenous.
Modified from Colburn B: personal communication, Sept 2, 2000; Arndt K: Inadvertent hypothermia in the OR, *AORN J* 70(2):204, 1999; Ensminger J, Moss R: Preventing inadvertent hypothermia—a success story, *AORN J* 70(2):298, 1999.

confirmed, and any patient allergies are elicited. Questions and concerns should be answered and clarified; however, patients may be hesitant to initiate a discussion that they feel might heighten their anxiety. Family members may be in attendance, and they should be included in these interactions.

Often the family will have been given an approximate time period for the anticipated length of surgery. The perioperative nurse should ask the family what they have been told. Occasionally the time frame provided by the surgeon (actual surgical time) needs to be expanded to include the activities performed immediately before the incision is made (e.g., insertion of monitoring lines, skin preparation) and actions after the skin is closed (e.g.,

application of dressings, attachment to portable monitors). These activities can add 1 to 2 hours to the original time estimate relayed to the family. There may be unnecessary concern when the initial time period has passed and the family is still waiting to receive word that the surgery is completed. Another consideration is that once the patient arrives in the ICU, admission procedures (e.g., checking vital signs, connecting monitoring lines and drainage tubes) must be performed. It may be as long as 1 hour before family members can first see the patient. Families tend to watch the clock closely, and offering a simple explanation of the various procedures that are performed in addition to the surgical repair itself can alleviate some of their emotional stress.

Another source of stress may be the cancellation of surgery because of an insufficient number of ICU beds or another patient's need for emergency surgery taking precedence over the scheduled operation. The increased anxiety and emotional stress accompanying the decision to cancel the operation may produce ischemic discomfort, dyspnea, and shortness of breath, and the nurse should be vigilant in observing the patient for these signs. Patients and families may be angry and feel a loss of control, but most accept the postponement, realizing that they themselves could be the ones needing an emergency operation. Perioperative nurses can reassure patients and family members that feelings of anger are understandable (and acceptable) and that the decision was made only after careful deliberation.

CHART REVIEW

The perioperative nurse reviews the hospital record for completion of laboratory work, operative permits, results of diagnostic studies, history and physical examination, medications, and other pertinent data. In the case of patients scheduled for coronary artery bypass grafting who underwent cardiac catheterization during a previous hospitalization, the old chart will be needed so that the test results can be reviewed. Special note should also be taken of abnormal laboratory values: prolonged bleeding times, elevated or low potassium levels (normal 3.5 to 5.5 mEq), cardiac enzymes, liver problems, and other results that may have a direct bearing on the surgical procedure.

The most recent chest x-ray films or digitized images (posteroanterior and lateral) should be available for evaluation of the heart and lungs, especially in patients undergoing repeat sternotomy whose pericardial adhesions may be against the sternum. In addition, the surgeon will want to view the cineangiogram of coronary artery bypass patients to note the location, size, and severity of coronary artery lesions; assess the pattern of coronary blood flow; and evaluate the contractile state of the heart. Portable cine viewers are often located near the OR, and the perioperative nurse may be responsible for obtaining these films before surgery.

MONITORING

Patients usually have peripheral intravenous (IV) lines inserted in the preinduction area; intraarterial blood pressure monitoring lines (A-lines) may also be started at this time or in the OR itself. A local anesthetic may be used at the insertion site and a sedative injected IV to allay the patient's anxiety. Additional central monitoring lines, such as a pulmonary artery catheter, are inserted in the OR (Table 6-3). Whether these are placed before or after anesthesia induction and intubation is decided by the anesthesiologist and varies from institution to institution. The nurse should remain close to the patient during induction and observe the monitors for signs of hemodynamic instability and cardiac rhythm disturbances (Fig. 6-1).

If the patient is intubated first, the nursing staff can apply the electrosurgical dispersive pads, catheterize the bladder, and position and wash the patient while the monitoring lines are being inserted. These nursing activities may have to be halted temporarily if assistance is needed to insert the central lines. The nurse should observe the electrocardiogram (ECG) and blood pressure monitors frequently for signs of hypotension or ventricular irritability, such as ectopy, tachycardia, or fibrillation. The defibrillator should be positioned near the patient and turned on so that it is readily available if needed.

In patients who are in cardiogenic shock there may be no time to establish invasive monitoring lines. The most important consideration for the anesthesiologist is to have a patent IV line so that medications and volume can be infused. Monitoring can be achieved with noninvasive methods: ECG, blood pressure cuff, pulse oximeter for arterial hemoglobin saturation, and capnography for end-tidal carbon dioxide measurements. Intravascular lines can be inserted after the patient has been stabilized (Hoffer, 1999).

If the anesthesiologist prefers to introduce the pulmonary (or central venous) pressure catheter before endotracheal intubation, most nursing activities should be delayed until the patient has been anesthetized. Padding of the hands and elbows can usually be performed at any time, but this and other interventions should be done in consultation with anesthesia personnel to prevent unnecessary stimulation of the patient. (Postponing padding of the hands may also enable the nurse to hold the hand of an anxious patient during induction.)

After the patient is intubated, a urinary drainage catheter is inserted to prevent bladder distension and to monitor renal function, especially during and after CPB. The catheter may contain a temperature probe; other temperature monitoring devices may be used in the esophagus, nasopharynx, or rectum. (CPB in-line sensors are used to measure blood temperatures, and ventricular septal temperature probes may be inserted during induced cardiac arrest.)

Transesophageal echocardiography (TEE) has enabled clinicians to make immediate perioperative anatomic and physiologic diagnoses. Not only is TEE frequently used to assess valvular repairs, but it is also increasingly being used to monitor signs of myocardial

TABLE **6-3**
Physiologic Monitoring

MONITORING DEVICE	LOCATION	ASSESSES/MEASURES
Cardiovascular System		
Electrocardiogram (ECG)	Electrodes placed on shoulders, hips, and left axillary line	Electrical activity of heart: lead II useful to monitor cardiac rhythm (good visualization of P wave and QRS) and myocardial ischemia (inferior surface); lead V5 useful to detect myocardial ischemia (anterior surface)
Intraarterial catheter	Radial artery (also femoral artery) aorta, bypass circuit, in children, may use superficial temporal or dorsalis pedis arteries; in neonates, may use umbilical artery	Direct arterial blood pressure (BP); blood gases; blood chemistries
Blood pressure cuff	Right or left arm	Indirect BP
Central venous pressure (CVP) line	Right atrium (RA)	RA pressure (CVP); right ventricular (RV) filling pressure; RV preload
Pulmonary artery (PA) catheter (addition of fiberoptics provides additional information about mixed venous oxygen saturation [Svo_2])	PA (proximal and distal)	PA pressures: systolic, diastolic, mean, wedge; pulmonary vascular resistance; left ventricular (LV) filling pressure; LV preload; cardiac output (CO); assessment of stroke volume, stroke work, systemic vascular resistance; mixed venous saturation (continuous indirect assessment of CO and reflection of tissue oxygenation); RV function
Left atrial (LA) catheter (when used)	LA	LA pressure (direct); LV filling pressure; LV preload
Transesophageal echocardiography (TEE)	Esophagus	Valve function before and after repair; LV wall motion, failure; intracardiac air bubbles
Urinary drainage catheter	Urinary bladder	Urinary output, renal perfusion; indirect measure of CO
Respiratory System		
Mass spectrometry	Anesthesia circuit	Inspired/expired O_2, CO_2, and anesthetic gases; used to avoid hypoxia, hypercarbia, anesthetic overdose
Pulse oximeter	Finger or toe cot; earlobe, nose	Oxygen saturation of arterial hemoglobin; tissue oxygenation
Capnography	Anesthesia circuit	End-tidal CO_2; used to detect integrity of anesthesia circuit; avoid disconnections of monitor, endotracheal tube; detect spontaneous ventilation, rebreathing, obstructive pulmonary disease
Central Nervous System		
Temperature	Esophagus, nasopharynx, urinary bladder, rectum, ventricular septum, bypass circuit, PA catheter	Core and peripheral temperature of heart, brain, and other organs
Electroencephalogram (when used)	Scalp electrodes	Detect cerebral ischemia, embolus; indication of depth of anesthesia
Renal System		
Urinary drainage catheter	Bladder	Urinary output; indirect measure of cardiac output

Modified from Charney JR: Cardiothoracic anesthesia. In Baumgartner FJ, editor: *Cardiothoracic surgery*, ed 4, Philadelphia, 1999, WB Saunders; Reich DL, Moskowitz DM, Kaplan JA: Hemodynamic monitoring. In Kaplan JA, editor: *Cardiac anesthesia*, ed 4, Philadelphia, 1999, WB Saunders.

ischemia, ventricular function, intracardiac air, and maldistribution of cardioplegia (Aronson and Dupont, 2000).

TEMPERATURE CONTROL

Cardiac surgery using CPB usually involves cooling the body to reduce tissue oxygen demand. Both ambient and patient body temperatures are purposely lowered during the operative repair and increased prior to the termination of CPB. Patients undergoing beating heart surgery are maintained at normothermia to reduce the risk of fibrillation and avoid the potentially harmful sequelae of hypothermia (e.g., impaired immune function and coagulopathy). Perioperative nursing interventions aimed at preventing and treating inadvertent hypothermia (Table 6-2) are important for maintaining homeostasis.

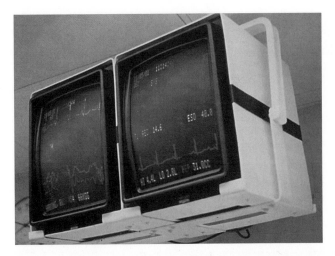

FIG. 6-1 Monitor screens can display electrocardiogram; systemic, pulmonary, and central venous pressures and waveforms; esophageal and rectal temperatures; high and low bypass flows; and name (obscured), age, weight, sex, and heparin dose. (Courtesy Doug Yarnold, CRNA.)

Intraoperative Medications

Numerous medications (Table 6-4) are used during surgery. Among these are drugs to maintain hemodynamic stability, maximize cardiac output, and promote metabolic homeostasis. Anesthesia, perfusion, and nursing services generally have specific patient drug needs, and the creation of individual medication exchange carts, jointly planned with pharmacy personnel, can be efficient and helpful. Nurses may wish to include heparin, topical antibiotics and hemostatic agents, 1% lidocaine (Xylocaine) (for topical anesthesia), calcium chloride, intracardiac epinephrine, papaverine, and other medications that may be needed by the sterile team. Perioperative nursing responsibilities for medications vary and should be reflected in the drug inventory maintained by the OR nursing staff.

Medications used before or during induction are selected with consideration given to their effects on myocardial oxygen supply and demand. In patients with obstructive coronary lesions, the supply of blood is relatively fixed, and interventions are aimed at minimizing or reducing myocardial oxygen demand. Drugs are used to control myocardial contractility, blood pressure and heart rate, ventricular wall tension, circulatory blood volume, and aortic pressure and coronary blood flow. Hypotension unresponsive to volume administration may be treated with vasoconstrictors and inotropic drugs; hypertension may respond to additional anesthetic drugs, vasodilators, beta blockers (e.g., propranolol hydrochloride [Inderal]), or a combination of these. Anesthesia is achieved with a combination of

agents to provide sleep, amnesia, analgesia, muscle relaxation, and blunting of autonomic nervous system reflexes (Belmont and Scott, 1999; Borill and Boer, 1999).

Positioning and Skin Preparation

POSITIONING

The supine position is the most commonly used position for cardiac surgery because it exposes the entire anterior chest, both groins for femoral artery access, and, when needed, the legs for saphenous vein excision. The surgeon can make a median sternotomy incision (see Chapter 9), which provides excellent exposure for surgery of the heart and great vessels and facilitates cannulation for a CPB. Patients in the supine position generally have their arms tucked along the side. Special caution should be taken when tucking the arms to prevent disruption of peripheral IV infusion lines and intraarterial blood pressure monitoring lines (A-lines). The nurse should confirm with anesthesia personnel that IV lines are infusing properly and that the arterial waveform has not been damped or otherwise adversely affected. The A-line is frequently placed in the radial artery; a splint may need to be applied to the wrist to maintain the correct position of the arterial catheter. If a radial artery graft is planned, the radial A-line is inserted into the contralateral artery. In obese patients the neck should be slightly extended so that the sternal notch can be incorporated into the field during draping and visualized for sternal splitting.

A modified anterolateral position may be required if a small thoracic incision is planned. A small roll can be placed under the left side of the chest to elevate it for exposure of the left ventricular apex. Small thoracotomy incisions are used less frequently than a full or partial median sternotomy for coronary bypass procedures, even when an off-pump operation is planned. The preference for sternotomy incisions is related to better exposure and less postoperative pain compared with thoracotomy incisions.

A left full-lateral or semilateral position in conjunction with a thoracotomy incision is used for operations requiring access to the descending thoracic aorta and for some procedures on the transverse aortic arch (see Chapter 14). Right lateral thoracotomies may be used for repeat mitral valve procedures. When the patient is positioned laterally, access to the legs and groin may be more difficult. With the right leg flexed, the right femoral artery is more easily accessible than the left in patients placed in the left full-lateral position. If femoral artery cannulation for bypass is planned, the nurse should provide an adequate area in which to insert and secure the cannula.

TABLE **6-4**

Medications Used in Adults During Cardiac Surgery

MEDICATION	PURPOSE/DESCRIPTION/DELIVERY
Analgesics and Anesthetics	
Thiopental	Induction, ultra-short-acting barbiturate, intravenous bolus
Fentanyl (Sublimaze)	Synthetic narcotic, intravenous bolus and/or infusion
Sufentanil (Sufenta)	Synthetic narcotic, intravenous bolus and/or infusion
Alfentanil (Alfenta)	Synthetic narcotic, intravenous bolus and/or infusion
Morphine	Narcotic, intravenous bolus
Halothane (Fluothane)	Inhalation anesthetic, maintenance
Enflurane (Ethrane)	Inhalation anesthetic, maintenance
Isoflurane (Forane)	Inhalation anesthetic, maintenance
Methohexital (Brevital)	Three times more potent and faster clearance than thiopental
Remifentanil (Ultiva)	Synthetic narcotic, intravenous bolus and/or infusion
Propofol (Diprivan)	Intravenous anesthetic; bolus and/or infusion; very fast acting
Sevoflurane (Ultane)	Inhalation anesthetic, maintenance
Desflurane (Suprane)	Inhalation anesthetic, maintenance
Muscle Relaxants	
Vecuronium (Norcuron)	Intubation, maintenance of muscle relaxation
Pancuronium (Pavulon)	Maintenance of muscle relaxation
Pipecuronium	Maintenance of muscle relaxation; relatively free of circulatory effects
Rocuronium (Zemuron)	Fast-acting muscle relaxant; allows hemodynamic stability
Amnesiacs	
Midazolam (Versed)	Hypnotic; anxiety-reducing sedative
Scopolamine	Sedative; amnesic
Lorazepam (Avitan)	Hypnotic sedative; premedication
Cardiovascular Agents	
ANTICHOLINERGICS	
Atropine	Decreases vagal tone; treats sinus bradycardia
Glycopyrrolate (Robinul)	Similar to atropine but has less incidence of dysrhythmias than atropine with slower onset
VASOPRESSORS	
Norepinephrine (Levophed)	Increases force and velocity of contraction; increases systemic and pulmonary vascular resistance
Phenylephrine (Neo-Synephrine)	Arteriolar and venous vasoconstriction; increases blood pressure and systemic vascular resistance
Vasodilators	
Nitroglycerin (Tridil)	Dilates coronary arteries; reduces preload
Phentolamine (Regitine)	Decreases systemic and pulmonary vascular resistance
Prostaglandin E 1 (Prostin VR)	Vascular smooth muscle dilator, potent pulmonary vascular dilator; used to maintain patency of ductus arteriosus in cyanotic neonates, patients with severe pulmonary hypertension
Nitroprusside (Nipride)	Arteriolar and venous vasodilation; reduces preload and afterload
Inotropic Agents	
Amrinone (Inocor)	Increases cardiac output, force and velocity of contraction
Calcium chloride	In ionized form, increases cardiac output, BP, and contractility
Dopamine (Intropin)	In low doses, increases renal and mesenteric perfusion; with moderate doses increases heart rate, contractility, and cardiac output; in higher doses increases systemic and pulmonary vascular resistance
Dobutamine (Dobutrex)	Increases contractility with less increase in heart rate than occurs with dopamine; has vasodilation effect on vascular bed
Ephedrine	Increases contractility, cardiac output, and BP
Epinephrine (Adrenalin)	Increases rate and strength of contraction, BP (effective bronchodilator)
Isoproterenol (Isuprel)	Increases heart rate, contractility, cardiac output; decreases systemic vascular resistance
Milrinone	Increases cardiac output, force and velocity of contraction

Modified from Larach DR: Cardiovascular drugs. In Hensley FA, Martin DE, editors: *The practice of anesthesia*, Boston, 1990, Little, Brown; Morrill P: Pharmacotherapeutics of positive inotropes, *AORN J* 71(1):173, 2000; Kervin MW and others: Nitric oxide: a primer for the practicing anesthetist, *CRNA* 9(3):93, 1998; Reves JC, Hill S, Berkowitz D: Pharmacology of intravenous anesthetic induction drugs. In Kaplan JA, editor: *Cardiac anesthesia*, ed 4, Philadelphia, 1999, WB Saunders.

TABLE 6-4
Medications Used in Adults During Cardiac Surgery—cont'd

MEDICATION	PURPOSE/DESCRIPTION/DELIVERY
Antidysrhythmics	
Lidocaine (Xylocaine)	Acts on ventricles; decreases automaticity of ischemic ventricular tissue
Bretylium (Bretylol)	Prolongs duration of action potential and refractory period; useful for ventricular dysrhythmias refractory to therapy
Digoxin (Lanoxin)	Decreases ventricular rate in atrial fibrillation or flutter and other supraventricular dysrhythmias; avoid in patients with Wolff-Parkinson-White syndrome and other accessory atrioventricular pathways
Nifedipine (Procardia)	Calcium channel blocker; reduces coronary artery spasm; produces coronary vasodilation; extremely light sensitive; must be given PO or via nasal or oral mucosa; antihypertensive
Procainamide (Pronestyl)	Decreases automaticity and conduction in all cardiac tissue (normal and ischemic); stabilizes cellular membranes
Quinidine	Similar to procainamide; atrial and ventricular dysrhythmias
Verapamil (Calan, Isoptin)	Calcium channel blocker; used to treat atrial dysrhythmias; slows ventricular rate in atrial fibrillation or flutter; can be given IV
Adenosine	Supraventricular dysrhythmias
Diuretics	
Furosemide (Lasix)	Decreases renal absorption of sodium and chloride; increases excretion of water and electrolytes, especially potassium, sodium, chloride, magnesium, and calcium
Mannitol	Osmotic diuretic; pulls free water out of organs (reducing cerebral edema); protects kidneys
Anticoagulants/Coagulants	
Heparin	Systemic anticoagulation during CPB; blocks activation of thrombin (and intrinsic clotting cascade)
Protamine sulfate	Heparin antagonist; NPH insulin-dependent diabetic patients may be at increased risk for protamine reaction
Antibiotics	
Cephalosporins (Mandol, Ancef, Keflex, Keflin, Cefadyl)	Broad-spectrum prophylaxis
Tobramycin (Nebcin)	Aerobic gram-negative and gram-positive bacteria
Vancomycin	Severe endocarditis
Bacitracin	Topical irrigation
Miscellaneous	
Diazepam (Valium)	Sedative, induction of anesthesia
Nitric oxide (NO)	Vascular (especially pulmonary) relaxation; inhaled; reduces pulmonary hypertension
Lidocaine 1% (plain)	Local anesthesia
Papaverine	Reduces arterial spasm (e.g., mammary artery)
Potassium	Replaces electrolyte loss
Sodium bicarbonate	Corrects acidosis
Insulin (NPH, etc.)	Corrects hyperglycemia in diabetic patients
Topical hemostatic agents	Intraoperative control of bleeding
Desmopressin (DDAVP)	Pharmacologic hemostatic agent

Additional nursing considerations related to positioning for median sternotomy and lateral incisions are given in Chapter 9. The reader is also referred to perioperative nursing texts for a fuller discussion of positioning techniques.

SKIN PREPARATION

Hair removal has been a subject of debate. In the past, cardiac patients often had full body shaves, but this practice has been largely abandoned. Most male patients, however, do have hair removed along the sternal midline from the sternal notch to just above the umbilicus. Female patients rarely require chest hair removal, and for cosmetic reasons the procedure is avoided. In coronary artery bypass patients, the skin along the inner aspect of the leg (in the path of the greater saphenous vein) is often clipped (or shaved). Hair in the inguinal region is also removed should entry into the femoral artery be required.

Numerous studies have demonstrated an increased incidence of skin damage and postoperative wound infection associated with shaving performed 24 hours or more before surgery. When hair removal is considered necessary, the use of depilatories or sterile skin clippers (rather than razors) has been suggested, although depilatories may cause hypersensitivity reactions. Ideally hair removal is done outside the OR (Mangram and others, 1999). However, patients admitted directly for emergency surgery require hair removal in the OR. Clippers should be immediately available for such occurrences.

Antimicrobial agents are applied to the skin as expeditiously as possible without jeopardizing antisepsis. Povidone-iodine is widely used for skin preparation and in gel form it can be applied rapidly to the anterior chest, abdomen, groin, legs, and feet. Chlorhexidine also is used widely for skin preparation. Both povidone-iodine and chlorhexidine have broad-spectrum antimicrobial activity; unlike iodophors, chlorhexidine is not inactivated by blood or serum proteins, although the former continues to exert a bacteriostatic effect as long as it is present on the skin (Mangram and others, 1999).

Skin preparation to the knees is recommended for all cardiac surgery patients because access to the femoral arteries may be required for intraaortic balloon or pressure monitoring line insertion. If saphenous vein is to be removed, a circumferential leg preparation (to and including the feet) is recommended. The feet can be placed on a "picket fence" (see Chapter 3) to elevate the legs.

It is also recommended that skin preparation solutions or gels routinely be readily available when patients enter the OR. Not infrequently a patient may suddenly become hemodynamically unstable, and precious time may be wasted organizing a table to wash the skin. In extreme emergencies antimicrobial solutions can be quickly sprayed onto the skin.

Draping

General principles based on the Association of periOperative Registered Nurses Recommended Practices (AORN, 2001) guide the cardiac nurse in maintaining a sterile field, with special consideration given to the draping of bypass lines and the multiple surgical sites that may exist (e.g., chest, legs, and groin for femoral access). Goals for draping the cardiac surgical patient include:

- Exposing the surgical sites—chest, legs, groin
- Maintaining sterility of the field, including instruments and equipment, and bypass lines
- Ensuring that the sterile end of bypass lines and other items passed off the field are securely attached to the drapes
- Ensuring that suction lines, bypass and cardioplegia infusion lines, electrosurgical pencils, defibrillator paddles, pressure monitoring lines, and pacemaker cables are easily and quickly accessible
- Creating a surface for instruments, such as needle holders, forceps, and suture tags, so that they do not slide off the field (e.g., using a magnetic mat or forming a flat surface with towels)
- Minimizing the potential for suture snagging on drapes, instruments, or other items (e.g., covering retractor handles with a towel or moist laparotomy tape)

Tangling of cords and tubing should be avoided; the nurse can arrange these so that there is an adequate length of cords and tubing to reach the area required on the field (e.g., the length of the defibrillator cable on the field should be sufficient for the attached paddle tips to reach the inside of the pericardium without the clinician's having to tug on the cords). Ceiling-mounted booms that incorporate suction, electrical, and medical gas outlets can minimize the floor clutter of cords and tubing.

Clear plastic adhesive drapes impregnated with iodophor or other bactericidal agents are often applied to the chest and occasionally to the legs. Some centers use stockinette to cover the feet and legs; the surgeon can cut through this material to expose the leg. The feet can be wrapped in towels secured with a towel clip.

Adhesive drapes are also useful for covering the exit site of catheters or pressure lines in the groin of patients who come to the OR with these in place. It is difficult to prepare these areas adequately, and they should be draped out of the sterile field. A catheter can be covered with a folded sterile towel, with the adhesive placed over this and the surrounding area to exclude it from the sterile field.

A "belly band" (incorporated into a disposable draping system [Fig. 6-2] or made from towels) can be placed across the umbilicus and attached to either side of the drape. Bypass lines can be securely attached to the band where it meets the side drape. The band should not be positioned so high as to cover the chest tube exit sites or so low as to obscure the common femoral artery.

Side pockets help to keep lines and other items readily available without cluttering the field. Drapes designed for cardiac surgery usually have a trough or pockets along each side. Individual pockets can also be made from towels and attached to the drapes with towel clips. To maintain sterility, nonpenetrating towel clips should be used if they are to be adjusted or removed during the procedure.

Drapes should be waterproof. They should extend below the level of the patient but not touch the floor. Draping of equipment and furniture (e.g., instruments tables, Mayo stand, slush machine, ring stands) should take into consideration their different heights. Drapes should be long enough (without touching the floor) so that if these items come into contact with each other, cross-contamination does not occur.

Many companies make disposable drape packs for cardiac surgery that combine a variety of drapes for the procedure. Customized drape packs can also be put together that include sheets, gowns, towels, and other desired items. Packs are advantageous in that they reduce setup time.

Infection Control Measures

Planning for infection control is outlined in Chapter 5. Implementing activities to minimize the risk of infection is affected by patient factors, by how team members perform, and by the environment in which they must work. Strict aseptic practices are mandatory, but small, cramped ORs present a challenge to perioperative cardiac nurses interacting with many persons, managing multiple pieces of equipment, and caring for surgical patients whose compromised cardiovascular system places them at risk for infection.

Traffic patterns should be established that reduce movement within the OR, and entering and exiting the room by personnel should be kept to a minimum. The arrangement of furniture and other items should be done in a way that protects the sterility of the instruments, supplies, and drapes. Consolidating equipment is one alternative. Carts can be constructed (or purchased) that allow stacking of equipment such as electrocautery devices and the defibrillator. Suspending items from the ceiling (with a handle that allows the nurse to adjust the height) is another option. The motor of an electric sternal saw may be attached to the surgeon's headlight power source; the air tanks of pneumatically powered saws can be moved to a peripheral area of the room once the chest has been opened, or a battery-operated saw is used. Extra-long electrical cords may allow other items (e.g., hypothermia/hyperthermia units) to be positioned farther away from the surgical field and thus provide more room for personnel to move around the operative area without contacting sterile areas.

Patient factors must be considered. In addition to the intrinsic cardiac disease, other physiologic alterations may predispose the patient to infection. In a study of 3027 patients (Saginur, Croteau, and Bergeron, 2000), deep wound infections were found more commonly in men and in patients who were elderly, diabetic, and obese. Infections were also more common in patients with longer preoperative lengths of stay and longer (e.g., more than 4 hours) surgical procedures. Patients with a colostomy or ileostomy require special interventions (e.g., using an adhesive antimicrobial drape) to exclude the stoma or ostomy device from the sterile field. Patients arriving in the OR with femoral artery catheters (intraaortic balloon pumps [IABPs], pressure lines) can be managed in a similar manner. IABPs and ventricular assist devices (VADs) pose challenges in addition to the potential for contamination. The integrity of the lines and catheters must also be protected, and

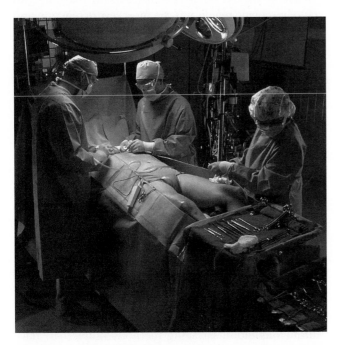

FIG. 6-2 Cardiovascular draping system provides exposure of the chest, groin, and legs. (Courtesy Kimberly-Clark Professional Health Care, Roswell, Georgia.)

team members must work in unison during transfer to the OR bed, positioning, skin preparation, and draping. Additional personnel may be needed to perform these activities safely.

For patients returning to the OR for control of postoperative bleeding, chest dressings should be removed with aseptic technique to avoid contamination of the incision. Other dressings are removed as necessary. The leg dressing in coronary artery bypass patients may remain and be covered with the sterile drapes. The contralateral groin may or may not be included in the operative site, depending on the surgeon's preference. Skin preparation and draping are influenced by the anticipated findings, and the nurse should discuss this with the surgeon before the skin is prepared.

Dressings applied to the internal jugular or subclavian venous exit sites for invasive pressure lines should be kept out of the sterile field. These dressings may have to be reapplied or their edges trimmed to achieve this.

Although postoperative cardiothoracic infections are relatively rare, the development of mediastinitis can be a life-threatening complication. Perioperative antibiotic prophylaxis has proved to be a consistent benefit as an adjunct to aseptic and antiseptic practices in avoiding postoperative wounds. Various antibiotic regimens using first- and second-generation cephalosporins may be followed. The cephalosporins cefazolin and cefuroxime, as well as vancomycin, are widely used antibiotics. However, the emergence of methicillin-resistant (gram-positive) *Staphylococcus aureus* and vancomycin-resistant organisms has made strict aseptic practices mandatory.

Transfusion Therapy and Blood Conservation

HOMOLOGOUS BLOOD

Although the indications for transfusion of homologous blood and blood products have undergone a change as a result of the risk of blood-borne diseases (Spiess, 2001; Ellison, 2001), blood transfusion can be a lifesaving measure in patients with reduced oxygen-carrying capacity, coagulopathies, or hypovolemia. Alternative measures such as volume expanders and artificial blood may not be suitable for the patient. Even with the popularity of bloodless surgery, blood availability remains a necessary aspect of cardiac surgery. The main indication for transfusion is to enhance the oxygen-carrying capacity of the blood; the decision is based on the hemoglobin and hematocrit count, as well as the clinical status of the patient.

Two to four units of packed red blood cells (RBCs) are generally ordered for cardiac surgery patients. The blood should be in the OR before the patient arrives. Many cardiac OR suites have their own blood refrigerator, which permits rapid access to the blood.

The units should be initially checked (e.g., patient's name and hospital record number, blood type, and unit number) when the blood is delivered to the OR and before it is stored in the blood refrigerator. Just before transfusion, it should be checked again by the person hanging the unit and by a witness. In large OR suites, blood refrigerators may contain the blood of more than one patient, and transfusion errors can be greatly reduced by confirming that patients are receiving the blood ordered for them. At the end of the procedure, any remaining units of blood should be promptly returned to the blood bank or sent to the ICU with the patient and stored in the ICU's blood refrigerator.

In addition to units of packed RBCs, fresh frozen plasma, platelets, and other blood products should be available, but these do not need to be prepared (e.g., thawed) and brought to the OR unless they are needed to enhance coagulation. These products, once ready, should not be refrigerated, and there is a time limit for their use. Wasting of blood products can be reduced by assessing the patient's hemodynamic and hemostatic status and by communication with the surgeon and anesthesia and blood bank personnel.

TRANSFUSION REACTION

The nurse should be alert to transfusion reactions. An acute hemolytic reaction is the most severe reaction and can be fatal. Bloody urine and hemodynamic alterations are notable signs that alert the clinician. Signs and symptoms usually associated with transfusion reactions, such as chills, anxiety, dyspnea, and pain, are of little use in the anesthetized patient. Even skin changes such as hives and rashes may not be readily apparent when surgical drapes cover most of the body. If such a complication occurs, the transfusion should be discontinued immediately and the institutional protocol implemented.

Occasionally, massive blood transfusions are required for severe bleeding. The importance of good working relationships with the blood bank cannot be overemphasized for rapidly acquiring large amounts of blood and having additional units prepared expeditiously. It is helpful if the blood bank is notified as soon in advance as possible of the blood needs of the patient.

AUTOLOGOUS BLOOD

Autologous blood salvaging methods (Table 6-5) have enhanced blood conservation and reduced (but not eliminated) the need for homologous banked blood. Autologous blood transfusions are now considered the safest form of transfusion therapy.

TABLE 6-5
Cellular Composition of Autologous Blood Collected by Various Methods

METHOD OF COLLECTION	RED BLOOD CELLS	PLATELETS	COAGULATION FACTORS	COMMENT
Preoperative deposit	+	−	+/−	Platelets and labile factors V and VIII decrease rapidly with storage time
Normovolemic hemodilution	+	+	+	High levels of platelet and coagulation factor activities are present if used on day of collection
Intraoperative salvage				
Unwashed	+	+/−	+	Platelets may be present, but functional activity is unknown
Washed	+	−	−	Platelets and coagulation factors are removed by washing
Postoperative salvage (unwashed)	+	+/−	+/−	Platelets and coagulation factors are consumed in the operative wound; levels may be severely reduced and are unlikely to be therapeutic

From Stack G, Snyder EL: Alternative to perioperative blood transfusion. In Stoelting RK, editor: *Advances in anesthesia,* vol 8, St Louis, 1991, Mosby; Valeri CR and others: Survival, function, and hemolysis of shed red blood cells processed as nonwashed blood and washed red blood cells, *Ann Thorac Surg* 72:1598, 2001; Andreasen AS and others: Autologous transfusion of shed mediastinal blood after coronary artery bypass grafting and bacterial contamination, *Ann Thorac Surg* 72:1327, 2001.

The first autologous transfusions were performed as early as 1921 when Dr. F.C. Grant collected a patient's blood preoperatively and later infused it during surgery. With the increased concern about the transmission of viral diseases, predeposit programs and intraoperative blood-salvaging techniques began to increase.

Predeposit donation can be considered in patients undergoing an elective procedure and whose condition allows phlebotomy; blood should be collected within 72 hours before surgery. Directed donation (by a specific individual known to the patient) is requested by some patients, but the safety of this technique over standard blood collection methods is questionable.

Another form of autotransfusion can be performed before the start of the operation. Blood is withdrawn from the patient and placed into collection bags to be reinfused later during the procedure. Blood removed is replaced with volume expanders. An advantage of this method is that it provides fresh whole blood with viable platelets and clotting factors. Autotransfusion can also be accomplished with the use of the cardiotomy suction during CPB. Blood from the surgical site is aspirated into the bypass machine and enters the CPB circuit, from which it can be infused back into the body (see Chapter 9).

BLOOD SALVAGING DEVICES

With autotransfusion devices the patient's blood (and other matter) is aspirated into a sterile collection system, where the blood is washed, concentrated, and reinfused as needed (some systems filter the aspirate and then reinfuse it without including a washing cycle). Anticoagulation is necessary to prevent clot formation in the circuit; heparin or citrate can be used.

Available commercial devices include those using suction cannisters, semicontinuous flow systems, or single-use disposable devices. Collected blood that has been heparinized may retain systemic anticoagulation if the blood is not adequately washed. To reduce hemolysis, these devices should be used to aspirate pools of blood rather than skimming tissue surfaces because this creates a traumatic blood-air interface.

Blood replacement in Jehovah's Witnesses presents a special challenge. Semiautomated centrifugal systems can be adapted so that the RBCs remain in a continuous circuit within the patient's intravascular space. In addition, present methods of CPB using crystalloid priming solution have been largely successful in avoiding blood transfusions. In many cases patients are able to tolerate the hemodilution and the reduction of circulating RBC mass (Despotis, Skubas, and Goodnough, 1999). In addition to the use of bloodless surgery protocols, pharmacologic and topical hemostatic agents (see later in chapter) can reduce bleeding and the need for transfusion.

Defibrillation

Whether beating heart or arrested heart surgery is performed, the perioperative nurse should be prepared to defibrillate the cardiac patient when ventricular tachycardia or fibrillation occurs. When beating heart/off-pump surgery is performed, normothermia is maintained as closely as possible; if the patient becomes hypothermic inadvertently, there is a risk of fibrillation. Alternatively, if a procedure is performed in the conventional manner with CPB, induced hypothermia, and cardioplegic arrest, the risk of fibrillation occurs before the heart is stopped with cardioplegia and after the heart resumes beating.

Current methods of myocardial protection (see Chapter 9), such as those using warm cardioplegia solution for initial and final infusion, have enhanced the global distribution of the solution. This has contributed to better preservation of the myocardial substrates that are necessary for the resumption of cardiac function once the aortic occlusion clamp is removed. Frequently the heart starts to contract spontaneously when the clamp is removed and warm blood enters the coronary circulation, washing out the residual cardioplegia solution.

Nevertheless, the heart is irritable and may fibrillate if inadvertently touched. If the heart starts to fibrillate, a shock of electrical current is delivered directly to the cardiac surface with internal defibrillator paddles. Both the sterile nurse and the circulating nurse should monitor the ECG for ventricular fibrillation and prepare to defibrillate the patient. (The sterile nurse can also observe the heart directly while the aortic cross-clamp is removed to detect fibrillation.) By monitoring the ECG and observing the sterile team members, circulating nurses will be aware of whether defibrillation will be required and can position themselves near the defibrillator to charge the power source and discharge the current when requested to do so by the surgeon. Although the heart can fibrillate at any time, especially critical periods during surgery with CBP are anesthesia induction, cannulation for CPB, rewarming, and coming off bypass. If the patient is having beating heart surgery, the nurse should anticipate that the heart can (and will) fibrillate at any time; because CPB is not available to perfuse the body's organs when this occurs, it is critically important to be vigilant in monitoring cardiac function and act quickly if the heart fibrillates.

The standard level of energy current for internal defibrillation in the adult is 10 to 20 joules; this dose will defibrillate more than 90% of fibrillating hearts. Lower settings often require repeat shocks; higher settings can cause myocardial necrosis (Mangano and others, 1999). The setting and the action of discharging should be confirmed with the surgeon in order to prevent injury to the patient or to staff. Internal paddles do not require additional lubrication because they are moistened by physiologic fluid. On discharging the defibrillator, the circulating nurse should recharge the machine immediately and then observe the ECG monitor for the return of a regular rhythm. If the patient is still fibrillating, the paddles can be activated without waiting; if the patient has been defibrillated, the energy can be "dumped" (see the individual manufacturer's instructions for performing this safely). Frequent monitoring of the ECG will alert the nurse to the development of fibrillation, which can occur at any time before or after the heart is purposely arrested. (Fibrillation oc-

curring during cardioplegic arrest is treated by reinfusing cardioplegia solution if continued standstill is desired). In some centers an anesthesiologist or anesthetist may be responsible for defibrillation. Some internal paddles contain the control button in the handle; these can be discharged by the surgeon.

Nurses activating the device for defibrillation should ensure that the device is in the "asynchronous" and not the "synchronous" mode. In the synchronous mode, the machine looks for an R wave or a QRS complex to synchronize the shock. Because there is no R wave or QRS complex in ventricular fibrillation, the machine will not discharge. It is recommended that the device be kept routinely in the asynchronous mode and that the other mode be instituted only for specific situations (e.g., converting atrial fibrillation to normal sinus rhythm). Conversely, if the patient requires cardioversion for recent-onset atrial fibrillation, then the synchronous mode is used to avoid shocking the patient during a vulnerable period that could produce ventricular fibrillation. To synchronize the shock, the defibrillator must be connected to the patient via ECG cables that are connected directly to the defibrillator. They may also be "slaved" into the anesthesia monitoring system. Without this ECG connection, the defibrillator is unable to detect existing R waves, and the shock cannot be timed properly.

Defibrillator failures can occur. The machine should be checked before every operative procedure, and a backup machine of the same manufacturer, design, and model should be available. The nurse must ensure that the internal paddles will connect into the defibrillator. The internal paddles of defibrillators made by different companies are not interchangeable, and paddles of different models of the same company are frequently not interchangeable. Additional sterile internal paddles should also be kept nearby in the event that those at the surgical field are contaminated.

Operator failures (Box 6-4) can also occur. In one study (Cummins and others, 1990) it was shown that such failures were related to maintenance and use of the device. Device-related failures were associated with malfunctioning components or poor design. The study concluded that adequate initial training and continuing education to ensure proper use of these devices were important for minimizing errors.

Sterile external paddles or adhesive defibrillator pads are necessary for certain procedures. In patients undergoing repeat sternotomy, pericardial or pleural adhesions can prevent insertion of internal paddles if the adhesions have not yet been dissected. Internal cardioverter defibrillator generator implantation may require external defibrillation (see Chapter 17) if the generator fails to defibrillate the patient during testing of the device. External settings can be from 200 joules up to 360 or more (internal settings are commonly between 10 and 20 joules).

Modified from Cummins RO and others: Defibrillator failures: causes of problems and recommendations for improvement, *JAMA* 264(8):1019, 1990.

Another method of internal defibrillation can be used in the presence of sternal adhesions. One paddle is placed on the anterior surface of the heart; the second paddle is placed through the peritoneum at the inferior end of the sternal incision and held against the cardiac portion of the diaphragm and above the left lobe of the liver. A single countershock of 50 joules is used to defibrillate the patient. Another method is to place one paddle on the anterior surface of the heart while the second paddle is placed in the left pleural cavity and held against the cardiac portion of the pleura.

Familiarity with various defibrillation methods can help the perioperative nurse to anticipate and prepare for alternative maneuvers. Because energy settings vary with the method used and the amount of tissue to be traversed, double-checking the setting and confirming it with the surgeon is an important safety consideration.

Temporary Epicardial Pacing

Temporary pacing is used to maintain optimum heart rate and atrioventricular (AV) synchrony in order to achieve an adequate cardiac output. (In patients with chronic atrial fibrillation, only ventricular pacing wires are inserted because atrial pacing is ineffective.) Pacing wires also can be used to suppress some dysrhythmias; atrial dysrhythmias may be treated with rapid atrial pacing (Dirks, 2000).

Pacing wires are generally inserted before the termination of bypass so that they will be available if needed to maintain a heart rate (e.g., 90 to 100 beats per minute) that will provide an adequate cardiac output. (Insertion is also easier during CPB, when the lungs are deflated and out of the way of the right atrium.)

The electrode (bare wire) end of the wire is sutured to the epicardial surface of the right atrium for atrial pacing (Fig. 6-3). A second wire is attached in a similar

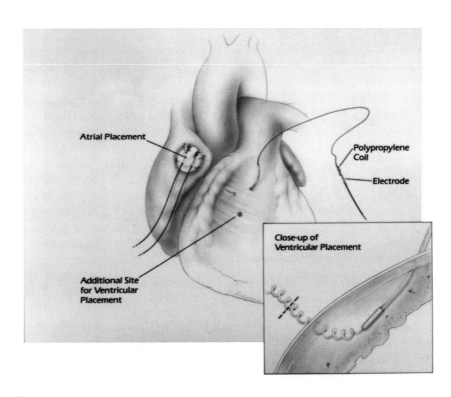

FIG. 6-3 Temporary pacing wires. The fixation coil can be positioned in the atrium or the ventricle. The fixation coil and the electrode are pulled into the myocardium with the needle at the end of the lead. When the electrode and a portion of the coil are in position *(inset),* the remaining coil and needle are cut and removed. For atrial placement a button *(shown)* can be used to fasten the leads to the heart. (Courtesy Medtronic, Inc.)

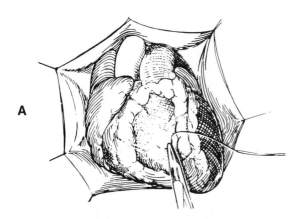

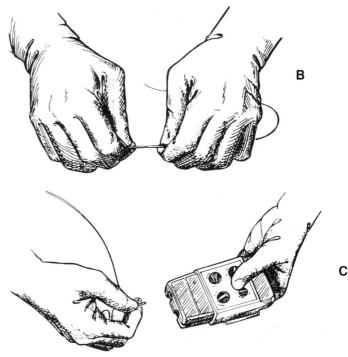

FIG. 6-4 **A,** A pacing wire is attached to the myocardium with the needle tip of the electrode. The wire is pulled until the electrode contacts the ventricle; the needle is then cut and removed. The electrode is fixed to the heart with a fine silk suture. A straight needle at the other end of the lead is used to bring the lead out through the chest wall. **B,** The straight needle is snapped at the scored portion. **C,** The needle is inserted into the temporary pacemaker generator. (Courtesy Ethicon, Inc., a Johnson & Johnson Company, Somerville, N.J.)

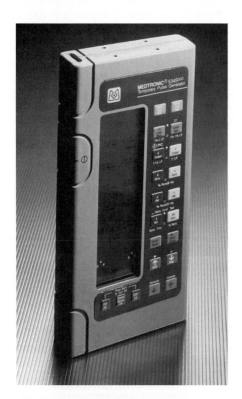

FIG. 6-5 Temporary external pacemaker generator that can pace and sense in both the atrial and the ventricular chambers to provide AV synchrony to maximize cardiac output during surgery. The generator also may be used in the short-term treatment of atrial dysrhythmias, heart block, and emergency pacing. (Courtesy Medtronic, Inc.)

manner near the first wire (but should not touch the first wire). A second pair of wires is sutured to the right ventricle for ventricular pacing (Fig. 6-4, *A*); in some cases one ventricular wire may be placed on the ventricle for pacing and a second (ground) wire sewn to the skin. All but the electrode end of each wire is insulated with plastic. A scored Keith needle at the other end of the wire is used to bring the wire out through the chest wall. (Some wires are positioned to exit at the base of the sternotomy skin incision.) The needle is broken at the scored section (Fig. 6-4, *B*), and that end of the wire is inserted directly into an external pacemaker generator (Fig. 6-4, *C*) or into a connecting cable that is then connected to the generator.

The needle tips are broken off at the scored portion and connected to the temporary pacer generator (Fig. 6-5). AV sequential generators have four openings for the two pairs of wires from the patient. Single-chamber generators (two openings for wires) are available, but dual-chamber pacing is performed when possible to maximize cardiac efficiency. By stimulating both the atrium and the ventricle to contract, AV sequential pacing enables the atrium to contribute to ventricular filling, thereby increasing stroke volume and cardiac output. Patients with rate-dependent cardiac output also benefit from temporary pacing at about 100 beats per minute (Dirks, 2000).

Because pacing obscures some ECG changes, it may need to be temporarily interrupted to assess ST segment elevations suggestive of myocardial ischemia. Occasionally pacemakers compete with the native heart rate, at which time the pacer can be discontinued. Not all patients require pacing during surgery, but postoperative dysrhythmias amenable to pacemaker therapy warrant the insertion of temporary leads. When not pacing, the wires should be wrapped with the bare wire/electrode end covered; these can be taped to the chest during transport. When external generators are in use, the box and attached cables and wires should also be secured with tape. Extreme caution should be taken when moving patients who are connected to a pacemaker generator to prevent disruption of connections or dislodgment of the wires.

The wires are removed on the third or fourth postoperative day (or earlier). The wires are firmly grasped and gently tugged to disengage the lead from the heart and pull it out through the chest wall. If there is resistance, pulling should be stopped and the surgeon notified. In such cases the wire may be cut where it exits the skin; this usually does not cause a serious problem.

Hemostasis

Hemostasis and blood salvaging have become even more important in recent years because of the risks involved with blood transfusions. Achieving hemostasis in cardiac surgery is influenced by a variety of factors. The patient assessment should include risk factors for increased intraoperative bleeding, such as a history of abnormal bleeding, liver dysfunction, aspirin use, or heparin or warfarin (Coumadin) therapy. CPB damages blood components and decreases or alters clotting factors; hypothermia retards clotting mechanisms; heparin inhibits coagulation; and tissue dissection injures blood vessels. Anastomoses on fibrotic or calcified sections of aorta may require adjunctive measures to ensure hemostasis.

Laboratory tests to screen for potential coagulation problems include the platelet count, prothrombin time (PT), and partial thromboplastin time (PTT). Deficiencies should alert the nurse to the possible need for platelets, fresh frozen plasma, or other blood products necessitated by the specific deficiency. Patients receiving warfarin (e.g., for prosthetic heart valves) usually have the medication stopped 4 to 5 days before surgery and heparin substituted until the night before the operation. PT and PTT are monitored during this period.

In the absence of preexisting bleeding disorders, hemostasis is related to the type of vascular injury and to the technical performance of the operation. (Reoperation requiring extensive dissection of adhesions also is associated with increased bleeding.) Constant surveillance of the operative field enables the sterile nurse to recognize sudden hemorrhage and be prepared to institute emergency measures. Depending on the situation, suction may be required first in order to expose the origin of the bleeding; direct manual pressure may be applied for temporary control of hemorrhage. Vascular clamps should be immediately available; their size and configuration depend on the size and location of the bleeding vessel. Sutures and pledget material (Fig. 6-6) to repair vessels are used once the bleeding site is determined. Smaller, discrete bleeding structures may be cauterized, clamped and tied, or suture ligated. (Cautery should not be used in close proximity to anastomoses sewn with polypropylene!) Bleeding from nonvascular sources may require other methods of hemostasis, such as pressure and topical hemostatic agents.

Persistent, generalized oozing may occur on raw surfaces (e.g., pericardial adhesions) or in vascular beds where extensive dissection has been performed (e.g., internal mammary artery [IMA] retrosternal bed). A number of topical hemostatic agents are available for use in those areas where capillary and small blood vessel bleeding persists (Table 6-6). These agents should be kept in a cup or towel and handled with clean, dry instruments. They should not be allowed to enter the bloodstream through opened, large blood vessels (which could lead to extensive intravascular clotting) and should not be aspirated into blood salvaging (autotransfusion) systems.

The use of epinephrine for hemostasis is not recommended for cardiac patients because of its sympathetic effects on the cardiovascular system. Bone wax, made from refined beeswax, is applied to the sternal edge to control bleeding from the marrow (see Fig. 6-6). It is pressed along the cut edge of the sternum, and excess wax is removed. Bone wax should be used sparingly.

"Fibrin glue" is another agent used topically for hemostasis. It is made by combining aprotinin with a mixture of thrombin and calcium chloride (CaCl). The aprotinin and thrombin/CaCl solutions must be placed in separate syringes (Fig. 6-7) until needed because combining the ingredients will rapidly produce a fibrin clot. When the contents of each syringe are sprayed onto the area desired, a coagulum forms that controls oozing. Sensitivity to the bovine aprotinin material should be determined before use (Katkhouda, 2001).

Pharmacologic agents are being used increasingly as alternatives or adjuncts to transfusion (Table 6-7). These are categorized as hemostatic agents (to reduce bleeding), platelet protective agents (to conserve clotting elements), and recombinant human erythropoietin (to stimulate the production of new RBCs). Two widely used drugs are desmopressin and aprotinin. Desmopressin (1 deamino-8-D-arginine vasopressin, or DDAVP) induces transient increases in factor VIII and von Willebrand's factor. It has been used to shorten

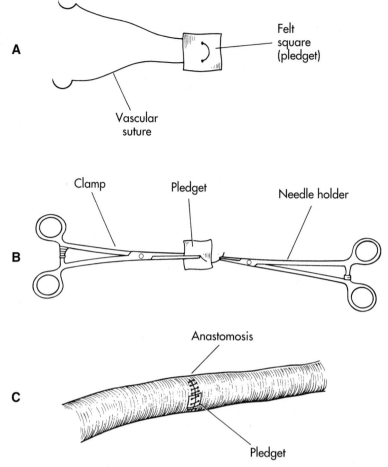

FIG. 6-6 Pledgeted suture. **A,** Double-armed vascular suture prepared with pledget. **B,** Technique for surgeon to add pledget to suture already in use. **C,** Appearance of suture line with pledget in place. (From Meeker MH, Rothrock JC: *Alexander's care of the patient in surgery,* ed 11, St Louis, 1999, Mosby.)

prolonged bleeding times and decrease blood loss in patients with or without intrinsic coagulopathies. Desmopressin does not always produce a consistent effect in hemostatically normal patients whose blood loss is not excessive, but it does offer some benefit when blood loss is greater.

Aprotinin, a 58-amino acid polypeptide, is derived mainly from bovine lung, parotid gland, or pancreas. It directly inhibits coagulation factors such as kallikrein and thrombin, preserves platelet function, and inhibits fibrinolysis during CPB (Levi and others, 1999). Because this pharmacologic agent is derived from bovine tissue, it has antigenic properties that can promote the formation of antibodies. If the patient is reexposed to the drug during a subsequent surgery, an anaphylactic reaction can occur (Dietrich and others, 2001).

Additional methods of achieving hemostasis are specific to the type of surgery performed. For instance, operations on the thoracic aorta (see Chapter 14) may require interventions such as anastomotic wraps made with small-caliber (e.g., 8- or 10-mm) tube grafts. The

harmonic scalpel is a device that cuts and cauterizes simultaneously by employing the principles of vibration and friction to reduce blood loss. Decreased surgical time is another factor that can reduce overall blood loss (Despotis, Skubas, and Goodnough, 1999), and nurses can play an important role by anticipating delays and implementing time-saving actions to control bleeding.

Chest Tube Insertion

Chest tube insertion during cardiac surgery has two purposes: (1) to remove fluid (e.g., blood) from the pericardial cavity in order to reduce the risk of cardiac tamponade and (2) to remove fluid and air from the pleural cavity in order to prevent pneumothorax, which would compromise ventilation and gas exchange. Although mediastinal drainage tubes are routinely inserted in patients who have had heart surgery via a median sternotomy or mini-thoracotomy, not all of these patients require pleural tubes unless the pleural space is entered. This commonly occurs with IMA dissection,

TABLE 6-6
Topical Hemostatic Agents

GENERIC NAME (TRADE NAME)	MODE OF ACTION	HOW USED	SPECIAL PRECAUTIONS
Thrombin (Thrombostat, Thrombogen)	Facilitates conversion of fibrinogen to fibrin (clot) through catalytic process	Spray, powder, or in combination with Gelfoam	Of bovine origin; may cause allergic reaction. Never inject into or allow to enter large vessels.
Aprotinin plus mixture of calcium chloride and thrombin (Hemaseel) ("fibrin glue")	Produces fibrin clot	Sprayed onto oozing tissue	Aprotinin is of bovine origin; may cause allergic reaction. Never inject into or allow to enter large vessels.
Absorbable gelatin sponge (Gelfoam, Gelfilm)	Provides physical matrix for clot formation through capillary action	Dry sponge moistened with saline or thrombin solution; cut sponge to desired size; also available as a powder, film, or prostatectomy cone	Do not use in the presence of infection or intestinal spillage. Do not use on skin edges. Possible increased incidence of wound infection if left in place. Increase in size of product caused by absorption of blood could cause unwanted pressure in confined space. Not to be used with menorrhagia or postpartum bleeding.
Microfibrillar collagen sheet hemostat (Avitene)	Provides web-type surface for aggregation of platelets	Loose powder or compacted form	Of bovine origin; may cause allergic reaction. Can provide focal point for infection. Do not moisten with saline or thrombin. Do not use with cell saver devices. Not for injection.
Absorbable collagen sheet hemostat (Instat)	Platelets aggregate on sheet and release coagulation factors, which combine with plasma factors to form a clot	Collagen sheet; applied to bleeding site with pressure	Of bovine origin; may cause allergic reaction. Do not use in contaminated wounds; may enhance infection.
Absorbable collagen sponge (Helistat)	Same as absorbable collagen sheet hemostat	Sponge applied to bleeding site with pressure	Of bovine origin; may cause allergic reaction. Not to be used in skin closure.
Oxidized cellulose (Oxycel); oxidized regenerated cellulose (Surgicel, Surgicel Nu-Knit)	Clotting process is initiated physically; forms gelatinous mass, which aids in clot formation and absorbs seven to eight times its weight in blood	Surgicel: sheet; Oxycel: pad, strips, pledgets; Nu-Knit: sheet; all of the above products work best when applied dry	May be left in situ, but advisable to remove after clot forms (may dislodge and migrate). Remove from confined spaces because swelling of product may exert unwanted pressure on surrounding tissue. Do not use to wrap around vascular anastomotic sites. Do not implant in bone defects.
Epinephrine	Topical; induces vasoconstriction	Added to local anesthetic agent	Be alert for systemic effects.
Bone wax	Physical action	Smeared on oozing bone surface	Remove excess bone wax.

Modified from Moak E: Hemostatic agents: adjuncts to control bleeding, *Todays OR Nurse* 13(11):6, 1991; Katkhouda N: The evolving role of fibrin sealants in surgery. In Medscape surgery treatment updates, http://www.medscape.com/Medscape/Surgery/TreatmentUpdate/2001/tu01/pnt-tu01.html (accessed July 30, 2001); Reger TB, Roditski D: Bloodless medicine and surgery for patients having cardiac surgery, *Crit Care Nurs* 21(4):35, 2001.

but it also can occur during sternal splitting if the lungs are not sufficiently deflated.

One straight mediastinal tube is positioned in the midline, and a second tube, straight or angled, may be placed as well. The tube size may be 32-French (although smaller Silastic drains are often used), which allows good drainage and a lesser chance of occlusion as compared with a smaller size. The tube is inserted by

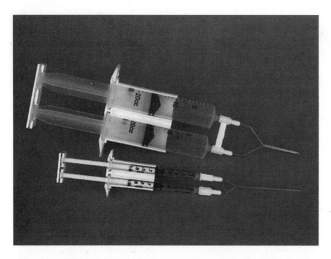

FIG. 6-7 Fibrin glue syringes contain cryoprecipitate in one syringe and a thrombin–calcium chloride mixture in another; a dual dispensing tip is used to prevent clogging within the tips. (Courtesy Haemacure Corp, Sarasota, Fla.)

making a stab wound in the epigastrium, placing the tip of a Kelly or tonsil clamp through the skin wound into the mediastinum, and pulling the tube out through the skin (Fig. 6-8). The exiting portion of the tube is sutured to the skin. When the chest is being closed (and handheld suction devices can no longer be used to aspirate blood from the pericardium), the drainage tube must be connected to suction to remove accumulating blood and fluid in order to avoid compression on the heart, which could lead to tamponade. An endotracheal suction (18-French) catheter attached to a suction line can be inserted into the chest tube to remove intrapericardial fluid quickly. Pleural tubes are inserted in a similar manner intraoperatively. The skin exit site is more lateral (under the breast), and the tube is often angled to conform to the anatomy and to drain behind the lung. The location of the pleural tube depends on whether the right or left (or both) pleura has been opened.

Postoperative pleural chest tube insertion (Fig. 6-9) is accomplished by inserting the internal end of the tube through a skin incision into the pleural cavity. This may be performed in the ICU.

In patients who have undergone operation with CPB or if blood in the pleural space has not been aspirated intraoperatively, the nurse can expect initially to see approximately 100 ml of blood (or more if irrigating solutions have spilled into the cavity) drain from the pleural tube once it has been connected to suction. Within a short time, however, this drainage should be significantly reduced. Persistent drainage from a pleural tube may be indicative of IMA bleeding and may require open exploration. This generally is performed only if other possible causes (such as coagulation deficiencies) have not been implicated. In patients undergoing off-pump surgery, less blood loss is anticipated.

The chest tubes may be attached to a collecting chamber that collects and reinfuses shed mediastinal blood (Andreason and others, 2001). This system was first described by Schaff and his associates (1978) as a method of salvaging postoperative shed blood. The patient's chest tubes are connected to the sterile drainage system. Anticoagulation is not required because the blood is mechanically defibrinated by the action of the heart and lungs against the blood cells (Martin and others, 2000).

Occasionally a cardiotomy reservoir is converted into a chest tube drainage system; the perfusionist removes the cardiotomy reservoir from the CPB circuit and modifies it to accept the chest tubes and be connected to wall suction. The distal end of the chest tube is inserted into the appropriate port. Before the patient's transfer to the surgical ICU, the reservoir is attached to the patient's bed and suction is discontinued; the patient is then transported. On admission to the ICU, suction is reestablished and transfusion initiated as indicated.

When three chest tubes are in place, a second collecting chamber (such as a PleurEvac) can be used for the third tube—preferably a pleural rather than a mediastinal tube. It is important to ensure that the system is connected to suction once the chest is closed so that blood accumulating in the pericardium does not tamponade the heart. Suction is discontinued just before the patient leaves the OR. Smaller blood collection systems that do not reinfuse shed blood are increasingly popular.

Completion of the Procedure

After CPB termination, heparin reversal, and achievement of hemostasis, the chest is closed (see Chapter 9) and chest tubes are connected to the drainage system. Dressings are applied. Before transferring the patient, the nurse telephones a report to the ICU; special concerns or fears verbalized by the patient preoperatively should be included, as well as operative details and physiologic alterations (Box 6-5). Perioperative documentation follows the standard protocol. It should include a complete description of the operation performed, the names of the surgical team members, identification of medications and prosthetic implants (with lot and serial numbers), the postoperative skin condition, and other pertinent data.

If there is a delay in transporting the patient to the ICU (e.g., because of sudden increased chest tube drainage or hemodynamic instability), the perioperative nurse can notify the unit and, if possible, revise the anticipated time of arrival. If arrival cannot be estimated at the time of the call, the OR nurse can call after the patient has been stabilized. Delays also should be communicated to waiting family members; the nurse should explain the delay honestly but in a reassuring manner so that the family's concern is not unnecessarily heightened.

TABLE 6-7
Pharmacologic Blood Conservation Agents

COMPOUND	CHEMICAL STRUCTURE	MECHANISM
Hemostatic agents		
Desmopressin acetate	Antidiuretic hormone analogue	Stimulates secretion of factor VIII and von Willebrand factor
ε-Aminocaproic acid ⎫ Tranexamic acid ⎬	Lysine analogue	Blocks plasmin; stabilizes clots
Platelet protective agents		
Aprotinin	Bovine polypeptide	Serine protease inhibitor; inhibits platelet aggregation; inhibits plasmin
Dipyridamole	Pyridopyrimidine	Inhibits platelet aggregation
Prostacyclin	Arachidonic acid metabolite	Inhibits platelet aggregation
Recombinant human erythropoietin	Recombinant protein	Stimulates erythropoiesis
Red blood cell substitutes		
Modified human hemoglobin	Polymerized, pyridoxylated stroma-free hemoglobin	Transports chemically bound oxygen
Perfluorochemicals	Emulsified perfluorocarbon compounds	Transports dissolved oxygen
Volume expanders	Hydroxyethyl starch; dextran polymers	Osmotically active agents increase intravascular volume and blood flow

From Stack G, Snyder EL: Alternative to perioperative blood transfusion. In Stoelting RK, editor: *Advances in anesthesia,* vol 8, St Louis, 1991, Mosby; Ellison N: Red blood cells: an analysis of risk versus benefit, *Ann Thorac Surg* 72:S1806, 2001.

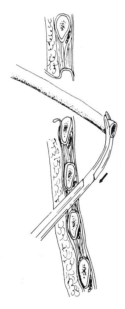

FIG. 6-8 Chest tube insertion. After the clamp has been passed through the skin incision into the pericardium, the distal end of the tube is grasped and pulled out through the skin until the desired length of tube remains in the pericardium. (From Gregory BS: Thoracic surgery. In Meeker MH, Rothrock JC: *Alexander's care of the patient in surgery,* ed 10, St Louis, 1995, Mosby.)

Before the patient is moved to the ICU bed for transfer, hemodynamic stability is reconfirmed and chest tube drainage (from mediastinal and pleural tubes, if present) assessed. Early drainage of 200 to 400 ml per hour is almost always "surgical" and requires explo-ration. Because of the possibility of having to reopen the chest, instruments, back tables, and internal defibrillator paddles should be kept sterile until the patient has reached the ICU or at least left the operating room. The patient is ventilated with an Ambu bag attached to an oxygen tank and is monitored during transport; a portable defibrillator accompanies the patient. The patient will remain intubated and mechanically ventilated in the ICU for a number of hours in order to reduce the metabolic demands imposed by breathing.

Fast-Track Cardiac Surgery

Some patients undergoing off-pump procedures may be extubated in the OR or early during the postoperative period. This is one component of what is popularly referred to as *fast-tracking* and is one of the methods to reduce length of hospital stay. Pressures to reduce costs and to maximize efficient resource use has made fast-tracking a clinical reality (Starr, Estafanous, and Roberts-Brown, 1999). In order to promote early extubation, anesthetic management is modified from a high-dose opioid technique to one that employs intravenous rapid-acting anesthetics such as propofol. High thoracic epidural analgesia facilitates immediate extubation in most patients. Contraindications to immediate extubation include prolonged CPB (e.g., more than 2.5 hours), hemodynamic instability, uncontrolled bleeding, morbid obesity, severe pulmonary hypertension, heart failure, and emergency surgery (Royse, Royse, and Soeding, 1999). When the patient is extubated in the OR, the nurse should monitor respiratory status and be

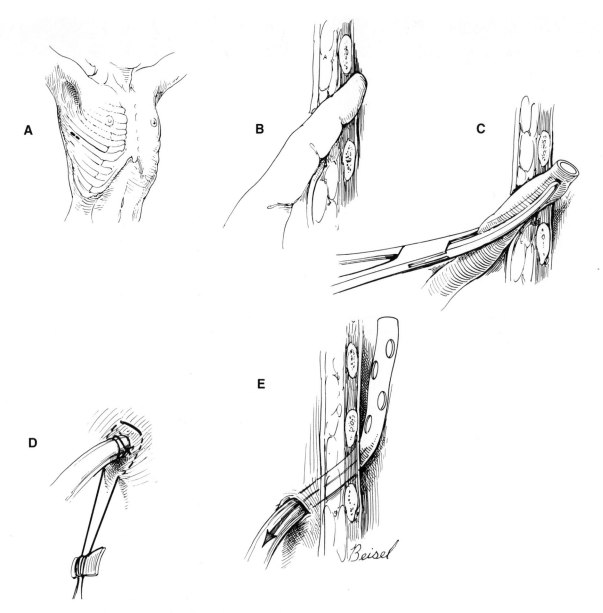

FIG. 6-9   Postoperative insertion of a right pleural chest tube. **A,** Incision. **B,** Finger dilation. **C,** Tube insertion with a clamp. **D,** Suture fixation of tube to skin. **E,** Completed procedure. (From Waldhausen JA, Pierce WS, Campbell DB: *Surgery of the chest,* ed 6, St Louis, 1996, Mosby.)

prepared to assist anesthesia personnel to reintubate the patient if necessary.

Postoperative Management

Postoperative management focuses on maintaining adequate cellular perfusion. Continuous monitoring of cardiac output, heart rate, systemic and pulmonary pressures, oxygen saturation of arterial hemoglobin, and mixed venous blood is performed. It is important to always treat the patient and not the "numbers" be-

cause laboratory and hemodynamic values are meaningful only in relation to the overall clinical picture (Weiland, 1994). It is also important to distrust the data displayed on monitors unless it can be confirmed by empiric evidence (e.g., warm, pink skin). This does not mean that monitoring technology is not useful, but it does need to be assessed in conjunction with the patient's clinical signs.

Chest tube drainage, urinary output, blood gases, temperature, and level of consciousness are assessed frequently and are frequently interrelated. For exam-

---

BOX 6-5
Patient Transfer Report

Procedure (include source of autogenous grafts and use of endoscopic vein harvest): _____
_____

Monitoring devices

CVP _____	Arterial line _____
Swan _____	Peripheral lines _____
CPB _____	off-pump _____

_____

Intraoperative occurrences

Blood loss _____	BP
Dysrhythmias_____	Bypass problems _____
Defib × _____	Lo temp_____
Setting _____	Hi temp_____
Cross-clamp time _____	Pump time_____
CO_____ CI_____	Urine_____

Blood: Given_____ Available_____
Autotransfusion totals: _____ ml _____ Units
Components: FFP_____ Platelets_____Cryo_____
Additional ordered (type) _____

Medications

Neo _____	Dopamine_____	Dobutamine _____
Lidocaine _____	Nitro_____	Levophed _____
Epinephrine_____	Nitroprusside_____	Inocor _____
DDAVP_____	Aprotinin_____	

Tubes/drains: Mediastinal _____Pleural _____

Epicardial leads: Atrial_____Ventricular_____
Pacing: Yes/No   Rate _____

Labs: K+_____ Na+ _____Glu _____Mg++_____
    Hgb _____ Hct _____ Other _____

Patient concerns _____
Additional information _____
ICU bed No. _____ ETA_____ Reported by_____
    To _____ Time _____

BP, Blood pressure; *CPB,* cardiopulmonary bypass; *CI,* cardiac index; *CO,* cardiac output; *cryo,* cryoprecipitate; *CVP,* central venous pressure line; *defib,* defibrillation; *ETA,* estimated time of arrival; *FFP,* fresh frozen plasma; *glu,* glucose; *Hct,* hematocrit; *Hgb,* hemoglobin; *hi/lo temp,* high and low temperatures; *K+,* potassium; *Mg++,* Magnesium; *Na+,* sodium; *neo,* neosynephrine; *nitro,* nitroglycerin; *Swan,* Swan-Ganz pulmonary artery catheter.

BOX 6-6
Postoperative Orders: Admission to the Cardiac Intensive Care Unit

Admit to the cardiac ICU_____
Status/post _____
Condition_____
Allergies_____
Vital signs q 15 min until stable, then q 1 hr _____
ECG on admission_____
Hemodynamic parameters STAT on admission then q 1 hr _

Continuous Sao_2 record q 1 hr_____
Hypothermia/hyperthermia blanket until temp 36° C (96.8° F)
Pacemaker: A _____ V_____ wires
Pacemaker settings_____
Ventilator settings: TV_____ SIMV_____ PEEP_____ Fio^2
Chest tubes to 20 cm suction _____
    Location _____
Splint chest when suctioning and coughing _____
Record chest drainage q 1 hr_____
NG to low continuous suction; record drainage q 8 hr _____

Foley to gravity with q 1 hr output _____
IV: D_5 lactated Ringer's at 20 ml/hr_____
Strict I&O _____   Daily weights _____
Labs: STAT CBC, basic metabolic panel,* Mg, ionized Ca,
PT/PTT on admission
ABGS on admission STAT and prn_____
Check K+ and H/H q 4 hr × 24 hrs_____
Portable chest x-ray examination on admission and in AM of
    POD 1_____
Keep 4 units packed RBCs on hold in blood bank _____
Meds: Cefuroxime (Zinacef)
    Vancomycin
    Then Levofloxacin after IV antibiotics are done _____
    Tylenol rectally/PO prn temp >38.3° C (101° F)
    Morphine IV prn pain
Keep 2 units PPF and 25% albumin on hold in unit
ECG _____

A, Atrial; *ABGs,* arterial blood gases; *Ca,* calcium; *CBC,* complete blood count; *Fio_2,* forced inspired oxygen; *H/H,* hemoglobin and hematocrit; *I&O,* intake and output; *K+,* potassium; *Mg,* magnesium; *NG,* nasogastric; *PEEP,* positive end-expiratory pressure; *PO,* orally; *POD,* postoperative day; *PPF,* plasma protein fraction; *prn,* as needed; *SIMV,* synchronized intermittent mandatory ventilation; *STAT,* immediately; *TV,* tidal volume; *V,* ventricular.
*Basic metabolic panel includes glucose, blood urea nitrogen (BUN), creatinine, CO_2 content, sodium, potassium, and chloride.
Courtesy John R. Garrett, MD.

---

ple, if the toes are warm and the patient is making urine, peripheral perfusion is adequate. If the chest tubes are draining and cardiac output is within normal limits, it is unlikely that there is cardiac tamponade (Box 6-6).

An important difference between a cardiac surgery patient and other patients in the ICU who have undergone surgery is that the former also is recovering from the effects of CPB (unless nonpump surgery has been performed). Postoperative management focuses on the temporary physiologic derangements that surgery and CBP produce, and cardiac perioperative nurses should be familiar with anticipated postoperative patient responses and ICU protocols. Knowledge of these factors enables the perioperative nurse to anticipate changes in the patient's status that may warrant, for example, surgical exploration for bleeding. It is also important to develop a strong professional relationship with critical care colleagues. This promotes communication and interaction, which is especially effective when emergencies arise.

References

Andreasen AS and others: Autologous transfusion of shed mediastinal blood after coronary artery bypass grafting and bacterial contamination, *Ann Thor Surg* 72:1327, 2001.

Arndt K: Inadvertent hypothermia in the OR, *AORN J* 70(2):204, 1999.

Aronson S, Dupont FW: Perioperative cardiac imaging, *Adv Cardiac Surg* 12:117, 2000.

Association of periOperative Registered Nurses (AORN): *Standards, recommended practices & guidelines,* Denver, 2001, AORN.

Belmont MT, Scott RPF: Muscle relaxants and the cardiovascular system. In Kaplan JA, editor: *Cardiac anesthesia,* ed 4, Philadelphia, 1999, WB Saunders.

Bovill JG, Boer F: Opioids in cardiac anesthesia. In Kaplan JA, editor: *Cardiac anesthesia,* ed 4, Philadelphia, 1999, WB Saunders.

Charney JR: Cardiothoracic anesthesia. In Baumgartner FJ, editor: *Cardiothoracic surgery,* Austin, Tex, 1997, Landes Bioscience.

Colburn B: Personal communication, Sept 2, 2000.

Cummins RO and others: Defibrillator failures: causes of problems and recommendations for improvement, *JAMA* 264(8):1019, 1990.

Despotis GJ, Skubas NJ, Goodnough LT: Optimal management of bleeding and transfusion in patients undergoing cardiac surgery, *Semin Thorac Cardiovasc Surg* 11(2): 84, 1999.

Dietrich W and others: Anaphylactic reactions to aprotinin reexposure in cardiac surgery: relation to antiaprotinin immunoglobulin G and E antibodies, *Anesthesiology* 95(1):64, 2001.

Dirks J: Cardiovascular therapeutic management. In Urden LD, Stacy KM, editors: *Priorities in critical care nursing,* ed 3, St Louis, 2000, Mosby.

Ellison N: Red blood cells: an analysis of risk versus benefit, *Ann Thorac Surg* 72:S1806, 2001.

Ensminger J, Moss R: Preventing inadvertent hypothermia—a success story, *AORN J* 70(2):298, 1999.

Esperson C: The RN first assistant in cardiac surgery. In Rothrock JC: *The RN first assistant: an expanded perioperative nursing role,* ed 3, Philadelphia, 1999, JB Lippincott.

Fox VJ: Patient education and discharge planning. In Meeker MH, Rothrock JC, editors: *Alexander's care of the patient in surgery,* ed 11, St Louis, 1999, Mosby.

Hoffer JL: Anesthesia. In Meeker MH, Rothrock JC, editors: *Alexander's care of the patient in surgery,* ed 11, St Louis, 1999, Mosby.

Kaempf G: Nursing considerations during surgery. In Seifert PC: *Cardiac surgery,* St Louis, 1994, Mosby.

Katkhouda N: The evolving role of fibrin sealants in surgery. In *Medscape surgery treatment updates,* http://www.medscape.com/Medscape/Surgery/TreatemntUpdate/2001/tu01/pnt-tu01.html (accessed July 30, 2001).

Kervin MW and others: Nitric oxide: a primer for the practicing anesthetist, *CRNA* 9(3):93, 1998.

Krucylak PE: Intraoperative considerations during minimal-access cardiac surgery, *Semin Thorac Cardiovasc Surg* 11(2):116, 1999.

Ladden CS: Concepts basic to perioperative nursing. In Meeker MH, Rothrock JC, editors: *Alexander's care of the patient in surgery,* ed 11, St Louis, 1999, Mosby.

Levi M and others: Pharmacological strategies to decrease excessive blood loss in cardiac surgery: a meta-analysis of clinically relevant endpoints, *Lancet* 354(9194)1940, 1999.

Mangano CM and others: Cardiopulmonary bypass and the anesthesiologist. In Kaplan JA, editor: *Cardiac anesthesia,* ed 4, Philadelphia, 1999, WB Saunders.

Mangram AJ and others: Guideline for the prevention of surgical site infection, 1999, *Am J Infect Control* 27:97, 1999.

Martin J, and others: Reinfusion of mediastinal blood after heart surgery, *J Thorac Cardiovasc Surg* 120(3):499, 2000.

Moak E: Hemostatic agents: adjuncts to control bleeding, *Todays OR Nurse* 13(11):6, 1991.

Morrill P: Pharmacotherapeutics of positive inotropes, *AORN J* 71(1):173, 2000.

Nierich AP: Anesthesia in beating heart CABG surgery. In *Minimally invasive cardiac surgery: information for associated professionals,* http://www.medtronic.com/cardiac/mics/phys_associates.html (accessed May 23, 2001).

Park KW and others: Effects of inhalation anesthetics on systemic hemodynamics and the coronary circulation. In Kaplan JA, editor: *Cardiac anesthesia,* ed 4, Philadelphia, 1999, WB Saunders.

Pfister AJ: Myocardial revascularization without cardiopulmonary bypass, *Adv Cardiac Surg* 11:35, 1999.

Reger TB, Roditski D: Bloodless medicine and surgery for patients having cardiac surgery, *Crit Care Nurs* 21(4):35, 2001.

Reich DL, Moskowitz DM, Kaplan JA: Hemodynamic monitoring. In Kaplan JA, editor: *Cardiac anesthesia,* ed 4, Philadelphia, 1999, WB Saunders.

Reves JC, Hill S, Berkowitz D: Pharmacology of intravenous anesthetic induction drugs. In Kaplan JA, editor: *Cardiac anesthesia,* ed 4, Philadelphia, 1999, WB Saunders.

Royse CF, Royse AG, Soeding PF: Routine immediate extubation after cardiac operation: a review of our first 100 patients, *Ann Thorac Surg* 68:1326, 1999.

Saginur R, Croteau D, Bergeron MG: Comparative efficacy of teicoplanin and cefazolin for cardiac operation prophylaxis in 3027 patients, *J Thorac Cardiovasc Surg* 120(6):1120, 2000.

Schaff HV and others: Autotransfusion of shed mediastinal blood after cardiac surgery: a prospective study, *J Thorac Cardiovasc Surg* 75(4):632, 1978.

Spiess BD. Blood transfusion: the silent epidemic, *Ann Thorac Surg* 72:S1832, 2001.

Starr NJ, Estafanous FG, Roberts-Brown M: Cost containment: anesthesia and cardiac surgery. In Kaplan JA, editor: *Cardiac anesthesia,* ed 4, Philadelphia, 1999, WB Saunders.

Watson D: Contemporary issues. In Meeker MH, Rothrock JC, editors: *Alexander's care of the patient in surgery,* ed 11, St Louis, 1999, Mosby.

Weiland AP: Postoperative assessment "pearls." In Seifert PC: *Cardiac surgery,* St Louis, 1994, Mosby.

7

Evaluating Outcome Achievement

Cardiac surgical nursing is challenging and demanding. The rapid progress being made in the medical and surgical treatment of heart disease makes constant evaluation of nursing care mandatory.

Maryann Powers, RN, and Frances Storlie, RN, 1969 (preface)

The assessment of quality begins with data.

Mark B. Orringer, 2001 (p. 2)

Evaluation is performed to judge the patient's progress toward the attainment of outcomes and to appraise the effectiveness of nursing interventions in achieving those outcomes (AORN, 2001). The evaluation process is systematic and ongoing; it supplies data for quality improvement efforts, enhances future planning, fosters more effective interventions, and establishes greater accountability for the perioperative nurse and other members of the team. When specified outcomes are not met, the nurse attempts to determine the reasons why. The nursing diagnosis may have been inaccurate, the plan incomplete, or the actions inappropriate or insufficient. Or the outcomes were unrealistic because the patient, family, and significant others were not involved in their development. Underlying patient factors, such as left ventricular dysfunction, renal failure, or hypertension may have contributed to less than optimal outcomes.

In some situations a problem may not be attributable to poor patient care management or preexisting patient factors. It may be created by existing structures or policies. Nurses may have difficulty meeting the Standards of Clinical Practice to provide nursing care or the Standards of Professional Performance to engage in professional role activities because of inadequate staff and material resources and support (AORN, 2001). A common impediment cited by many nurses is the lack of sufficient time (or encouragement) to interview patients preoperatively and postoperatively; this problem is becoming particularly evident with the increasing number of patient admissions occurring on the morning of surgery.

Another consideration is the multidisciplinary nature of cardiac care, necessitating cooperation and col-laboration between members of the health care team. Rarely can the achievement of outcomes be attributed solely to the interventions of one person. A more comprehensive and accurate evaluation of patient outcomes is likely when there are formal and informal joint reviews by nurses, physicians, and other members of the cardiac team.

Although collaborative working relationships often reflect the interdependent nature of many nursing activities, the importance of sound nursing judgment is no less critical when actions are generated from medical orders or are supervised directly by physicians. Preparing a patient for emergency surgery and performing in the RN first assistant (RNFA) role are just two examples of interdependent practice that require the nurse to have well-developed critical thinking skills.

Another method of evaluating outcome achievement is through the use of local, regional, and national databases. The Society of Thoracic Surgeons' (STS; http://www.sts.org) Cardiac National Database (managed by the Duke Clinical Research Institute) provides comparative information on the clinical outcomes of cardiac surgical patients. The STS database has evolved in response to the demand by patients, payers, and administrators for improved patient care (Harlan, 2001; Orringer, 2001). Institutions participating in the database document the characteristics and interventions performed on every patient undergoing cardiac surgery, submit the data to STS, and receive reports comparing the submitting institution's outcomes with regional and national standards. (A similar database for cardiologists performing cardiac catheterization and percutaneous coronary intervention [PCI] is managed by the American College of Cardiology [ACC; http://www.acc.org].)

Changes in the health care system also have had an impact on the nurse's role in evaluating patient care. Reimbursement issues and regulatory mandates have increased the nurse's accountability for the human, material, and fiscal resources used in the delivery of care. Factors related to safety, effectiveness, efficiency, environmental concerns, and cost are now an integral part of the evaluation process (AORN, 2001). Nurses must be able to demonstrate the cost effectiveness of their interventions and the cost-benefit derived from the services provided (Beyea and Nicoll, 2000).

Research

Evaluation methods can also be used to identify problems and errors amenable to the research process. The process may include a situation that seems wrong or needs a solution or an area that requires improvement or modification. If the problem is to become a researchable question, the "who," "where," "what," and "when" must be clearly defined so that the specific "why" and "how" can be determined. Such evidence-based research plays an important role in quality improvement. Although not all perioperative nurses can develop and implement research studies, they can base their practice on research findings and support scientific investigations by serving as study participants or expert reviewers of content areas. Nursing interventions based on research results create a planned, evidence-based process rather than one based on conjecture and assumption.

EVIDENCE-BASED PRACTICE

The shift toward using evidence from scientific research has become a powerful and relevant trend in the current health care market (Walshe and Rundall, 2001). Prompted by the wide variations in clinical practice patterns, Sackett and Rosenberg (1995) popularized the concept of evidence-based clinical practice in order to distinguish therapies of known effectiveness from those known to be ineffective.

The Institute of Medicine (IOM, 1999) described three categories of problems relating to this gap between research and practice: overuse, underuse, and misuse of health care interventions. *Overuse* can be exemplified by poorly designed patient satisfaction questionnaires that produce data infrequently employed. *Underuse* can be seen in the relatively small percentage of individuals with heart disease who participate in cardiac rehabilitation. *Misuse* is illustrated most often by medication errors: wrong drug, dose, route, or time (Becher and Chassin, 2001). Organizations should fos-

ter a culture that attempts to learn from research; such a culture promotes innovation, experimentation, data collection and analysis and the development of critical thinking skills. Relevant research is reviewed and incorporated into institutional systems (Walshe and Rundall, 2001).

Other factors that complicate the implementation of evidence-based practices include the dramatic increase in the amount of data and information that must be managed, increasingly complex systems that tend to breed errors, educational programs that assume there is a finite body of knowledge that can be mastered and used to answer all clinical questions, and professional practice models that undervalue the contributions of all members of the health care team (Becher and Chassin, 2001).

Improvements in outcomes as a result of evidence-based initiatives have been demonstrated for patients undergoing coronary artery bypass grafting (CABG) and other types of cardiac surgery. The Northern New England Cardiovascular Disease Study Group is a regional consortium that has improved its mortality rates by regular and frequent feedback among participating institutions, structured site visits, organized efforts to better understand the processes contributing to mortality, and determination of the causes of mortality (Nugent, 1999; O'Connor and others, 1996, 1998). This multiinstitutional model for continuous improvement in cardiac surgery has been adopted by other cooperative groups in Alabama (Holman and others, 2001), Washington (Goss and others, 2000), and Minnesota (Arom and others, 1997), as well as other areas of the country (Harlan, 2001).

Managers and administrators benefit from research activities because these can provide accurate information for developing clinical and administrative policy and initiating quality improvement and cost-saving initiatives. Joint efforts by members of health care facilities and educational institutions combine operational and theoretical expertise to promote access to ideas and resources. Nursing managers can facilitate this process by nurturing an environment that welcomes questions from practicing nurses and fosters critical thinking (Box 7-1). In the perioperative arena research activities can be used by managers to study not only patient-related needs but also other factors such as calculation of the staffing and supply costs of surgical procedures, determination of the most efficient scheduling system, and evaluation of new products.

SOCIETY OF THORACIC SURGEONS DATABASE

Institutional tracking of patient outcomes provides a valuable source of data that can stimulate quality improvement initiatives. The Society of Thoracic Sur-

BOX **7-1**
Ideas for Quality Improvement

- Create multidisciplinary teams
- Involve all staff
- Break down barriers between departments
- Map processes
- Approach problems from multiple aspects
- Make site visits with multidisciplinary teams
- Call colleagues at other institutions with questions or problems
- Share data and ideas
- Learn from others
- Be open to fresh perspectives
- Standardize protocols and processes
- Attend multidisciplinary conferences
- Institute an ongoing forum to pose questions and seek answers and solutions

Modified from O'Connor GT and others: A regional intervention to improve the hospital mortality associated with coronary artery bypass graft surgery, *JAMA* 275(11):841, 1996; O'Connor GT and others: Results of a regional study of modes of death associated with coronary artery bypass grafting, *Ann Thorac Surg* 66:1323, 1998.

geons (STS) database was conceived in the mid-1980s by surgeons interested in comparing their institutional clinical data with that of their colleagues in other local, regional, and national cardiac programs (Orringer, 2001). Applications of the database include individual assessment of risk, quality improvement, responses to managed care requests for operative results, state regulatory requirements, and research.

In assessing risk, the purpose of the database is not to *predict* survival or death; it is intended to *estimate* the probability of operative death based on the aggregate experience of the national database participants. The database model tells the surgeon how a patient with specific comorbidities (e.g., renal disease, heart failure, diabetes) can be expected to fare based on a national standard of care (Edwards and Grover, 2000).

When an institution's outcomes differ from the national comparative sample, examination of the institution's practices may be warranted to determine if changes are indicated. Clinical reviews promote quality improvement initiatives and also provide data on patient outcomes to managed care organizations, who compare health care providers based on clinical results as well as costs.

In those states that have regulatory requirements for submission of morbidity and mortality data, the STS format has provided valid information in a format that does not require a separate (and cumbersome) reporting format. In those states that have their own different reporting system, the STS Database Liaison Committee has developed a program to assist in adopting the STS system. Finally, the STS database is a rich source of information for research studies, and subjects such as the impact of gender and race on outcome have been investigated (Edwards and Glover, 2000). Congenital cardiac surgery and thoracic surgery databases are almost completed (Ferguson and others, 2000).

Patient Care Management

The primary objective of patient care management is to assist the patient in achieving optimum surgical outcomes (see Chapter 5). Goal attainment is demonstrated by the patient's progress toward the expected outcome (and the absence of injury or harm or other complications) during the preoperative, intraoperative, and postoperative periods. The evaluation process can be concurrent or retrospective, objective or subjective. Concurrent evaluation is performed while the activities are being performed and the patient responses can be monitored continuously. Retrospective reviews provide a cumulative picture of nursing care and can be used to measure the overall effectiveness of nursing interventions in achieving patient outcomes (AORN, 2001). Objective evaluations of outcomes are based on data collection; subjective evaluations rely on observation of patient responses. Regardless of the type of process, information should be communicated to appropriate team members and documented in a retrievable form (AORN, 2001). The nurse can evaluate responses from patients themselves or solicit information from significant others, clinical colleagues, and others directly or indirectly involved in providing care. Among the indicators supporting goal achievement are expected physiologic signs and symptoms, expected psychologic and emotional responses, behavioral expectations, patient statements, and laboratory and diagnostic test results (AORN, 2001).

As a result of the review process, the nurse identifies opportunities to improve care that can be incorporated into future patient situations. The nurse investigates whether outcomes identified by the caregiver were congruent with the patient's expectations and whether the goals of patient care were realistic (Rothrock, 1996).

To evaluate interventions and outcomes, the nurse should possess the knowledge and skill to develop individualized outcomes and criteria to measure their achievement. Data from internal quality improvement programs and external bench marks (e.g., the STS database) must be collected to provide consistent measurement of responses and analyzed to determine whether the outcomes were met. Additional or alternate nursing actions that are necessary can be identified, and the status of goal achievement communicated appropriately.

Evaluation activities can be performed at any time during the perioperative period, but certain outcomes may require review specifically in the preoperative, intraoperative, or postoperative period, depending on the time frame established for their accomplishment. Outcomes related to knowledge and emotional well-being, for example, may be evaluated preoperatively and postoperatively when patient communication is necessary for confirmation. Outcomes affected by intraoperative variables but appearing (or absent) in the postoperative period, such as infection, are evaluated after the completion of surgery. Outcomes related to more immediate physiologic responses, such as those relating to patient safety and hemodynamic status, are likely to be monitored continuously throughout the perioperative period.

PREOPERATIVE PERIOD

Anxiety

Anxiety reduction during the preoperative period is a common goal of nursing care. Feelings of anxiety are aroused by generalized, nonspecific fears of the unknown, in contrast to specific fears of death, pain, or body image disturbances. Interventions to reduce fear focus on the provision of information that addresses the known threat and on the creation of a supportive environment that allows the patient to benefit from the information (Koivula and others, 2001).

The vague, undefined sense of apprehension or uneasiness that characterizes the feeling of anxiety can range from mild to panic level. Some degree of anxiety is common in most if not all patients awaiting cardiac surgery, and a moderate degree of anxiety may be adaptive and even therapeutic when arousal is appropriate to the situation. In its more severe form, however, anxiety provokes a powerful adrenergic response that can create additional stress for an already jeopardized myocardium. Studies have shown that either low or high levels of anxiety produce poorer outcomes (Lenz and Perkins, 2000, Bergmann and others, 2001).

Including family members in preoperative interviews is beneficial because they can have a positive effect on the patient's recovery. The family (or significant others) often provides the primary support for the patient and can enhance patient coping mechanisms. If family members themselves have unmet needs, unrealistic expectations, or excessive fear and anxiety, transference of these feelings to the patient may increase the patient's own stress level. Thus meeting the family's needs may be closely linked to meeting the patient's needs (Leske, 1986).

Better preparation of family members before their witnessing the condition and appearance of the patient can be beneficial. Immediately postoperatively, for example, families should be aware that the patient may be intubated and sedated, appear pale, feel clammy, and have multiple indwelling lines and catheters.

Whenever possible, family members should be included in the interactions between perioperative nurse and patient. These can provide an opportunity to explain or clarify what the planned treatment is and why and how it will be implemented. In addition, periodic communication with family members or significant others during the intraoperative period can foster feelings of hope, provide reassurance, and enhance coping mechanisms, which in turn can help family members to support and encourage the patient during recuperation.

To determine the effectiveness of interventions for anxiety, the nurse compares the physiologic and psychologic characteristics of the anxious behavior with the patient's responses to interventions. Physiologic manifestations often include rapid breathing and increased heart rate; successful outcome achievement could be measured in terms of (1) respiratory rate within 5 breaths of the patient's normal respiratory rate and (2) heart rate within 10 beats of the patient's normal pulse. Psychologic cues to anxiety may include withdrawal, crying, poor eye contact, increased muscle tension, and urinary frequency. The support of family members and friends often can ease some of the stress felt by patients.

Restlessness and agitation also may be present, but the nurse should first determine whether these are signs of emotional or physiologic distress (such as hypoxia or some other physical alteration). The appropriate intervention is then instituted and evaluated.

The nurse also can judge patient needs and identify a variety of possible interventions by discussing anxiety-reducing techniques (and the educational needs of patients) with members of The Mended Hearts, Inc., a support group for patients who have undergone cardiac surgery. Members make preoperative and postoperative visits or communicate by telephone to provide moral support and education about the impending surgery. Because they have experienced cardiac surgery, The Mended Hearts members have great insight into patient needs; they are a valuable resource to nurses and to patients (especially patients displaying excessive levels of anxiety preoperatively).

Evaluation can be performed postoperatively as well. The nurse can solicit suggestions from the patient (and significant others) about which interventions were most effective and apply these to future situations.

Knowledge

Knowledge about the physiologic and psychologic responses to the cardiac disorder and its treatment helps patients to cope with the disease, participate in the therapy and recuperation, and promote healthy behaviors that contribute to a successful outcome with fewer complications.

The informational needs of families of critically ill patients have been studied by a number of researchers (Leske, 1986; Reeder, 1991), and the findings have been consistent in demonstrating the importance of the following:

- To feel there is hope
- To receive information about the patient once a day
- To be called at home about changes in the patient's condition
- To know why things are being done for the patient
- To be assured that the best care possible is being given to the patient
- To know exactly what is being done for the patient
- To have questions answered honestly

Preoperatively the patient should have a sufficient understanding of the effects of the illness and the treatment to participate in preoperative activities (such as intravascular catheter insertion and application of electrocardiographic electrodes. The use of humor may enhance knowledge retention in cardiac surgery patients (Schrecengost, 2001). Postoperatively, outcome achievement is also evaluated with regard to recovery and rehabilitation (see later section).

Cardiac surgical patients often request information about mechanical ventilation, suctioning procedures, use of an endotracheal tube, deep breathing and coughing, and chest tube removal. Patients may not appreciate fully the type, degree, and location of pain and discomfort postoperatively. This may be related to insufficient time for comprehensive teaching or to differing expectations between nurses and patients regarding which information should be provided.

INTRAOPERATIVE PERIOD

Injury

Intraoperatively the patient is at risk for injuries related to positioning, retained foreign objects, and physical, chemical, electrical, and thermal hazards. For example, immediately after positioning, the nurse should determine that pressure areas are properly padded. When arms and hands are tucked along the side of a supine patient, the nurse and anesthesia personnel jointly ensure that intravenous solutions are infusing properly and that intraarterial monitoring lines have not been disturbed and are recording the blood pressure accurately. Patients in the lateral position are evaluated to ensure that circulation of dependent body parts is not jeopardized, that ventilation of the dependent lung is adequate, that musculoskeletal injury is avoided, and that pressure points are protected. Patients with limited range of motion, back problems, or joint pain require special precautions during positioning.

When the arms must be flexed, the nurse should consider the potential risk of neuropathy. Nerve injury tends to occur in the arms more frequently than in the legs. Ulnar nerve compression neuropathy may occur with extreme elbow flexion; the longer the elbow is maintained in that position, the more likely it is that injury will occur.

Brachial plexus nerve injury during cardiac surgery can occur, and somatosensory evoked potential (SEP) monitors to measure ulnar and median nerve SEPs may be used. Retraction of the sternum and retraction of the chest wall for internal mammary artery exposure can produce peripheral nervous system injury. Using the SEP technique may provide an early warning to the surgeon to modify the surgical technique.

In the immediate postoperative period and a few hours after surgery, the effects of positioning can be evaluated when the patient is awake and able to describe symptoms of neuromuscular discomfort. The nurse will want to confirm that joint problems were not aggravated by the positioning techniques and that patients with fragile skin or little adipose tissue were adequately protected against pressure sores or tissue necrosis.

Injury also can be caused by retained foreign bodies; their absence usually is confirmed by documentation of correct counts. When needles or other small objects are missing, an x-ray film is taken, and review of the film should rule out the presence of the missing object. When counts are incorrect, it may be helpful to review the method used to keep track of these objects during surgery. For example, anchoring bulldog clamps and free needles not in use can help to avoid their misplacement; pill (Kittner) sponges can be kept in a container or placed in a clamp; hypodermic needles can be placed in a cup or a needle boat, or attached to a syringe. Inattentiveness or feeling pressured to hurry may be the cause of misplaced items in the majority of cases, but how one arranges supplies and instruments also may increase the possibility of missing items.

Chemical injury is best prevented by instituting preventive measures such as avoiding known patient allergy–producing substances, labeling fluids, and placing only physiologic solutions near the surgical site. Toxic substances (such as glutaraldehyde valve storage solution) should be kept away from topical solutions. Allergic reactions or tissue injury should be absent throughout the intraoperative period. Exposure to ethylene oxide can be another hazard to both patients and staff. Ethylene oxide should be limited to sterilization of items that cannot be sterilized in another manner. Adequate aeration of ethylene oxide–sterilized supplies should be confirmed; if items have not been fully aerated, they should not be used. In dire emergencies, institutional policy should be followed.

Physical hazards include malfunctioning or missing instruments (which result in prolonging ischemic time), supplies, or equipment. For example, malaligned jaws on vascular clamps can tear blood vessels and cause severe bleeding; torn vessels are also more difficult to repair than those that are surgically incised. Unsafe medical devices are another concern; nurses more than any other health care professionals encounter the majority of problems. Because they provide direct patient care, nurses may be among the first to detect a malfunction in a medical device. Nurses play an important role in medical device surveillance by complying with the requirements of the Food and Drug Administration (FDA) for reporting malfunctioning devices. Patient safety is enhanced with consistent implementation of the regulations.

Electrical injuries producing redness, blistering, and other signs of burning are another potential hazard. Misuse of electrical equipment also can place the patient at risk for developing lethal dysrhythmias and conduction disturbances. Evaluation should demonstrate absence of these signs of injury.

Absence of thermal injuries from excessive heat is confirmed by the absence of reddened or burned areas. Mechanical warming pads, blankets from a warming unit, and heated solutions should all be tested before being placed in contact with the patient's skin or internal organs. Heat lamps should be kept a safe distance from the patient to avoid injury.

Cold injuries are also a potential problem. The very young and the elderly are at increased risk because of immature and less efficient internal temperature regulatory mechanisms, respectively. To generate heat, the body shivers. Shivering increases the metabolic rate and oxygen consumption, which, in cardiac patients with depressed ventricular function, can compromise cardiac output. Although neuromuscular blocking medications prevent shivering, the patient is at risk for sudden cardiac decompensation during the period before administration of the paralyzing agent. Inadvertent hypothermia can become a problem again after the termination of cardiopulmonary bypass (when the patient has been made normothermic). If the temperature drifts down significantly after bypass or during off-pump procedures, hypothermia can impair coagulation processes and predispose the patient to irregularities in the heartbeat. Interventions such as increasing the room temperature, using warm topical solutions, and reactivating the thermia blanket can retard this process.

Some patients have "cold allergies" that cause red blood cell agglutination at low temperatures. The presence of this allergy should be communicated to the cardiac team by the blood bank; intraoperatively the patient's temperature may not be reduced as much as it would be in other patients undergoing similar surgery.

It is especially important to avoid delays during the period of cross-clamping, when higher temperatures pose a risk of ischemic injury. Another cold-related injury can result from ice in contact with the phrenic nerve. Nerve injury can impair movement of the diaphragm and affect breathing; this becomes apparent when the patient attempts to breathe independently. Normothermic off-pump techniques may be indicated.

Fluid and electrolyte status

Preoperatively the nurse assesses the patient's status: mental state, skin turgor, blood pressure, pulses, temperature, renal status, intravenous (IV) infusion rate, and laboratory results—especially hematocrit and potassium (K^+) level. Intraoperatively fluid and electrolyte status commonly is evaluated by frequent monitoring of urinary output, volume status via intravascular pressure catheters, and pulmonary and systemic blood pressures and by laboratory tests to determine arterial blood gases, blood counts, and electrolyte levels. In addition, the electrocardiogram (ECG) is used to detect rhythm disturbances associated with electrolyte imbalances, particularly potassium. Perioperative nursing interventions focus on preparation (e.g., having blood and blood products available, being aware of preexisting bleeding disorders), implementation (e.g., using suction devices safely and appropriately, salvaging blood), communication (e.g., with surgical team members and blood bank personnel), and monitoring (e.g., laboratory results, ECG, blood loss, intravascular pressures, urinary output). Volume status can change suddenly, as when acute hemorrhage occurs, and the importance of planning becomes evident in these situations.

Although decisions relating to replacement therapy are generally not within the scope of the perioperative nurse (AORN, 2001) monitoring fluid and electrolyte balance, instituting safety mechanisms (e.g., avoiding excessive aspiration of either topical crystalloid solutions or hyperkalemic cardioplegia solutions into the CPB circuit), and anticipating therapeutic interventions (e.g., blood administration for a low hematocrit) are important nursing considerations. During cardiac surgery, fluctuation of K^+ levels is common and should alert the nurse to the possible development of cardiac dysrhythmias.

Nursing interventions applicable to the perioperative nurse are those related to monitoring and observing for signs and symptoms of fluid and electrolyte imbalance, having replacement therapy available, consulting with physicians about the fluid and electrolyte status of the patient, and teaching patients about therapy.

Perioperative nurses also should be aware that banked blood stored for more than 3 days has elevated plasma K^+ concentration levels because the electrolyte leaks out of the red blood cells over time. Multiple transfusions of old blood may produce significantly elevated K+ levels, which can lead to intraoperative cardiac arrest. Whenever possible, the perioperative nurse should ensure that patients at high risk (e.g., trauma patients, patients undergoing repeat sternotomy) receive fresh blood. Hypokalemia is another potential risk that can result from induced hypothermia, CPB, and intraoperative diuresis.

Skin integrity

Freedom from skin breakdown or alteration during surgery is affected by multiple factors. Immobility during surgery is a major risk factor, but patients who are obese, malnourished, dehydrated, diabetic, infected, very old or young, or who have circulatory impairment have an even greater risk of skin impairment.

Because positioning changes and direct skin care are unfeasible during surgery, the perioperative nurse relies on preventive measures so that the effects of body pressure and immobility do not result in impairment or worsen preexisting conditions. Careful removal of residual adhesives (e.g., from previously applied ECG electrodes or dressing tape) can reduce direct trauma to the skin, as can the use of nonallergenic skin preparation solutions. Skin preparation fluids should not be allowed to drip down under the buttocks and other dependent body areas. Adequate padding of dependent and peripheral areas of the body, patient transfer onto and off of the OR bed without shearing trauma, and use of nonreactive dressings and adhesive tape are among the interventions that can reduce the incidence of impaired skin integrity. After surgery, the nurse evaluates the skin, giving special attention to the sites of dispersive pads and bony prominences. Patient teaching interventions include proper wound care, signs and symptoms of incisional disruption or infection, the need for proper nutrition and adequate rest, and notification of health care personnel when problems arise. Documentation of a patient's skin condition should reflect preoperative and postoperative status, interventions, and patient outcome (AORN, 2001).

Tissue integrity

Maintaining the integrity of various organ systems depends on their being adequately perfused and on reducing ischemic injury from particulate and air emboli, as well as preventing avoidable delays during surgery. Body organs require sufficient oxygen, nutrients, and other metabolic substrates for cellular metabolism. The delivery and use of these substances is affected by preexisting conditions, notably cardiac disease, and induced circulatory alterations such as CPB, hypothermia, and cardioplegic arrest. Perioperative nursing interventions that decrease myocardial oxygen demand, protect myocardial integrity, enhance the safety of extracorporeal circulatory techniques, and promote wound healing can minimize renal, cerebral, cardiopulmonary, gastrointestinal, and peripheral tissue impairment.

Pharmacologic manipulation of vasomotor tone with vasoconstrictors and vasodilators is one method of enhancing organ perfusion. Hypothermia and cardioplegic arrest reduce metabolic needs and conserve energy resources. Among the nursing interventions are assessing the patient's clinical status and comparing it with baseline values. For example, preexisting neurologic deficits should be included in the report to the surgical intensive care unit (SICU) nurses so that postoperatively the SICU nurse can distinguish between prior deficits and those acquired perioperatively.

Intraoperatively the nurse monitors the patient's status (e.g., assessing urinary output as an indicator of kidney perfusion) and institutes measures to promote a safe CPB run (e.g., using bypass circuit components appropriately). Preparation for and implementation of defibrillation, cardioversion, cardiac pacing, and antidysrhythmia therapy are activities related to protecting and maintaining cardiac function. Keeping surgical debris off of instruments and supplies is another important action that can reduce tissue injury related to embolization of particulate matter.

Cardiac output

A decreased cardiac output can be caused by a variety of mechanical (e.g., preload, afterload, contractility), structural (e.g., valve dysfunction), or electrical (alterations in heart rate and/or rhythm) factors that affect the pumping ability of the heart. Decreased cardiac output also may be caused by an inadequate circulating blood volume (e.g., hypovolemia). To implement the most appropriate therapy, it is helpful to differentiate between cardiogenic, ischemic, and hypovolemic causes, but often these factors are interrelated, making precise identification of the problem difficult.

Independent nursing activities for perioperative nurses include monitoring hemodynamic status, promoting rest, providing pain relief, positioning for comfort and ease of breathing, instituting warming measures to prevent shivering, teaching patients and families, and monitoring pacemaker activity. Applicable collaborative interventions include assisting with insertion and monitoring of an intraaortic balloon pump and a ventricular assist device. Performing these activities can help prevent myocardial ischemia or depression and promote a cardiac output consistent with patient needs.

Specific perioperative interventions also can focus on problems caused by cardiogenic or hypovolemic factors. Instituting safety measures to minimize myocardial injury is covered earlier in this section under the subheading injury. Treatment for bradydysrhythmias includes having pacemaker lead and generators available and assisting with their insertion; tachydys-rhythmias can be treated by defibrillation, cardiover-sion, or antidysrhythmic drugs and by correcting un-derlying problems (e.g., ischemia, hypovolemia).

When a decreased cardiac output is caused by hypo-volemia (e.g., from bleeding or fluid shifts), correction of the volume deficit and control of the bleeding site (if indicated) can increase preload and the subsequent cardiac output. Ensuring an adequate supply of blood and blood products is a collaborative activity that con-tributes to a successful outcome.

The performance of RNFA activities also can have a direct impact on cardiac function and surgical outcome. Collaborative RNFA–surgeon interactions not only en-hance the technical results of surgery but also foster greater cohesiveness among cardiac team members (Seifert, 1999). RNFAs can enhance the knowledge and skill of fellow staff members by sharing what has been learned at the field about specific anatomic factors, in-strument use, surgeon preferences, and specific opera-tive techniques. Avoiding injury and promoting patient safety are fundamental RNFA concerns. For example, the RNFA can reduce the risk of myocardial injury by us-ing instruments appropriately and cautiously and by avoiding overzealous manipulation of tissue. Archie's (1992) study comparing MD first assistants and RNFAs during abdominal aortic aneurysm surgery showed that equally satisfactory surgical repair was achieved with ei-ther first assistant and that morbidity and mortality were independent of the type of assistant.

POSTOPERATIVE PERIOD

Early extubation

Older age has been associated with prolonged mechan-ical ventilation after CABG, but Bezanson and col-leagues (2001) have shown that many older adults can be extubated easily in the early postoperative period with good outcomes. The presence of comorbid condi-tions and severity of illness were better predictors of the need for prolonged ventilation than age alone.

Although the increased interest in early extubation for cardiac surgical patients has been driven primarily by economic pressures, the shift to more rapid discontinua-tion of mechanical respiratory support is consistent with general principles. These principles include the presence of adequate cardiopulmonary reserves for spontaneous ventilation, acceptable laboratory results, and the ab-sence of clinical indicators contraindicating cessation of respiratory support (Shapiro and Lichtenthal, 1999).

Other factors promoting early extubation include anesthetic management that employs short-acting anes-thetic agents, reduces the amount of narcotics (which are respiratory depressants), avoids hypothermia and shiver-ing, maintains hemodynamic stability, and reduces pain. Contraindications are prolonged CPB, hemodynamic in-stability, uncontrolled bleeding, morbid obesity, severe pulmonary disease, congestive heart failure, and emer-gent operation (Royse, Royse, and Soeding, 1999).

Bleeding

Excessive mediastinal bleeding (e.g., greater than 500 ml for the first hour postoperatively) usually is mechanical and caused by bleeding from suture lines but may result from coagulopathy. Coagulation panels should be ob-tained and any coagulation deficiencies corrected. If bleeding persists, reexploration and control of bleeding may be indicated to prevent the development of cardiac tamponade. When tamponade develops, blood in the pericardium compresses the heart and prevents adequate filling of the ventricles (preload); this in turn reduces the cardiac output required for cellular perfusion. If the tam-ponade is unrelieved, organ ischemia and acidosis occur, resulting in death (Ledoux and Luikart, 2000). Emer-gency reexploration in the surgical intensive care unit (SICU) may be necessary if the patient is too unstable to transport to the operating room (see Chapter 19).

Pain

Considered the fifth vital sign, pain after CABG (and other forms of cardiac surgery) is common because many pain-sensitive structures in the skin, muscle, bone, and viscera are incised, cauterized, or manipu-lated. Poststernotomy and postthoracotomy pain can impair pulmonary function (Lichtenberg and others, 2000), and pain in the leg vein graft harvesting site can retard ambulation necessary for cardiovascular recov-ery. Patients with internal mammary artery (IMA) grafts report more pain than those who did not receive an IMA graft (Cohen and others, 1993; Watt-Watson and Stevens, 1998). Unrelieved pain generates a sympa-thetic response that can cause an imbalance between myocardial oxygen supply and demand.

Adequate analgesia (via intermittent injection, con-tinuous IV infusion, epidural infusion, intercostal block, or oral medications) is an important factor in pain relief, but patients may not request pain medica-tion. Nurses can help patients by assessing and manag-ing pain more effectively and implementing educa-tional programs for both patients and colleagues (Watt-Watson and Stevens, 1998).

Nonpharmacologic pain management in combina-tion with analgesics can enhance the effect of pain-relieving drugs. Direct interventions include using de-vices (e.g., a pillow) that splint the chest when cough-ing, repositioning, deep breathing, and massage. Cog-nitive, behavioral, or affective measures such as distraction, imagery, and relaxation also may be employed. Van Kooten (1999) found that 70% of patients reported decreased perception and sensation of pain with the use of nonpharmacologic interventions. Massage, distraction, and repositioning were the most helpful interventions, according to Van Kooten.

Atrial fibrillation

Atrial fibrillation (AF) is common after cardiac surgery and affects more than 30% of patients; it is the major reason for hospital stays longer than 4 days after CABG (Cox, 1999). Once considered little more than a nuisance, AF currently is considered a potentially serious complication because it can lead to deterioration in cardiac output and blood pressure. There are also substantial increased costs associated with the need for additional diagnostic tests, medications, and time spent in the hospital (Creswell, 1999).

Risk factors for the development of postoperative AF include increasing patient age, preoperative history of AF, preoperative use of digoxin, history of rheumatic heart disease, chronic obstructive pulmonary disease, and prolonged aortic cross-clamp (e.g., ischemic) time (DeJong and Morton, 2000). It has been theorized that atrial ischemia during the period of cardioplegic arrest may be a significant cause of AF, although atrial chemical imbalance, fibrosis or stretch of the atrial tissue, sinoatrial nodal artery disease, or a defective gene may be implicated (Cox, 1999; Al-Shanafey and others, 2001).

The treatment for postoperative AF continues to evolve. Beta blocker drugs have been used prophylactically in some patients at risk for AF; when AF develops, atrial pacing and cardioversion in combination with antidysrhythmic medications may be employed (Kern, 1998; Borzak and Silverman, 1999). The postoperative withdrawal of beta blocker drugs should be avoided in patients who received this medication preoperatively (Hogue and Hyder, 2000).

Neurologic outcomes

Neurologic problems after CPB can be divided into two types. Type I are those that result in various forms of clinical stroke. More common are the type II injuries that affect memory and cognition (Murkin, 2001). Long-term (5-year) follow-up has shown that 42% of patients who have undergone CABG continue to have cognitive decline. Patients with cardiac dysfunction may be at increased risk for cognitive difficulties after surgery (Newman and others, 2001). The genesis of central nervous system injury after cardiac surgery is not clear, but it is considered to be an interplay among cerebral embolization, hypoperfusion, and both local and systemic inflammatory processes (Salazar and others, 2001). Women have more neurologic events (and a higher mortality rate) after cardiac surgery compared

with men (3.8% versus 2.4%, respectively) (Hogue and others, 2001). Women are more likely to have diabetes and hypertension, but these factors (along with smaller coronary arteries) do not explain the overall increased susceptibility to new stroke during the perioperative period. Interest in the role of estrogen as a neural protector has stimulated research (Hogue and others, 2001).

Atheroemboli account for the majority of type I outcomes. Advanced age, diabetes, and vascular disease, which are predictors of advanced systemic arteriosclerosis, are important risk factors for stroke. Aortic manipulation, cannulation, and clamp application and removal can dislodge arteriosclerotic and atherosclerotic material, which can subsequently embolize to the brain.

Significant contributors to type II neurologic injury are microemboli (air and particulate matter) associated with CPB. Arterial line filters, CPB equipment modifications, and avoidance of reinfusion of blood collected in the cardiotomy suction can reduce the amount of microemboli. Another contributing factor is the systemic inflammatory response that occurs when platelets and leukocytes are activated during CPB. Administration of aprotinin (a nonspecific serine protease enzyme inhibitor with broad-spectrum anti-inflammatory properties) has been shown to decrease white blood cell activation and systemic dissemination (Murkin, 2001).

To lower the risk of stroke, different approaches during cardiac surgery employing CPB have been recommended (Engelman, 2001): less hemodilution (to enhance the oxygen-carrying capacity of the blood), higher pump flow and pressure (to increase cerebral perfusion), shorter CPB pump times (to reduce the period of lower blood flow), use of epiaortic imaging (to identify a calcified aorta and plan alternative aortic cannulation and proximal bypass graft sites), fewer aortic clamp applications and removals, and possibly the use of off-pump CABG (to avoid manipulation and incision of a calcified or sclerotic aorta) (Engelman, 2001; Salazar and others, 2001).

Perioperative nurses play a role in reducing the risk for perioperative neurologic injury by avoiding unnecessary surgical delays, monitoring blood pressure and cardiac rhythm, keeping instruments free of blood and particulate debris, using the cardiotomy suction judiciously, avoiding aspiration of blood containing visible fat particles or other debris, and monitoring inflow CPB/cardioplegia lines for air (and alerting the surgeon before infusion begins). RN first assistants should be especially cautious when touching, retracting, or manipulating the aorta.

Knowledge

Outcomes related to knowledge may be evaluated preoperatively, especially when they pertain to learning needs that lessen the patient's fear and anxiety and enhance intraoperative care. In the postoperative period patient teaching activities are directed toward maximizing recovery and rehabilitation. Confirmation that outcomes have been achieved can be made by patient observation, chart review, consultation with colleagues, demonstration of activities that have been taught (such as deep breathing and coughing, use of incentive spirometry, leg exercises), and verbalization of what has been learned by the patient (AORN, 2001). Discharge concerns requiring immediate attention are listed in Box 7-2.

Patients with coronary artery disease (CAD), valvular heart disease, and other cardiovascular disorders have specific learning needs that should be addressed. Teaching can be performed by the cardiac perioperative nurse, but often critical care nurses, unit nurses, and others participate in the educational process. Teaching protocols vary among institutions, but the perioperative nurse can provide valuable information directly to the patient or indirectly by providing inservices to patient educators about the short-term and long-term implications of surgery.

In patients with CAD, the nurse needs to confirm that the patient is aware of the progressive nature of the atherosclerotic process, the purpose of surgery, and possible lifestyle modifications that can have both a physical and a psychologic impact on the patient. In patients with valve disease, implantation of a mechanical prosthesis that requires chronic anticoagulation may have a substantially different impact on the patient's lifestyle as compared with reparative procedures that do not subject the patient to the risks of bleeding complications associated with warfarin therapy.

The nurse can assess patient outcomes by using the criteria established (or other measurable indicators) to determine the degree of goal attainment. The nurse

can appraise the level of patient satisfaction, identify occurrences that posed risk management concerns, and determine whether there were areas that could have been strengthened or improved. Monitoring these areas and making necessary adjustments based on the findings contribute to quality improvement efforts.

Differences between women and men during recovery also may be a factor in evaluating outcomes. Women have a higher mortality after CABG than men and are more likely to experience perioperative myocardial infarction (MI) and hemorrhage. Women also have less likelihood of freedom from angina and return to work. Rates of long-term survival, infarction, and reoperation are similar between men and women (Douglas, 2001).

Women and young men also tend to exhibit more anxiety and depression than older men before and after surgery. Women have longer lengths of stay in the intensive care unit and report poorer cardiac functional status. Because psychologically distressed patients have higher rates of rehospitalization for cardiovascular disorders and a higher risk of MI, cardiac arrest, and death, they should be identified and given psychologic support (McCrone and others, 2001).

Infection

Surgical site infections make up a significant portion of nosocomial infections. In the cardiac surgery patient infections can be lethal, especially if mediastinitis develops. Aseptic technique and infection control practices are critical interventions, but they are only as effective as the level of compliance demonstrated by team members. Controlling the movement of personnel and supplies in and out of the OR can reduce infection. Complete hair covering is recommended because bacteria harbored in the hair can be a source of contamination (CDC, 1999).

Other factors can contribute to a successful outcome. Classen and associates (1992) found that prophylactic antibiotics given up to 2 hours before the surgical incision, compared with infusion more than 2 hours before or after skin incision was made, led to a decrease in the incidence of postoperative wound infections. The perioperative nurse can help to ensure that the antibiotic has been given by reviewing the patient's record to verify infusion of the medication. If it has not been given, the anesthesiologist and surgeon should be notified and the antibiotics ordered and infused before the start of the operation.

Rehabilitation

The goal of cardiac rehabilitation is to assist the patient to take responsibility for maximizing his or her own physical and emotional wellness. The phases of cardiac rehabilitation begin in the hospital setting and extend into the outpatient setting. *Phase I* begins early after surgery (myocardial infarction or other cardiac event)

BOX **7-2**
Discharge Concerns Requiring Immediate Attention

Chest pain (angina-like) similar to preoperative pain
Heart rate faster than 150 beats per minute with shortness of breath or new irregular heart rate
Shortness of breath not relieved by rest
Chills or fever
Coughing up bright red blood
Sudden numbness or weakness in arms or legs
Sudden, severe headache
Fainting spells
Severe abdominal pain
New episodes of nausea, vomiting, or diarrhea
Bright red stool

Modified from the Society of Thoracic Surgeons: patient information [On-line], 1999. Available:http://www.sts.org/doc/3563 (accessed November 2, 1999).

and includes light supervised exercise and education about cardiovascular disease, risk factors, diet, sexual activity, exercise, and other activities. *Phase II* occurs early after discharge (2 to 6 weeks) from the hospital and builds on phase I activities; phase II also focuses on exercising (with telemetry monitoring) to improve functional capacity and endurance, reducing fear and anxiety about increased activity or exercise, and providing education about lifestyle changes. *Phase III* provides an ongoing exercise program, offers support for making lifestyle changes, and assists in retarding progression of heart disease. *Phase IV* is a wellness program for individuals who have completed any of the other rehabilitation phases. Exercise is performed 3 or 4 times per week with minimal staff supervision (STS, 1999). Although the emphasis of rehabilitation has been largely on physical health, the promotion of mental and psychologic well-being has gained more attention with evidence linking coronary artery disease with personality factors (anger, hostility), depression, chronic stress, anxiety, and lack of a social support network (AACPR, 1999).

Human Resource Management

The process of evaluation also can be used to assess how effectively human resources have been used and how well individual team members have performed.

EVALUATION OF NURSING CARE

Performance reviews identify the current level of practice and particular areas of strength and weakness. The level of intellectual and technical skill is appraised in light of the complexity and demands of the patient population and the surgical procedures. As a result of the appraisal process, teaching and learning opportunities can be provided to strengthen deficient areas.

The evaluation of a nurse's performance includes the supervisor's review, peer review, preceptor appraisal, and self-assessment; patients and medical colleagues also may contribute to the assessment process. Methods of evaluation include verbal reports, needs assessments, and written appraisals.

Evaluation commonly is accomplished through direct observation of the nurse's clinical performance based on competency-based skills (see Chapter 2) and standards of practice. However, limited staffing or time may necessitate supplemental or alternative options such as written examinations. The staff should participate in deciding how evaluations are to be performed. If the decision is to use a written examination, it should be comprehensive and include material from the unit competency skills list, as well as from articles, lectures, standards and recommended practices, and audiovisual materials. A passing grade should be established. Basic competencies may require a 100% passing grade because the stated skills are essential for safe patient care. Tests used to evaluate nurses being considered for promotion would measure advanced nursing practice and would not necessarily require a 100% passing grade. Based on the test results, additional learning needs may become apparent.

Peer review evaluations are performed by perioperative colleagues with the same role expectations and job descriptions as the nurse being evaluated. One way to implement the process is for the supervisor to select two or three colleagues who demonstrated knowledge, skill, and objectivity and then allow the nurse being evaluated to select his or her evaluator from this group. Self-assessments are also useful because they can provide an opportunity for the nurse to identify personal strengths and weaknesses, specify learning needs, set goals, and confirm (or deny) that expectations of performance are congruent with those of the supervisor.

INTERPERSONAL RELATIONSHIPS

Labor-management relations and the stress of the cardiac surgical environment can affect staff performance and subsequently patient outcomes. Excessive staff turnover and increased use of sick time may be an indication of low morale affecting the cohesiveness of the team. Dissatisfaction among team members impedes communication and productive working relationships. Staff nurses may need to ventilate frustrations or discuss concerns that affect the group in an open and honest manner. Nurse managers who listen to employees ventilate frustrations and offer advice are more likely to be perceived by the staff nurses as supportive (Farrell, 2001).

Aiken and her colleagues (2001), addressing nursing care in five countries (including the United States), have shown that problems in work design and workforce management threaten the provision of care. Not surprisingly, their study demonstrates a link between the shortage of nurses and high dissatisfaction among nurses in the workplace. The potential impact of large numbers of dissatisfied and emotionally exhausted nurses on the quality of patient care and patient outcomes (and the increased likelihood of clinical error) is notable, according to the researchers.

Although more than half the nurses studied reported that hospital management was not responsive to their concerns, the vast majority of those surveyed believed that both their physician and nurses colleagues were clinically competent and provided high-quality care. The authors recommended management interventions that can reduce job dissatisfaction, burnout, and intent to leave. Specific interventions include responding to nursing staff concerns, providing opportunities for participation in decision making, and acknowledging nurses' contributions to patient care (Aiken and others, 2001). Additional strategies include self-scheduling, creating opportunities for advancement, and retaining front-line nursing management positions so that responsibilities for managing operational, fiscal, and staffing issues (which take time away from direct patient care) are not added to the staff nurse's workload.

If team members become physically and emotionally drained, particularly after prolonged periods of long workdays or multiple emergencies, they may require additional support and consideration in the form of time off or formal recognition of their efforts. Visiting recuperating patients can be an especially gratifying experience for the perioperative nurse because, in addition to providing an opportunity for patient evaluation, the patient's comments often reaffirm the important contribution that the nurse has made to the patient's well-being.

Interpersonal relationships between nurses, physicians, technologists, and others can be evaluated. If the interactions are constructive and reflective of respect for one another and if there is cooperation among the team members, team function is more likely to be efficient and mutually rewarding. Collaboration enhances job satisfaction, which in turn promotes retention and reduces turnover costs (Seifert, 1999). Cooperation among perioperative nurses and nurses in other specialty units is another factor that can impact communication and patient care.

Espin and Lingard (2001) studied communication patterns between nurses and surgeons and described patterns and sites of tension. Five categories were identified: time, resources, roles and relationships, safety and sterility, and situations (e.g., temperature regulation and recording activities). The issue of time, especially patient scheduling and room turnover, was the source of greatest controversy and tension. Among the recommendations listed by the authors are educational strategies for novice (and experienced) nurses to recognize and deal with communication tensions, instruction to enhance communication skills, and promotion of interchange among different disciplines so that alternative perspectives can be appreciated and better understood.

Evaluation of Fiscal and Material Resources

Patient outcomes are increasingly linked to the cost of achieving those outcomes. The most beneficial nursing interventions are those that provide quality care in the most cost-effective manner. Consideration of cost, especially in resource-intensive cardiac services, has become an integral component of care, and the nurse must be able to justify the expenses and the clinical benefits of care. Nurses can participate more fully in unit decision-making activities when they are familiar with the financial and operational components of the cardiac service. Service efficiency can be improved by standardizing processes and supplies (Kirshner, 2000). Costs can be analyzed in relation to revenue by tracking both patient-related costs (e.g., staffing, supplies) and overhead costs (e.g., administration, laundry) (Mishea and others, 2001). Working collaboratively with representatives of all personnel involved in cardiac care (including finance administrators) is another mechanism for problem identification and shared problem solving (Cohn, Rosborough, and Fernandez, 1997).

Chiang (2001) describes a system of activity-based benchmarking that calculates individual cardiac surgeon procedure times, the types of procedures (e.g., CABG, valve), and equipment/supply use. This system can enable physicians and staff members to have a clearer picture of how practices correlate to costs, how cost effectiveness can be improved, and which practices are most effective.

Supply costs in particular have come under intense scrutiny. Prosthetic grafts and valve supply levels should be determined according to projected caseloads and in consultation with the surgeon. When surgeons express a preference for a different or new item, the nurse responsible for purchasing and maintaining the inventory can discuss possible options for using existing models to reduce shelf stock; when an old item is used, it can be replaced with the new, preferred model. Rarely used sizes of valves and grafts should be kept to a minimum. Negotiating with manufacturers to exchange unneeded inventory or to place items such as valve prostheses on consignment can reduce capital expenditures for newer, preferred devices. In the event of emergencies, alternate sources for prostheses should be available (e.g., from colleagues in other institutions with whom an agreement to share has been established).

Customized supply packs consolidate numerous items and can produce cost savings from decreased time to collect supplies, reduced turnover, and faster set up in the operating room. To be cost effective, the selection and evaluation of bundled pack contents should consider preference, use, storage, and cost; packs are cost effective only if the contents serve a specific purpose (e.g., routinely used chest closure supplies) and are fully used. Pack contents should be reviewed periodically, and items rarely or no longer used should be deleted or replaced as necessary with appropriate new supplies (Raab, 2001).

Because nurses are most familiar with the material resources required, they are the best qualified to assume a proactive role in cost containment efforts. RNFAs also can contribute to cost savings because their familiarity with surgeons' preferences and rationales for the use of specific supplies and equipment can promote a more judicious use of material resources. If perioperative nurses themselves do not initiate and develop expense-reduction initiatives, it is likely that externally imposed restraints will be established for them by those without an understanding of the clinical aspects of care.

Minimal amounts of suture should be opened, and other cost-containment measures should be taken. Because nurses are most familiar with the material resources required, they are the best qualified to assume a proactive role in cost-containment efforts. RNFAs also can contribute to cost-savings because their familiarity with surgeons' preferences and rationales for the use of specific supplies and equipment can enhance more judicious use of material resources. If perioperative nurses themselves do not initiate and develop expense-reduction measures, it is likely that externally imposed restraints will be established for them by those without an understanding of the clinical aspects of care.

Additional Methods of Evaluation

Patient satisfaction questionnaires and the interaction with colleagues, administrators, and professional and community organizations provide additional opportunities to evaluate patient care and human and material resources. Members of the health care team, such as surgeons, perfusionists, anesthesiologists, nurses in other specialty areas, and cardiologists, are important sources of information and opinion concerning the patient's response to surgery. Whether formally (as in grand rounds) or informally (as in private discussion), members of the health care team can provide valuable insights into patient needs and offer additional or alternative interventions. National organizations such as the American Heart Association* and The Mended Hearts† and their local affiliations can be important allies in helping patients to achieve desired outcomes.

Conclusion

Meeting the needs of patients undergoing cardiac surgery is as challenging and demanding today as it was when Powers and Storlie (1969) wrote about the care of these patients. As technology has become more complex, a greater variety of methods have become available to evaluate patient care; these can enhance a deeper understanding of the impact that cardiac surgery has on patients and identify opportunities to continually improve care. Evaluation of past performance is the initial step in future planning.

---

*7272 Greenville Ave., Dallas, TX 75231.
†7320 Greenville Ave., Dallas, TX 75231.

References

Aiken LH and others: Nurses' reports on hospital care in five countries, *Health Aff* 20(3):43, 2001.

Al-Shanafey S and others: Nodal vessels disease as a risk factor for atrial fibrillation after coronary artery bypass graft surgery, *Eur J Cardiothorac Surg* 19(6):821, 2001.

American Association of Cardiovascular and Pulmonary Rehabilitation (AACPR): *Guidelines for cardiac rehabilitation and secondary prevention programs*, ed 3, Champaign, Ill, 1999, Human Kinetics.

Archie JP: Influence of the first assistant on abdominal aortic aneurysm surgery, *Tex Heart Inst J* 19(1):4, 1992.

Arom KV and others: Establishing and using a local/regional cardiac surgery database, *Ann Thorac Surg* 64(5):1245, 1997.

Association of periOperative Registered Nurses (AORN): *Standards, recommended practices & guidelines*, Denver, 2001, AORN.

Becher EC, Chassin MR: Improving quality, minimizing error: making it happen, *Health Aff* 20(3):68, 2001.

Bergmann P and others: The influence of medical information on the perioperative course of stress in cardiac surgery patients, *Anesth Analg* 93(5)1093, 2001.

Beyea SC, Nicoll LH: Evaluating patient care programs, *AORN J* 71(1):228, 2000.

Bezanson JL and others: Predictors and outcomes associated with early extubation in older adults undergoing coronary artery bypass surgery, *Am J Crit Care* 10(6):383, 2001.

Borzak S, Silverman NA: Treatment of postoperative atrial fibrillation, *Semin Thorac Cardiovasc Surg* 11(4):314, 1999.

Centers for Disease Control and Prevention (CDC): Guideline for the prevention of surgical site infection, 1999, *Am J Infec Cont* 27:97, 1999.

Chiang B: Activity-based benchmarking in cardiac surgery, *Surg Serv Manag* 7(1):30, 2001.

Classen DC and others: The timing of prophylactic administration of antibiotics and the risk of surgical-wound infection, *N Engl J Med* 326(5):281, 1992.

Cohen AJ and others: Effect of internal mammary harvest on postoperative pain and pulmonary function, *Ann Thorac Surg* 56(5):1107, 1993.

Cohn LH, Rosborough D, Fernandez J: Reducing costs and length of stay and improving efficiency and quality of care in cardiac surgery, *Ann Thorac Surg* 64(6 suppl):S58, 1997.

Cox JL: A perspective on postoperative atrial fibrillation, *Semin Thorac Cardiovasc Surg* 11(4):299, 1999.

Creswell LL: Postoperative atrial arrhythmias: risk factors and associated adverse outcomes, *Semin Thorac Cardiovasc Surg* 11(4):303, 1999.

De Jong MJ, Morton PG: Predictors of atrial dysrhythmias for patients undergoing coronary artery bypass grafting, *Am J Crit Care* 9(6):388, 2000.

Douglas PA: Coronary artery disease in women. In Braunwald E, Zipes DP, Libby P, editors: *Heart disease: a textbook of cardiovascular medicine* ed 6, vol 2, Philadelphia, 2001, WB Saunders.

Edwards FH, Grover FL: Surgical risk assessment, *Adv Card Surg* 12:77, 2000.

Engelman R: Review of Hogue and others, 2001, Sex differences in neurological outcomes and mortality after cardiac surgery: a Society of Thoracic Surgery National Database report [On-line], 2001. Available: http://ctdigest.com/Jun01/rev3/rev3.asp (accessed June 20, 2001).

Espin SL, Lingard LA: Time as a catalyst for tension in nurse-surgeon communication, *AORN J* 74(5):672, 2001.

Farrell V: Employees make a difference, *Surg Serv Manag* 7(3):30, 2001.

Ferguson TB Jr and others: The STS National Database: current changes and challenges for the new millennium, *Ann Thorac Surg* 69(3):680, 2000.

Goss JR and others: Washington state's model of physician leadership in cardiac outcomes reporting, *Ann Thorac Surg* 70(3):695, 2000.

Harlan BJ: Statewide reporting of coronary artery surgery results: a view from California, *J Thorac Cardiovasc Surg* 121(3):409, 2001.

Hogue CW Jr, Hyder ML: Atrial fibrillation after cardiac operation: risks, mechanisms, and treatment, *Ann Thorac Surg* 69(1):300, 2000.

Hogue CW Jr and others: Sex differences in neurological outcomes and mortality after cardiac surgery: a Society of Thoracic Surgery National Database report, *Circulation* 103(17):2133, 2001.

Holman WL and others: Alabama coronary artery bypass grafting project: results of a statewide quality improvement initiative, *JAMA* 285(23):3003, 2001.

Institute of Medicine (IOM): *The national round-table on health care quality: measuring the quality of care,* Washington, DC, 1999, IOM.

Kern LS: Management of postoperative atrial fibrillation, *J Cardiovasc Nurs* 12(3):57, 1998.

Kirshner R: Standardization is the key to streamlining cardiac surgery, *Surg Serv Manag* 6(9):18, 2000.

Koivula M and others: Fear and anxiety in patients awaiting coronary artery bypass grafting, *Heart Lung* 30(4):302, 2001.

Ledoux D, Luikart H: Cardiac surgery. In Woods SL, Froelicher ES, Motzer SA: *Cardiac nursing,* ed 4, Philadelphia, 2000, JB Lippincott.

Lenz ER, Perkins S: Coronary artery bypass graft surgery patients and their family member caregivers: outcomes of a family-focused staged psychoeducational intervention, *Appl Nurs Res* 13(3):142, 2000.

Leske JS: Needs of relatives of critically ill patients: a follow-up, *Heart Lung* 15(2):189, 1986.

Lichtenberg A and others: Effects of minimal invasive coronary artery bypass on pulmonary function and postoperative pain, *Ann Thorac Surg* 70(2):461, 2000.

McCrone S and others: Anxiety and depression: incidence and patterns in patients after coronary artery bypass graft surgery, *Appl Nurs Res* 14(3):155, 2001.

Mishea V and others: Cost analysis of cardiothoracic procedures, *Surg Serv Manag* 7(3):44, 2001.

Murkin JM: Attenuation of neurologic injury during cardiac surgery, *Ann Thorac Surg* 72(5):S1838, 2001.

Newman MF and others: Longitudinal assessment of neurocognitive function after coronary-artery bypass surgery, *N Engl J Med* 344(6):395, 2001.

Nugent WC: Innovative uses of a cardiothoracic database, *Ann Thorac Surg* 68(2):359, 1999.

O'Connor GT and others: A regional intervention to improve the hospital mortality associated with coronary artery bypass graft surgery, *JAMA* 275(11):841, 1996.

O'Connor GT and others: Results of a regional study of modes of death associated with coronary artery bypass grafting, *Ann Thorac Surg* 66(4):1323, 1998.

Orringer MB: STS database activities and you: "What's in it for me?" *Ann Thorac Surg* 72(1):1, 2001.

Powers M, Storlie F: *The cardiac surgical patient; pathophysiologic considerations and nursing care,* New York, 1969, Macmillan.

Raab J: Creating custom packs, *Surg Serv Manag* 7(1):53, 2001.

Reeder JM: Family perception: a key to interpretation. In Leske JS, editor: Family interventions, *AACN Clin Issues Crit Care Nurs* 2(2):188, 1991.

Rothrock JC: The relationship of outcomes management and performance assessment to improvement. In *Perioperative nursing care planning,* ed 2, St Louis, 1996, Mosby.

Royse CF, Royse AG, Soeding PF: Routine immediate extubation after cardiac operation: a review of our first 100 patients, *Ann Thorac Surg* 68(4):1326, 1999.

Sackett DL, Rosenberg WM: The need for evidence-based medicine, *J R Soc Med* 88(11):620, 1995.

Salazar JD and others: Stroke after cardiac surgery: short- and long-term outcomes, *Ann Thorac Surg* 72(4):1195, 2001.

Schrecengost A: Do humorous preoperative teaching strategies work? *AORN J* 74(5):683, 2001.

Seifert PC: The RN first assistant and collaborative practice. In Rothrock JC, editor: *The RN first assistant: an expanded perioperative nursing role,* ed 3, Philadelphia, 1999, JB Lippincott.

Shapiro BA, Lichtenthal PR: Postoperative respiratory management. In Kaplan JA, editor: *Cardiac anesthesia,* ed 4, Philadelphia, 1999, WB Saunders.

Society of Thoracic Surgeons (STS): Patient information: what to expect after your heart surgery [On-line], 1999. Available: http://www.sts.org/doc/3563 (accessed November 2, 1999).

Van Kooten ME. Non-pharmacologic pain management for postoperative coronary artery bypass graft surgery patients, *Image: J Nurs Scholarship* 31(2):157, 1999.

Walshe K, Rundall TG: Evidence-based management: from theory to practice in health care, *Milbank Q* 79(3):429, 2001.

Watt-Watson J, Stevens B: Managing pain after coronary artery bypass surgery, *J Cardiovasc Nurs* 12(3):39, 1998.

8

Anatomy and Physiology

The motion of the heart is as follows: first of all, the auricle contracts, and . . . throws the blood . . . into the ventricle, which, being filled, the heart raises itself straightway, makes all its fibres tense, contracts the ventricles, and performs a beat, by which beat it immediately sends the blood supplied to it by the auricles into the arteries.

William Harvey, 1628 (Cited in Clendening, 1942, p. 161)

The concept that the heart can function as a neuroendocrine organ must be considered seriously.

Eugene Braunwald, 1964 (p. 1)

It is only a matter of time before the results of gene identification studies for complex [cardiovascular] disease lead to improvement in the diagnosis and treatment for individuals with these diseases.

Elizabeth Hauser and Margaret Pericak-Vance, 2000 (p. S42)

The radical notion of the heart as an endocrine organ, proposed by Braunwald in 1964, has become a reality. No longer viewed as merely a pump, the heart now is known to be capable not only of sensing its pressure and volume but also of regulating these parameters through the production and release of hormones (norepinephrine and natriuretic peptides) affecting the kidneys, the vascular and endocrine systems, and the heart itself (Chen and Burnett, 1999).

Similarly striking advances have been made in the discovery of the sequencing of the human genome and its relationship to acquired and congenital heart diseases and to peripheral vascular disorders (Meyerson and Schwartz, 1999; Winkelmann and others, 2000). Although it is not within the scope of this chapter to discuss these advances in detail, it is important to be aware that gene-related and other discoveries will expand the study of cardiovascular anatomy and physiology by placing greater emphasis on the underlying basis of disease at the cellular level.

Location of the Heart

The heart and the origins of the great vessels are commonly approached through a median sternotomy incision (Fig. 8-1). The sternum consists of three parts: the bony *manubrium* and *sternal body,* attaching at the second costal cartilage (angle of Louis), and the cartilaginous *xiphoid process* (Fig. 8-2). The superior edge of the sternum is known as the *suprasternal notch.* Coursing behind and parallel to the lateral border of the sternum are the right and left *internal mammary* (thoracic) *arteries,* which can be used as conduits during coronary revascularization procedures.

PERICARDIUM

When the sternum is divided, it exposes the *pericardial sac,* which is situated within the middle portion of the mediastinal compartment of the thorax. The pericardium is fused inferiorly to the central tendon of the diaphragm, partially overlapped laterally by the lungs in their pleural sacs, and protected anteriorly by the sternum and the costal cartilages of the third, fourth, and fifth ribs. Behind the pericardium are the esophagus, posterior mediastinum, descending aorta, and vertebral column.

The pericardium consists of serous and fibrous layers (Fig. 8-3). The *visceral pericardium* is a serous layer that is closely adherent to the outer surface of the heart. It extends superiorly onto the great vessels, where it is reflected forward to form the *parietal pericardium,* which fuses to the fibrous pericardial wall. The area between the visceral and parietal serous layers, the pericardial cavity, contains about 50 ml of clear, thin, lubricating fluid that enables the heart to move freely within the space. Adhesions from prior surgery or inflammatory processes can produce thickening of the

187

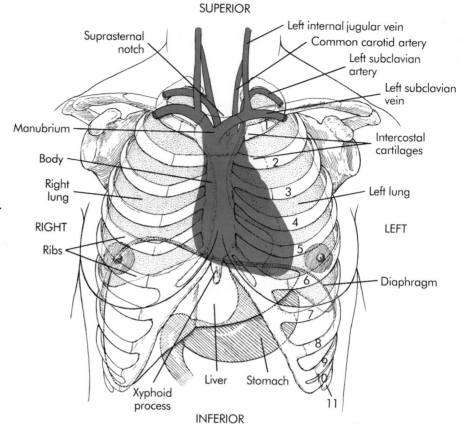

FIGURE 8-1 Location of the heart. (Drawing by Peter Stone.)

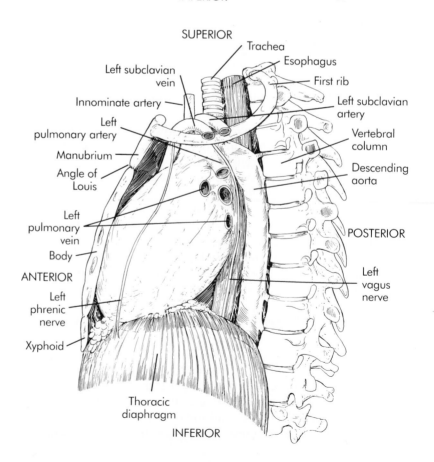

FIGURE 8-2 Lateral view of the pericardium within the mediastinum. (Drawing by Peter Stone.)

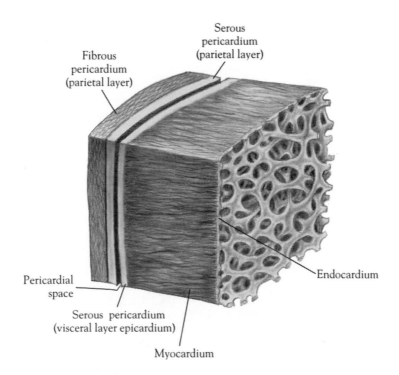

Serous
pericardium
(parietal layer)

Fibrous
pericardium
(parietal layer)

Endocardium

Pericardial
space

Serous pericardium
(visceral layer epicardium)

Myocardium

FIGURE 8-3 Cross section of the layers of the pericardium and the heart (epicardium, myocardium, and endocardium). (From Thompson JM and others: *Mosby's clinical nursing,* ed 4, St Louis, 1998, Mosby.)

pericardium or obliteration of the cavity, which, in extreme cases, may constrict the ventricles and impair diastolic filling. When the pericardium is incised during surgery, care is taken to avoid the underlying structures, which include the innominate vein, ascending aorta, proximal pulmonary artery, and right ventricle.

Running vertically along the lateral pericardium are the right and left *phrenic nerves,* which innervate the diaphragm. Identifying these nerves is important for protecting the diaphragm during procedures in which the lateral pericardium is incised or excised.

Size and Position of the Heart

The heart itself is about the size of a person's fist. Depending on the age, sex, height, nutritional status, and amount of epicardial fat, the weight of the heart is variable, but in the average man it is about 325 g, and in the average woman, it is about 275 g (Schlant, Sonnenblick, and Katz, 1998).

The cardiac wall is composed of three layers (see Fig. 8-3). The outermost layer is the *epicardium* (visceral pericardium); the *myocardium* is the functional muscular layer; and the innermost layer, the *endocardium,* covers the inside of the cardiac chambers and is continuous with the lining of the blood vessels.

Approximately two thirds of the heart is to the left of the midline. It is tilted forward and to the left, with the *apex,* the lower tip of the left ventricle, anterior to the rest of the heart (Fig. 8-4). The apex is located in the fifth intercostal interspace, about 3½ inches from the left sternal border. From the front, one sees the right ventricle in the center with the aorta and the pulmonary artery above it; the superior vena cava, right atrium, and atrial appendage on the right; and a sliver of the left ventricle on the left with the tip of the left atrial appendage high on the left border of the heart. Thus the right ventricle lies anteriorly, and the greater portion of the left ventricle is situated posteriorly. When the cardiac silhouette is viewed on a chest x-ray film, the right cardiac border is formed by the right atrium, the inferior border is formed by the right ventricle; and the left border is almost entirely formed by the apex of the left ventricle (Fig. 8-5).

The *base,* or upper portion, of the heart is fixed by attachment of the right and left atria to the superior and inferior venae cavae and the pulmonary veins, respectively (Fig. 8-6). The outflow portion of the right ventricle is attached superiorly to the pulmonary artery, and the outflow tract of the left ventricle is connected to the aorta. The apex is free, which enables the surgeon to elevate the heart for surgical exposure.

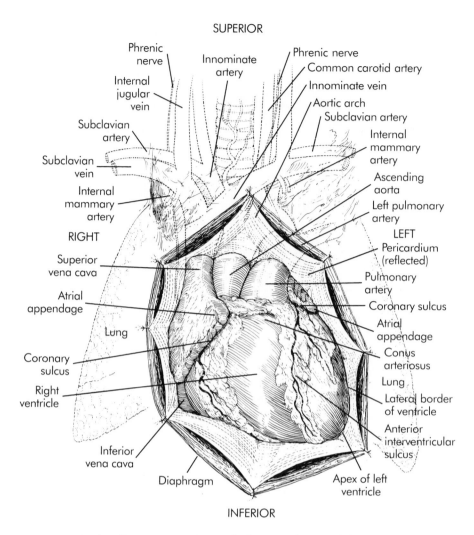

FIGURE 8-4 Pericardium open to expose the heart and roots of the great vessels. (Drawing by Peter Stone.)

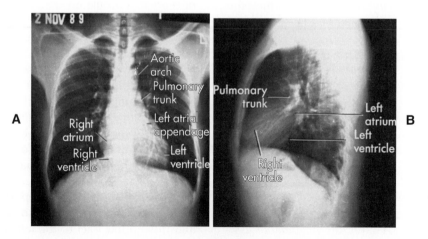

FIGURE 8-5 Normal chest x-ray films. **A,** Anteroposterior. **B,** Lateral. (From Canobbio MM: *Cardiovascular disorders,* St Louis, 1990, Mosby.)

SUPERIOR

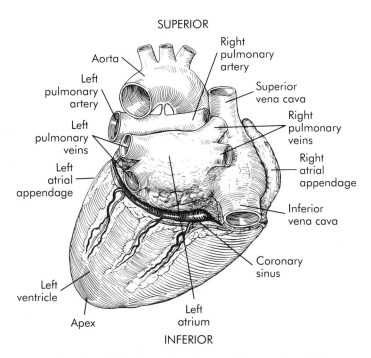

FIGURE 8-6   Posterior view of the heart showing attachment of cardiac structures. (Drawing by Peter Stone.)

External Features of the Heart

Externally the atria are separated from the ventricles by the *coronary sulcus,* also called the *atrioventricular groove.* The proximal portions of the right coronary artery and the left circumflex coronary artery can be found within this groove. The right and left ventricles are divided by the *interventricular sulcus,* which lies over the interventricular septum. It descends from the coronary sulcus toward the apex and often is obscured by epicardial fat in the adult.

Just to the left side of the anterior interventricular groove is the left anterior descending coronary artery, which courses down to the apex, where it curves around to the posterior interventricular groove on the diaphragmatic surface of the heart.

The posterior interventricular groove is the pathway for the posterior descending coronary artery, which is commonly the distal branch of the right coronary artery or, less commonly, the terminal portion of the left circumflex artery.

In the area where the posterior atrioventricular groove meets the posterior interventricular groove is the *crux.* It is at this point internally that the atrial septum meets the ventricular septum. It is an important landmark for the surgeon performing coronary bypass grafting because it is at this point that the posterior descending (interventricular) coronary artery turns to course downward toward the apex.

Cardiac Chambers

RIGHT ATRIUM

Internally the right atrium contains both a smooth surface and a rough area formed by the *pectinate muscles.* The two areas are separated by a muscular bundle called the *crista terminalis.* Externally this corresponds to the *sulcus terminalis,* which extends vertically from the superior vena cava to the inferior vena cava (Fig. 8-7).

The smoother posterior and medial (septal) walls contain the orifices of venous channels. The *superior vena cava (SVC)* enters the atrium superiorly, and the *inferior vena cava (IVC)* enters inferiorly. Both cavae receive systemic venous drainage. The IVC is guarded by the *eustachian valve;* occasionally this valve impedes cannulation of the IVC for cardiopulmonary bypass (Kirklin and Barratt-Boyes, 1993).

Medial to the IVC, coronary venous return drains through the coronary sinus, which is guarded by a flap of tissue called the *thebesian valve.* Cardioplegia solution for intraoperative myocardial protection (see Chapter 9) may be infused in a retrograde manner through a cannula inserted directly (or indirectly via the right atrium) into the sinus. The thebesian valve may partially obstruct the entrance to the coronary sinus, making retrograde cannula insertion difficult.

Also within the septal wall is the *atrioventricular (AV) node* of the conduction pathway. The node is located

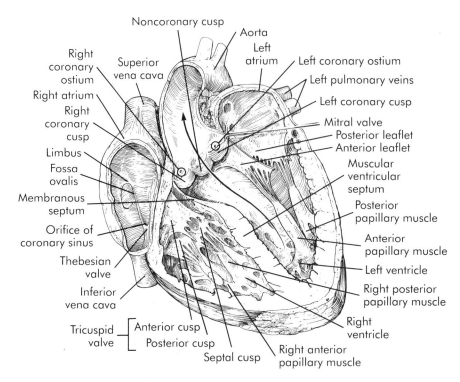

FIGURE 8-7   Interior of the heart (pulmonary artery removed). (Drawing by Peter Stone.)

anterior and medial to the coronary sinus and above the septal leaflet of the tricuspid valve. Because the AV node is not grossly visible, extreme caution is used to avoid injury to the node and other conduction tissue during surgical manipulation of the atrial septum. The atrial septum additionally contains what was the fetal *ostium secundum* and the *foramen ovale,* surrounded anteriorly by a thickened ridge called the *limbus.*

Protruding anteromedially and overlapping the aortic root is the triangular *right atrial appendage.* For the surgeon the appendage is a convenient entry point for venous cannulation and can be severed without functional impairment of the heart (Bharati, Lev, and Kirklin, 1983).

The lower portion of the right atrial wall is occupied by the tricuspid valve orifice. During ventricular systole the tricuspid valve is closed, and the right atrium functions as a holding chamber for blood. During ventricular diastole blood from the right atrium flows through the opened valve into the right ventricle.

RIGHT VENTRICLE

The right ventricle, normally the most anterior of the cardiac chambers, is located directly behind the sternum. It is a crescent-shaped chamber with a wall 4 to 5 mm thick. The inflow portion, originating at the tricuspid valve, contains numerous thick, muscular tissue

bands, called *trabeculae carneae.* From these arise two to four *papillary muscles* and multiple threadlike *chordae tendineae,* which attach to the tricuspid valve. The outflow portion of the right ventricle, called the *infundibulum,* or *conus arteriosus,* is relatively smooth walled and exits at the *pulmonary valve* (Fig. 8-8).

A number of prominent muscular bands form the demarcation between the inflow and outflow portions: the *crista supraventricularis,* the *parietal band,* the *septal band,* and the *moderator band.* The right bundle branch of the conduction system travels through the moderator band toward the right ventricular endocardium. The moderator band, crossing from the lower ventricular septum to the anterior wall, joins the anterior papillary muscle projecting from the inner ventricular wall. Attached to this muscle are the anterior chordae tendineae, which anchor the tricuspid valve leaflets and prevent them from everting into the right atrium during ventricular systole.

LEFT ATRIUM

Desaturated blood flows from the right ventricle through the pulmonary valve orifice to the right and left branches of the *pulmonary artery* and into the lungs (see Fig. 8-7). From the lungs, oxygenated blood drains into the left atrium by way of the *pulmonary veins,* usually two on either side of the left atrium. Like the right

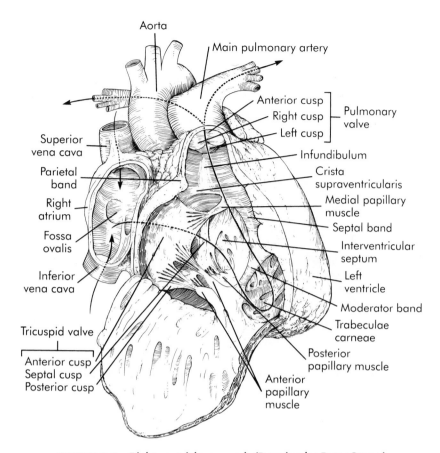

FIGURE 8-8 Right ventricle opened. (Drawing by Peter Stone.)

atrium, the left atrium serves as a collecting chamber for blood during ventricular systole and as a conduit during ventricular diastole.

The left atrium is superior and posterior to the other cardiac chambers and as a result is not normally seen in the frontal chest x-ray film. If, as a consequence of the increased pressure or volume associated with severe mitral stenosis or regurgitation, it becomes massively dilated, the enlarged lateral borders of the left atrium will be evident on the roentgenogram.

The endocardial surface is smooth, with the exception of the *left atrial appendage,* which is lined with pectinate muscles. This appendage, like the one on the right atrium, can be sacrificed with little consequence to myocardial function. In the left atrium the *fossa ovalis* (the remnant of the foramen ovale) is a central shallow area in the atrial septum.

LEFT VENTRICLE

The left ventricle receives blood from the left atrium via the orifice of the mitral valve, whose leaflets create a funnel-shaped inflow tract into the left ventricle (Fig. 8-9). The exit of the outflow tract, the aortic valve, is ad-

jacent to the mitral valve. The aortic and mitral valves are separated by a fibrous band from which originates most of the anterior leaflet of the mitral valve and portions of the left and posterior (noncoronary) cusps of the aortic valve. This intimate relationship is important during procedures on the mitral or aortic valve.

The left ventricular chamber is conical and is surrounded by thick muscular walls between 8 and 15 mm thick, approximately three times the thickness of the right ventricular wall. The tip of the apex may be thin, measuring 2 mm or less. The left ventricle is posterior to and to the left of the right ventricle and inferior to, anterior to, and to the left of the left atrium.

The ventricular *septum* forms the medial wall and normally bulges into the right ventricle. It is almost entirely muscular except for the superiorly located *membranous septum* just below the right and posterior (noncoronary) cusps of the aortic valve. On the left ventricular side the demarcation between the membranous septum and the *muscular septum* is called the *limbus marginalis.*

The membranous septum is both interventricular and atrioventricular. The former portion lies between the left ventricle and the right ventricle (behind the

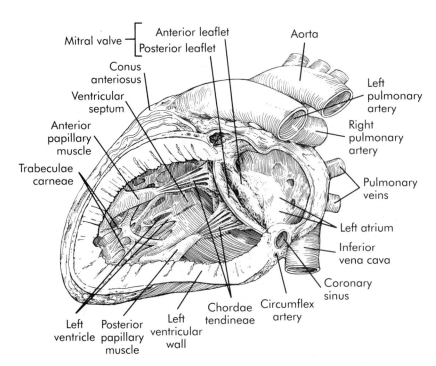

FIGURE 8-9 Left ventricle opened. (Drawing by Peter Stone.)

supraventricular crest). The latter, superior part of the membranous septum lies between the left ventricle and the right atrium.

Trabeculae carneae are found in the left ventricle, but they are finer and more numerous than those of the right ventricle. Arising from the trabeculae are two papillary muscles, which, with their attached chordae, anchor the mitral valve. These papillary muscles are stronger than those on the right and, with the chordae, help to maintain coaptation of the valve leaflets during ventricular systole. Because the papillary muscles receive their blood supply from the distal portion of the coronary arterial system, impaired blood flow as a result of coronary artery disease may produce ischemia with subsequent papillary muscle dysfunction.

Cardiac Valves

The four valves within the base of the heart are designed to maintain forward blood flow and prevent regurgitation into the originating chamber (Fig. 8-10). Essentially this is a passive process that depends on changing pressure gradients. As blood accumulates behind the valve, the pressure increases to a point where it becomes greater than the pressure in front of the valve. The valve then opens to allow transvalvular flow. Increasing pressure beyond the valve forces the leaflets to close.

The atrioventricular *mitral valve* and the *tricuspid valve* are structurally and functionally similar to each

other. The two semilunar valves, the *aortic valve* and the *pulmonary valve,* are also similar to each other and are located at the exits of their respective left and right ventricular outflow tracts.

A consistently uniform relationship exists between the four valves, with the aortic valve centrally wedged between the tricuspid and mitral valves (Fig. 8-11). The pulmonary valve is located anterior to, to the left of, and superior to the aortic valve. The merger of the valve annuli forms the *central fibrous skeleton* of the heart. This fibrous body, also known as the *right fibrous trigone,* is pierced by the conduction *bundle of His.* A *left fibrous trigone* is formed by connective tissue coursing from the central fibrous body to the left, posteroinferiorly and anteriorly.

MITRAL VALVE

Situated at the entrance to the left ventricle, the mitral valve allows blood from the right atrium to enter the lower chamber. The area of the mitral valve orifice in adults is 4 to 6 cm² and will permit insertion of the tips of two fingers. The valve consists of two fibroelastic leaflets that originate from the annulus fibrosus encircling the left atrioventricular orifice (see Fig. 8-9). The leaflets are pale yellow, thin, glistening membranes whose atrial surface is relatively smooth. The ventricular surface is very irregular because of the attachment of the chordae tendineae (Hurst, 1988).

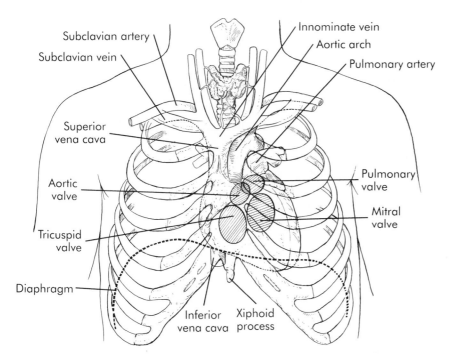

FIGURE 8-10 Position of the cardiac valves in the chest. (Drawing by Peter Stone.)

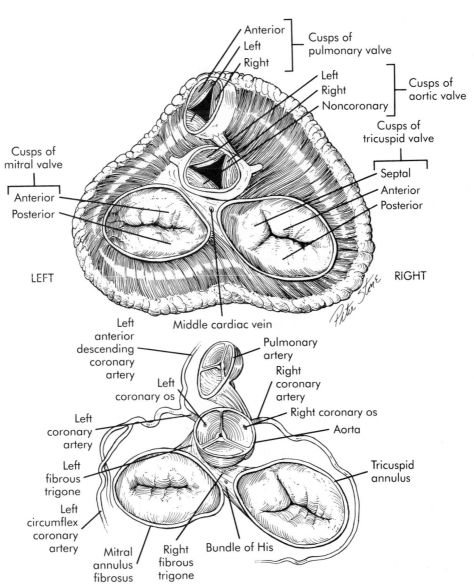

FIGURE 8-11 Superior view of the valves (atria, pulmonary trunk, and aorta removed). (Drawing by Peter Stone.)

The triangular *anterior leaflet*, also called the *anteromedial, septal,* or *aortic leaflet,* stretches across the ventricular cavity from the septum to the anterolateral wall of the left ventricle. The leaflet is continuous with the supporting tissues of the posterior aortic valve cusp lying above it and is visible during surgery on the aortic valve.

The quadrangular *posterior leaflet,* otherwise known as the *posterolateral* or *mural leaflet,* is longer and less mobile than the anterior leaflet. It encircles about two thirds of the valve circumference from the anterolateral to the posteromedial ventricular wall. Although differing in shape, both leaflets have similar surface areas, with the combined leaflet area being twice that of the mitral orifice. This provides a large area of approximation, or coaptation, during ventricular systole.

Mitral valve function during ventricular diastole and systole is regulated by the interaction of an intricate system consisting of not only the valve leaflets and their annular attachment but also the chordae tendineae, the papillary muscles, and the ventricular wall (see Fig. 8-9). These components form the *mitral apparatus,* or *mitral complex,* and contribute to maintaining the normal geometry and mechanical function of the left ventricle (Kirklin and Barratt-Boyes, 1993; Spotnitz, 2000).

At the end of ventricular systole, when the pressure of accumulated blood in the left atrium exceeds the pressure in the left ventricle, the mitral valve leaflets are forced open, allowing blood to enter the ventricular chamber. Near the end of ventricular filling, the atrium contracts, increasing ventricular volume by an additional 30%. Left ventricular systole then begins with the contraction of the papillary muscles. These muscles, as well as the chordae tendineae, which insert into the valve leaflets, prevent the leaflets from everting into the atrium. As intraventricular pressure rises, the free edges of the valve leaflets coapt along their atrial surfaces to form a tight closure. If chordae rupture as a result of infection or ischemia, severe valvular regurgitation with heart failure ensues. Dilation of either the valve annulus or the left ventricle also can impair valve closure.

TRICUSPID VALVE

The orifice of the right atrioventricular valve is larger than that of the mitral valve and will permit entry of three fingertips in the adult—approximately 10 cm^2 (see Fig. 8-8). The tricuspid valve has three leaflets, the *anterior, posterior,* and *medial (septal) leaflets,* which are unequal in size. The *anterior papillary muscle* and the *medial papillary muscle* are the two main attachments for the tricuspid valve; the medial (conal) papillary muscle also may be well developed. The proximity of the septal leaflet to the His bundle of the conduction system warrants special consideration to avoid heart block during surgery on the tricuspid valve or the septal walls.

Although similar in form and function to the mitral valve, the leaflets and chordae of the tricuspid valve complex (see Fig. 8-8) are thinner and more translucent. The anterior leaflet stretches downward from the infundibulum to the inferolateral wall of the right ventricle. The posterior leaflet is usually the smallest, with its chordae originating from the posterior and anterior papillary muscles. The septal (medial) leaflet attaches to the membranous septum and the muscular septum; it may obscure small ventricular septal defects.

AORTIC VALVE

Each of the semilunar valves is composed of three cusps, which open passively when the pressure behind them exceeds that in front of them. They are similar in form except that the aortic valve cusps are thicker than the pulmonary valve cusps. The normal adult aortic orifice area is 3 to 4 cm^2. The cusps are suspended from the annulus, a fibrous ring that encircles the proximal portion of the aorta, known as the *aortic root* (see Fig. 8-9). Within the root and behind each cusp the vessel wall forms pouchlike dilations called the *sinuses of Valsalva* (Fig. 8-12). Because the openings, or ostia, of the right and left coronary arteries originate in two of the sinuses, the cusps are designated the *right, left,* and *noncoronary (posterior) cusps.* During ventricular systole, when blood pushes the cusps upward into the aorta, obstruction of the coronary ostia is prevented by the sinus of Valsalva dilations. The right and noncoronary sinuses are proximal to the medial wall of the right atrium (see Fig. 8-7) (Waller and Schlant, 1998).

PULMONARY VALVE

The pulmonary valve cusps are called *anterior, right,* and *left cusps* (see Fig. 8-8). The valve orifice area is usually about 4 cm^2. During ventricular diastole, when pulmonary artery pressure exceeds right ventricular pressure, the valve cusps fall passively backward and coapt to support the column of blood above. This closing mechanism is similar to that of the aortic valve. A discrete annulus is absent in the pulmonary valve.

Coronary Arteries

Oxygen and nutrients are supplied to the myocardium by the *right* and *left coronary arteries* (Fig. 8-13; see Fig. 8-12), originating in the aortic root. The *left main coronary artery* (whose ostium is slightly higher than the right coronary ostium), passes between the main pulmonary artery and the left atrial appendage before di-

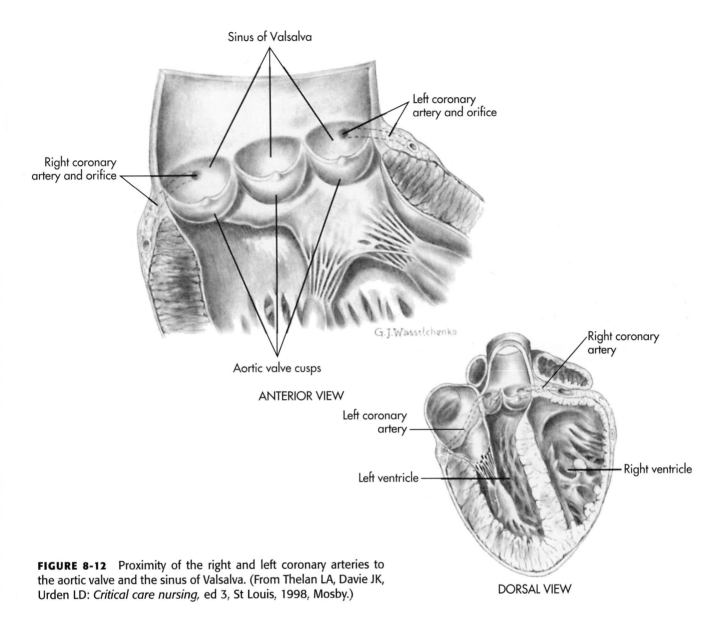

Sinus of Valsalva

Left coronary
artery and orifice

Right coronary
artery and orifice

G.J.Wasstlchenko

Aortic valve cusps

ANTERIOR VIEW

Right coronary
artery

Left coronary
artery

Left ventricle

Right ventricle

DORSAL VIEW

FIGURE 8-12 Proximity of the right and left coronary arteries to the aortic valve and the sinus of Valsalva. (From Thelan LA, Davie JK, Urden LD: *Critical care nursing,* ed 3, St Louis, 1998, Mosby.)

viding into the *left anterior descending (LAD) coronary artery* and the *circumflex coronary artery.* Obtuse marginal branches of the circumflex artery supply blood to the left lateral wall of the heart. LAD branches perforate the septum and the free walls of the left atrium and left ventricle, and they supply portions of the conduction system and the anterior papillary muscle of the mitral valve. Other branches between the left coronary artery and the right coronary artery provide anastomotic connections to supply parts of the anterior right ventricular wall; in the presence of coronary atherosclerosis, these anastomoses are a source of collateral circulation.

The right coronary artery travels within the right atrioventricular groove before branching into the sinus node and acute marginal arteries to perfuse the right side of the heart. The *posterior descending coronary artery,* which supplies the posterior interventricular septum, is commonly the terminal branch of the right coronary artery. When this is the case, patients are said to have a *right dominant* system. When the posterior descending branch is a continuation of the (left) circumflex coronary artery, the patient is said to be *left dominant;* when both arteries supply the posterior septum, coronary distribution is said to be *balanced.*

Dominance assumes significance in patients with ischemic heart disease affecting the dominant coronary distribution. Thus obstructive lesions of the left main coronary artery are especially critical in those patients with left dominant systems because so much of the myocardium (particularly the anterior and posterior portions of the "workhorse" left ventricle) is dependent on flow from branches of the left coronary artery.

The LAD, circumflex, and right coronary arteries represent the three main vessels of the coronary artery

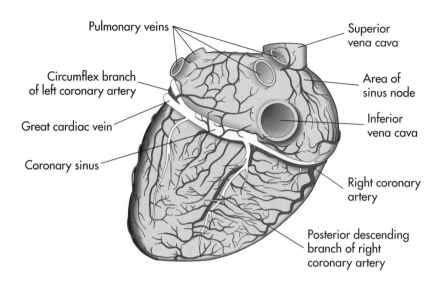

POSTERIOR VIEW

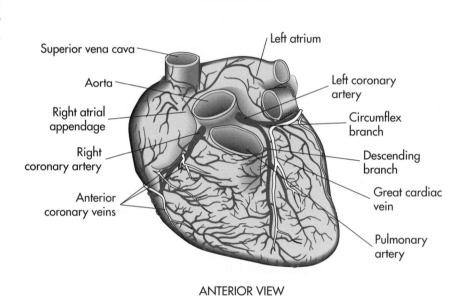

ANTERIOR VIEW

FIGURE 8-13 Anterior and posterior surfaces of the heart, illustrating the location and distribution of the principal coronary vessels. (From Berne RM, Levy MN: *Cardiovascular physiology*, ed 8, St Louis, 2001, Mosby.)

system. *Triple-vessel* coronary artery disease refers to the presence of obstructive lesions in all three of these arteries.

Variations in the branching pattern of the coronary arteries are common. Occasionally only one coronary artery originates from the aortic root, and anomalies of the coronary system are not uncommon in pediatric cardiac patients (O'Brien and Nathan, 1999).

CORONARY BLOOD FLOW

In contrast to the other vascular beds of the body, myocardial blood flow is greater during diastole than it is during systole. The epicardial segment of the coronary ar-

teries is perfused during systole, but the blood vessels within the myocardium are subject to compression by the left ventricular muscle during contraction (Fig. 8-14). This compression is especially evident in the subendocardium, where there is almost a total lack of flow during systole. When the heart relaxes in diastole, intramyocardial vessels fill with blood. In the presence of obstructive coronary artery disease, subendocardial perfusion suffers most. If there is concomitant heart failure and if rising left ventricular diastolic pressures further compress the inner ventricular wall, blood flow is further jeopardized and can result in cellular death (Guyton and Hall, 2000).

Another factor affecting myocardial blood flow is aortic pressure, which is generated by the heart itself. When

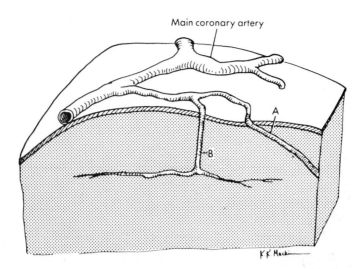

Main coronary artery

FIGURE 8-14 Myocardial distribution of the coronary arteries. *A,* Epicardial arteries arise at acute angles from the main coronary vessels to supply the surface of the heart. *B,* Smaller vessels branch from the main vessels and epicardial arteries to penetrate deeper into the myocardium and endocardium. (From Quaal SJ: *Comprehensive intra-aortic balloon pumping,* St Louis, 1984, Mosby.)

diastolic pressure is low, coronary perfusion suffers. This is evident in patients with an aortic valve that does not completely close; regurgitating blood causes the aortic pressure to drop and the intraventricular pressure to increase, creating a double threat to the myocardium.

Cardiac Veins

Blood enters the cardiac venous system after the exchange of oxygen and other substances in the dense capillary network of the heart. The principal cardiac veins, the *greater* and *middle cardiac veins* and the *posterior left ventricular vein,* enter the right atrium via the coronary sinus.

The veins of the anterior right ventricular wall enter the right atrium independently of the coronary sinus. This is an important consideration when cardioplegia solution is infused in a retrograde manner through the coronary sinus because theoretically the right side of the heart would not be adequately permeated by the solution and therefore would not be sufficiently protected. This hypothesis has been challenged, however, because there is an extensive network of venous collateral vessels that could allow a sufficient amount of cardioplegia to be delivered (Rankin and Sabiston, 1995).

Although the coronary sinus is the major venous drainage pathway, it is one of a number of drainage routes. Individual variability and a large network of venous interconnections provide routes. A number of

small venous channels (*thebesian veins*) within the atrial and ventricular septal walls open directly into the cardiac chambers, most often the right atrium.

Veins draining into the left side of the heart create a mixing of unoxygenated blood with freshly oxygenated blood from the lungs to produce a physiologic shunt. Deoxygenated bronchial blood also drains into the pulmonary veins. This is normal and explains why the expected oxygen saturation of blood leaving the left ventricle is slightly less than 100%. (Abnormal shunts occur when there is a defect producing communication between the right and left sides of the heart.)

Conduction System

Excitation, conduction, and contraction are characteristic of cardiac tissue (see Chapter 17). The ability to initiate a beat *(automaticity)* and to generate it on a regular basis *(rhythmicity)* are properties of the excitation mechanism that begins on about the twenty-second day of gestation (Keller and Markwald, 1998).

Once these electrical impulses are generated, they are conducted rapidly throughout the heart via specially differentiated muscle fibers. The initiation and propagation of electrical impulses precedes (and controls) the mechanical activity of contracting myocardial cells, enabling the heart to function as a pump.

The conduction system consists of the *sinoatrial (SA) node,* the *atrioventricular (AV) junction,* the *bundle of His,*

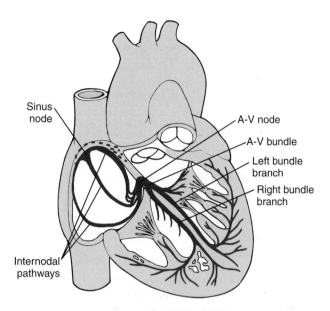

FIGURE 8-15 Sinus node and the Purkinje system of the heart, showing also the AV node, atrial internodal pathways, and ventricular bundle branches. (From Guyton AC, Hall JE: *Textbook of medical physiology,* ed 9, Philadelphia, 1996, WB Saunders.)

the right and left *bundle branches,* and the *Purkinje fibers* (Fig. 8-15).

The SA node, known as the natural pacemaker of the heart, demonstrates self-excitation to the greatest degree. Although all conduction tissue possesses the property of automaticity, the SA node initiates impulses at a faster rate and ordinarily controls the rate of the heartbeat. It lies within the sulcus terminalis of the right atrial wall at the junction of the superior vena cava. There is little risk to the node during venous cannulation unless a clamp is placed too low on the appendage (Bharati, Lev, and Kirklin, 1983).

It is theorized that internodal pathways spread the electrical impulses between the SA node and the AV junction. Branches of these pathways conduct impulses to the left atrium. As the impulse spreads, the atria depolarize and contract (seen as the P wave on an electrocardiogram [ECG]).

Conduction slows momentarily when the impulse reaches the *AV node* within the AV junction, which is situated between the upper part of the coronary sinus and the septal (medial) leaflet of the tricuspid valve. This brief pause, reflected on the ECG by the PR interval (Fig. 8-16), allows sufficient time for atrial contraction (atrial "kick") to contribute to ventricular filling. AV nodal delay also protects the ventricle by limiting the transfer of abnormally excessive impulses associated with atrial fibrillation or atrial flutter. If every atrial fibrillation or atrial flutter

impulse produced ventricular contraction, the increased workload and reduced cardiac output eventually would produce cardiac failure and cellular death.

On emerging from the AV node, the impulse is conducted rapidly through the bundle of His, penetrating the central fibrous body (right trigone). His bundle fibers travel down the right side of the intraventricular septum for approximately 1 cm and then divide into the right and left bundle branches. The right bundle branch extends almost to the apex of the right ventricle, where it becomes a profuse terminal network of Purkinje fibers to supply the right ventricular endocardium. The thicker left bundle branch arises almost perpendicularly from the bundle of His and crosses the septum to enter the left ventricle. It then subdivides into anterior and posterior branches, or *fascicles,* terminating in Purkinje fibers throughout the ventricular subendocardium (Berne and Levy, 2001).

The impulse spreads uniformly throughout the Purkinje fibers and at a high rate of velocity throughout the ventricular cells; the ventricles depolarize and contract, forming the electrocardiographic QRS complex. Ventricular relaxation (the T wave) occurs with repolarization and a return to the resting electrical state. When one of the fascicles of the left bundle branch does not conduct impulses properly, it is referred to as a hemiblock. Conduction defects affecting the bundle branches are termed bundle-branch blocks.

It should be emphasized that the ECG does not provide direct information about the mechanical activity of the heart; it simply reflects the course of the cardiac impulse by recording variations in electrical potential from various locations on the body (Berne and Levy, 1996). The ECG also provides an indication of the adequacy of coronary perfusion. For example, in the presence of ischemia, changes in the ECG tracing, such as ST segment elevation or depression, are often apparent.

Innervation of the Heart

Although a denervated heart will continue to beat (as evidenced by the success of cardiac transplantation), it cannot adjust its rate efficiently without the influence of the *autonomic nervous system (ANS).* The ANS plays an important role in regulating the rate and vigor of each contraction to meet the moment-to-moment metabolic demands of the body.

Sensory nerves are found in the pericardium, ventricular walls, coronary vessels, and major blood vessels. These transmit impulses to the *central nervous system*

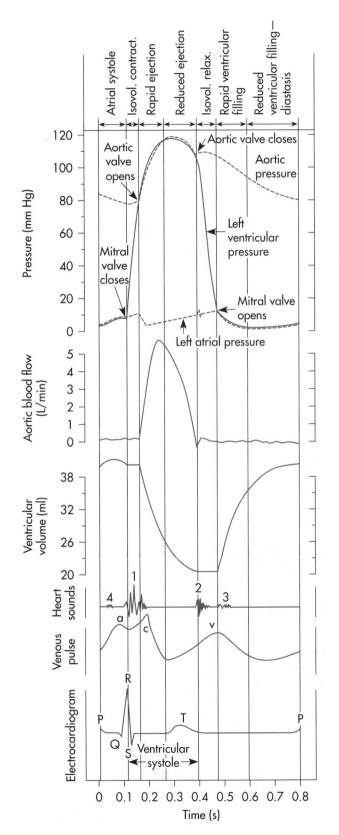

FIGURE 8-16 Left atrial, aortic, and left ventricular pressure pulses correlated in time with aortic flow, ventricular volume, heart sounds, venous pulse, and the electrocardiogram for a complete cardiac cycle in a dog. (From Berne RM, Levy MN: *Cardiovascular physiology*, ed 8, St Louis, 2001, Mosby.)

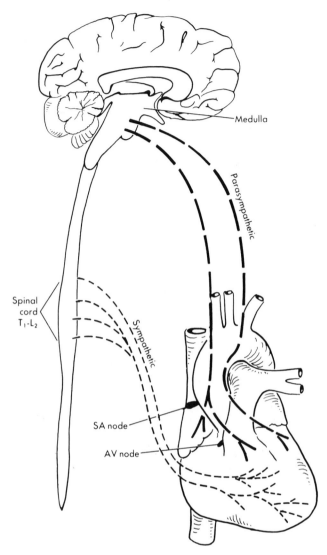

FIGURE 8-17 Autonomic nervous system innervation of nodal tissue and myocardium by parasympathetic vagus nerve fibers and sympathetic chains. (From Quaal S: *Comprehensive intraaortic balloon pumping,* ed 3, St Louis, 1998, Mosby.)

(CNS). Autonomic motor fibers of the *sympathetic nervous system* stimulate increased contractility *(inotropy),* as well as heart rate *(chronotropy)* (Fig. 8-17). Stimulation of the right and left *vagus nerves* of the *parasympathetic nervous system* produces a slower (bradycardic) heart rate and prolonged conduction through the AV node. Ordinarily, parasympathetic tone predominates in healthy, resting persons. Blocking parasympathetic influences with atropine generally results in an increased heart rate, although reducing the effects of sympathetic influences (e.g., with propranolol) usually has only a slight effect on the heart rate. When both the sympathetic and parasympathetic divisions are blocked in a young, healthy adult, the heart reverts to an intrinsic

heart rate of approximately 100 beats per minute (Opie, 1997; Berne and Long, 2001).

The cardiac parasympathetic fibers originate in the *medulla oblongata* of the brain, and the sympathetic fibers originate in the thoracic and cervical segments of the *spinal cord.* Fibers from both divisions combine to create a complex network of nerves that travel to the heart. Sympathetic fibers also are found within the adventitia of the great vessels at the base of the heart (Berne and Levy, 2001).

Cardiac function also is regulated by receptors found in the walls of the aortic arch and the carotid sinus, which sense changes in blood pressure. Other receptors in various parts of the body respond to changes in the chemical composition of the blood (e.g., levels of oxygen, carbon dioxide, or hydrogen). These changes initiate impulses to the cardiovascular center of the brain, which responds by adjusting pressure, rate, flow, and contractility within the cardiovascular system (Thelan and others, 1998).

Another control mechanism is found in certain cells of the cardiac atria. These secrete a hormone, called *atrial natriuretic factor (ANF),* into the blood in response to increased atrial volumes. This produces a marked increase in urinary sodium and water excretion and acts as a potent vasodilator. The body can rid itself of excess extracellular volume and enable the veins to restore intravascular blood volume (Chen and Burnett, 1999).

The higher centers of the brain also affect heart activity, as evidenced by the cardiovascular responses to intense emotions such as fear and anxiety. These responses are probably initiated by the hypothalamus and the limbic system.

Excitation-Contraction of the Cardiac Cell

Although extracardiac factors affect cardiac function, it is at the cellular level in the cardiac myocyte that excitation-contraction occurs. The conduction system typifies one kind of cardiac tissue. Contractile units comprise the second major group of cells. These two types of cells are related in that conducted electrical impulses are converted into the mechanical work of myocardial contraction. The cardiac myocyte is the basic unit of the heart's contraction mechanism.

CARDIAC MYOCYTE

The cardiac myocyte (Fig. 8-18) is composed of a basement membrane, the *sarcolemma,* containing pumps and channels involved in the contractile process and receptor systems that modulate excitation-contraction mecha-

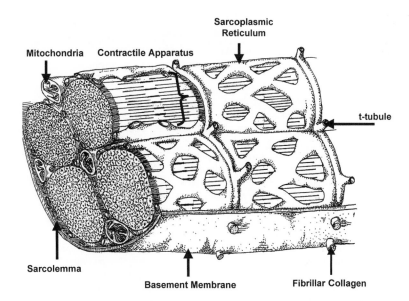

FIGURE 8-18 Longitudinal cross section of an individual cardiac myocyte. The sum of the integral parts of the cardiac myocyte are shown here, moving from outward in. The basement membrane, which is composed of collagen, glycoproteins, and proteoglycans, provides an interface for myocyte adhesion, as well as continuity with the extracellular matrix. The basement membrane serves as an anchoring site for the collagen fibrils. The sarcolemma, which enfolds the myocyte, contains integrins that bind the myocyte to the extracellular matrix and integral proteins that contribute to the action potential. Invaginations of the sarcolemma, which contains a high density of L-type calcium (Ca^{++}) channels, are the transverse (T) tubules. This specialized region of the sarcolemma allows for the close apposition of the L-type Ca^{++} channel to the Ca^{++} release channels of the sarcoplasmic reticulum. The sarcoplasmic reticulum serves both as a source and an internal store of cytosolic Ca^{++} required for excitation-contraction coupling. The contractile apparatus is a highly organized array of myofilament proteins composed primarily of thick myosin and thin actin filaments. The overlapping of these proteins form the dark and light bands as shown in this illustration. Shown in cross section are the numerous mitochondria, which are in close proximity to the myofilament apparatus. (From Walker CA, Spinale FG: *The structure and function of the cardiac myocyte: a review of fundamental concepts, J Thorac Cardiovasc Surg* 118(2): 376, 1999.)

nisms, and the *cytoskeleton,* which actively maintains the shape of the cell and contributes to the alignment of the *sarcomeres* (see following). The myocyte also contains the *sarcoplasmic reticulum,* an intracellular membrane network that regulates calcium concentration in conjunction with the sarcolemma and the transverse (T) tubular system, which conducts impulses to the interior of the cells (Walker and Spinale, 1999). The fundamental contractile unit in the cardiac myocyte is the sarcomere, which contains the components of the contractile apparatus: myosin, actin, tropomyosin, and the troponin complex (troponin C, troponin I, and troponin T) (Walker, Crawford, and Spinale, 2000).

Most of the energy (in the form of high-energy phosphates—adenosine triphosphate [ATP] and phosphocreatine) necessary for normal cardiac function is produced in the myocyte (see Fig. 8-18) by the *mitochondria,* which consume more than 95% of available oxygen molecules (Robinson and others, 2000). It is notable that normal cardiac mitochondria turn over the energy pool supplied by ATP and phosphocreatine four times per minute and can stockpile only 15 seconds of energy reserve (Robinson and others, 2000). Because the myocardium is unable to effectively store either oxygen or energy, a continuous supply of oxygen to the mitochondria is needed. When oxygen delivery is reduced, the cardiac myocyte reduces its contractile work in order to regain the balance between energy supply and demand (Little, 2001). Depending on the degree of damage to the cardiac myocyte from reduced blood flow and oxygen delivery, a variety of injuries can occur (Table 8-1) (Cook and Poole Wilson, 1999).

TABLE 8-1

Functional Conditions of Ischemic Myocardium

CONDITION	DESCRIPTION	CHARACTERISTICS
Transient ischemia	Short (2-5 minute) period of inadequate oxygen and metabolic substrate supply to normothermic myocardium. Prolonged ischemia can lead to more severe injury	Contractile dysfunction (e.g., reduced contractility, dysrhythmogenesis) relieved by resumption of oxygen/substrate delivery. Promotes protective mechanism of cardiac "preconditioning" (Robinson and others, 2000), which increases tolerance to subsequent ischemia
Stunned myocardium	Moderate ischemia lasting many minutes to many hours; return of normal function can take hours or days. Multiple stunning events lead to hibernation and apoptosis (Little and Braunwald, 2001).	Extracellular release of oxygen free radicals and excess calcium; ATP and phosphocreatine decreased. Interventions to reduce stunning include antioxidants and calcium channel antagonists
Hibernating myocardium	Chronic ischemia producing hypocontractility; condition may be temporary if sufficient blood supply restored; otherwise, permanent impairment occurs	Temporary hypocontractility; reversal possible with resumption of blood supply. Contractile reserve evident with sympathomimetic agents; nearly normal levels of ATP and phosphocreatine
Apoptosis	Ischemia-induced, permanently impaired contractile function (Cook and Poole-Wilson, 1999)	Cell destruction; energy-dependent form of cell "suicide" (Robinson and others, 2000). Some ATP remaining; inflammation and fibrosis associated with necrosis not present
Necrosis	Permanently impaired contractile function; cell death	Cell death with inflammatory and late fibrotic response to cell death. Irreversible myocardial contractile dysfunction; depletion of ATP

Modified from Robinson TN and others: Therapeutically accessible clinical cardiac states, *J Am Coll Surg* 191(4):452, 2000; Cook SA, Poole-Wilson PA: Cardiac myocyte apoptysis, *Eur Heart J* 20:1619, 1999; Little WC: Assessment of normal and abnormal cardiac function. In Braunwald E, Zipes DP, Libby P, editors: *Heart disease: a textbook of cardiovascular medicine,* ed 6, Philadelphia, 2001, WB Saunders.

CELLULAR CONTRACTION

Cell depolarization producing cellular contraction is initiated when an electrical impulse passes over the cell membrane (sarcolemma) and the T tubules and enters the interior of the cell. The passage of the electrical impulse is facilitated by the electrolytes (which become ions when dissolved in fluid) inside and outside the cellular membranes. Sodium (Na^+) and calcium (Ca^{++}) are more concentrated in the extracellular fluid, whereas potassium (K^+ is more highly concentrated within the intracellular fluid. This electrical gradient is maintained by the cell membrane, which prevents the equalization of these ions by pumping sodium out of and potassium back into the cell via the sodium-potassium pump.

When the electrical impulse passes over the myocyte, the cell membrane becomes more permeable to both Na^+ and Ca^{++} ions entering the cell through selective channels, thereby producing an action potential (Fig. 8-19).

During the early phase of depolarization, sodium rushes in via the *"fast" sodium channel* and neutralizes some of the negative charges inside the cell. This allows even more sodium to enter until the fast sodium channels are inactivated, contraction ceases, and the cell becomes refractory to further excitation. Until the cell has repolarized, the heart is unable to contract again, thereby preventing sustained, tetanic myocardial contraction (Berne and Levy, 2001).

After the opening of the fast sodium channels, the *"slow" sodium channels* open and allow Ca^{++} (and some Na^+) to enter the cell after the initial fast entry of Na^+. Activation, inactivation, and recovery of the slow channels is slower than that of the fast channels. Calcium channel–blocking medications reduce Ca^{++} inflow and thereby diminish cardiac contractility. Conversely, catecholamines increase the inward current of Ca^{++} and enhance contractility (Berne and Levy, 2001).

During this period of repolarization, potassium diffuses out of the cell, a process that culminates in the restoration of the resting membrane potential. The sodium-potassium pump restores Na^+ and K^+ to their appropriate concentration inside and outside the cell membrane, and the cycle is ready to start again.

Cardiac Cycle

Depolarization stimulates muscles to contract, producing the systolic phase of the cardiac cycle, whereas repolarization allows the myocardium to relax, producing the diastolic phase of the cardiac cycle. With each heartbeat the ventricles propel blood through the vascular system. (See Fig. 8-16 for the relationship between the successive electrical and mechanical events during one cardiac cycle.) Approximately 70% of the ventricular volume flows directly into the ventricles from the atria. Atrial systole contributes another 30%

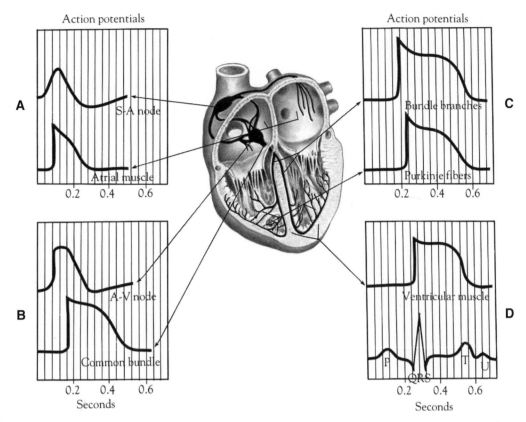

FIGURE 8-19 Normal cardiac conduction pathways and transmembrane action potential of **(A)** SA node, **(B)** AV node, **(C)** bundle branches, and **(D)** ventricular muscle. (From Thompson JM and others: *Mosby's clinical nursing,* ed 4, 1998, Mosby.)

to the total volume of blood in the ventricle at the end of ventricular diastole. Although atrial contraction is not essential in the normal heart, it contributes significantly to left ventricular filling in the presence of a narrowed (stenotic) mitral valve.

The onset of ventricular contraction (systole) is termed *isovolumic contraction.* During this brief period, ventricular volume is constant, but ventricular pressure rises and closes the mitral (and tricuspid) valve. When the pressure within the ventricle is sufficient to open the aortic and pulmonary valves, the *ejection phase* begins. Ejection of blood into the aorta (or pulmonary artery) is rapid at first and then is reduced. In the systemic circulation, aortic pressure declines as blood flow is transmitted to the vascular periphery. Left ventricular pressure also decreases, and a gradient develops, with the relatively higher aortic pressure closing the aortic valve. The ventricle does not completely empty during systole. Approximately 40% of the end-diastolic volume remains; the amount of blood ejected is called the *ejection fraction* and is commonly used to indicate ventricular function (Table 8-2).

Isovolumic relaxation is the period between closure of the semilunar valves and opening of the atrioventricular valves. Ventricular volume remains constant, but

ventricular pressure drops dramatically (Guyton and Hall, 2000).

Atrial pressure rises with the blood accumulated during the previous systolic period to open the AV valves and cause rapid filling of the relaxed ventricles. The *rapid filling phase* is followed by the period of *diastasis,* during which there is slow filling of the ventricles by venous return from the lungs and the periphery. An increase in ventricular volume and pressure initiates the repetition of the cycle.

Cardiac Output

The cardiac output is the volume of blood pumped by the heart per minute. It is determined by multiplying the *stroke volume* (the amount of blood ejected with each contraction) by the *heart rate.* Thus the cardiac output of a subject who ejects 70 ml of blood 80 times a minute is 5600 ml/min or 5.6 L/min. Because patients vary in size, the metabolic requirements for blood differ. The cardiac output can be corrected for differences in body size by dividing it by the body surface area to compute the *cardiac index.* (The *stroke volume index* can be computed by dividing the stroke volume by the body surface area.)

TABLE 8-2
Concepts Related to Cardiac Output

CONCEPT	DEFINITION	DETERMINANTS
Cardiac output (CO)	Amount of blood (in liters) ejected by left ventricle per minute; product of heart rate multiplied by stroke volume; 4.5-7 L/min (adult)	Heart rate, stroke volume
Cardiac index (CI)	Cardiac output per square meter of body surface area; used to compare CO of different-sized persons; 2.5-4.2 L/min/m^2 (adult)	CO divided by body surface area
Ejection fraction	Percentage of end-diastolic volume ejected into (systemic) circulation; indicator of left ventricular function; 60%-70% (adult)	Preload, afterload, contractility
Heart rate	Number of contractions, or beats, per minute (bpm); chronotropy; 70-100 bpm (adult)	Autonomic nervous system; chemical/pharmacologic stimulation
Stroke volume	Amount of blood ejected per heartbeat; 60-130 ml/beat (adult)	Preload, afterload, contractility
Preload	Volume of blood in ventricle at end of diastole. Right-sided heart preload: measured by central venous pressure; mean 0-8 mm Hg (adult). Left-sided heart preload: measured by pulmonary artery wedge pressure; mean 1-10 mm Hg	Total blood volume, body position, intrathoracic pressure, intrapericardial pressure, venous tone, skeletal muscle contraction, atrial contribution to ventricular filling
Afterload	Impedance to contraction; vascular resistance the heart must overcome to pump blood into the circulation; wall tension/stress during systole. Right ventricular afterload is reflected by pulmonary vascular resistance; 0.5-1.5 Wood units (WU) (adult) Left ventricular afterload is reflected by systemic vascular resistance; 12-18 WU (adult)	Ventricular volume, ventricular wall thickness, systolic intraventricular pressure, systemic arterial pressure, pressure gradient across outflow valve (e.g., impact of aortic contraction) stenosis of left ventricular outflow
Contractility	Ability of ventricle to pump; inotropic state of the heart. Difficult to measure in clinical setting; intraoperative echocardiography increasingly employed to assess contractility (in addition to visual estimation)	Availability of intracellular Ca^{++}; sympathetic (increase) and parasympathetic (decrease) stimulation effects, inotropic (positive/negative) drugs; hypoxia, acidosis, ischemia, myocardial disease

Modified from Thys DM, Dauchot P, Hillel Z: Advances in cardiovascular physiology; Chambers CE, Skeehan TM, Hensley FA: The cardiac catheterization laboratory: diagnostic and therapeutic procedures in the adult patient. In Kaplan JA, editor: *Cardiac anesthesia,* ed 4, Philadelphia, 1999, WB Saunders. Gauthier DK: Anatomy and physiology of the heart. In Kinney MR, Packa DR, editors: *Comprehensive cardiac care,* ed 8, St Louis, 1996, Mosby.

Normally the right and left ventricles eject equal amounts of blood per minute, but individual stroke outputs may vary. If the right ventricle momentarily pumps more blood than the left ventricle, the minute output will equalize because the increased right ventricular volume will increase left ventricular filling and thereby increase the left ventricular stroke volume (Schlant, Sonnenblick, and Katz, 1998).

DETERMINANTS OF CARDIAC OUTPUT

Depending on the needs of the body, cardiac output is increased or decreased by four interrelated factors: heart rate, preload, afterload, and contractility.

Heart rate

Heart rate refers to the frequency of contraction, reflected by the pulse rate. Although the sinus node usually determines the heart rate, neural and humoral factors also play a role in determining the heart rate. A change in the heart rate will alter the following three factors.

Preload

Preload is the amount of blood in the ventricle before it contracts. It is also known as the *left ventricular end-diastolic volume (LVEDV)*. Because it is technically easier to measure pressure than it is to measure volume, *left ventricular end-diastolic pressure (LVEDP)* is commonly used to measure preload (although it is not synonymous with LVEDV (Berne and Levy, 2001). The greater the preload, within physiologic limits, the more the myocardial fibers stretch and subsequently the more forcefully the fibers shorten to produce an increase in stroke volume. The relationship between volume, stretch, and subsequent contraction is known as the *Frank-Starling law.*

Because the heart is composed of two pumps, it is necessary to distinguish between right and left ventricular preload. Venous return to the right atrium, measured with a central venous pressure (CVP) catheter, represents the right filling pressure, or preload. The preload of the left ventricle is inferred with a pulmonary artery catheter containing an inflatable balloon at its tip. The balloon can be inflated and wedged temporarily in a branch of the pulmonary artery. Because there are no valves between the pulmonary artery and the left atrium, this *pulmonary artery wedge pressure (PAWP),* measured when the mitral valve is open, reflects both left atrial pressure and LVEDP.

Preload also is dependent on the amount of circulating blood and its distribution throughout the body. Conditions that decrease blood volume (e.g., hemorrhage) decrease venous return and cardiac output. The distribution of blood can be affected by contracting external muscles, body position, and venous tone. Veins are capable of dilating and sequestering large amounts of blood in dependent portions of the body.

Finally, ventricular wall compliance plays a role in diastolic filling of the ventricle. When the heart is relaxed, rapid diastolic filling can be achieved. However, a stiff or thickened ventricle, found in patients with left ventricular hypertrophy, coronary artery disease, or cardiac tamponade, is less compliant and impairs diastolic filling (Thys and others, 1999).

Afterload

Afterload is the ventricular wall tension created during ejection; it is the resistance the ventricles must overcome during contraction. Resistance is created by aortic distensibility, the systemic vascular bed, and blood volume and viscosity. Left ventricular or right ventricular outflow tract obstructions (such as aortic valve stenosis or pulmonary valve stenosis) also increase the workload of the heart. Calculation of the systemic vascular resistance commonly is performed to indicate afterload. Because of the great energy requirements of the left ventricle, pharmacologic manipulation of the afterload is frequently performed in the operating room and the critical care setting to decrease the workload of the ventricle.

When left ventricular function is impaired and the ventricle cannot eject adequately, blood backs up in the lungs. This raises pulmonary vascular pressure and hence pulmonary vascular resistance, which increases right ventricular afterload. In very young patients with congenital lesions producing increased blood flow to the lungs, pulmonary hypertension and elevated right ventricular afterload can produce heart failure in a short period.

Contractility

Contractility refers to the inotropic state of the ventricle, independent of changes in heart rate, preload, or afterload. Sympathetic stimulation or inotropic agents such as digitalis, calcium, and dobutamine hydrochloride increase contractility and cardiac output. When pharmacologic agents such as barbiturates, halothane, beta blockers, or calcium channel blockers are given or

when there is a loss of functioning ventricular muscle, as in myocardial infarction or left ventricular aneurysm, contractility is decreased.

Whether extrinsic or intrinsic, manipulation of the heart rate, preload, afterload, and contractility to achieve optimum cardiac output helps to ensure adequate perfusion of the tissues.

Myocardial Oxygen Consumption

Closely related to the determinants of cardiac output is *myocardial oxygen consumption (MVo$_2$).* Oxygen is required to do the work associated with contraction and relaxation. When the oxygen demand exceeds the supply, hypoxemia results. Mechanisms are instituted to return the myocardium to a balanced state by either reducing the oxygen demand or increasing the oxygen supply. In patients with ischemic heart disease (where reduced blood flow produces a decrease in oxygen supply), beta-blocking drugs can reduce the demand, whereas surgical revascularization of the myocardium increases the supply. Without surgery, the ability to increase the oxygen supply is limited because of the obstructive lesions and the already high rate of myocardial oxygen extraction from the blood. In patients with left ventricular hypertrophy, the increased thickness of the myocardial wall (without a commensurate increase in the vascular network supplying the tissue) adversely affects the distribution of coronary blood flow to the subendocardium. When the supply of oxygen cannot be readily increased via coronary artery blood flow, balancing the supply and demand equation focuses on reducing the demand.

MVo$_2$ is primarily determined by heart rate, wall tension, and contractility—all factors associated with cardiac output. Myocardial wall tension is affected by conditions that increase pressure (aortic stenosis) or volume (aortic regurgitation) loads on the heart. Both pharmacologic and psychologic interventions are warranted in decreasing myocardial oxygen demands.

Circulatory System

The heart pumps blood to the tissues to provide nourishment and to remove the waste products of metabolism. The transportation route for the distribution and exchange of these substances is formed by the circulatory system.

SYSTEMIC CIRCULATION

The systemic circulation supplies all the tissues of the body except the lungs. Blood is ejected from the left ventricle into the aorta, from which arteries branch off to perfuse the head, upper extremities, abdominal organs, and lower extremities (Fig. 8-20).

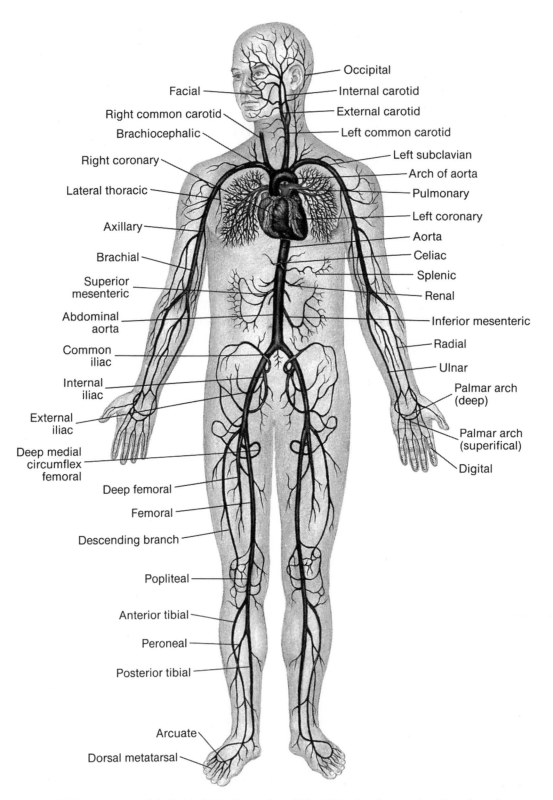

FIGURE 8-20 Arterial circulation. (From Canobbio MM: *Cardiovascular disorders,* St Louis, 1990, Mosby.)

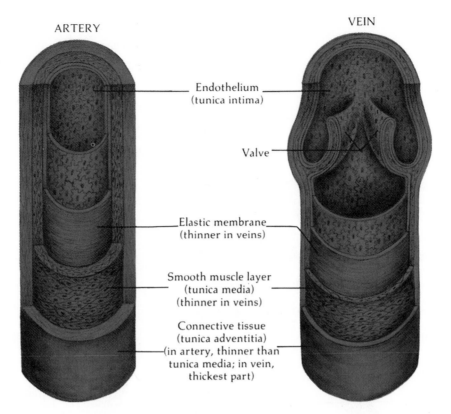

ARTERY

VEIN

Endothelium
(tunica intima)

Valve

Elastic membrane
(thinner in veins)

Smooth muscle layer
(tunica media)
(thinner in veins)

Connective tissue
(tunica adventitia)
(in artery, thinner than
tunica media; in vein,
thickest part)

FIGURE 8-21 Cross section of an artery and vein showing the three layers: tunica intima, tunica media, and tunica adventitia. Larger veins and arteries have their own blood supplies provided by tiny blood vessels (vasa vasorum) distributed throughout the vessel walls. (From Thompson JM and others: *Mosby's clinical nursing,* ed 4, St Louis, 1998, Mosby.)

Arteries transport blood under high pressure and have strong muscular walls (Fig. 8-21).

Arteries subdivide into *arterioles,* whose function is to control the release of blood into the capillaries. Internal respiration occurs in the *capillaries,* where fluids, nutrients, electrolytes, oxygen, and other substances are exchanged through their single-layer walls for the end products of cellular metabolism. Blood then collects in the *venules* and flows into progressively larger veins to return to the right atrium (Fig. 8-22). Flap valves within the veins help to maintain unidirectional blood flow. Contracting external muscles propel venous blood toward the heart.

PULMONARY CIRCULATION

In the pulmonary circulation, blood is pumped from the right ventricle into the main pulmonary artery, which divides into the right and left pulmonary arteries. These further subdivide into the arterioles and capillaries of the lungs. External respiration occurs in the capillary beds, where carbon dioxide is exchanged for oxygen. Oxygenated blood from the lungs flows

through the pulmonary veins into the left atrium. Following birth, direct contact between blood from the right side of the heart and blood from the left side occurs only at the capillary level.

FETAL CIRCULATION

In utero there is mixing of blood from both sides of the heart through the *foramen ovale,* which becomes the fossa ovalis (Fig. 8-23). In addition, there is a communication between the aorta and the pulmonary artery, called the *ductus arteriosus.* In fetal life deoxygenated blood is oxygenated in the placenta (rather than the lungs). The lungs are relatively nonfunctional; thus perfusion of this organ is not critical. At birth, however, the lungs assume responsibility for oxygenation. Expansion of the lungs with air decreases pulmonary vascular resistance and therefore resistance to flow from the right atrium and the right ventricle. Studies by Rudolph (1970) have shown that pulmonary vascular resistance decreases mainly in response to the elevated oxygen levels within the pulmonary vessels.

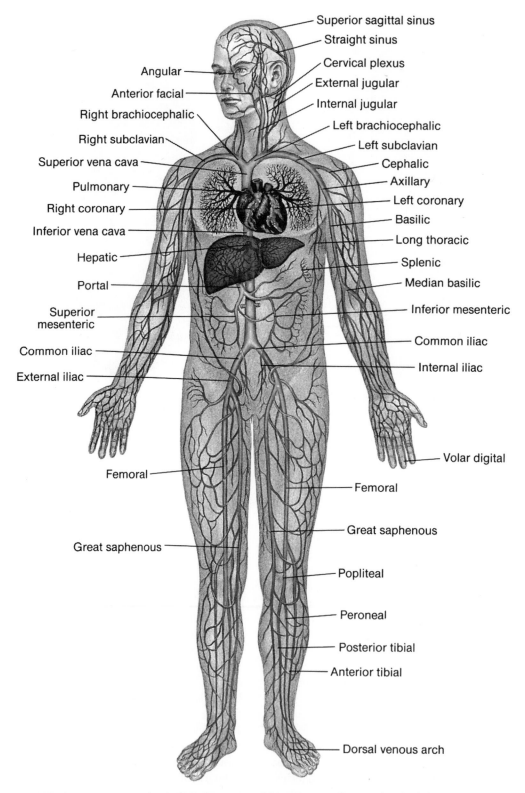

FIGURE 8-22   Venous circulation. (From Canobbio MM: *Cardiovascular disorders,* St Louis, 1990, Mosby.)

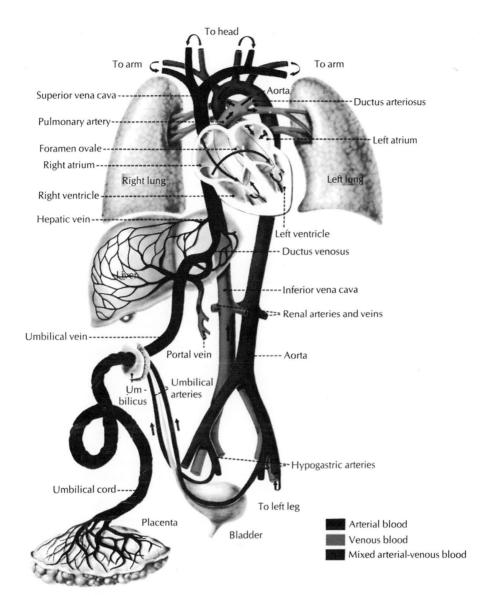

FIGURE 8-23 Fetal circulation. The mother's blood is circulated to the placenta, where oxygen and nutrients are exchanged for the fetus's metabolic products. From the placenta, blood flows through the umbilical vein, fetal ductus venosus, and inferior vena cava to the right atrium. This blood is directed through the foramen ovale into the left atrium, bypassing the fetal lungs. From the left atrium blood flows into the left ventricle, which pumps it into the aorta and the umbilical arteries and then back to the placenta. The greater portion of the blood returning to the right atrium from the superior vena cava is directed through the tricuspid valve into the right ventricle. From there it is pumped into the pulmonary artery. Pulmonary blood flow is shunted through the ductus arteriosus into the aorta. A small amount of pulmonary blood flow enters the fetal lungs and returns to the left atrium via the pulmonary veins. (Courtesy Ross Laboratories, Columbus, Ohio.)

At the same time systemic vascular resistance and aortic pressure increase because the tremendous blood flow through the placenta ceases. This increased pressure is reflected in the left ventricle and the left atrium. Because blood flows from areas of higher pressure to areas of lower pressure, blood preferentially travels from the right side of the heart into the lower-pressure right ventricle and pulmonary bed rather than into the higher-pressure region of the left side of the heart. Increased left atrial pressure closes the flap that lies over the foramen ovale on the left atrial wall.

Cessation of flow through the ductus arteriosus is not related to pressure gradients, however. It is caused by changes in the muscular wall of the ductus that cause it to constrict. Over the next few months, fibrous ingrowth occludes the lumen altogether; the remaining structure is called the *ligamentum arteriosum*. Occasionally a ductus remains patent, causing excessive pulmonary blood flow. The ductus can be ligated to close the communication; surgery can be performed in the neonatal intensive care unit or the operating room (see Chapter 18).

References

Berne RM, Levy MN: *Cardiovascular physiology,* ed 8, St Louis, 2001, Mosby.

Bharati S, Lev M, Kirklin JW: *Cardiac surgery and the conduction system,* New York, 1983, John Wiley & Sons.

Braunwald E, Harrison DC, Chidsey CA: The heart as an endocrine organ, *Am J Med* 36:1, 1964.

Chambers CE, Skeehan TM, Hensley FA: The cardiac catheterization laboratory: diagnostic and therapeutic procedures in the adult patient. In Kaplan JA, editor: *Cardiac anesthesia,* ed 4, Philadelphia, 1999, WB Saunders.

Chen HH, Burnett, Jr, JC: The natriuretic peptides in heart failure: diagnostic and therapeutic potentials, *Proc Assoc Am Phys* 111(5):406, 1999.

Clendening L: *Sourcebook of medical history,* New York, 1942, PB Hoeber.

Cook SA, Poole-Wilson PA: Cardiac myocyte apoptosis, *Eur Heart J* 20(22):1619, 1999.

Guyton AC, Hall JE: *Textbook of medical physiology,* ed 10, Philadelphia, 2000, WB Saunders.

Hauser ER, Pericak-Vance MA: Genetic analysis for common complex disease, *Am Heart J* 140(4):S36, 2000.

Hurst JW, editor: *Atlas of the heart,* New York, 1988, Gower.

Keller BB, Markwald RR: Embryology of the heart. In Alexander RW, Schlant RC, Fuster V, editors: *Hurst's the heart, arteries and veins,* ed 9, vol 1, New York, 1998, McGraw-Hill.

Kirklin JW, Barratt-Boyes BG: *Cardiac surgery: morphology, diagnostic criteria, natural history, techniques, results, and indications,* ed 2, Vol II, New York, 1993, Churchill Livingstone.

Little WC: Assessment of normal and abnormal cardiac function. In Braunwald E, Zipes DP, Libby P, editors: *Heart disease: a textbook of cardiovascular medicine,* ed 6, Philadelphia, 2001, WB Saunders.

Meyerson SL, Schwartz LB: Gene therapy as a therapeutic intervention for vascular disease, *J Cardiovasc Nurs* 13(4):91, 1999.

O'Brien ER, Nathan HJ: Coronary physiology and atherosclerosis. In Kaplan JA, editor: *Cardiac anesthesia,* ed 4, Philadelphia, 1999 WB Saunders.

Opie LH: Mechanisms of cardiac contraction and relaxation. In Braunwald E, Zipes DP, Libby P, editors: *Heart disease: a textbook of cardiovascular medicine,* ed 6, Philadelphia, 2001, WB Saunders.

Rankin JS, Sabiston DC: Physiology of coronary blood flow, myocardial function, and intraoperative myocardial protection. In Sabiston DC, Spencer FC, editors: *Surgery of the chest,* ed 6, vol 2, Philadelphia, 1995, WB Saunders.

Robinson TN and others: Therapeutically accessible clinical cardiac states, *J Am Coll Surg* 191(4):452, 2000.

Rudolph AM: The changes in the circulation after birth: their importance in congenital heart disease, *Circulation* 41(2):343, 1970.

Schlant RC, Sonnenblick EH, Katz AM: Normal physiology of the cardiovascular system. In Alexander RW, Schlant RC, Fuster V, editors: *Hurst's the heart, arteries and veins,* ed 9, vol 1, New York, 1998, McGraw-Hill.

Spotnitz HM: Macro design, structure, and mechanics of the left ventricle, *J Thorac Cardiovasc Surg* 119(5):1053, 2000.

Thelan LA and others: *Critical care nursing: diagnosis and management,* ed 3, St Louis, 1998, Mosby.

Thys DM, Dauchot P, Hillel Z: Advances in cardiovascular physiology. In Kaplan JA, editor: *Cardiac anesthesia,* ed 4, Philadelphia, 1999, WB Saunders.

Walker CA, Crawford FA Jr, Spinale FG: Myocyte contractile dysfunction with hypertrophy and failure: relevance to cardiac surgery, *J Thorac Cardiovasc Surg* 119(2):388, 2000.

Walker CA, Spinale FG: The structure and function of the cardiac myocyte: a review of fundamental concepts, *J Thorac Cardiovasc Surg* 118(2):375, 1999.

Waller BF, Schlant RC: Anatomy of the heart. In Alexander RW, Schlant RC, Fuster V, editors: *Hurst's the heart, arteries and veins,* ed 9, vol 1, New York, 1998, McGraw-Hill.

Winkelmann BR and others: Genetics of coronary heart disease: current knowledge and research principles, *Am Heart J* 140(4):S11, 2000.

9 Basic Cardiac Procedures

The ultimate object of my work in this field has been to be able to operate inside the heart under direct vision. From the beginning, I have not only been interested in the substitution of a mechanical device for the heart, but also for the lung.

John H. Gibbon, Jr., MD, 1954 (p. 171)

Safe and effective cardiac surgery is possible because of the technologic developments that have enabled surgeons to work on the heart without injuring it or the other major organs of the body. The use of endotracheal anesthesia in thoracic surgery by Elsberg in the early twentieth century allowed surgeons to enter the thorax without causing a pneumothorax, with its accompanying pulmonary collapse and asphyxia (Westaby, 1999). Cardiopulmonary bypass (CPB), introduced into clinical use by Gibbon (1954), provided a method for operating on a quiet, bloodless field, unobscured by the lungs, while at the same time perfusing the brain and the rest of the body. Methods to protect the heart itself—reported by Melrose and others (1955); Sealy, Brown, and Young (1958); Gay and Ebert (1973); Buckberg (1979); and others—helped to minimize the dangers associated with intraoperatively induced cardiac arrest. The rapid growth of *minimal access surgery* (also referred to as *minimally invasive surgery*) that employs percutaneous bypass techniques, or no CPB, continues to change the landscape of cardiac surgery. This chapter describes the types of incisions used to expose the heart and other thoracic structures, CPB, and methods to protect the myocardium during cardiac procedures with or without the use of CPB.

Thoracic Incisions

The incision should allow adequate exposure of the operative site. Depending on the particular anatomic and physiologic problem, a variety of incisions are available to expose the heart and other thoracic structures (Table 9-1). Increasingly, smaller incisions are used to produce better cosmetic results and less postoperative pain and morbidity (Anderson and Milano, 2001).

The median sternotomy is the most common incision used for cardiac surgery; partial upper or lower sternotomy and a transverse sternal incision (clamshell) also can be employed for selected procedures. A variety of thoracic incisions also are used for myocardial revascularization, mitral valve repair or replacement, and reoperation.

Sternotomy also produces the least respiratory impairment and causes less discomfort for the patient than do other thoracic incisions. Unlike the various lateral thoracotomy incisions, sternotomy requires no muscle division, and the sternal bones can be closed firmly together. Postoperatively, coughing and deep breathing do not create the same degree of pain encountered by patients with thoracotomy because of moving ribs and incised chest muscles. This facilitates the performance of postoperative breathing exercises, which enhance pulmonary function (Rusch and Ginsberg, 1999).

Injury to the brachial plexus can result from excessive spreading of the sternal retractor blades (Rusch and Ginsberg, 1999) or extreme abduction of the arms during median sternotomy or thoracotomy (Waldhausen, Pierce, and Campbell, 1996). Preventive measures include avoiding overstretching the sternum, positioning the retractor as caudally as possible, and preventing overabduction of the arms.

MEDIAN STERNOTOMY

Median sternotomy remains the most popular incision for acquired cardiac disorders because it provides the best access to the heart and mediastinum and optimum exposure for the institution of CPB. It is also the incision of choice for pericardiectomy, thymectomy, and anterior mediastinal tumors (Waldhausen, Pierce, and Campbell, 1996). Many surgeons have maintained a preference for the median sternotomy approach in

TABLE 9-1
Thoracic Incisions

INCISION	POSITION	INDICATIONS	SPECIAL PATIENT NEEDS
Median sternotomy: Incision down center of sternum	Supine	Most adult cardiac procedures except those on branch pulmonary arteries, distal transverse aortic arch, and descending thoracic aorta	Padding for hands, elbows, feet, back of head, dependent bony prominences
Mini-sternotomy: Partial upper or lower sternal incision starting either from sternal notch or xiphoid process and extending to midportion of sternum; lower-end sternal splitting (LESS)	Supine	MAS, on- or off-CPB procedures	Same as median sternotomy
Parasternotomy: Resection of right or left costal cartilages (from second to fifth cartilage, depending on surgical target)	Supine; small roll may be placed under affected side	Left: MAS CABG Right: MAS CABG, valve procedures	Same as median sternotomy; risk of postoperative chest wall instability
Anterolateral thoracotomy: Curvilinear incision along subpectoral groove to axillary line	Supine with pad or pillow under operative site; arm supported in sling or overarm board; arm on unaffected side may be tucked along side	MAS, MIDCAB, trauma to anterior pericardium and left ventricle; repeat sternotomy	Padding for extremities; pillow or other device to elevate affected side; armboard or sling for arm on affected side
Left anterior small thoracotomy (LAST), right anterior mini-thoracotomy: Curvilinear incision along subpectoral groove, right or left side	Supine with small roll under affected side	Left: MAS, MIDCAB Right: MAS valve procedures or CABG	Same as anterolateral thoracotomy
Lateral thoracotomy: Curvilinear incision along costochondral junction anteriorly to posterior border of scapula	Placed on side with arms extended and axilla and head supported; knees and legs protected	Lung biopsies; first-rib resection; lobectomy	Armboard, overarm board, axillary roll, padding for extremities, pillow between legs; sandbags, straps, wide tape, or other devices to support torso
Posterolateral thoracotomy: Curvilinear incision from subpectoral crease below nipple, extended laterally and posteriorly along ribs almost to posterior midline below scapula (location of intercostal incision depends on surgical site); used less frequently with availability of VATS techniques	Lateral with arms extended and axilla and head supported; knees and legs protected	First-rib resection; lobectomy	Similar to needs for lateral thoracotomy
Transsternal bilateral anterior thoracotomy (clamshell): Submammary incision extending from one anterior axillary line to the other across sternum at fourth interspace	Supine	Lung transplant; emergency access to heart when sternal saw not available	Same as median sternotomy; requires transsection of left and right IMA
Subxiphoid incision: Vertical midline incision from over xiphoid process to about 10 cm inferiorly (may divide lower portion of sternum to enhance exposure)	Supine	Pericardial drainage, pericardial biopsy, attachment of pacemaker electrodes, MAS	Same as median sternotomy
Thoracoabdominal incision: Low curvilinear incision on left side, extended to anterior midline, continued vertically down abdomen	Anterior thoracotomy with chest at 45-degree angle to table; abdomen supine	Thoracoabdominal aneurysm	Same as anterolateral thoracotomy

CPB, Cardiopulmonary bypass; *CABG,* coronary artery bypass grafting; *MAS,* minimal access surgery; *MIDCAB,* minimal access direct coronary artery bypass; *IMA,* internal mammary artery; *VATS,* video-assisted thoracoscopic surgery.
Modified from Rusch VW, Ginsberg RJ: Chest wall, pleura, lung, and mediastinum. In Schwartz SI editor: *Principles of surgery,* ed 7, New York, 1999, McGraw-Hill; Waldhausen JA, Pierce WS, Campbell DB: *Surgery of the chest,* ed 6, St Louis, 1996, Mosby; Arom KV, Emery RW: Ministernotomy for coronary artery bypass surgery. In Yim APC and others: *Minimal access cardiothoracic surgery,* Philadelphia, 2000, WB Saunders; Arom KV, Emery RW: Alternative incisions for cardiac surgery. In Yim APC and others: *Minimal access cardiothoracic surgery,* Philadelphia, 2000, WB Saunders.

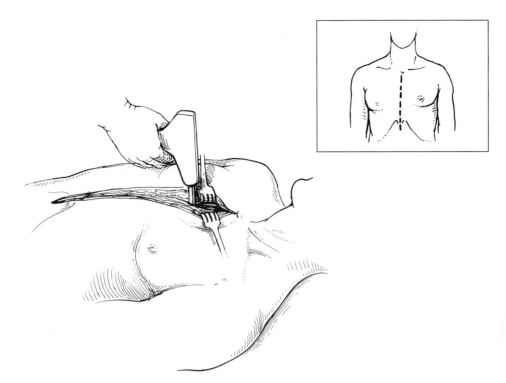

FIGURE 9-1 Median sternotomy with a power saw. (From Waldhausen JA, Pierce WS, Campbell DB: *Surgery of the chest,* ed 6, St Louis, 1996, Mosby.)

comparison with other smaller incisions, even with the rapid growth of minimally invasive surgery (MIS); for some surgeons the concept of minimally invasive often pertains to the avoidance of CPB (and its deleterious sequelae) rather than to the size of incisions.

STERNAL INCISION

The skin incision is made from the sternal notch to the xiphoid process. Waldhausen, Pierce, and Campbell (1996) have stressed the importance of not extending the incision into the suprasternal space for physiologic, as well as cosmetic, reasons. For instance, if tracheostomy is anticipated, the tracheal opening should be placed as far from the sternotomy incision as possible because of the risk of cross-contamination and infection.

The sternal bone is divided with an air-driven or electrically powered saw (Fig. 9-1). Battery-powered saws are also available. Manual sternotomy with a Lebsche knife and mallet is performed rarely unless a saw is unavailable. The saw should be checked and tested before it is needed, and a backup saw should be readily available. Registered nurse first assistant (RNFA) considerations are listed in Box 9-1.

The use of *mini-sternotomy* incisions for myocardial revascularization (and some valve procedures) has overcome some of the limitations posed by small thoracotomy incisions employed for minimal access surgery.

The skin incision (starting either at the sternal notch or the xiphoid process) is approximately 10 to 12 cm long (compared with approximately 30 cm for complete sternotomy), and the partially divided sternum is spread apart about 6 to 8 cm (compared with approximately 25 cm for complete sternotomy). Mini-sternotomy variations include the reverse J and the C incisions (Fig. 9-2). Compared with complete sternotomy, patients with a partial sternotomy have fewer postoperative complications from stretching or damaging of the ribs, shoulder joints, and cartilages (Arom and Emery, 2000a, 2000b).

Operative procedure: sternotomy

1A. For median sternotomy the skin incision is made from the sternal notch to the linea alba, 1 to 2 cm below the xiphoid process (see Fig. 9-1) (Waldhausen, Pierce, and Campbell, 1996).

1B. For mini-sternotomy the skin incision starts below either the sternal notch or the xiphoid process (depending on the location of the planned sternotomy and the surgical site target) and continues toward the midsternum (see Fig. 10-11). A modification of the mini-sternotomy is the partial sternotomy, which creates a reverse J incision or a C incision (see Fig. 9-2) (Arom and Emery, 2000B); an inverted T also may be made to provide, for example, additional right lateral access for mitral valve procedures (Cosgrove and Gillinov, 1998).

BOX 9-1
RN First Assistant Considerations Related to the Incision

- Retract skin edges manually with a laparotomy pad to expose subcutaneous and periosteal bleeders; handheld retractors can be used initially to expose the retrosternum and the upper end of the incision, or the pleura or lungs, for sternotomy or thoracotomy, respectively.
- Suction cautery plume when chest is opened.
- Avoid retracting sternum too vigorously during repeat sternotomy to prevent tearing the heart or great vessels; identify existing coronary bypass grafts to avoid laceration.
- If sudden, copious bleeding is seen during repeat (or initial) sternotomy, follow surgeon's specified commands; for example, RNFA may be requested to suction (autotransfusion and discard suction both may be necessary to clear field adequately) or to compress both sides of the chest together to tamponade bleeding while surgeon accesses femoral artery for CPB cannulation.
- Look for bleeding vessels at upper end of median sternotomy (or thoracotomy) incision before retractor is inserted; once retractor is opened, it may stretch tissue and close bleeders, concealing their presence and making it difficult to find them during chest closure after the retractor is removed.
- After initial incision into pericardium is made, place a suction tip under the pericardium to elevate it off the heart and prevent injury to underlying myocardium while the pericardial incision is extended with cautery (the surgeon may perform this maneuver with the fingers).
- Provide countertraction during insertion of chest wires or rib sutures.
- Ensure that pacing wires, chest tubes, and bypass grafts are not caught in the sternal wires or pinched between the reapproximated sternal edges.

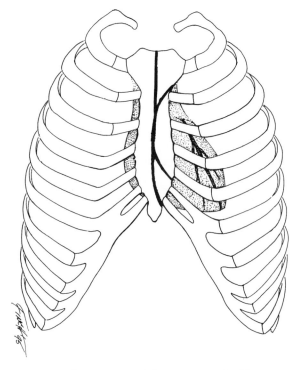

FIGURE 9-2 Common partial sternotomy incisions to expose the left coronary artery system. A reverse J incision starts from the left fifth or sixth costosternal angle and extends upward to the sternal notch. A C incision starts from the last costoxiphoid angle and extends upward, exiting at the first left intercostal space. (Arom KV, Emery RW: Ministernotomy for coronary artery bypass surgery. In Yim APC and others, editors: *Minimal access cardiothoracic surgery*, Philadelphia, 2000, WB Saunders.)

1C. For parasternotomy (see Fig. 10-11), the right or left costal cartilages (from the second to the fifth costal cartilage, depending on the desired access) are removed with bone rongeurs (Cohn, 1998).

1D. For transsternal incisions (clamshell) (Fig. 9-3), a bilateral submammary incision is made and the sternum is divided transversely; both thoraces are entered through the fourth or fifth interspace.

2. The periosteum along the manubrium and the sternal body is coagulated to mark the midline. The fibrous bands between the two clavicular heads are divided, and the xiphoid process is cut in the middle. The distal retrosternal space is bluntly dissected with the finger. Bleeding points are coagulated.

3. The sternum is divided along the midline with a reciprocating saw (see Fig. 9-1) or an oscillating saw. The anesthesiologist may deflate the lungs momentarily just before the sternum is divided to reduce the risk of opening the pleural spaces and injuring the lungs.

Depending on surgeon preference, the bone is incised from the upper end of the incision to the lower end, or the reverse. A handheld retractor (such as an Army-Navy or rake retractor) can be placed along the sides and at the upper end of the incision to protect the skin and subcutaneous tissue.

4. The upper and lower edges of the sternal periosteum are cauterized to control bleeding from the marrow. Bone wax may be applied to the sternal edges for excessive bleeding, but it is used sparingly as a result of reports noting impaired osseus wound healing, possible embolization of the wax to the lungs, and bacterial contamination (Francel and Kouchoukos, 2001b).

Additional bleeding points along the incision are cauterized. Occasionally, bilateral suture ligatures are required for large venous bleeders at the upper end of the incision; this is more common in patients with engorged veins from systemic venous hypertension.

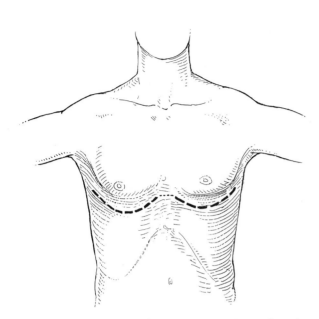

FIGURE 9-3   Bilateral submammary incision; referred to as the *clamshell.* (From Waldhausen JA, Pierce WS, Campbell DB: *Surgery of the chest,* ed 6, St Louis, 1996, Mosby.)

5. The sternal retractor is inserted and opened gradually to avoid sternal fractures. Before insertion of the retractor, the sternal edges may be covered with laparotomy pads or surgical towels.

Sternal closure

1. After hemostasis has been achieved, stainless steel wire sutures (No. 5 or 6) are passed around or through the bone (Fig. 9-4). Generally, five or six wires are inserted (fewer for partial sternotomy). A simple or mattress suture technique or a combination technique may be performed. Countertraction on the sternum by the assistant may make passage of the wire through the bone easier. Heavy suture is used to reapproximate ribs.
2. The surgeon and assistant evaluate the sternum for bleeding from branches of the internal mammary artery or other blood vessels, and hemostasis is achieved.
3. The wires are twisted closed tightly enough to immobilize the sternum. Excess wire is cut, and the ends are buried in the periosteum. Some surgeons prefer a wire closure device (Fig. 9-5) that uses locking plates and a crimper to close the wires. When this is used, it is important to avoid entangling temporary pacing wires and drapes in the device.
4. Linea alba fascia is closed with nonabsorbable suture in an interrupted stitch. Subcutaneous tissue and skin are closed with absorbable suture; occasionally staples may be used on the skin (a staple remover must accompany the patient).

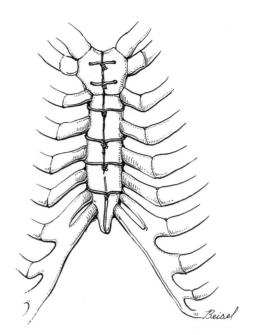

FIGURE 9-4   Sternal closure with stainless steel wire. The first wire is placed through the manubrium, and remaining wires are placed around the sternal body. Wires may also be placed through the sternum. (From Waldhausen JA, Pierce WS, Campbell DB: *Surgery of the chest,* ed 6, St Louis, 1996, Mosby.)

Weak sternums

In osteoporotic or otherwise weak, unstable sternums, additional methods may be employed to bolster the closure. Nylon bands (Parham bands) or wide metal bands (Fig. 9-6) may be passed around the sternum and secured with metal plates. Another technique is to thread extra-long sternal wires vertically down and back along the lateral sternal borders (Fig. 9-7). The transverse wires are then inserted around the vertical wires so that when the sternum is approximated, the transverse wires do not cut through the sternum because they are buttressed by the vertical wires (Robicsek, Daugherty, and Cook, 1977; Waldhausen, Pierce, and Campbell, 1996). A third technique to reduce the possibility of cutting through the bone is to place two or more heavy (No. 5) polyester sutures between the wires. (If these patients require emergency sternotomy, scissors, as well as wire cutters, will be necessary to open the sternum.)

Delayed sternal closure

Delayed sternal closure may be indicated in patients with a distended heart that is unable to tolerate compression, causing hypotension and reduced cardiac output. Occasionally, delayed closure is also necessary in patients whose impaired clotting mechanisms pose a risk of cardiac tamponade in the early postoperative period. When the decision to delay closure is made in the

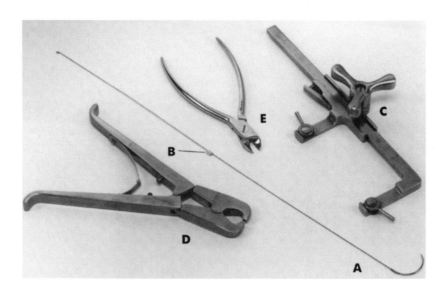

FIGURE 9-5 Pilling-Wolvek sternal approximator and fixation system. The sternal wire **(A)** is inserted into each side of the sternum and the needle is removed with wire cutters **(E).** Each end of the wire is placed through a locking plate **(B)** so that the wires are crossed over the outer sternum. The ends of the wires are then separately secured into an arm of the approximator **(C).** As the knob is turned clockwise, the arms move wider apart, tightening the wire around the bone. The crimper **(D)** is applied to the locking plate and closed tightly to crimp the plate and secure the wires. The excess wire is removed with the wire cutter. (Courtesy Pilling Co., Fort Washington, Pa.)

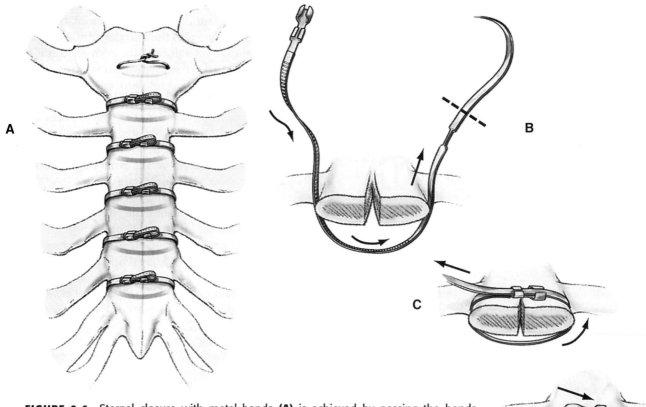

FIGURE 9-6 Sternal closure with metal bands **(A)** is achieved by passing the bands around the sternum **(B).** The metal loop is tightened **(C)** and the end of the band is secured **(D).** (From Buxton B and others: Basic surgical techniques. In Buxton B, Frazier OH, Westaby S, editors: *Ischemic heart disease: surgical management,* London, 1999, Mosby.)

operating room (OR), the sternum is left open, but the overlying skin edges are sutured together. In some cases an oval patch cut from a sterile Esmarch rubber bandage is sewn to the skin edges to cover the open wound, or a sterile adhesive drape is applied over the sternal opening. Previously placed anterior mediastinal tubes drain the pericardium.

The patient is transferred from the OR to the surgical intensive care unit (SICU). After cardiac function improves and the heart size decreases or correction of

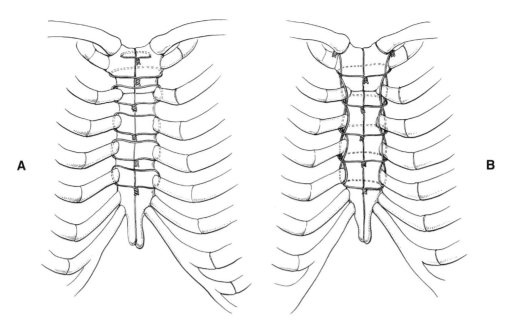

FIGURE 9-7 Two methods of wire closure for brittle, thin, or fragile sternums. **A,** Box wiring distributes the force of the wires more diffusely and limits the possibility of the wires cutting through the bone. **B,** To prevent or correct sternal separation, the sternal wires are threaded along each side of the sternum. Transverse wires are placed around the vertical wires, which act as a bolster to prevent the transverse wires from cutting through the bone. (From Waldhausen JA, Pierce WS, Campbell DB: *Surgery of the chest,* ed 6, St Louis, 1996, Mosby.)

the bleeding diathesis has been achieved, the patient is returned to the OR for chest closure.

Repeat sternotomy

The number of patients, especially those with coronary artery disease who have had coronary artery bypass grafting (CABG), undergoing repeat sternotomy is increasing, largely because of the progression of their atherosclerotic heart disease in both the native coronary arteries and the bypass grafts (Lytle, 1999). Reoperation is associated with an increased morbidity and mortality, which is in part the result of the dangers encountered during reopening of the sternum (Buxton, Goldblatt, and Komeda, 1999). To avoid reopening the sternum in patients with limited grafting requirements (e.g., the need to revascularize a right coronary artery or a circumflex coronary artery), the surgeon may employ a right or left anterior thoracotomy (Anderson and Milano, 2001).

As part of the healing process after initial sternotomy, dense adhesions form between the pericardium, the great vessels, the retrosternum, and, in CABG patients, the bypass conduits. The severity of these adhesions is usually apparent on the lateral chest x-ray film (which should be available in the operating room for review by the surgeon). Occasionally there is a retrosternal space that will allow passage of a sternal saw such as that shown in Fig. 9-1, but very often dense adhesions necessitate

the use of an oscillating saw to divide the sternum from the anterior table down to the posterior table. Another technique used by some surgeons anticipating repeat operation (e.g., in young patients undergoing open mitral commissurotomy) is partial closure of the pericardium at the time of the first operation. This technique can reduce the amount of adhesions that form without obstructing pericardial drainage.

Procedural considerations

Because there is a risk of massive hemorrhage from laceration of the structures below the sternum (in particular, the right ventricle, great vessels, and patent bypass grafts), both sides of the groin should be prepared and draped as part of the sterile field. The surgeon may then expose the femoral vessels for cannulation. Bypass lines should be ready so that CPB can be instituted quickly if necessary. If extensive bleeding is encountered, the patient can be placed on femoral bypass (described later in this chapter). The patient must be given heparin before CPB is instituted. Femoral bypass can reduce blood loss and the risk of myocardial ischemia and allow shed blood to be reinfused; it also decompresses the heart and facilitates dissection of the pericardial adhesions.

Operative procedure

1. The skin incision is made along the previous incision; scar tissue may be excised.

2. Cautery is used to dissect the subcutaneous tissue and to expose the sternal wires. The lower fascial closure is reopened, and the retrosternal area is evaluated.

3. The exposed wires are cut or untwisted.

4A. The wires are removed with a wire twister (or Kocher clamp). A reciprocating saw (see Fig. 9-1) or an oscillating saw is used to divide the sternum.

4B. The wires are not removed, and the free ends of the wire are retracted upwardly to elevate the sternum away from mediastinal structures. An oscillating saw is used to divide the sternum; the retained wires serve as a barrier to the saw blade as it cuts through the posterior table of the sternum (Buxton, Goldblatt, and Komeda, 1999). The wires are removed after the bone is divided.

5. After the bone is cut, the sternal edges are retracted gently with rakes (or other preferred retractors) and the tissue between the retrosternum and the pericardium is divided with a knife or scissors. The sternal retractor is not inserted until the heart is freed from the sternum to lessen the risk of tearing attached cardiac structures.

6. Once the heart is freed from the sternum, dissection proceeds along the diaphragmatic surface of the heart, where a relatively free plane may be found. Dissection then continues around the right atrium and the right ventricle and over the aorta and pulmonary artery (Fig. 9-8). If serious bleeding is encountered, CPB can be instituted.

7. After the heart is freed sufficiently, the surgeon can cannulate for CPB (see later section). After CPB is instituted and the heart is decompressed, left ventricular adhesions can be dissected more easily.

Sternal infection

Infection of the sternum may range from suprasternal soft tissue infection, which is usually responsive to debridement, antibiotics, drainage, and superficial wound care, to deep wound infection causing mediastinitis and requiring more extensive treatment.

The development of wound complications is related to repeat sternotomy, surgical technique, reoperation for bleeding, off-midline sternotomy, excessive use of cautery or bone wax, duration of operation, prolonged CPB, external cardiac massage, prolonged mechanical ventilation, infected hospital personnel, and contaminated hospital equipment (ventilators). Other predisposing factors include a history of diabetes (associated with poor wound healing), bilateral internal mammary artery (IMA) harvest (the IMA provides the primary blood supply to the sternum), preexisting infection, immunosuppression (e.g., steroids or other antirejection transplantation medications), age over 60 years, obesity, postoperative low car-

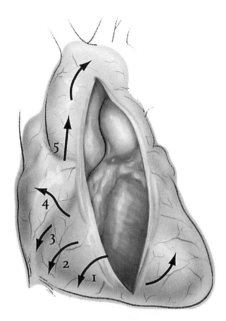

FIGURE 9-8 Mobilization of the pericardium during repeat sternotomy. Dissection begins at the diaphragmatic surface and continues over the right ventricle, right atrium, and aorta. (From Buxton B, Goldblatt J, Komeda M: Reoperation. In Buxton B, Frazier OH, Westaby S, editors: *Ischemic heart disease: surgical management,* London, 1999, Mosby.)

diac output, and chronic pulmonary insufficiency (Francel and Kouchoukos, 2001b).

Staphylococcus species (*S. aureus, S. epidermis*) are responsible for the majority of sternal infections (Combes and others, 2001; Risnes and others, 2001); wound contamination by skin flora during or just after surgery has been identified as the main route of sternal infection in this setting (Combes and others, 2001). Other infecting agents include *Pseudomonas, Acinetobacter,* and *Candida albicans.*

Superficial wound complications occur in approximately 2% of patients undergoing sternotomy (Francel and Kouchoukos, 2001b). Presenting symptoms often include local tenderness, erythema, or serous drainage; the presence of fever, chills, and leukocytosis suggest a deeper infection. Minor infections involve only the subcutaneous tissues, and in some cases they can be managed by drainage, antibiotics, and dressings (Flood and Johnstone, 1999). If patients have an undiagnosed fever, an unstable sternum, or a retrosternal collection of fluid (as seen on computed tomography [CT] scan), the sternum should be reopened and assessed to determine if more serious infection is present. Fig. 9-9 represents a decision tree for determining the care of patients with wound problems.

The presence of purulent drainage and mobile sternal fragments often signals deep mediastinal infection. Mediastinitis occurs in approximately 1% to 4% of procedures, and it may be seen within the first postoperative week or 2 weeks or more after the initial operation (Francel and Kouchoukos, 2001b). Signs and symptoms include sternal pain (or pain with breathing), fever, leukocytosis, erythema, tenderness, and wound drainage. Although the incidence of mediastinitis is low, mortality (20% to 50%) and morbidity (approximately 50%) is high. The additional cost of hospitalization for mediastinitis can be more than $60,000 (Francel and Kouchoukos, 2001b).

The patient is brought to the OR. Loose sternal wires are removed, and debridement of all infected bone and

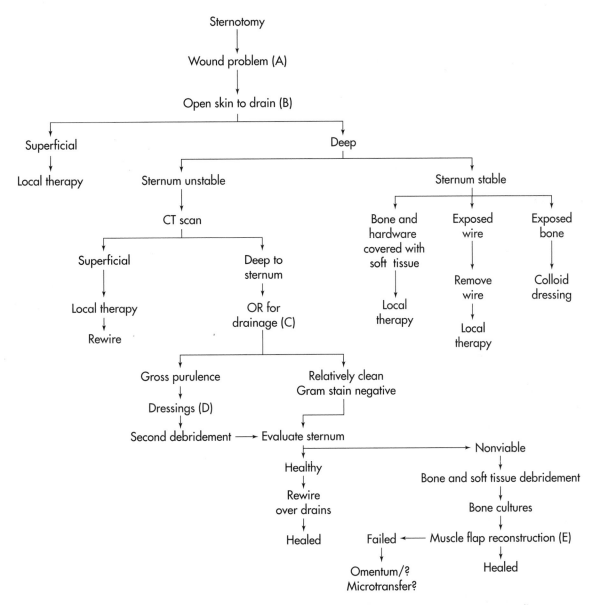

FIGURE 9-9 Decision tree that diagrams the evaluation process for a patient postmediasternotomy. The diagram shows the importance of sternal stability in the eventual care of the patient. *A,* Wound problems include localized erythema and drainage or systemic signs (increased white blood cells, fever, chills, lethargy). *B,* Culturing all drainage helps dictate correct antibiotic therapy. *C,* Requires debridement, cultures, and evaluation of mediastinum for area of undrained sepsis. *D,* Beware of risk for right ventricular laceration. *E,* Choice of donor muscle is dependent on the volume of the mediastinal defect, except ipsilateral rectus, which may not be immediately available after internal mammary artery harvest. (From Francel TJ, Kouchoukos NT: A rational approach to wound difficulties after sternotomy: the problem, *Ann Thorac Surg* 72:1411, 2001.)

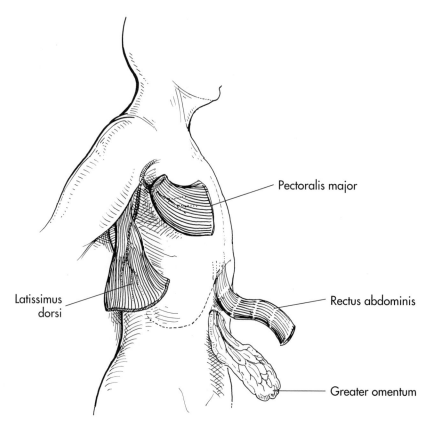

Pectoralis major

Rectus abdominis

Latissimus dorsi

Greater omentum

FIGURE 9-10 Chest wall and abdominal muscles and omentum, each of which can be rotated into the chest on a vascularized pedicle to repair sternal wound defects. (From Waldhausen JA, Pierce WS, Campbell DB: *Surgery of the chest*, ed 6, St Louis, 1996, Mosby.)

surrounding tissue of questionable viability is performed. Complete debridement of infected and necrotic bone and tissue must be performed to avoid the risk of recurrent infection (Rand and others, 1998). Careful inspection of the mediastinum is performed, cultures of tissue and fluid are obtained, and appropriate antibiotic therapy is instituted. Closed chest catheter irrigation with vancomycin or betadine antibiotic solutions (for staphylococcal or mixed bacterial cultures, respectively) may be used (Francel and Kouchoukos, 2001a). A catheter connected to the antibiotic solution is placed in the pericardium to infuse the medication (at a rate of approximately 100 ml per hour), and two drainage tubes are placed in the pericardium to drain the irrigation solution into a discard fluid container (De Feo and others, 2001). Chest closure must be secure; the method originally developed by Robicsek (Robicsek, Daugherty, and Cook, 1977) and shown in Fig. 9-7, *B* may be used.

If there is excessive remaining dead space separating the mediastinal structures and the posterior table of the sternum, it should be obliterated so that healing can occur. Patients with prosthetic material (whether pledgets

or prosthetic vascular grafts) pose special challenges. Excess pledget material can be trimmed; prostheses incorporated into healthy tissue can remain undisturbed. In cases of mediastinitis involving foreign material (such as that incorporated into an aortic root or ascending aortic aneurysm repair), removal of the prosthetic material may be impossible; Francel and Kouchoukos (2001b) recommend irrigating the prosthetic material with vancomycin antibiotic solution and wrapping the vascular graft with an omental pedicle flap (described later) to encase the graft with healthy, vascularized tissue.

Tissue flap wound closure

The pectoralis, rectus abdominus, and latissimus dorsi muscles and the omentum have been used as flaps individually or in combination to eradicate mediastinal dead space and to close sternal wounds (Fig. 9-10; Table 9-2). Latissimus dorsi muscle generally is used only if other muscles have failed or are unavailable (Francel and Kouchoukos, 2001a). The pectoralis muscle may be the only suitable graft in patients who have had ab-

TABLE 9-2
Flap Selection

FLAP	ADVANTAGES/INDICATIONS	DISADVANTAGES/CONTRAINDICATIONS
Pectoralis turnover	Large bulk of muscle Fills upper and lower defects Can be used after ITA taken Minimal donor site effects	Muscle flap may be less reliable and lateral intercostal perforators must be preserved if the ITA has been harvested as a conduit
Pectoralis advancement	Fills central defects Independent of ITA	Does not reach lower half
Rectus abdominis	Adequate for lower half Upper end may be bipedicled with pectoralis	Less vascular if ITA taken Weakens abdominal wall Doubles wound dimensions Restricts ventilation
Omentum	Fills defect wall (reaches neck) Independent of ITA	Abdominal wound Variable bulk (thinner patients)
Latissimus dorsi free flap	Excellent bulk and vascularity Minimal donor site defect	Patients must be turned Microsurgical anastomosis

ITA, Internal thoracic artery.
From Buxton B, Frazer OH, Westaby S: *Ischemic heart disease: surgical management,* London, 1999, Mosby.

dominal surgery involving the rectus muscles and omentum. The use of one or both IMAs for CABG also affects the choice of muscle flaps.

An important consideration in the selection of reconstructive techniques is the depth of the mediastinal defect. The omentum and the rectus flaps provide greater bulk; less deep defects may be filled with either a rectus muscle alone or with a pectoralis muscle flap detached from the humerus to enable rotation into the defect.

Operative procedure: flap closure of the sternum (Francel and Kouchoukos, 2001a; Flood and Johnstone, 1998)

1. The patient is placed in the supine position with the arms at the sides.
2. The entire chest and abdomen are prepared.
3. Skin edges and subcutaneous tissue of the sternotomy are debrided, and approximately 1 to 2 mm of tissue along the edges is excised.
4. Sternal bone edges are debrided with rongeurs and curettes until bleeding from healthy tissue is encountered. Exposed costal cartilages are resected to prevent their becoming a nidus for infection.
5. Fibrinous exudate is removed from the surface of the heart.
6. The wound is irrigated and hemostasis is achieved.
7. The surgical team changes gowns and gloves, and a new set of instruments replaces those used during the first part of the procedure.
8A. Pectoralis muscle flap (Fig. 9-11): The skin and subcutaneous tissue are elevated off the pectoralis major muscle digitally and with cautery. The subpectoral plane can be opened laterally over the pectoralis minor to mobilize the pectoralis major.

The pectoralis major is advanced to cover the sternal defect. When bilateral pectoralis muscle flaps are used, they remain inserted on the humerus, and the muscle origins are advanced into the sternal defect.

8B. Rectus abdominus flap (Fig. 9-12): The midline sternal incision is extended inferiorly over the rectus muscle to be harvested.

The anterior rectus sheath is divided and peeled back to expose the rectus muscle. The muscle is elevated digitally from the posterior sheath, and the inferior epigastric pedicle is ligated and divided. An absolute contraindication to the use of the rectus muscle includes previous subcostal incisions, which, in combination with inferior epigastric artery ligation, produce an avascular rectus muscle that cannot heal (Francel and Kouchoukos, 2001a).

The inferior portion of the muscle is rotated superiorly up to the chest; intercostal bundles are ligated as encountered.

The flap is attached to the wound, and the rectus sheath is repaired carefully with heavy nonabsorbable suture in order to avoid subsequent hernia formation (Flood and Johnstone, 1999).

8C. Omental flap (Fig. 9-13): Omentum is useful when both IMAs have been used, when the sternal defect is extensive, and when exposed prosthetic great vessel grafts need to be covered (Francel and Kouchoukos, 2001a).

The midline sternal incision is extended, and the omentum is mobilized. Omental attachments to the transverse colon are divided. Gastroepiploic artery continuity is maintained to provide a blood supply to the flap.

The flap is transferred subcutaneously or transdiaphragmatically into the mediastinum.

A nasogastric tube is inserted to decompress the stomach and duodenum, to avoid compression of the pedicle, and to avoid gastric outlet obstruction.

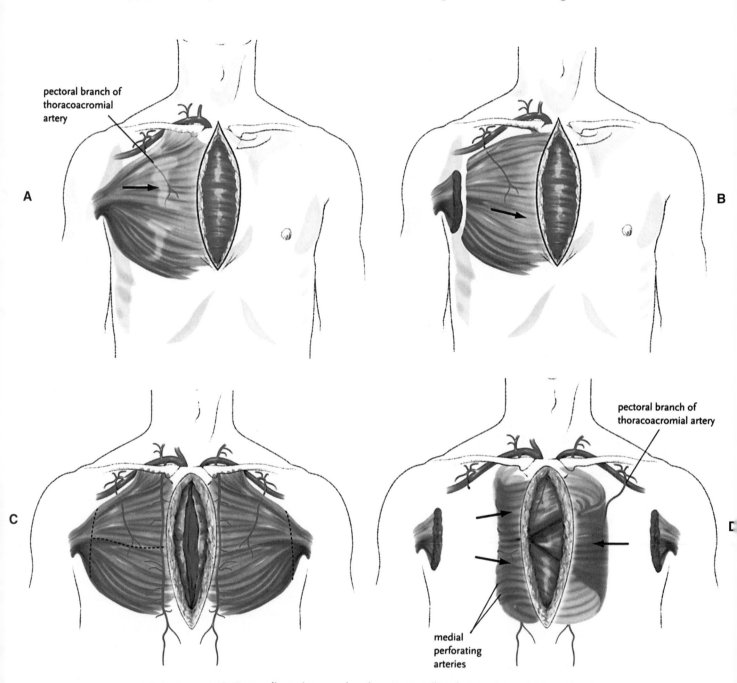

FIGURE 9-11 **A,** Pectoralis major muscle advancement flap, leaving humeral insertion intact. **B,** Pectoralis island flap. **C,** Lines of division for pectoralis major muscle flaps. **D,** The right pectoralis major is pedicled on medial perforators, split along the line of its fibers, and turned over into the sternotomy defect. The left pectoralis major has been pedicled on the thoracoacromial artery to fill the central defect before skin closure. (From Flood S, Johnstone B: Reconstruction of the sternum. In Buxton B, Frazier OH, Westaby S, editors: *Ischemic heart disease surgical management,* London, 1999, Mosby.)

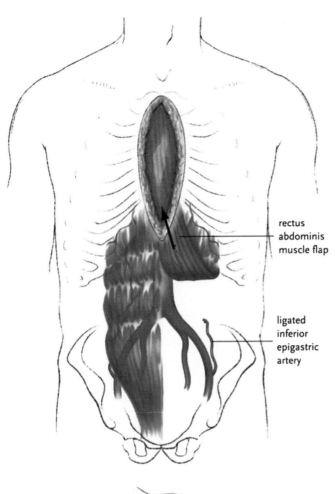

FIGURE 9-12 Rectus abdominus muscle flap is rotated superiorly to fill the sternal defect. (From Flood S, Johnstone B: Reconstruction of the sternum. In Buxton B, Frazier OH, Westaby S, editors: *Ischemic heart disease: surgical management,* London, 1999, Mosby.)

rectus abdominis muscle flap

ligated inferior epigastric artery

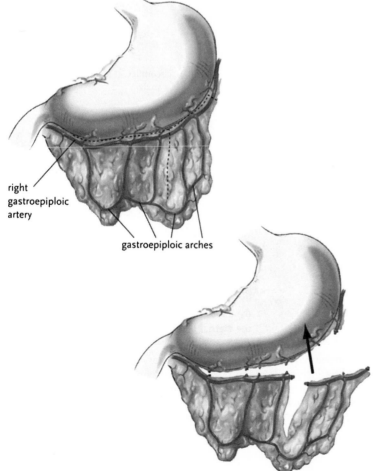

right gastroepiploic artery

gastroepiploic arches

FIGURE 9-13 The omentum is freed from its attachment to the gastroepiploic vessels, the greater curvature of the stomach, the transverse colon, and the mesocolon. The omentum may be lengthened, maintaining its viability, using the incisions shown *(below).* (From Flood S, Johnstone B: Reconstruction of the sternum. In Buxton B, Frazier OH, Westaby S, editors: *Ischemic heart disease: surgical management,* London, 1999, Mosby.)

9. The subcutaneous tissue of the chest wall is elevated, and the flaps are secured in position with absorbable interrupted sutures.

10. Soft drainage tubes are placed to drain the flaps and the donor beds.

11. The skin is closed primarily. Occasionally skin grafting may be necessary to close the incision.

Postoperatively, early cessation of mechanical ventilation encourages more rapid healing because there is less positive pressure and chest movement. Shoulder activity (e.g., pushing against the bed railing) should be limited in patients with pectoralis flap; bending or lifting should be avoided in patients with rectus flaps. Nutrition is especially important for adequate healing (Francel and Kouchoukos, 2001a).

OTHER THORACIC INCISIONS

Although median sternotomy is the most widely used incision, other thoracic approaches are necessary for certain lesions (see Table 9-1). These include the anterolateral (Fig. 9-14), lateral, posterolateral (Fig. 9-15), subxiphoid, and thoracoabdominal incisions (see Chapter 14 on surgery for the thoracic aorta).

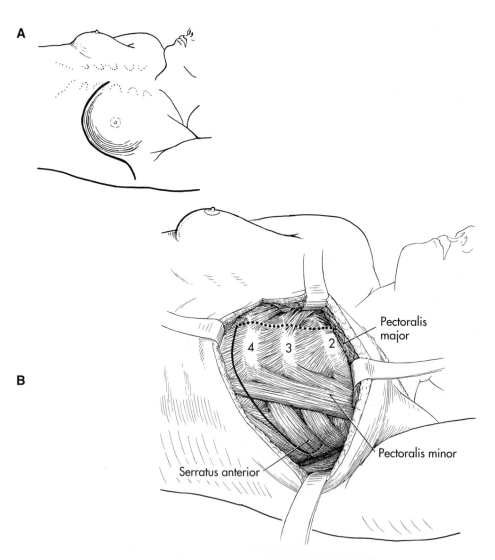

FIGURE 9-14 Anterolateral thoracotomy. Incision: **A,** In women a submammary incision is preferable to avoid breast scars. In men the incision is made over the interspace to be entered. For minimal access surgery the skin flap and incision are less extensive than shown. **B,** The major muscles and the ribs *(numbered)* are shown. (From Waldhausen JA, Pierce WS, Campbell DB: *Surgery of the chest,* ed 6, St Louis, 1996, Mosby.)

Continued

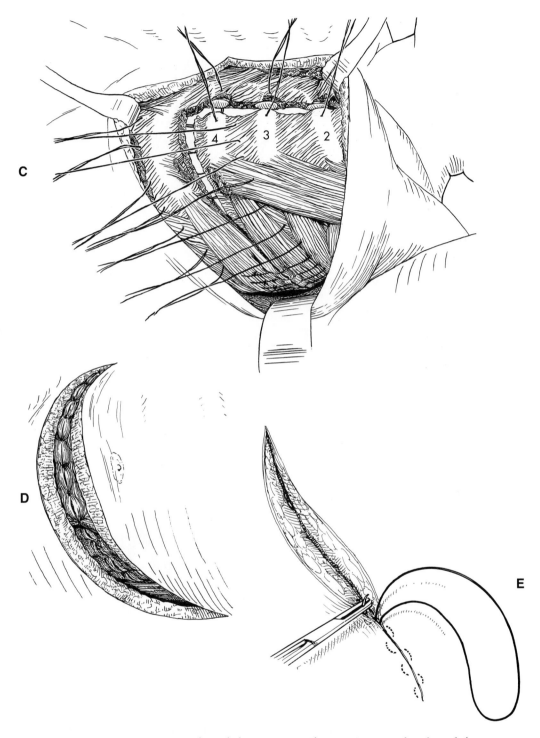

FIGURE 9-14, cont'd Anterolateral thoracotomy. Closure: **C,** Approximation of the pectoralis major is performed with interrupted or running sutures. **D,** Superficial fascia and subcutaneous tissue are closed. **E,** The skin is closed with a running *(shown)* or a subcuticular technique. (From Waldhausen JA, Pierce WS, Campbell DB: *Surgery of the chest,* ed 6, St Louis, 1996, Mosby.)

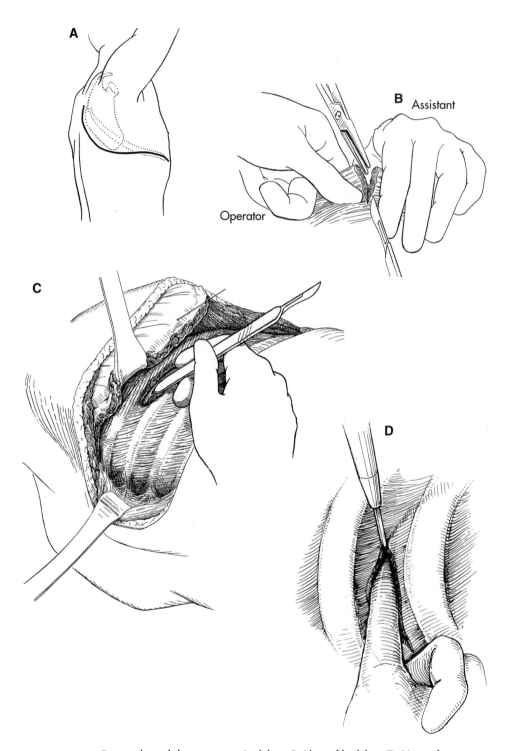

FIGURE 9-15 Posterolateral thoracotomy. Incision: **A,** Line of incision. **B,** Manual pressure is used to control bleeding while the surgeon incises through the chest muscles. **C,** The chest is entered through the fourth or fifth intercostal space. **D,** Scissors are used to open the interspace. The index finger is inserted to protect the lung. (From Waldhausen JA, Pierce WS, Campbell DB: *Surgery of the chest,* ed 6, St Louis, 1996, Mosby.)

Continued

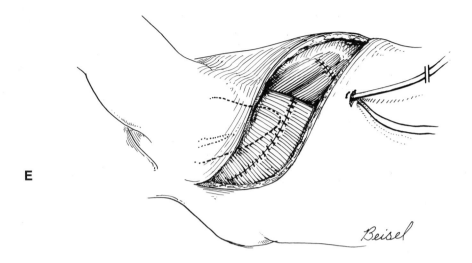

E

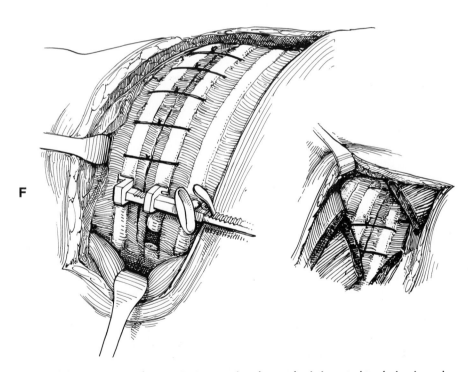

F

FIGURE 9-15, cont'd Closure: **E,** An anterior chest tube is inserted to drain air, and a posterior tube is inserted to drain fluid. A rib approximator can be used to assist with tying of the pericostal sutures. **F,** The chest wall muscles are closed in layers. (From Waldhausen JA, Pierce WS, Campbell DB: *Surgery of the chest,* ed 6, St Louis, 1996, Mosby.)

Exposure of the distal portion of the transverse aortic arch and the descending thoracic aorta is achieved best with a left posterolateral incision. Aneurysms of the distal thoracic aorta extending into the abdominal aorta may be approached with the left side of the chest tilted at a 45-degree angle (antero-lateral position) and the lower portion of the torso supine. Subxiphoid incisions have been used for peri-cardial drainage and the insertion of pacemaker electrodes.

Cardiopulmonary Bypass

Most cardiac operations rely on extracorporeal circulation to perfuse the body so that the heart is stopped for precise and accurate repair. Relying on a beating heart to pump blood to the kidneys and the brain is unfeasible for surgeries, such as mitral valve replacement, that require opening one or more of the cardiac chambers. For procedures that do not require opening the heart (such as CABG), nonbypass (off-pump) procedures have become popular; however, the steep learning curve associated with nonbypass techniques prevents the widespread adoption of off-pump procedures. Consequently, CABG continues to be performed with the use of CPB. Undoubtedly the use of off-pump techniques will continue to grow, but it is likely that for patients with complex, ischemic lesions of the coronary arteries, as well as valvular, congenital, and aneurysmal lesions, there will continue to be an important and necessary role for cardiopulmonary bypass.

The idea that blood could be infused into organs to maintain their viability had been suggested in the early part of the nineteenth century. But the development of the modern-day heart-lung machine could not have become a reality without the work of researchers whose discoveries provided the theoretic and scientific basis for extracorporeal circulation (Table 9-3). The most notable achievement was Gibbon's (1954) development of the first heart-lung machine to be used in humans.

Gibbon's contribution was to provide a method of perfusing the organs without relying on the heart and the lungs. By diverting venous return to a device that could remove carbon dioxide and add oxygen, and then propel the oxygen-saturated blood back into the body, the use of CPB enabled clinicians to isolate the heart and lungs from the rest of the body. In addition, because oxygenation and ventilation (removal of carbon dioxide) were achieved with a mechanical lung, the patient's own lungs could be deflated and allowed to fall back out of the way of the surgical site.

The heart and the other organs of the body are more tolerant of anoxia than is the brain. With a method to perfuse the brain while the heart was arrested, surgeons were no longer limited to a 6-minute period or less of

TABLE 9-3
Selected Advances and Discoveries Facilitating the Development of Cardiopulmonary Bypass

ADVANCE/DISCOVERY	PERIOD
Blood transfusion	Early 1800s
Antiseptic surgery	1860s
Mechanical oxygenation of blood	1860s
Direct suture of heart	1890s
ABO blood compatibility	1900
Endotracheal thoracic anesthesia	Early 1900s
Blood vessel surgery	Early 1900s
Development of plastics	Early 1900s
Discovery of heparin	1916
Elucidation of acid-base balance	1920s
Discovery of antibiotics	1920s
Elucidation of shock	1930s
Titration of protamine sulfate	1940s
Defibrillation (internal)	1940s
Measurement of intracardiac pressures	1940s
Clinical use of hypothermia	1940s
Understanding of metabolic effects of surgery	Early 1950s
First clinical use of a heart-lung machine	1953
Use of cross-circulation (using parent to act as biologic oxygenator for child)	Early 1950s
Azygos (low-flow) principle: heart and brain can be sustained with reduced blood flow (e.g., when SVC and IVC are occluded and only azygos venous return contributes to preload and cardiac output)	1950s

Modified from Johnson SL: *The history of cardiac surgery 1896-1955,* Baltimore, 1970, Johns Hopkins Press; Shumacker HB: *The evolution of cardiac surgery,* Bloomington, 1992, Indiana University Press; Westaby S: *Landmarks in cardiac surgery,* Oxford, UK, 1997, Isis Medical Media. *IVC,* Inferior vena cava; *SVC,* superior vena cava.

cerebral anoxia during which they had to complete intracardiac repairs. Gibbon (1954) demonstrated this by using CPB in an 18-year-old girl who underwent a 26-minute period of normothermic cardiac arrest—considerably longer than the 6-minute period tolerated by the ischemic brain—while the operation was performed. By combining the already-familiar technique of hypothermia with CPB, other researchers were able to prolong safely the period of ischemia.

HYPOTHERMIA

Before the introduction of CPB, topical hypothermia was used to arrest the heart during surgery. Studies by Bigelow, Lindsay, and Greenwood (1950) had shown that, like hibernating animals, humans could lower their metabolic rate and oxygen consumption when their body temperature was reduced. Hypothermia alone, however, proved unreliable because of the attendant risks of ventricular fibrillation and the relatively short period during which surgery could be performed

TABLE **9-4**
Components of the Bypass System

COMPONENT	PURPOSE/MECHANISM
Pump	Move fluid throughout extracorporeal circuit
Roller pump	Uses positive displacement with rotating roller head to propel fluid; amount of flow is dependent on degree that tubing is occluded and on number of revolutions per minute; additional roller heads are used for cardiotomy suctions and venting catheters
Centrifugal pump	Transforms potential energy generated by electromagnetic forces into kinetic energy; vortex principle
Pneumatic and electrical pumps	Used primarily as cardiac assistive or replacement devices (see Chapter 15)
Oxygenator	Performs gas exchange functions; provides oxygen, removes carbon dioxide; contains an arterial reservoir
Membrane	Uses a semipermeable membrane through which oxygen diffuses into and carbon dioxide diffuses out of desaturated blood; no direct blood-gas interface exists; less trauma to blood than with bubble method; preferred method, especially for long bypass runs
Bubble	Injects oxygen directly through a column of blood; direct blood-gas interface exists, and gas bubbles are formed that must be removed in defoaming section; traumatic to blood elements; contributes to protein denaturation and formation of microemboli
Heat exchanger	Used to alter temperature of blood by principle of conduction; may be freestanding or, more commonly, incorporated into oxygenator system
Venous reservoir	Collects venous return and stores excess volume; may be incorporated into oxygenator system
Blood filters	Inserted into arterial line to remove gas and particulate emboli
Cardiotomy suction/venting devices	Suction used to aspirate blood from operative site and return to cardiotomy reservoir; intracardiac vent used to decompress cardiac chambers and to aspirate air and blood that is returned to cardiotomy reservoir; aspirated blood is filtered and returned to venous reservoir and oxygenator
Cardioplegia infusion system	Used to cool and deliver cardioplegia solution; uses a separate roller head; when blood cardioplegia is used, system is connected to arterial blood supply
Ultrafiltration device	Removes excess water from perfusate
Bypass tubing	Made from polyvinylchloride or Silastic; thickness and caliber of tubing vary depending on its use (e.g., arterial or venous lines, suction lines); heparin-coated tubing has advantage of making inner surfaces of bypass circuit more blood compatible and reducing inflammatory responses associated with bypass
Priming solution	Often a balanced salt solution, pH corrected, that will produce hemodilution with a hematocrit of 20% to 25%; extra heparin, albumin, and various other ingredients may be added; whole blood is not used unless patient is small or severely anemic
Safety mechanisms	To reduce or prevent complications and injury; include air bubble detectors, filters, arterial and venous oxygen saturation sensors, vents, pressure sensors, shutoff valves
Monitoring devices	To measure blood pressure, flow rates, blood oxygen and carbon dioxide levels, pH, electrolytes, temperature

Modified from Bell PE, Diffee GT: Cardiopulmonary bypass, *AORN J* 53(6):1480, 1991; Westaby S: Cardiopulmonary bypass for coronary artery surgery. In Buxton B, Frazier OH, Westaby S: *Ischemic heart diseases: surgical management,* London, 1999, Mosby.

without incurring irreversible cerebral anoxia. Sealy, Brown, and Young (1958) were among the first to combine the use of hypothermia with extracorporeal circulation, and their work, along with that of many others, enhanced the safety of CPB and paved the way for the techniques of hypothermic circulatory arrest and myocardial preservation.

CARDIOPULMONARY BYPASS CIRCUIT

Even though there are adverse effects associated with its use, present-day CPB is safer and more efficient than the early heart-lung machines. Components of the CPB system are listed in Table 9-4. Venous blood is drained from the right side of the heart via the superior vena cava (SVC) and the inferior vena cava (IVC), arterial-

ized in the oxygenator, and pumped back into the systemic circulation (Fig. 9-16). To prevent thrombosis within the bypass circuit from exposure of the blood to foreign surfaces, the circulatory system is anticoagulated with heparin. Heparin-coated circuits may reduce the amount of additional heparin required, but the safety of reducing heparin levels has not been established; heparin-coated circuits lessen the activation of complements (Galloway and others, 1999a).

Heparin and protamine sulfate

Heparin. Heparin, made from bovine lung tissue or porcine intestinal mucosa, prevents the formation of blood clots by producing a conformational change in antithrombin III and converting it to a rapid inhibitor of factor V and factor VIII. This in turn inhibits the

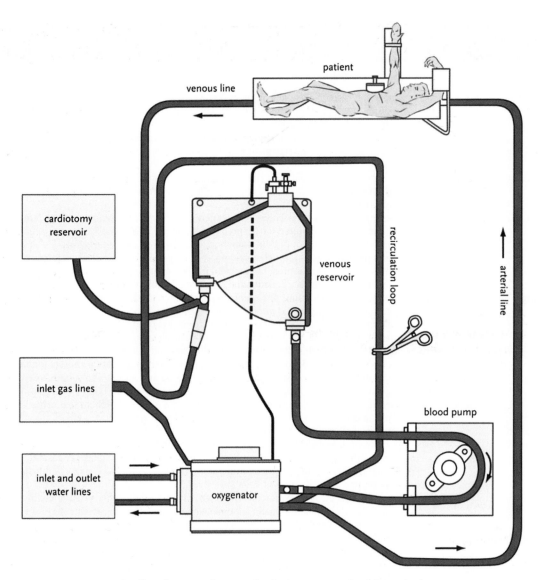

FIGURE 9-16 Cardiopulmonary bypass circuit (see text and Table 9-4). (From Buxton B, Frazier OH, Westaby S, editors: *Ischemic heart disease: surgical management,* London, 1999, Mosby.)

conversion of prothrombin to thrombin and fibrinogen to fibrin (see Fig. 4-14).

Heparin prolongs whole-blood clotting time, thrombin time, partial thromboplastin time, and prothrombin time and has a platelet-inhibiting effect. It is given before cannulation for CPB or before clamping of blood vessels (e.g., for CPB or during harvesting of the IMA). The initial bolus is approximately 300 international units (IU) per kg (100 units = approximately 1 mg). Thus a patient weighing 70 kg would receive a heparin dose of 21,000 units (or approximately 210 mg). Heparin may be given by the surgeon directly into the right atrium or by the anesthesiologist through a central venous line. Peripheral venous infusion is not recommended because if CPB must be instituted rapidly, thereby curtailing the time required to measure the blood anticoagulation levels, there is less certainty that the heparin has reached the central circulation (Waldhausen, Pierce and Campbell, 1996).

To determine whether the blood is adequately heparinized, the activating clotting time (ACT) is measured about 3 minutes after heparin infusion but before CPB is initiated. A baseline ACT, taken at the start of surgery, often is used for comparison, especially in the presence of coagulation abnormalities. (Because the ACT monitors coagulation but not heparin levels, some clinicians also measure heparin concentration.) Although there is some controversy over the appropriate ACT necessary to initiate CPB safely, a minimum ACT of 400 seconds (four times normal) generally is considered necessary. During bypass, periodic ACTs are measured, and additional heparin is given to maintain the ACT between 400 and 600 seconds (Westaby, 1999). When aprotinin is used, a longer ACT should be achieved.

Occasionally it is difficult to achieve adequate anticoagulation with heparin. Some patients on prolonged preoperative heparin regimens demonstrate heparin resistance; the reasons for this are not entirely clear, but increasing the heparin level is usually effective. Inadequate anticoagulation also may be the result of significantly depressed antithrombin III levels; this produces an insufficient amount of the factor for the heparin to affect. Infusion of fresh frozen plasma (FFP) may be necessary to increase the antithrombin III levels.

Protamine sulfate. In the absence of heparin, protamine sulfate acts as a mild anticoagulant, but in the presence of heparin, it acts as an antidote to the anticoagulant. Protamine is strongly basic, and it combines with the strongly acidic heparin to form a stable complex. A dosage of 3 mg/kg of protamine usually is administered. The ACT and the calculated heparin dose response are used to guide additional protamine infusion.

Protamine infusion, especially when bolused, is associated with systemic hypotension, thought to be caused by arterial vasodilation and decreased systemic vascular resistance. In the worst cases a full anaphylactic reaction may occur. Some surgeons may prefer not to remove the arterial cannula before or immediately after the initiation of protamine infusion so that, if necessary, volume may be given to maintain an adequate blood pressure or CPB can be resumed if myocardial function is too depressed (additional heparin may be required to reinstitute bypass). If a serious protamine reaction is going to occur, it is usually apparent shortly after the infusion is started. When minimal or no reaction is evident and the blood pressure is stable, the arterial cannula is removed.

Total and partial cardiopulmonary bypass

Total CPB exists when all the systemic venous drainage is returned to the oxygenator. This necessitates individual cannulation of the SVC and IVC, with the addition of a tourniquet or caval clamp placed around each of these vessels and tightened against the cannulas within them. This forces all returning systemic venous blood to enter the distal ends of the cannulas. Coronary sinus drainage and bronchial return entering the heart can be removed with an intracardiac venting catheter.

Partial CPB exists when some venous return is allowed to enter the right atrium. This can occur when only one (e.g., two-stage) cannula is placed in the right

atrium, or when bicaval cannulas are inserted into the SVC and IVC but tourniquets or caval clamps are not used, allowing some returning blood to drain around the distal ends of the cannulas and into the right atrium. Coronary sinus blood drains into the holes in the mid-portion of the two-stage venous cannula.

Pumps and oxygenators

Various types of pumps have been designed to propel blood, but the roller pump (a positive displacement pump) and the centrifugal pump (a constrained vortex pump) are the most widely used. Unlike the body's normal hemodynamics, nonpulsatile (i.e., no systolic or diastolic phases) flow usually is produced by these pumps. (The roller pump can be modified to provide pulsatile flow.) Although there does not seem to be a significant increase in morbidity from nonpulsatile flow, the potential advantages of pulsatile flow have increased interest in its use. Among these advantages are increased flow in the microcirculation, reduced volume overloading, and improved renal, cerebral, and pancreatic blood flow.

Membrane oxygenators have largely replaced bubble oxygenators because of the absence of a direct blood-gas interface. This offers the advantages of less blood cell trauma, reduced incidence of air emboli (especially microemboli), and independent control of oxygenation and ventilation. The absence of a direct blood-gas interface also reduces complement activation (Galloway and others, 1999a).

Suction devices

Aspiration of blood and other fluids is an important component of any surgical procedure, and the ability to reuse shed blood is what makes CPB possible. A variety of suctioning devices are used during cardiac surgery. Indications for their use differ, and a safe and efficient operation is dependent in part on the proper use of these devices (Table 9-5). Some of these are an integral part of the bypass circuit; others that are not also are described in this section.

Cardiotomy suction. One or more cardiotomy suction lines (see Fig. 9-16) aspirate blood directly back to the pump, where it is filtered, oxygenated, and reinfused with the rest of the bypass volume into the arterial circulation. Because blood is returned directly to the pump, the patient must be given systemic heparin before the cardiotomy sucker can be used. Often the perfusionist will "protect" the pump from thrombus formation by not activating the cardiotomy suction until adequate heparin administration has been confirmed.

Blood trauma can result from excessive negative pressure and shear forces. The amount of negative

TABLE 9-5
Safety Considerations During Cardiopulmonary Bypass

POTENTIAL DANGER	CAUSE	SAFETY MEASURES
Embolism Air	Air in arterial line	Constant vigilance Minimum distraction (avoid loud talking or music) Before connecting arterial cannula to arterial line and during connection, check for air (look at highest point) Ensure that tubing clamps are tight; do not use clamps too small for caliber of tubing Notify surgeon and perfusionist immediately of air in arterial line or cannula Test venting catheters before use to ensure they are suctioning (and not infusing) Be aware that perfusion circuit air sensors may trigger shutoff valve if air is detected Be aware that left side of heart should never be opened before aorta is cross-clamped Ensure identification of outflow (e.g., venous and venting lines) and inflow (e.g., arterial and cardioplegia lines) tubing; label if necessary
Thrombus	Inadequate heparin; old blood clots entering opened arterial line; coagulation agents introduced into circuit	Ensure that proper heparin dose is given before initiating CPB Keep field free of formed blood clots, especially before arterial line is connected to cannula Avoid aspiration of coagulation agents into pump via cardiotomy suction; discontinue use of cardiotomy suction shortly after protamine has been started Monitor ACT; additional heparin is given as needed If CPB must be reinstituted after heparin reversal with protamine sulfate, ensure that heparin is given before reinitiating CPB Note and notify perfusionist of existing cold antibodies, which promote agglutination of red blood cells at low temperatures (determined by laboratory blood testing)
Particulate debris	Free bone fragments, bone wax, suture pieces, calcium particles, fat globules	Keep field free of loose debris; monitor lines
Inadequate venous return	Cannulas too small for adequate venous drainage; cannulas clogged by caval or atrial tissue; table too low; cannulas malpositioned or compressed	Discuss size of cannulas with perfusionist/surgeon to ensure sufficient size for adequate drainage Establish good venous return before instituting hypothermia (e.g., adjust cannulas, tighten tourniquets/ pursestring sutures, increase CVP, change heart position) Note that right atrium is decompressed (collapsed) and CVP is 0-3 mm Hg when venous return is adequate Anticipate adjusting patient volume if flow is too low Use cardiotomy suction whenever possible to return volume to pump
Interruption of venous return	Tubing kinked or clamped; air lock; tubing/cannulas disrupted or dislodged	If holding heart, avoid compression of right atrial lines Avoid clamping lines (during CPB), or stepping or leaning on lines Avoid large amounts of air in venous line; be able to "chase air" down venous line (raising and lowering line to move air toward pump); refill venous line if necessary During open right-sided heart cases (atrial septal defect, tricuspid valve surgery), be prepared to use double venous cannulation, caval clamps, or tourniquets to avoid sucking air into venous circuit Use caution when walking near lines
Interruption of arterial inflow	Arterial line occluded or kinked (can cause rupture of bypass circuit); tubing/cannula dislodged	Do not occlude arterial line with clamp Avoid kinks in line Refrain from leaning on line Protect line during pleural chest tube insertion
Contamination of circuit	Contaminants introduced into CPB circuit	Monitor location of cardiotomy suction tip; suction must be turned off immediately if tip falls off field Ensure that components of circuit are assembled aseptically Ensure that additives (e.g., fluids, drugs) are administered aseptically Fill venous lines only with appropriate solutions; discuss with perfusionist/surgeon Avoid aspiration of topical antibiotics or other contraindicated fluids Maintain sterility of lines when OR table is raised or lowered
Excessive hemodilution	Excess volume aspirated into circuit	Avoid aspirating excessive amounts of irrigating or topical hypothermic solutions into circuit; use discard suction or autotransfusion
Cellular destruction	Trauma to red blood cells, platelets, and other blood cells	Use cardiotomy suction gently and sparingly Avoid unnecessary connectors in bypass tubing Position bypass lines in gentle curves; avoid tight angles or kinks

Modified from Pae WE and others: Prevention of complications during cardiopulmonary bypass. In Waldhausen JA, Orringer MB: *Complications in cardiothoracic surgery,* St Louis, 1991, Mosby.
CVP, Central venous pressure.

pressure can be regulated by the perfusionist, and the tip of most cardiotomy suckers has multiple holes (similar to a small Poole tip), which also reduces the negative pressure. The suction should be used to aspirate pools of blood rather than skimming blood away from specific surgical sites (e.g., anastomoses). Another danger occurs when the suction falls off the sterile field and contaminated material is aspirated into the system, increasing the risk of infection. If this happens, the perfusionist should be informed immediately and suction temporarily halted while new tubing is set up.

Cardiotomy suction is used throughout CPB and then terminated once heparin reversal with protamine has been started. Aspiration of irrigating fluids should be avoided because it can cause excessive hemodilution with a significant drop in the hematocrit of the pump volume. Aspiration of particulate matter should be avoided when possible; even with inline microfilters, it is safer to minimize the risk of potential emboli entering the circuit. Pleural effusate, pericardial fluid, topical antibiotic solutions, and hemostatic agents should be avoided as well.

Autotransfusion suction. Although not part of the bypass circuit, autotransfusion systems conserve red blood cells (RBCs) by returning them to a reservoir from which they can be processed and reinfused back into the patient. Because of the time required for processing, blood return to the patient cannot be achieved as quickly as it can with the cardiotomy sucker. Thus it is always preferable to use cardiotomy suction for large amounts of blood.

Irrigating solutions containing a significant amount of blood can be aspirated back to the reservoir, where processing removes the excess volume. When the fluid is mostly asanguineous, use of the discard suction is preferable to avoid overloading the autotransfusion reservoir. Other fluids contraindicated for cardiotomy suction (e.g., antibiotic solutions, fibrin glue) are similarly contraindicated with this system.

The system also can be used in conjunction with the CPB circuit. After termination of CPB, blood remaining within the circuit can be pumped over to the autotransfusion reservoir by connecting the arterial CPB line to the autotransfusion suction tubing.

Discard suction. The standard discard suction system used for many noncardiac procedures is used to rapidly aspirate fluid that cannot or should not be reinfused. This includes crystalloid irrigating solutions, hypothermic lavage fluid, and the fluids and debris contraindicated for cardiotomy aspiration and autotransfusion.

The T & A tip is used often. With the addition of a microsuction tip, the discard suction can be used to aspirate blood from anastomotic sites; the small amount of

blood involved (a few milliliters) does not appreciably affect circulating blood volume. Discard suction with an open-ended tip (debridement tip) is valuable for aspirating calcium debris during heart valve procedures.

Venting devices and methods to deair the heart

One of the most serious complications associated with cardiac surgery is air embolism, especially to the brain, where it can cause a cerebrovascular accident. Air embolism can occur in a number of ways. The risk is most pronounced when the heart has been opened and trapped air is introduced into the arterial circulation when the aortic occlusion clamp is removed. During CABG, air is introduced into the coronary arteries, and if it is not aspirated, it can cause transient (or permanent) myocardial dysfunction. Patients with intracardiac shunts are also at risk because air within peripheral or central venous lines can be shunted to the left side of the heart and can embolize to the brain.

Because the danger of air embolism is ever present, the surgical team must be vigilant in preventing entry of air, detecting its presence, and instituting measures to remove it. One of the safest ways to protect the brain is to avoid opening the left side of the heart before the aortic occlusion clamp has been applied. After the heart has been opened, Kirklin and Barratt-Boyes (1993) stress four principles for deairing the heart: (1) the heart is filled with fluid before it is closed to minimize air entrapment; (2) residual air is aspirated from the heart before it is allowed to eject; (3) the lungs are intermittently inflated to remove air from the pulmonary veins and cardiac chambers; and (4) there is continuous suction on a needle vent or catheter in the ascending aorta as the heart begins to eject so that residual air in the heart or pulmonary veins is aspirated.

Venting catheters provide two other benefits: decompression of the ventricles and prevention of rewarming from blood entering the cardiac chambers. Aspiration of blood within the cardiac chambers, especially the left ventricle, decompresses the ventricle and avoids overdistension, and aspiration of returning systemic, bronchial, and coronary venous drainage (which is relatively warmer than myocardial temperature) minimizes temperature gradients within the heart. Rewarming is avoided when possible because it makes the ventricle and in particular the subendocardium less tolerant of ischemia.

Cardiac venting catheters. Cardiac venting catheters are placed within the heart or aorta to remove air. The most common venting device is a needle or catheter placed in the ascending aorta that is connected to suction tubing that aspirates air and blood

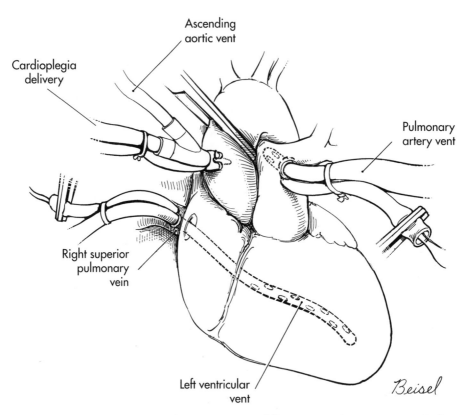

Cardioplegia delivery

Ascending aortic vent

Pulmonary artery vent

Right superior pulmonary vein

Left ventricular vent

Beisel

FIGURE 9-17 Types of venting devices. (From Waldhausen JA, Pierce WS, Campbell DB: *Surgery of the chest,* ed 6, St Louis, 1996, Mosby.)

back to the pump (Fig. 9-17). The same catheter can be used to infuse cardioplegia solution when the inflow line is connected via Y line into the suction line. During infusion the suction line is clamped, and during aspiration the infusion line is clamped. Before the aortic cross-clamp is removed, the vent is turned on slowly to avoid cavitation of the aorta, and then the clamp is opened slowly to allow blood to fill the aortic root.

Additional maneuvers. Additional maneuvers are used to supplement venting devices because air may be entrapped in the pulmonary veins, the left atrium, the ventricular trabeculations, or other areas of the heart not directly accessible to the venting catheters. Before the aortic cross-clamp is removed, the patient is placed in steep Trendelenberg's position so that air within the aorta travels preferentially out through the needle vent rather than to the brain; this occurs because air rises and the aortic vent is now in a higher position than the aortic arch vessels.

Another method to dislodge and aspirate air within the cardiac chambers is to pull the heart forward gently and insert a large-bore needle (e.g., 18 gauge) into the left ventricular apex (Fig. 9-18). This may be accompanied by gentle massage of the cardiac chambers. CPB can be slowed temporarily to fill the heart with blood

(the venous line is partially clamped to allow some venous return to enter the heart); the anesthesiologist hyperinflates the lungs to allow air in the pulmonary veins to be displaced into the cardiac chambers, where it can be aspirated.

The heart should not be allowed to eject blood while the presence of air is evident in the aortic vent tubing or air bubbles are seen exiting the left ventricular apical needle. Some surgeons purposely fibrillate the heart so that it cannot pump potential emboli into the aorta.

When the aorta has been opened, blood and air are allowed to escape through the aortotomy before the incision is completely closed; the aortic vent is not turned on until the aorta has been closed in order to avoid sucking air into the aorta through the aortotomy. During CABG the proximal anastomosis may be allowed to bleed while the suture is being tied, and completed vein grafts may be aspirated with a small-gauge needle (e.g., 27 gauge).

Bypass tubing

Bypass tubing is made most often from polyvinylchloride (PVC). At very low temperatures this plastic can become stiff and does not compress well. In the past, when very low temperatures were anticipated, silicone was used in portions of the circuit where flexibility is desired (e.g., in

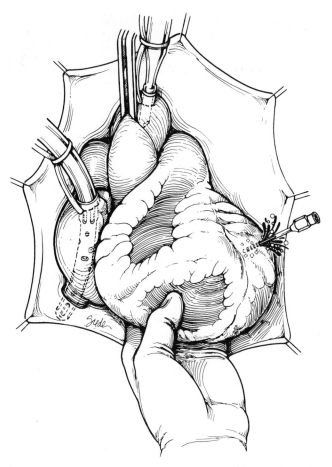

FIGURE 9-18 Deairing of the left ventricle. Massage and ballottement of the cardiac chambers with the apex tilted slightly allows air to escape through an apical or aortic vent needle. CPB is slowed to let the heart fill with blood; the anesthesia care provider inflates the lungs to dispel remaining air into the heart, and a needle is inserted into the apex of the left ventricle to aspirate air and blood. (From Mills NL, Morris JM: Air embolism associated with cardiopulmonary bypass. In Waldhausen JA, Orringer MB: *Complications in cardiothoracic surgery,* St Louis, 1991, Mosby.)

the roller pump head). Recent refinements in the durameter (degree of stiffness or hardness) of PVC tubing have lessened these problems, and silicone inserts are used mainly for infusion or venting lines.

Heparin-coated CPB circuits are available; they are most effective when blood is kept in constant circulation. They may slightly reduce the amount of heparin needed but do not supplant it entirely because areas of stagnant or low flow (within the CPB circuit) require anticoagulation to prevent clot formation. A greater advantage may be related to the immune response that accompanies blood exposure to foreign surfaces. The CPB circuit consists of numerous synthetic materials—plastics and metals—and these also can activate

platelets, granulocytes, and proteins associated with the coagulation pathways; heparin-coated circuits have been shown to reduce the immune system response.

Priming solution

Early bypass systems were primed with whole blood. Current perfusates consist of a balanced electrolyte solution with a near-normal pH and an ionic content similar to that of plasma. Bank blood is rarely used now because of cost considerations, availability, and concern about blood-borne pathogens. Such a policy is usually favorable to patients with religious objections to the use of blood products. Because asanguineous perfusates reduce the hematocrit and hemoglobin (H & H), a unit of packed RBCs may be required occasionally to achieve an adequate, albeit reduced, H & H in patients with relatively small blood volumes compared with the total CPB circuit volume (e.g., small women and children).

Hemodilution is advantageous during hypothermia, which increases blood viscosity. Generally a hematocrit of 20% to 22% (normal is 40% to 50% in the adult) during moderate hypothermia provides a sufficient number of blood cells for oxygen transport, and it lowers the viscosity and shear rates of blood cells (Galloway and others, 1999a). During rewarming, a higher hematocrit may be needed to meet increased oxygen demands; this can be achieved with ultrafiltration devices, the addition of packed RBCs or pharmacologically induced diuresis. Although some hemodilution is well tolerated, hematocrits less than 19% are associated with a higher mortality (De Foe and others, 2001).

Other additives to the prime may include albumin or hetastarch, which are similar to glycogen and raise the plasma colloid oncotic pressure), diuretics such as mannitol and furosemide (to draw fluid from the interstitial space into the vascular space), and vasodilators (to counteract the vasoconstriction produced by catecholamines). Steroids also may be added to improve tissue perfusion and lessen the increases in extracellular water (Canver and Nichols, 2000).

Safety considerations

Many perfusionists use a written prebypass checklist to ensure that the CPB circuit is assembled properly and its integrity tested before CPB is initiated. Although the conduct of CPB is controlled primarily by the perfusionist in close collaboration with the surgeon and the anesthesiologist, the perioperative nurse also has a vital role in protecting the patient and maintaining a safe operative environment. Among the most important safety considerations (see Table 9-5) are preventing disruption of the bypass circuit, using the various suctioning devices appropriately, and protecting the patient against air or particulate embolism. Perioperative

BOX 9-2
RN First Assistant Considerations During Cardiopulmonary Bypass

Prebypass

If end of arterial line has been cut at the field, do not allow any particulate matter (e.g., bone wax, fat debris) to enter open end of line. Do not unclamp arterial line (may allow entry of air) until necessary.

Ensure that heparin has been given; if you do not either (1) witness surgeon injecting it or (2) hear anesthesia personnel verbalize that it has been (or is being) infused, alert surgeon before any blood vessels are clamped; be especially aware of this when CPB must be reinstituted rapidly and heparin reversal with protamine has been started.

When surgeon attaches arterial cannula to arterial line, look for air—especially at highest point in tubing circuit; if air is noted, ensure immediately that surgeon is aware of it.

Use cardiotomy suction both to retract and to aspirate blood during venous cannulation.

Test intracardiac venting catheters to confirm they are suctioning (and not infusing) before they are inserted into the heart.

Bypass

Do not lean on bypass lines or cause them to kink; be especially alert to perfusionist's warnings that venous return is low or that there is an excessively high pressure in the CPB circuit.

Know purpose and direction of flow of all CPB lines on the field.

Do not clamp any bypass lines except under direct orders from surgeon; never clamp arterial line.

Avoid aspirating significant amounts of irrigating solutions with cardiotomy sucker; avoid aspiration of contraindicated substances (e.g., topical antibiotics, hemostatic agents, surgical debris).

Postbypass

Do not use cardiotomy suction after heparin has been reversed with protamine.

Remove venous cannula quickly (but carefully) to prevent excess blood loss from atriotomy; salvage blood with cardiotomy suction.

Remove arterial cannula with part of your hand covering aortotomy so that blood is not splashed all over the field.

Avoid excess tension when tightening aortic cannula pursestring.

TABLE 9-6
Blood Elements Activated During Cardiopulmonary Bypass

PROTEIN SYSTEMS	BLOOD CELLS
Contact	Platelets
Intrinsic circulation	Neutrophils
Extrinsic coagulation	Monocytes
Complement	Endothelial cells
Fibrinolysis	Lymphocytes

From Edmunds LH Jr: Why cardiopulmonary bypass makes patients sick: strategies to control the blood-synthetic surface interface, *Adv Card Surg* 6:131, 1995.

All patients respond physiologically to CPB to one degree or another. Significant adverse reactions can occur—especially in the very young and the very old—producing what Kirklin (1991) called *postperfusion syndrome*. This is evidenced by prolonged pulmonary insufficiency, excessive accumulation of extravascular water, elevated temperature, vasoconstriction, coagulopathy, and variable degrees of renal and other organ dysfunction.

The proposed mechanism for these damaging effects is the exposure of blood to the abnormal surfaces of the CPB circuit, as well as conditions such as hypothermia and altered blood flow, which initiate a systemic inflammatory response. This inflammatory response produces, releases, or alters a host of vasoactive substances that react with specific receptor proteins throughout the body. The resulting vascular smooth muscle and endothelial cell contractions are responsible for many of the morbid complications associated with CPB (Edmunds, 1995).

CPB activates at least five plasma protein systems and five kinds of blood cells during perfusion of heparinized blood (Table 9-6). When these blood elements are activated, they produce a defense reaction called the "whole body inflammatory response" (Edmunds, 1995, p. 132) (Fig. 9-19). Interaction of blood elements with foreign surfaces of the CBP circuit activate the contact system, which directly and indirectly stimulates the intrinsic coagulation pathway, complement, and neutrophils. Platelets, endothelial cells, and the fibrinolytic system also are activated. The extrinsic coagulation pathway and monocytes also may be activated (Edmunds, 1995).

Platelets are activated by interaction with the plastic surfaces of the bypass tubing. Platelet activation is also stimulated by the injury and hemolysis that occur from the turbulence and high shear stress induced by venting and suctioning devices. Endothelial cells produce tissue plasminogen activator (t-PA), which activates the fibrinolytic system.

Activation of the complement pathways, described almost two decades ago by Kirklin (Kirklin and others,

nurses who assist during cardiac procedures may have additional opportunities to ensure a safe and effective procedure (Box 9-2).

ADVERSE EFFECTS OF CARDIOPULMONARY BYPASS

Although CPB has made possible the repair of congenital and acquired cardiac disorders with relatively low morbidity and mortality, it is not a totally benign intervention.

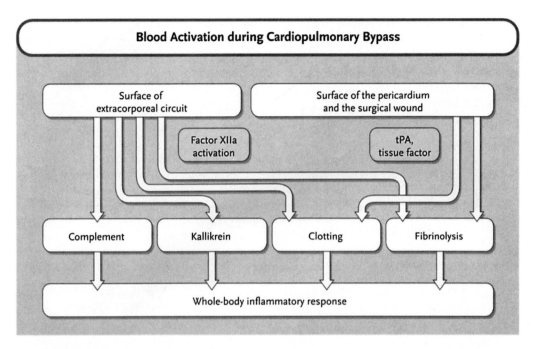

FIGURE 9-19 Blood activation during cardiopulmonary bypass leads to a whole-body inflammatory response. (From Buxton B, Frazier OH, Westaby S, editors: *Ischemic heart disease: surgical management,* London, 1999, Mosby.)

1983), releases the anaphylatoxins C3a and C5a that initiate the whole-body inflammatory response and can produce postoperative organ system dysfunction. Neutrophils, triggered by C5a, aggregate in the pulmonary microcirculation and release protease enzymes; neutrophils also generate oxygen free radicals, which can damage capillary membranes. In addition to the lungs, the brain, kidneys, and coagulation processes also are affected by the inflammatory response, which produces microvascular permeability and leads to fluid retention and weight gain (Westaby, 1999).

The use of membrane oxygenators (versus bubble oxygenators) and the use of the less traumatic centrifugal pumps have been shown to minimize injury to the blood (Galloway and others, 1999a). Controlling the length of the pump time (longer than 4 hours substantially increases the number and severity of complications) and reducing the inflammatory response by coating CPB circuits with biocompatible materials and inflammation-reducing medications (steroids and protease inhibitors such as aprotinin) also can minimize the damaging effects of CPB (Mojcik and Levy, 2001). Even with the adverse effects of CPB, the great majority of adult patients have excellent outcomes and can be extubated shortly after surgery. Thus the overall significance of the inflammatory response is not fully apparent (Westaby, 1999).

CARDIOPULMONARY BYPASS PROCEDURES

Cannulation of the aorta for arterial inflow and of the IVC and SVC (or the right atrium) for venous drainage is the most common form of CPB. Other arteries (e.g., the femoral or, rarely, the subclavian) can be cannulated for arterial inflow. The femoral vein can be used to drain venous blood, but venous return may be limited (which then limits arterial flow to the body).

Aortocaval cannulation bypasses both the right and left sides of the heart. Occasionally, left-sided heart bypass or right-sided heart bypass is used to support a failing left or right ventricle, respectively. Left-sided heart bypass may be used during repair of descending thoracic aneurysms. Right- or left-sided heart bypass also may be used during off-pump surgery to maintain hemodynamic stability. Left-sided heart bypass does not require an oxygenator because oxygenated blood is being withdrawn (from the left atrium) and reinfused (into a systemic artery) without its being desaturated. Right-sided heart bypass (e.g., right atrium to pulmonary artery) does not require an oxygenator either because the lungs will perform that function. However, whenever desaturated blood is removed from the body, it cannot be infused back into the systemic circulation without prior oxygenation (and ventilation). Doing so would create a shunt and produce hypoxia with cyanosis.

The following procedures are commonly used to achieve CPB.

Operative procedures: arterial cannulation for cardiopulmonary bypass
Cannulation of the aorta

1. After the sternum has been opened, a longitudinal incision is made in the pericardium with scissors and cautery from the pericardial reflection at the aorta to the diaphragmatic portion of the pericardium. The pericardium often is incised laterally at its ends to enhance exposure of the heart. The pericardial edges are sewn to the chest wall. Heparin is given.
2. The aorta is dissected partially from the pulmonary artery.
3. A pursestring double-armed suture is inserted in the ascending aorta just below the great vessels. The needles are removed from the suture, the loose ends of which are threaded with a stylet through a plastic or red rubber catheter. The catheter is clamped with a hemostat so that it does not slide off the suture (but the pursestring is not tightened).
4. A second pursestring suture is placed around the first as described in step 3 (Fig. 9-20).
5. The adventitia inside the pursestring is divided, and a stab wound is made in the aorta (some surgeons use a partial-occlusion clamp on the aorta).

6. The aortic cannula (occluded near the proximal end with a vented cap or a tubing clamp) is inserted into the aorta (Fig. 9-21). The pursestring tourniquets are tightened and held to the cannula with a heavy tie (Fig. 9-22). If a tubing clamp is used, it is opened momentarily to fill the cannula with blood from the aorta. If there is a cap over the cannula, blood will fill the cannula, displacing any air; the cannula then is clamped, and the cap is removed.
7. While the perfusionist slowly pumps priming solution out the end of the arterial line (to remove any

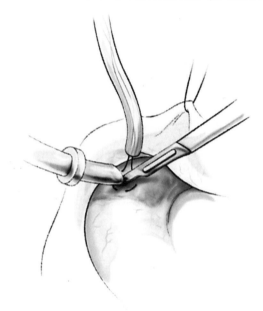

FIGURE 9-21   After the stab wound is made in the aorta, the arterial cannula is inserted. (From Buxton B, Frazier OH, Westaby S, editors: *Ischemic heart disease: surgical management,* London, 1999, Mosby.)

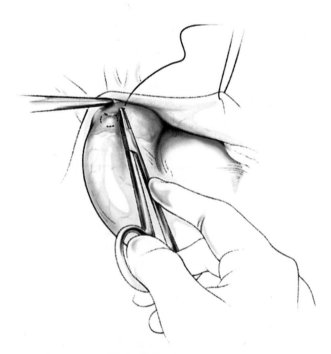

FIGURE 9-20   The pursestring suture is placed on the anterior surface of the aorta. A second pursestring is often placed. (From Buxton B, Frazier OH, Westaby S, editors: *Ischemic heart disease: surgical management,* London, 1999, Mosby.)

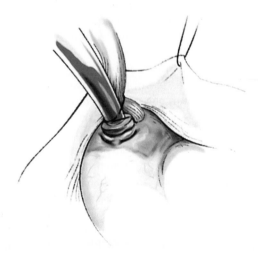

FIGURE 9-22   The tourniquet is tightened (two tourniquets may be used) and tied to the arterial cannula. (From Buxton B, Frazier OH, Westaby S, editors: *Ischemic heart disease: surgical management,* London, 1999, Mosby.)

air), the surgeon connects the proximal end of the aortic cannula to the arterial line, taking care to avoid letting air enter the system. The perfusionist then stops infusing any more solution.

The tubing clamp is removed from the cannula, and the circuit is inspected for air. If any air bubbles are noted, the cannula is reclamped, the connection is opened, priming solution is infused, air is allowed to escape, and the connection is reestablished. The cannula also may be allowed to fill with blood from the aorta. The arterial line is then attached to the chest with a towel clip or a suture.

Cannulation of the femoral artery

1. A vertical or oblique incision is made in the femoral triangle, and the common femoral artery is exposed (Fig. 9-23).
2. Umbilical tapes are passed around the vessel above and below the planned arteriotomy, and tourniquet catheters are threaded over the tapes. The artery is occluded proximally and distally with femoral artery clamps.
3. An incision is made in the artery and extended with Potts scissors.
4. The arterial catheter (clamped at the proximal end) is inserted into the artery retrogradely as the proximal femoral clamp is removed (Fig. 9-24). The proximal tourniquet is tightened around the cannula in the artery and tied to the cannula (Fig. 9-25).

5. The cannula is attached to the arterial inflow line as described in step 7 and is secured to the drapes. The arterial line should be kept longer to reach the cannula without tension. The distal artery remains occluded with the tourniquet or the femoral artery clamp.

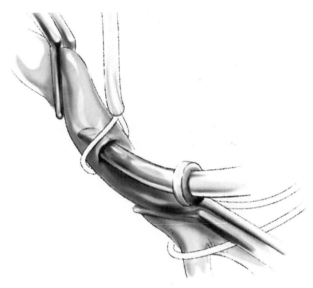

FIGURE 9-24 The femoral cannula is inserted into the artery. (From Buxton B, Frazier OH, Westaby S, editors: *Ischemic heart disease: surgical management,* London, 1999, Mosby.)

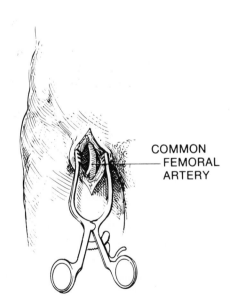

COMMON FEMORAL ARTERY

FIGURE 9-23 Exposure of the femoral artery for cannulation. A Weitlaner self-retaining retractor is shown. (From Waldhausen JA, Pierce WS, Campbell DB: *Surgery of the chest,* ed 6, St Louis, 1996, Mosby.)

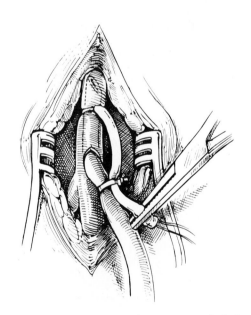

FIGURE 9-25 After the femoral artery cannula is inserted, the tourniquet is tightened and tied to the cannula. The femoral vein is adjacent and, when necessary, can be cannulated in a similar manner for venous drainage. (From Waldhausen JA, Pierce WS, Campbell DB: *Surgery of the chest,* ed 6, St Louis, 1996, Mosby.)

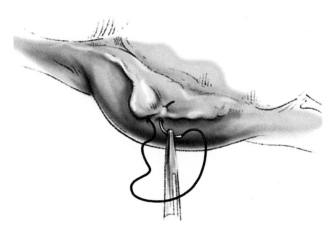

FIGURE 9-26 A pursestring suture is placed in the right atrial appendage. (From Buxton B, Frazier OH, Westaby S, editors: *Ischemic heart disease surgical management,* London, 1999, Mosby.)

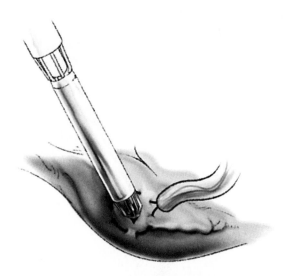

FIGURE 9-27 The two-stage venous cannula is inserted into the right atrium. (From Buxton B, Frazier OH, Westaby S, editors: *Ischemic heart disease surgical management,* London, 1999, Mosby.)

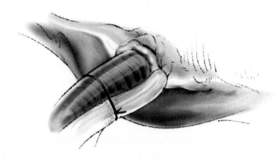

FIGURE 9-28 The tourniquet is tied to the wire-reinforced venous cannula. (From Buxton B, Frazier OH, Westaby S, editors: *Ischemic heart disease surgical management,* London, 1999, Mosby.)

Operative procedure: cannulation for venous return

The two-stage venous cannula is used for most procedures. When entry into the right side of the heart is planned, bicaval cannulation of the IVC and SVC is performed. Occasionally the femoral vein is cannulated when very large thoracic aneurysms obscure the right atrium or pose too great a risk of rupture; the femoral vein is exposed and cannulated in a manner similar to that of femoral artery cannulation. Because femoral venous return drains only the lower body, an SVC cannula is inserted and Y'd into the venous line after the aneurysm is controlled.

Cannulation of the right atrium with a two-stage catheter

1. A partial-occlusion clamp is applied to the right atrial appendage.
2. A single pursestring suture is inserted (Fig. 9-26) around the appendage, and tourniquets are applied loosely as described in step 3 of the procedure for cannulation of the aorta.
3. The tip of the appendage is excised, and the surgeon and assistant grasp either side of the cut edges. Atrial trabeculations are divided sharply with scissors.
4. With the other hand, the surgeon inserts the venous cannula (with obturator) into the atriotomy and advances the distal fenestrated end into the IVC (Fig. 9-27). The proximal openings of the cannula are positioned in the right atrium. The obturator is removed, and the cannula is allowed to fill with blood. The proximal end is occluded with a tubing clamp.
5. The tourniquet is tightened and attached to the cannula with a tie (Fig. 9-28). The cannula is connected to the venous drainage line. The venous line should be of sufficient length to create a gentle curve on the field.
6. The tubing clamp is removed, and venous drainage is allowed to commence (Fig. 9-29). The perfusionist begins to slowly pump arterial inflow, and CPB is established. Venous return is assessed, and if it is found to be inadequate, the pump is turned off, the tourniquet is loosened, and the venous cannula is repositioned. The tourniquet is retightened and again tied to the cannula.

Bicaval cannulation of the right atrium. Two venous cannulas are used: one to cannulate the SVC and the other to cannulate the IVC (Fig. 9-30). For procedures in the right side of the heart (e.g., tricuspid valve disorders or atrial septal defects) when maximum exposure is required, a right-angle SVC cannula may be used (see Fig. 13-12).

Operative procedure

1. A partial-occlusion clamp may be placed on the right atrial appendage, and a pursestring suture is placed as described for single venous cannulation. If not already

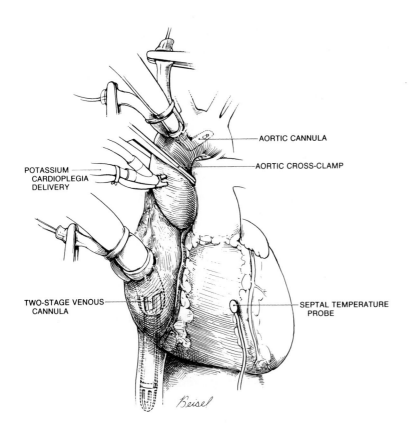

AORTIC CANNULA

AORTIC CROSS-CLAMP

POTASSIUM
CARDIOPLEGIA
DELIVERY

TWO-STAGE VENOUS
CANNULA

SEPTAL TEMPERATURE
PROBE

FIGURE 9-29 A two-stage venous cannula is shown. The distal openings drain the IVC, and the proximal openings drain venous return from the SVC and the heart via the coronary sinus in the right atrium. The antegrade cardioplegia delivery catheter and the aortic cross-clamp are in place. A temperature probe is shown in the interventricular septum. (From Waldhausen JA, Pierce WS: Johnson's surgery of the chest, ed 5, St Louis, 1985, Mosby.)

in place, a partial-occlusion clamp is placed on the appendage (outside the pursestring suture). The appendage is excised, and as the assistant opens the clamp, the surgeon inserts the venous cannula; the assistant then tightens the tourniquet. The cannula may be placed in the SVC or the IVC, depending on the surgeon's preference. When the right atrium is to be opened, the cannula is placed in the SVC so that it does not obscure the operative field. The tourniquet is tightened and tied to the cannula. The proximal end of the cannula is occluded with a tubing clamp.

2. A second pursestring suture is similarly placed lower in the right atrium, and the tourniquet is applied. A partial-occlusion clamp may or may not be used; if it is not used, the surgeon makes a stab wound into the atrium and enlarges it with a tonsil hemostat. The cannula is inserted and (usually) threaded to the IVC; the tourniquets are tightened and tied to the cannula.

3. The cannulas are attached to the openings of a Y connector at the end of the venous line. The tubing clamp is removed, and venous drainage is started.

Discontinuation of cardiopulmonary bypass

After the surgical repair has been completed, the surgeon prepares to discontinue bypass. The patient will have been rewarmed to normothermia (rewarming is started before the cross-clamp is removed), and the

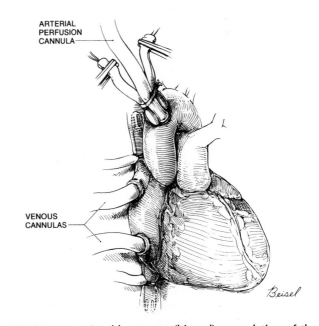

ARTERIAL
PERFUSION
CANNULA

VENOUS
CANNULAS

FIGURE 9-30 Double venous (bicaval) cannulation of the IVC and SVC. When tourniquets are placed around the cavae and tightened, all systemic venous return is forced into the cannulas, producing total CPB. (From Waldhausen JA, Pierce WS, Campbell DB: *Surgery of the chest*, ed 6, St Louis, 1996, Mosby.)

heart will be contracting in a regular manner. The anesthesiologist starts to ventilate the lungs, and the surgeon (or perfusionist) gradually occludes the venous line, allowing blood to enter the right atrium. At the same time, the perfusionist reduces the arterial inflow to equal the venous drainage to the pump. As the heart gradually is allowed to accept all the venous return, the surgeon assesses cardiac contractility by monitoring the systemic and pulmonary blood pressures and visually inspecting the heart. When heart action is judged to be sufficient and systemic blood pressures are stable, the venous line is clamped completely, and the heart resumes responsibility for maintaining the circulation. Pump volume remaining in the oxygenator is infused gradually and in increments as necessary to maintain optimum filling pressures (preload) and systemic blood pressure.

Removal of the aortic cannula. After bypass has been discontinued and heparin reversal with protamine sulfate begun, the CPB cannulas are removed. Generally the venous cannula is removed before the arterial cannula so that blood can continue to be infused if necessary. It is also safer to keep the arterial cannula in place during the beginning of protamine infusion in the event there is a hypotensive reaction to the protamine.

Operative procedure

1. The towel clip or tie attaching the arterial line to the chest is removed, and the tourniquets are freed from the cannula and loosened.
2. While the surgeon stabilizes the cannula, the assistant removes the tourniquet from one pursestring and makes a throw in the suture, tightening it around the cannula. The assistant holds this stitch taut with one hand and takes the cannula from the surgeon with the other hand.
3. The surgeon then removes the other tourniquet and makes a throw in the stitch. As the assistant removes the cannula, the surgeon tightens the stitch to close the arteriotomy. The assistant hands the cannula to the scrub nurse and then tightens the first pursestring. The surgeon ties his or her pursestring, followed by the pursestring held by the assistant.
4. The incision site is inspected for hemostasis, and additional sutures are placed if necessary.

Removal of the femoral artery cannula

1. Tourniquets are detached from the cannula and loosened.
2. As the surgeon slides the cannula out of the arteriotomy, the assistant tightens the tourniquet around the artery. A femoral artery clamp may be placed on the artery proximally, and the umbilical tape is removed.
3. The artery is closed with two 4-0 or 5-0 polypropylene sutures; one suture is started on one side and the other on the opposite side of the incision. The stitches

are tied at the middle. Tourniquets and clamps are removed, and the incision is checked for hemostasis.

Removal of the venous cannulas. The tourniquet is freed from the cannula and removed from the pursestring. As the assistant removes the cannula, the surgeon tightens the pursestring and then finishes tying the suture. Another pursestring may be placed to achieve hemostasis. If there is a second cannula, it is removed in the same manner.

PERCUTANEOUS CARDIOPULMONARY BYPASS

Different forms of percutaneous CPB are available for emergency salvage, as well as for preplanned surgical procedures.

Emergency extracorporeal support

In the past, portable extracorporeal circulation systems were developed that could be wheeled to the emergency department or the critical care unit for patients with massive pulmonary embolus, accidental hypothermia, or cardiac arrest. These systems employed femoral cannulation (as described previously) with the addition of smaller, mobile pump oxygenators. Modifications to the bypass cannulas systems have enabled percutaneous femoral vein–femoral artery insertion in patients undergoing high-risk percutaneous coronary interventions (PCI) in the cardiac catheterization laboratory. These patients may require immediate extracorporeal support if acute vessel closure occurs and transfer to the OR is delayed (Dukovcic, Daleiden-Burns, and Shawl, 1998).

Operative procedure

1. After the heparin has been administered, large-bore, thin-walled cannulas are inserted into the femoral artery and femoral vein.
2. A small cutdown incision may be required for arterial insertion; venous insertion may be performed through a small incision or percutaneously (Loulmet and others, 1998).
3. One type of venous cannula (Fig. 9-31) is long enough to extend into the SVC; openings in the distal tip drain the upper body, and openings in the right atrial section of the cannula drain venous return from the IVC. This two-stage venous cannula is inserted percutaneously via Seldinger technique (see Fig. 15-6).
4. The arterial and venous cannulas are connected to a circuit containing an oxygenator and heat exchanger.
5. A centrifugal pump is used to actively drain venous return (passive drainage would not allow adequate venous return through the cannula). Blood is then propelled through the membrane oxygenator into the systemic circulation. Because suction is used to drain the heart, the central venous vascular system is

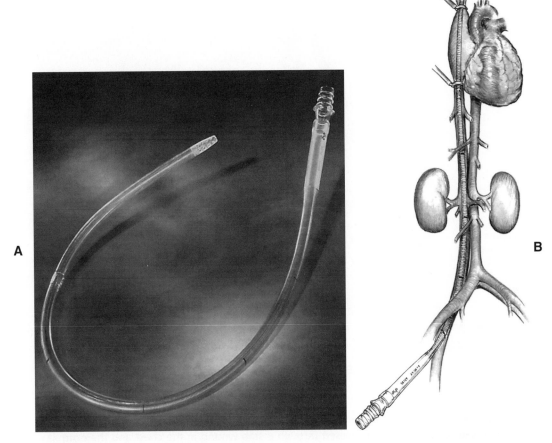

FIGURE 9-31 The venous cannula **(A)** is inserted into the femoral vein and threaded to the right atrium **(B).** The distal tip is positioned in the SVC to drain the upper body. (Courtesy Medtronic, Inc.)

under negative pressure; this can cause intravenous (IV) drip rates to speed up, and there is a risk of air entering the perfusion system via open central venous pressure or IV lines.

6. Once assisted perfusion is no longer needed, CPB is terminated, the cannulas are removed, and incisions are closed.

Complications are those associated with other forms of CPB; these include air embolus, hemolysis with subsequent renal injury, protamine reaction, and aortic dissection.

Endovascular systems

Further refinement of percutaneous bypass technology has led to endovascular systems that complement minimal access surgery through small chest incisions or ports for CABG, valve procedures, and other cardiac operations (see also Chapters 3 and 10). This approach is based on the technique for insertion of intraaortic balloon pump cannulas (Galloway and others, 1999b).

Components of the system include femoral arterial and venous cannulas and endovascular catheters that vent the pulmonary artery, infuse cardioplegia into the coronary sinus, and perform endovascular occlusion of the aorta. The arterial and venous cannulas are inserted into the femoral artery and vein, respectively. Occasionally a second venous cannula is inserted into the SVC under direct vision via a small lateral incision in the chest (Fig. 9-32) and Y'd into the main venous line.

Aortic occlusion and cardioplegia infusion to arrest the heart (described more fully later) are achieved with endovascular catheters. The aortic occlusion catheter is inserted into the femoral artery and threaded to the ascending aorta. The correct position of the catheter balloon tip is confirmed with transesophageal echocardiography (TEE) or fluoroscopy, and the balloon is inflated to occlude the aorta (Fig. 9-33). The aortic catheter contains additional lumens through which a cardioplegic solution can be infused antegradely to arrest the heart and through which air can be vented.

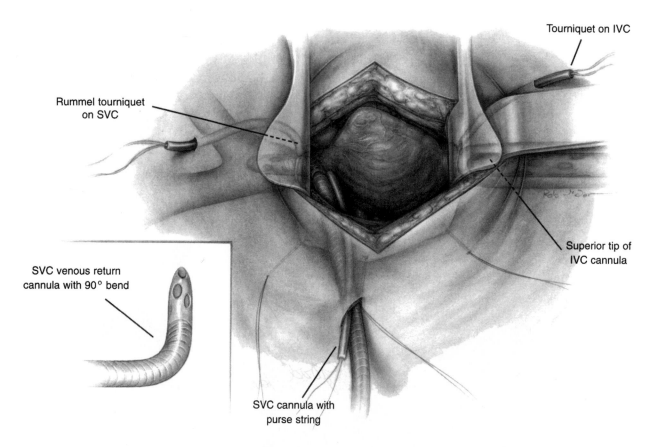

Tourniquet on IVC

Rummel tourniquet on SVC

Superior tip of IVC cannula

SVC venous return cannula with 90° bend

SVC cannula with purse string

FIGURE 9-32 Cannulation for minimal access surgery through a submammary incision. An angled venous cannula is passed through a stab wound in the chest and the cannula tip is inserted into the SVC. The tourniquet is brought out through the cannula stab wound. (From Cox JL: The minimally invasive Maze III procedure, *Op Tech Thorac Cardiovasc Surg* 5(1):79, 2000.)

Temperature and blood pressure sensors also are incorporated into the catheter tip (Pavelka and Park, 1998).

Another catheter can be inserted into the jugular vein and threaded into the right atrium (RA) to the entrance of the coronary sinus. A cardioplegic solution can be infused retrogradely into the coronary circulation via the venous catheter positioned inside the coronary sinus. After the catheters are positioned and the heart is arrested, the surgical repair is performed either through small incisions (and direct vision) or by video-assisted endoscopic techniques.

The endovascular system has the potential for the performance of a totally endoscopic cardiac procedure, but there are complications that must be considered, including aortic dissection (which is a concern with any retrograde arterial perfusion system) and inadequate removal of intracardiac air. Caution in the placement of guidewires for the introduction of the femoral arterial cannula, preoperative vascular screening of patients with suspected atherosclerotic aortoiliac disease, and

conversion to a standard CPB technique if cannulas cannot be easily introduced have reduced some of the complications associated with dissection. Endovascular venting catheters passed into the left ventricle can be used to deair the heart. The placement of external defibrillation pads make defibrillation possible if the patient's heart arrests.

VENTRICULAR ASSISTANCE FOR BEATING HEART SURGERY

Partial right- or left-sided heart assistance devices also may be used during beating heart (i.e., off-pump) CABG to provide hemodynamic stability to the heart when it is elevated to expose posterior or lateral coronary arteries. Displacement of the ventricle produces mainly right-sided heart dysfunction because of right ventricular outflow obstruction. One device that has been experimentally studied is a cannula pump that transfers blood from the right atrium to the pulmonary

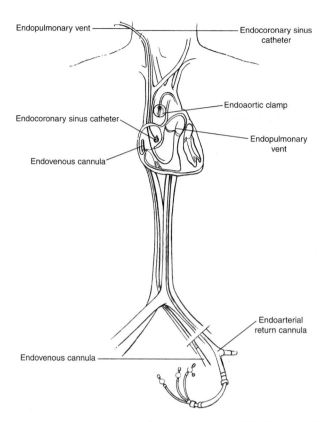

FIGURE 9-33 Endovascular port-access CPB (see text). (From Fann JI and others: Port-access multivessel coronary artery bypass grafting, *Op Tech Card Thorac Surg* 3(1):16, 1998.)

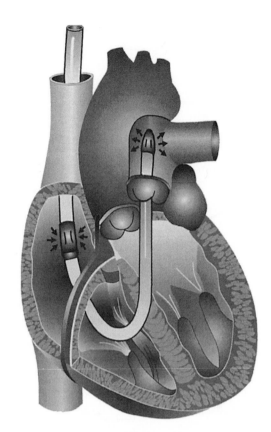

FIGURE 9-34 Right-sided heart support device expels blood from the right atrium into the main pulmonary artery. (From Porat E and others: Hemodynamic changes and right heart support during vertical displacement of the beating heart, *Ann Thorac Surg* 69(4):1188, 2000.)

artery (Fig. 9-34); the catheter is inserted percutaneously into the jugular vein and threaded to the pulmonary artery (PA) in a manner similar to the insertion of a Swan-Ganz pulmonary artery catheter. Openings in the atrial portion of the catheter allow blood to enter and to be expelled into the PA through the distal openings of the catheter (Porat and others, 2000).

EXTRACORPOREAL LIFE SUPPORT

The development of membrane oxygenators and their success in minimizing hemolysis for prolonged periods has allowed additional applications of CPB. *Extracorporeal membrane oxygenation* (ECMO), now referred to as *extracorporeal life support* (ECLS), has been used largely to support patients with potentially reversible respiratory failure, but ECLS has been used also for cardiac support. With the improvement in ventricular assist devices, ECLS is used more often for temporary pulmonary support in neonates and adults.

In neonates, acute respiratory failure (ARF) is usually secondary to abnormal pulmonary vasculature, immaturity of the surfactant system, or chemical pneumonitis

from meconium aspiration. Adults with ARF from destructive primary lung disease or from acute respiratory distress syndrome (ARDS) causing severe parenchymal injury and fibrosis may derive less benefit from ECLS therapy because the underlying disease is less likely to be reversible (Anderson, 1998; Bartlett, 1990). These individuals may require lung transplantation.

Types of ECLS

ECLS is achieved by draining venous blood, removing carbon dioxide, adding oxygen, and returning the blood to the circulation via an artery (venoarterial bypass) or a vein (venovenous bypass). In venoarterial bypass (Fig. 9-35, *A*) the function of both the heart and the lungs is replaced by an artificial organ (e.g., the extracorporeal pump). In the neonate the internal jugular vein and the common carotid artery may be cannulated for venous return and arterial inflow, respectively.

Venovenous bypass (Fig. 9-35, *B*) is the preferred mode of support for patients with pure respiratory failure. In venovenous ECLS the oxygenated venous blood

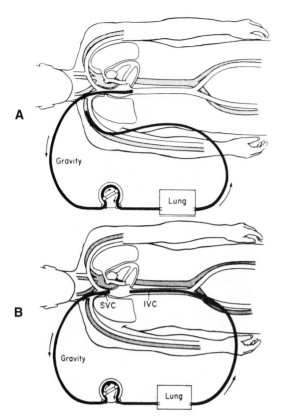

FIGURE 9-35 Two modes of long-term extracorporeal circulation. **A,** Venoarterial circuit. Blood is removed from the right atrium, and oxygenated blood is pumped into the subclavian artery. **B,** Venovenous circuit (provides only respiratory support). Blood is removed from the SVC, and oxygenated blood is pumped into the IVC. Other vascular sites can be used. (From Bartlett RH: Extracorporeal life support for cardiopulmonary failure, *Curr Probl Surg* 27[10]:621, 1990.)

is returned to the venous circulation, where it raises the oxygen content and lowers the carbon dioxide level of the venous blood. The right internal jugular and the femoral vein may be cannulated for inflow and outflow. Among the clinical advantages of this method over venoarterial ECLS is that it is less invasive and as a result can be instituted earlier. Lower flow rates can be used (resulting in less trauma to blood cells), the carotid artery need not be sacrificed, and the potential risk of arterial emboli is avoided (Anderson, 1998). Subsequently, less aggressive ventilator support (i.e., lower airway pressures and a reduced percentage of oxygen) can be used.

Systemic heparin administration is required; the ACT is maintained from 160 to 200 seconds (Anderson, 1998). As with other CPB circuits, complement and other inflammatory agents are activated. The duration of ECLS is a function of the patient's rate of recovery

from the intrinsic disease, improvement in lung compliance, and diagnostic imaging evidence of pulmonary improvement. Complications are similar to those for CPB (Table 9-7).

POSTOPERATIVE CONSIDERATIONS RELATED TO EXTRACORPOREAL CIRCULATION

Postoperative management of cardiac surgery patients includes assessing not only structural and functional changes associated with the operation and the specific cardiac disease (e.g., coronary artery disease, valvular disorders) but also the clinical sequelae of CPB (see Table 9-7). Hemodilution, hypothermia, inflammation, altered blood flow patterns, and changes in capillary membrane permeability are just some of the contributing factors that can produce temporary or permanent organ system dysfunction.

The major considerations during postoperative care are (1) hemodynamic evaluation and maintenance of adequate cardiac output, (2) electrocardiographic assessment and management of dysrhythmias, (3) blood loss and conservation, (4) ventilation and pulmonary care, and (5) general care that focuses on the assessment of fluid and electrolytes, nutrition, wound care, neurologic and renal function, and rehabilitation (Galloway and others, 1999a).

DEEP HYPOTHERMIA WITH CIRCULATORY ARREST

The technique of deep hypothermia with circulatory arrest is useful for complex procedures in which cerebral flow must be temporarily interrupted or in which adequate surgical exposure is hampered by the size of the patient or the location of the lesion. In neonates and other small patients this technique allows removal of both aortic and venous catheters to provide an uncluttered operative field during circulatory arrest; the catheters are reinserted for resumption of CPB and rewarming.

In adults with aneurysms of the distal ascending aorta, the transverse arch, or the descending thoracic aorta, application of a cross-clamp on the arch vessels may be difficult or may pose an increased risk of injury to friable aortic tissue (see Chapter 14 on surgery on the thoracic aorta). Moreover, clamping these vessels interrupts cerebral blood flow.

Past experiences with selected cannulation of the arch vessels to perfuse the brain have been disappointing. Current methods to protect the brain use hypothermia (approximately 22° to 24° C [72° to 76° F] or lower) to further reduce cerebral metabolic requirements, as well as circulatory arrest to provide a relatively

---

TABLE 9-7
Effects of Cardiopulmonary Bypass

EFFECTS	CONTRIBUTING FACTORS
Cardiovascular System	
Perioperative myocardial infarction	Inadequate myocardial protection and emboli
Low cardiac output syndrome after surgery	Preexisting heart disease, inadequate myocardial protection; alteration in colloidal osmotic pressure, left ventricular dysfunction, hypoperfusion injury, hypothermia, long pump run
Increased afterload	Catecholamine release
Hypertension	Elevated renin, angiotensin, and aldosterone levels
Hypotension	Postoperative diuresis, sudden vasodilation, (rewarming), third spacing
Pulmonary System	
Respiratory insufficiency	Alterations in colloidal osmotic pressure, interstitial pulmonary edema, decreased perfusion, alterations in ventilatory patterns, decreased surfactant production, pulmonary microemboli
Atelectasis	Complement activation and inflammatory response, emboli, alveolar-capillary membrane damage
Neurologic System	
Cerebrovascular accident	Cerebral emboli
Transient motor deficits	Decreased cerebral blood flow
Cerebral hemorrhage	Systemic heparin administration
Neuropsychologic deficits	Microemboli, ischemia, altered perfusion flow of bypass
Gastrointestinal System	
Gastrointestinal bleeding	Hormonal stress and coagulation diatheses
Intestinal ischemia or infarction	Emboli and decreased perfusion
Acute pancreatitis	Pancreatic vasculature emboli
Renal System	
Acute renal failure	Decreased renal blood flow, microemboli, and myohemoglobin release
Hemoglobinuria	Red blood cell hemolysis
Fluid and Electrolyte Balance	
Interstitial edema, weight gain	Increased extravascular fluid and organ dysfunction, fluid shifts, decreased plasma protein concentration, increased capillary permeability
Intravascular hypovolemia	Decreased intravascular volume, bleeding, and interstitial edema
Hypokalemia	Dilution, polyuria, intracellular shifts of potassium ions
Hyperkalemia	Potassium cardioplegia and increased intracellular exchange of glucose and potassium, cellular destruction
Hyponatremia, hypocalcemia, and hypomagnesmia	Dilution, fluid shifts, diuresis
Endocrine System	
Water and sodium retention	Increase in antidiuretic hormone
Hypothyroidism	Increased levels of thyroxine (T_4) and decreased levels of triiodothyronine (T_3) and thyroid-stimulating hormone
Hyperglycemia	Depressed insulin response, stimulation of glycogenesis
Immune System	
Infection	Exposure to multiple pathogens, decreased immunoglobin levels, and hypothermia
Postperfusion syndrome	Release of anaphylactic toxins, complement activation
Hematologic Factors	
Bleeding	Blood cell hemolysis, heparin rebound, reduction in platelet count and coagulation factors, coagulopathy, systemic heparin administration, depressed liver function from hypothermia

Modified from Edmunds LH Jr: Why cardiopulmonary bypass makes patients sick: strategies to control the blood-synthetic surface interface, *Adv Card Surg* 6:131, 1995; Thelan LA and others: *Critical care nursing: diagnosis and management,* St Louis, 1998, Mosby.

bloodless field. At 18° C (65° F) the safe period is up to 60 minutes (Griepp and others, 2000).

Additional cerebral protection is provided with ice bags placed around the patient's head. The ears and nose should be padded to avoid frostbite injury (Oliver, Nuttall, and Murray, 1999).

Operative procedure

1. CPB is instituted with right atrial venous cannulation, and femoral arterial cannulation for inflow. The patient's body temperature is cooled to 18° to 24° C (65° to 76° F), depending on the surgeon's preference.
2. When the desired temperature is reached, the venous line is occluded and arterial flow discontinued.
3. Operative repair: An incision is made (e.g., into the aortic arch; distal and arch anastomoses are completed). Aspiration of blood is limited to that required to visualize the operative site.
4. After sufficient completion of the repair to allow placement of a cross-clamp on the proximal transverse aortic prosthetic graft, arterial perfusion is resumed slowly, and the aorta and arch vessels are filled with blood. Air is allowed to escape from the arch vessels.
5. Arterial perfusion is continued, and rewarming is started at a rate of 3 minutes for each degree Centigrade. The proximal anastomosis is completed during rewarming (see Chapter 14 for additional discussion).

CEREBROPLEGIA

Circulatory arrest poses additional risk to the brain. Cerebral protection, cerebroplegia (see Fig. 14-20), is provided by the infusion of oxygenated blood (from the arterial pump circuit) to the brain in a retrograde fashion via the superior vena cava cannula. The venous drainage line is occluded and the cerebroplegia line connecting the arterial inflow line and the SVC venous line is opened so that arterialized (i.e., oxygenated) blood flows in a retrograde manner from the SVC line into the head and cerebral circulation. The cerebroplegia solution drains out through the arterial arch vessels.

Because CPB is temporarily halted, the vena cava cannula is not needed to drain venous blood and can be connected to the source of oxygenated blood for cerebral infusion. After the repair is completed, the venous cannula can be used again to drain venous return when CPB is reestablished (Safi, Petrik, Miller, 2001).

Myocardial Protection

At one time early postoperative cardiac failure and death were assumed to be primarily the result of the patient's own disease. It became apparent, however, that diminished left ventricular function and acute cardiac failure also might be caused by operative myocardial ischemia or necrosis. Although periods of ischemia and hypoxia are necessary to provide a motionless operative field, ventricular function should not be impaired because protective measures were not taken intraoperatively. Myocardial damage can be minimized by interventions that reduce ischemic time, lower metabolic requirements, conserve energy stores, and maintain an appropriate cellular environment (Kay and others, 1978; Buckberg, 1995).

When the aorta is cross-clamped, blood flow to the myocardium is interrupted, producing hypoxia and ischemia. Deprived of sufficient oxygen, cardiac cells must use alternative methods of energy production if they are to remain viable. These energy demands are determined primarily by myocardial electromechanical work and secondarily by wall tension and temperature (Beuren, Sparks, and Bing, 1958). The energy available in high-energy phosphates—adenosine triphosphate (ATP) and creatine phosphate (CP)—must be provided by anaerobic metabolism, which is itself energy dependent and requires the use of glucose and oxygen. Anaerobic metabolism is less efficient, however, producing far fewer high-energy phosphates per unit of glucose.

The effects of ischemia are even more deleterious than those of hypoxia because inadequate coronary blood flow not only impairs oxygen delivery but also prevents adequate removal of accumulated metabolic waste products. Increased lactate levels lower intracellular pH, which interferes with vital enzyme functions. Glycolysis is eventually inhibited, resulting in energy depletion. Insufficient ATP is available for resumption of excitation-contraction coupling and for energizing the sodium and potassium pumps. Increased levels of intracellular calcium potentiate the use of high-energy phosphates, further depleting the energy pool. Without protection, irreversible myocardial damage can occur, the most dramatic being irreversible ischemic contracture, which Cooley, Reul, and Wakasch (1972) termed the *stone heart.*

Even when measures are instituted to reduce ischemic time and the accumulation of waste products, ischemia and its adverse consequences cannot be avoided entirely. Some cells will die; others will be damaged slightly, and some will be "stunned" (see Chapter 10). To protect potentially viable cells, corrective measures are necessary to prevent extension of the injury when the cross-clamp is removed and the heart is reperfused (Mangano and others, 1999). Reperfusion injury includes structural, biochemical, electrical, and mechanical abnormalities (Box 9-3).

To minimize the damaging effects of hypoxia and ischemia during cross-clamping, researchers have focused on two factors that have become the basis of myocardial protection and preservation: hypothermia and

BOX 9-3
Abnormalities Encountered During Reperfusion

Structural
- Myocardial edema
- Platelet deposition
- Neutrophil activation
- Vascular injury
- Vascular compression

Biochemical
- Acidosis
- Decreased oxygen use
- Decreased high-energy phosphate production
- Increased catecholamines
- Complement activation
- Increased intracellular calcium
- Increased free radicals

Electrical
- Dysrhythmias
- Increased automaticity

Mechanical
- Impaired systolic/diastolic function

From Mangano CM and others: Cardiopulmonary bypass and the anesthesiologist. In Kaplan JA, editor: *Cardiac anesthesia,* ed 4, Philadelphia, 1999, WB Saunders.

immediate cardiac arrest. The first reduces the metabolic rate and consequently the workload of the heart (Bigelow, Lindsay, and Greenwood, 1950; Sealy, Brown, and Young, 1958; O'Dwyer, Prough, and Johnston, 1996). The second conserves existing energy stores because an arrested heart requires less energy than either a nonworking heart (i.e., one that is not volume loaded, as occurs during CPB) or a fibrillating heart. The sooner a heart achieves cardiac standstill, the fewer energy resources are used in maintaining the contraction and fibrillation that precede arrest induced by ischemia and hypothermia alone.

Measures to minimize reperfusion injury focus on structural and functional recovery. Reestablishing homogeneous flow to the coronary vascular bed expedites the delivery of reparative substrates and therapeutic agents (Esmailian, Athanasuleas, and Buckberg, 1999).

HYPOTHERMIA FOR MYOCARDIAL PROTECTION

Systemic hypothermia is used during CPB to reduce the metabolic rate, and subsequently the energy demands, of the systemic organs. (Shivering, however, must be prevented pharmacologically because it increases the work and energy demands of the heart.) Cooling the myocardium itself achieves the same goals, but additional methods must be used when the heart is separated from the systemic circulation during cross-clamping. Cold solutions can be applied topically, or they can be infused directly into the heart antegradely via the aortic root or retrogradely via the coronary sinus. Because antegrade transmural cooling is especially difficult in the presence of left ventricular hypertrophy and coronary artery disease, which can retard or obstruct an even distribution of the infusate, all three methods— topical, antegrade, and retrograde—may be used in conjunction with prior systemic hypothermia to achieve homogeneous myocardial cooling.

Topical solutions consist of lactated Ringer's solution or normal saline solution that has been chilled in a refrigerator or a device specifically designed for this purpose. The solution should not be allowed to form large ice particles because they can injure the phrenic nerves running along the lateral pericardium; some surgeons use an insulating pad between the heart and the pericardium to protect the nerves. Other surgeons do not routinely use topical hypothermic irrigation, relying instead on the hypothermic benefits of direct antegrade or retrograde infusion. Topical hypothermia is used adjunctively only when portions of the heart may not be adequately protected with other methods (e.g., because of left ventricular hypertrophy).

Direct antegrade and retrograde myocardial infusion is accomplished with delivery systems consisting of catheters and tubing incorporated into the bypass circuit (Fig. 9-36). Antegrade infusion is achieved by placing a needle-tipped catheter into the aorta proximal to the aortic CPB cannula and the anticipated site of the aortic cross-clamp. With the aorta clamped, infusion of the solution under sufficient pressure closes the aortic valve, forcing the solution into the right and left coronary ostia and the coronary vascular bed. When aortic valve incompetence is present, antegrade infusions are contraindicated because the solution would enter the left ventricle and distend the ventricular wall. In this situation the surgeon relies on retrograde cardioplegia infusion through a catheter placed in the coronary sinus via the right atrium. Another, less common method is to open the aorta and infuse the solution directly into each coronary os. Selective infusion of coronary bypass grafts also can be performed.

Warm heart surgery
Because there are disadvantages associated with hypothermia, notably adverse effects on enzymatic function, energy generation, and cellular integrity, some researchers have used continuous hyperkalemic infusions of warm (or tepid) blood for cardioplegic arrest during

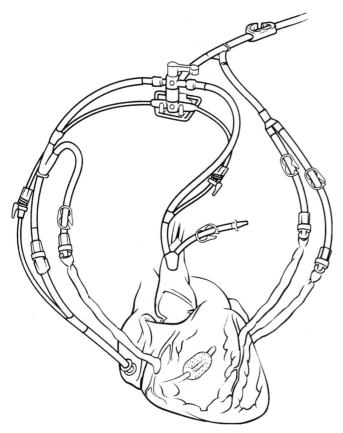

FIGURE 9-36 Cardioplegia setup for coronary grafting and valve replacement. The stopcock *(top)* allows simultaneous cardioplegia delivery and monitoring of arterial or coronary sinus pressure. The system also allows simultaneous perfusion of coronary bypass grafts and retrograde infusion of cardioplegia through the coronary sinus. The vein graft limbs can be perfused separately. (From Buxton B, Frazier OH, Westaby S, editors: *Ischemic heart disease: surgical management,* London, 1999, Mosby.)

cardium. Studies have shown no superior myocardial protection with warm continuous retrograde infusion, as compared with antegrade/retrograde, cold-blood cardioplegia, and concerns about inferior cerebral protection warrant further investigation (Esmailian, Athanasuleas, and Buckberg, 1999).

CARDIOPLEGIA

Although hypothermia reduces oxygen consumption, metabolic requirements can be lowered further by reducing, or nearly avoiding altogether, the ventricular fibrillation that commonly occurs between the period that the cross-clamp is applied and when hypothermic cardiac standstill is achieved. Fibrillation wastes energy resources that could be used when the cross-clamp is removed and the heart must resume beating.

The addition of chemical agents that could quickly arrest the heart with little or no fibrillation has been attempted (Melrose and others, 1955), but results were poor. Gay and Ebert (1973) demonstrated improved results using components similar to Melrose's but altering the composition of the ingredients of the arresting solution, notably potassium and other ions such as sodium, calcium, and magnesium. Buckberg (1979) proposed a solution to the issue of myocardial protection that has become the foundation for cardioplegia management.

The infusion of hyperkalemic solutions inhibits membrane depolarization and propagation of the action potential. The resulting cardiac paralysis, cardioplegia, produces a reversible diastolic arrest that allows the surgeon to perform delicate procedures on a quiet field. Multidose infusions are needed because the cardioplegia solution eventually washes out and the myocardium rewarms. The solution is reinfused about every 20 to 30 minutes (Galloway and others, 1999a); if cardiac activity is visualized directly or noted on the electrocardiographic (ECG) monitor before this time period has elapsed, another bolus is given (when the heart is arrested, the ECG is a flat line). Table 9-8 lists the objectives of cardioplegic management.

Cardioplegia solutions may be one of two types: blood or crystalloid. The advantages of blood cardioplegia solutions include providing oxygen to the heart while it is arrested, allowing reoxygenation when the perfusate is replenished, and providing a buffering effect from the plasma. Repeat infusions of blood cardioplegia solution help to maintain hypothermic arrest, remove accumulated acid wastes, treat evolving edema, and provide additional substrate. The cardioplegia solution consists of oxygenated blood (4 parts blood to 1 part cardioplegia solution) from the arterial line of the bypass pump, which is separately cooled to 3° to 4° C (38° to 40° F). Potassium (K^+) is the most common arresting agent, but

CABG (Engelman and Verrier, 2001). The arrested heart is perfused continuously, thereby obviating the need for hypothermia. With this method of "aerobic arrest," some studies have shown no difference in mortality rates between the warm-blood groups and the cold-blood groups, and myocardial function was improved (e.g., less perioperative myocardial infarction, low-output syndrome, and use of the intraaortic balloon pump) in the warm-blood group. Moreover, the authors propose that this method eliminates reperfusion injury (Engelman and Verrier, 2001).

One of the disadvantages of this method cited by the authors is that anastomotic sites are obscured by blood, necessitating temporary discontinuation of the infusion of the warm cardioplegia solution. This makes the technique cumbersome and may produce ischemic injury, especially to the more vulnerable areas of the myo-

TABLE 9-8	
Objectives of Cardioplegia Management	
OBJECTIVE	POTENTIAL AGENTS
Immediate arrest to lower energy demands and avoid ATP, glycogen, and other substrate depletion	Potassium, magnesium, lidocaine
Temperature reduction and maintenance	Hypothermia CPB; topical, intramyocardial hypothermia
Substrate provision for metabolic activity that remains, especially at lower temperatures (less than 20° C [68° F])	Infusion of blood cardioplegia, glucose, oxygen, lactate, Krebs cycle intermediates
Buffering capacity to maintain appropriate myocardial pH	Sodium bicarbonate, tromethamine, phosphate, blood
Cellular membrane stabilization	Exogenous additives such as calcium antagonists, steroids, local anesthetics, oxygen free radical scavengers
Ideal osmolality with physiologic colloidal oncotic pressure	Blood, albumin
Minimal reperfusion injury	Normothermic cardioplegia induction; warm cardioplegia administration before removal of cross-clamp

Modified from Esmailian F, Athanasuleas CL, Buckberg GD: Myocardial preservation. In Buxton B, Frazier OH, Westaby S, editors: *Ischemic heart disease: surgical management*, London, 1999, Mosby.

others, such as magnesium (Mg^{++}), also may be used. The solution is adjusted for pH and osmotic pressure.

Crystalloid cardioplegia solution, once widely used, also contains K^+ and some of the components contained in sanguineous cardioplegia solution (e.g., sodium chloride, sodium bicarbonate). Because of the advantages associated with blood cardioplegia solutions, many surgeons limit the use of crystalloid solutions to special situations. One of these occurs when a patient has a significantly elevated level of cold antibodies that can stimulate RBC agglutination in vital organs during hypothermia. Measures to protect the patient, in addition to the use of crystalloid cardioplegia solution, include maintaining temperatures above the critical point and infusing the heart with warm crystalloid solution before allowing blood to reenter the coronary circulation.

Reperfusion management

Reperfusion injury can be reduced by measures taken before, during, and after the heart is arrested. Initial infusion of a warm hyperkalemic bolus of cardioplegia solution with substrate-enriched blood is considered advantageous in hearts that are already energy depleted and have reduced ejection fractions (less than 40%) preoperatively. The warm blood enhances global distribution of the cardioplegia solution, especially to the subendocardium. Subsequent boluses are cooled to take advantage of the beneficial effects of hypothermia.

To lower cardiac energy demands, a warm bolus of cardioplegia solution with reduced levels of K^+ is infused antegradely and retrogradely for a few minutes before the cross-clamp is removed to add substrates, buffer acidosis, and limit the calcium load. This bolus is followed by warm, noncardioplegic blood to wash out the cardioplegia solution. When the cross-clamp is removed (or even before), the heart often resumes con-

traction. If asystole continues, the surgeon may initiate contraction by gently tapping the heart with the finger; temporary pacing may be helpful when asystole is more persistent. If ventricular fibrillation is noted, the heart is defibrillated immediately because fibrillation interferes with adequate distribution of coronary blood flow (Buckberg, 1995).

ANTEGRADE/RETROGRADE BLOOD CARDIOPLEGIA INFUSION

The blood cardioplegia solution is cooled to the desired temperature via the heat exchanger incorporated into the cardioplegia delivery system. Antegrade infusion is performed first, followed by retrograde infusion. The initial bolus contains a higher concentration of K^+ than later doses, so prompt cardiac arrest can be achieved. Later infusions have a lower K^+ level.

Retrograde infusion alone may be used in the presence of significant aortic insufficiency. When only retrograde cardioplegia is used, right ventricular protection is less predictable than left ventricular protection. Pericardial lavage with hypothermic solutions can be used to provide additional protection to the right ventricle (Buckberg, 1995). (See Box 9-4 for RNFA considerations.)

Operative procedure: insertion of the antegrade/retrograde cardioplegia infusion catheter
Antegrade cannulation

1. After the aortic cannula has been inserted and connected to the arterial CPB line, a double-armed pursestring suture is placed in the aorta proximal to the aortic cannula, leaving enough space between the two catheters for future placement of the aortic cross-clamp. The pursestring may be pledgeted to buttress the suture.

BOX 9-4

RN First Assistant Considerations Related to Myocardial Protection

Be sure cardioplegia infusion line is clamped before it is attached to antegrade (aortic) cardioplegia catheter (to prevent introduction of air into systemic circulation).

Use cardiotomy suction both to retract and to aspirate blood during retrograde cardioplegia catheter insertion.

Alert surgeon to presence of air in cardioplegia line before cardioplegia infusion is initiated; when saphenous vein grafts are selectively infused, flush cardioplegia line before attaching it to bypass graft.

When retrograde cardioplegia is being infused, verify that aortic vent is turned on (a momentary delay is acceptable); monitor coronary sinus pressure to determine whether it is too high (greater than 50 mm Hg).

If retrograde cardioplegia catheter requires manual inflation and deflation, ensure that balloon is inflated during infusion and deflated during antegrade infusion (occasionally surgeon will maintain balloon inflation during initial stages of antegrade infusion to enhance myocardial distribution of solution, but balloon must be deflated shortly thereafter); do not overinflate balloon (which can injure coronary sinus).

If topical hypothermic solutions are used, remove large ice particles to prevent phrenic nerve injury.

Monitor electrocardiogram and observe heart directly for cardiac activity to anticipate reinfusion of cardioplegia solution.

Use discard sucker to aspirate cardioplegia solution that may have collected in pericardial well.

---

2. The needles are removed, and a tourniquet is threaded over the free ends of the suture. A hemostat is placed on the free ends of the suture (or over the tourniquet around the suture).

3. The cardioplegia catheter containing a needle obturator is inserted into the aorta, and the obturator is then removed. The surgeon places a finger over the opened end of the catheter to prevent excessive blood loss from the catheter. The tourniquet is tightened by the assistant.

4. The cardioplegia tubing is handed to the surgeon, who connects the tubing to the cardioplegia catheter. The tubing must be clamped so that air in the cardioplegia system is not drawn into the aorta.

5. With the clamp still occluding the tubing where it is attached to the cardioplegia catheter, the cardioplegia circuit is deaired by circulating cardioplegia solution into the infusion tubing and out the vent (suction) tubing integrated into the circuit (see Fig. 9-36).

6. After the circuit is deaired, the cardioplegia inflow line is clamped. The suction line is kept open so that when the clamp between the cardioplegia catheter and the rest of the circuit is removed, remaining air is aspirated back to the pump.

7. The suction line is then clamped, and the cardioplegia line is opened to infuse the cardioplegia. The aortic cross-clamp is placed on the aorta between the aortic cannula and the cardioplegia catheter. The initial bolus of cardioplegia is 300 to 350 ml per minute at an aortic pressure ranging from 60 to 80 mm Hg. This is infused over a 2-minute period. Coronary venous drainage exiting through the coronary sinus combines with systemic venous return going back to the pump.

8. Cardiac arrest should be achieved within 1 minute. Failure to obtain arrest within this time may be caused by (1) an inadequate rate of flow (increase flow up to 500 ml per minute), (2) subtotal occlusion of the aorta (the surgeon can readjust the clamp or replace it with another), (3) aortic insufficiency (switch to retrograde infusion), (4) inadequate venous drainage (readjust the venous cannula), or (5) no K^+ in the cardioplegia solution or an inadequate amount of K^+ in the solution (add K^+).

Retrograde cannulation

1. After venous cannulation (but before CPB is initiated), a double-armed pursestring or mattress suture is placed in the lower right atrium. The needles are removed, and a tourniquet is applied as described in step 2 of the procedure for antegrade cannulation. (A full right atrium facilitates insertion of the cannula.)

2. A stab wound is made within the right atrial pursestring, and the opening is enlarged with a tonsil hemostat.

3. The retroplegia catheter with a stylet in place is inserted through the atrial incision, and the tip of the catheter is advanced to the coronary sinus (Fig. 9-37). The stylet is removed, and blood is aspirated from the cannula to displace air. Correct placement is confirmed by palpating the undersurface of the heart. The tourniquet is tightened and tied to the catheter with a heavy silk tie.

4. The proximal end of the catheter is attached to the cardioplegia infusion tubing.

5. The pressure port of the catheter is connected to a pressure-monitoring line (often passed off the surgical field to a transducer maintained by anesthesia personnel or cardiopulmonary technologists). The coronary sinus pressure is measured.

The catheter may be self-inflating, in which case the infusion of cardioplegia solution automatically inflates the balloon surrounding the distal opening of the catheter and wedges it into the entrance of the coronary sinus; when cardioplegia infusion is stopped, coronary venous drainage deflates the balloon. If the catheter requires manual inflation and deflation, a small (3-ml) syringe is attached to an in-

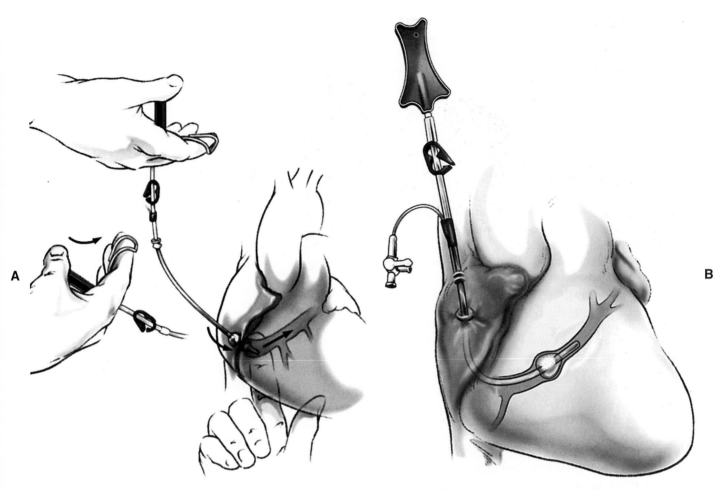

FIGURE 9-37 **A,** Method of introducing the retroplegia catheter. **B,** Position of the retroplegia catheter within the coronary sinus. (From Buxton B, Frazier OH, Westaby S, editors: *Ischemic heart disease: surgical management,* London, 1999, Mosby.)

flation port; once the infusion is stopped, the balloon should be deflated to reduce the possibility of injury to the coronary sinus.

6. Back bleeding from the coronary sinus is allowed to fill the cardioplegia line back to its connection to the main cardioplegia circuit, or blood is aspirated. Once the air is displaced, the retroplegia line is clamped.

7. Infusion of the cardioplegia solution is initiated at a rate of 200 to 250 ml per minute; coronary sinus pressure should remain between 30 and 50 mm Hg. If the coronary sinus pressure is below 20 mm Hg, the coronary sinus balloon may not be inflated sufficiently to occlude the sinus. When the self-inflating balloon is used, the surgeon may compress the coronary sinus–right atrial junction to increase the pressure (Esmailian, Athanasuleas, and Buckberg, 1999).

8. The aortic vent is turned on to aspirate blood exiting via the coronary ostia so that the ventricle is not distended by the retroplegia solution. Blood exits via

the aortic cardioplegia catheter and vent tubing connected to it. The aortic (antegrade) cardioplegia infusion line should be clamped.

Removal of cardioplegia catheters

1. The antegrade catheter tourniquet is removed, and one throw is placed in the pursestring. The surgeon holds the stitch taut with one hand and removes the catheter with the other; as this is done, the assistant places a finger over the aortotomy to prevent excessive blood loss. After the surgeon makes a second throw in the suture, the assistant removes the finger, and the surgeon completes the tie. Another stitch can be placed if necessary to achieve hemostasis.

2. After the tourniquet is removed, the retrograde catheter is withdrawn (the balloon should be deflated before removal of the catheter), and one throw is placed in the pursestring suture. The surgeon finishes tying the stitch, the wound is assessed for hemostasis, and another stitch is inserted if necessary.

Myocardial protection for beating heart surgery

It may appear counterintuitive to be concerned about myocardial protection during beating heart surgery, but the issue is important because there are periods of selective myocardial ischemia during off-bypass CABG. Specifically, during coronary anastomosis the artery is occluded with a small tourniquet or a clamp for a brief period. Additionally, when the heart is manipulated or retracted, injury can occur to the muscle from excessive pressure of the stabilizer (see Chapter 10) or from manually holding the heart too tightly.

Monitoring the status of the heart is a team responsibility and requires constant vigilance of physiologic parameters. The electrocardiogram and the V_5 lead, frequently used during traditional procedures, is less reliable when the heart is beating, so pulmonary artery and systemic blood pressures and transesophageal echocardiography are used to monitor both left ventricular function and electrical activity. Blood gases and pH status need to be monitored closely, especially during coronary occlusion for bypass graft anastomosis. External defibrillator pads are recommended for all patients, and prophylactic lidocaine may be infused before unclamping the coronary anastomosis to minimize reperfusion dysrhythmias (Kaplan and Wynands, 1999).

Occasionally an assist device is required, especially when the heart is displaced and cardiac output is diminished suddenly. Ventricular assist devices successfully support patients and avoid CPB and artificial oxygenation because the patient's own lungs are functioning. Decompression is also effective and allows the surgeon to reach the target vessels. A variety of assistive pumps have been employed for right-sided (see Fig. 9-34) and left-sided heart support. The axial flow pump (Lonn and Casimir-Ahn, 2000) also has been used for left-sided heart support during off-pump surgery, using the principle of the Archimedes screw to move liquid through a small pump inserted into the aorta and threaded into the left ventricle (LV). The pump sucks blood out of the LV and expels it into the systemic circulation to maintain organ perfusion.

As off-pump, beating heart procedures continue to evolve, the repair of more complex lesions in older and sicker patients challenges perioperative clinicians. The basic principles deairing of the heart, avoiding reperfusion injury, minimizing macroemboli and microemboli, preserving ventricular function, and maintaining homeostasis will continue to guide the surgical team.

References

Anderson HL 3rd: Extracorporeal life support for cardiorespiratory failure, *Adv Surg* 31:189, 1997.

Anderson RW, Milano CA: Acquired heart disease: coronary insufficiency. In Townsend CM, editor: *Sabiston's textbook of surgery: the biological basis of modern surgical practice*, ed 16, Philadelphia, 2001, WB Saunders.

Arom KV, Emery RW: Alternative incisions for cardiac surgery. In Yim APC and others, editors: *Minimal access cardiothoracic surgery*, Philadelphia, 2000a, WB Saunders.

Arom KV, Emery RW: Ministernotomy for coronary artery bypass surgery. In Yim APC and others, editors: *Minimal access cardiothoracic surgery*, Philadelphia, 2000b, WB Saunders.

Bartlett RH: Extracorporeal life support for cardiopulmonary failure, *Curr Probl Surg* 27(10):621, 1990.

Beuren A, Sparks C, Bing RJ: Metabolic studies on arrested and fibrillating perfused heart, *Am J Cardiol* 1:103, 1958.

Bigelow WG, Lindsay WK, Greenwood WF: Hypothermia: its possible role in cardiac surgery: an investigation of factors governing survival in dogs at low body temperatures, *Ann Surg* 132:849, 1950.

Buckberg GD: Update on current techniques of myocardial protection, *Ann Thorac Surg* 60(3):805, 1995.

Buckberg GD: A proposed "solution" to the cardioplegic controversy, *J Thorac Cardiovasc Surg* 77(6):803, 1979.

Buxton B, Goldblatt J, Komeda M: Reoperation. In Buxton B, Frazier OH, Westaby S, editors: *Ischemic heart disease: surgical management*, London, 1999, Mosby.

Buxton B and others: Basic surgical techniques. In Buxton B, Frazier OH, Westaby S, editors: *Ischemic heart disease: surgical management*, London, 1999, Mosby.

Canver CC, Nichols RD: Use of intraoperative hetastarch priming during coronary bypass, *Chest* 118(6):1616, 2000.

Cohn LH: Parasternal approach for minimally invasive aortic valve surgery, *Op Tech Card Thorac Surg* 3(1):54, 1998.

Combes A and others: Is it possible to cure mediastinitis in patients with major postcardiac surgery complications? *Ann Thorac Surg* 72(5):1592, 2001.

Cooley DA, Reul GJ, Wukasch DC: Ischemic contracture of the heart: "stone heart," *Am J Cardiol* 29(4):575, 1972.

Cosgrove DM, Gillinov AM: Partial sternotomy for mitral valve operations, *Op Tech Card Thorac Surg* 3(1):62, 1998.

Cox JL: The minimally invasive Maze III procedure, *Op Tech Thorac Cardiovasc Surg* 5(1):79, 2000.

De Feo M and others: Deep sternal wound infection: the role of early debridement surgery, *Eur J Cardiothorac Surg* 19(6):811, 2001.

DeFoe GR and others: Lowest hematocrit on bypass and adverse outcomes associated with coronary artery bypass grafting, *Ann Thorac Surg* 71(3):769, 2001.

Dukovic AL, Daleiden-Burns A, Shawl FA: Percutaneous cardiopulmonary support for high-risk angioplasty, *Crit Care Nurs Q* 20(4):16, 1998.

Edmunds LH Jr: Why cardiopulmonary bypass makes patients sick: strategies to control the blood-synthetic surface interface, *Adv Card Surg* 6:131, 1995.

Engelman RM, Verreir ED: Optimal temperature for routine cardiopulmonary bypass, *Adv Card Surg* 13:121, 2001.

Esmailian F, Athanasuleas CL, Buckberg GD: Myocardial preservation. In Buxton B, Frazier OH, Westaby S, editors: *Ischemic heart: disease surgical management*, London, 1999, Mosby.

Fann JI and others: Post-access multivessel coronary artery bypass grafting, *Op Tech Card Thorac Surg* 3(1):16, 1998.

Flood S, Johnstone B: Reconstruction of the sternum. In Buxton B, Frazier OH, Westaby S, editors: *Ischemic heart disease: surgical management,* London, 1999, Mosby.

Francel TJ, Kouchoukos NT: A rational approach to wound difficulties after sternotomy: reconstruction and long-term results, *Ann Thorac Surg* 72(4):1419, 2001a.

Francel TJ, Kouchoukos NT: A rational approach to wound difficulties after sternotomy: the problem, *Ann Thorac Surg* 72(4):1411, 2001b.

Galloway AC and others: Acquired heart disease. In Schwartz SI, editor: *Principles of surgery,* ed 7, vol 2, New York, 1999, McGraw-Hill.

Galloway AC and others: First report of the Port Access International Registry, *Ann Thorac Surg* 67(1):51, 1999b.

Gay WA Jr, Ebert PA: Functional, metabolic, and morphologic effects of potassium-induced cardioplegia, *Surgery* 74(2): 284, 1973.

Gibbon JH Jr: Application of a mechanical heart and lung apparatus to cardiac surgery, *Minn Med* 37:171, 1954.

Griepp RB and others: Cerebral protection in aortic surgery, *Adv Card Surg* 12:1, 2000.

Johnson SL: *The history of cardiac surgery 1896-1955,* Baltimore, 1970, Johns Hopkins.

Kaplan JA, Wynands JE: Anesthesia for myocardial revascularization. In Kaplan JA, editor: *Cardiac anesthesia,* ed 4, Philadelphia, 1999, WB Saunders.

Kay HR and others: Effects of cross-clamp time, temperature and cardioplegic agents on myocardial function after induced arrest, *J Thorac Cardiovasc Surg* 76(5):590, 1978.

Kirklin JK: Prospects for understanding and eliminating the deleterious effects of cardiopulmonary bypass, *Ann Thorac Surg* 51(4):529, 1991.

Kirklin JW, Barratt-Boyes BG: *Cardiac surgery: morphology, diagnostic criteria, natural history, techniques, results, and indications,* ed 2, vol 2, New York, 1993, Churchill Livingstone.

Kirklin JW and others: Complement and the damaging effects of cardiopulmonary bypass, *J Thorac Cardiovasc Surg* 86(6):845, 1983.

Lonn U, Casimir-Ahn H: Axial flow pumps: an alternative to cardiopulmonary bypass for coronary surgery. In Yim APC and others, editors: *Minimal access cardiothoracic surgery,* Philadelphia, 2000, WB Saunders.

Loulmet DF and others: Less invasive techniques for mitral valve surgery, *J Thorac Cardiovasc Surg* 115(4):772, 1998.

Lytle B: Results of coronary artery bypass surgery. In Buxton B, Frazier OH, Westaby S, editors: *Ischemic heart disease: surgical management,* London, 1999, Mosby.

Mangano CM and others: Cardiopulmonary bypass and the anesthesiologist. In Kaplan JA, editor: *Cardiac anesthesia,* ed 4, Philadelphia, 1999, WB Saunders.

Melrose DG and others: Elective cardiac arrest: preliminary communication, *Lancet* 2:21, 1955.

Mills NL, Morris JM: Air embolism associated with cardiopulmonary bypass. In Waldhausen JA, Orringer MB: *Complications in cardiothoracic surgery,* St Louis, 1991, Mosby.

Mojcik CF, Levy JH: Aprotinin and the systemic inflammatory response after cardiopulmonary bypass, *Ann Thorac Surg* 71(2):745, 2001.

O'Dwyer C, Prough DS, Johnston WE: Determinants of cerebral perfusion during cardiopulmonary bypass, *J Cardiothorac Vasc Anesth* 10(1):54, 1996.

Oliver WC, Nuttall G, Murray MJ: Thoracic aortic disease. In Kaplan JA, editor: *Cardiac anesthesia,* ed 4, Philadelphia, 1999, WB Saunders.

Pae WE and others: Prevention of complications during cardiopulmonary bypass. In Waldhausen JA, Orringer MB: *Complications in cardiothoracic surgery,* St. Louis, 1991, Mosby.

Pavelka C, Park M: Heartport: providing an alternative to conventional heart surgery, 1998, http://www.clininfo.health.nsw.gov.au/hospolic/stvincents/stvin98/a11.html (accessed July 9, 2001).

Porat E and others: Hemodynamic changes and right heart support during vertical displacement of the beating heart, *Ann Thorac Surg* 69(4):1188, 2000.

Rand RP and others: Prospective trial of catheter irrigation and muscle flaps for sternal wound infection, *Ann Thorac Surg* 65(4):1046, 1998.

Risnes I and others: Sternal wound infections in patients undergoing open heart surgery: randomized study comparing intracutaneous and transcutaneous suture techniques, *Ann Thorac Surg* 72(5):1587, 2001.

Robicsek F, Daugherty HK, Cook JW: The prevention and treatment of sternum separation following open heart surgery, *Coll Works Cardiopulm Dis* 21:61, 1977.

Rusch VW, Ginsberg RJ: Chest wall, pleura, lung, and mediastinum. In Schwartz SI, editor: *Principles of surgery,* ed 7, vol 2, New York, 1999, McGraw-Hill.

Safi HJ, Petrik PV, Miller CC: Brain protection via cerebral retrograde perfusion during aortic arch aneurysm repair: updated 2001, *Ann Thorac Surg* 71:1062, 2001.

Sealy WC, Brown IW, Young WG: A report on the use of both extracorporeal circulation and hypothermia for open heart surgery, *Ann Surg* 147:603, 1958.

Shumacker HB: *The evolution of cardiac surgery,* Bloomington, 1992, Indiana University Press.

Thelan LA and others: *Critical care nursing: diagnosis and management,* St Louis, 1998, Mosby.

Waldhausen JA, Pierce WS, Campbell DB: *Surgery of the chest,* ed 6, St Louis, 1996, Mosby.

Waldhausen JA, Pierce WS: *Johnson's surgery of the chest,* ed 5, St Louis, 1985, Mosby.

Westaby S, Bosher C: *Landmarks in cardiac surgery,* Oxford, UK, 1997, Isis Medical Media.

Westaby S: Cardiopulmonary bypass for coronary artery surgery. In Buxton B, Frazier OH, Westaby S, editors: *Ischemic heart disease: surgical management,* London, 1999, Mosby.

10 Surgery for Coronary Artery Disease

In certain cases of angina pectoris, when the mouth of the coronary arteries is calcified, it would be useful to establish a complementary circulation for the lower parts of the arteries.

Alexis Carrel, MD, 1910 (p. 83)

The success of off-pump CABG is truly dependent on a team effort.

Albert J. Pfister, MD, 1999 (p. 40)

Surgery for ischemic heart disease was proposed in the late nineteenth century by Francois Franck, a French physiologist, whose suggestion to divide the cardiac sympathetic pain fibers was based on the theory that the patient would be unable to perceive angina pectoris. Thoracic sympathectomy did relieve angina in many patients, but it did not alter the underlying disease nor ameliorate its adverse effects. More direct efforts to treat ischemia by increasing the myocardial blood supply, suggested by Carrel in 1910, were attempted by Claude Beck in the 1930s. Beck's belief that the heart could be perfused by surrounding tissue led him to devise various techniques whereby pectoral muscle, pericardial tissue, or omentum was grafted to the denuded epicardium of patients. Eventually these procedures were abandoned, but they did set the stage for Vineberg's 1948 implantation of the bleeding end of an internal mammary artery into the myocardium of a patient. This indirect method of revascularizing the myocardium remained popular until Favaloro's large-scale success with direct revascularizing using aortocoronary bypass grafts (and extracorporeal circulation) superceded previous techniques for the surgical treatment of coronary artery disease (Westaby, 1997).

In the 1970s there was a renewed interest in myocardial revascularization without the use of cardiopulmonary bypass (CPB). This interest was driven both by financial concerns and by the realization that some of the adverse sequelae of CPB could be avoided with off-pump coronary artery bypass grafting (CABG). Pfister and others (1992), among the first in the United States to publish their results, concluded from their revascularization of 220 patients off bypass that CABG could be successfully performed and that left ventricular (LV) function was better preserved than after cold cardioplegic arrest. The technical difficulty of performing perfect coronary anastomoses on a beating heart was largely overcome with the subsequent introduction of stabilizing devices that isolate the anastomotic site to provide a motionless target for suturing (Mack, 2000).

A parallel trend has been the growth of minimally invasive surgical (MIS) approaches, reflecting a desire both to avoid CPB and to reduce the size of surgical incisions. These changes have been motivated not only by cost and cosmetic considerations but also by a greater understanding of the adverse effects of CPB (Edmunds, 1995; see Chapter 9 for basic cardiac procedures) and by the desire to avoid median sternotomy. Among the various forms of coronary artery bypass (Table 10-1), perhaps the most minimally invasive incisional approach to date has been the port-access robotic operation for revascularization; the technique employs three to four small incisions for the percutaneous endoscopic equipment. The precision possible with robotic retraction and anastomoses suggests many future opportunities for port-access surgery. Additionally the number of off-pump procedures continues to increase, but the use of small (technically challenging) incisions has declined. The median sternotomy has been repopularized in large part because of the excellent exposure it provides.

Coronary Artery Disease

Endothelial injury has been established as a factor in generating atherosclerosis, a chronic and progressive process that produces coronary artery disease (CAD) (Futterman and Lemberg, 2001). CAD is the leading cause of morbidity and mortality in the United States,

TABLE 10-1
Types of Coronary Artery Bypass

NAME	INCISION	INDICATION
Minimally invasive direct coronary artery bypass (MIDCAB)	Left anterolateral thoracotomy	Single left anterior descending (LAD) coronary artery anastomosis with left internal mammary artery (LIMA)
Lateral anterior thoracotomy coronary artery bypass (LATCAB)	Anterolateral thoracotomy	Saphenous vein or radial artery from descending aorta to circumflex coronary artery system
Off-pump coronary artery bypass (OPCAB)	Median sternotomy with full or limited skin incision	Multiple anastomoses
Totally endoscopic coronary artery bypass (TECAB); endoscopic coronary artery bypass graft (ECABG)	Thoracic ports	Multiple anastomoses; on or off bypass
Port-access coronary artery bypass (PACAB [also called Port-access CAB])	Thoracic ports	Multiple anastomoses; robot may or may not be used
MIS employing robotic assistance (Robotic CAB)	Thoracic ports, small incisions	Multiple anastomoses
Combined surgery and percutaneous coronary intervention (PCI) (Hybrid)	Sternotomy (usually)	CABG: LAD coronary artery PCI: posterior coronary arteries

Modified from Mack M: Coronary surgery: off-pump and port access, *Surg Clin North Am* 80(5):1575, 2000; Mohr FW and others: Computer-enhanced "robotic" cardiac surgery: experience in 148 patients, *J Thorac Cardiovasc Surg* 121:824, 2001.

affecting 12.4 million persons (American Heart Association, 2001). Atherosclerosis is a multifactoral process represented by a wide spectrum of histopathologic lesions (Table 10-2). Vascular injury caused by physical trauma or other insults, such as viruses, homocysteine, nicotine, or low-density lipoproteins (LDL), stimulates vascular smooth muscle cell proliferation (Fig. 10-1). This process distorts the vessel architecture, producing vascular remodeling, and is characterized by endothelial accumulations of fatty and fibrous tissue (particularly in the epicardial portions of the coronary arteries). The resulting atheromatous plaques gradually decrease the cross-sectional area of the affected coronary artery (Selzman, Miller, and Harken, 2001).

As the atherosclerotic process continues, perfusion is reduced to the coronary bed distal to the stenotic portion of the artery. When the eventual reduction in myocardial blood flow becomes inadequate to meet the heart's oxygen demand (determined by heart rate, contractility, preload, and afterload) and hinders the adequate removal of metabolic waste products, myocardial ischemia results (Box 10-1). This may be well tolerated at rest, when the myocardial oxygen supply is sufficient to meet the demands of the heart (and collateral circulation provides alternate routes for blood flow), but during periods of physical exertion or emotional stress (Rozanski, Blumenthal, and Kaplan, 1999; Krantz and others, 2000), the blood supply to the myocardium (and in particular the innermost layer of the myocardium, the subendocardium) becomes insufficient to meet cellular oxygen demands (Ganz and Ganz, 2001). The imbalance that is created between myocardial oxy-

TABLE 10-2
Histopathologic Classification of Atherosclerosis*

TYPE	LESION	HISTOPATHOLOGY
I	Initial	Adaptive intimal thickening at lesion-prone locations; aberrant smooth muscle cells and isolated macrophages
II	Fatty streak	Intracellular accumulation of lipids; macrophages form foam cells
III	Intermediate	Continued accumulation of lipids with small pools of extracellular lipids
IV	Atheroma	Coalescence of extracellular lipid pools into a lipid core with a thin fibrous cap
V	Fibroatheroma	Accelerated proliferation of smooth muscle and collagen synthesis; multiple lipid cores and fibrotic layers, with or without calcification
VI	Complicated	Surface defect with hemorrhage into plaque and subsequent thrombosis

*As endorsed by the American Heart Association.
From Selzman CH and others: Therapeutic implications of inflammation in atherosclerotic cardiovascular disease, *Ann Thorac Surg* 71:2066, 2000.

gen supply and myocardial oxygen demand (MVo_2) requires therapy to restore the balance by either decreasing the demand for or increasing the supply of oxygen and nutrients.

Decreasing the myocardial oxygen demand by reducing the workload of the heart is the goal of medical

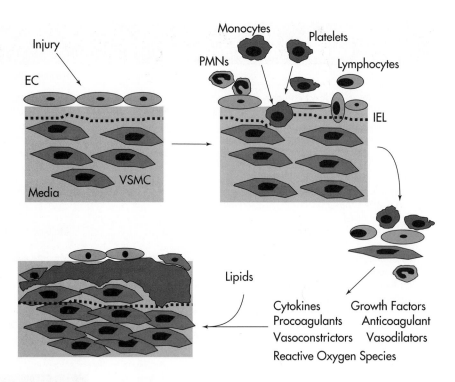

FIGURE 10-1 Atherogenesis as a response to vascular injury. Therapeutic approaches target one or more points within this model (*EC,* Endothelial cells; *IEL,* internal elastic lamina; *PMNs,* polymorphonuclear neutrophils; *VSMC,* vascular smooth muscle cell) (From Selzman CH and others: Therapeutic implications of inflammation in atherosclerotic cardiovascular disease, *Ann Thorac Surg* 71[6]:2066, 2000.)

BOX 10-1
Myocardial Oxygen Deprivation: Consequences and Considerations

Hypoxia/ hypoxemia	Reduced oxygen supply to myocardial tissues despite adequate perfusion (e.g., anemia, congenital cyanotic lesions, right-to-left shunts)
Anoxia	Absence of oxygen supply despite adequate adequate perfusion (e.g., carbon monoxide poisoning)
Ischemia	Oxygen deprivation and inadequate removal of metabolic products as a result of reduced perfusion; leads to lactic acid accumulation and decrease in intracellular pH (e.g., obstructive coronary artery disease, myocardial infarction)
Reactive hyperemia	Marked increase in coronary flow after release of coronary occlusion; the response is driven in part by need to repay myocardial oxygen debt
Myocardial stunning	After brief episode of severe ischemia, period of prolonged myocardial dysfunction with gradual return of contractual activity
Myocardial hibernation	Temporarily impaired left ventricular function, secondary to reduced coronary blood flow, that can be restored to normal by revascularization; hibernation is thought to be a protective mechanism of ischemic myocardium to balance its oxygen demand to reduced oxygen supply produced by ischemia; recovery may take days to months

Modified from Ganz P, Ganz W: Coronary blood flow and myocardial ischemia. In Braunwald E, Zipes DP, Libby P: *Heart disease: a textbook of cardiovascular medicine,* ed 6, Philadelphia, 2001, WB Saunders.

---

therapy in treating ischemia. Treatment includes rest, risk factor modification, and pharmacologic therapy. Among the medications employed are beta blocking agents (which decrease heart rate and contractility), calcium channel blocking agents (which reduce wall tension and heart rate), antihypertensive medications (such as angiotensin converting enzyme [ACE] inhibitors that decrease afterload), antidysrhythmic drugs (to treat conduction disturbances), and nitrates (which alter preload and afterload). Platelet antagonists that reduce platelet aggregation (e.g., occurring during acute coronary events such as unstable angina and myocardial infarction) include aspirin, ticlopidine, clopidogrel, and abciximab. Statins are another a family of drugs that reduce cholesterol and are given to lower the risk of coronary heart disease (CHD) (Eagle and others, 1999).

Increasing the myocardial oxygen supply can be achieved with surgery such as CABG and by percutaneous coronary interventions (PCI) such as percutaneous transluminal coronary angioplasty (PTCA), stent insertion, and atherectomy, as well as fibrinolytic and antiplatelet therapy. These procedures revascularize the myocardium by increasing the blood supply to the heart via conduits that bypass the obstructions (CABG), enlarge the artery (PCI), or lyse clots and prevent platelet aggregation. Without surgery or interventional procedures, increasing the myocardial oxygen supply is difficult because the heart already removes approximately 65% of the oxygen from the blood it receives at rest and 80% during strenuous exercise (Berne and Levy, 2001).

TABLE 10-3
Cardiac Structures and their Coronary Supply

STRUCTURE	CORONARY ARTERY
Sinus node	Sinus node artery from right coronary artery (RCA), 55%
	Sinus node artery from left circumflex artery, 45%
Right atrium	Sinus node artery from RCA, 55%
	Sinus node artery from left circumflex artery, 45%
Atrioventricular (AV) node	RCA, 90%; left circumflex, 10%
Bundle of His	RCA, 90%; left circumflex, 10%
Right ventricle	
Anterior	Major supply from RCA; minor supply from left anterior descending (LAD) coronary artery
Posterior	Major supply from RCA and posterior descending branch of RCA; minor supply from distal LAD
Left atrium	Major supply from left circumflex
Left ventricle	
Anterior	Left coronary artery (LCA), left circumflex and LAD
Posterior (diaphragmatic)	Major supply from left circumflex; posterior descending branch of RCA (90%) or left circumflex (10%); minor supply from distal LAD
Apex	Major supply from LAD
Left ventricular papillary muscles	
Anterior	Diagonal branch of LAD; other branches of LAD and left circumflex
Posterior	RCA and left circumflex
Interventricular septum	Major supply from the septal perforating branches of the LAD; minor supply from the posterior descending branch of the RCA and the AV nodal branch of the RCA

Modified from Popma JJ, Bittl J: Coronary angiography and intravascular ultrasonography. In Braunwald E, Zipes DP, Libby P, *Heart disease,* ed 6, Philadelphia, 2001, WB Saunders.

ISCHEMIA AND ANGINA PECTORIS

Angina pectoris is the precordial chest discomfort associated with myocardial ischemia. Patients presenting with angina undergo a history and physical examination and have an electrocardiogram (ECG) performed. An exercise stress test, echocardiogram, and other diagnostic studies are used to evaluate the extent and severity of the disease. Cardiac catheterization may be ordered to identify the affected arteries and myocardial tissue at risk (Table 10-3; Fig. 10-2). Wall motion abnormalities *(asynergy)* and other signs of left ventricular malfunction (Box 10-2) may be diagnosed with echocardiography and nuclear studies.

In some patients with ischemic heart disease, anginal symptoms are not always present. This condition, known as *silent ischemia,* places patients at increased risk because they do not have pain, one of the important warning signals that would prompt them to seek medical attention. Ambulatory ECG (Holter) monitoring may be used to identify ischemic episodes. The presence of traditional risk factors can alert the clinician to the possibility of ischemic heart disease. These established risk factors cannot fully account for atherogenesis, and newly identified risk factors (Table 10-4), such as chronic infection, may play a role in plaque formation and disruption (Harjai, 2000; Benitez, 1999). Myocardial infarction (MI) may be the first manifestation of CAD.

Anginal syndromes can be classified as stable or unstable. The symptoms of *stable angina* are predictable and recurrent and tend to be consistent in pattern and severity. Symptoms usually subside within 15 minutes and often disappear with rest (which reduces MVO_2) and the administration of nitroglycerine. Typical symptoms include tightness or pressure in the chest that radiates to the jaw and the left arm; atypical symptoms include fatigue, indigestion, and dizziness.

Unstable angina refers to pain that increases in frequency, intensity, and duration and often occurs at rest. This syndrome has been given various names, such as *preinfarction angina, rest angina, increasing angina,* and *intermediate anginal syndrome.* A major feature of unstable angina is the rupture of vulnerable atheromatous plaques. These plaques may have been weakened by the presence of inflammatory cells, proteolytic enzymes, low-density lipoproteins, and mechanical stress. Another mechanism not yet fully understood may be the genetically programmed death *(apoptosis)* of smooth muscle cells (Colucci and Braunwald, 2001; White, 2000).

The difference between apoptosis and *necrosis* of cardiac myocytes is that the former process is associated with intact cellular membranes and requires energy, whereas necrosis involves the loss of cellular integrity and the subsequent inability of the cells to manufacture energy. This distinction is important because apoptosis, which is seen in patients with heart failure (or cardiac transplant rejection), can lead to progressive myocardial failure and cellular death (necrosis). Apoptosis is also thought to have a role in remodeling mechanisms that produce accelerated atherosclerosis of saphenous vein grafts (Rodriguez and others, 2000). Developing treatment regimens that target apoptosis has the potential to forestall further myocardial injury (Ganz and Ganz, 2001).

If there is disruption of the plaque, thrombogenic material is exposed, which can lead to myocardial infarction. Attempts to stabilize the plaque include decreasing the lipid core of the plaque with statins (lipid-lowering drugs) and antithrombotic therapy (e.g.,

aspirin and other platelet antagonists). Invasive strategies (e.g., surgery or PCI) are often advantageous for patients at high risk (e.g., those who have persistent ischemia or an ejection fraction less than 50%). Low-risk patients (e.g., with normal electrocardiogram and negative enzymes) may not benefit from surgery or PCI (Miller and Reeder, 2001).

In addition to angina, myocardial ischemia can lead to depressed ventricular function and other forms of ventricular asynergy. Decreased ventricular compliance, tachydysrhythmias and other conduction disturbances, and systemic embolization from thrombi originating within the left ventricular cavity can also develop. In severe cases, MI with irreversible cellular injury occurs

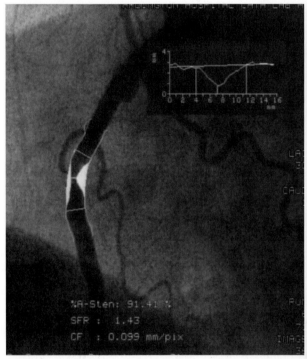

A

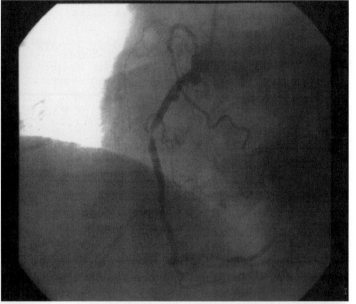

B

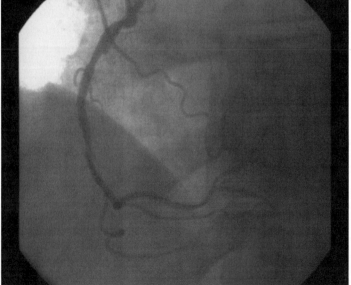

C

FIGURE 10-2 A, Quantitative coronary analysis is used to measure the percentage of narrowing within the lumen of the right coronary artery *(shown here).* Using electronic calipers, the interventionalist has calculated a 91.41% stenosis in the artery shown here **(B). C,** Artery shown after stent insertion. (Courtesy Warren S. Levy, MD.)

(Fig. 10-3). In survivors of MI the mechanical sequelae are related to the location of the blockage and the area of the heart perfused by the blocked artery. Sequelae include left ventricular aneurysm, ventricular septal perforation, left ventricular rupture, and acute mitral valvular insufficiency caused by rupture of chordae tendineae or a papillary muscle. The prognosis is poor for patients in whom these mechanical lesions have acutely and severely compromised ventricular function, and emergency surgical repair is indicated.

Thrombolytic/Antiplatelet Therapy

Patients with emergent symptoms of acute coronary thrombosis (e.g., intense, unrelieved chest pain; overwhelming weakness; diaphoresis; nausea and vomiting) are candidates for interventional therapy. The standard treatment for acute MI has been fibrinolytic therapy and PCI. Fibrinolytic agents, such as streptokinase and urokinase, and tissue plasminogen activators (e.g., alteplase, anistreplase, and reteplase) degrade fibrin clots and restore vessel patency after infarct, especially in patients receiving treatment within 6 hours after the onset of symptoms (Gylys and Gold, 2000). The tissue plasminogen activators (e.g., t-PA) are more clot selective than streptokinase and urokinase. Additionally, the newest plasminogen activator drug, reteplase, can be given as a double bolus and is easier to administer; how-

ever, reteplase has a lower affinity for fibrin, which can lead to reocclusion. A more recent approach to treating MI is to combine reteplase with platelet inhibitors (especially *abciximab*, a platelet membrane glycoprotein IIb/IIIa inhibitor, and aspirin).

The administration of abciximab during percutaneous coronary procedures has reduced the incidence of MI, the need for subsequent revascularization, and

---

BOX 10-2
Types of Ventricular Asynergy

Uniform ventricular wall motion depends on the cooperative and sequential contraction of the heart muscle. This coordinated contraction is termed *synergy;* disturbances in wall motion patterns are termed *asynergy.* Types of asynergy include the following:

Hypokinesis	Weak or poor contractions in part of the ventricular wall; motion is diminished but not absent
Asynersis	Disrupted and uncoordinated ventricular contraction (e.g., cardiomyopathy)
Akinesis	No motion in part of the ventricular wall; contraction is absent
Dyskinesis	Paradoxic motion of part of the ventricular wall during systole; abnormal bulging during contraction (e.g., left ventricular aneurysm)

Modified from Kern MJ, editor: *The cardiac catheterization handbook,* ed 3, St Louis, 1999, Mosby.

TABLE 10-4
New and Established Cardiovascular Risk Factors

NEW RISK FACTOR	ESTABLISHED RISK FACTOR	ASSOCIATION BETWEEN NEW AND ESTABLISHED RISK FACTORS
Homocysteine: High levels may be associated with cardiovascular disease	Male gender, postmenopausal status	Higher levels seen in older men and postmenopausal women
Left ventricular hypertrophy (LVH): Increases myocardial workload, dysrhythmias, ischemia	Older age, hypertension, obesity	LVH increases with age, hypertension, obesity
Lipoprotein(a): A form of LDL cholesterol that inhibits fibrinolysis, increases cholesterol deposition in arterial walls, and promotes smooth muscle cell proliferation	Postmenopausal status	Lipoprotein(a) levels higher in postmenopausal women
Oxidative stress: Oxidized LDL cytotoxic to subendothelial and smooth muscle cells	Smoking, diabetes, LDL cholesterol, hypertension	Increased susceptibility of LDL to oxidation in presence of smoking, diabetes, hypertension
Fibrinogen: High levels of fibrinogen linked to recurring ischemia, platelet aggregation, increased blood viscosity	Hypertension, diabetes, high levels of LDL, increased age, family history, obesity, smoking, low levels of high-density lipoproteins (HDL)	Higher fibrinogen levels associated with established risk factors listed
Infectious pathogens: Helicobacter pylori, Chlamydia pneumoniae, and cytomegalovirus may promote atherogenesis	Low levels of HDL, increased triglycerides	C-reactive protein and fibrinogen (markers for inflammation) are elevated and may enhance increased adhesion and procoagulant activity, especially in presence of low HDL and high triglyceride levels

Modified from Harjai KJ: New paradigms in preventive cardiology: unconventional coronary risk factors, *Ochsner J* 2(4):209, 2000; Benitz RM: Atherosclerosis: an infectious disease? *Hosp Pract* (Sept 1):79, 1999.

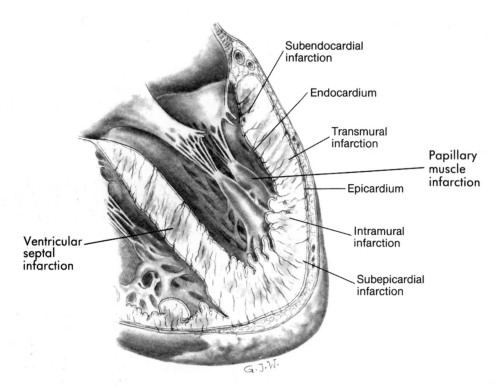

FIGURE 10-3 Location of myocardial infarctions in the left ventricle and septum. (From Thelan L, Urden L, Davie J: *Textbook of critical care nursing: diagnosis and management,* St Louis, 1990, Mosby.)

death. Although the use of abciximab during PCI reduces the incidence of urgent or emergent CABG by 50%, some patients do require surgery while under the effect of the drug, and there is a potential for serious bleeding complications. In stable patients CABG can be delayed for 12 to 24 hours; in patients with ongoing ischemia, surgery should not be delayed solely because of concern about bleeding (Levy and others, 2000). These patients should receive the full standard heparin dose for anticoagulation during CPB; after bypass is discontinued, donor platelet transfusion can reverse the abciximab effect (although not all abciximab-treated patients require platelet transfusion) (Lemmer, 2000).

Percutaneous Coronary Intervention

The demonstrated benefit of primary percutaneous coronary intervention over thrombolysis has stimulated a growing number of catheter-based perfusion techniques (Weaver and others, 1997). Among the interventional procedures performed in the cardiac catheterization laboratory, PTCA (Fig. 10-4) with stent insertion (Fig. 10-5) is the most common (Kereiakes, 2000). Other revascular-

ization procedures include atherectomy and laser vaporization of plaque.

PERCUTANEOUS TRANSLUMINAL CORONARY ANGIOPLASTY

Percutaneous transluminal coronary angioplasty was the earliest catheter-based method of revascularization. An estimated 539,000 procedures were performed in 1998 in the United States; this number represents an increase of 248% in the number of PTCAs performed since 1987 (AHA, 2001).

The concept of PTCA was first described by Dotter, Rosch, and Judkins in 1968, when they suggested the use of mechanical force to dilate atherosclerotic vascular obstructions by inserting progressively larger catheters through a stenosed coronary artery. In 1977 Gruentzig refined the process by developing a small catheter with an inflatable balloon at the tip, which he used to perform the first transluminal coronary angioplasty (Gruentzig, Senning, and Siegenthaler, 1979).

PTCA consists of positioning the inflatable balloon across a stenosed segment of coronary artery and inflating the balloon, thereby exerting pressure against the atheromatous plaque, causing fracture and splitting of the lesion. Balloon dilation stretches and thins the medial wall, thereby enlarging the lumen and enhancing perfusion of the distal coronary vascular bed (see Fig. 10-4) (Kern, 1999).

The procedure is performed in the cardiac catheterization laboratory under local anesthesia. It may be coincident with a diagnostic catheterization, or PTCA may be performed at a later date. Surgical standby for PTCA may be available because of the possibility of dissection of the artery and subsequent acute coronary occlusion. Increased operator expertise combined with cost-saving initiatives have reduced the number of mandatory surgical standby policies. Whether standby is mandated or not, frequent communication between the surgical team and the cardiac catheterization laboratory team, especially when unstable patients are undergoing PCI, is important for anticipating and preparing for emergency surgical care. Emergent bypass surgery may be performed to prevent or minimize myocardial infarction; it is required in less than 5% of PTCA procedures (Kern, 1999).

Much of the subsequent popularity of angioplasty and other PCI has been attributed to an acceptable level of success, greater procedure-related comfort for the patient (compared with CABG), shorter hospital stays, and lower initial cost than CABG. However, restenosis of the repaired coronary arteries is necessary in more than 30% of patients within 6 months (Anderson, 2000; Kern, 1999), and repeat cardiac catheterization and additional PTCAs or other interventional procedures make the difference in cost (compared with surgery) less pronounced. PTCA can be performed in patients with single-vessel or multivessel disease, with numerous lesions, and with stenosed coronary bypass grafts. It also can be used adjunctively with thrombolytic therapy in the emergency treatment of patients with acute myocardial infarction.

Because restenosis is the main problem limiting the benefits of balloon angioplasty, additional treatment options have been employed (Fischman and others, 1994). Efforts to reduce the 30% to 40% restenosis rate include intracoronary stenting (see later discussion) and the application of beta (and gamma) radiation (*brachytherapy*). Brachytherapy has been shown to reduce the vascular neointimal proliferation and constrictive remodeling that are considered the main causes of coronary restenosis (Verin and others, 2001). The radioactive material is delivered via catheter on a "ribbon" containing radioactive seeds. The ribbon is placed at the site of the coronary stenosis for a short time after PTCA revascularization and then removed (Sheppard and Eisenberg, 2001).

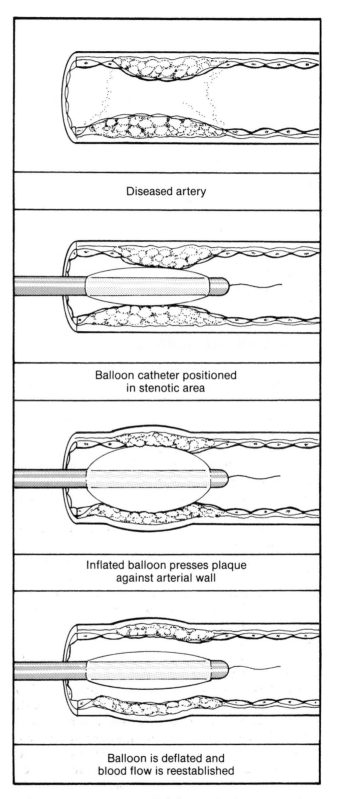

FIGURE 10-4 Coronary balloon angioplasty procedure. (From Canobbio M: *Cardiovascular disorders*, St Louis, 1990, Mosby.)

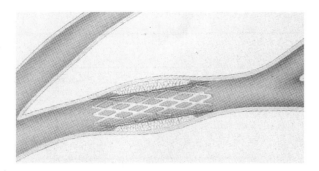

FIGURE 10-5 Intracoronary stent in place at the site of the lesion. Newer stents may incorporate atheroma-inhibiting drugs into the device. (Courtesy Cordis Corp. Johnson & Johnson Co.)

Safety issues (e.g., potential aneurysm formation, oncogenesis) associated with the use of ionizing radiation continue to be addressed (Sapirstein, Zuckerman, and Dillard, 2001).

INTRACORONARY STENTING

Because of the restenosis rate for PTCA, insertion of an intracoronary stent was introduced to maintain the patency of the angioplastied vessel. The device is a coil-like (usually) metal device implanted within the artery lumen to support the diseased vessel wall; stents are generally balloon expandable, although self-expanding stents are also available (Popma, 2001). Sizes range from 8 to 38 mm in length and from 2.5 to 4 mm in diameter (Suwaidi, Berger, and Holmes, 2000). Stents are reportedly used in approximately 525,000 procedures annually (Sapirstein, Zuckerman, and Dillard, 2001).

Stent insertion is also performed to repair angioplasty-induced dissection, which can lead to MI. Before the introduction of intracoronary stents, urgent CABG was usually required to treat dissection; CABG remains an important treatment option but is required less frequently for this complication.

Restenosis after stenting has been a persistent problem, occurring in 20% to 30% of patients (Fischman and others, 1994). Brachytherapy has also been applied to inhibit restenosis after stenting (Leon and others, 2001). Additional options to reduce restenosis of stented vessels include the development of biodegradable stents made of various polymers (Tamai and others, 2000) and coated stents (Yoshitomi and others, 2001). The newer polymer, biodegradable stents tend to be bulkier than metal stents; most are prothrombotic and create an inflammatory response (Sigwart and others, 2001). Biologically active coatings can elute compounds that reduce cellular mitosis, inflammation, and thrombosis.

In one study comparing bare stents with stents coated with sirolimus (an immunosuppressive drug used by kidney transplant patients), the coated stents were reported to have a 0% restenosis rate at 6 months, compared with a 26% restenosis rate in the control group (Wood and Lowry, 2001). Coated stents that reduce the inflammatory, proliferative process leading to restenosis are under intense scrutiny. Locally administered antiinflammatory gene therapy to retard restenosis is also under investigation (Sigwart and others, 2001).

Stenting for stenotic saphenous vein grafts is also performed and accounts for up to 10% of PCIs (Barsness and others, 2000). (Thrombolytic therapy alone in occluded saphenous vein grafts has not been very effective in establishing reperfusion [Brodie, 2001; Suwaidi and others, 2001].) Post-CABG vein graft stenosis differs from that of primary (de novo) native coronary stenosis in that vein graft lesions demonstrate multiple patterns of disease and diffuse degeneration throughout the graft that is difficult to modify by selective stent implantation (Lincoff, 2000). After stent insertion, the saphenous vein graft failure rate can be 50% after 2 years. However, stenting has demonstrated greater success than balloon angioplasty, which is associated with distal embolization, as well as restenosis (Suwaidi, Berger, and Holmes, 2000).

PCI and CABG

Numerous studies have compared the clinical outcomes and the costs of PCI and CABG. In one randomized study, Serruys and colleagues (2001) compared CABG with stenting for the treatment of multivessel disease. The authors found that at 1 year there was no significant difference between the two groups in terms of *death, stroke,* or *MI.* Of those in the stent group, 16.8% underwent a second revascularization, compared with 3.5% in the surgery group. Event-free survival at 1 year was 73.8% for the stent group and 87.8% for the CABG group. Costs for the initial stent procedure was $4212 less than that for CABG; but the difference was reduced to $2973 as a result of the increased need for repeat revascularization in patients receiving stents. The study also reinforced other findings (e.g., Detre and others, 1999) that patients with diabetes who undergo PCI have more adverse clinical outcomes compared with surgery.

Debate continues over the comparative advantages of catheter interventions (e.g., PTCA, stent) and coronary bypass grafting, but available data suggest that within subsets of patients there are differences in survival and recurrence of angina. With respect to survival, CABG provides greater benefit to patients with left main and three-vessel coronary disease; some patients with two-vessel disease receive considerable comparative benefit. Fewer patients with single-vessel disease receive comparative benefit from CABG, and many of these patients undergo PCI (Eagle and others, 1999). CABG patients demonstrate greater freedom from angina compared with stenting (Serruys and others, 2001).

HYBRID PROCEDURES

Combined surgical-interventional procedures to treat patients with multivessel coronary disease have been employed. These *hybrid* procedures can overcome some of the inherent limitations of performing beating heart surgery on patients with lateral or posterior coronary lesions.

The enthusiasm for beating heart (e.g., off-pump) surgery was generated by the desire to avoid CPB (Pfister and others, 1992; Bennetti and others, 1991), but early procedures were performed to revascularize easily accessible anterior coronary arteries, such as the left anterior descending (LAD) coronary artery and occasionally the right coronary artery (RCA). Bypass grafting to other coronary arteries has been technically challenging because retraction of the heart, necessary for exposing the target lateral or posterior anastomotic sites, carries a number of risks. Risks include performing bypass grafting to the back of the heart while the heart is filled with blood ("loaded") and beating, the potential for hemodynamic deterioration from inadequate venous return to the heart, and rhythm disturbances that can accompany the manual retraction required to expose the posterior surface.

MIDCAB

The introduction of the minimally invasive direct coronary artery bypass (MIDCAB) (Subramanian and others, 1995), with its left anterior thoracotomy incision placed over the LAD anastomotic site, further limited the usefulness of off-pump CABG to patients with single-vessel disease. Although the MIDCAB operation has advantages over standard approaches (e.g., lower cost, better cosmesis, avoidance of CPB), wound complications (especially in patients with large, pendulous breasts or obese body habitus) have not been insignificant (Ng and others, 2000). Patient selection and surgeon experience are important predictors of excellent clinical results (Mehran and others, 2000).

Accessing the posterior wall is nearly impossible with the left anterior thoracotomy incision that is used for MIDCAB. Even with the increased use of median sternotomy for off-pump CABG, the risks of apical retraction remain (although they are reduced with newer retraction techniques; see the following). For patients with additional critical lesions in the circumflex and right coronary systems, complete revascularization often requires CPB.

When CPB is used, the heart is decompressed as venous return is diverted away from the heart and into the pump circuit; during beating heart surgery, the heart receives venous return and pumps it into the circulation. The heart is not decompressed with off-pump surgery.

Broader application of off-pump CABG to patients with multivessel disease has been possible with stabilizers and LV apical retractors that expose formerly inaccessible arteries; the use of right-sided heart assist devices is another technique that facilitates bypass grafting of posterior vessels (Mack, 2000).

The hybrid procedure provides another option for patients with multivessel disease by combining surgery and percutaneous revascularization. The left IMA is anastomosed to the LAD coronary artery during surgery; lesions in the circumflex or right coronary artery systems are stented (either at time of surgery or, more often, postoperatively). Hybrid procedures are especially useful in patients with (1) LAD disease not amenable to angioplasty or stenting and (2) non-LAD disease treatable by PCI (Mack, 2000).

Surgery for Coronary Artery Disease

Coronary artery bypass grafting is the attachment of conduits, most commonly the internal mammary artery (IMA) or other arteries, and greater saphenous vein directly to the coronary artery at a point distal to the narrowed artery. Mammary arteries may be as small as 1 mm, and surgeons and their assistants must be able to perform the delicate anastomoses with dexterity and in the least possible time (Favaloro, 1991), regardless of whether CABG is performed with or without CPB.

GROWTH OF NEW TECHNIQUES

The explosion of technical options for performing myocardial revascularization has led to considerable confusion over the meaning of terms such as *on-*and-*off-pump, beating* and *nonbeating (arrested) heart surgery,* and *minimally invasive surgery.* Numerous (and creative) acronyms (see Table 10-1) further challenge the perioperative clinician. Box 10-3 attempts to bring a reasonable understanding to this situation with the caveat that changes, modifications, and varying interpretations will continue.

What is certain and unchanging is that cellular demands for oxygen, nutrients, and waste removal remain basic needs that must be met no matter what form the surgical procedure may take.

BOX 10-3

Concepts, Techniques, Implications, and Innovations: Minimally Invasive and Beating Heart Surgery

Minimally invasive surgery is interpreted in different ways; the following reflect some of the most common interpretations of the concept of MIS:

1. *MIS* most often refers to the use of incisions smaller than conventional median sternotomy or full-length incisions for conduit retrieval. Examples include the following:

CHEST INCISIONS

- Small (less than 8 cm) right or left anterior thoracotomy incision
- Mini-sternotomy (half or less of the sternum is divided)
- Full sternotomy with limited skin incision
- Parasternal incision
- Intercostal ports

CONDUIT INCISIONS

- Conduit removal (e.g., internal mammary artery, greater saphenous vein, radial artery) via small incisions with or without endoscopic, video-assisted techniques

2. The concept of *minimally invasive* also reflects an attempt to reduce the physiologic disturbances attributed to cardiopulmonary bypass, prompting the use of *beating heart surgery* (see Implication 6) regardless of incision size.
3. A third aspect of the concept reflects a growing demand for more cosmetically appealing incisions.

Implication 1

Smaller incisions reduce operator visibility and require adjunctive techniques to ensure an adequate view of the surgical site. Innovations include the following:
- Lighted endoscopes
- Lighted retractors
- Magnification (loupes, cameras, microscope)
- Video monitors
- Three-dimensional video imaging
- Blower/mister/suction devices that kept the field clear of blood
- Three-dimensional reconstruction of coronary angiograms that can be fused with the intraoperative videoscopic image (Mohr and others, 2001)

Implication 2

Smaller incisions limit the operator's ability to dissect, sew, retract, and control the position of tissues and organs. Innovations to assist the operator include the following:
- Robots to provide precision in retracting tissue and sewing blood vessels with remote, tremor-free control that mimics wrist and hand action (e.g., degrees of freedom)
- Computerized systems to facilitate visualization, tissue manipulation, anatomoses
- Endoscopic instrumentation especially designed to manipulate tissue effectively and without obscuring the surgical field
- Automatic anastomotic devices

Implication 3

Smaller incisions reduce the maneuverability of traditional instruments. Innovations in technique, instrument design, and newer devices include the following:
- Emphasis on location of incision ports and patient position
- Double-action handles that reduce the opening angle of the instrument shaft
- Single long arms (instead of dual arms) on instruments with proximal control of the jaws
- Longer handles to permit insertion of the instrument through a narrow incision
- Robotic arms
- Computer-enhanced instrumentation systems
- Lack of tactile feedback or visualization (conventionally used to determine the anastomotic site) overcome in part with endoscopic Doppler ultrasonography (Mohr, 2001)

Implication 4

Smaller incisions require new techniques to perform anastomoses in constricted spaces. Innovative suturing techniques, currently available or under development, include the following:
- Staples, clips, tissue glue, laser tissue welding, ventricle-to-coronary artery shunts, and other anastomotic techniques/devices
- Endoscopic manual suturing with intracorporeal knotting
- Robotic technology to minimize tremor
- Stabilizers to limit cardiac motion at anastomotic site

Implication 5

Smaller incisions create challenges to organ viability for ensuring adequate oxygenation, sufficient energy substrate, and metabolic waste removal. Historically, cardiopulmonary bypass (CPB) was developed in order to maintain organ viability while the heart is arrested so that complex intracardiac procedures can be performed. Innovations in minimally invasive extracorporeal perfusion techniques *(nonbeating heart surgery, arrested heart surgery)* include the following:

SYSTEMIC PERFUSION/PROTECTION

- Percutaneous CPB systems that employ transfemoral venous and arterial catheters; endoluminal balloon aortic occlusion
- Percutaneous chest insertion of venous and arterial catheters directly into the right atrium and ascending aorta, respectively

MYOCARDIAL PERFUSION/PROTECTION

- Percutaneously inserted intracardiac retrograde and intraaortic antegrade cardioplegia infusion systems
- Intracardiac and intraaortic venting catheters
- Intraluminal balloon devices that occlude the aorta

Modified from Pfister AJ: Myocardial revascularization without cardiopulmonary bypass, *Adv Cardiac Surg* 11:35, 1999; Reichenspurner H: Port-access surgery: pros and cons, *Adv Cardiac Surg* 13:1, 2001; Mohr FW and others: Computer-enhanced "robotic" cardiac surgery: experience in 148 patients, *J Thorac Cardiovasc Surg* 121(5):842, 2001; Mack MJ: Coronary surgery: off pump and port access, *Surg Clin North Am* 80(5):1575, 2000; Szabo and others: Suturing and knotting techniques for thoracoscopic cardiac surgery, *Surg Clin North Am* 80(5):1555, 2000.

BOX 10-3

Concepts, Techniques, Implications, and Innovations: Minimally Invasive and Beating Heart Surgery—cont'd

Implication 6

For some authors (Mack, 2000) the term *minimally invasive* is interpreted to mean that the most invasive component of conventional CABG is the use of cardiopulmonary bypass, not necessarily the size or location of the incision. The detrimental effects of CPB (e.g., inflammatory response, air/particulate emboli) have prompted the dramatic increase in the number of beating heart procedures in order to minimize the physiologic invasiveness of CPB. This has not only prompted techniques to avoid the use of CPB, but it also has repopularized the use of full median sternotomy (albeit with a limited skin incision) in order to optimize visualization and manipulation of the heart.

The use of CPB provides organ perfusion and at the same time allows the heart to be arrested with cardioplegia to produce a motionless and relatively bloodless field. When CPB is not employed, the heart remains responsible for organ perfusion and serves as the power source for delivering blood and nutrients and for removing waste products from the cells.

Innovations that enable *beating heart* surgery to be performed include the following:

- Stabilizer systems positioned around the target coronary artery anastomotic site to reduce local cardiac movement
- Left ventricular apical suction devices to elevate the LV so that posterior coronary artery anastomoses can be performed
- Preconditioning techniques to test the heart's ability to withstand temporary ischemia (e.g., during anastomosis)
- Doppler and echocardiography technology to monitor and test hemodynamic status and left ventricular function
- Right ventricular assist devices to augment flow to the right side of the heart (as needed)
- Double-lumen endotracheal tubes to selectively ventilate one lung while the other lung is deflated to enhance surgical exposure
- Coronary tourniquets (e.g., using a silastic tape with a blunt needle) to interrupt temporarily blood blooding the field
- Special retractors with attachable components for illumination, suction, retraction, and so on
- Ability to convert to a sternotomy incision (when other incisions initially are used) or to CPB if patient becomes hemodynamically destabilized

---

INDICATIONS

Pioneered in 1969 by Favaloro (Box 10-4) and his colleagues, coronary artery bypass grafting with reversed autogenous saphenous vein conduits has become one of the most widely performed operations in the United States, with 553,000 procedures performed in 1998 (AHA, 2001). There is now general agreement that surgery is appropriate for patients with significant (1) left main coronary artery stenosis, (2) triple vessel disease (left anterior descending, circumflex, and right coronary systems), (3) severe double-vessel disease involving the proximal left anterior descending and dominant right coronary arteries, and (4) persistent and unacceptable symptoms after maximal medical therapy or failure of medical therapy. Usually major arteries and secondary branches with 50% or greater stenosis and at least 1 mm in size are anastomosed; the arteries should have relatively good distal blood flow (Eagle and others, 1999).

CONDUITS

Use of the internal mammary artery (also known as the *internal thoracic artery*) and other arterial grafts has increased dramatically since the publication of results (Cosgrove, Loop, and Sheldon, 1982; Lytle and others, 1983; Loop and others, 1986; Cameron and others, 1996) demonstrating improved long-term patency and minimal atherosclerosis of the IMA compared with vein grafts. More than 80% of IMA grafts are patent 10 years

---

BOX 10-4

Comments on Coronary Artery Bypass Grafting

Rene G. Favaloro, MD[†]
Instituto de Cardiologia y Cirugia Toracica y Cardiovascular
Buenos Aires, Argentina

I believe that for this delicate type of surgery, even more precise since the application of the internal mammary–coronary anastomosis, the nurse is of paramount significance in our work. If the nurse is not acquainted with every single step and is not ready to help us, especially in difficult situations, our work will be impossible to accomplish.

Even though the extracorporeal circulation has improved very much, I always say that when the patient is connected to the pump, really the patient is dying, because extracorporeal circulation is far from being close to our normal circulation. As a consequence, we have to organize the operation; simplification and standardization are the most important steps to be able to perform the operation with dexterity using the least possible time. In this respect the work of the nurses is really significant. Without their help in an organized manner it would be impossible to carry out the complicated myocardial revascularization combination that we are doing at present.

[†]Deceased.

---

postoperatively, compared with approximately 40% of saphenous vein grafts. The use of the IMA has increased substantially. In 1990, 48.5% of patients had an IMA graft, and in 1997, 80% of patients had an IMA graft, according to the Society of Thoracic Surgeons' (see www.STS.org) national database (see Chapter 7).

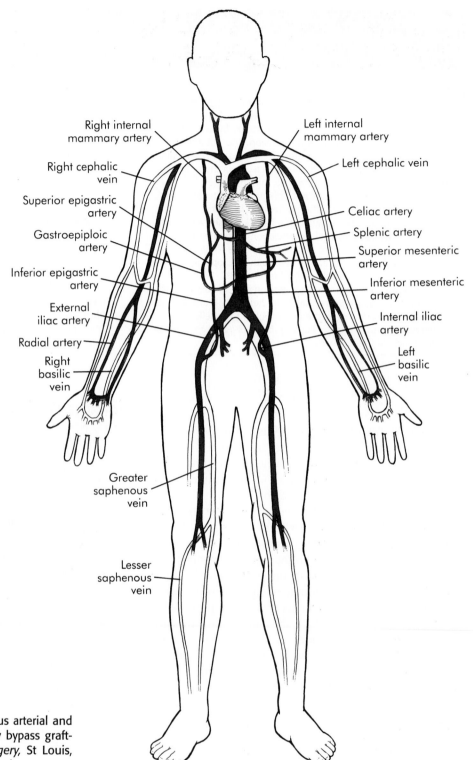

FIGURE 10-6 Alternative autologous arterial and venous conduits for coronary artery bypass grafting. (From Seifert PC: *Cardiac surgery,* St Louis, 1994, Mosby. Drawing by Peter Stone.)

Routine use of the left IMA for LAD coronary artery grafting (and the right IMA for right coronary artery grafting) and supplemental grafting with other arteries (e.g., radial, gastroepiploic) and saphenous vein has become the standard grafting technique (Eagle and others, 1999). Bilateral IMA grafts are increasingly used except in obese or diabetic patients, who are at greater risk for deep sternal infection (Lytle and others, 1986). The 5-year patency rate for *radial artery* grafts is approximately 85%, compared with nearly 90% for IMA grafts (Parolari and others, 2000). Suma and his colleagues (2000) have reported a 5-year patency rate of 80.5% for the GEA.

In addition to autologous arterial and venous conduits (Fig. 10-6), allograft (cadaver) saphenous veins, bovine umbilical veins, and synthetic (e.g., Dacron) grafts have been used. Long-term patency has not been acceptable in synthetic grafts, and their use generally is reserved for patients undergoing re-repeat operations and in whom there are few remaining autologous conduits.

Because early graft closure of vein grafts is commonly caused by thrombosis, patients may be placed on early postoperative antiplatelet regimen with aspirin to retard this process; antilipid (e.g., ticlopidine or clopidogrel) treatment may be instituted if the patient is allergic to aspirin (Limet and others, 1987; Eagle and others, 1999). Surgical technique in the preparation of bypass conduits and their anastomosis to the coronary arteries are also critical to surgical outcome, as is adequate blood flow through the newly constructed grafts. Extremes in temperature and distension pressure should be avoided during dissection and preparation of the saphenous vein.

Late closure of grafts is attributed to progressive atherosclerosis (Lytle and others, 1992; Gersh, Braunwald, and Bonow, 2001). Dietary adjustments, pharmacologic treatment with statin therapy to lower lipid levels and antiplatelet agents to prevent graft closure, and cardiovascular risk factor modification are aimed at decelerating the atherosclerotic process and reducing postop-erative morbidity and mortality. Other strategies include preoperative carotid screening and the perioperative use of drugs to reduce the inflammatory response to CPB, dysrhythmogenesis, surgical site infection, and blood transfusion requirements (Table 10-5).

SEQUELAE OF CORONARY ARTERY DISEASE

Other procedures developed to repair the mechanical sequelae of coronary ischemia and myocardial infarction include repair of left ventricular aneurysm, repair of postinfarction ventricular septal defect (see p. 298), and surgery for ischemia-related mitral valve regurgitation (see Chapter 11 on mitral valve surgery). Operations to treat electrical disturbances include insertion of pacemakers, resection or ablation of dysrhythmogenic tissue, and antitachycardia devices (see Chapter 17 on cardiac dysrhythmia procedures).

In otherwise healthy patients with good left ventricular function, 30-day mortality for CABG is less than 1% (Eagle and others, 1999). Mortality rates increase in high-risk and older patients with complex multivessel lesions receiving coronary artery bypass grafting. The most common predictors of mortality after CABG are priority of operation, age, prior heart surgery, sex, left ventricular ejection fraction (EF), percent stenosis of the left main coronary artery, and number of major coronary arteries with significant stenosis (Eagle and others, 1999).

TABLE 10-5

Proven Management Strategies to Reduce Perioperative and Late Morbidity and Mortality

TIMING	CLASS INDICATION	INTERVENTION	COMMENTS
Preoperative			
Carotid screening	I	Carotid duplex ultrasound in defined population	Carotid endarterectomy if stenosis ≥80%
Perioperative			
Antimicrobials	I	Prophylactic antimicrobials	
Antifibrinolytics	IIa	Aprotinin in selected groups	Significant reduction in blood transfusion requirement
Antiarrhythmics	I	Beta blockers to prevent postoperative atrial fibrillation	Propafenone or amiodarone are alternatives if contraindication to beta blocker
Antiinflammatory drugs	IIa	Minimize diffuse inflammatory response to cardiopulmonary bypass	
Postoperative			
Antiplatelet agents	I	Aspirin to prevent early vein-graft attrition	Ticlopidine or clopidogrel are alternatives if contraindications to aspirin
Lipid-lowering therapy	I	Cholesterol-lowering agent plus low-fat diet if low-density lipoprotein cholesterol >100 mg/dl	3-Hydroxy-3-methylglutaryl/coenzyme A reductase inhibitors preferred if elevated low-density lipoprotein is major aberration
Smoking cessation	I	Smoking cessation education, and offer counseling and pharmacotherapies	

Modified from Eagle KA and others: ACC/AHA guidelines for coronary artery bypass graft surgery, *J Am Coll Cardiol* 34(4):1263, 1999.

TRANSMYOCARDIAL REVASCULARIZATION

Transmyocardial revascularization (TMR) or transmyocardial laser revascularization (TMLR) employing carbon dioxide or Holmium: yttrium-aluminum-garnet (YAG) laser energy may be useful for patients with angina that is refractory to medical treatment and who are unsuitable for standard surgical revascularization, PCI, or heart transplant (Box 10-5). A series of small-bore, transmural channels are created with the laser from the epicardial to the endocardial surface of the heart. This process allows oxygenated blood from the LV to perfuse the myocardium (Horvath and others, 1997). Percutaneously inserted intracardiac laser catheters create channels from the endocardium to the epicardial portion of the heart.

The mechanism by which angina improves with TMLR has not been fully clarified. One theory is that relief of angina is less the result of a reduction in ischemia and more the result of denervation secondary to the destruction of cardiac afferent fibers during TMLR. Other theories suggest a placebo effect or that new blood vessels are formed (angiogenesis) within the myocardium (Eagle and others, 1999). Allen and colleagues (2000) reported on a randomized study using TMLR as an adjunct to coronary artery grafting; their results demonstrated improved clinical status for patients who would not be revascularized completely by CABG alone. Additional randomized studies are needed before the efficacy of TMLR can be confirmed (Gersh, Braunwald, and Bonow, 2001).

SURGERY FOR END-STAGE HEART DISEASE

The *Batista* procedure (Batista and others, 1997) and the *Dor* (1997) procedure are two techniques that have been developed for end-stage heart disease refractory to conventional therapy. Although left ventricular assist devices and heart transplantation are the traditional interventions for end-stage disease, these options may not be viable because of the lack of availability of ventricular assistance technology or the shortage of donor organs. Both the Batista and the Dor techniques are attempts at anatomic remodeling, but their effectiveness requires further study to determine the role of *cellular* function in the context of ventricular gross anatomic pathologic conditions (Frazier and others, 2000; Weber, 2000).

Batista procedure

Pioneered by Brazilian heart surgeon Randas J.V. Batista and introduced into the United States in 1995, the Batista procedure was developed to help patients in remote sections of Brazil where modern technology is not readily available and where Chagas disease (caused by a protozoan parasite that infects up to 20 million people in Latin America) is the leading cause of heart disease and death in young adults in areas in which the parasite is endemic.

The procedure involves the removal of a triangular portion of the enlarged left ventricle. The rationale for this cardiac volume reduction surgery (partial left ventriculotomy) is that reducing the size of the heart enhances ventricular function by producing a more efficiently shaped pumping organ. There has been limited success with the procedure in the United States, in part because of the lack of well-defined guidelines for patient selection and because the myocyte abnormalities commonly seen in heart failure may not be amenable to surgical remodeling. Patients selected for partial left ventriculotomy before cellular function becomes seriously deranged may be better candidates for the procedure (Frazier and others, 2000).

Dor procedure

The Dor procedure, also referred to as the *endoventricular circular patch plasty* procedure, reshapes the ventricle

---

BOX 10-5

Comments on Transmyocardial Revascularization

Renee Dodge RN, MSN, CNOR, RNFA
Cardiovascular Specialty Service Coordinator
Sutter Memorial Hospital
Sacramento, California

Transmyocardial revascularization uses the holmium laser to bore tiny holes through the heart muscle and into the left ventricle. The bored holes fill with blood each time the heart beats, thereby oxygenating the heart muscle. TMR has become an alternative to those coronary patients with myocardial ischemia in which angioplasty or bypassing with a graft is not an option. This procedure can be performed in conjunction with coronary bypass or done via a mini thoracotomy incision. If no bypasses are performed and a thoracotomy incision is made, a thoracotomy tray is needed. Sterile internal paddles (preferably pediatric size) are highly recommended on the scrub nurse's back table, and external defibrillator paddles applied to the patient for this approach. No additional instrumentation is needed if this procedure is performed in conjunction with bypasses and cardiopulmonary bypass.

From a nursing standpoint, the procedure is rather simple and adds only minutes to the surgical procedure. The circulating nurse is responsible for making sure that all team members have protective eyewear and the patient's eyes are covered with a moistened sponge, posting "Do Not Enter" signs on all entry doors, and operating the holmium laser machine. The circulating nurse also records the number of channels created, how many pulses the laser emitted, and the region of the heart lasered. The scrub nurse hands the laser probe to the surgeon and prevents it from being contaminated between channels. Both the circulating and scrub nurse keep a running count of the number of channels created for accuracy. Lasering is performed just prior to the patient being weaned from cardiopulmonary bypass.

It is imperative that the company whose holmium laser they are using properly train the nursing staff.

by excising scarred LV myocardium and repairing the remaining defect with a Dacron patch. The procedure resembles repair of a left ventricular aneurysm (see p. 296). Long-term results are not yet available (Weber, 2000).

WOMEN AND CORONARY ARTERY DISEASE

Adverse surgical outcomes and hospital mortality tend to be higher in women than men. Studies have suggested that women tend to have more comorbid conditions preoperatively and tend to present for surgery at an older age than men. Referral to surgery later in the course of heart disease, when LV function is more likely to be impaired, could account for some of the differences in outcome. CABG should not be delayed (or denied) to women who have appropriate indications (Eagle and others, 1999).

Anatomic factors may also play a role in outcomes and contribute to the technical difficulties encountered in CABG surgery for women. Hearts and coronary arteries in women are generally smaller than those in men, and this can affect anastomotic techniques. Graft patency is lower in women; smaller vessels, thin-walled saphenous veins, and a higher percentage of diabetes, obesity, and hypertension have also been cited as possible reasons (Edwards and others, 1998). Long-term survival, myocardial infarction, and reoperation rates in women are similar to those in men (Douglas, 2001).

PATIENT TEACHING CONSIDERATIONS

Teaching considerations focus on the nature of the disease, the selection of which surgical intervention to employ, expected perioperative events, and postoperative activities designed to enhance the recuperative process. Many of these considerations are applicable to all cardiac procedures, but the nurse can specify certain aspects, such as the care of incisions, the progressive nature of the atherosclerotic process, and modification of coronary risk factors. In particular, questions about minimally invasive procedures are asked by patients (Table 10-6). Many patients have used the Internet to learn about cardiac procedures that they or their loved ones plan to undergo; nurses can be especially helpful in clarifying confusing information and correcting misinformation.

TABLE 10-6
Patient Teaching Considerations for Minimally Invasive Surgery (On/Off Pump)

	BEATING HEART/OFF PUMP	ARRESTED HEART
Definition	CABG without CPB or induced cardiac arrest; heart rate and contractile force may be pharmacologically reduced; stabilizer used at anastomotic site	CABG with CPB and endovascular technique for CPB and induced cardiac arrest
Indications	Single-, double-vessel disease, angioplasty contraindicated, medical problems, poor anatomy, accessible target arteries (LAD), previous CABG with blocked grafts	Single-, double-vessel disease, angioplasty contraindicated, need to stop the heart to enhance technical precision, accessible target arteries, mitral valve disease
Contraindications	Complex lesions, posterior targets	Highly complex lesions, posterior targets
Incisions	One to three small right or left rib or submammary incisions, mini-sternotomy (cephalad or caudad)	One to three or four small rib incisions, one to two groin incisions, one to two neck incisions
CPB	No, available on standby	Yes
Cardioplegia	No	Yes
Procedure time	2 to 3 hours or more	2 to 3 hours or more
Hospital LOS	3 to 5 days (versus 5 to 7 for sternotomy)	3 to 5 days (versus 5 to 7 for sternotomy)
Advantages	Avoids CPB, ischemic arrest, and hypothermia; may enable more complete revascularization with postoperative insertion of intracoronary stents into the posterolateral coronary arteries in cardiac catheterization laboratory (hybrid procedure)	Allows repair of more complex lesions without the technical challenge of a moving heart; better able to produce more complete revascularization
Potential complications and disadvantages	Learning curve, technically more challenging, may cause VF, may have to revert to standard sternotomy with CPB and induced arrest	Learning curve, technically more challenging, may have to revert to standard sternotomy, potential for endovascular injury to cannulated blood vessels
Discharge planning	Anticipated faster recovery of 1 to 2 weeks (versus 4 to 12 weeks for sternotomy), earlier ambulation, need to identify reportable signs and symptoms (angina, difficulty breathing, infection)	Anticipated faster recovery of 1 to 2 weeks (versus 4 to 12 weeks for sternotomy), earlier ambulation, need to identify reportable signs and symptoms (angina, difficulty breathing, infection)

CABG, Coronary artery bypass grafting, *CPB,* cardiopulmonary bypass; *LAD,* left anterior descending; *LOS,* Length of stay; *VF,* ventricular fibrillation.
Modified from Mack M: Coronary surgery, *Surg Clin North Am* 80(5):1575, 2000; Reichenspurner H: Port-access surgery: pros and cons, *Adv Cardiac Surg* 13:1-19, 2001.

TABLE 10-7
Cardiac Surgery Early Extubation Protocol

Definition	Extubation within 4 hr after surgery
Patient selection	
Inclusion criteria	All patients ≤80 yr old, LV ejection fraction >25%
Exclusion criteria	High inotropic requirement, postoperative bleeding or ischemia
Anesthetic management	
Intraoperative	Low-dose synthetic narcotics and inhalation agents
Postoperative	Muscle relaxant reversal Propofol 0.1 ml/kg/hr Minimize narcotic use
Ventilatory management	
Postoperative	SIMV mode Check ABGs and decrease ventilatory support every 20 min Always keep pH between 7.35 and 7.45 Always keep Po_2 >75 mm Hg
Extubation guidelines	
Oxygenation	Po_2 >75 mm Hg at an Fio_2 ≤0.50
Respiratory drive	Pco_2 <45 mm Hg and pH >7.35 Spontaneously breathing
Mechanics	Respiratory rate <25 breaths/min Negative inspiratory pressure >20 cm H_2O Tidal volume >8 cc/kg Vital capacity >10 cc/kg
Airway protection	Alert with gag reflex Absence of heavy secretions
Cardiovascular	Cardiac index >2.0 liters/min/m² MAP >80 and <120 mm Hg

ABG, Arterial blood gas; *LV,* left ventricular; *MAP,* mean arterial pressure; *SIMV,* synchronized intermittent mandatory ventilation.
From Braunwald E, Zipes DP, Libby P, editors: *Heart disease: a textbook of cardiovascular medicine,* ed 6, Philadelphia, 2001, WB Saunders.

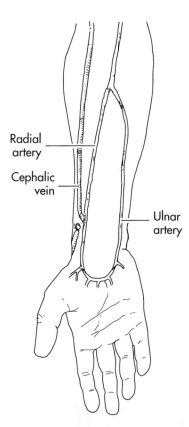

FIGURE 10-7 Arteries and vein of the lower arm. The basilic vein (not shown) runs parallel to the ulnar artery; both the basilic and the cephalic veins extend into the upper arm. (From Meeker MH, Rothrock JC: *Alexander's care of the patient in surgery,* ed 11, St Louis, 1999, Mosby.)

Some patients may be "fast-tracked" and be extubated in the immediate postoperative period (Table 10-7); some patients are extubated in the operating room (OR). Advantages of extubation include improved patient mobility, with early transfer to a nursing step-down unit; patients with excessive postoperative bleeding or those requiring high inotropic drug support are excluded (Adams and Antman, 2001). Patients expected to be extubated in the early postoperative period should have the process explained so that they can cooperate in their care.

Additional considerations may be included in the teaching plan, including information about the decision to perform surgery on or off pump, as well as the proposed conduits (see Fig. 10-6). For example, use of the gastroepiploic artery (described later in this chapter) is associated with increased postoperative pain and gastrointestinal discomfort. This information is useful both to the patient and to the postoperative caregivers. When the use of the radial artery is considered, the clinician must confirm that there will be sufficient perfusion to the lower arm and hand by the ulnar artery (Fig. 10-7).

Before the radial artery is excised, the ulnar collateral blood supply to the hand must be confirmed. Traditionally, Allen's test (see Box 4-5) has been performed to determine adequate ulnar artery blood flow. Jarvis and his colleagues (2000) found that the diagnostic accuracy of Allen's test for determining adequate collateral flow was low, and they recommend the use of Doppler ultrasound as a more reliable test.

Use of one or both cephalic or basilic arm veins affects postoperative arm movement, and potential self-care deficits should be incorporated into patient care planning. The risks and benefits of CPB should be clarified if the patient is unclear about which technique is planned and why. Perioperative nurses should contact the surgeon if there are specific questions concerning the surgeon's plan of operation.

In emergency situations (e.g., for failed PTCA or coronary dissection) when patients are unstable, the surgeon usually makes a median sternotomy and uses only saphenous vein as a conduit because an assistant can dissect and prepare the leg vein while the surgeon is opening the sternum and cannulating for cardiopulmonary bypass. Dissecting the IMA may delay cannulation for bypass, although if the patient is sufficiently stable, generally there is time for IMA dissection.

PREOPERATIVE EVALUATION

Minimum requirements for preoperative evaluation of patients with ischemic heart disease include the following (Mangano, 1999):

- History and physical examination (including functional and anginal classification—see Chapter 4)
- Chest roentgenogram (size, shape, position of thoracic structures)
- Echocardiography (carotid artery stenosis; aortic calcification)
- Urinalysis (e.g., creatinine level to assess kidney function)
- Electrocardiogram (signs of ischemia)
- Cardiac catheterization (coronary arteries, other cardiac structures)
- Blood typing and cross-matching (for homologous transfusion or autologous donation)
- Blood analysis for complete blood cell count, platelet count, chemistries, bleeding times, other diseases (diabetes) and cardiac enzymes (to rule out MI)
- Blood gas analysis
- Assessment of nutritional status
- Medical consultation as indicated

If an off-pump procedure is planned, LV function may be further assessed to determine whether normothermic periods of ischemia can be tolerated. Before anastomosis the coronary artery to be grafted may be occluded for a few minutes to test the heart's ability to withstand the longer period of interrupted blood flow when the anastomosis is actually performed. If there is substantial hemodynamic decline, conversion to traditional CABG with CPB may be indicated. As in many new techniques, different cardiac teams are at different points on the learning curve; teams with extensive experience may have fewer conversions to traditional techniques. Additionally, patient selection is important in identifying the most suitable candidates for off-pump procedures.

PROCEDURAL CONSIDERATIONS

Perioperative management focuses on preventing myocardial ischemia by maintaining oxygen supply while reducing oxygen demand. This principle holds true for all types of revascularization (e.g., on pump and off pump).

ECG leads II and V5 are commonly employed to detect signs of ischemia in the left ventricle. Tachycardia and hypotension also alert the clinician to suspect ischemia, but these hemodynamic alterations may not always be present during ischemic episodes.

Nitroglycerine acts as a coronary vasodilator, and if patients come to the operating room with nitroglycerine tablets or dermal patches, nurses should wear gloves to remove these patches so that the medication does not contact the nurse's skin (and possibly cause a hypotensive episode). The patches can be removed after consulting with the anesthesia care provider and before the skin preparation.

Before surgery the surgeon again reviews cardiac catheterization data to assess the patient's coronary anatomy and to determine the severity and location of coronary lesions. Coronary angiography also identifies whether circulation to the posterior aspect of the left ventricle is supplied by the right coronary artery (right dominant), by the circumflex branch of the left coronary artery (left dominant), or by both right and left arteries (balanced system). This knowledge is used by the surgeon to select anastomotic sites. The surgeon also will want to evaluate the function of the left ventricle and the mitral apparatus, especially in patients who have sustained an MI and whose ventricular wall motion may be impaired (Sweeney, Frazier, and Cooley, 2000). Transesophageal echocardiography (TEE) is used to monitor LV function (Heckman, 2001).

Procedural considerations for CABG are listed in Box 10-6. Coronary artery instruments (see Chapter 3) are added to the basic setup for cardiac surgery; these include delicate blades to incise the coronary artery, fine forward and backward Potts scissors to extend the incision, and forceps and needle holders for the anastomoses. Additional supplies may include one or more blunt-tipped cannulas that are inserted into the distal ends of the saphenous vein. Syringes inserted into the vein can be used to distend the vessel; and blunt-tip needles may be used to infuse papaverine (to reduce spasm) in the IMA and radial and gastroepiploic arteries. If coronary endarterectomy is to be performed, dissectors and endarterectomy loops may be required (Fig. 10-8). Cotton gloves help the assistant to grasp the arrested heart securely during CABG with CPB for circumflex marginal and posterior descending coronary artery anastomoses. For beating heart procedures, LV apical suction devices (see Chapter 3) may be used for retracting the heart to expose the lateral and posterior coronary arteries.

BOX 10-6
Myocardial Revascularization: Procedural Considerations

Instrumentation and equipment

Internal mammary artery (IMA) retractor and table parts
Arm holder for radial artery (or arm vein) excision
Epicardial retractor
Balfour or other abdominal retractor for gastroepiploic artery exposure
Artery/vein excision instruments (dissecting instruments)
Coronary anastomosis instruments (needle holders, forceps, scissors)
Endarterectomy instruments (spatulas, dilators, clamps)
Coronary, IMA dilators
For minimally invasive/off pump procedures: endoscopic or robotic devices and instruments, video systems, coronary stabilizers, LV apical suction retractors, special anterior thoracotomy or mini-sternotomy retractors

Supplies

Coronary anastomotic suture (5-0, 6-0, 7-0, 8-0)
Micro-bulldogs
Blunt-tipped needles for irrigation/infusion
Vein cannulas and syringes to irrigate vein
25- and 27-gauge needle to deair bypass grafts
Cotton glove(s) for assistant to retract heart
If resection/repair of left ventricular aneurysm or repair of postinfarction ventricular septal defect to be performed, have felt strips and pledgets, heavy suture, and Dacron graft/patch material available
For minimally invasive/off-pump procedure: silastic tourniquets, coronary shunts, endovascular bypass supplies, intraaortic balloon occlusion devices

Medications

Label syringes and containers of solutions, medications:
　　Papaverine
　　Heparin, heparinized saline
　　Topical antibiotic irrigating solution

Positioning

Supine, legs slightly everted
Leg holder for prep; raise and lower legs simultaneously
Pillows or positioning pad for legs
If arm veins used, place arms on boards without overextending to avoid injury to brachial plexus; tuck arms after dissection completed
If lesser saphenous vein used, position leg to expose posterior aspect of calf (may need to suspend leg)
If anterior thoracotomy incision, small roll placed under left side to enhance exposure of anterolateral section of heart

Skin preparation

Shave midline chest, inner aspect of both legs
Wash anterior chest, abdomen and groin, side to side
Wash legs and feet circumferentially

For minimally invasive procedure: shave (if needed) midline or anterolateral chest, leg incision sites

Draping

Anterior chest exposed
Legs exposed from groin to ankle; feet wrapped
For minimally invasive procedure: for thoracotomy incisions, expose anterior and lateral chest on affected side (usually left side)

Special infection control measures

Confine and contain groin and leg instruments
Change gown and gloves before moving from groin to chest
Change gown and gloves if contaminated by team member's back (e.g., during retraction of heart)
Apply dressing to leg incisions, then wrap elastic bandage around leg from ankle to groin to avoid venous stasis and seroma formation
If table height is adjusted for exposure of IMA, protect sterility of drapes and bypass lines; add additional drapes if necessary

Safety considerations

Insulate all but distal tip of long cautery pencil
Place IMA retractor so as to avoid injury to arms; if retractor impinges on arm, remove immediately after IMA dissection
Prevent topical cold solutions from contacting IMA
Avoid use of ice chips (can injure phrenic nerve)
Account for all bulldogs, IMA infusion needles, vein cannulas, blades, dilators, epicardial retractors
Remove coronary atheromatous material from field to reduce possibility of emboli
Prepare for selective infusion of cardioplegic solution into coronary grafts; have appropriate tubing, connectors, and so on
Observe for electrocardiographic signs of ischemia (ST segment changes) denoting possible incomplete revascularization; if noted, prepare for revision of grafts or additional grafts
Monitor presence of ventricular failure and possible need for mechanical ventricular support (intraaortic balloon or ventricular assist device)

Documentation/Report to Cardiac Surgical Intensive Care Unit*

Procedure; bypass grafts: number, type, location, endoscopic saphenous vein harvest
Incision: location, number
On pump/off pump
Chest tubes: number, location (mediastinal and pleural)
Monitoring lines: type, location
Epicardial pacemaker lead placement (single, dual) and if being paced
Patient problems, concerns related to coronary heart disease, surgery
Preoperative left ventricular function (e.g., ejection fraction); previous coronary bypass surgery

*In addition to standard documentation/postoperative report (see Chapter 6).

Much of the dissecting instrumentation for beating heart surgery is similar to that used for traditional coronary bypass surgery; stabilizers and devices to maintain a clear operative field are shown in Chapter 3. Port-access, minimally invasive surgery employs endoscopic instruments specially made for working within the chest cavity (Fig. 10-9). The working end of these instruments provides great flexibility that mimics the human manual dexterity required for complex dissection and sewing (Fig. 10-10).

Standards of nursing care for myocardial revascularization (Table 10-8) include hair removal (with electric clippers or depilatories) along the center of the anterior chest, the groin, and the inner aspect of both legs (along the path of the greater saphenous vein). For endoscopic vein harvest (see p. 283) shaving may be restricted to the smaller vein incision access sites. Chest hair removal is often not required in women. For median sternotomy the patient is placed in the supine position and standard precautions are taken to avoid nerve/pressure injury. The legs and feet are washed circumferentially.

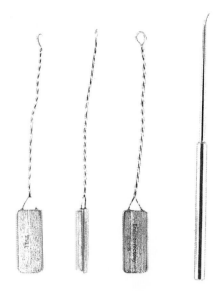

FIGURE 10-8 Endarterectomy loops *(left)* and Penfield dissector *(far right)* used for coronary endarterectomy procedures. (From Brooks Tighe SM: *Instrumentation for the operating room: a photographic manual,* ed 3, St Louis, 1989, Mosby.)

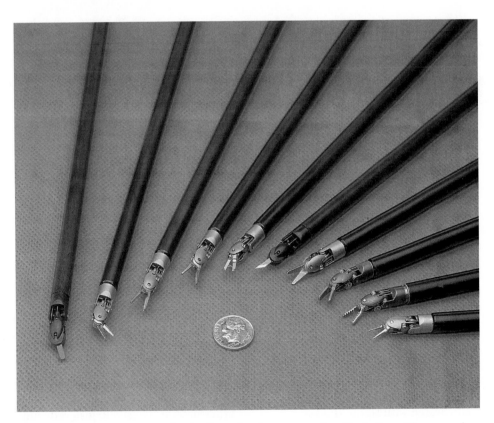

FIGURE 10-9 Port-access robotic dissecting instrument tips illustrate cutting, grasping, and suturing functions. (Copyright 1999, Intuitive Surgical Inc.)

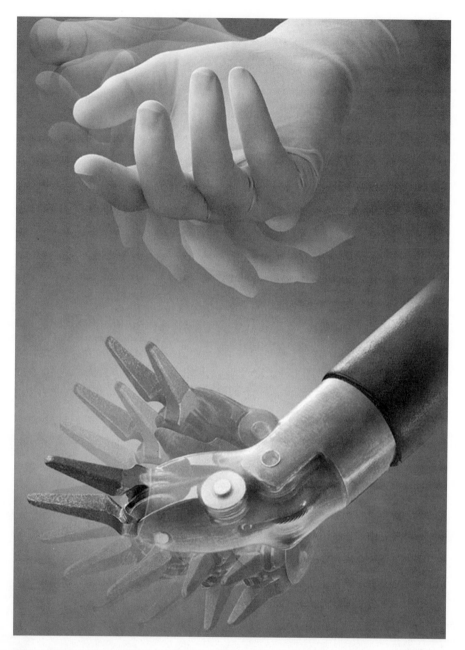

FIGURE 10-10 Wrist and hand action is mimicked by the robotic grasping forcep. (Copyright 1998, Intuitive Surgical, Inc.)

Draping for median sternotomy or a parasternal incision (Fig. 10-11) is accomplished to expose the anterior chest, the groin, and the legs; the feet are covered with towels, stockinette, or other material. The legs are everted slightly with folded sterile towels or drapes, or they are placed onto a special positioning device (Fig. 10-12) that has been covered with sterile sheets.

In patients requiring grafts only to the RCA or the LAD coronary artery (and in particular those patients with heavily calcified aortas, in whom there is an in-creased risk of dissection, rupture, or embolization), CABG without cardiopulmonary bypass may be indicated. These patients may undergo median sternotomy or have an anterolateral thoracotomy incision, in which the patient's affected side is slightly elevated with a roll, and drapes are placed to expose the left (or right) anterolateral chest. Registered nurse first assistant (RNFA) considerations are listed in the Box 10-7; RNFAs play an important role in addressing patients' psychosocial concerns about the planned surgery,

TABLE 10-8
Standards of Nursing Care for Myocardial Revascularization

NURSING DIAGNOSIS	PATIENT OUTCOME	NURSING ACTIONS
Anxiety/fear of death, changes in life-style or quality of life, ability to modify risk factors	Patient verbalizes concerns/fears and demonstrates a reduction in level of apprehension	Describe perioperative routine that patient will encounter while awake: transport to OR, insertion of intravascular lines, description of OR (size, color, temperature, number of people and their roles, etc.) Provide comfort measures (warm blankets, etc.) Answer questions to patient's (and family's) level of understanding; respect coping mechanisms (such as denial) if they do not interfere with ability to cooperate with therapeutic regimen Allow patient to verbalize any concern; if necessary, refer to appropriate person
Knowledge deficit related to inadequate knowledge of planned surgery and perioperative events	Patient demonstrates knowledge of physiologic and psychologic responses to myocardial revascularization	Determine patient's understanding of chronic and progressive nature of CAD Determine patient's understanding of surgical procedure (e.g., on- or off-pump, minimally invasive vs standard incisions); describe (briefly) immediate preoperative events (that will take place while patient is awake); reinforce or clarify what patient (and family) has been told by surgeon; reconcile conflicting time frames given to family (make family aware of preparation and transport time) Assess patient's understanding of planned conduits for bypass grafts (e.g., greater saphenous vein, internal mammary artery, alternative conduits); answer questions or refer as needed If saphenous vein is to be used, inform patient of leg incisions, leg discomfort, and adequacy of venous drainage even with removal of saphenous vein; clarify difference between standard and minimally invasive technique as indicated If additional myocardial revascularization procedures are to be performed (resection or repair of left ventricular aneurysm, coronary endarterectomy, closure of post–myocardial infarction ventricular septal defect), assess patient's understanding and clarify as necessary Determine where family will be waiting during and immediately after surgery; inform them of patient's appearance postoperatively (chest and leg dressings in addition to drains and invasive lines; pallor, cool skin)
Risk for infection related to surgery	Patient is free of infection related to aseptic technique	Perform hair removal on anterior chest, groin, and inner aspect of both legs, as needed Perform circumferential skin preparation of legs and feet Confine and contain instruments and supplies used to excise saphenous vein Change gown and gloves before moving from groin/leg to chest or radial artery-arm to chest and if contaminated Wrap dressing around leg from ankle to groin to avoid venous stasis and seroma formation If table height is adjusted for exposure of mammary artery, protect sterility of drapes and bypass lines; use additional drapes if necessary
Risk for injury related to positioning, use of mammary retractor	Patient is free of injury related to surgical positioning or use of retraction devices	Place IMA retractor so as to avoid injury to brachial plexus; do not overextend; have all table parts available If IMA retractor post impinges on arm, remove after completion of dissection; pad arms Use caution when elevating legs to perform circumferential skin preparation; raise and lower legs simultaneously; have additional personnel if required If arm veins or artery are to be used, place arms on boards without overextending (to avoid injury to brachial plexus) If lesser saphenous vein is to be used, expose posterior aspect of leg using caution to avoid injury to leg or contamination of field
Risk for injury related to: Retained foreign objects	Patient is free of injury related to: Retained foreign objects	Account for bulldog clamps, IMA infusion needles, coronary artery knives or blades, saphenous vein or radial artery cannulas, coronary dilators, epicardial retractors and other items, remove coronary plaque from field to reduce possibility of becoming emboli
Chemical hazards	Chemical hazards	Label syringes containing papaverine, heparinized saline, or other solutions; use only physiologically compatible solutions to distend conduits.

Modified from Seifert PC: Cardiac surgery. In Rothrock JC: *Perioperative nursing care planning*, ed 2, St Louis, 1996, Mosby.

Continued

TABLE 10-8
Standards of Nursing Care for Myocardial Revascularization—cont'd

NURSING DIAGNOSIS	PATIENT OUTCOME	NURSING ACTIONS
Physical hazards	Physical hazards	If left ventricular aneurysm is to be resected, have felt strips and pledgets, suture, patch material, and vents available as needed
		If coronary endarterectomy is to be performed, have dilators, spatulas, and clamps as needed
		If postinfarction ventricular septal defect is to be performed, have felt strips and pledgets, suture, and patch material available
		If reoperation is to be performed, have lateral and posteroanterior chest x-ray films taken to determine location of mediastinal structures relative to sternum and to count number of chest wires; be prepared to cannulate femoral artery for cardiopulmonary bypass if necessary
Electrical hazards	Electrical hazards	Place unused cautery or ultrasonic pencil where it cannot be inadvertently discharged; test defibrillator paddles before start of procedure; if using long cautery tip during IMA dissection, insulate all but distal end to avoid injury to retrosternal structures
Thermal injury	Thermal injury	Avoid pouring ice chips on IMA; test warm solutions before application
		Avoid inadvertent hypothermia
Risk for decreased cardiac output/decreased tissue perfusion related to coronary artery disease	Patient's fluid and electrolyte balance is maintained	If reoperation, anticipate need for additional blood/blood products; on all cases monitor blood loss
		If patient has had bypass surgery with IMA, have bulldog clamp available to clamp IMA when cardioplegia infusion is initiated (persistent IMA flow will prevent cardioplegic arrest)
		Insert urinary drainage catheter to monitor urinary drainage, renal perfusion (cardiac output)

as well as participating in the operative procedure (Espersen, 1998).

CABG WITH ARTERIAL AND VENOUS CONDUITS

Operative procedure

1. A median sternotomy, mini-sternotomy (Fig. 10-13), or anterolateral thoracotomy is performed.
2. Conduit preparation
    a. IMA: If a median sternotomy incision is used, the left and the right IMA are dissected free from the retrosternal bed after the sternal incision is made. A special retractor (see Chapter 3) can be used to expose the IMA within its pedicle in the retrosternal bed, and cautery, ultrasonic scalpel, or scissors used to dissect a sufficient length of the vessel (Fig. 10-14). Small vascular ligating clips are used on the arterial branches, and venous tributaries are sealed with hemostatic clips, ultrasonic scalpel, or electrocautery. Before the artery is divided, the patient is given heparin to prevent thrombosis of the artery. The IMA then is divided distally and the blood flow assessed. A bulldog is placed across the artery to control blood flow. The distal artery remaining in the chest wall is ligated with a heavy tie.

    A small dilator (1 mm) may be inserted into the end of the artery to dilate the opening, after which a solution of papaverine may be injected into the IMA to distend it and to reduce arterial spasm (the assistant opens the bulldog while this is done). The pedicle may be sprayed with the solution as well. Connective tissue surrounding the distal end of the artery is removed. The pedicle is placed in the ipsilateral pleural cavity until needed; the pedicle may or may not be wrapped in a sponge moistened with papaverine.

    For MIDCAB using a left anterior thoracotomy, IMA dissection is performed with a retractor (Fig. 10-15) inserted into the left anterior thoracic incision at the level of the fourth intercostal space. A light source (e.g., endoscope of lighted retractor) is usually required to visualize the proximal IMA. Ligation of arterial branches and venous tributaries is performed as described above.

    b. Arm vessels: One or both arms are placed on arm boards; the skin is prepared from the upper arm to the hand for radial artery excision and from the shoulder to the hands for vein excision. Whenever possible, no intravascular lines are inserted into the affected arm; if lines must be inserted, they are draped out of the field with towels, stockinette, or other material.

    Radial artery: A longitudinal incision is made 3 cm distal to the elbow crease lateral to the biceps

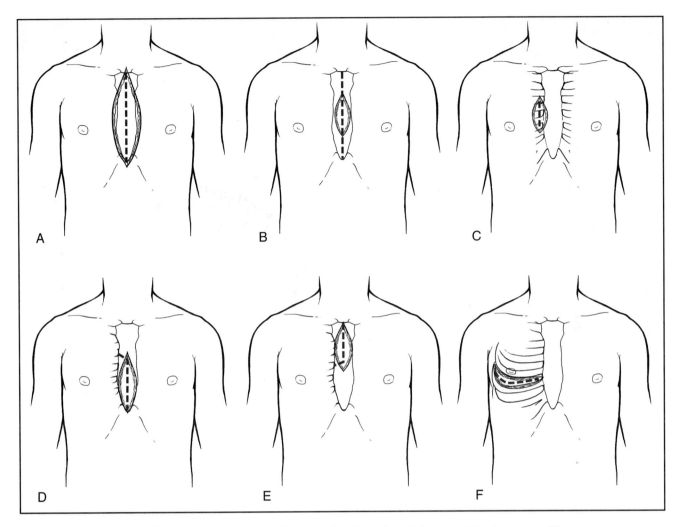

FIGURE 10-11 Traditional and less invasive thoracic incisions used for bypass grafting; *dotted lines* represent chest wall incisions. **A,** Traditional sternotomy with full skin incision. **B,** Limited skin incision with full sternotomy is increasingly popular because of improved cosmetics and reduced trauma from the limited chest wall retraction. **C,** The parasternal incision, once popular, is used less often because of the residual chest wall defect. **D** and **E,** Partial lower and upper sternotomy incisions may be used mainly for valve procedures. **F,** Right *(shown)* anterior thoracotomy incision may be used for mitral valve operations; left anterior thoracotomy can be used predominantly for single internal mammary artery–to–left anterior descending coronary artery anastomosis. (From Braunwald E, Zipes DP, Libby P, editors: *Heart disease,* ed 6, Philadelphia, 2001, WB Saunders.)

tendon, stopping 1 cm before the wrist crease (Fig. 10-16). The artery is exposed and mobilized with a vessel loop and harvested as a free graft with adjacent veins and fatty tissue. The artery is ligated distally after heparin is administered systemically. Papaverine or nitroglycerine may be injected into the lumen to reduce spasm. The arm is closed over a small suction drain (Green and Malias, 2001).

Endoscopic, minimally invasive excision of the radial artery can be performed with a lighted retractor or endoscope to dissect the radial artery

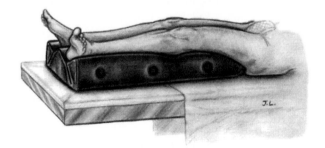

FIGURE 10-12 Padded support that elevates and externally rotates legs to improve exposure of saphenous vein. (Courtesy Tony Rodono, Leatherette Specialty, Cleveland Heights, Ohio.)

BOX **10-7**
RN First Assistant Considerations for Myocardial Revascularization

General Considerations

Know the sequence of steps in the cardiac procedures

Know the preferences of the individual surgeon

Learn the rationale for the surgeon's preferences

Share the knowledge learned with other members of the cardiac team

Dissection of Internal Mammary Artery

Suction away cautery plume during IMA dissection

Avoid touching endothelium of IMA (may cause arterial spasm)

Retract lung with ribbon or other retractor

If pericardium incised to provide a window for the IMA, note location of and avoid injury to phrenic nerve

In emergency situations with unstable patient, there may be insufficient time to dissect the IMA; saphenous vein only may be used

During anterior thoracotomy IMA harvest, avoid tension on ribs

Dissection of Radial Artery

Perform Allen's test or use Doppler to ensure sufficient perfusion by ulnar artery

Alert anesthesia personnel of intended radial artery harvest so that peripheral intravascular lines can be inserted on opposite side

During positioning on arm board, avoid overextension of arm

Clip arterial branches in a manner that avoids compromising vascular lumen

Irrigate conduit with vasodilator of surgeon's choice

Close and dress arm incisions and retuck arm, per surgeon's preference; change gown and gloves

Dissection of Saphenous Vein

Clamp tributaries on vein side, leaving a pedicle, or "neck," to tie without causing adventitial constriction of the vein lumen

Clip tributaries on leg side close to leg to avoid impinging on vein

Avoid excessive distension of vein with irrigating solution

During endoscopic vein harvest, avoid hitting head against sterile field

Close leg incisions as soon as possible to minimize risk of surgical infection

Coronary Anastomoses

Anticipate and avoid suture snagging on instrument handles, pericardial stitch or cannulation suture knots, sternal edges, fingers, coronary stabilizer, etc.

Cover protruding items with damp lap sponge or towels

Keep fingers moist (but not dripping wet) to allow suture to slip easily

If retracting heart and it begins to slip, notify surgeon before the heart slips; avoid digging fingertips into myocardium (keep hands as flat as possible)

Suction coronary artery with caution, avoid contact with endothelium, avoid obstructing surgeon's view

Use humidified gas (e.g., CO_2) to prevent drying of endothelium

Prevent twisting of bypass graft

Avoid excessive tension on snares encircling coronary artery during off-pump CABG

Repair Left Ventricular Aneurysm

Stabilize and maintain alignment of tissue and prosthetic material with forceps

When following suture to close infarctectomy, maintain sufficient tension to prevent leaking from suture line, but avoid excessive tension that may cause myocardial tearing

Repair Ventricular Septal Defect (VSD)

If retracting heart for closure of posterior VSD, use cotton glove to maintain secure grasp of ventricle (repair may be lengthy)

Assist surgeon to maintain alignment of felt pledgets, felt strips, and prosthetic patch

Keep interrupted stitches in order

Modified from Espersen C: The RN first assistant in cardiac surgery. In Rothrock JC, editor: *The RN first assistant: an expanded perioperative role*, ed 3, Philadelphia, 1998, JB Lippincott.

pedicle from the surrounding tissue (Lewis and Hammon, 2001).

Cephalic or basilic veins: Arm veins are rarely used, but they may be required if few other conduits are available. The necessary length of cephalic vein is excised from the radial aspect of the wrist to the inner aspect of the antecubital space up to the deltopectoral groove; basilic vein is taken from the ulnar aspect of the wrist to the elbow and upper arm where it courses toward the axilla. Variations in the venous patterns are common and numerous.

Tributaries are ligated with 3-0 silk ties and vascular clips on the vein and arm sides, respectively. The distal (hand) end is cannulated with a blunt-tipped needle. The cephalic vein is prepared in a manner similar to saphenous vein, but because the arm vein is more thin walled, it may be more difficult to handle. Subcutaneous tissue and skin are closed with absorbable suture; staples may be used on the skin. Dressings are applied to the arm.

If the abducted position of the arms interferes with the surgeon's or the assistant's access to the chest, the arms may be tucked along the patient's side after the dressings are applied. Additional drapes may be placed along the lateral borders to maintain the sterility of the field.

Arm vein graft anastomoses are similar to those employing saphenous vein.

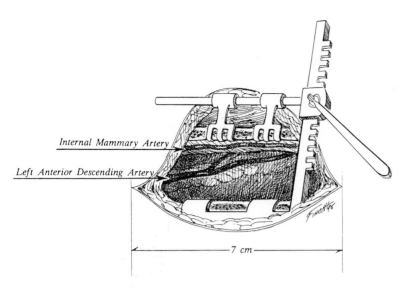

Internal Mammary Artery

Left Anterior Descending Artery

—————— 7 cm ——————

FIGURE 10-13 Mini-sternotomy incision with retractor in place. Sponges may be placed behind the heart in order to expose the entire length of the left anterior descending coronary artery. (From Arom K and others: Mini-sternotomy for CABG, *Ann Thorac Surg* 61:1271, 1996.)

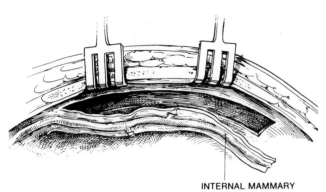

INTERNAL MAMMARY
ARTERY

FIGURE 10-14 Dissection of the left internal mammary artery from the retrosternal bed. The artery is dissected proximally from the subclavian artery and distally to the costal margin. The artery and accompanying vein are dissected out together within the pedicle; bleeding from the vein (and its tributaries) and the arterial branches is controlled with electrocautery, ultrasonic energy, or ligation clips. (From Waldhausen JA, Pierce WS, Campbell DB: *Surgery of the chest,* ed 6, St Louis, 1996, Mosby.)

c. Greater saphenous vein: The necessary length of greater saphenous vein is harvested from the medial aspect of one or both legs (Fig. 10-17). The initial skin incision can be made proximally at the saphenous bulb in the groin or distally at the medial malleolus. The incision is then extended as far as necessary to expose a sufficient length of vein. Tributaries are identified and ligated with 3-0 silk ties and vascular clips on the vein and the leg sides, respectively.

The distal (ankle) end of the vein is identified and cannulated with a blunt-tipped needle to which is attached a syringe of flush solution. The vein is flushed with heparinized (10,000 units per liter) physiologic solution (usually blood) to distend it and inspect it for leaks. Tears in the vein may be repaired with a figure-of-eight suture (usually 6-0 or 7-0 polypropylene; Fig. 10-18). The vein should be kept moist.

Caution is taken to reverse the vein so that the semilunar valves do not interfere with the flow of blood: the proximal (groin) end of the vein will be attached to the coronary artery to become the distal anastomosis, and the distal (ankle) end of the vein will become the proximal (aortic) anastomosis. (The vein is not turned inside out.)

d. Lesser saphenous vein: Also known as the short saphenous vein, this vessel may be used to augment available venous conduits. The vein runs along the posterior aspect of the lower leg, which can make exposure difficult. The patient may be placed in the prone position to expose the vein (requiring the patient to be rolled over and a new sterile field created) or the leg may be elevated by an assistant or suspended in a sling. A sterile mammary retractor can be used to hold the sling. The vein is removed and prepared in a manner similar to that of the greater saphenous vein, although the lessor saphenous vein tends to have more tributaries than the greater saphenous vein. Caution is taken during dissection to avoid injury to the sural nerve and the posterior cutaneous nerve.

Minimally invasive saphenous vein harvesting is performed through one to three incisions over the vein at the knee and at the ankle and the groin if necessary (Fig. 10-19). The vein is located under direct vision; the remaining length of vein is excised via video assistance with endoscopic scissors. An endoscopic clip applier is used to clip

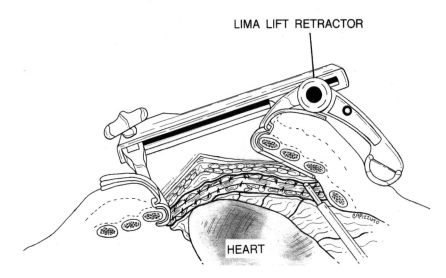

LIMA LIFT RETRACTOR

HEART

FIGURE 10-15 Lateral view of a left internal mammary artery (LIMA)–access retractor that is introduced into the left fourth intercostals space. The retractor pushes the fifth rib downward, thereby creating a wide space for direct access to the LIMA. (From Subramanian VA: MIDCAB approach for single vessel coronary artery bypass graft, *Op Tech Cardiac Thorac Surg* 3(1):2, 1998.)

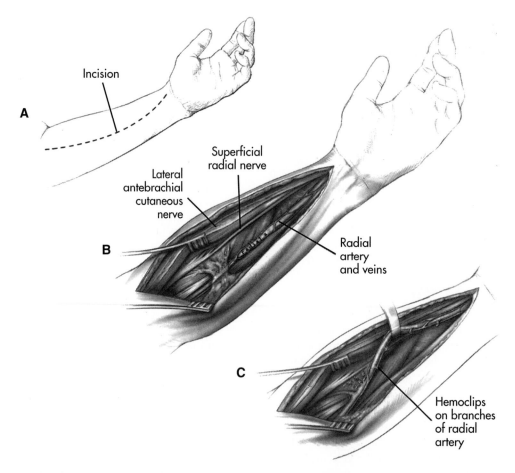

A Incision

Lateral antebrachial cutaneous nerve

Superficial radial nerve

B

Radial artery and veins

C

Hemoclips on branches of radial artery

FIGURE 10-16 Dissection of the radial artery. Before removal of the radial artery, Allen's test (see text) or a Doppler study is performed to ensure that the ulnar artery will provide sufficient blood flow to the hand if the radial artery is excised. **A,** Incision line. **B,** Deep forearm dissection exposes the radial artery and vein pedicle. **C,** Radial artery pedicle is mobilized, and multiple side branches are clipped on the arm and artery side. The artery is removed and may be irrigated with a vasodilator. (From Meeker MH, Rothrock JC: *Alexander's care of the patient in surgery,* ed 11, St Louis, 1999, Mosby.)

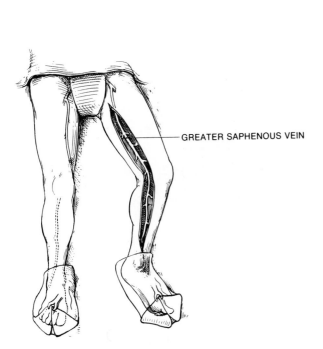

GREATER SAPHENOUS VEIN

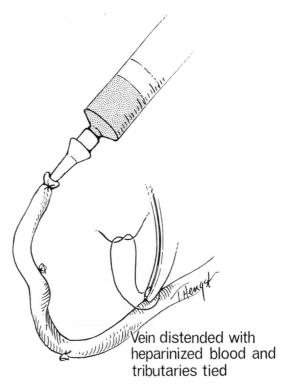

Vein distended with
heparinized blood and
tributaries tied

FIGURE 10-17 Dissection of the greater saphenous vein, which runs along the medial aspect of the leg. A cannula is inserted into the distal (ankle) end and the vein gently dilated with physiologic solution. Tributaries are ligated. (From Waldhausen JA, Pierce WS, Campbell DB: *Surgery of the chest,* ed 6, St Louis, 1996, Mosby.)

FIGURE 10-18 The saphenous vein is distended with heparinized blood, and the tributaries are tied. (From Cooley DA: *Techniques in cardiac surgery,* ed 2, Philadelphia, 1984, WB Saunders.)

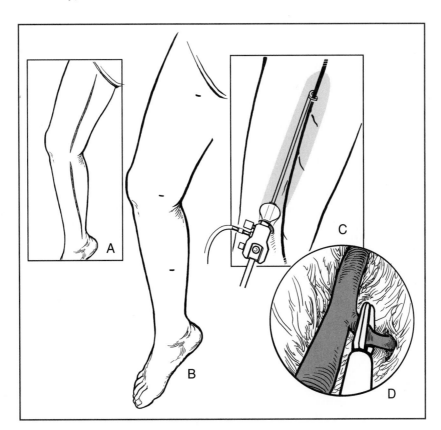

FIGURE 10-19 Minimally invasive approach to saphenous vein harvesting. **A,** Traditional leg incision. **B,** Small leg incisions allow insertion of a **(C)** videoscopic dissecting cannula. **D,** Vein tributaries are clipped on the leg and vein sides and divided. (From Braunwald E, Zipes DP, Libby P, editors: *Heart disease: a textbook of cardiovascular medicine,* ed 6, Philadelphia, 2001, WB Saunders.)

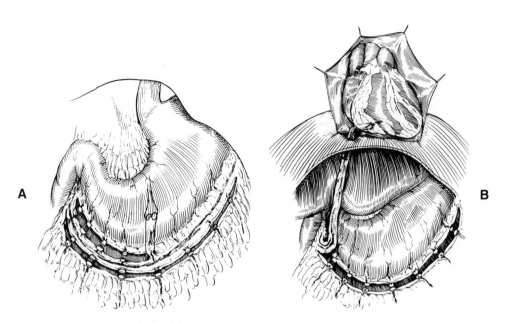

FIGURE 10-20   Use of the right GEA for coronary artery bypass grafting. **A,** Staples are used to divide omental branches of the GEA, and branches to the stomach are ligated with silk ties. **B,** The right GEA is brought through the diaphragm and anastomosed to the right coronary artery. (From Lytle BW and others: Coronary artery bypass grafting with the right gastroepiploic artery, *J Thorac Cardiovasc Surg* 97[6]:826, 1989.)

tributaries on the leg side; tributaries on the vein side may be clipped or ligated with suture after removal from the leg. To reduce postoperative tunnel dead space and minimize fluid accumulation, the leg is wrapped with a pressure bandage (Allen and Shaar, 1997).

e.   Gastroepiploic artery: The median sternotomy incision is extended along the midline abdominal fascia to a point just above the umbilicus. An abdominal retractor, such as a Balfour, may be inserted.

The peritoneal cavity is entered, and the right gastroepiploic artery (GEA) is identified along the greater curvature of the stomach. Branches to the omentum are ligated with silk ties or clipped with staples (Fig. 10-20, *A*); branches to the stomach are ligated with silk ties (Fig. 10-20, *B*). The GEA is isolated from the greater curvature of the stomach (to a point where the artery becomes less than 1 mm in diameter) back to the level of the pylorus, just distal to its takeoff from the gastroduodenal artery. The patient is given heparin before the GEA is divided. Papaverine can be injected into the distal (cut) end of the GEA to reduce arterial spasm.

If the GEA is to be used in situ, the vessel is divided distally and brought through an opening made into the diaphragm to the site of the coronary anastomosis. In situ grafts commonly are performed on the main right coronary artery and its posterolateral branches and the posterolateral branches of the circumflex coronary artery (Fig. 10-20, *C*). They also can be attached to the LAD if there is sufficient length to reach the planned anastomotic site.

Free GEA grafts may be used. They allow greater versatility, but early results are not as good as they are for in situ grafts. Anastomotic techniques are similar to those for the IMA free graft. When used as a free graft, the GEA is divided at both the distal and proximal ends and remaining portions of the artery tied off with heavy ties.

The abdominal incision is closed in layers.

f.   Other coronary artery bypass conduits: Although the IMA, radial artery, and saphenous vein are the vessels of choice, there are situations that preclude their use. The increasing number of reoperations for coronary artery disease has been a major factor in the use of alternative conduits. Also, patients with previous bilateral vein stripping, extensive varicosities, or vessels too small, too short, or too fragile are candidates for alternative conduits. Alternative autologous venous and arterial conduits include the cephalic vein, basilic vein, splenic artery, and inferior epigastric artery (IEA) (Hlozek and Zacharias, 1997). Draw-

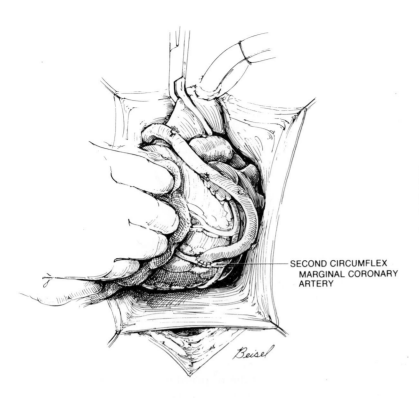

SECOND CIRCUMFLEX
MARGINAL CORONARY
ARTERY

FIGURE 10-21 Retraction of the heart to expose the obtuse marginal arteries of the circumflex system; a completed anastomosis is shown. (From Waldhausen JA, Pierce WS, Campbell DB: *Surgery of the chest,* ed 6, St Louis, 1996, Mosby.)

backs to the use of arm veins include a higher failure rate than saphenous vein or IMA, cumbersome and difficult positioning for access to the upper portion of the arm veins, and the disfiguring skin incision. The splenic artery and the IEA involve abdominal incisions that are technically more difficult and (like the GEA) are associated with additional postoperative discomfort.

Among the allografts that have been used are human umbilical vein and greater saphenous vein. Synthetic grafts made of Dacron or polytetrafluoroethylene (PTFE) have been used on occasion as well.

3a. When used, cardiopulmonary bypass is instituted as previously described. Usually, mild to moderate hypothermia (28° to 32° C) is employed; cooling may be initiated either before or after the cross-clamp is applied. The aorta is cross-clamped and antegrade or retrograde cardioplegia infused (through the aortic root or the coronary sinus, respectively). Both distal (coronary) and proximal (aortic) anastomoses may be performed during a single cross-clamping (with the heart arrested), or all distals are performed with the cross-clamp, the heart is defibrillated, and proximals are performed with a partial occlusion clamp (and a beating heart). Some surgeons prefer to perform the proximal anastomoses first.

3b. Beating heart surgery: When CPB is not employed, the heart (and body) need to remain normothermic. Maintenance of normal body requires active

interventions such as the use of warming blankets, increasing ambient temperature, and irrigating with warmed solutions.

4. Coronary anastomosis: The surgeon assesses the heart and identifies the arteries to be bypassed, comparing anatomic findings with the cineangiograms taken during cardiac catheterization. Infusion of cardioplegia allows the surgeon to visualize the artery and note a suitable incision site.

Left anterior descending, diagonal coronary arteries: Cold laparotomy pads are placed under the left side of the heart; additional retraction may be provided by the assistant. If there is a great deal of epicardial fat obstructing the coronary artery, a small spring (epicardial) retractor may be used to improve exposure.

Circumflex obtuse marginal coronary arteries: Cold laparotomy pads may be used to elevate the heart; more commonly the assistant holds the heart (Fig. 10-21). Wearing a cotton glove provides greater traction and allows the heart to be held securely; a special sling may be used.

Right coronary artery: The proximal or mid-right coronary artery may be exposed with a suture around the artery and tagged to the drapes to elevate the heart. An assistant may provide additional retraction.

Posterior descending coronary arteries: The assistant holds the heart (with a cotton glove), or a retention suture is used (Fig. 10-22), to expose the artery.

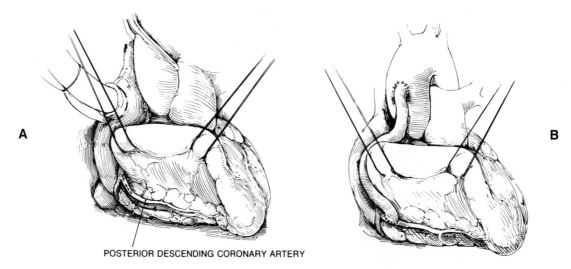

POSTERIOR DESCENDING CORONARY ARTERY

FIGURE 10-22 **A,** Use of retention sutures to expose the posterior descending coronary artery. **B,** Completed anastomosis. (From Waldhausen JA, Pierce WS, Campbell DB: *Surgery of the chest,* ed 6, St Louis, 1996, Mosby.)

a. The coronary artery is incised with a fine blade; the cardioplegia is turned off and suction turned on. The incision is extended forward and backward with delicate angled scissors, and a probe is inserted to measure and dilate the arterial lumen. External pressure with small bulldogs or a pill sponge may be applied proximally or distally to the arteriotomy to prevent bleeding during the anastomosis, although suctioning through the aortic venting needle usually provides a sufficiently dry field. Placement of the coronary suction tip within the artery should be done carefully (if at all) to avoid injury to the vascular intima.

b. The distal end of the vein or artery is beveled with scissors to approximate the coronary incision for the end-to-side anastomosis, which can be performed with a continuous suture technique (Fig. 10-23) or with interrupted stitches.

    If a side-to-side (Fig. 10-24) sequential graft is to be performed, a venotomy or arteriotomy is made with a blade and extended with scissors.

c. The anastomosis is made with fine cardiovascular suture. With the continuous technique a 6-0 or 7-0 monofilament is used commonly; an interrupted suture technique is performed by some surgeons with fine silk stitches.

    Before each distal anastomosis is completed, the coronary artery may be probed to ensure patency. The stitch is tied carefully to avoid compromising the size of the lumen. Physiologic solution may be injected into the conduits to detect leaks, to assess distal flow into the coronary bed, or to unravel a twisted graft. Cardioplegia may be selectively infused into the completed graft to protect the myocardium beyond the stenosis (or retrograde cardioplegia is infused).

A small bulldog clamp may be placed on the proximal portion of the vein to prevent air from entering the coronary artery. The proximal anastomosis can be performed at this time or after all of the distal anastomoses are completed.

IMA grafts to the LAD artery and its branches require little manipulation of the heart and usually are performed last to minimize disruption of previously placed grafts and so that tension on the IMA graft is avoided. The IMA pedicle is brought out of the pleura with the bulldog in place (to prevent blood flow from obscuring the field and rewarming the heart). The distal end of the IMA is beveled and sewn to the coronary artery; the adventitia is tacked to the epicardium (Fig. 10-25). No aortic proximal anastomosis is required because the IMA remains attached to its takeoff from the subclavian artery (Fig. 10-26).

Occasionally, IMA free grafts are used, with the IMA proximal anastomosis made on the aorta. Sequential side-to-side anastomoses also may be performed; these are accomplished in a manner similar to that used for vein grafts.

After completion of the anastomosis, the pedicle is tacked to the epicardium with a fine suture. The pericardium may be incised at the point where the IMA crosses it to allow sufficient room for the IMA graft once the lungs are reinflated; caution is taken to avoid injuring the phrenic nerve running along the lateral borders of the pericardium.

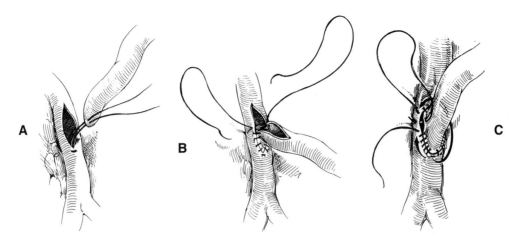

FIGURE 10-23 **A,** Continuous end-to-side anastomosis begins distally at the "toe" and **(B)** continues along the edge of the arteriotomy toward the "heel." **C,** The anastomosis is almost completed. After the knot is tied, cardioplegia is infused through the graft to test for leaks, assess distal flow, and deliver cardioplegic solution to the myocardium distal to the coronary blockage. (From Waldhausen JA, Pierce WS, Campbell DB: *Surgery of the chest,* ed 6, St Louis, 1996, Mosby.)

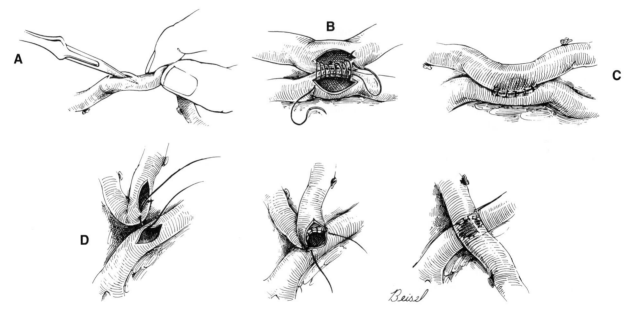

FIGURE 10-24 Continuous side-to-side anastomosis for sequential grafts. **A,** Longitudinal incision of the vein. **B,** The anastomosis is started at the distal end. **C,** Completed anastomosis. **D,** Diamond anastomosis. (From Waldhausen JA, Pierce WS, Campbell DB: *Surgery of the chest,* ed 6, St Louis, 1996, Mosby.)

Beating heart/arrested heart minimally invasive anastomoses. Beating heart procedures are most often indicated for patients with lesions in the LAD, diagonal, and occasionally the right coronary arteries. The heart is not arrested, and hypothermia is not used. Bleeding from the arteriotomy can be controlled with small clamps or tourniquet snares (or gentle pressure with the blunt end of an instrument). Often a silastic tape may be placed around the coronary artery (distally or proximally) and tightened to reduce blood flow into the field. Saline or lactated Ringer's solution misting, suction, and carbon dioxide blown over the anastomotic site also keep the field clear.

Maintaining a bloodless field without injuring the coronary artery endothelium (which can

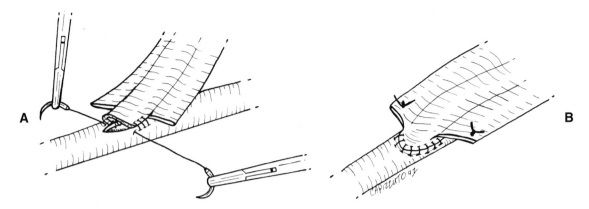

FIGURE 10-25 **A,** The distal end of the IMA pedicle is beveled and connective tissue trimmed back from the vessel tip. A double-armed suture is used for the anastomosis. **B,** The completed anastomosis. The two "ears" of the pedicle are tacked to the epicardium with a fine suture. Before the lung is inflated, the pericardium adjacent to the IMA is incised in order to minimize stretching of the IMA. (From Subramanian VA: MIDCAB approach for single vessel coronary artery bypass graft, *Op Tech Cardiac Thorac Surg* 3[1]:2, 1998.)

produce postoperative graft occlusion) was studied by Okazaki and colleagues (2001), who compared (1) the use of elastic (e.g., silastic) sutures versus nonelastic (e.g., polypropylene) sutures to snare the coronary artery and (2) the use of humidified gas insufflation (e.g., with carbon dioxide) versus nonhumidified gas blowing for 20 minutes. They found that elastic sutures and humidified gas blowing produced less injury to the coronary endothelium than nonelastic sutures and dry gas, and they recommend that techniques to maintain a dry field reflect these findings.

A coronary stabilizer (Fig. 10-27), placed around the target coronary artery, minimizes cardiac motion and allows the surgeon to perform the anastomosis. One of the earliest stabilizers was introduced by Borst and his colleagues (1996). Called the *octopus,* the device consisted of two arms (the underside of which look like octopus tentacles with their suction cups used for grasping). The stabilizer arms are connected to wall suction. When the device is placed over the target portion of the heart and the suction activated, the tissue is held in place against stabilizer arms. One advantage of this system is that stabilization does not exert pressure on the myocardium (which can injure tissue); rather, the tissue is controlled by pulling the tissue to the stabilizer. The device has been modified and is currently available (see Chapter 3).

Additional exposure is achieved with gentle traction and with moist, warm laparotomy pads, a saline-filled glove, or other similar device placed under the heart. With the introduction of LV api-

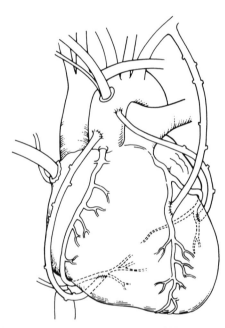

FIGURE 10-26 Completed internal mammary artery and vein graft anastomoses. (From Seifert PC: *Cardiac surgery,* St Louis, 1994, Mosby.)

cal retractors, posterior coronary arteries are increasingly being accessed as well. Monitoring the ECG for ischemia, using TEE to monitor LV function, and maintaining adequate volume status are essential. If the heart becomes ischemic, the team should be prepared to institute cardiopulmonary bypass.

Unlike on-pump cases, when beating heart procedures are performed, the IMA anastomosis is performed before the other conduits are at-

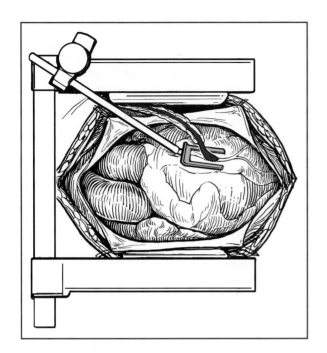

FIGURE 10-27 Off-pump coronary artery bypass on the beating heart has been facilitated by the development of stabilizer systems to provide isolated immobilization during the performance of distal anastomoses. The left anterior descending artery is the most amenable to stabilization, in contrast to the lateral and posterior coronary circulations. (From Braunwald E, Zipes, DP, Libby P, editors: *Heart disease*, ed 6, 2001, Philadelphia, WB Saunders.)

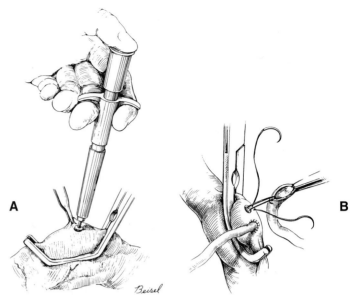

FIGURE 10-28 **A,** A partial occlusion clamp is placed on the anterior aorta (away from areas that are calcified or sclerotic) for the proximal anastomosis. A small incision is made in the aorta with a knife, and the aortic punch is then used to create the aortotomy (4.5 mm). **B,** Anastomosis of the vein graft (or radial artery) is performed with 5-0 or 6-0 polypropylene. (From Waldhausen JA, Pierce WS, Campbell DB: *Surgery of the chest*, ed 6, St Louis, 1996, Mosby.)

tached. The reason for this is that the LV can be perfused immediately after the IMA is attached; IMA perfusion also allows the heart to tolerate periods of ischemia when subsequent grafts are attached (Mack, 2000).

5. Aortic anastomoses: The proximal conduit anastomoses may be performed while the aorta is still cross-clamped and the heart arrested or with the clamp removed and the heart beating. In the latter case, an angled, partial-occlusion clamp, such as a Beck or Cooley clamp, is used to isolate a segment of aorta (Fig. 10-28, *A*).

   a. A small segment of aorta is resected, approximately the diameter of the vein graft. A knife blade (e.g., No. 11 or No. 15) is used to incise the aorta and a punch inserted into the aortotomy to create an oval opening (Fig. 10-28, *A*).

   b. The proximal end of the vein or artery is anastomosed to the side of the aorta with 5-0 vascular suture (Fig. 10-28, *B*). The site may be marked with a radiopaque ring or clip for future identification of the graft.

   c. The partial-occlusion clamp, or the cross-clamp, is removed and the suture lines checked. Air is removed from the vein graft using a fine hypodermic

needle (25- or 27-gauge) and the bulldogs removed. The IMA bulldog also is removed at this time.

Sutureless anastomoses. New anastomotic devices for proximal attachments that can be employed without cross-clamping the aorta are under development, as are mechanical devices to perform distal anastomoses. One of these extraluminal devices is in the form of a cylinder that deploys an inner and outer row of metal (Nitinol) pins, which penetrate the everted segment of the vein. The vein is mounted on the delivery system before making the aortotomy with the punching component of the system. The distal end of the vein in the carrying handle is released inside the aortic lumen, the inner row of pins attach the conduit to the inner aortic lumen, and the outer row of pins connect the conduit to the outer wall of the aorta. The vein delivery system is extracted, leaving the completed anastomosis (Calafiore and others, 2001).

Other sutureless techniques under study include stapling, clipping, coupling, pasting, gluing, and laser welding. A "one-shot" anastomotic device for end-to-side coronary anastomoses also has been designed (Heijmen and others, 1999). According to Shennib (2001), it is only a question of time before many if not most anastomoses are performed with these sutureless techniques.

6. Closing:
   a. A chest tube is inserted to drain one or both pleural cavities that may have been opened during the IMA dissection (or the distal end of the straight mediastinal drainage tube can be inserted into the pleural cavity).
   b. Pacing wires are inserted.
   c. Hemostasis is achieved.
   d. Cardiopulmonary bypass is discontinued, and the sternum is closed.

Port-access and robotic surgery

Port access. The combination of port-access technology (Fig. 10-29) with or without robotic assistance has expanded the minimally invasive options for working on the beating or arrested heart with less trauma. Arrested heart MIS can be performed through small sternal or thoracic incisions or ports using endoscopic video-assisted technology. Port-access systems (Fig. 10-30) for extracorporeal perfusion (e.g., bypass) include the following components (Reichenspurner, 2001; Fann and others, 1998):

- A femoral arterial inflow cannula
- A femoral venous return cannula
- An endopulmonary venting catheter
- A multilumen endoaortic balloon occlusion catheter that serves as an endoaortic clamp, a left ventricular venting catheter, a pressure monitoring line, and an antegrade cardioplegia infusion catheter
- An endocoronary sinus catheter for infusion of retrograde cardioplegia

These components are inserted percutaneously (or through small incisions) through peripheral arteries and veins (usually the femoral vessels); TEE and fluoroscopy are used to guide insertion. Modifications that allow direct cannulation include arterial and venous catheters that can be percutaneously inserted through small parasternal (thoracic) incisions directly into the aorta for antegrade arterial inflow and into the right atrium for venous drainage.

After confirmation of placement of the catheters, CPB is initiated. A small sternal incision is made to dissect the IMA with video-assisted endoscopic techniques and to access the target coronary artery. After the IMA is dissected, the surgical site is identified, and the endoaortic balloon occlusion catheter is inflated. Right radial artery pressure is monitored closely to ensure that the balloon has not occluded the bracheocephalic artery. Antegrade or retrograde cardioplegia is infused, and the coronary anastomoses are performed.

Robotic surgery. Robotic techniques for CABG include a computerized console (Fig. 10-31) where the

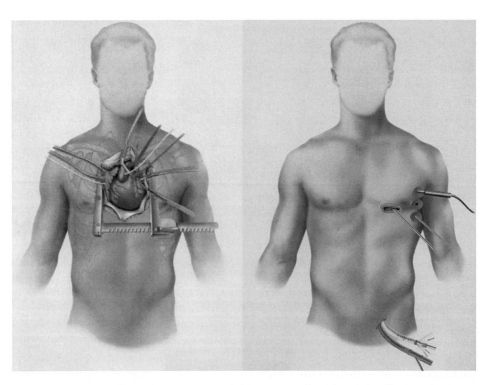

FIGURE 10-29 Traditional sternotomy *(left)* compared with minimally invasive/port-access incisions *(right)* that provide access to the heart and to the femoral artery and vein. (Courtesy CARDIOVATIONS, a division of ETHICON, Inc.)

surgeon sits to manipulate the robotic arms to perform the anastomoses (Fig. 10-32). A high-resolution, three-dimensional videoscopic image allows the surgeon to sew from a remote site through the robotic arms. The computerized system minimizes hand tremor, provides a sense of touch (haptic feedback), and correlates what is seen on the monitor with the surgeon's movements (Box 10-8) (Damiano and others, 2001).

The following is one technique for totally endoscopic robotic coronary artery bypass (Mohr and others, 2001). (Exclusion criteria include known contraindications to port-access percutaneous CPB, LV dilation, and diffuse target coronary artery disease.)

1. The patient is placed in the supine position with the left side slightly elevated and the left arm lowered.
2. A double-lumen endotracheal tube is inserted and the left lung deflated for IMA harvesting.

3. A 30-degree angled thoracoscope is inserted (facing cephalid) through the fourth intercostal space, and the instrument ports are inserted at the third and sixth intercostal spaces to allow insertion of the dissecting instruments.
4. The IMA is dissected under videoscopic guidance.
5. A pericardial window is made in the region of the LAD, and the target artery anastomotic location is marked with a clip.
6. The patient is given heparin, and a vascular clamp is inserted to occlude temporarily the IMA. The IMA is clipped, cut, and trimmed for the anastomosis.
7. Femoral vein–femoral artery bypass is initiated, and cardioplegia is infused via the endovascular system described previously.
8. The same ports used for IMA dissection are employed for the anastomosis, but the 30-degree scope

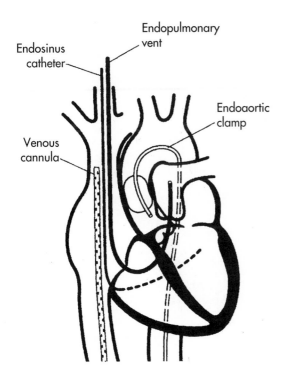

FIGURE 10-30 Schematic diagram of endovascular CPB system. Venous cannula: drains mixed blood into the CPB circuit. Endosinus catheter: distal tip placed in coronary sinus is used to deliver retrograde cardioplegia. Endopulmonary venting catheter: distal tip placed in main pulmonary artery is used to suction blood and air from the heart; may also be used to monitor pulmonary artery pressures. Endoaortic clamp: (1) Distal balloon inflated to occlude aorta acts as an internal cross-clamp. (2) Catheter can be used either to infuse antegrade cardioplegia or to suction blood and air from the heart. On/off clamps control direction of flow. (3) Catheter tip may be used to monitor aortic root pressures. (From Pompili MF and others: Port access mitral valve replacement in dogs, *J Thorac Cardiovasc Surg* 112(5):1268, 1996.)

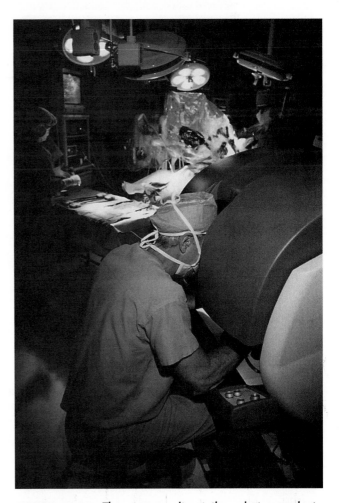

FIGURE 10-31 The surgeon sits at the robot console to perform coronary anastomoses. Note that the surgeon is not sterile and the patient is approximately 10 feet from the surgeon. (Courtesy Edward A. Lefrak, MD; from *Kardia*, Fall 2001, Inova Fairfax Hospital, Falls Church, Va.)

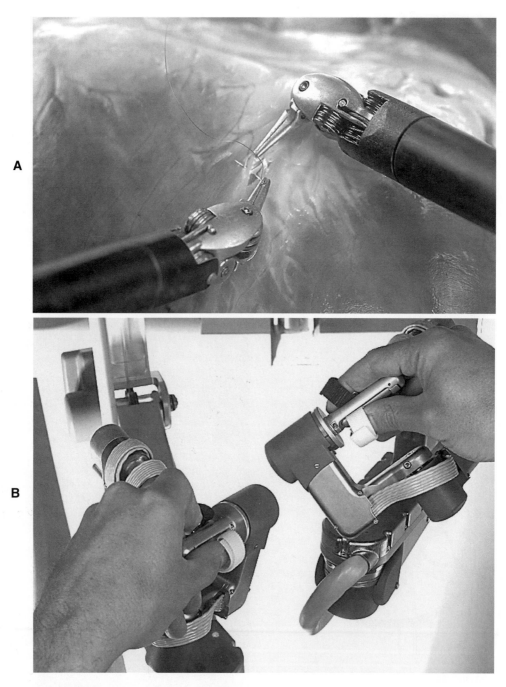

FIGURE 10-32 A, Port-access robotic anastomosis replicates the surgeon's natural hand and wrist movements. **B,** The surgeon's hands at the computerized robot console. (Copyright 2000, Intuitive Surgical, Inc.)

is turned downward to expose the LAD anastomotic site.

9. The anastomosis is performed by the surgeon at the console with robotic instrumentation.

10. After completion of the anastomosis and confirmation of hemostasis, the surgeon inserts a small drain

and removes the instruments and the robotic arms and closes the incisions.

According to Mohr and associates (2001), advantages of computer-enhanced robotic instrumentation over conventional endoscopic include more favorable ergonomics, more natural hand-eye alignment, less trans-

---

Controller: transforms the spatial motion of the robotic tools into the camera frame of reference to achieve hand-eye coordination.

Degrees of freedom: the robotic arms' ability to produce the different motions by the human hand, wrist, elbow, and arm, such as the following:
- Outer pitch—moving your hand by moving your elbow up and down
- Inner pitch—moving your wrist up and down
- Outer yaw—moving your elbow right to left
- Inner yaw—moving your wrist right and left
- In/out—putting the instrument into the body and extending it farther; moving your elbow in front and in back
- Roll—rolling your forearm/wrist to roll your hand
- Combination—holding your wrist steady and moving your hand in a clockwise or counterclockwise movement

Input/output devices:
- **input device:** surgeon's console with display system, input handles, user interface, and electronic controller
- **output device:** robotic manipulator

Manipulator: tool handles that are high-resolution (input) devices capable of reading the position, orienting the surgeon to the field, and providing grip commands from the surgeon; they also serve as haptic displays (i.e., they provide a sense of touch). Three manipulators are positioned around the body by three passive multiple-link arms mounted to a fixed base.

Scaling: the ability to view the field in a 2:1 ratio. In other words, the field appears on the video console screen as twice as big as it really is; however, the surgeon's hand movements do not need to be twice as large (as they would have to be during "open" surgery). Larger ratios (e.g., 3:1, 3 times the normal size, and 5:1, 5 times the normal size and higher) are possible for very small areas.

Modified from Mohr FW and others: Computer-enhanced "robotic" cardiac surgery: experience in 148 patients, *J Thorac Cardiovasc Surg* 121:824, 2001; Damiano RJ and others: Initial prospective multicenter clinical trial of robotically-assisted coronary artery bypass grafting, *Ann Thorac Surg* 72:1263, 2001; Lyndel Thompson, Intuitive Surgical, Inc., personal communication, Oct 2, 2001.

mission of hand tremor, more degrees of freedom, and less force required to manipulate instrument tips.

Beating heart, port-access robotic surgery (using a fourth port in the subxiphoid position for insertion of a coronary stabilizer) is still in the initial stages of clinical development, but early successes support additional investigation (Mohr and others, 2001). (Refer to Web sites for two of the leading manufacturers of robotic technology: Computer Motion, Inc., at www.computermotion.com, and Intuitive Surgical, Inc., at www.intuitivesurgical.com.)

Coronary endarterectomy

Coronary endarterectomy usually is reserved for removal of plaque from the right coronary artery system

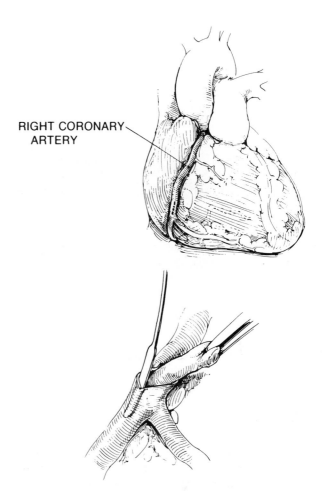

RIGHT CORONARY ARTERY

FIGURE 10-33 Endarterectomy of the right coronary artery. An endarterectomy spatula is used for blunt dissection of the atheromatous inner core. (From Waldhausen JA, Pierce WS, Campbell DB: *Surgery of the chest,* ed 6, St Louis, 1996, Mosby.)

in situations where the right coronary artery is occluded and no distal branches are available for anastomosis. Endarterectomy of the left coronary system is performed rarely.

Operative procedure

1. An arteriotomy is made above the plaque, commonly at the bifurcation of the right coronary artery and the posterior descending coronary artery.
2. An endarterectomy spatula is used to bluntly dissect the atheromatous intimal core from the inner wall of the artery (Fig. 10-33).
3. The atheroma (Fig. 10-34) is freed circumferentially as far as possible from each separate branch of the artery and removed by gentle traction with a small clamp. The distal ends should be feathered, indicating complete removal of the plaque.

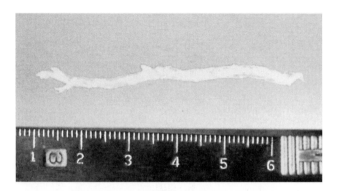

FIGURE 10-34 Native coronary atheroma is shown. In contrast to a saphenous vein bypass graft atheroma (which is friable and not well organized), the native atheroma tends to be firm and amenable to excision as a unit. (Courtesy Alan M. Speir, MD; Kip Seymour, photographer.)

4. A probe can be inserted distally to ensure patency.
5. The arteriotomy site is then used for anastomosing a bypass graft.

Combined procedures

If concomitant mitral or aortic valve replacement or mitral valve ring annuloplasty is performed (see Chapters 11 and 12), the coronary anastomoses are performed first, followed by the valve surgery. The procedure is done in this order so that cardioplegia can be infused into the grafts to protect the distal myocardium and so that during manipulation of the heart for anastomoses, injury does not occur to perivalvular tissue from the valve prosthesis.

REPAIR OF A LEFT VENTRICULAR ANEURYSM

A left ventricular aneurysm is one of the complications of acute myocardial infarction (AMI) and occurs in approximately 8% to 15% of patients with AMI (Waldhausen, Pierce, and Campbell, 1996). Anterolateral and anteroseptal aneurysms are seen more often than diaphragmatic or posterior aneurysms. An aneurysm occurs in the muscular area where the artery supplying that portion of the myocardium has been occluded and where there is an absence of significant collateral circulation. Without treatment, patients generally succumb to heart failure or recurring dysrhythmias and are at risk for embolization of endoventricular thrombus or rupture of the ventricle.

The aneurysmal tissue, often clearly delineated from the surrounding myocardium, appears as a thinned-out transmural scar devoid of the trabeculations normally seen in the ventricular endocardium. A large mural thrombus may be present; over time the thrombus may break into pieces, which can embolize; the remaining thrombus may calcify. The overlying pericardium may be densely adherent to the epicardial surface of the aneurysm, and this also may calcify. Chest x-ray films demonstrate existing calcification and show enlargement of the left ventricle. Cardiac cineangiography, echocardiography, or other imaging techniques may reveal akinesis or dyskinesis (e.g., paradoxic motion with bulging of the affected area) during systole (see Box 10-2).

The 3-year *survival* rate for untreated patients with an aneurysm from the time of infarction is as low as 25%. Operative mortality can range from 3% to 30% depending on the patient's age, general status, concomitant disease, and extent of myocardial involvement (Waldhausen, Pierce, and Campbell, 1996).

The goal of surgical repair is to remove the dysfunctional tissue while retaining the geometry of the left ventricle as much as possible in order to optimize LV function. Early reparative techniques produced distortion of the cardiac anatomy because the repair produced a linear rather than a circular or elliptic suture line. Patients often required early postoperative support with an intraaortic balloon pump (IABP).

The technique of ventricular endoaneurysmorrhaphy described by Jatene (1985) and refined by Cooley (1989) was developed to preserve the surface anatomy and restore the internal contour of the ventricle. Endoaneurysmorrhaphy, as well as conventional repair that involves resecting and plicating ventricular tissue, are described here.

Procedural considerations

The patient is placed in the supine position. The aneurysm usually is adherent to the pericardium, which increases the risk of bleeding during sternal opening. It may not be possible to fully dissect away the adhesions until cardiopulmonary bypass has been established (when the decompressed ventricle creates a better plane for dissection).

Teflon felt strips to bolster the suture line, pledgets, patch material (woven Dacron, PTFE, or pericardium), and additional sutures (1-0, 2-0, 3-0) of polypropylene or polyester with large needles are needed in addition to instruments and supplies for coronary artery bypass. The left side of the heart is vented with a catheter placed in the ventricle via the right superior pulmonary vein or through the ventriculotomy. The superior and inferior vena cavae are cannulated for venous return.

Operative procedure: apical ventricular aneurysm patch repair

1. A median sternotomy is performed, and CPB is instituted as previously described. Moderate

hypothermia (28° to 30° C [82.4° to 86° F]) is generally used. The aorta is cross-clamped, and the heart is arrested with cardioplegia. To reduce the possibility of dislodging a mural thrombus, the aneurysm is not palpated until the cross-clamp is applied and the heart arrested. Adhesions between the left ventricular apex and the pericardium are sharply divided.

2. The aneurysm is identified and inspected. A circular incision is made in the aneurysmal tissue over the apex. A pursestring suture with felt pledgets is placed around the scar edge (Fig. 10-35, *A*).

3. Scar tissue of the ventricle is excised and any clot removed carefully. A cuff of fibrotic scar tissue is left, through which heavy cardiovascular sutures reinforced with Teflon felt pledgets are passed. The mitral apparatus is inspected.

4. An oval patch of woven Dacron or pericardium is cut to duplicate the infarcted area in the ventricular cavity (Fig. 10-35, *B*). The patch is secured with continuous sutures of 3-0 polypropylene placed in the fibrotic tissue that forms the boundary between infarcted and healthy myocardium (Fig. 10-35, *C*). Care is taken not to damage the LAD or the mitral papillary muscles.

5. The ventriculotomy edges may be reapproximated over the patch by direct suture or buttressed with felt strips using heavy suture.

6. If CABG is planned, it often is performed after the aneurysm is repaired.

Operative procedure: conventional repair of a left ventricular aneurysm (Waldhausen, Pierce, and Campbell, 1996).

Linear closure of the defect, described here, is performed less often than patch repair.

1. Median sternotomy, CPB, and hypothermic cardioplegic arrest are instituted. Adhesions are dissected free.

2. The central portion of the aneurysm is incised, and existing clot is removed (Fig. 10-36, *A* and *B*). Boundaries of viable myocardium are identified, and the endocardium and mitral apparatus are inspected.

3. Clamps (such as straight Kocher clamps) are placed along the edges of the aneurysm (Fig. 10-36, *B*), and the thinned-out scar tissue is excised, leaving a rim of fibrous tissue to close the aneurysm. Normal tissue should not be compromised in the repair.

4. Two strips of Teflon felt (approximately 2 cm × 15 cm) are fashioned and placed along each side of the incision (one strip along each edge); (Fig. 10-36, *C*). The needle of a double-armed heavy (No. 1, 0, 2-0)

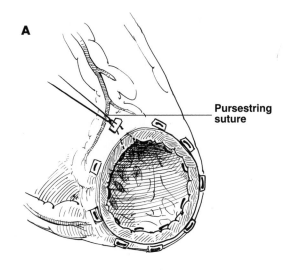

Pursestring suture

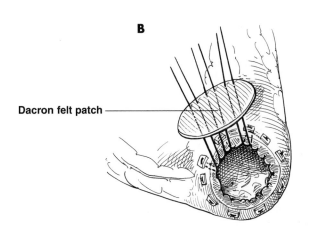

Dacron felt patch

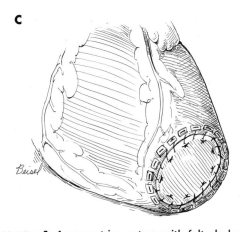

FIGURE 10-35 **A,** A pursestring suture with felt pledgets is placed around the rim of the scar. **B,** A patch is inserted with interrupted sutures. **C,** The stitches are tied and the suture edge may be reinforced with a running suture. (From Waldhausen JA, Pierce WS, Campbell DB: *Surgery of the chest,* ed 6, St Louis, 1996, Mosby.)

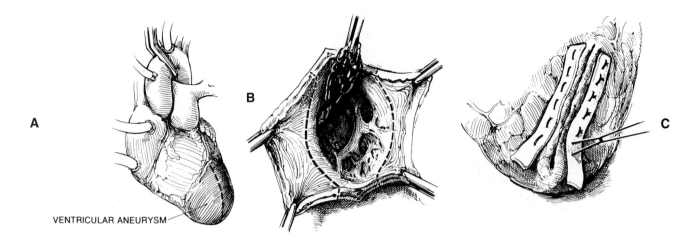

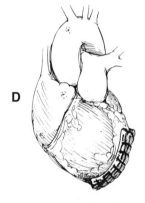

FIGURE 10-36 Conventional repair of a left ventricular aneurysm. **A,** The apex is incised. **B,** Thrombus is removed. The mitral apparatus is inspected. **C,** The ventriculotomy edges are plicated with buttressing felt strips using an interrupted suture technique, followed by **(D)** oversewing with a continuous suture. (From Waldhausen JA, Pierce WS, Campbell DB: *Surgery of the chest,* ed 6, St Louis, 1996, Mosby.)

suture is passed through the edge of one felt strip, through the edge of the fibrous tissue below the felt, across to the other edge of the tissue, and up through the opposing felt strip. The needles are cut off, and the suture ends are tagged. A series of these interrupted stitches is made along the length of the ventriculotomy.

5. A venting catheter may be placed at the apex of the incision.
6. The interrupted stitches are tied.
7. A secondary, continuous suture of polyester or polypropylene is run down and back the length of the incision to oversew the repair (Fig. 10-36, *D*). An additional felt strip may be placed over the middle of the incision to prevent leakage of the fibrous walls. Additional pledgeted suture may be placed as necessary to achieve hemostasis.
8. Air is removed from the left ventricle, after which the apical catheter is removed and the incision is closed.

REPAIR OF A POSTINFARCTION VENTRICULAR SEPTAL DEFECT

Ventricular septal defect (VSD) or free wall rupture is a catastrophic complication of myocardial infarction that originates in the zone of necrotic myocardium. Free wall ruptures with immediate cardiac tamponade and cardiovascular collapse are almost uniformly fatal because there is insufficient time to close the left ventricle. Ruptures tend to occur in older patients with hypertension (greater than 140/90 mm Hg), diabetes, and a smaller heart and after the first episode of MI (Chaux and others, 1998).

Ventricular septal ruptures represent a surgical emergency, and the principles enumerated by Daggett in 1994 (Box 10-9) remain pertinent in the current environment. Septal ruptures often are located in the anterior septum near the apex of the heart, although posterior septal ruptures occur with increasing frequency (Chaux and others, 1998). Defects also may appear in the midseptum. Postinfarction VSDs usually occur within 2 weeks of infarction.

Incidence and pathophysiology

Septal ruptures are rare (1% to 2% incidence), but they are often lethal, with a 40% mortality in the first 48 hours (Killen and others, 1997). A growing percentage of patients are older and sicker, which is typical of the cardiac surgical population in general (Daggett, 1998). Clinical manifestations include dyspnea, pulmonary hypertension, pulmonary edema, and often cardiogenic shock (e.g., systolic blood pressure below 80 mm Hg, oliguria or anuria, elevated creatinine level, and cool, clammy skin).

BOX 10-9
Comments on the Repair of Postinfarction Ventricular Septal Defects

Willard M. Daggett, MD
Massachusetts General Hospital
Boston, Massachusetts

Increasingly we view the patient with a postinfarction ventricular septal rupture as a surgical emergency, not dissimilar to the patient with a leaking abdominal aortic aneurysm. We tend to operate on patients with postinfarction septal rupture as they present. Operations in these patients will occur at odd hours and, of course, on weekends as well. This has a lot of meaning for cardiac surgical nursing, as this type of operation is complex in its planning and execution and, paradoxically, relatively infrequent in its occurrence. This means that experience with this type of procedure needs to be concentrated in the hands of highly trained cardiac surgical nurses who will be on call for this type of emergent procedure nights and weekends.

It is our distinct impression that each of these defects is in some way anatomically unique; therefore the repair to be instituted in a given patient may in itself be unique, requiring flexibility in the conduct of the operation both for the surgeon and the cardiac perioperative nurse. A wide variety of suture material may be used in these repairs, again requiring some flexibility. The first priority to achieve success for these patients is complete closure of the defect itself, this repair being accomplished without tension on the adjacent muscle to prevent recurrence of the defect or free wall left ventricular rupture.

Each of these operations is a little like "weaving a rug" in that different locations of the defect, the extent of muscle loss, and the extent of coronary artery disease require flexibility in both the planning and the execution of the operation.

This is the type of procedure wherein operative outcome will depend a great deal on the specific knowledge, experience, and planning of the operating room team. Reading appropriate articles and discussion with all of the surgical staff will aid greatly in making sure that all possible contingencies have been covered and thought out in advance.

There is an increase or step-up in the oxygen content of the blood in the right ventricle and pulmonary artery after septal rupture because of the left-to-right shunting of oxygenated blood from the left ventricle through the defect into the right ventricle. Pulmonary flow may be twice that of systemic flow. Blood returning to the right atrium may reflect a lower than normal oxygen saturation because of the body's extraction of more oxygen in the presence of lowered cardiac output. A loud holosystolic murmur can be heard at the lower left sternal border. Color Doppler echocardiography and a pulmonary artery catheter are useful for confirming the diagnosis. Cardiac catheterization and cineangiography remain important techniques for diagnosing coronary artery disease. Left-to-right shunts and valve anatomy and function are best assessed by two-dimensional echocardiography (Chaux and others, 1998).

Preoperative care

Patients may require ventricular support with an intraaortic balloon pump or a left ventricular assist device (LVAD) during diagnostic testing, after which they are transported directly to the operating room. Because of the critical nature of post-MI ventricular septal defect, patients and families are extremely frightened and anxious. This fear and anxiety may be aggravated by the lack of preanesthetic medication in patients too unstable to tolerate the depressive effects of these drugs. Although detailed teaching or instruction is unrealistic, it is possible (and important) to reduce some of the fear and anxiety through a calm and caring manner that is at the same time efficient. The family can be directed to the waiting area and kept informed of the patient's progress by the perioperative nurse or a designated person such as a case manager or a patient representative.

Perioperative nursing considerations

Once the patient enters the OR, intravascular lines and a urinary drainage catheter are inserted (if not already in place). Skin preparation and draping are performed as soon as possible; the sternum is incised, and CPB is instituted (VSD repair involves opening the heart, which requires extracorporeal circulation). The aim of surgery is to excise infarcted tissue and close the defect with a patch of prosthetic material or pericardium (bovine or autologous). Concomitant valve repair (or replacement) or coronary artery bypassing of documented coronary obstructions is performed as indicated. Saphenous vein grafts may be the required conduit if there is insufficient time to dissect the IMA.

The mortality from ventricular septal rupture is largely the result of multisystem failure resulting from hypoperfusion of peripheral organs. Thus one of the main considerations is to avoid delay in operating on the patient. CPB (with bicaval cannulation and systemic cooling to 20° to 24° C [68° to 75° F]) should be instituted expeditiously, and meticulous attention should be given to myocardial protection. Surgical mortality may range from 25% to 40%, although in females and in patients with past MIs, mortality can reach 70% (Chaux and others, 1998).

Implications for the perioperative nurse include having necessary instruments and supplies immediately available, including basic sternotomy, valve and coronary instruments, heavy suture such as that used for left ventricular aneurysms (0 to 2-0 polyester, double-armed), felt strips, felt pledgets (1 cm × 1 cm or smaller), patch material, and woven graft material. Cold topical solutions for pericardial lavage should be available. Fibrin glue may be used on the suture lines.

Freshly infarcted myocardial tissue tends to be friable and does not hold sutures securely. For this reason, suture lines often are buttressed with felt strips or felt pledgets to prevent disruption of the repair and to distribute stresses more evenly along the suture line. Strips of felt and individual pledgets may be cut from prepackaged felt squares (6 inches × 6 inches). Some repairs use multiple strips (e.g., four) and multiple individually pledgeted sutures (e.g., 20 or more). Antegrade cardioplegia is commonly used.

Operative procedure: repair of a postinfarction ventricular septal defect

Cooley and associates (1957) were the first to report a successful repair of a postinfarction VSD. Since then, a number of techniques have evolved. Notable has been the work of Daggett and colleagues (1977; Box 10-10; see Box 10-9), who are credited with developing a number of reparative techniques for this complication. Among Daggett's and other's refinements that have improved survival are (1) aggressive early therapy, (2) expeditious preoperative definition of coronary anatomy, (3) assessment of ventricular and valvular anatomy and function with color Doppler two-dimensional echocardiography, (4) repair of associated coronary and valve disease, (5) use of Teflon felt to buttress suture lines of friable myocardium, (6) repair of larger defects with patch material to reduce tension on tissue edges and produce a more normal ventricular geometry, (7) insti-

---

BOX 10-10
Principles of Repair of Postinfarction Ventricular Septal Defects

1) Expeditious establishment of total cardiopulmonary bypass with moderate hypothermia and meticulous attention to myocardial protection.
2) Transinfarct approach to ventricular septal defect with the site of ventriculotomy determined by the location of the transmural infarction.
3) Thorough trimming of the left ventricular margins of the infarct back to viable muscle to prevent delayed rupture of the closure.
4) Conservative trimming of the right ventricular muscle as required for complete visualization of the margins of the defect.
5) Inspection of the left ventricular papillary muscles and concomitant replacement of the mitral valve only if there is frank papillary muscular rupture.
6) Closure of the septal defect without tension, which in most instances will require the use of prosthetic material.
7) Closure of the infarctectomy without tension with generous use of prosthetic material as indicated and epicardial placement of the patch to the free wall to avoid strain on the friable endocardial tissue.
8) Buttressing of the suture lines with pledgets or strips of Teflon felt or similar material to prevent sutures from cutting through friable muscle.

From Madsen JC, Daggett WM: Repair of postinfarction ventricular septal defects, *Semin Thorac Cardiovasc Surg* 10(2):117, 1998.

---

tution of left or right ventricular support, and (8) incision of the ventricle through infarcted rather than normal tissue, thereby sparing functional myocardium (Madsen and Daggett, 1998; Waldhausen, Pierce, and Campbell, 1996; Cooley, 1998).

Each defect is anatomically unique, with the condition of the tissue uncertain. Therefore the surgeon may not be sure of the precise technique needed until the tissue can be inspected. After cardiopulmonary bypass is instituted and the heart arrested, the nurse should anticipate a period of inspection of the anatomy before the final surgical plan is formulated. Repair of anterior, apical, and posteroinferior defects are described in the following.

Procedure

1. Bicaval CPB is established, and the heart is arrested with antegrade cardioplegia.
2. An incision is made through the infarcted left ventricular wall, and intracavitary thrombus is removed.
3. Infarcted LV tissue is trimmed to viable myocardium (rarely is there fibrotic tissue between viable and nonviable muscle because there has been insufficient time for healing and scar formation after AMI).
4. The mitral apparatus is inspected. If there is a ruptured papillary muscle, valve repair or replacement is performed through a conventional left atrial approach. This avoids tearing friable myocardium that could occur with ventricular exposure of the valve (Cooley, 1998).
5a. Repair of anterior defects: The heart is elevated with cold laparotomy pads to expose the left anterior coronary artery.
   a. Occasionally, small defects beneath anterior infarcts can be closed without a patch by approximating the septal margin of the defect to the right ventricular free wall. Horizontal mattress sutures with felt pledgets are placed and then tied.
   b. Larger anterior defects (Fig. 10-37) require a patch to reduce tension on the suture line. Excessive tension can contribute to postoperative rupture of the repair. Interrupted 3-0 felt pledgeted sutures are placed through the edge of the defect and then into the VSD patch. When all the sutures are placed, the patch is seated against the left ventricular side of the VSD and an additional pledget is attached to each suture. The needles are cut and all the stitches tied. The ventriculotomy is closed by patching or by approximation of the edges with felt-buttressed sutures (Fig. 10-38; see Fig. 10-37).
5b. Repair of apical defects: The principles of closing anterior VSDs also are applied to apical defects (see Fig. 10-37).

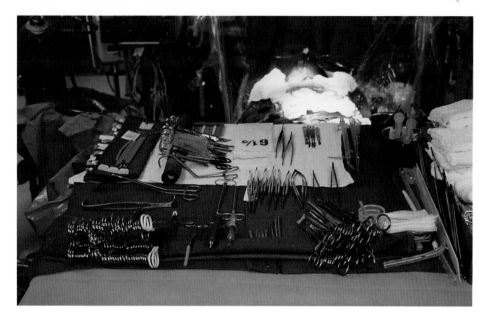

PLATE 1 Elevated back table with instruments and supplies for cardiac surgery. Setups may vary among institutions according to experience, preference, and operative needs, but all setups should promote easy access to items and maintain a consistent arrangement so that items can be readily located. (Courtesy John R Garrett, MD; Howard Kaye, photographer.)

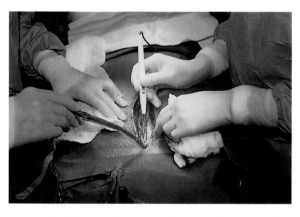

PLATE 2 Incision and cautery of the periosteum. The RN first assistant *(left)* retracts the skin edges and aspirates and retracts with the suction tip. (Courtesy John R Garrett, MD; Howard Kaye, photographer.)

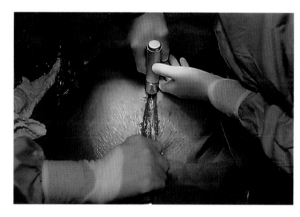

PLATE 3 Sternal division with a saw. The RN first assistant is holding a retractor at the upper end of the incision *(bottom of picture)*. (Courtesy John R Garrett, MD; Howard Kaye, photographer.)

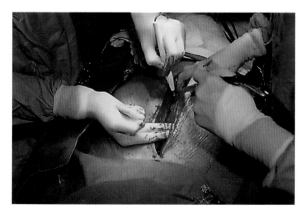

PLATE 4 While the RN first assistant elevates the sternal bone, the surgeon cauterizes to control bleeding. (Courtesy John R Garrett, MD; Howard Kaye, photographer.)

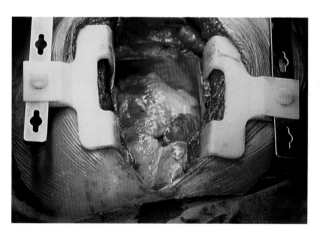

PLATE 5 The sternal retractor is used to expose the heart within the pericardium; the aorta arises from the left ventricle *(bottom of picture)*. (Courtesy John R Garrett, MD; Howard Kaye, photographer.)

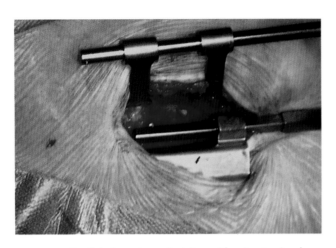

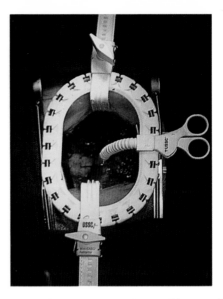

PLATE 6   Partial sternotomy incision with retractor in place. Both right and left internal mammary arteries may be exposed. (From Yim APC and others: *Minimal access cardiothoracic surgery,* Philadelphia, 2000, WB Saunders.)

PLATE 7   Partial sternotomy incision with sternal spreader. Attachments can provide suction, retraction, illumination, and coronary stabilization. (From Yim APC and others: *Minimal access cardiothoracic surgery,* Philadelphia, 2000, WB Saunders.)

PLATE 8   Anterior thoracotomy incision; useful for accessing left anterior descending (LAD) coronary artery for single LAD bypass graft. (From Buxton B, Frazier OH, Westaby S: *Ischemic heart disease surgical management,* London, 1999, Mosby.)

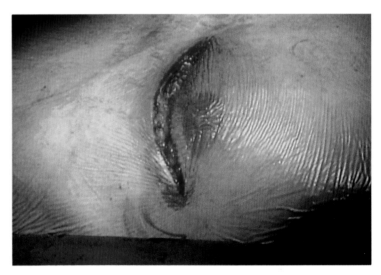

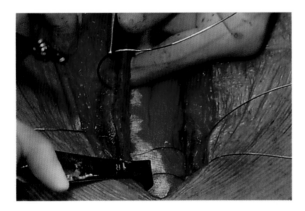

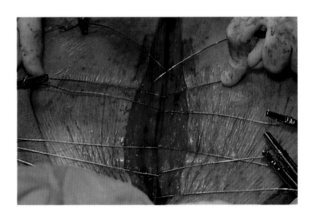

PLATE 9   The RN first assistant provides countertraction while the surgeon inserts wire sutures into the sternum. (Courtesy John R Garrett, MD; Howard Kaye, photographer.)

PLATE 10   The sternal wires are crossed and then twisted manually. Note the Kocher clamps attached to the ends of the wires to facilitate their manipulation. (Courtesy John R Garrett, MD; Howard Kaye, photographer.)

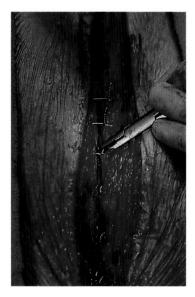

PLATE 11 After excess wire is cut, the wire needle holder is used to completely tighten the wires. The wire ends are then buried into the subcutaneous tissue. (Courtesy John R Garrett, MD; Howard Kaye, photographer.)

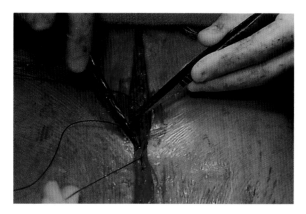

PLATE 12 Subcutaneous tissue closure with absorbable suture. (Courtesy John R Garrett, MD; Howard Kaye, photographer.)

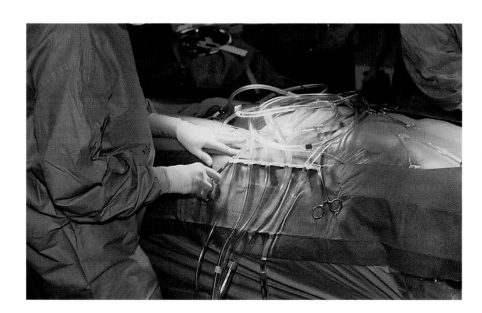

PLATE 13 Bypass tubing is connected to the drapes. The perioperative nurse and other sterile team members ensure that bypass lines remain securely attached, inflow lines are clearly distinguished from outflow lines, and precautions are taken to avoid air and particulate matter from entering inflow (i.e., arterial) lines and embolizing within body organs. (Courtesy John R Garrett, MD; Howard Kaye, photographer.)

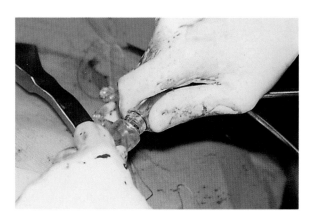

PLATE 14 Connecting a cannula to bypass tubing. (Courtesy John R Garrett, MD; Howard Kaye, photographer.)

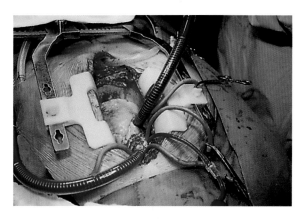

PLATE 15 Bypass circuit with an arterial cannula in the ascending aorta and a two-stage venous cannula *(right)* in the right atrium. (Courtesy John R Garrett, MD; Howard Kaye, photographer.)

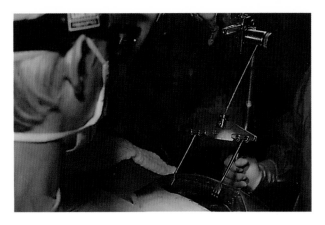

PLATE 16 IMA retractor positioned to elevate the left chest wall. (Courtesy John R Garrett, MD; Howard Kaye, photographer.)

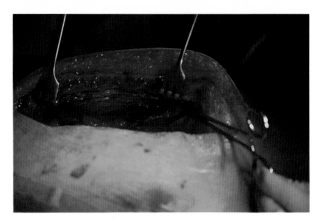

PLATE 17 The left sternal border is elevated with the internal mammary artery (IMA) retractor to expose the artery. The tonsil clamp *(right)* is applied to the IMA just below. (Courtesy John R Garrett, MD; Howard Kaye, photographer.)

PLATE 18 The left leg is positioned for excision of the greater saphenous vein through small incisions. Note Weitlaner retractor in one incision below the knee. (Courtesy John R Garrett, MD; Howard Kaye, photographer.)

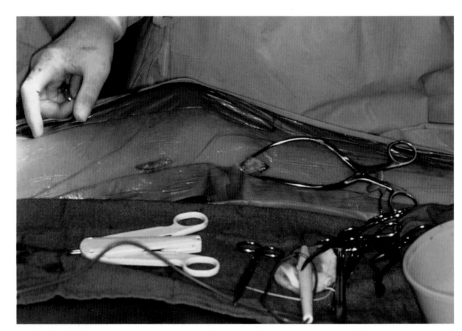

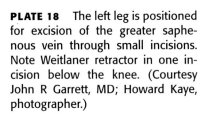

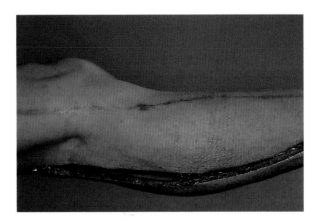

PLATE 19 Dissection of the lesser (posterior) saphenous vein. The incision is made posterior to the lateral malleolus and extended up over the calf. Note the incisional scar where the greater saphenous vein has been excised. (Courtesy Edward A Lefrak, MD.)

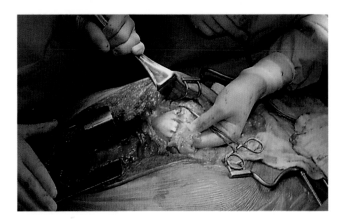

PLATE 20 Dissection of the right gastroepiploic artery (GEA). The surgeon is holding the GEA pedicle; the clamp is placed on the distal portion of the right GEA. Branches of the GEA can be seen penetrating the stomach wall (pale smooth area). A Balfour retractor is in the abdomen; a Cooley sternotomy retractor is in the chest. (Courtesy John R Garrett, MD; Howard Kaye, photographer.)

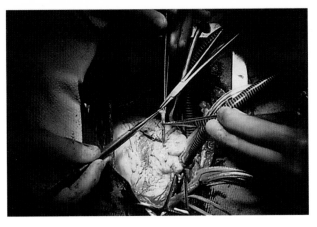

PLATE 21 Proximal anastomosis. The assistant holds apart the edges of the proximal vein graft while the surgeon places stitches into the vein and then into the aortotomy. The vein will be seated onto the aorta, and the anastomosis will be completed. (Courtesy Edward A Lefrak, MD; Doug Yarnold, CRNA, photographer.)

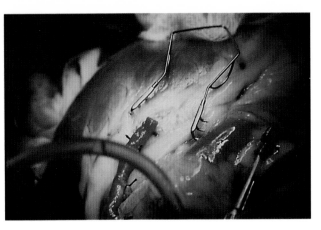

PLATE 22 A coronary epicardial retractor improves exposure of the left anterior descending coronary artery embedded in adipose tissue. Note the silk ties on tributaries of the vein graft. (Courtesy Edward A Lefrak, MD; Doug Yarnold, CRNA, photographer.)

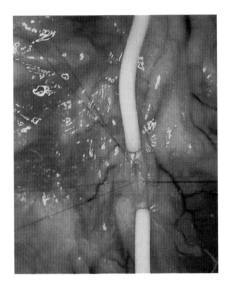

PLATE 23 During beating heart surgery anastomoses, tourniquets may be placed around the coronary artery proximally and distally to prevent bleeding into the anastomotic site. (From Yim APC and others: *Minimal access cardiothoracic surgery,* Philadelphia, 2000, WB Saunders.)

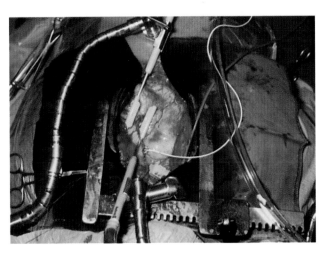

PLATE 24 Octopus retractor positioned to stabilize the target coronary artery through median sternotomy incision. (From Yim APC and others: *Minimal access cardiothoracic surgery,* Philadelphia, 2000, WB Saunders.)

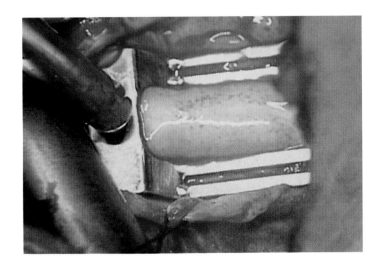

PLATE 25 Close-up of coronary artery stabilized by octopus retractor. (From Buxton B, Frazier OH, Westaby S: *Ischemic heart disease surgical management,* London, 1999, Mosby.)

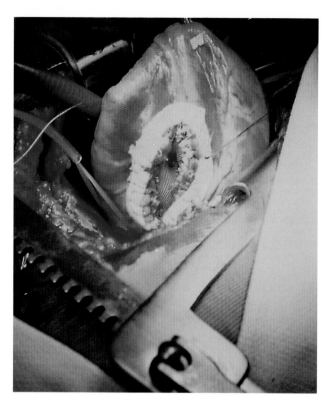

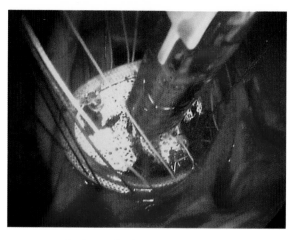

PLATE 27 Mitral annuloplasty ring (attached to prosthetic ring holder and handle) is lowered into the mitral annulus. The stitches *(shown)* will be tied and cut. (From Yim APC and others: *Minimal access cardiothoracic surgery,* Philadelphia, 2000, WB Saunders.)

PLATE 26 Completed repair of a posterior ventricular septal defect. The ventricular free wall has been closed with an elliptic patch of graft material and buttressed with a strip of felt. The left ventricular apex is elevated to expose the posterior wall. (Courtesy Edward A Lefrak, MD.)

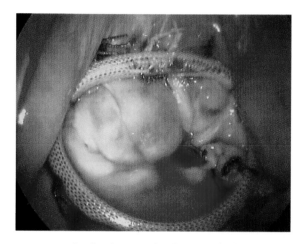

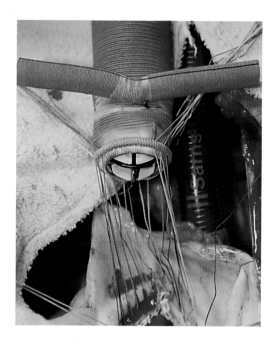

PLATE 28 Mitral valve repair. The annuloplasty ring has been attached with interrupted sutures; note that a portion of the posterior leaflet has been excised and the remaining edges reapproximated with polypropylene suture. (From Yim APC and others: *Minimal access cardiothoracic surgery,* Philadelphia, 2000, WB Saunders.)

PLATE 29 The Cabrol technique for aortic root replacement procedure. One way to revascularize the heart during a Bentall procedure for repair of an ascending aortic dissection is to anastomose a prosthetic graft perpendicular to the ascending aortic graft. Each end of the smaller graft is anastomosed to a major right and left coronary artery. When blood is ejected from the heart and enters the aortic graft, a portion of the blood flows into the perpendicular graft to perfuse the heart. (From Buxton B, Frazier OH, Westaby S: *Ischemic heart disease surgical management,* London, 1999, Mosby.)

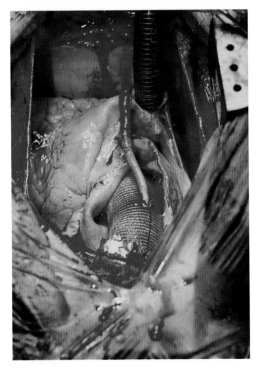

PLATE 30 Bentall procedure with bypass graft. In patients with documented coronary artery disease, bypass grafts can be anastomosed to the target coronary artery distally, and to the prosthetic graft proximally. (From Buxton B, Frazier OH, Westaby S: *Ischemic heart disease surgical management,* London, 1999, Mosby.)

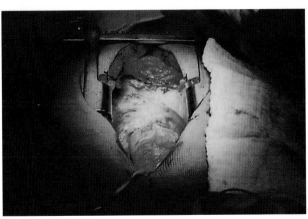

PLATE 31 Plates 32 to 39 show steps in performing a modified Bentall–deBono procedure. Here, the aneurysm is exposed through a median sternotomy (patient's head is at bottom of picture). (Courtesy Edward A Lefrak, MD; Doug Yarnold, CRNA, photographer.)

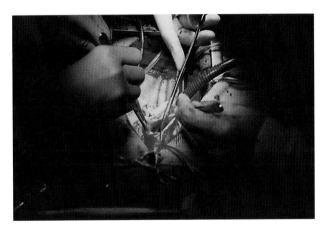

PLATE 32 The aneurysm is incised. (Courtesy Edward A Lefrak, MD; Doug Yarnold, CRNA, photographer.)

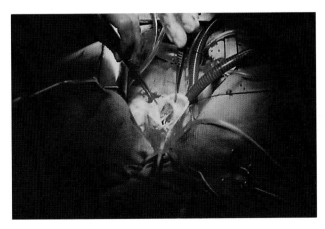

PLATE 33 The aortic valve is inspected. (Courtesy Edward A Lefrak, MD; Doug Yarnold, CRNA, photographer.)

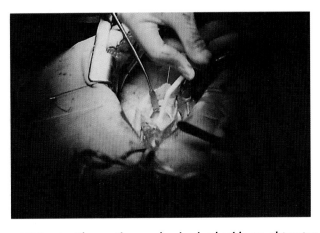

PLATE 34 The aortic annulus is sized with an obturator. Note the aortic leaflet retractor. (Courtesy Edward A Lefrak, MD; Doug Yarnold, CRNA, photographer.)

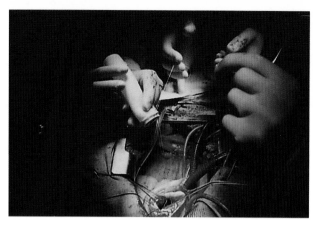

PLATE 35 After stitches have been inserted into the aortic annulus, sutures are placed in the sewing ring of the valve end of the conduit. Another technique is to place sutures into the annulus and prosthesis sewing ring at the same time. (Courtesy Edward A Lefrak, MD; Doug Yarnold, CRNA, photographer.)

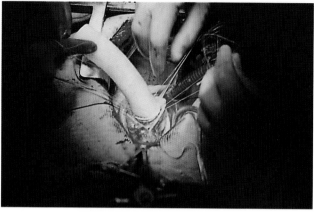

PLATE 36 After all the sutures have been inserted, the prosthesis is seated and the stitches are tied. (Courtesy Edward A Lefrak, MD; Doug Yarnold, CRNA, photographer.)

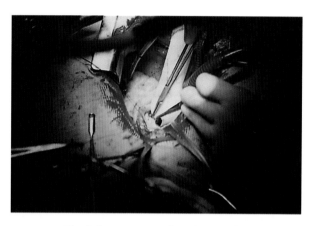

PLATE 37 The left coronary ostium is reimplanted into the graft. (Courtesy Edward A Lefrak, MD; Doug Yarnold, CRNA, photographer.)

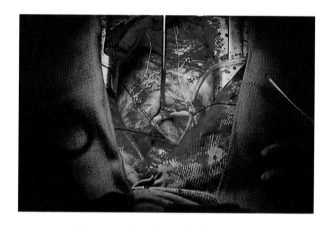

PLATE 38 The completed repair. The aortic wall will be closed around the graft after protamine has been infused to reverse the effects of heparin and hemostasis has been achieved. Note that the patient is off bypass and that the venous cannulas have been removed. (Courtesy Edward A Lefrak, MD; Doug Yarnold, CRNA, photographer.)

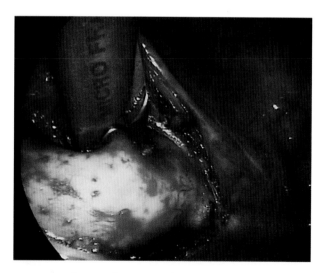

PLATE 39 Patent ductus arteriosus (PDA) repair. A vascular clip is placed on the pulmonary side of the ductus. (From Yim APC and others: *Minimal access cardiothoracic surgery,* Philadelphia, 2000, WB Saunders.)

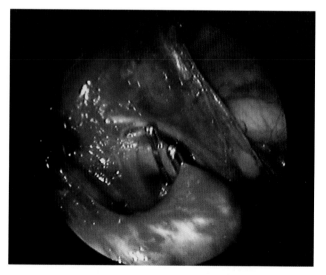

PLATE 40 The completed PDA repair. A second clip has been placed on the aortic side of the ductus. (From Yim APC and others: *Minimal access cardiothoracic surgery,* Philadelphia, 2000, WB Saunders.)

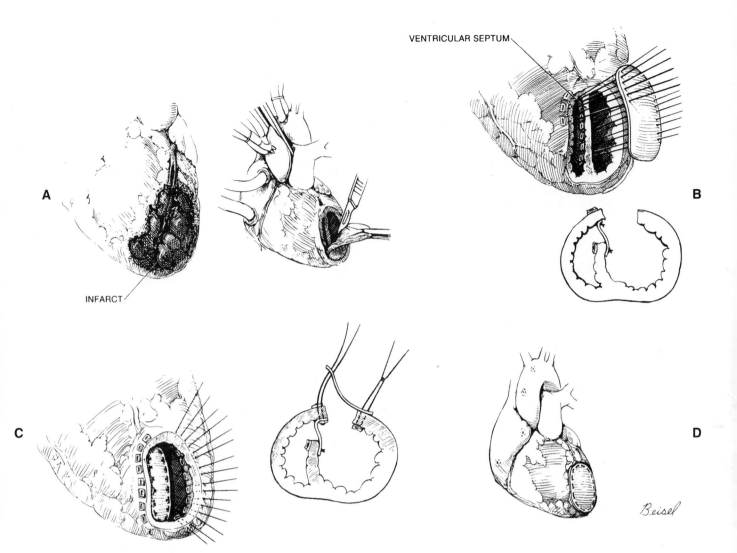

FIGURE 10-37 Technique for closing apical and anterior post-myocardial infarction ventricular septal defects. **A,** The apex is incised and necrotic tissue is excised. **B,** Pledgeted sutures are placed in the right ventricular septum and the right ventricular wall. The stitches are inserted into the edges of a patch that is placed against the left ventricular side of the septum and the endocardial side of the right ventricular free wall. **C,** The ventriculotomy is closed with another felt-buttressed patch. **D,** Completed repair. (From Waldhausen JA, Pierce WS, Campbell DB: *Surgery of the chest,* ed 6, St Louis, 1996, Mosby.)

a. The LV apex is elevated and the infarcted tissue incised. Necrotic myocardium is debrided.

b. Closure of the remaining apical portion of the left and right ventricular free wall and the apical septum is accomplished with felt strips and pledgets sandwiched between the layers.

c. Interrupted mattress sutures are placed through felt pledgets into the ventricular septum and the edge of the right ventricular anterior wall. The sutures are placed into the edges of a patch (Dacron, PTFE, or autologous or bovine pericardium) that is placed against the septum and the right ventricular free wall. The needles are cut and the stitches

tied. The ventriculotomy is closed with a woven patch that may be buttressed with felt.

5c. Inferoposterior septal defects (Madsen and Daggett, 1998): In patients with posterior VSDs, infarction of the right ventricle (RV) is more extensive compared with patients with anterior VSDs who have more extensive LV infarction (David and Armstrong, 1998). Posterior defects commonly are associated with mitral regurgitation (Madsen and Daggett, 1998).

a. The surgeon may identify the margins of the infarct before clamping the aorta and note whether the infarct involves the diaphragmatic aspect of the left ventricle or both ventricles.

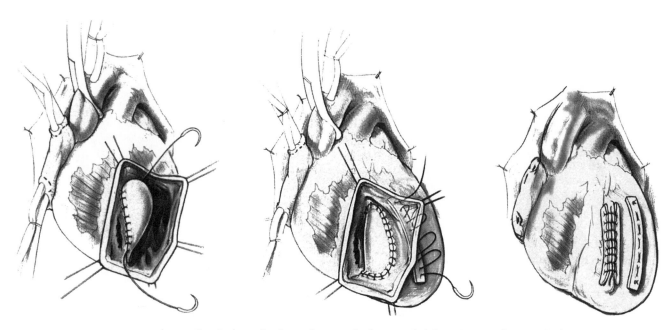

FIGURE 10-38 Surgical repair of anterior ventricular septal defect. An anterior ventriculotomy is performed and a pericardial patch is sutured to the endocardium of the left ventricle to exclude the infarct from the left ventricular cavity. (From David TE, Armstrong S: Repair of postinfarction VSD, *Semin Thorac Cardiovasc Surg* 10[2]:105, 1998.)

b. The heart is arrested and the apex retracted to expose the posterior descending coronary artery.

c. The septal defect is exposed through a left ventricular infarctectomy. (The surgeon may stand on the patient's left for better visualization of the defect.)

d. The mitral valve is inspected and repaired or replaced if indicated.

e. Infarcted right and left ventricular tissue is debrided. Right ventricular muscle is conservatively trimmed as necessary to identify the margins of the defect.

f. If the defect is small, it may be closed by approximating the edge of the septum to the right ventricular free wall with mattress sutures buttressed with felt strips. Larger defects require a patch inserted with running (Fig. 10-39) or individually pledgeted mattress sutures. The patch is seated against the septum, and the sutures are tied.

g. The ventricular wall is closed using another patch (to avoid excessive tension and subsequent hemorrhage from the suture line). The epicardial technique developed by Daggett (Madsen and Daggett, 1998) is used. Pledgeted mattress sutures are inserted on the endocardial surface and brought out through the epicardial surface around the circumference of the ventriculotomy. In the region of the septal repair, the sutures are passed through the edge of the

septal patch and exit on the epicardial surface of the right ventricle.

h. A woven, double-velour, collagen-impregnated Dacron patch is cut to overlap the perimeter of the ventriculotomy. The previously placed sutures (step g) are passed through the edges of the patch and then through individual pledgets. The patch and overlying pledgets are seated, and the stitches are tied.

6. Coronary artery bypass grafting may be performed after infarctectomy and repair.

7. Air is removed from the heart, and the cross-clamp is removed. The surgeon assesses ventricular and valve function and confirms with TEE that the shunt is closed.

The most common problems associated with weaning from CPB are low cardiac output and bleeding (Madsen and Daggett, 1998). IABP and pharmacologic support that balances inotropic and vasodilatory properties can enhance cardiac output. A ventricular assist device may be necessary for persistent low cardiac output. Treatment for coagulopathy includes preoperative infusion of antifibrinolytic therapy with aprotinin or aminocaproic acid (the latter preferred in patients receiving bypass grafts, those who are diabetic, and those with renal dysfunction) before initiation of CBP. Intraoperatively, monitoring the activated clotting time (ACT) and applying fibrin glue to the suture line can enhance hemostasis. Postoperatively, early diuresis and

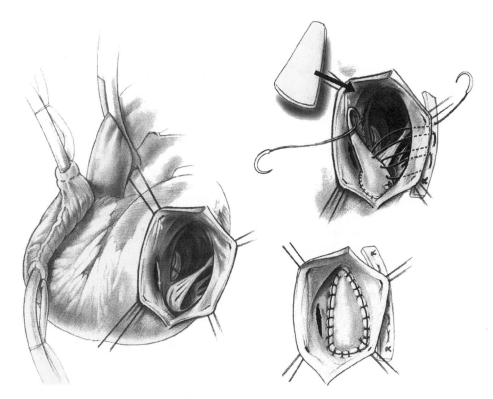

FIGURE 10-39 Surgical repair of posterior ventricular septal defect. An incision is made in the posterior part of the septum and a pericardial patch is sutured to the mitral annulus, endocardium of the septum, and posterior wall. (From David TE, Armstrong S: Surgical repair of postinfarction ventricular septal defect infarct exclusion, *Sem Thorac Cardiovasc Surg* 10[2]:105, 1998.)

positive end-expiratory pressure ventilation are used to decrease intravascular pulmonary water. Intractable ventricular dysrhythmias that are not amenable to standard treatment may require intravenous amiodarone.

Completion of Procedures

After the bypass grafting is completed and a stable rhythm resumes, the surgeon assesses the anastomoses, conduits, and additional repairs for hemostasis. Bleeding from IMA branches or venous tributaries can be controlled with clips or cautery. Occasionally a stitch may be required on the conduit or at the anastomotic site. The proximal anastomosis can be marked with radiopaque rings or metal clips for future reference.

If a vein graft is too long, a number of options are available. Topical collagen hemostatic agents can be used to tack the graft to the heart, or a fine suture can be used to attach the adventitia of the conduit to the epicardium. Usually the graft is attached in at least two places so that it lies in a gentle curve rather than at an acute angle, which could cause occlusion of the graft. Another method is to resect excess tissue. This can be accomplished with a small, curved partial-occlusion clamp

placed over the graft and the excess tissue pulled into the jaws. While an assistant steadies the clamp, the surgeon excises the excess vein and reanastomoses the cut ends. Air is removed from the graft, and the clamp is removed. Usually this can be performed on a beating heart.

Temporary epicardial pacing wires are attached and the pacemaker set to 90 to 100 beats per minute (if the native rhythm is lower). Maintaining an adequate blood pressure is especially critical for perfusing the conduits. Transient hypotension caused by decreased contractility or volume is treated accordingly.

After weaning the patient from CPB, the surgeon inserts one or two chest tubes into the pericardial cavity and into the pleura that was opened during IMA dissection. Smaller (e.g., 19-French) fluted silicone drains are preferred increasingly over the standard 36-French polyvinyl chloride (PVC) tubes, in part because they are less painful for the patient. These tubes may be connected to a small suction reservoir rather than to the conventional chest drainage system.

After hemostasis is achieved, the incisions are closed and dressings applied. The leg incision is dressed and the leg wrapped from ankle to thigh with an elastic pressure dressing (in many cases even when a minimally invasive approach has been used). The perioperative nurse can assess the pedal pulse and the capillary refill of the toes to determine perfusion to the affected leg.

Postoperative Considerations and Complications

The goals of postoperative care are to maintain hemodynamic stability and avoid complications. For the patient who has undergone myocardial revascularization, major considerations include monitoring the ECG for dysrhythmias and signs of ischemia or perioperative infarction; maintaining adequate blood pressure to ensure sufficient flow through arterial and venous conduits; treating bradycardia, which can decrease cardiac output and tissue perfusion; and monitoring for tamponade resulting from excessive bleeding into the pericardium without adequate drainage (Table 10-9).

CLINICAL OUTCOMES AND QUALITY OF LIFE

Long-term survival and freedom from cardiac-related complications after CABG are related to completeness of the revascularization, the progression of the patient's native coronary artery disease, and the maintenance of bypass graft patency (Ascione and others, 2001). Complete revascularization in patients with three-vessel coronary artery disease, for example, consists of performing bypass grafts to the three main vessels involved (e.g., LAD, circumflex, and RCA) and their major branches. In this case, bypassing one or two vessels, rather than all three vessels, results in incomplete revascularization. Additionally, a survival benefit has been shown in patients with more arterial grafts and in particular bilateral versus single IMA conduits (Taggart, D'Amico, and Altman, 2001; Lytle and others, 1999).

After 5 years, 66% of bypass patients are symptom free, compared with 38% of medically treated patients. By 10 years these differences are not statistically significant, partly because of the failure of venous grafts and the crossover of medically treated patients to bypass surgery (Eagle and others, 1999).

The results of off-pump bypass grafting, compared with on-pump CABG, have shown improved renal function, less neurologic dysfunction (stroke or coma), and less blood loss (related to fewer coagulation factor abnormalities) (Cleveland and others, 2001). Worse outcomes are seen in women after CABG performed on or off pump. Women undergoing revascularization tend to be older and have more comorbidities than men. Capdeville, Chamogeogarkis, and Lee (2001) compared women undergoing off-pump revascularization via median sternotomy (OPCAB) with men, who have improved recovery when CPB is avoided. The female

subjects in the study did not demonstrate a comparable improvement in recovery, and the authors suggest that biochemical, hormonal, or pharmacokinetic factors in women may neutralize the beneficial effect of avoiding CPB that is seen in men.

The effect of increasing age on functional recovery and quality of life after myocardial revascularization has received greater scrutiny with the aging surgical population. Older patients undergoing elective CABG have reported functional benefits similar to those reported in younger patients (Sakamoto and others, 2001). Quality of life is improved in patients who have undergone surgery versus medical therapy: Patients have greater relief of symptoms, fewer activity limitations, less requirement for medications, and improved functional capacity (Eagle and others, 1999).

Reoperation for Coronary Artery Disease

An increasing number of CABG patients require reoperation a second or a third time because of progressive atherosclerotic heart disease and graft failure. Native atherosclerotic coronary artery lesions tend to be focal, eccentric, and proximal, with encapsulated plaques. In contrast, saphenous vein atherosclerotic lesions are more diffuse and concentric and do not have a fibrous cap; intimal debris from these lesions may embolize. These friable and fragile lesions are more prone to embolization and should be manipulated with extreme caution during reoperation. Although percutaneous coronary intervention (e.g., stenting or angioplasty) of saphenous vein grafts has been attempted in the hope of reducing the need for reoperation, results have been considerably less satisfactory than PCI on native coronary vessels (Keely, Velez, and Safian, 2001).

Although the patency of IMA grafts is significantly greater than vein graft patency (Lytle and others, 1999), many patients undergoing a second reoperation may not have IMA graft conduits because the initial surgery was performed at a time when IMA use was not widespread. In addition, vein grafts often are needed to supplement the conduits required for complete revascularization. Even with the increased use of single and double IMA grafts and the use of radial artery grafts, vein conduits frequently are required to provide sufficient conduits.

When reoperation is indicated, previous chest wires are exposed and removed. Occasionally the sternum is divided with an oscillating saw (see Chapter 9), and care is taken to avoid lacerating previously placed IMA or other grafts that may be lying under the sternum. Off-pump techniques have gained popularity for reoperation, and excellent results have been reported in carefully selected patients (Arom and others, 2001). Some

TABLE 10-9
Postoperative Complications of Myocardial Revascularization

COMPLICATION	INTERVENTIONS
Bleeding	Monitor chest tube drainage, inspect wounds for bleeding
	Report excessive bleeding (greater than 200-400 ml/hr)
	Investigate, report sudden cessation of chest tube drainage
	Monitor laboratory values: PT, PTT, platelet count, H&H, DIC screen, ACT
	Administer blood, blood products, fluids as indicated
	Monitor VS and hemodynamics for hypotension, tachycardia, hypovolemia, tamponade
	Promote normothermia with warming blankets, warmed solutions
	If cardiac tamponade occurs, be prepared to open chest to evacuate hematoma and perform cardiac massage; anticipate return to OR (see Box 3-4 for list of emergency supplies for sternotomy in intensive care unit)
Respiratory complications	Monitor for fluid shifts and left ventricular dysfunction during transition from mechanical to spontaneous ventilation
	Evaluate gas exchange and respiratory parameters: breath sounds, respiratory rate, vital capacity, tidal volume
	Monitor skin color, ABGs, restlessness, decreased LOC
	Promote expansion of atelectasis by deep breathing and coughing, incentive spirometry, suctioning, mobilizing the patient
	Monitor for phrenic nerve injury reducing the strength of respiratory efforts
	Monitor for signs and symptoms of pneumothorax, pneumonia, hemothorax, mediastinal shift, asymmetric chest movement
Neurologic complications	Assess for signs and symptoms: pain, peripheral neuropathy, stroke, coma, abnormal reflexes
	Avoid air in intravascular lines
	Assess for postoperative delirium: agitation, disorientation, hallucinations, paranoia; orient to person, place, and time
	Initiate interventions to maintain mental stability and foster orientation to environment
	Use alternative communication techniques as needed
	Relieve discomfort/agitation caused by pain, hypoxia, full bladder, fear, anxiety
Cardiac complications	
Graft closure	Give aspirin as ordered to reduce early graft thrombosis
Myocardial failure	Monitor peripheral pulses, foot and toe temperatures, urinary output, arterial blood pressure, central venous pressure, pulmonary artery pressure, thermodilution, CO/CI measurements, systemic/pulmonary vascular resistance
	Report MAP below 65 mm Hg, especially in presence of IMA graft
	Manipulate determinants of CO to optimize perfusion:
	Increase preload—institute volume replacement
	Decrease afterload—administer vasodilators
	Augment contractility—administer inotropic drugs
	Regulate heart rate—institute cardiac pacing
	Augment ventricular function with mechanical assistance (IABP, LVAD, RVAD)
Myocardial infarction	Assess ECG changes, significant increase in cardiac enzymes (creatine kinase–MB fraction)
Dysrhythmia	Institute cardiac pacing for bradycardia, atrial fibrillation, and other supraventricular dysrhythmias
	Administer antidysrhythmic drugs
	Monitor potassium levels
	Cardiovert, ventricular tachycardia or fibrillation
	If cardiac arrest occurs, be prepared to open chest and perform internal chest massage; anticipate return to OR
Infection & wound disruption	Monitor temperature, report if above 38° C
	Inspect incisions for evidence of swelling, redness, exudate, and tenderness
	Administer antibiotics as prescribed
	Wash hands often and before and after contact with patient
	May require return to OR for sternal debridement and rewiring; mediastinitis may require muscle flap repair
Renal complications	Assess urine output, BUN, creatinine, color, and urine specific gravity
	Measure weight daily
	Assess CO, central venous pressure, electrolyte levels, acid-base balance
	Maintain adequate volume, reduce afterload
	Promote adequate renal blood flow (dopamine) and fluid management (diuretics)
Gastrointestinal complications	Assess nasogastric tube drainage and stool, bowel sounds, gastric pH, signs of abdominal distension
	Assess for signs and symptoms of gastroduodenal ulcer, cholecystitis, pancreatitis, intestinal ischemia, perforation, bleeding, abdominal distension
	In patients with gastroepiploic grafts, anticipate increased pain, abdominal discomfort
	Administer vasopressors judiciously, avoid aspirin

ABG, Arterial blood gases; *ACT,* activated clotting time; *BUN,* blood urea nitrogen; *CI,* cardiac index; *CO,* cardiac output; *DIC,* disseminated intravascular coagulopathy; *H&H,* hemoglobin and hematocrit; *IABP,* intraaortic balloon pump; *LOC,* level of consciousness; *LVAD,* left ventricular assist device; *MAP,* mean arterial pressure; *PT,* prothrombin time; *PTT,* partial thromboplastin time; *RVAD,* right ventricular assist device; *VS,* vital signs.
Modified from Thelan LA and others: *Critical care nursing: diagnosis and management,* ed 3, St Louis, 1998, Mosby.

authors (Noyez and others, 2000) prefer to cannulate the groin before dividing the sternum in case the patient requires immediate circulatory support, especially when the patient is undergoing a re-reoperation. If the lateral chest x-ray film does not show severe adhesions between the heart and the sternum, the initial aortic cannulation site may be used.

CONDUITS

At reoperation, if one or both IMAs or the radial artery are available, they are the preferred conduits; greater saphenous vein can supplement arterial grafts. Other conduits (see Fig. 10-6) are used as necessary. The position of a pre-existing IMA graft may make exposure of the marginal arteries in the left lateral wall difficult; careful retraction of the IMA is mandatory for protecting that graft. When CPB is employed, an IMA graft may require temporary occlusion with a small bulldog clamp so that blood flow through the IMA does not rewarm the heart and prevent cardioplegic arrest during the period of cross-clamping. When reoperation is performed off bypass, the IMA is not clamped; bleeding from the anastomotic site can be controlled with snares, suctions, or humified gas misting.

References

Adams DH, Antman EM: Medical management of the patient undergoing cardiac surgery. In Braunwald E, Zipes DP, Libby P, editors: *Heart disease*, ed 6, Philadelphia, 2001, WB Saunders.

Allen KB, Shaar CJ: Endoscopic saphenous vein harvesting, *Ann Thorac Surg* 64(1):265, 1997.

Allen KB and others: Transmyocardial laser revascularization combined with coronary artery bypass grafting: a multicenter, blinded, prospective, randomized, controlled trial, *J Thorac Cardiovasc Surg* 119(3):540, 2000.

American Heart Association (AHA): *2001 heart and stroke statistical update*, http://www.americanheart.org/statistics/cvd.html (accessed Sept 14, 2001).

Anderson HV: Percutaneous coronary interventions for stable angina pectoris. In Willerson JT, Cohn JN, editors: *Cardiovascular medicine*, ed 2, New York, 2000, Churchill Livingstone.

Arom KV and others: Mini-sternotomy for CABG, *Ann Thorac Surg* 61:1271, 1996.

Arom KV and others: OPCAB surgery: a critical review of two different categories of pre-operative ejection fraction, *Eur J Cardiothorac Surg* 20(3)533, 2001.

Ascione R and others: Clinical and angiographic outcome of different surgical strategies of bilateral internal mammary artery grafting, *Ann Thorac Surg* 72(3)959, 2001.

Barsness GW and others: Reduced thrombus burden with abciximab delivered locally before percutaneous intervention in saphenous vein grafts, *Am Heart J* 139(5):824, 2000.

Batista RJV and others: Partial left ventriculectomy to improve left ventricular function in end-stage heart disease, *J Card Surg* 11(2)96, 1996.

Benitez RM: Atherosclerosis: an infectious disease? *Hosp Pract* 34(9):79, 1999.

Benetti FJ and others: Direct myocardial revascularization without extracorporeal circulation, *Chest* 100(2):312, 1991.

Berne RM, Levy MN: *Cardiovascular physiology*, ed 8, St Louis, 2001, Mosby.

Borst C and others: Coronary artery bypass grafting without cardiopulmonary bypass and without interruption of native coronary flow using a novel anastomosis site restraining device ("Octopus"), *J Am Coll Cardiol* 27(6):1356, 1996.

Braunwald E, Zipes DP, Libby P, editors: *Heart disease: a textbook of cardiovascular medicine*, ed 6, Philadelphia, 2001, WB Saunders.

Brodie BR: Reperfusion therapy for acute myocardial infarction in patients with prior bypass surgery, *Am Heart J* 142(3)381, 2001.

Calafiore AM and others: Early clinical experience with a new sutureless anastomotic device for proximal anastomosis of the saphenous vein to the aorta, *J Thorac Cardiovasc Surg* 121(5):854, 2001.

Cameron A and others: Coronary bypass surgery with internal-thoracic-artery grafts—effects on survival over a 15-year period, *N Engl J Med* 334(4):216, 1996.

Capdeville M, Chamogeogarkis T, Lee JH: Effect of gender on outcomes of beating heart operations, *Ann Thorac Surg* 72(3)S1022, 2001.

Carrel A: On the experimental surgery of the thoracic aorta and the heart, *Ann Surg* 52:83, 1910.

Chaux A and others: Postinfarction ventricular septal defect, *Semin Thorac Cardiovasc Surg* 10(2):93, 1998.

Cleveland JC Jr and others: Off-pump coronary artery bypass grafting decreases risk-adjusted mortality and morbidity, *Ann Thorac Surg* 72(4):1282, 2001.

Colucci WS, Braunwald E: Pathophysiology of heart failure. In Braunwald E, Zipes DP, Libby P, editors: *Heart disease*, ed 6, Philadelphia, 2001, WB Saunders.

Cooley DA: *Techniques in cardiac surgery*, ed 2, Philadelphia, 1984, WB Saunders.

Cooley DA: Postinfarction ventricular septal rupture, *Semin Thorac Cardiovasc Surg* 10(2):100, 1998.

Cooley DA: Ventricular endoaneurysmorrhaphy: results of improved method of repair, *Tex Heart Inst J* 16(2):72, 1989.

Cooley DA and others: Surgical repair of ruptured intraventricular septum following acute myocardial infarction, *Surgery* 41:930, 1957.

Cosgrove DM, Loop FD, Sheldon WC: Results of myocardial revascularization: a 12-year experience, *Circulation* 65(Suppl 2):37, 1982.

Daggett WM: Postinfarction ventricular septal defects: Introduction, *Sem Thorac Cardiovasc Surg* 10(2):92, 1998.

Daggett WM and others: Surgery for post-myocardial infarction ventricular septal defect, *Ann Surg* 186(3):260, 1977.

Damiano RJ and others: Initial prospective multicenter clinical trial of robotically-assisted coronary artery bypass grafting, *Ann Thorac Surg* 72(4):1263, 2001.

David TE, Armstrong S: Surgical repair of postinfarction ventricular septal defect infarct exclusion, *Sem Thorac Cardiovasc Surg* 10(2):105, 1998.

Detre KM and others: Coronary revascularization in diabetic patients: a comparison of the randomized and observational components of the Bypass Angioplasty Revascularization Investigation (BARI), *Circulation* 99(5):633, 1999.

Dodge R: Personal communication, 2001.

Dor V: Left ventricular aneurysms: the endoventricular circular patch plasty, *Semin Thorac Cardiovasc Surg* 9(2):123, 1997.

Dotter CT, Rosch J, Judkins MP: Transluminal dilatation of atherosclerotic stenosis, *Surg Gynecol Obstet* 127(4):794, 1968.

Douglas PS: Coronary artery disease in women. In Braunwald E, Zipes DP, Libby P, editors: *Heart disease*, ed 6, Philadelphia, 2001, WB Saunders.

Eagle KA and others: ACC/AHA Guidelines for Coronary Artery Bypass Graft Surgery: executive summary and recommendations, *J Am Coll Cardiol* 34(4):1262, 1999.

Edmunds LH: Why cardiopulmonary bypass makes patients sick: strategies to control the blood-synthetic surface interface, *Adv Card Surg* 6:131, 1995.

Edwards FH and others: Impact of gender on coronary bypass operative mortality, *Ann Thorac Surg* 66(1):125, 1998.

Espersen C: The R.N. first assistant in cardiac surgery. In Rothrock JC, editor: *The RN first assistant: an expanded perioperative role*, ed 3, Philadelphia, 1999, JB Lippincott.

Fann JI and others: Port-access multivessel coronary artery bypass grafting. In Cox JL, Sundt TM, editors: *Op Tech Card Thorac Surg: A Comparative Atlas* 3(1):16, 1998.

Favaloro RG: Personal communication, 1991.

Fischman DL and others: A randomized comparison of coronary-stent placement and balloon angioplasty in the treatment of coronary artery disease, *N Engl J Med* 331(8):496, 1994.

Frazier OH and others: Partial left ventriculectomy: which patients can be expected to benefit? *Ann Thorac Surg* 69(6):1836, 2000.

Futterman LG, Lemberg L: The critical role of the endothelial cell in acute coronary events, *Am J Crit Care* 10(3):191, 2001.

Ganz P, Ganz W: Coronary blood flow and myocardial ischemia. In Braunwald E, Zipes DP, Libby P, editors: *Heart disease*, ed 6, Philadelphia, 2001, WB Saunders.

Gersh BJ, Braunwald E, Bonow RO: Chronic coronary artery disease. In Braunwald E, Zipes DP, Libby P, editors: *Heart disease*, ed 6, Philadelphia, 2001, WB Saunders.

Gylys K, Gold M: Acute coronary syndrome: new developments in pharmacological treatment strategies, *Crit Care Nurse* (Suppl):3, April 2000.

Green MA, Malias MA: Arm complications after radial artery procurement for coronary bypass operation, *Ann Thorac Surg* 72:126, 2001.

Gruentzig AR, Senning A, Siegenthaler WE: Non-operative dilatation of coronary artery stenosis—percutaneous transluminal coronary angioplasty, *N Eng J Med* 301:61, 1979.

Harjai KJ: New paradigms in preventive cardiology: unconventional coronary risk factors, *Ochsner J* 2(4):209, 2000.

Heckman R: Ultrasound use in cardiothoracic surgery, *AORN J* 73(1):144, 2001.

Heijmen RH and others: A novel one-shot anastomotic stapler prototype for coronary bypass grafting on the beating heart: feasibility in the pig, *J Thorac Cardiovasc Surg* 117(1):25, 1999.

Hlozek CC, Zacharias WM: The RN first assistant's role during inferior epigastric artery harvesting, *AORN J* 65(1):26, 1997.

Horvath KA and others: Transmyocardial laser revascularization: results of a multicenter trial with transmyocardial laser revascularization used as sole therapy for end-stage coronary artery disease, *J Thorac Cardiovasc Surg* 113(4):645, 1997.

Jarvis MA and others: Reliability of Allen's test in selection of patients for radial artery harvest, *Ann Thorac Surg* 70(4):1362, 2000.

Jatene AD: Left ventricular aneurysmectomy: resection or reconstruction. *J Thorac Cardiovasc Surg* 89(3):321, 1985.

Keeley EC and others: Long term clinical outcome and predictors of major adverse cardiac events after percutaneous interventions on saphenous vein grafts, *J Am Coll Cardiol* 38(3)659, 2001.

Kereiakes DJ: ACC/AHA PTCA guidelines. *Report of the American College of Cardiology Scientific Session 2000*, March 15, 2000, http://www.medscape.com/medscape/CNO/2000/ACC/story.cfm?story_id=1112 (accessed April 30, 2000).

Kern MJ: *The cardiac catheterization handbook*, ed 3, St Louis, 1999, Mosby.

Killen DA and others: Early repair of postinfarction ventricular septal rupture, *Ann Thorac Surg* 63(1):138, 1997.

Krantz DS and others: Effects of mental stress in patients with coronary artery disease: evidence and clinical implications, *JAMA* 283(14):1800, 2000.

Lemmer JHJ: Clinical experience in coronary bypass surgery for abciximab-treated patients, *Ann Thorac Surg* 70(2 Suppl):S33, 2000.

Leon MB and others: Localized intracoronary gamma-radiation therapy to inhibit the recurrence of restenosis after stenting, *N Engl J Med* 344(4):250, 2001.

Levy JH and others: Group recommendations, *Ann Thorac Surg* 70:S43, 2000.

Lewis K, Hammon JW: Technique for the minimally invasive harvest of the radial artery, *Surg Phys Assist* 7(7):18, 2001.

Limet R and others: Prevention of aorta-coronary bypass graft occlusion: beneficial effect of ticlopidine on early and late patency rates of venous coronary bypass grafts: a double-blind study, *J Thorac Cardiovasc Surg* 94(5)773, 1987.

Lincoff AM: Stent scrutiny, *JAMA* 284(14):1839, 2000.

Loop FD and others: Influence of the internal-mammary-artery graft on 10-year survival and other cardiac events, *N Engl J Med* 314(1):1, 1986.

Lytle BW and others: Two internal thoracic artery grafts are better than one, *J Thorac Cardiovasc Surg* 117(5):855, 1999.

Lytle BW and others: Vein graft disease: the clinical impact of stenosis in saphenous vein bypass grafts to coronary arteries, *J Thorac Cardiovasc Surg* 103(5):831, 1992.

Lytle BW and others: Coronary artery bypass grafting with the right gastroepiploic artery, *J Thorac Cardiovasc Surg* 97(6):826, 1989.

Lytle BW and others: Perioperative risk of bilateral internal mammary artery grafting: analysis of 500 cases from 1971 to 1984, *Circulation* 74(2):37, 1986.

Lytle BW and others: Multivessel coronary revascularization without saphenous vein: long-term results of bilateral internal mammary artery grafting, *Ann Thorac Surg* 36(5):540, 1983.

Mack MJ: Coronary surgery: off pump and port access, *Surg Clin North Am* 80(5):1575, 2000.

Madsen JC, Daggett WM: Repair of postinfarction ventricular septal defects, *Semin Thorac Cardiovasc Surg* 10(2):117, 1998.

Mangano DT: Preoperative assessment of cardiac risk. In Kaplan JA, editor: *Cardiac anesthesia,* ed 4, Philadelphia, 1999, WB Saunders.

Mehran R and others: One-year clinical outcome after minimally invasive direct coronary artery bypass, *Circulation* 102:2799, 2000.

Miller WL, Reeder GS: Adjunctive therapies in the treatment of acute coronary syndromes, *Mayo Clin Proc* 76(4):391, 2001.

Mohr FW and others: Computer-enhanced "robotic" cardiac surgery: experience in 148 patients, *J Thorac Cardiovasc Surg* 121(5):842, 2001.

Ng PC and others: Anterior thoracotomy wound complications in minimally invasive direct coronary artery bypass, *Ann Thorac Surg* 69(5):1338, 2000.

Noyez L and others: Third-time coronary artery bypass grafting, *Ann Thorac Surg* 70(2):483, 2000.

Okasaki Y and others: Coronary endothelial damage during off-pump CABG related to coronary-clamping and gas insufflation, *Eur J Cardio-Thorac Surg* 19:834, 2001.

Parolari A and others: The radial artery: which place in coronary operation? *Ann Thorac Surg* 69(4):1288, 2000.

Pfister A: Myocardial revascularization without cardiopulmonary bypass, *Adv Cardiac Surg* 11:35, 1999.

Pfister AJ and others: Coronary artery bypass without cardiopulmonary bypass, *Ann Thorac Surg* 54(6):1085, 1992.

Pompili MF and others: Port-access mitral valve replacement in dogs, *J Thorac Cardiovasc Surg* 112(5):1268, 1996.

Popma JJ: Stent selection in clinical practice: have clinical trials provided the evidence we need? *Am Heart J* 142(3):378, 2001.

Reichenspurner H: Port-access surgery: pros and cons, *Adv Cardiac Surg* 13:1, 2001.

Rodriguez E and others: Contractile smooth muscle cell apoptosis early after saphenous vein grafting, *Ann Thorac Surg* 70(4):1145, 2000.

Rozanski A, Blumenthal JA, Kaplan J: Impact of psychological factors on the pathogenesis of cardiovascular disease and implications for therapy, *Circulation* 99(16):2192, 1999.

Sakamoto S and others: Coronary artery bypass grafting in octogenarians, *Cardiovasc Surg* 9(5):487, 2001.

Sapirstein W, Zuckerman B, Dillard J: FDA approval of coronary-artery brachytherapy, *N Engl J Med* 344(4):297, 2001.

Selzman CH, Miller SA, Harken AH: Therapeutic implications of inflammation in atherosclerotic cardiovascular disease, *Ann Thorac Surg* 71(6):2066, 2001.

Serruys PW and others: Comparison of coronary-artery bypass surgery and stenting for the treatment of multivessel disease, *N Engl J Med* 344(15):1117, 2001.

Sheppard R, Eisenberg MJ: Intracoronary radiotherapy for restenosis, *N Engl J Med* 344(4):295, 2001.

Shennib H: A renaissance in cardiovascular surgery: endovascular and device-based revascularization, *Ann Thorac Surg* 72(3):S993, 2001.

Sigwart U and others: Stent coatings, *J Invas Cardiol* 13(2):141, 2001.

Subramanian VA: MIDCAB approach for single vessel coronary artery bypass graft, *Op Tech Cardiac Thorac Surg* 3(1):2, 1998.

Subramanian VA and others: Minimally invasive coronary bypass surgery: a multicenter report of preliminary clinical experience, *Circulation* 92(Suppl):1645, 1995.

Suma H and others: Late angiographic result of using the right gastroepiploic artery as a graft, *J Thorac Cardiovasc Surg* 120(3):496, 2000.

Suwaidi JA, Berger PB, Holmes DR: Coronary artery stents, *JAMA* 284(14):1828, 2000.

Suwaidi JA and others: Primary percutaneous coronary interventions in patients with acute myocardial infarction and prior coronary artery bypass grafting, *Am Heart J* 142:452, 2001.

Sweeney MS, Frazier OH, Cooley DA: Surgical treatment. In Kaplan JA, editor: *Cardiac anesthesia,* ed 4, Philadelphia, 2000, WB Saunders.

Szabo Z and others: Suturing and knotting techniques for thoracoscopic cardiac surgery, *Surg Clin North Am* 80(5):1555, 2000.

Taggart DP, D'Amico R, Altman DG: Effect of arterial revascularization on survival: a systematic review of studies comparing bilateral and single internal mammary arteries, *Lancet* 358(9285):870, 2001.

Tamai H and others: Initial and 6-month results of biodegradable poly-l-lactic acid coronary stents in humans, *Circulation* 102(4):399, 2000.

Verin V and others: Endoluminal beta-radiation therapy for the prevention of coronary restenosis after balloon angioplasty, *N Engl J Med* 344(4)243, 2001.

Waldhausen JA, Pierce WS, Campbell DB: *Surgery of the chest,* ed 6, St Louis, 1996, Mosby.

Weaver WD and others: Comparison of primary coronary angioplasty and intravenous thrombolytic therapy for acute myocardial infarction: a quantitative review, *JAMA* 278(23):2093, 1997.

Weber MM: Surgical management of unstable angina and symptomatic coronary artery disease, *J Cardiovasc Nurs* 15(1):27, 2000.

Westaby S: *Landmarks in cardiac surgery,* Oxford, UK, 1997, Isis Medical Media.

White H: Acute ischemic syndromes: an interventional perspective. In Shah PK and others: *Review of the American College of Cardiology Scientific sessions,* March 14, 2000, http://www.medscape.com/medscape/cno/2000/ACC/Story.cfm?story _id=1085 (accessed April 30, 2000).

Wood S, Lowry F: RAVEL results: sirolimus-coated stent may usher in "a new era." In Report on the XXIII Congress of the European Society of Cardiology, http://www.theheart.org/documents/page.cfm?from=590001200&doc_id =25050 (accessed Sept 10, 2001).

Yoshitomi Y and others: Does stent design affect probability of restenosis? A randomized trial comparing Multilink stents with GFX stents, *Am Heart J* 142(3):445, 2001.

11 *Mitral Valve Surgery*

I anticipate that with the progress of cardiac surgery some of the severest cases of mitral stenosis will be relieved by slightly notching the mitral valve.

DW Samways, MD, 1898

A quarter century after Samways' prediction, Cutler and Levine (1923) performed the first effective operative procedure for the treatment of valvular heart disease with a closed mitral commissurotomy on an 11-year-old girl suffering severe mitral stenosis. Although this initial experience was successful, subsequent attempts by Cutler and others were failures, largely because of the mitral insufficiency created by resecting portions of the valve. The resulting controversy diminished enthusiasm for direct valvular surgery, which was not reintroduced until after World War II (Lefrak and Starr, 1979). The next era of valve surgery was stimulated by the efforts of Harken and colleagues (1948) and Bailey (1949), who promoted greater understanding of the underlying pathophysiology and the importance of mobilizing the leaflets without creating mitral insufficiency during commissurotomy. The introduction of cardiopulmonary bypass and the development of biologically compatible prosthetic materials enabled further advances in technology and operative technique, which culminated in the first mitral valve replacement in 1960 by Starr (Starr and Edwards, 1961).

Atrioventricular Valves

Heart valves enable efficient cardiac function by providing unimpeded forward blood flow and preventing backflow into the originating chamber. Unlike the more simple aortic and pulmonary semilunar valves, the atrioventricular mitral and tricuspid valves reflect a complex interplay among the valve leaflets, annulus fibrosis, chordae tendineae, papillary muscles, and intraventricular wall (see Chapter 3). Structurally and functionally the mitral valve (Fig. 11-1) is similar to the tricuspid valve, the atrioventricular valve found in the right side of the heart. Differences are that the mitral valve is slightly smaller and is composed of two leaflets or cusps (Fig. 11-2), whereas the tricuspid valve has three cusps.

Mitral Valve Apparatus

The larger anterior (septal or aortic) mitral leaflet is roughly triangular, inserting into approximately one third of the annulus. It is in fibrous continuity with the aortic valve and forms one boundary of the left ventricular outflow tract. The posterior (mural or ventricular) leaflet is narrower and has a scalloped appearance; it inserts into approximately two thirds of the annulus (Kirklin and Barratt-Boyes, 1993; Sakai and others, 1999).

Valvular opening and closing is related to pressure changes between the atria and ventricles. Opening of the valve leaflets occurs during ventricular diastole after the left atrium has filled with blood, and the pressure in the atrium exceeds the pressure in the left ventricle. The valve leaflets then are forced open. Near the completion of ventricular filling, the atrium contracts, providing an additional 20% to 30% to the left ventricular end-diastolic volume.

At the beginning of ventricular systole, the papillary muscles contract. As the innerventricular pressure rises, these muscles and the attached chordae tendineae, which insert into the valve leaflets, prevent the leaflets from everting into the atrium. Each leaflet receives chordae from both the anterolateral and the posteromedial papillary muscles. The chordae, which tether the leaflets to the papillary muscles, are divided into three categories: primary chordae insert into the leaflet edges, secondary chordae insert into the leaflet undersurface, and tertiary chordae (arising from trabeculations within the posterior left ventricular wall) are prominent in the ventricular aspect of the posterior leaflet (Harlan, Starr, and Harwin, 1980). The free edges of the valve leaflets coapt firmly along their atrial surface, with the remainder of each leaflet bulging somewhat toward the atrium like a parachute. The annulus decreases in size and becomes more elliptical, thereby reducing the area the leaflets must cover. Abnormalities in any of these components (Table 11-1) affect the ability of the mitral

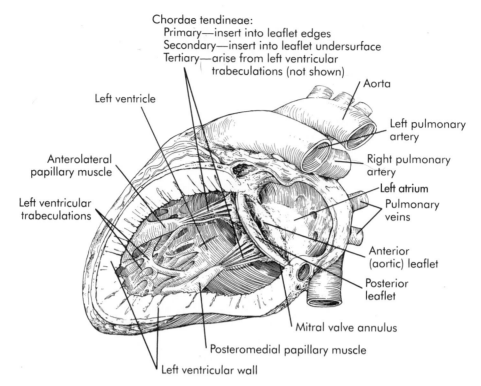

Chordae tendineae:
  Primary—insert into leaflet edges
  Secondary—insert into leaflet undersurface
  Tertiary—arise from left ventricular
    trabeculations (not shown)

FIGURE 11-1   The mitral valve apparatus consists of the valve leaflets, chordae tendineae, papillary muscles, valvular annulus, and left ventricle. (Drawing by Peter Stone.)

apparatus to act in synchrony to regulate blood flow between the left atrium and the left ventricle.

Mitral Valve Disease

Commonly, mitral valve disease is a disorder of the valve and its related components. It is not primarily a disorder of the myocardium (although an important exception is mitral valve incompetence caused by ischemic coronary artery disease). The two most common functional anomalies affecting the opening and closing motions of the valve are increased leaflet motion and restricted or diminished leaflet motion (Carpentier, 1983). Not infrequently the two conditions coexist because the diminished leaflet opening (producing obstructed flow) often is accompanied by incomplete leaflet closing (resulting in regurgitation). Occasionally there is impaired blood flow even in the presence of normal leaflet motion, such as occurs with leaflet perforation or cleft mitral valve.

Impedance to flow from the left atrium to the left ventricle is caused by mitral stenosis, a narrowing of the valve orifice (normally 4 to 6 cm²). This process usually occurs gradually. Mitral valve regurgitation (or incompetence or insufficiency) occurs when the valve leaflets do not coapt properly and thus are unable to prevent backflow into the left atrium during ventricular systole.

This process may be gradual or may occur suddenly when the chordae or the papillary muscles supporting the valve leaflets rupture. Either of these conditions, stenosis or regurgitation, creates hemodynamic alterations that impose a progressively greater myocardial workload to maintain a sufficient cardiac output. The aim of surgery is to correct existing mechanical derangements in order to restore valve function as close to normal as possible (Carpentier, 1983).

Mitral valve disease in adulthood is often attributable to rheumatic fever in childhood, although it also can result from coronary artery disease, infection, degenerative changes, trauma, tumors, congenital anomalies, or failure of a previously implanted prosthesis. It is thought that the initial injury to the valve is aggravated further by the higher pressures in the left side of the heart and greater mechanical trauma to the valve, particularly when it is closed, compared with the other valves of the heart.

An awareness of the cause is helpful to perioperative nurses because they can anticipate and prepare for adjunctive procedures and interventions. These may include culturing infected valve tissue, debriding calcified leaflets, repairing a septal defect created by excision of an atrial tumor, performing a valve replacement if it becomes apparent that valve repair cannot be achieved, or planning for concomitant coronary artery bypass grafting in patients with ischemic coronary heart disease.

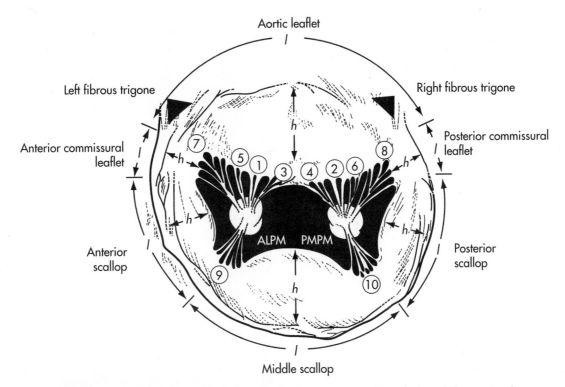

FIGURE 11-2 Surgeon's view of the mitral valve apparatus. Knowledge of the anatomic locations of the elements of the mitral apparatus facilitates precise valve repairs. *ALPM,* Anterolateral papillary muscle; *PMPM,* posteromedial papillary muscle; *hP,* height of a leaflet; *l,* length of the attachment of a leaflet; *1,* anterior main chorda; *2,* posterior main chorda; *3,* anterior paramedial chorda; *4,* posterior paramedial chorda; *5,* anterior paracommissural chorda; *6,* posterior paracommissural chorda; *7,* anterior paracommissural chorda; *8,* posterior commissural chorda; *9,* anterior cleft chorda; *10,* posterior cleft chorda. (From Sakai and others: Distance between mitral annulus and papillary muscles: anatomic study in normal human hearts, *J Thorac Cardiovasc Surg* 118[4]:235, 1999.)

MITRAL STENOSIS

Mitral stenosis occurs when deformities of the valve leaflets or other components of the apparatus produce narrowing of the mitral valve orifice and create an impedance to blood flow across the valve. These deformities produce turbulent blood flow, which can result in further injury to the valve itself (e.g., calcification) or promote the formation of thrombus. The most common causes of mitral stenosis include rheumatic fever, bacterial vegetations, and tumors.

Rheumatic fever

The most common cause of mitral stenosis remains rheumatic fever. Although it has become less common in the United States, new outbreaks continue to occur (Pezzella, Utley, and Salm, 1998). As one of the sequelae of beta-hemolytic streptococcal infection, rheumatic fever is a systemic immune process that can be self-limiting but may lead to progressive valvular deformity. Rheumatic fever may be associated with pericarditis and congestive heart failure; presenting signs include cardiomegaly and mitral or aortic murmurs.

The isolated mitral valve is affected in the majority of cases; aortic valve lesions are seen less commonly, and tricuspid valve involvement is usually seen only in association with mitral or aortic valve disease. The pulmonary valve is affected rarely.

When rheumatic carditis affects the mitral valve, the valve cusps become rigid and deformed; this is often accompanied by varying amounts of calcification. The commissures fuse, and the chordae tendineae thicken and shorten. The fixed stenotic orifice often is described as having a "fish mouth" appearance (Fig. 11-3). Mobilization of the valve leaflets by commissurotomy is often effective during the earlier stages of the rheumatic process, when there is some leaflet pliability and heavy calcification is absent.

Over years or decades the turbulence in blood flow produced by the fibrosis and calcification of the valve tissue causes further thickening of the leaflets and chordae tendineae. Leaflet motion is restricted and the valve

TABLE 11-1
Abnormalities of the Mitral Apparatus Producing Stenosis and Regurgitation

STENOSIS	REGURGITATION
Valve Leaflets	
Fibrosis	Retraction of cusps
Calcification (preventing leaflet opening)	Calcification (preventing leaflet closure)
Thickening	Perforation, tearing
Rigidity	Myxomatous degeneration
Commissural fusion	Congenital deformity (cleft leaflet)
Annulus	
Fibrosis	Dilation
Calcification (impinging on orifice)	Calcification (preventing annular contraction)
Chordae Tendineae	
Shortening	Elongation
Fusing	Rupture
	Shortening
	Fusing
Papillary Muscle	
Thickening	Rupture (head or body)
	Dysfunction (ischemia or infarction)
	Congenital malformation
Innerventricular Wall	
—	Dilation of left ventricle
	Hypokinetic left ventricle
	Cardiomyopathy

Modified from Braunwald E: Valvular heart disease. In Braunwald E, Zipes DP, Libby P, editors: *Heart disease: a textbook of cardiovascular medicine*, ed 6, Philadelphia, 2001, WB Saunders.

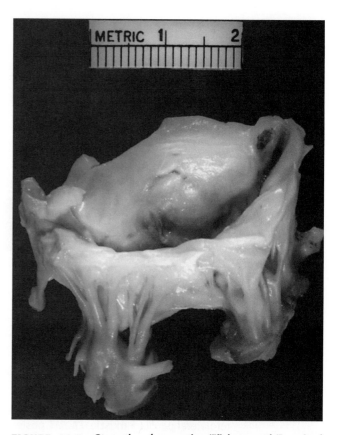

FIGURE 11-3 Stenotic, rheumatic ("fish mouth") mitral valve. Note the typical, smooth thickened leaflets and the shortened and fused chordae tendineae arising from the tips of the papillary muscles. (Photograph courtesy William C. Roberts, MD. Michael Spencer, photographer.)

orifice narrows, in severe cases to less than 1 cm². Valve replacement is usually necessary at this stage, particularly when the valve is heavily calcified.

Bacterial endocarditis

The infectious process of bacterial endocarditis attacks the valve leaflets and may extend to the perivalvular tissue (annulus, chordae tendineae, and papillary muscles). Often there are vegetations composed of bacterial colonies, fibrin, white blood cells, and red blood cells. When the destruction of the valve and adjacent tissue is severe, surgery is performed to remove infected tissue and to reconstruct the annulus so that a prosthetic valve can be anchored securely. Mitral insufficiency accompanies stenosis when endocarditis causes perforation of the leaflets.

Other causes

Left atrial thrombus or tumor, such as atrial myxoma, may obstruct left ventricular inflow. Degenerative processes may cause calcification of the leaflets and annulus.

PATHOPHYSIOLOGY OF MITRAL STENOSIS

The various physiologic derangements of mitral stenosis have similar clinical manifestations. The most significant effects are seen in the left atrium and the pulmonary vasculature. In severe cases the right ventricle may be affected (Fig. 11-4).

As the mitral and subvalvular orifices narrow, left atrial pressure increases to maintain normal flow across the valve, and a pressure gradient is created between the left atrium and ventricle throughout diastole. When increased left atrial pressure becomes sustained as a result of impedance to forward flow, the pulmonary vessels become congested, producing pulmonary edema. The patient may complain of dyspnea, especially when in the supine position or when the legs are elevated. Chronic pulmonary congestion leads to an increased volume and pressure load on the right side of the heart, which compensates by increasing the heart rate. The problem is exacerbated by exercise, which increases venous return to the right side of the heart in addition to causing tachycardia, shortening the period for diastolic

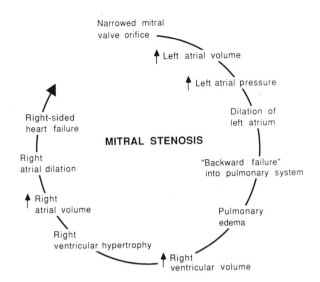

FIGURE 11-4 Pathophysiology of mitral stenosis. (From Kinney MR and others: *Comprehensive cardiac care,* ed 8, St Louis, 1996, Mosby.)

filling. This results in a reduced cardiac output and insufficient peripheral perfusion, which in turn produces dyspnea and fatigue.

With long-standing pulmonary venous hypertension, medial thickening and fibrosis of the pulmonary arterioles occurs and pulmonary artery pressures are increased, often to systemic levels. Because the right side of the heart must then work against nearly systemic pressures, the right ventricle enlarges, dilates, and eventually fails.

The majority of patients also develop transient or chronic atrial fibrillation as the left atrium dilates and enlarges in response to chronic atrial overloading. Because atrial fibrillation is not as effective as normal sinus rhythm in providing an adequate left ventricular preload, cardiac output is reduced. Another problem associated with atrial fibrillation is venous stasis, which increases the risk of thrombus formation and embolization. The 30% to 40% of patients who come to surgery with chronic atrial fibrillation often remain in atrial fibrillation after surgery (and require chronic anticoagulation). This has prompted some surgeons to perform a *Maze* procedure (see Chapter 17) in addition to the mitral valve repair. The Maze procedure ablates the atrial fibrillation conduction pathways to restore normal sinus rhythm. According to Handa and others (1999), other potential benefits include a reduction in stroke and anticoagulation-related bleeding.

Although pathologic changes in the left atrium, the lungs, and the right-sided heart chambers are typical, pure mitral stenosis (unlike mitral regurgitation) does not stress the left ventricle (LV) itself, yet impeded flow from the left atrium (LA) to the LV does limit the ventricle's preload. Thus the LV may be normal in config-

uration and not demonstrate hypertrophy or dilation. However, there may be more subtle changes in left ventricular function related to the reduction in LV filling volume (secondary to the mitral valve stenosis). Moreover, because the LV has not been stimulated to hypertrophy, when faced with an increased load (pressure or volume), LV contractility may be depressed (Jackson and Thomas, 1999).

MITRAL REGURGITATION

When valvular regurgitation exists, the heart must eject the regurgitant fraction of blood and its normal volume. Valvular and subvalvular abnormalities of the mitral apparatus (see Table 11-1) producing mitral regurgitation may have inflammatory, degenerative, infective, structural, or congenital causes (Braunwald, 2001).

Rheumatic fever remains a significant but less frequent cause. More common are mitral valve prolapse, fibroelastic degeneration, infective endocarditis, dilation of the annulus or the left ventricle, trauma, and coronary heart disease. Valve leaflets that have become thickened, noncompliant, and retracted as a result of the inflammatory process of rheumatic carditis may fail to coapt. These valves commonly display symptoms of both stenosis and regurgitation.

Mitral valve prolapse

Mitral valve prolapse (Box 11-1) is an increasingly recognized clinical syndrome known by various names: Barlow's syndrome, floppy valve syndrome, billowing mitral valve syndrome, and systolic click–murmur syndrome. It is common in women and in its milder form may not cause mitral regurgitation.

The multiple names given to the syndrome, the diverse causes, the nonspecific findings, and the lack of consistent definitions in the terminology occasionally create difficulty in describing the syndrome and planning

---

> ### BOX 11-1
> ## *Terms Associated with Mitral Valve Prolapse*
>
> **Billowing mitral valve:** ballooning or protruding of leaflet tissue into the left atrium; the valve edges coapt and regurgitation does not occur unless complicated by prolapse
> **Floppy mitral valve:** exaggerated billowing
> **Prolapse of the mitral valve:** billowing without leaflet coaptation; produces regurgitation
> **Flail mitral valve:** produced when chordae (or papillary muscle) rupture and the untethered leaflet is flung into the left atrium; produces acute regurgitation

Modified from Carpentier A: Cardiac valve surgery—the "French correction," *J Thorac Cardiovasc Surg* 86(3):323, 1983. Barlow JB: Idiopathic (degenerative) and rheumatic mitral valve prolapse: historical aspects and an overview, *J Heart Valve Dis* 1(2):163, 1992.

treatment. For surgeons the term *prolapse* refers to valve leaflets that do not coapt and by definition are incompetent (dysfunctional) when they prolapse into the left atrium. Prolapsed leaflets require repair (or replacement) to regain functional valve performance (Barlow, 1992; Carpentier, 1983).

Changes in the fibroelastic components of the valvular tissue, such as myxomatous proliferation (Fig. 11-5), produce thinning, elongation, and redundancy of valve leaflet tissue, which prolapses into the atrium during systole. Numerous mechanisms are thought to produce the syndrome, including hereditary disorders, thoracic deformities, coronary heart disease, and, most commonly, abnormal collagen metabolism and other connective tissue disorders that produce degenerative changes. Severe hemodynamic disturbances result from extensive calcification, elongation of the chordae, and asymmetric dilation of the annulus (Braunwald, 2001).

Other leaflet disorders

Valve leaflets may become perforated or chordae may rupture as a result of infective endocarditis or trauma, producing sudden regurgitation that requires emergency surgery. Rarely, congenital clefts, organized thrombus, or tumors prevent secure leaflet closure. Previously implanted bioprostheses may degenerate, causing tears or perforations of the leaflets and producing regurgitation (Fig. 11-6).

Chordal dysfunction

Ruptured chordae tendineae to a prolapsed posterior mitral leaflet are the most common entity seen in mitral valve reparative surgery (Cohn, 1998). When attacked by bacterial endocarditis, they may rupture, resulting in sudden prolapse of the untethered leaflet. Chordal rupture also may result from trauma or acute ventricular dilation. Chordae tendineae affected by rheumatic disease restrict leaflet closure when they are shortened and fused.

Annular dilation

Another abnormality of the mitral valve annulus is primary dilation of the annulus. Annular dilation also may be produced secondary to the dilation of the left ventricle surrounding the annulus, which normally constricts during left ventricular contraction. In the elderly, severe idiopathic calcification of the annulus may be a common cause of regurgitation and may be accelerated by systemic hypertension, aortic stenosis, diabetes, chronic renal failure, and fibrous skeletal diseases (Braunwald, 2001).

Papillary muscle dysfunction

Papillary muscle dysfunction secondary to coronary artery disease is an increasingly common cause of mitral regurgitation. Papillary muscles are especially vulnerable to ischemia because of their terminal position in the coronary vascular bed. In severe cases papillary muscle necrosis and rupture create acute, severe regurgitation. Trauma to the muscles is a less common but important cause of regurgitation.

Left ventricular aneurysm and left ventricular dilation occurring with increased volume loads or cardiomyopathy alter the ventricular geometry. Stretching of the chordae and the papillary muscles prevents leaflet coaptation.

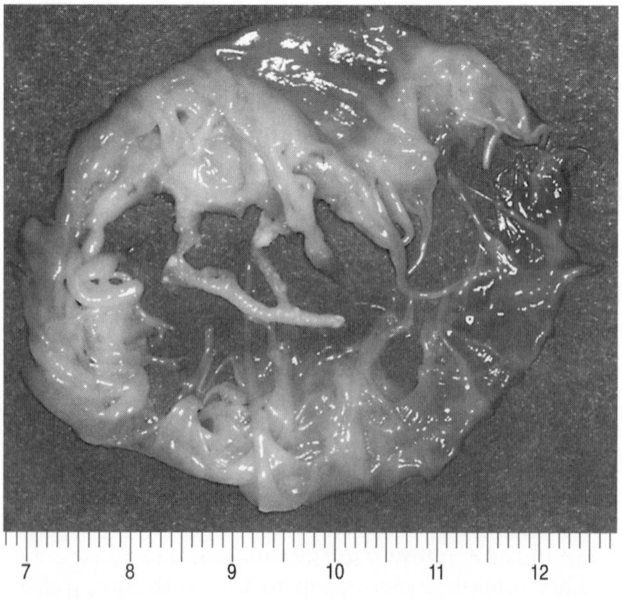

FIGURE 11-5 Myxomatous mitral valve producing regurgitation. The degenerative process causes the leaflets to become thinned and elongated. (Courtesy Edward A. Lefrak, MD.)

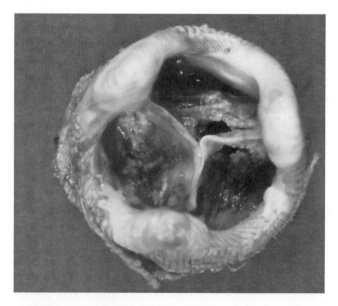

FIGURE 11-6 Explanted porcine mitral valve prosthesis; note the tears and calcification of the leaflet tissue. (Courtesy Edward A. Lefrak, MD.)

PATHOPHYSIOLOGY OF MITRAL REGURGITATION

An incompetent valve is incapable of preventing the backflow of blood into the left atrium during ventricular systole. Left atrial pressure rises from the additional regurgitant volume; the left atrial chamber dilates and may then hypertrophy to overcome the additional volume (Fig. 11-7). Enlargement of the left atrium is not necessarily proportional to the degree of regurgitation, however, and only a slight increase in size may be seen in patients with significant disease, whereas a giant left atrium may be present in others with less severe disease. Pulmonary vascular changes appear later in the course of the disease process as compared with the changes seen in mitral stenosis, depending on the ability of the atrium to dilate and adjust to gradual increases in volume over time. When mitral regurgitation occurs suddenly (e.g., rupture of a papillary muscle), the heart is unable to compensate for the acutely increased volume load presented to it, and heart failure ensures rapidly. Acute regurgitation requires immediate surgical treatment.

When the ventricle contracts, more than 50% of its volume can be preferentially ejected into the left atrium, thereby significantly reducing the amount of blood entering the aorta. As the amount of regurgitation increases and the volume overload becomes progressively greater, the left ventricle attempts to maintain an adequate cardiac output by the compensatory mechanisms of an increased heart rate, hypertrophy, and dilation (Jackson and Thomas, 1999).

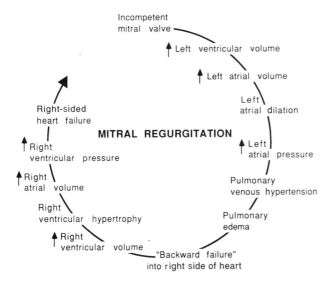

FIGURE 11-7 Pathophysiology of mitral regurgitation. (From Kinney MR and others: *Comprehensive cardiac care,* ed 8, St Louis, 1996, Mosby.)

Diagnostic Evaluation of Mitral Valve Disease

Chronic valvular stenosis and regurgitation develop gradually but often are first detectable by a murmur after about 10 years (Table 11-2). The electrocardiogram commonly shows abnormalities of the left atrium, including atrial fibrillation. The chest roentgenogram often demonstrates an enlarged left atrium and, in advanced states, pulmonary artery and right ventricular enlargement; occasionally calcium is seen on the mitral valve.

Preoperative diagnostic ultrasound methods with two-dimensional echocardiography, Doppler echocardiography, and color flow imaging provide detailed anatomic and functional information about the cardiac valves. Chest wall deformities or marked obesity may impede the penetration of ultrasound waves, necessitating cardiac catheterization and angiography. Transesophogeal echocardiography (TEE) and Doppler color flow imaging often are employed during the intraoperative period to provide immediate structural and functional assessment of valvular function after repair or replacement (Figs. 11-8 and 11-9).

In patients with concomitant coronary artery disease requiring myocardial revascularization, selective coronary arteriography remains the most accurate method for delineating the coronary arterial anatomy and the location of obstructive lesions. Coronary angiography also may be done to evaluate pulmonary hypertension, mitral insufficiency, aortic valve disease, and left ventricular function.

Surgery for Mitral Valve Disease

Surgical options, particularly for mitral regurgitation, have increased dramatically since the 1960s when only commissurotomy and prosthetic replacement were technically feasible. Perioperative nurses, including registered nurse first assistants (RNFAs; Box 11-2) can actively participate in the development and implementation of these procedures.

Carpentier and his colleagues (1971, 1983) are credited with many of the technical advancements associated with mitral valve repair and bioprosthetic replacement. Their description and categorization of the anatomic changes that occur with mitral (and tricuspid) insufficiency and the clinical application of their research findings have led to a number of improvements. These include the creation of the annuloplasty ring to correct annular dilation (see Chapter 3) and the development of an array of procedures to repair not only the annulus but also the leaflets, the chordae tendineae, and the papillary muscles. Carpentier also introduced the glutaraldehyde-treated

---

TABLE 11-2

Signs, Symptoms, and Findings of Mitral Valve Disease

MITRAL STENOSIS	MITRAL REGURGITATION
Signs	
Atrial fibrillation	**CHRONIC**
Low-pitched, rumbling diastolic murmur	Atrial fibrillation
Opening snap (unless leaflets are immobile)	High-pitched, blowing systolic murmur
Hepatomegaly, ascites	Atrial pulsation at third left intercostal space
Jugular venous distension	Jugular venous distension
Peripheral edema	Hepatomegaly
	Point of maximal impulse downward and to left
	ACUTE
	Signs of infective endocarditis
	Sinus tachycardia
	High-pitched, blowing systolic murmur at apex
Symptoms	
Dyspnea	**CHRONIC**
Orthopnea	Fatigue, exhaustion
Paroxysmal nocturnal dyspnea	Palpitations
Hemoptysis	Atypical chest pain
Hoarseness	Dysphagia
	ACUTE
	Pulmonary edema
Chest X-Ray Film	
Large LA indenting esophagus	Enlarged LA and LV
Large RV and PA with pulmonary hypertension	
Calcification (occasionally)	
Echocardiography	
Restricted valve movement	Prolapsed, flail leaflet
Thickened, immobile annulus and leaflets	Enlarged LV
LA enlargement	Vegetations on leaflets
Subvalvular fibrosis	Regurgitant flow mapped (color Doppler)
Prolonged flow across valve	
Cardiac Catheterization	
Confirms valve lesion	Confirms valve lesion
Assesses LV function	Assesses degree of regurgitation, LV function, PA pressures
Detects coronary artery disease	Detects coronary artery disease
Measures valve orifice, pressure gradient	

Modified from Braunwald E: Valvular heart disease. In Braunwald E, Zipes DP, Libby P, editors: *Heart disease: a textbook of cardiovascular medicine,* ed 6, Philadelphia, 2001, WB Saunders. Jackson JM, Thomas SJ: Valvular heart disease. In Kaplan JA, editor: *Cardiac anesthesia,* ed 4, Philadelphia, 1999, WB Saunders.

porcine heterograft in 1969, thereby expanding the number and type of valvular prostheses (Westaby, 1997).

At present, patients can benefit from a variety of possible interventions. Decisions regarding the timing and selection of the procedure (repair or replacement) are determined on an individual basis and are influenced by the lesion and associated cardiac anatomy, the age of the patient, the medical history, and the patient's lifestyle. Heavily calcified and deformed valves may not be amenable to repair; bulky valves may ob-

struct blood flow in a small ventricle. Ideally, if a prosthetic valve is inserted, it should last the expected lifetime of the patient without degeneration or significant complications.

The medical history provides information about the status of the left ventricle (functional class), previous surgery, thromboembolic episodes, atrial fibrillation, and disease processes (e.g., hepatic disease, gastric ulcers, and coagulopathies) that could contraindicate the use of valve prostheses requiring continuous anticoagulation. Aspects of the patient's lifestyle influencing the

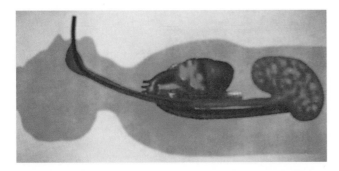

FIGURE 11-8 Diagram of transesophogeal echocardiography probe in position, demonstrating the orientation of the TEE probe and the esophagus, heart, lungs, diaphragm, and stomach. The close proximity between the probe tip and the structures of the heart facilitates intraoperative assessment of cardiac function. (Courtesy Hewlett-Packard Co.)

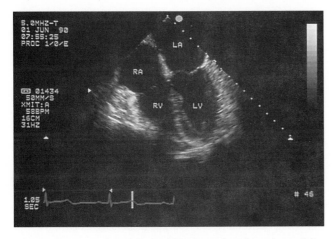

FIGURE 11-9 Echocardiographic four-chamber view of the heart. In addition to evaluating ventricular and valvular function, TEE also is useful to detect air in the chambers and within the trabeculations of the ventricle. Air bubbles appear as light specks. (Courtesy Hewlett-Packard Co.)

selection of a prosthesis include the ability and desire to comply with prescribed medication regimens. In addition, the prosthetic orifice should be large enough to accommodate a stroke volume commensurate with the activity level and size of the patient.

Increasingly patients are considered for surgery before symptoms become severe and permanent myocardial damage develops. Surgery for patients with symptomatic mitral insufficiency often is indicated earlier after onset of symptoms compared with patients with mitral stenosis because of the greater risk to left ventricular function seen in insufficiency. Surgery becomes necessary when left ventricular function deteriorates to a point that activities of daily living are curtailed.

BOX 11-2

Registered Nurse First Assistant Considerations for Mitral Valve Surgery

- Keep sutures from tangling: use suture holder or tag with small clamps and arrange in orderly fashion around operative site, or tag and hold each stitch
- Keep running count of stitches in each leaflet (or annular segment) and total count
- Be alert to calcium particles, thrombus, pieces of resected chordae, or other debris that could be retained and subsequently embolize; notify surgeon and remove from field
- Use open-tip suction to remove calcium pieces and other large pieces of debris
- Keep bioprostheses moist with frequent saline irrigation (with bulb syringe); prevent drying of prosthesis
- Monitor instruments and wipe clean of debris with moist sponge
- Assist in keeping suture pledgets from twisting
- Hold prosthesis (annuloplasty ring or valve) securely with handle (or manually); do not twist prosthetic rings
- Avoid excess pressure on tissue when using handheld retractors
- Avoid aggressive manipulation of rigid suction tip or venting catheter (may tear endocardial ventricular wall)
- If heart must be elevated to inspect suture lines and anastomoses, do so cautiously to avoid puncturing ventricle with prosthetic struts
- Avoid having prosthesis handle or other long instruments touch surgeon's head when surgeon is leaning over the field to see the operative site
- Avoid damage to prosthetic valves from instruments and other sharp objects
- Monitor venous drainage, especially if percutaneous femoral cannula is used
- During closure of parasternal incision, be alert for possible lung herniation; alert surgeon

---

MITRAL VALVE REPAIR

Reparative procedures that preserve the native valve are popular because the complications associated with prosthetic replacement and anticoagulation can be avoided. The availability of reparative techniques, their lower rate of complications compared with valve replacement, and the improved results seen with preservation of the native valve have made mitral valve repair especially attractive.

Procedures to reconstruct incompetent valves may not always be curative. Reoperation may be required in patients who have undergone initial commissurotomy at a younger age if commissural fusion recurs. Biologic or synthetic material used in the repair of the valve may degenerate, and patients should be informed of this possibility when their informed consent for surgery is granted. In addition, reparative procedures often require more time (and additional training) than a standard valve replacement. These considerations necessitate excellent myocardial protection (Kirklin and Barratt-Boyes, 1993).

Patient teaching considerations

Patient teaching considerations focus on the disease and the surgical intervention and their effects on the patient's ability to adapt physiologically and psychologically. Including the family in the teaching process reinforces patient learning, enhances postoperative compliance with prescribed therapy, and provides a supportive social structure. Patient teaching focuses on the disease, its causes, anticipated treatment, associated complications, and information about the postoperative course. The patient should be aware of the possibility of valve replacement and be prepared accordingly.

The use of reparative techniques generally obviates the need for long-term anticoagulation (unless the patient has a history of chronic atrial fibrillation). This is significant in children, women of childbearing age, and patients with bleeding tendencies, for whom anticoagulation poses increased risk of hemorrhagic complications. Patients who do receive anticoagulant medications postoperatively need to be aware of reportable signs and symptoms of bleeding, such as pink urine, black stools, excessive nose bleeds, unusual vaginal or anal bleeding, purple or red skin discoloration, and bleeding gums (Ansell, Hirsh, and Wenger, 1999; Box 11-3).

Prevention of infective endocarditis is another important teaching areas. Patients benefit from understanding the importance of antibiotic prophylaxis and the need to inform dentists and physicians about their history of valve disease and its medical and surgical treatment.

Procedural considerations

The terms *annuloplasty* and *valvuloplasty* often are used to categorize the type of repair. The former designates procedures performed on the valve annulus; valvuloplasty is a broad category that refers to reconstruction of the leaflets, chordae, or papillary muscles. Very selective repairs such as chordal replacement fall under this category.

Because the technique selected must be tailored to the unique pathophysiologic findings, a careful evaluation of the leaflets and the subvalvular mechanism is performed before deciding which technique to employ. If damage to the valve is more extensive than anticipated, valve replacement may become necessary. Consequently the nurse should be ready with instruments, prostheses, and related supplies to excise the valve and implant a mechanical or biologic prosthesis.

In preparation for surgery, mitral valve instruments (Box 11-4) are added to the basic setup. Standard vein retractors may be used, or special self-retaining retrac-

---

BOX 11-3
Warfarin (Coumadin) Anticoagulation Therapy

Indications
Thromboembolic complications associated with:
- Atrial fibrillation
- Cardiac valve replacement (especially mechanical prostheses)

Prevention and treatment of cardiac embolism

Major Adverse Effects
Hemorrhage, risk of bleeding; related to:
- Intensity of anticoagulation
- Concomitant clinical disorders (e.g., cerebral aneurysm, impaired clotting)
- Concomitant use of other medications
- Quality of management

Special Considerations in Elderly Patients
Increased risk of bleeding related to:
- Increased sensitivity to usual doses
- Comorbidity
- Increased drug interactions

Low initial doses of warfarin recommended for elderly (and for frail, liver-diseased, or malnourished) patients

Clinical Testing for Warfarin Therapy
PROTHROMBIN TIME (PT)
- Historically most relied on; range of 1.5 to 2 times normal clotting time
- Variety of thromboplastin reagents used to measure PT
- Laboratory results are variable
- Affected by diet, liver disease, gut absorption
- High percentage of PT outside therapeutic range

INTERNATIONAL NORMALIZED RATIO (INR)
- Currently the standard method for reporting PT; range of 2 to 3.5
- Calculated from the PT, taking into account reagent used to measure PT
- Allows comparison of results between laboratories
- Recommended values individualized according to clinical factors and type and position of prosthesis
- Indication for mechanical prosthetic heart valve: INR range of 2.5 to 3.5 (target 3.0)
- Monitor INR every 1 to 4 weeks and adjust as necessary
- Efficacy of warfarin diminishes rapidly below INR of 2; no efficacy below INR of 1.5
- Safety compromised (e.g., risk of severe bleeding) above INR of 4
- Calculation: $INR = \left(\dfrac{\text{patient's PT in seconds}}{\text{mean normal PT in seconds}} \right) ISI$

Modified from Ansell J, Hirsh J, Wenger NK: Management or oral anticoagulant therapy, 1999, American Heart Association [On-line]. Available: http://www.americanheart.org/Scientific/slideset/oat/index/html (accessed 4/19/01); Finkelmeier BA: *Cardiothoracic surgical nursing,* ed 2, Philadelphia, 2000, JB Lippincott.
ISI, International sensitivity index.

BOX 11-4
Special Considerations for Mitral Valve Surgery

Instrumentation

Self-retaining mitral valve retractor with changeable blades
Handheld mitral valve retractors
Small dental mirror (to assess subvalvular structures)
Mitral valve hook
Longer scissors, forceps, needle holders, and other instruments
Long, angled Babcock clamp to grasp valve leaflets for retraction
Double-action long lamps for transthoracic approach
Video-assisted and robotic instruments, when indicated

Valve Prostheses and Accessories

Annuloplasty rings
Mechanical heart valves
Bioprostheses (porcine or bovine pericardium)
Sizers (obturators), range of sizes, specific to prosthesis
Sizer (obturator) handles
Prosthetic valve holders and handles (some prostheses are packaged with an attached holder); the sterile nurse applies the handle into the holder

Supplies

Valve suture, single and multipack (multicolored)
Pledgeted
Nonpledgeted
Suture organizer (if used)
French-eye needles (to adjust suture after needle has been removed)
Free pledgets, precut or cut to size
18G, 19G needle to deair ventricle
Long (spinal) 18G needle for transseptal deairing of ventricle
Additional basins for bioprosthetic saline rinse (3), antibiotic solutions, or glutaraldehyde preparation of autologous pericardium
Culture tubes (for valve tissue, suture, rinse solutions)
Small urinary catheter for transvalvular insertion to allow air to escape
Venting lines for deairing left ventricle
Separate venous cannula for inferior and superior vena cava (or femoral venous drainage cannula)
Umbilical tapes and tourniquets to isolate cavae
ECG cables for cardioversion (patients with atrial fibrillation)

Positioning

Supine
If coronary bypass grafts to be performed, position as for removal of leg vein (see Chapter 10)

Skin Preparation

Shave midline chest, inner aspect of both legs
Wash anterior chest (side to side) and legs at least to knees

Draping

Anterior chest exposed; include right parasternal area if this incision used
Legs exposed from groin to knees (can be covered with a towel if access is not required)
Place anesthesia screen over lower legs to keep drapes off feet

Special Infection Control Measures

Confine and contain tissue and instruments from infected tissue
Culture valve tissue, rinse solutions, and other items as requested by surgeon
Place mechanical prostheses in antibiotic solution before insertion as requested by surgeon
Keep instruments free of debris
Document lot and serial numbers of all implants

Special Safety Measures

Label syringes and containers of solutions, medications, such as
• Antibiotic solution
• Heparinized saline
• Glutaraldehyde
Account for all sizers, handles, and holders used to size and insert a prosthesis; pledget material, suture needles, hypodermic needles, retractor parts
Monitor presence of ventricular failure and possible need for mechanical ventricular support (intraaortic balloon or ventricular assist device)
Keep prostheses stored in a cool, dry, contamination-free location
Have at least two of each size valve available
Follow institutional policy/procedure for complying with Safe Medical Devices Act

Documentation/Report to Cardiac Surgical Intensive Care Unit (in Addition to Standard Documentation/Postoperative Report)

Procedure: repair or replacement, type of prosthesis
Serial and lot numbers of prostheses
Preoperative diagnosis (stenosis, regurgitation, or both; onset)
Epicardial pacemaker lead placement (single, dual) and if being paced
History of atrial fibrillation
Patient problems, concerns related to valvular heart disease, surgery
Preoperative left ventricular function (e.g., ejection fraction)
Completion of valve implant card (also send copy to manufacturer)

---

tors designed for exposure of the mitral valve may be employed (see Chapter 3). Because the decision regarding the most appropriate reparative technique is made only after careful inspection, nurses should have available a variety of sutures and prosthetic materials.

Some surgeons may use autologous pericardium treated with glutaraldehyde solution to patch or repair leaflets. Discussing possible surgical options preoperatively guides the nurse and helps to avoid delay once a definitive repair is selected.

TABLE 11-3
Standards of Nursing Care for Mitral Valve Surgery

NURSING DIAGNOSIS	PATIENT OUTCOME	NURSING ACTIONS
Anxiety related to disease, surgery, and postoperative events	Patient demonstrates acceptable level of anxiety and is able to cooperate with therapeutic regimen	Elicit questions and concerns about disease and proposed treatment Identify and reinforce effective coping mechanisms; respect some denial Provide comfort measures; identify perceived needs and expectations
Knowledge deficit related to inadequate knowledge of planned surgery and perioperative events	Patient demonstrates knowledge of physiologic and psychologic responses to mitral valve surgery	Determine patient's understanding of mitral valve disease; possible surgical interventions (annuloplasty, valvuloplasty, commissurotomy, valve replacement); types, benefits, and risks of prostheses; and preferences if any Determine patient's understanding of surgical procedure; describe (briefly) immediate preoperative events (while patient is awake); reinforce or clarify what patient (and family) has been told by surgeon; elicit expected outcome of surgery Assess patient's lifestyle (exercise limits, geographic location, proximity to laboratory facilities, community resources, support groups); note age and, if female, ability or desire to have children If additional myocardial revascularization procedures are to be performed (coronary artery bypass grafts), assess patient's understanding and clarify as necessary Assess patient's ability to comply with possible anticoagulation regimen Assess family support mechanism
Risk for infection related to surgery	Patient is free of infection related to aseptic technique	Culture excised valve and suture as requested Confine and contain instruments and supplies used to excise infected valve tissue Place mechanical prosthesis in antibiotic solution before implantation as requested by surgeon Keep instruments free of debris Document lot and serial numbers of implants
Risk for impaired skin integrity	Patient's skin integrity is maintained	In severely thin and malnourished patients (cardiac cachexia), use additional padding to protect skin, joints, and bony prominences
Risk for injury related to use of valve retractor	Patient is free of injury from use of retraction devices	Use handheld valve retractors with caution to avoid injury to perivalvular tissue (e.g., conduction tissue)
Risk for injury related to: Retained foreign objects	Patient is free of injury related to: Retained foreign objects	Account for valve sizers, holders, and handles, and other items Keep instruments free of tissue, suture, and calcium debris
Chemical hazards	Chemical hazards	Label syringes containing antibiotic solutions, heparinized saline, or other solutions; use only physiologically compatible solutions to rinse bioprosthetic valve; do not place bioprosthesis in antibiotic solution; follow

ECG, Electrocardiogram.
Modified from Seifert PC: Cardiac surgery. In Rothrock JC: *Perioperative nursing care planning,* ed 2, St Louis, 1996, Mosby.

Continued

Patient care standards for mitral valve surgery (Table 11-3) include skin preparation on the supine patient from chin to knees. Access to the femoral artery should be retained in the event that arterial pressure monitoring lines or an intraaortic balloon must be inserted or if a segment of saphenous vein is needed for revascularization.

Patients receiving oral (warfarin [Coumadin]) anticoagulation medications preoperatively will have them discontinued. Patients often are switched to heparin before surgery because heparin can be given intravenously, acts more rapidly, and has a shorter half-life than warfarin. Heparin is the anticoagulant of choice during cardiopulmonary bypass because it can be reversed quickly with its antagonist, protamine sulfate (Ansell, Hirsh, and Wenger, 1999).

The choice of incisions has expanded with the growth of minimally invasive techniques (and has raised issues such the importance of cosmetic results, the learning curve, and the ability to achieve an optimal repair). Most of the newer approaches employ some form of sternotomy or thoracotomy. For mitral valve procedures a median sternotomy (or ministernotomy), right parasternal incision, or limited (e.g., submammary) thoracotomy have been used. Carpentier, Loulmet, and their colleagues (Loulmet and others, 1998); Cooley (2000); and

TABLE 11-3
Standards of Nursing Care for Mitral Valve Surgery—cont'd

NURSING DIAGNOSIS	PATIENT OUTCOME	NURSING ACTIONS
Chemical hazards—cont'd	Chemical hazards—cont'd	protocol for removing glutaraldehyde from bioprostheses (rinsing in three baths of saline for at least 2 minutes each); keep bioprostheses moist with saline during implantation
Physical hazards	Physical hazards	Have available type and sizes of valvular prostheses desired by surgeon; store valves in cool, dry location; have appropriate accessories to size and insert valve; have necessary suture available (pledgeted, nonpledgeted, multicolored); be prepared with needles and venting catheters to deair left ventricle
Electrical hazards	Electrical hazards	Have appropriate ECG cables and confirm defibrillator setting with surgeon if cardioversion is planned for patients with atrial fibrillation
Thermal injury	Thermal injury	Avoid pouring ice chips directly on phrenic nerve (in lateral pericardium)

Risk for self-care deficit related to inadequate knowledge of rehabilitation period	Patient demonstrates knowledge of rehabilitation period as it relates to self-care abilities	Assess patient's knowledge of signs/symptoms of valve failure
		Assess patient's understanding of medications prescribed; signs/symptoms of anticoagulation-related hemorrhage, thrombosis, emboli; need for antibiotic prophylaxis before invasive procedures; need for follow-up laboratory work (prothrombin time)
		Identify signs/symptoms of anticoagulation-related hemorrhage (notify physician):
		  Nosebleeds, bleeding gums
		  Red or brown urine
		  Red or black bowel movements
		  Bleeding from cuts that cannot be stopped, bruises that get larger
		  Severe and persistent headaches
		  Abdominal pain
		  Faintness, dizziness, or unusual weakness
		  Excessive menstrual flow
		Identify signs/symptoms of suboptimal anticoagulation (notify physician):
		  Stroke, transient ischemic attacks
		  Closing sound of prosthesis no longer audible; absent "click"
		  Sudden-onset congestive heart failure
		List precautions for patients on anticoagulants:
		  Use a soft-bristled toothbrush
		  Use electric shavers rather than razors
		  Wear gloves when gardening
		  Do not go barefoot
		  Trim nails with a soft emery board instead of scissors or clippers
		  Avoid sports in which skin may be broken or internal injuries may occur
		Provide patient with name of person to contact if questions/problems arise
		Wear medical alert bracelet

Cosgrove and his associates (Gillinov and Cosgrove, 1999; Gillinov, Casselman, and Cosgrove, 2000) have described their selection of ministernotomy (over thoracotomy) as the minimally invasive incision of choice (although these authors all note that the ministernotomy—versus full sternotomy—approach to the mitral valve can be challenging). Reasons cited for ministernotomy include less pain, preservation of the (right) internal mammary artery, prevention of damage to the intercostal nerve, improved exposure of the cardiac chambers, minimal likelihood of lung herniation on chest closure, and less risk of chest wall instability. Another advantage is that standard instruments can be used. Others (Byrne and others, 1999; Cohn, 1998) have used the parasternal approach with few complications. It should be noted that smaller incisions make standard defibrillation with internal paddles (even with pediatric-size paddles) difficult; the preoperative application of external defibrillation pads is recommended.

The choice of cardiopulmonary bypass (CPB) techniques has similarly expanded. In addition to the standard methods of right atrial-aortic ("central") cannulation and femoral vein–femoral artery CPB (with superior vena cava cannulation), a combination of ascending aortic cannulation with percutaneous femoral venous drainage (with vacuum assistance) has demonstrated some advantages (Loulmet and others, 1998). There are also port-access techniques (with video assistance and robotics) that use percutaneous CPB systems (Chitwood, 1999; Reichenspurner, Boehm, and Reichart, 1999; Vanermen and others, 1999). Standard cannulation for CPB requires no additional special cardiac instrumentation, which is required for port-access procedures.

TEE with color flow Doppler is performed to establish a baseline for later comparison, to test repairs, and to monitor for residual intracardiac air.

Operative procedures
Incision, cannulation, and closure techniques (Cohn, 1998)

Median sternotomy and standard cardiopulmonary bypass

1. After sternotomy, both the inferior vena cava (IVC) and superior vena cava (SVC) are cannulated to completely decompress the right side of the atrium and facilitate exposure of the left atrium (Fig. 11-10). Antegrade and retrograde cardioplegia are used to arrest the heart. If there is aortic insufficiency, retrograde cardioplegia through the coronary sinus is mandatory for myocardial protection.
2. Exposure of the mitral valve (Fig. 11-11, *A*) is achieved by incising the interatrial groove along the left atrial side. A self-retaining retractor is inserted (Fig. 11-11, *B*), and the reparative procedure is performed.
3. On completion of the surgical repair, the repair is tested for residual regurgitation (usually with a bulb syringe of saline squirted into the LV to assess the amount of regurgitating fluid). The left atrium is

closed with a continuous cardiovascular suture technique. Two sutures are commonly used; one suture is started at one end of the atrial incision, and the second suture is started at the other end. The sutures are left untied where they join until deairing has been completed. The left atrium is allowed to fill with blood, the aortic cross-clamp is removed, and air is actively dislodged (e.g., by jiggling the heart or rotating the OR bed). The sutures are then tied. TEE is employed to look for air (see Fig. 11-9), to evaluate residual valvular insufficiency, and to confirm the effectiveness of the repair.

4. Temporary pacing wires are attached to the ventricle.
5. The heart returns to regular rhythm spontaneously or with defibrillation, and the patient is weaned from CPB.
6. Chest tubes are inserted, the sternum is reapproximated with wires, and the subcutaneous layers and skin are closed.

Parasternal incision

1. Minimally invasive parasternal incision is used (Fig. 11-12, *A*).
2. Cannulation of the femoral vein and artery (Fig. 11-12, *B*) is performed through an incision placed parallel to the groin crease.
3. A small portion of the third and fourth costal cartilage is resected (Fig. 11-13, *A*).
4. A modification of the CPB technique uses an SVC cannula, a flexible wire-reinforced transaortic cannula inserted through a stab wound in the skin and inserted into the aortic arch, and a percutaneous transfemoral IVC cannula (Fig. 11-13, *B*). A smaller

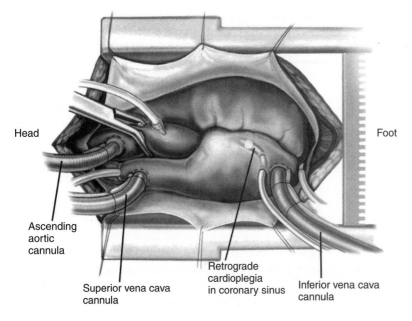

Head

Ascending aortic cannula

Superior vena cava cannula

Retrograde cardioplegia in coronary sinus

Inferior vena cava cannula

Foot

FIGURE 11-10 Standard incision for median sternotomy with bicaval cannulation for venous drainage and ascending aortic cannula for arterial inflow. (From Cohn LH: Mitral valve repair, *Oper Techn Thorac Cardiovasc Surg* 3[2]:109, 1998.)

femoral venous cannula can be used when vacuum/suction is added to assist venous drainage.

5. The right atrium is incised to expose the atrial septum (Fig. 11-14). The septum is incised in the area of the fossa ovalis, exposing the mitral valve (Fig. 11-15). Retraction sutures are placed in the atrial and septal walls to enhance exposure of the valve.

6. The atrial septum is closed with a running suture (Fig. 11-16, *A*); the right atrium is similarly closed

(Fig. 11-16, *B*). The parasternal incision edges are reapproximated as closely as possible over the small area of intercostal cartilage that has been removed; the pectoral fascia is closed tightly over this area to prevent lung herniation.

7. The repair is performed and the procedure completed as described previously.

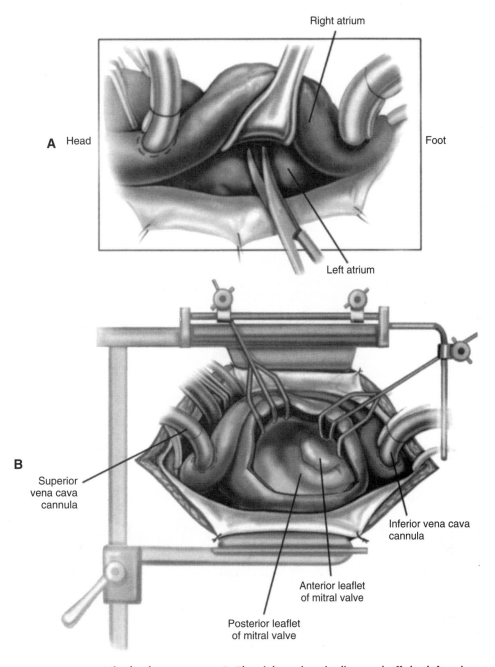

FIGURE 11-11 Mitral valve exposure. **A,** The right atrium is dissected off the left atrium before incising the interatrial groove to expose the mitral valve **(B).** (From Cohn LH: Mitral valve repair, *Oper Techn Thorac Cardiovasc Surg* 3[2]:109, 1998.)

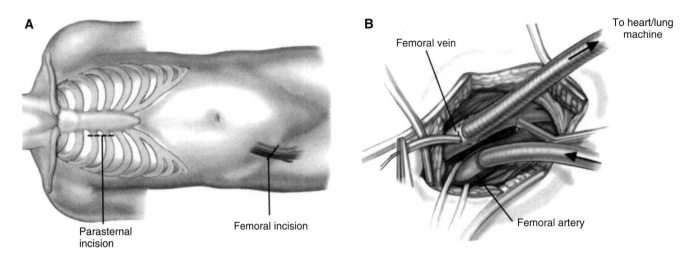

A

Parasternal
incision

Femoral incision

B

Femoral vein

To heart/lung
machine

Femoral artery

FIGURE 11-12 **A,** Right parasternal incision with resection of a small portion of the third and fourth costal cartilage. Groin cannulation may be used for CPB. (From Cohn LH: Mitral valve repair, *Oper Techn Thorac Cardiovasc Surg* 3[2]:109, 1998.)

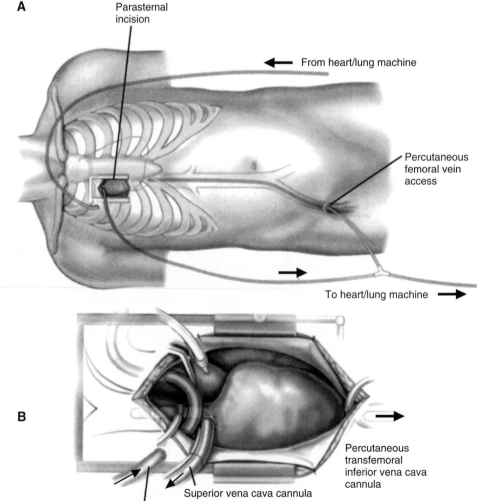

A

Parasternal
incision

From heart/lung machine

Percutaneous
femoral vein
access

To heart/lung machine

B

Aortic
cannula in
stab incision

Superior vena cava cannula

Percutaneous
transfemoral
inferior vena
cava
cannula

FIGURE 11-13 **A,** Parasternal incision with percutaneous femoral venous drainage. **B,** A second venous cannula is placed in the SVC to drain the upper body, and an aortic cannula is inserted through a stab wound in the right side of the chest. (From Cohn LH: Mitral valve repair, *Oper Techn Thorac Cardiovasc Surg* 3[2]:109, 1998.)

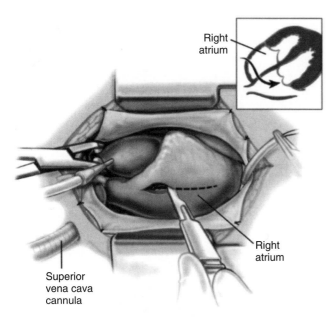

FIGURE 11-14 Right atrial incision. (From Cohn LH: Mitral valve repair, *Oper Techn Thorac Cardiovasc Surg* 3[2]:109, 1998.)

Mitral commissurotomy for mitral stenosis.
Closed mitral commissurotomy was the first effective surgical technique for treating valvular heart disease. The operation is now performed less often because of the drawbacks associated with the procedure—most importantly, lack of direct visualization and inadequate access to all cardiac structures. For example, in patients with severe mitral valve disease, the tricuspid valve may be affected. Adequate repair of the tricuspid valve cannot be performed with a closed mitral commissurotomy.

Although there are disadvantages to the closed technique, it is of great value in less technologically advanced countries where open procedures may not be feasible (Waldhausen and others, 1996). Closed commissurotomy generally is performed with a Tubbs dilator, which mechanically dilates the commissures and enlarges the valve orifice (Fig. 11-17).

Open mitral commissurotomy, first performed in 1956 by Lillehei (1958), is the separation of fused, adherent leaflets (Fig. 11-18) under direct vision. It is effective in patients without serious mitral regurgitation, left atrial thrombus, calcification, or severe

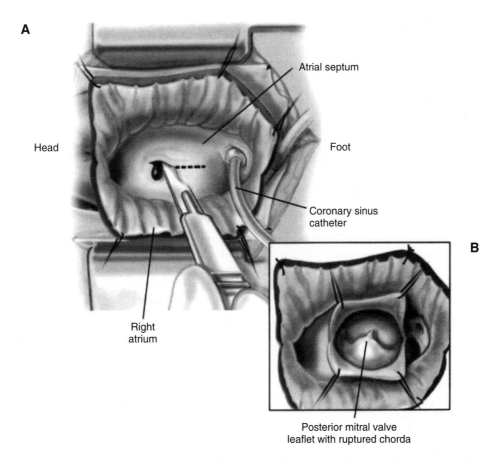

FIGURE 11-15 **A,** To gain access to the mitral valve, the atrial septum is incised. **B,** The exposed mitral valve. (From Cohn LH: Mitral valve repair, *Oper Techn Thorac Cardiovasc Surg* 3[2]:109, 1998.)

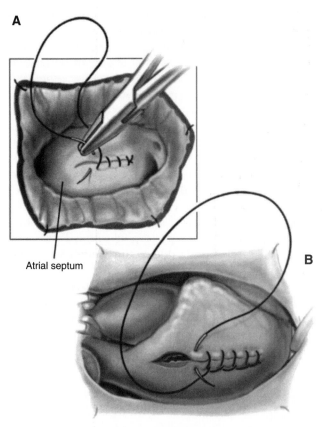

FIGURE 11-16 **A,** Closure of the atrial septum is performed with a running suture. **B,** Right atrial closure. (From Cohn LH: Mitral valve repair, *Oper Techn Thorac Cardiovasc Surg* 3[2]:109, 1998.)

chordal fusion and shortening. Operative results are best if the procedure is performed before the onset of chronic atrial fibrillation or heart failure (Braunwald, 2001).

Procedural considerations. Depending on surgeon preference, the patient is positioned for sternotomy, parasternotomy, or in some cases submammary thoracotomy. Mitral valve instruments are added to the basic sternotomy setup, including instruments and supplies not only for valve repair but also valve replacement, should this be necessary (see Box 11-4).

Procedure

1. After the incision of choice and exposure of the right atrium, the surgeon may place a finger through the right atriotomy before cannulation for bypass to determine whether functional tricuspid valve insufficiency is present.

2. The left atrium is incised, and a self-retaining or handheld retractor is inserted. A wet laparotomy pad may be placed under the left ventricular apex to facilitate exposure of the valve (if there is sufficient access to the LV).

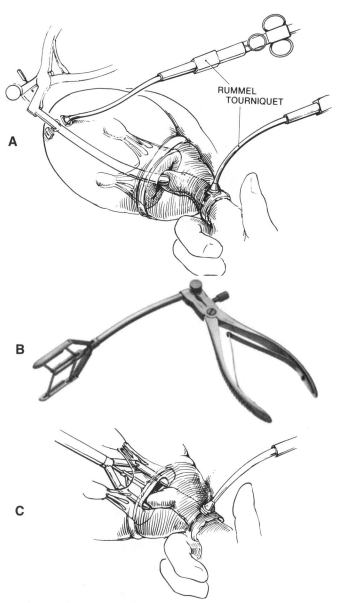

FIGURE 11-17 Closed mitral commissurotomy. **A,** A tourniquet is applied to the atrial pursestring and the surgeon's finger inserted through the atriotomy. A Rummel tourniquet is applied over a heavy polyester suture, buttressed with felt pledgets, and placed near the left ventricular apex. **B and C,** The Tubbs dilator is inserted through the ventriculotomy and advanced into the mitral valve orifice. (**A and C,** from Waldhausen JA and others: *Surgery of the chest,* ed 6, St Louis, 1996, Mosby; **B,** courtesy Baxter Healthcare, V. Mueller Division.)

3. The valve is grasped with forceps and inspected. A retraction suture may be placed into the anterior cusp to mobilize the leaflet.

4a. The fused leaflets are separated at the commissures with scissors or a knife and a long clamp such as a tonsil (Fig. 11-18). The mitral valve dilator (see Fig.

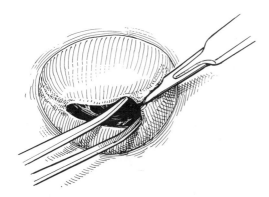

FIGURE 11-18 Open mitral commissurotomy. A knife is used to incise the fused commissures. The commissurotomy is extended with a tonsil clamp. (From Waldhausen JA and others: *Surgery of the chest,* ed 6, St Louis, 1996, Mosby.)

11-17, *B*) may be used to spread apart the leaflets and to measure the orifice.

4b. Fused chordae can create obstruction within the subvalvular apparatus. To improve flow, the chordae inserting into the leaflets may be divided at the commissural level, with the longitudinal incision extending to the head of the papillary muscles.

5. The valve is tested for competency, and the left atrium is closed with continuous cardiovascular suture.

Mitral annuloplasty for mitral regurgitation. Mitral annuloplasty is the reduction in size of a dilated annulus using a suturing technique or, more commonly, through application of a prosthetic ring. Placement of the annuloplasty ring is performed to correct dilation of the mitral annulus, to increase leaflet coaptation by reforming the deformed annulus, to reinforce the annular sutures when part of the valve leaflet has been resected, and to prevent further dilation of the annulus (Gillinov and Cosgrove, 1998).

Procedural considerations. Annuloplasty rings may be relatively rigid ("classic" ring; Carpentier, 1983), semirigid (Carpentier "physio" ring), or flexible (Duran and others, 1980). A semicircular annuloplasty system (Gillinov and Cosgrove, 1998) is also available.

Proponents of the preshaped, rigid ring (see Chapter 3) stress the importance of restoring the shape and the size of the dilated orifice. Flexible rings offer the advantage of not compromising the ability of the annulus to change size and shape throughout the cardiac cycle. The Cosgrove flexible semicircular ring (annuloplasty system) is sewn to the annular portion of the posterior leaflet; the advantage of this ring is that it repairs annular dilation, which occurs mainly in the posterior leaflet.

Annuloplasty rings reduce the annular circumference by gathering excess posterior leaflet tissue and redistributing it toward the larger anterior leaflet to produce a competent valve. The size of the ring is determined by measuring the anterior leaflet with special sizing obturators. Carpentier (even-numbered) ring sizers (also used for Cosgrove rings) have metal holders that fit into the middle of the sizer. Duran (odd-numbered) ring sizers do not have their own holder and must be grasped through a central opening with a tonsil or Kelly clamp from the nurse's basic instrument set. The side of the obturator displaying the letter *M* (for mitral) should be facing the operator (the reverse side with *T* is used for tricuspid sizing).

Ring sizes of 27/28 to 31/32 mm are appropriate for most female patients, and sizes 29/30 to 33/34 mm are common for male patients.

Prostheses may be handheld or attached to a holder with a separate handle for insertion of the stitches. Flexible rings require that they be grasped firmly (even though they are attached to the ring holder) during insertion of stitches into the prosthesis. The method of suture insertion is similar for all kinds of rings.

Children are generally poor candidates for ring annuloplasty because of the risk of evolving valvular stenosis as growth occurs. Suture techniques may be employed in younger age groups and in women wishing to become pregnant. Development of an absorbable (biodegradable) prosthetic ring would be useful to reduce the problem of secondary stenosis in younger patients.

The size of the left atrium may influence the selection of incision. Patients with chronic mitral insufficiency often have large atria, facilitating exposure of the mitral apparatus. When insufficiency is of acute onset, the atrium has not had time to dilate, and exposure may be difficult. This also may be a problem in the presence of dense adhesions from previous surgery, calcification, thrombosis, or chest deformities. In these situations exposure can be enhanced by incising the right atrium and the atrial septum to expose the mitral valve, as first described by Dubost and colleagues (1966) and subsequently modified by others (Cohn, 1998; Byrne and others, 1999).

Procedure

1. The chest is opened, cardiopulmonary bypass with double venous cannulation is instituted, and the heart is arrested. For patients who have undergone previous surgery through a median sternotomy, a right or left thoracotomy may be performed.

2. The left atrium is opened, and the mitral valve is exposed. In patients with small left atria, right atriotomy and right septotomy may be preferred for adequate exposure (see Fig. 11-16).

Cardiotomy suction tips are inserted into the atrium. Special handheld or self-retaining atrial retractors may be inserted to expose the valve.

3. The valve annulus, leaflets, and related structures are identified and inspected. Annular dilation is evaluated.

4a. *Resection and plication:* Redundant posterior leaflet tissue may be resected and the cut edges approximated and sewn together; the corresponding annular segment is plicated (Fig. 11-19).

4b. *Sliding technique for systolic anterior motion (SAM):* If the residual height of the plicated section of the posterior leaflet is too high, it can produce systolic anterior motion of the valve, which can cause some impedance to blood flow during LV ejection (systole).

To reduce the height of the posterior leaflet (Fig. 11-20), the annular portion of the remaining posterior leaflet segments are incised for a short distance. These segments are advanced toward the excised portion of the posterior leaflet and reattached to the annulus with a 4-0 polypropylene suture (Fig. 11-21). The cut edges of the leaflet are then sewn together with another 4-0 polypropylene suture. This sliding maneuver also reduces the tension on the posterior leaflet segments to be approximated and plicated.

5. *Ring annuloplasty:* An annuloplasty ring is inserted (step 6) to reinforce the repair and correct the annular dilation commonly seen in the posterior (mural) leaflet. Annuloplasty with a ring (Figs. 11-22 and 11-23) or a semicircular ring (Fig. 11-24) is performed. A sizing obturator is used to measure the area of the anterior leaflet (Fig. 11-22, *A* and *B*; Fig. 11-24, *A*), and the comparable annuloplasty ring is delivered to the field.

6. For Carpentier (Fig. 11-22) and Duran (Fig. 11-23) rings, interrupted sutures are placed around the circumference of the annulus and then into the ring. Because the anterior leaflet is less dilated than the posterior leaflet, spacing of the sutures is done so that when the stitches are tied, the excessive posterior leaflet tissue is evenly drawn up against the prosthesis, and the anterior leaflet retains its original shape and size.

7. For a Cosgrove ring (Fig. 11-24, *B*), stitches are placed in the posterior leaflet from fibrous trigone to fibrous trigone (see Fig. 11-2).

8. *Commissuroplasty:* If there is residual mitral regurgitation (or a large floppy valve), a commissural stitch may be inserted (Fig. 11-25) in the anterior commissure to take a tuck in the prolapsed segment.

9. Competency of the repair is tested with a bulb syringe (Fig. 11-22, *D*).

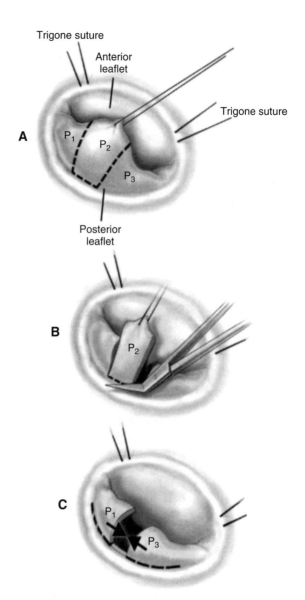

FIGURE 11-19 Repair of ruptured chordae to prolapsed posterior leaflet. **A,** The posterior leaflet is divided mentally into three anatomic segments: P (posterior) 1, P2, and P3. **B,** Segment P2, containing the ruptured chordae, is resected. **C,** The remaining segments of the posterior leaflet are reapproximated. (From Cohn LH: Mitral valve repair, *Oper Techn Thorac Cardiovasc Surg* 3[2]:109, 1998.)

10. The left atrial appendage may be excised and oversewn to reduce the risk of thrombus formation and subsequent embolization.

11. The atrial incision is closed partially to allow air to exit the left ventricle. The heart is allowed to resume beating. TEE is used before and after the discontinuation of cardiopulmonary bypass to evaluate ventricular function and valve performance.

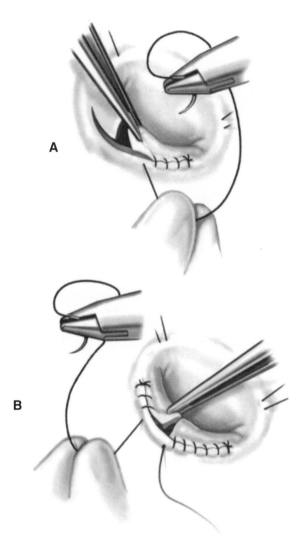

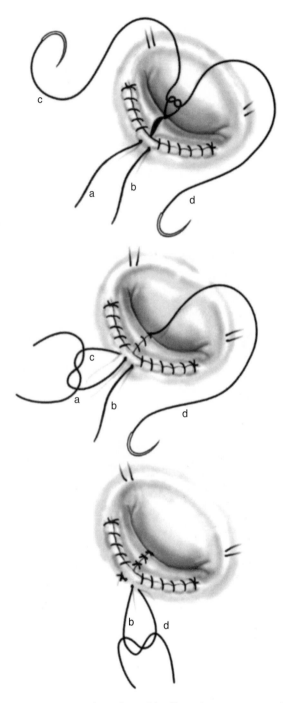

FIGURE 11-20 To reduce the height of the residual leaflet (and avoid the creation of systolic anterior motion, which can create left ventricular outflow tract obstruction) **(A)**, the remaining segments are incised for a short distance toward their respective commissures. **B,** The annular leaflet edges are sewn to the annulus, and then the segment edges are sewn to each other. (From Cohn LH: Mitral valve repair, *Oper Techn Thorac Cardiovasc Surg* 3[2]:109, 1998.)

FIGURE 11-21 Continuation of leaflet advancement technique (see text). (From Cohn LH: Mitral valve repair, *Oper Techn Thorac Cardiovasc Surg* 3[2]:109, 1998.)

Mitral valvuloplasty for mitral regurgitation

Procedural considerations. Valvuloplasty represents an array of techniques to repair the valve leaflets and related structures. Not infrequently there are abnormalities in one or more components of the apparatus, such as a dilated annulus with elongated chordae.

Procedure

1. After the atrium is opened and the valve exposed, a thorough evaluation of the valvular and subvalvular structures is made.

2a. *Patch repair:* Perforations of the anterior or posterior leaflets may be patched with autologous pericardium (Fig. 11-26) that has been treated by immersion in glutaraldehyde solution (available from pharmaceutical companies). Resection of the torn portion of the leaflet and annular plication with annuloplasty may be used to repair the posterior

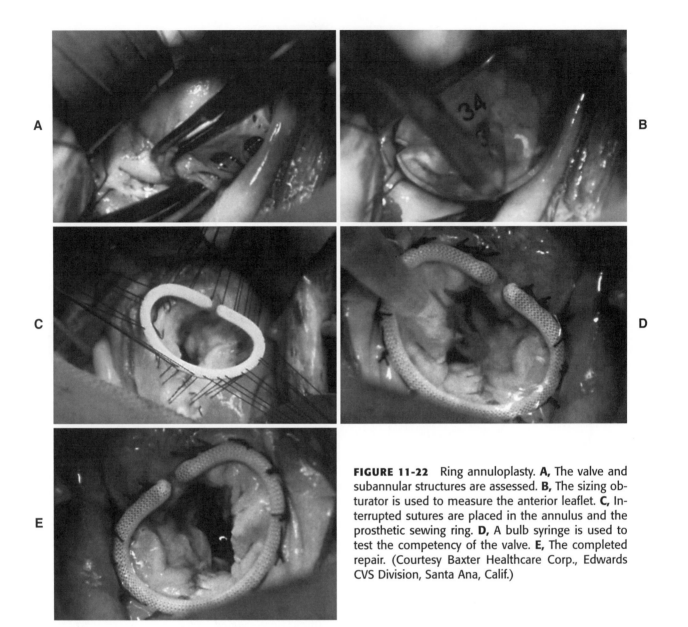

FIGURE 11-22 Ring annuloplasty. **A,** The valve and subannular structures are assessed. **B,** The sizing obturator is used to measure the anterior leaflet. **C,** Interrupted sutures are placed in the annulus and the prosthetic sewing ring. **D,** A bulb syringe is used to test the competency of the valve. **E,** The completed repair. (Courtesy Baxter Healthcare Corp., Edwards CVS Division, Santa Ana, Calif.)

leaflet. This technique is generally not used for the anterior leaflet, which does not tolerate repair of its free edge as well as does the posterior leaflet.

2b. *Debridement:* Leaflets with discrete areas of calcification may be debrided. If the calcium extends through the leaflet, the remaining defect in the leaflet after excision of the calcium may be patched with pericardium (Fig. 11-26), as described previously. In some situations extensive calcification can be removed by debridement.

2c. *Mobilization:* Shortened, fused chordae tendineae can be mobilized and lengthened by their division into secondary chordae or by incising the tip of the papillary muscle.

2d. *Chordal replacement:* Chordal replacement (Fig. 11-27) is less traumatic and more reproducible (David,

1998; David and others, 1998) than the technique of chordal shortening (in which redundant tissue of elongated chordae are implanted into an incised papillary muscle head or folded over itself and secured with a suture).

Two to four 5-0 expanded polytetrafluoroethylene (PTFE) sutures are attached in multiple locations to the posterior medial and anterior lateral papillary muscles; they are then inserted into the leading edge of the anterior leaflet and tied. It is important not to tie the sutures too tightly (which can occur in the flaccid heart) so that leaflet incompetence is not created (Cohn, 1998).

2e. *Chordal transfer:* This technique is also less popular as a result of the use of chordal replacement with PTFE sutures, but it is useful in certain situations. A

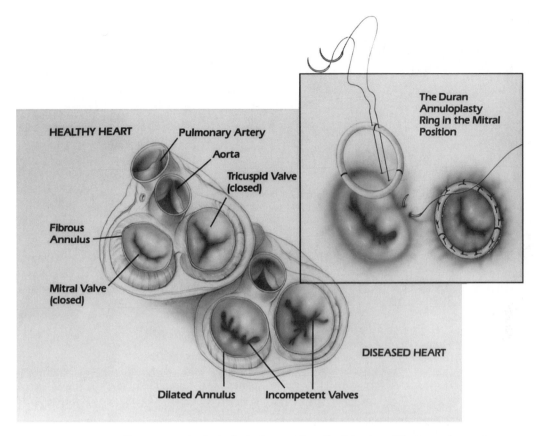

FIGURE 11-23 Duran annuloplasty technique with a flexible ring. (Photograph courtesy Medtronic, Inc.)

section of intact chordae are transferred from a portion of the posterior leaflet to the unsupported segment of the anterior leaflet. The transferred chordae are sutured to the free edge of the anterior leaflet. An alternative method is to transfer a healthy secondary chord to the free edge of the anterior leaflet and have the transferred chord thereby take on the function of a primary chord (Gillinov and Cosgrove, 1998).

2f. *Papillary muscle repair:* Occasionally one head of a ruptured papillary muscle can be sutured to an immediately adjacent papillary muscle.

MITRAL VALVE REPLACEMENT

Mitral valve replacement is the excision of one or both mitral valve leaflets, supporting chordae, and papillary muscle heads, and replacement with a mechanical or biologic prosthesis. There is evidence that preserving the posterior (mural) leaflet and associated chordae minimizes impaired postoperative left ventricular function by maintaining the normal geometry and mechanics of the left ventricle.

Replacement is indicated for patients in whom extensive valvular damage precludes repair. Patients may

be moderately or severely symptomatic (functional class 3 or 4). Impaired ventricular function should be documented by diagnostic evaluation with echocardiography or nuclear studies.

Patient Teaching Considerations

In addition to patient-related factors (Box 11-5), prosthetic valve–related factors (Box 11-6) must be considered when replacement is performed. This includes not only anticoagulation-related hemorrhage and endocarditis but other complications related to prosthetic performance (Vongpatanasin, Hillis, and Lange, 1996).

Signs of prosthetic failure vary according to the prosthesis inserted. A thrombosed disk valve will no longer be audible if the opening and closing mechanism is impaired. A perforated bioprosthetic leaflet (see Fig. 11-6) may produce sudden regurgitation, as can a valve that has a dehisced sewing ring. Periprosthetic leaks resulting from detachment of part of the sewing ring from the annulus are suggested by the presence of new murmurs, varying degrees of regurgitation, and signs of hemolysis secondary to blood trauma from being squeezed between the prosthesis and the annulus.

Thromboembolism is a risk with all prostheses, but there is a higher incidence in patients who have had

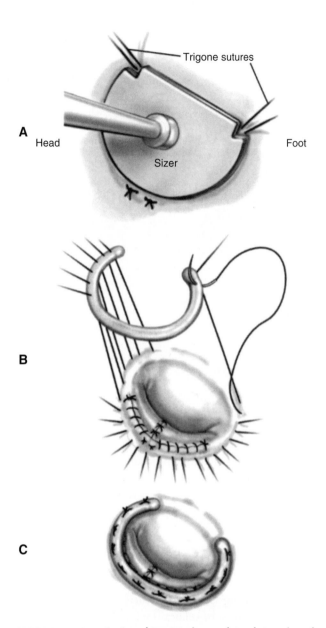

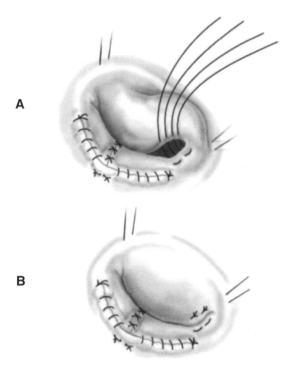

FIGURE 11-25 **A,** Residual mitral regurgitation can be repaired with commissural stitches **(B).** (From Cohn LH: Mitral valve repair, *Oper Techn Thorac Cardiovasc Surg* 3[2]:109, 1998.)

FIGURE 11-24 **A,** An obturator is used to determine the correct size for the annuloplasty ring by measuring the anterior leaflet of the mitral valve. **B,** A series of interrupted stitches are inserted into the annulus and then into the annuloplasty ring. **C,** The completed ring. (From Cohn LH: Mitral valve repair, *Oper Techn Thorac Cardiovasc Surg* 3[2]:109, 1998.)

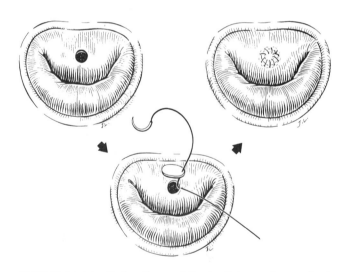

FIGURE 11-26 Perforations of the leaflet may be patched with autologous pericardium. (From Cosgrove DM, Stewart WJ: Mitral valvuloplasty, *Curr Probl Cardiol* 14[7]:353, 1989.)

mechanical valves implanted and whose bleeding times are not sufficiently prolonged with anticoagulants (see Box 11-5). The risk increases significantly in patients with a history of chronic atrial fibrillation. Warfarin therapy is used to maintain an individualized dose according to the patient's response as indicated by the international normalized ratio (INR). Regular laboratory follow-up is necessary to adjust and maintain warfarin levels in a range that causes neither bleeding nor increased risk of thrombus formation (Ansell, Hirsh, and Wenger, 1999).

Plans for patient teaching (see Table 11-1) during the perioperative, recuperative, and rehabilitative periods incorporate information related to risks and complica-

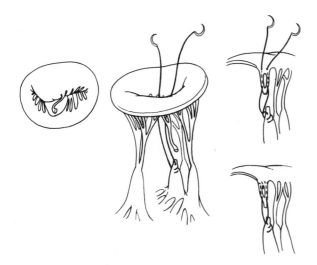

FIGURE 11-27 Chordal replacement with polytetrafluoroethylene suture (see text). (From David TE and others: Long-term results of mitral valve repair for myxomatous disease with and without chordal replacement with expanded polytetrafluoroethylene, *J Thorac Cardiovasc Surg* 115[6]:1279, 1998.)

tions, diet, lifestyle, and living environment (Finkelmeier, 2000).

The decision regarding which prosthesis to use should be a joint effort among the surgeon, the cardiologist, and the patient. The perioperative nurse can assist the patient by clarifying the reasons for the selection of a particular prosthesis and providing information about the possible effects of such a choice on the patient's future lifestyle.

Procedural Considerations

Since the introduction of a prosthetic valve in the 1960s, many prostheses have been developed with a variety of configurations and closing mechanisms (Box 11-7; Figs. 11-28 and 11-29). Although these early prostheses are no longer approved by the U.S. Food and Drug Administration (FDA) for implantation, patients who present for reoperation may have one of these valves. Knowledge of their design may be helpful for radiologic identification and surgical excision.

Mechanical and bioprosthetic valves currently approved for implantation are listed in Table 11-4, along with considerations for use, advantages, and disadvantages. The choice of a mechanical or biologic prosthesis is complicated by the fact that each type of prosthesis has drawbacks. Increased risk of thromboembolism is associated with mechanical valves, and durability can be a problem with biologic valves (Campbell and Grover, 1995). Additionally, all prosthetic heart valves are inherently stenotic because attachment of the sewing ring to the annulus takes up a portion of the na-

---

BOX 11-5
Patient-Related Factors and Risks Associated With Mitral Valve Surgery

Left ventricular function (e.g., functional class, coronary artery disease, congestive heart failure)
Age
Sex
Residence
Preoperative endocarditis
History of atrial fibrillation
Connective tissue disorders (e.g., Marfan syndrome)
Congenital anomalies (e.g., cleft mitral valve)
Enlarged left atrium
Left atrial thrombus
History of transient ischemic attacks
Anticoagulation compliance
Preexisting health problems (e.g., diabetes mellitus, pulmonary or systemic hypertension, hepatic or renal disease)
Valve lesion
Previous cardiac surgery

Modified from Braunwald E: Valvular heart disease. In Braunwald E, Zipes, DP, Libby P, editors: *Heart disease: a textbook of cardiovascular medicine,* ed 6, Philadelphia, 2001, WB Saunders.

BOX 11-6
Valve-Related Risks and Complications

Anticoagulation-related hemorrhage
Thromboembolism
Prosthetic valve endocarditis
Periprosthetic leak
Prosthetic failure
Left ventricular outflow tract obstruction

Modified from Werly JA, Crawford MH: Choosing a prosthetic heart valve, *Cardiol Clin* 16:491, 1998.

---

tive orifice. Proper selection includes considerations related to patient age, lifestyle, and activity level and the safety of anticoagulation.

Patient age is a factor because biologic valves deteriorate. The durability of mechanical valves is important, especially in patients who may have to face reoperation because their life expectancy is longer than that of a bioprosthesis (Moon and others, 2001). In children and young adults degenerative calcification occurs at an accelerated rate and is thought to be related to the active calcium metabolism within this age group. In adults the reasons for the calcific stenosis are less clear, but it is thought to be associated with altered metabolism of calcium and other substances. In addition, this may be a factor in patients with renal disease who also demonstrate accelerated bioprosthetic failure.

Leaflet calcification is considered the most important reason for the reduced viability of bioprostheses. Investigational studies (Duarte and others, 2001) on

BOX 11-7
Cardiac Valve Prostheses Developed Since the 1960s

A variety of prosthetic valves have been designed and developed. The opening and closing mechanism of synthetic valves is usually one of two configurations: the ball and cage or the single- or double-tilting disk. The prostheses that follow are listed under their respective heading; they are no longer available in the United States.

Ball and Cage
Braunwald-Cutter
Braunwald-Morrow
Cooley-Bloodwell-Liotta-Cromie
DeBakey-Surgitool
Harken ball and cage (see Fig. 12-1)
Hufnagel (see Fig. 12-2)
Magovern-Cromie
Smeloff-Cutter
Smeloff-Cutter-Davey-Kaufman
Starr-Edwards (1260, 6120 models still available; (see Fig. 11-28)

Tilting Disk
Bjork-Shiley
Hufnagel trileaflet
Lillehei-Kastor
Wada-Cutter

Caged Disk
Barnard-Goosen
Beall-Surgitool
Cooley-Bloodwell-Cutter
Cooley-Cutter
Cross-Jones
Hufnagel-Brunswick
Kay-Shiley
Kay-Suzuki
Starr-Edwards disk

Bileaflet Disk
Carbomedics
Edwards-Duromedics
Gott-Daggett
Kalke (see Fig. 11-29)

Modified from Akins CW: Mechanical cardiac valvular prostheses, *Ann Thorac Surg* 52:161, 1991; Lefrak EA, Starr A: *Cardiac valve prostheses,* Norwalk, Conn, 1979, Appleton-Century-Crofts.

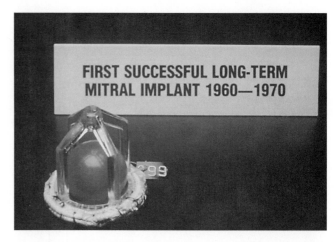

FIGURE 11-28 Original Starr-Edwards ball-and-cage valve (explanted 10 years after implantation when the patient died from an accident). (Courtesy Baxter Healthcare Corp., Edwards CVS Division, Santa Ana, Calif.)

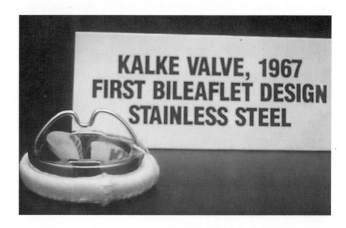

FIGURE 11-29 Kalke double-leaflet valve was a forerunner of modern-day bileaflet prostheses. (Courtesy Baxter Healthcare Corp., Edwards CVS Division, Santa Ana, Calif.)

porcine bioprostheses treated with alpha-amino oleic acid (AOA) have demonstrated reduced leaflet calcification. The potential benefits of bioprostheses with a lower incidence of calcification include prolonged durability, greater freedom from reoperation, and more effective function.

An active lifestyle may warrant selection of a prostheses with optimal hemodynamics. Hemodynamic function is comparable for most mitral prostheses, especially in the larger sizes. There may be some differences in patients with a small native mitral valve (less than 29 mm), but the small valve orifice is more often a problem in aortic valve surgery (see Chapter 12).

The risk of anticoagulation-related complications increases if laboratory follow-up is not consistent or if there are preexisting bleeding tendencies. In one long-term study (Hammermeister and others, 2000) comparing valve-related complications in mechanical and biologic valves, researchers found that although thromboembolic rates were similar between the two prostheses, bleeding was more common with the mechanical valve. This latter finding is not surprising because patients with mechanical valves are almost always on warfarin therapy (with its attendant risk for bleeding);

TABLE 11-4
Commonly Used Mechanical and Biologic Valve Prostheses

| | MECHANICAL | |
| BALL AND CAGE | TILTING DISK | |
STARR-EDWARDS	MEDTRONIC-HALL, OMNISCIENCE	ST. JUDE MEDICAL, CARBOMEDICS
Model/Description		
6120 Mitral	Spherical tilting disk	Bileaflet tilting disk
1260 Aortic		
Advantages		
Long-term durability	Long-term durability	Long-term durability
Good hemodynamics	Good hemodynamics in all sizes	Good hemodynamics in all sizes
Inaudible	Low profile	Low TE rate for a mechanical valve
Least risk of sudden thrombosis		Low profile
Disadvantages		
Anticoagulation required	Anticoagulation required	Anticoagulation strongly recommended
Higher incidence of TE than disk valves	Sudden thrombosis	Sudden thrombosis
Suboptimal hemodynamics in small aortic sizes (less than 23 mm)	Noisy	Some noise
	Higher risk of TE in mitral position	Higher risk of TE in mitral position
High profile not optimal in small LV or aortic root	If warfarin must be discontinued, there is increased risk of catastrophic thrombosis	If warfarin must be discontinued, there is increased risk of catastrophic thrombosis
Higher risk of TE in mitral position		
Special considerations		
Sizers and handles specific to prosthesis; must be sterilized	Sizers and handles specific to prosthesis; must be sterilized	Sizers and handles specific to prosthesis; must be sterilized
Poppet of aortic valve removable to facilitate tying sutures; replaced before aorta closed. Mitral poppett not removable		Frequently used in children needing prosthetic valve
Aortic model has three struts; mitral has four		
Resterilization		
Follow manufacturer's instructions. All prostheses should be stored in a cool, dry, contamination-free area.		

*Modified from Fullerton DA, Grover FL: Complications from cardiac prostheses: I. Prosthetic valve endocarditis; and Campbell DN, Grover FL: Complications from cardiac prostheses: II. Thrombosis and thromboembolisms of prosthetic cardiac valves and extracardiac prostheses. In Sabiston DC, Spencer FC, editors: *Surgery of the chest*, ed 6, Philadelphia, 1995, WB Saunders. Hammermeister K and others: Outcomes 15 years after valve replacement with a mechanical versus a bioprosthetic valve: final report of the Veterans Affairs randomized trial *J Am Coll Cardiol* 36(4):1152, 2000. Doty BD, Dilip KA, Millar RC: Mitral valve replacement with homograft and Maze III procedure *Ann Thorac Surg* 69:739, 2000.
TE, Thromboembolism; *EO,* ethylene oxide; *AVR,* aortic valve replacement.

Continued

patients with bioprostheses are less likely to be taking anticoagulants unless there are other factors, such as atrial fibrillation, that indicate a need for warfarin.

Patients who have a history of atrial fibrillation (and have been on anticoagulants) are expected to continue their anticoagulant regimen because the dysrhythmia rarely reverts to normal sinus rhythm. In these patients it has been logical to implant the more durable, mechanical valve rather than a potentially less durable biologic valve. Advances in dysrhythmia management and the application of allograft technology to mitral valve surgery (Acar and others, 1996) have been combined by Doty and his colleagues (2000). They replaced a patient's native mitral valve with a mitral valve (cadaver)

allograft. Concomitantly they performed a Maze procedure (see Chapter 17) to correct the atrial fibrillation.

Perioperative considerations

A complete range of prostheses with sizers should be available, as well as pledgeted and nonpledgeted sutures. Obturators can be arranged in order of size on the back table (and the size written on the table cover next to each obturator). Individual obturator and prosthetic valve holders may appear similar; the nurse can identify these quickly with labels or by writing the name of the corresponding prosthesis next to each one.

Three basins capable of holding at least 500 ml of normal saline for rinsing glutaraldehyde-stored bioprostheses

TABLE **11-4**
Commonly Used Mechanical and Biologic Valve Prostheses—cont'd

	BIOLOGIC	
HETEROGRAFT (XENOGRAFT)		**ALLOGRAFT (HOMOGRAFT)**
CARPENTIER-EDWARDS; HANCOCK STENTLESS PORCINE BIOPROSTHESIS.	CARPENTIER-EDWARDS PERICARDIAL VALVE	
Model/Description		
Porcine heterograft (from excised pig aortic valves)	2700 aortic Bovine pericardium (cut and shaped into a trileaflet valve)	Aortic valve allograft (cadaver, organ donor, excised cardiomyopathic heart from transplant recipient (mitral valve allograft also available)
Advantages		
Incidence of TE very low	Incidence of TE very low	Incidence of TE very low
Anticoagulation rare after AVR	Anticoagulation rare after AVR	Anticoagulation rare
No hemolysis	No hemolysis	Used for AVR and MVR
Good hemodynamics	Good hemodynamics in all sizes	No hemolysis
Central flow	Central flow	Excellent hemodynamics (especially with stentless technique)
Gradual failure allows elective reoperation	Gradual failure allows elective reoperation	Central flow
Durability good after age 60	Residual gradient minimal	Gradual failure allows elective reoperation
Stentless graft has many advantages of allograft valves		No residual gradient
Disadvantages		
Durability less than 15 years	Durability not yet established	Limited durability
Accelerated fibrocalcific degeneration in children, patients with hypertension or on chronic renal dialysis	Available only for AVR	Limited availability
Stentless valve available only for AVR	Accelerated calcification may be a problem in children, renal patients, or those with hypertension	
Suboptimal hemodynamics (except stentless model) and residual gradient in smaller sizes (less than 23 mm aorta or 29 mm mitral)		
May be contraindicated in small, hypertrophied LV		
Special Considerations		
Sizers and handles specific to prosthesis; must be sterilized before insertion; must be rinsed in saline to remove storage solution	Sizers and handles specific to prosthesis must be sterilized before insertion, must be rinsed in saline to remove storage solution	No specific sizers; may use sizers for heterografts
Before insertion, frequent irrigation recommended to prevent drying	Before insertion, frequent irrigation recommended to prevent drying	Cryopreserved allograft must be thawed per protocol
Diets low in calcium recommended for children, renal patients	Diets low in calcium recommended for children, renal patients	Used for aortic or mitral valve replacement; stent can be attached if indicated for use in other positions
Resterilization		
Not recommended.	Not recommended.	Not recommended.

should be arranged on the back table cover or on a separate sterile field. Forceps, suture scissors, one to three syringes (10 ml), and one to four culture tubes are added. Biologic valves require rinsing for at least 2 minutes in each of the three basins. They should be kept moist with frequent saline irrigation during implantation but should not be moistened with topical antibiotic solution.

Additional basinware may be needed for heparinized saline and other solutions.

Operative procedures

1. Cardiopulmonary bypass with double-venous cannulation is instituted (Fig. 11-30, *A*). Umbilical tapes with tourniquets may be placed around the

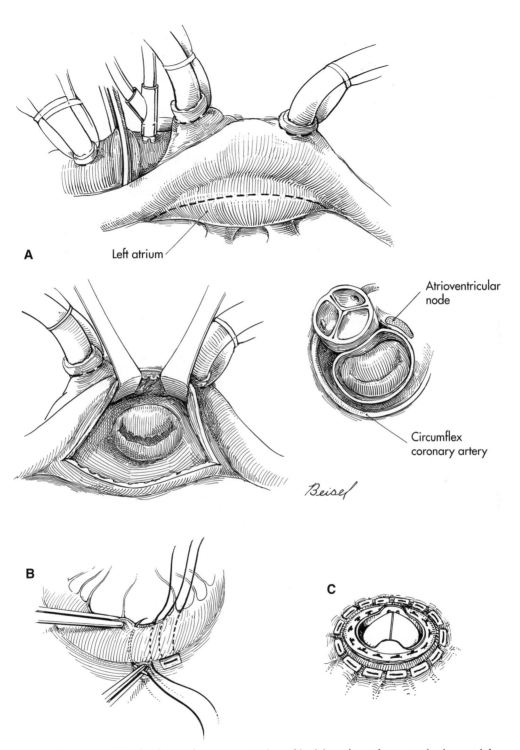

FIGURE 11-30 Mitral valve replacement. **A,** Line of incision along the posterior interatrial groove. Handheld retractors in the left atrium expose the mitral valve. Note the relationship between the mitral valve and aortic valve. The valve is excised; the posterior leaflet and chordae may be retained. **B,** Insertion of interrupted stitches into annulus and prosthetic sewing ring. Felt pledgeted suture helps reduce the risk of perivalvular leaks when there is a fragile or calcified annulus. The pledget is positioned in the subannular position. **C,** Completed valve insertion. (From Waldhausen JA and others: *Surgery of the chest,* ed 6, St Louis, 1996, Mosby.)

IVC and SVC to isolate the heart from any venous return.

2. The left atrium is incised, blood suctioned away, and the incision enlarged to expose the mitral valve (Fig. 11-30, *A*). The atrium is inspected and any thrombotic material removed.

3. Retraction stitches may be placed in the anterior leaflet for exposure and the valvular apparatus inspected. Stitches may be placed in each commissure.

4. The valve leaflets, along with their respective chordae tendineae and tips of the papillary muscle heads, are excised with a blade and scissors. Increasingly, only the anterior leaflet and subvalvular structures are removed; the posterior leaflet and attached chordae (and occasionally part of the anterior leaflet and associated chordae) are left intact as support structures for the left ventricle.

A fibrous margin of the valve annulus is left for insertion of fixation sutures to the valve prosthesis (Fig. 11-30, *B*). Caution is taken not to transect too much of the papillary muscle because this can weaken the ventricular wall and lead to rupture. The valvular tissue may be sent to the laboratory for bacterial examination and culturing (even if infected carditis is not suspected). Some surgeons have abandoned this practice because the incidence of false positive results from native valve cultures is high (Campbell, Tsai, and Mispireta, 2000).

Rongeurs may be used to debride calcium particles; the rongeur tips should be rinsed in saline and wiped clean with a wet sponge. The atrium and ventricle are inspected and all loose debris removed.

5. The valve annulus is sized with obturators corresponding to the specific prosthesis desired; the appropriate size valve is selected, verified by the circulating nurse and the sterile nurse, and delivered to the field.

   a. *Mechanical valve:* The sterile nurse attaches the appropriate handle, cuts the identification label, and places the prosthesis in a protected area of the field until needed. (Some surgeons request that the prosthesis be wrapped in a sponge moistened with heparinized saline or antibiotic solution.)

   b. *Biologic valve:* The sterile nurse attaches the appropriate handle and removes any packing material from the prosthesis. The identification tag is cut and removed before beginning the rinsing procedure (agitation of the prosthesis with the tag attached could lacerate the prosthetic leaflets).

   The bioprosthesis is then rinsed for at least 2 minutes in each of three basins of normal saline (total minimum time: 6 minutes). Five to ten ml of the rinse solution from the third basin is placed in a tube and sent for culture; cultures may be taken from all three of the basins if requested. The bioprosthesis is wrapped in a saline-moistened sponge and placed in a protected area of the field until needed. It should not be allowed to dry or come into contact with antibiotic solutions (which can damage the tissue).

6. Nonabsorbable, alternately colored individual cardiovascular sutures (approximately 20) are placed in the retained fibrous annular margin (avoiding the muscular wall, which can tear when the sutures are tied) (Fig. 11-30, *B*) and then into the prosthetic sewing ring. The needles then are removed.

Some surgeons prefer to insert stitches into the prosthetic sewing ring only after all the annular stitches are in place.

7. The sutures are held taut as the prosthesis is guided into position. Sprinkling normal saline on the sutures makes them slide more easily through the sewing ring. (Surgeons also may want to keep their fingers moist to facilitate tying each stitch.) The sutures are tied and cut (Fig. 11-30, *C*), and the surgeon confirms that no stitches are entangled in the prosthetic struts. A small dental mirror (prewarmed in saline to prevent fogging) can be used to assess the subvalvular placement of stitches in bioprostheses.

8. A catheter may be placed through the orifice of a mechanical valve to keep the valve incompetent, thereby allowing air to escape from the left ventricle. This maneuver is used cautiously if at all in a bioprosthesis because the leaflets could be injured.

9. In patients with an enlarged left atrium or history of embolic episodes, the atrial appendage is often ligated to prevent the subsequent formation and embolization of thrombus.

10. The atriotomy is closed partially (around the transvalvular catheter) with nonabsorbable sutures. The patient is placed in Trendelenburg's position so that residual air in the left ventricle exits preferentially through the venting needle placed in the anterior ascending aorta (rather than traveling to the brain and causing an air embolus).

Air also is aspirated from the left ventricle with a handheld hypodermic needle (or, less frequently, an apical venting catheter). Caution is taken to avoid excessive elevation of the ventricle, which could produce a ventricular wall tear or rupture. In reoperations in which ventricular apical adhesions remain, a spinal needle can be placed transseptally from the right ventricle to the left ventricle to remove air. If bleeding from the needle holes persists, a stick tie may be used for repair.

11. Additional venting measures may be employed (e.g., moving the table from side to side, gently jiggling the heart, inflating the lungs). The cross-clamp is removed and the heart allowed to fibrillate. The ventricle is not allowed to eject blood until the surgeon is assured that sufficient air is evacuated. After adequate venting, the heart is defibrillated. The transvalvular catheter (if used) is removed and the atrial closure completed.

12. Rewarming is completed, and the patient is weaned from cardiopulmonary bypass. TEE may be used to assess ventricular function (and detect the presence of residual air).

ADDITIONAL PROCEDURES

Reoperation for mitral valve disease

Patients with a prior commissurotomy may require reoperation for recurring mitral stenosis. If the initial approach was via thoracotomy, few if any sternal adhesions will be present. If repeat sternotomy is planned, additional dissecting time and increased bleeding can be anticipated. Some surgeons may elect to use a right or left thoracotomy approach for repeat valve replacement in patients who had an initial sternotomy. Exposure is critical, and the surgeon will use the approach that allows optimal visualization of the operative site (Loulmet and others, 1998). Operative risk is increased with repeat valve replacement (Kirklin and Barratt-Boyes, 1993).

The nurse can anticipate some difficulty in removing the prosthetic valve. Reconstruction of the annulus with autologous or bovine pericardium may be necessary.

Infective endocarditis

Infective endocarditis of the native valve or a prosthetic valve is an indication for surgery when there is heart failure, septic emboli, conduction disturbances, prosthetic valve dysfunction, or persistent signs of infection. Repair may be feasible in some native valves, but replacement is necessary with infections involving the sewing ring or annulus or when the valve is severely damaged (Moon and others, 2001; Fullerton and Grover, 1995).

Multiple valve surgery

When concomitant aortic valve disease is serious enough to warrant surgical correction (see Chapter 12), valve replacement is performed during the same operation. Both valves may be excised first. Mitral valve replacement is then performed, with the prosthesis seated and the sutures tied, followed by aortic valve replacement (Fig. 11-31). Performing the surgery in this order avoids injury to aortic structures from a rigid

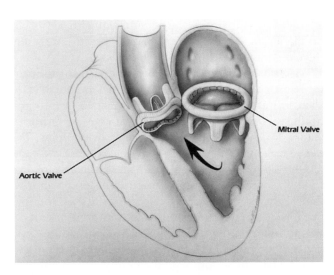

FIGURE 11-31 Double valve replacement with bioprostheses in the mitral and aortic positions. (Courtesy Medtronic, Inc.)

prosthesis during manipulation of the mitral valve. Closure of the atrial incision can be completed after the aortic valve has been implanted and the aorta closed (Mueller and others, 1998).

Tricuspid valve surgery is performed after mitral valve replacement. Generally suture or ring annuloplasty is performed for tricuspid regurgitation and commissurotomy for stenotic lesions. Valve replacement is uncommon (see Chapter 13). Multiple valve surgery poses an increased risk to the patient.

Coronary artery disease

The proportion of patients undergoing mitral valve replacement who also have catheterization documented coronary artery disease has increased over the past years, as has the number of patients undergoing concomitant mitral valve replacement and coronary artery bypass grafting (Thourani and others, 2000). When both procedures are performed, the distal coronary artery bypass grafts are performed first, followed by valve replacement, and then proximal anastomoses. If resection of an apical left ventricular aneurysm is planned, the mitral valve can be replaced through the ventriculotomy, after which the aneurysm is resected and the ventricle closed.

Completion of the Procedure

At the completion of the surgical repair, the surgeon inspects the suture line for hemostasis. In patients with recent onset of atrial fibrillation, the heart may return to normal sinus rhythm; cardioversion may be attempted if atrial fibrillation is present. Warfarin therapy is initiated a few days postoperatively in patients with chronic atrial fibrillation (and those with mechanical prostheses) after the danger of surgical bleeding has passed.

Surgical manipulation and local edema may produce transient conduction disturbances, so temporary ventricular and atrial pacing wires are attached prophylactically. (Atrial pacing is ineffective in converting fibrillation to sinus rhythm; ventricular wires may be necessary to maintain an adequate heart rate.)

One or two mediastinal drainage catheters are inserted; pleural drainage tubes are unnecessary unless the pleura has been opened. Occasionally the superior portion of the pericardium is closed to prevent extensive adhesions from developing. This is helpful in patients for whom there is a high probability of reoperation at a later time. Although the pericardium generally is left open (to preclude the risk of tamponade when mediastinal blood cannot drain properly), it may be partially closed over the base of the heart and the great vessels so that fewer adhesions form after surgery. This may be considered in patients who are expected to require reoperation, such as young patients or recipients of bioprostheses who have a greater than 10- to 15-year life expectancy.

Postoperative Considerations

COMPLICATIONS

Complications of mitral valve surgery are related to valve repair or replacement, the insertion and function of the particular prosthesis, and patient factors that affect the outcome of surgery. Patients with long-standing mitral valve disease preoperatively, for example, may be at increased risk for multiorgan dysfunction postoperatively as a result of their chronic low cardiac output. These patients tend to be sicker and may not recover as rapidly as the patient with acute onset valvular dysfunction.

Table 11-5 lists complications associated with mitral valve surgery. Among the most serious complications are valve thrombosis and cardiac free wall rupture. Cardiac valve thrombosis may be treated initially with thrombolytic therapy (Manteiga and others, 1998). Rupture of the left ventricle may occur intraoperatively (usually after the termination of cardiopulmonary bypass, when the heart resumes its pressure-volume work and is loaded with blood) or in the immediate postoperative period. Rupture is associated with a high

---

TABLE 11-5
Postoperative Complications of Mitral Valve Surgery

COMPLICATION	INTERVENTIONS
Rupture of the left ventricular free wall or the atrioventricular groove	If chest is still open, reinstitute cardiopulmonary bypass to decompress the heart and control hemorrhage with fingers. If prosthesis is implicated in rupture, replace with different valve. Repair perforation with heavy suture in manner similar to repair of left ventricular aneurysm.
	If chest is closed, sudden massive chest tube drainage will be noted. Perform immediate sternotomy and proceed as above.
	Repair may compromise circumflex coronary, producing ischemic changes or infarction. Coronary artery bypass grafting should be anticipated.
Prosthetic failure; thrombosed occluder (disk or ball) or degeneration of bioprosthesis	Cessation of valve noise alerts the patient or clinician. Sternotomy, assessment of valve, and replacement are required; thrombolytic therapy may be initially attempted.
	If bioprosthesis is damaged, a new murmur will appear with elevated pulmonary pressures. Replacement is indicated.
Prosthetic dehiscence; perivalvular leak	A new murmur with elevated pulmonary pressures alerts the clinician. Surgical exploration may necessitate insertion of additional stitches or prosthetic replacement. Hemolysis producing a decreased hematocrit may be apparent.
Prosthetic valve endocarditis	Elevated temperature and positive blood cultures alert the clinician. Valve replacement often indicated, especially if annulus is affected.
Anticoagulation-related hemorrhage	Readjust warfarin dosage; recommend more frequent lab studies until prothrombin time is within acceptable range.
	Refer for additional teaching and family support.
Thromboembolism, embolism related to surgical intervention	Anticoagulation dosage adjusted to prolong prothrombin time. Neurologic deficits should be reported. Meticulous Intraoperative cleaning of instruments and removal of particulate debris can reduce risk of surgical emboli.
Residual regurgitation after valve repair	Echocardiographic assessment, new murmurs, or congestive heart failure may indicate suboptimal repair. Surgical exploration required to revise repair or perform valve replacement.

Modified from Ansell J, Hirsh J, Wenger NK: Management or oral anticoagulant therapy, 1999, American Heart Association [On-line]. Available: http://www.americanheart.org/scientific/slideset/oat/index/html (accessed April 19, 2001). Fullerton DA, Grover FL: Complications from cardiac prostheses: I. prosthetic valve endocarditis; Campbell DN, Grover FL: Complications from cardiac prostheses: II. thrombosis and thromboembolisms of prosthetic cardiac valves and extracardiac prostheses. In Sabiston DC, Spencer FC, editors: *Surgery of the chest,* ed 6, Philadelphia, 1995, WB Saunders.

mortality; a number of causes have been suggested. Anatomic factors may predispose the ventricle to injury (e.g., ischemic or weakened myocardium), or rupture may be related to the technique of native valve excision and prosthetic valve insertion (Bjork, Henze, and Rodriguez, 1977; Karlson, Ashraf, and Berger, 1988; Seifert and Speir, 1990). Other factors may include excessive tilting of the ventricle during venting (which pushes the valve struts into the ventricular endocardial wall) and aggressive manipulation of rigid suction or venting catheters. When the complication is detected (by the appearance of sudden, massive hemorrhage), the location of the rupture guides the type of repair employed (Figs. 11-32 and 11-33).

In the postoperative period clinicians should be aware that external chest compressions during cardiac resuscitation may produce injury as a result of the prosthesis' pushing against the ventricle and causing it to rupture. Immediate sternotomy is performed to repair the ventricle.

Complications related to prostheses, such as anticoagulation-related hemorrhage and endocarditis, may be modified by the patient's and family's ability to anticipate problems and seek help when signs and symptoms arise (see Table 11-5). Patient teaching is critical in avoiding many of these risks (Ansell, Hirsh, and Wenger, 1999).

References

Acar C and others: Homograft replacement of the mitral valve: graft selection, technique of implantation, and results in forty-three patients, *J Thorac Cardiovasc Surg* 111(2):367, 1996.

Akins CW: Mechanical cardiac valvular prostheses, *Ann Thorac Surg* 52:161, 1991.

Ansell J, Hirsh J, Wenger NK: Management or oral anticoagulant therapy, 1999, American Heart Association [On-line]. Available: http://www.americanheart.org/Scientific/slideset/oat/index/html (accessed April 19, 2001).

Bailey CP: The surgical treatment of mitral stenosis (mitral commissurotomy), *Dis Chest* 15:377, 1949.

Barlow JB: Idiopathic (degenerative) and rheumatic mitral valve prolapse: historical aspects and an overview, *J Heart Valve Dis* 1(2):163, 1992.

Bjork VO, Henze A, Rodriguez L: Left ventricular rupture as a complication of mitral valve replacement, *J Thorac Cardiovasc Surg* 73(1)14, 1977.

Braunwald E: Valvular heart disease. In Braunwald E, Zipes DP, Libby P, editors: *Heart disease: a textbook of cardiovascular medicine* ed 6, Philadelphia, 2001, WB Saunders.

Byrne JG and others: Minimally invasive direct access mitral valve surgery, *Semin Thorac Cardiovasc Surg* 11(3):212, 1999.

Campbell DN, Grover FL: Complications from cardiac prostheses: II. Thrombosis and thromboembolisms of prosthetic cardiac valves and extracardiac prostheses. In Sabiston DC, Spencer FC, editors: *Surgery of the chest,* ed 6, Philadelphia, 1995, WB Saunders.

Campbell WN, Tsai W, Mispireta LA: Evaluation of the practice of routine culturing of native valves during valve replacement surgery, *Ann Thorac Surg* 69(2):548, 2000.

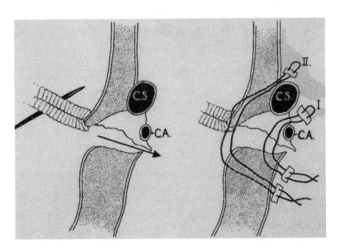

FIGURE 11-32 Type I rupture of the left ventricle occurs at the atrioventricular junction. The repair is performed with a double layer of buttressed sutures penetrating the left atrial wall on each side of the coronary sinus and left ventricular myocardium. The circumflex coronary artery is avoided; sutures are passed through the prosthetic sewing ring. Occasionally the prosthesis must be replaced with another that is smaller or of a different configuration. (From Bjork VO, Henze A, Rodriquez L: Left ventricular rupture as a complication of mitral valve replacement, *J Thorac Cardiovasc Surg* 73:14, 1977.)

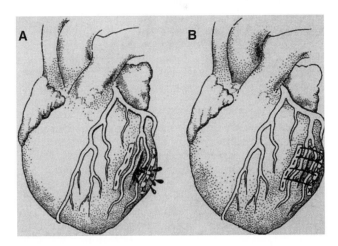

FIGURE 11-33 Type II rupture of the left ventricle occurs in the ventricular wall near the location of an excised papillary muscle. The repair consists of a first layer of isolated mattress sutures buttressed with felt strips **(A)**. These may not be able to hold friable myocardium. **B,** A second, reinforcing layer of isolated over-and-over sutures may be required to achieve hemostasis. (Note the similarity to conventional repair of left ventricular aneurysm [see Chapter 10]). (From Bjork VO, Henze A, Rodriquez L: Left ventricular rupture as a complication of mitral valve replacement, *J Thorac Cardiovasc Surg* 73:14, 1977.)

Carpentier A: Cardiac valve surgery—the "French correction," *J Thorac Cardiovasc Surg* 86(3):323, 1983.

Carpentier A and others: A new reconstructive operation for correction of mitral and tricuspid insufficiency, *J Thorac Cardiovasc Surg* 61(1):1, 1971.

Chitwood, Jr, WR: Video-assisted and robotic mitral valve surgery: toward an endoscopic surgery, *Semin Thorac Cardiovasc Surg* 11(3):194, 1999.

Cohn LH: Mitral valve repair, *Op Tech Thorac Cardiovasc Surg* 3(2):109, 1998.

Cooley DA: Commentary on Arom KV and Emery RW: alternative incisions for cardiac surgery. In Yim AP and others, editors: *Minimal access cardiothoracic surgery,* Philadelphia, 2000, WB Saunders.

Cutler EC, Levine SA: Cardiotomy and valvulotomy for mitral stenosis: experimental observations and clinical notes concerning an operated case with recovery. *Boston Med Surg J* 188:1023, 1923.

David TE: Chordal replacement with expanded polytetrafluoroethylene sutures in mitral valve repair, *Op Tech Thorac Cardiovasc Surg* 3(2):126, 1998.

David TE and others: Long-term results of mitral valve repair for myxomatous disease with and without chordal replacement with expanded polytetrafluoroethylene, *J Thorac Cardiovasc Surg* 115(6):1279, 1998.

Doty DB, Dilip KA, Millar RC: Mitral valve replacement with homograft and Maze III procedure, *Ann Thorac Surg* 69(3):739, 2000.

Duarte IG and others: In vivo hemodynamic, histologic, and antimineralization characteristics of the Mosaic bioprosthesis, *Ann Thorac Surg* 71(1):92, 2001.

Dubost C and others: Nouvelle technique d'ouverture de l'oreillette gauche en chirurgie a coeur ouvert: l'abord bi-auriculaire transseptal, *Techn Chirurg* 74(30):1607, 1966.

Duran CG and others: Conservative operation for mitral insufficiency: critical analysis supported by postoperative hemodynamic studies of 72 patients, *J Thorac Cardiovasc Surg* 79(3):326, 1980.

Finkelmeier BA: *Cardiothoracic surgical nursing,* ed 2, Philadelphia, 2000, JB Lippincott.

Fullerton DA, Grover FL: Complications from cardiac prostheses: I. prosthetic valve endocarditis. In Sabiston DC, Spencer FC, editors: *Surgery of the chest,* ed 6, Philadelphia, 1995, WB Saunders.

Gillinov AM, Cosgrove DM: Minimally invasive mitral valve surgery: ministernotomy with extended transseptal approach, *Semin Thorac Cardiovasc Surg* 11(3)206, 1999.

Gillinov AM, Cosgrove DM: Mitral valve repair, *Op Tech Thorac Cardiovasc Surg* 3(2):95, 1998.

Gillinov AM, Casselman FP, Cosgrove DM: Minimally invasive heart valve surgery: operative technique and results. In Yim AP and others, editors: *Minimal access cardiothoracic surgery,* Philadelphia, 2000, WB Saunders.

Hammermeister K and others: Outcomes 15 years after valve replacement with a mechanical versus a bioprosthetic valve: final report of the Veterans Affairs randomized trial, *J Am Coll Cardiol* 36(4):1152, 2000.

Handa N and others: Outcome of valve repair and the Cox maze procedure for mitral regurgitation and associated atrial fibrillation, *J Thorac Cardiovasc Surg* 118(4):628, 1999.

Harkin DE and others: The surgical treatment of mitral stenosis: valvuloplasty. *N Engl J Med* 239:801, 1948.

Harlan BJ, Starr A, Harwin FM: *Manual of cardiac surgery,* vol 1, New York, 1980, Springer-Verlag.

Jackson JM, Thomas SJ: Valvular heart disease. In Kaplan JA, editor: *Cardiac anesthesia,* ed 4, Philadelphia, 1999, WB Saunders.

Karlson KJ, Ashraf MM, Berger RL: Rupture of left ventricle following mitral valve replacement, *Ann Thorac Surg* 46(5):590, 1988.

Kirklin JW, Barratt-Boyes BG: *Cardiac surgery: morphology, diagnostic criteria, natural history, techniques, results, and indications,* ed 2, New York, 1993, Churchill Livingstone.

Lefrak EA, Starr A: *Cardiac valve prosthesis,* New York, 1979, Appleton-Century-Crofts.

Lillehei CW and others: The surgical treatment of stenotic or regurgitant lesion of the mitral and aortic valves by direct vision utilizing a pump oxygenator, *J Thorac Surg* 35:154, 1958.

Loulmet DF and others: Less invasive techniques for mitral valve surgery, *J Thorac Cardiovasc Surg* 115(4)772, 1998.

Manteiga R and others: Short-course thrombolysis as the first line of therapy for cardiac valve thrombosis, *J Thorac Cardiovasc Surg* 115(4):780, 1998.

Mueller XM and others: Long-term results of mitral-aortic valve operations, *J Thorac Cardiovasc Surg* 115(6):1298, 1998.

Moon MR and others: Treatment of endocarditis with valve replacement: the question of tissue versus mechanical prosthesis, *Ann Thorac Surg* 71(4):1164, 2001.

Pezzella AT, Utley JR, Salm TJ: Operative approaches to the left atrium and mitral valve: an update, *Op Tech Thorac Cardiovasc Surg* 3(2):74, 1998.

Reichenspurner H, Boehm D, Reichart B: Minimally invasive mitral valve surgery using three-dimensional video and robotic assistance, *Semin Thorac Cardiovasc Surg* 11(3):235, 1999.

Sakai T and others: Distance between mitral anulus and papillary muscles: anatomic study in normal human hearts, *J Thorac Cardiovasc Surg* 118(4):636, 1999.

Samways DW: Cardiac peristalsis: its nature and effects, *Lancet* 1:927, 1898. In Lefrak EA, Starr A: *Cardiac valve prosthesis,* New York, 1979, Appleton-Century-Crofts.

Seifert PC: Cardiac surgery. In Rothrock JC: *Perioperative nursing care planning,* ed 2, St Louis, 1996, Mosby.

Seifert PC, Speir AM: Left ventricular rupture: a collaborative approach to emergency management, *AORN J* 51(3):714, 1990.

Starr A, Edwards ML: Mitral replacement: clinical experience with a ball-valve prosthesis, *Ann Surgery* 154:726, 1961.

Thourani VH and others: Ten-year trends in heart valve replacement operations, *Ann Thorac Surg* 70(2):448, 2000.

Vanermen H and others: Video-assisted port-access mitral valve surgery: from debut to routine surgery. Will trocar-port-access cardiac surgery ultimately lead to robotic cardiac surgery? *Semin Thorac Cardiovasc Surg* 11(3):223, 1999.

Vongpatanasin W, Hillis LD, Lange RA: Prosthetic heart valves, *N Engl J Med* 335(6):407, 1996.

Waldhausen JA, Pierce WS, Campbell DB: *Surgery of the chest,* ed 6, St Louis, 1996, Mosby.

Werly JA, Crawford MH: Choosing a prosthetic heart valve, *Cardiol Clin* 16:491, 1998.

Westaby S, Bosher C: *Landmarks in cardiac surgery,* Oxford, UK, 1997, Isis Medical Media.

12

Aortic Valve Surgery

Diseases of the aortic valve present many anatomic and clinical syndromes. Aortic insufficiency with a dilated left ventricle in failure has been totally refractory to surgical intervention. Because of the clear diagnosis and grave prognosis of these patients, we are not only eager to intervene but have an obligation to undertake whatever we may regard as the most reasonable therapy. It is to this group that we address ourselves here.

Dwight E. Harken, MD, and associates, 1960 (p. 744)

As always, we need to listen to our patients. We also need to look directly at the valve.

Catherine M. Otto, MD, 2000 (p. 654)

When Harken and his co-workers (1960) performed the first successful subcoronary aortic valve replacement with a ball valve prosthesis (Fig. 12-1), they introduced an era of rapid development in the treatment of aortic valve disease. The stage for this accomplishment had been set during the previous decade.

In the year before Gibbon (1954) introduced the first successful clinical application of a mechanical heart-lung machine, Hufnagel and Harvey (1953) had inserted a prosthetic ball valve (Fig. 12-2) into the descending aorta of a patient with aortic regurgitation. Although providing only partial hemodynamic relief, this accomplishment stimulated further research into the development of valvular prostheses, which led to Harken's (Harken and others, 1960) subcoronary aortic valve replacement. Ironically, Harken and Starr (Starr and Edwards, 1961) independently developed the ball valve at the same time, and each used his own prosthesis to perform the first aortic valve replacement and the first mitral valve replacement, respectively.

Although there have been many technologic and scientific advances since Harken's (and others') early achievement, Otto (2000) reminds clinicians 40 years later that listening to the patient remains a cornerstone of therapy.

Anatomy and Physiology of the Aortic Valve

The aortic valve (see Figs. 8-7 and 8-12), normally tricuspid morphologically, is located at the junction of the left ventricle and the origin of the ascending aorta (the aortic root). The valve is composed of fibrous leaflets that insert into a fibrous annular skeleton and the sinuses of Valsalva, which are slightly dilated pouches between the valve cusps and the aortic wall. The valve annulus and attached leaflets are located below the openings to the right and left coronary arteries. The area between adjacent cusps is called a *commissure*. The sinuses of Valsalva and corresponding valve cusps are respectively named after the right and left coronary arteries that originate within the sinuses. The third cusp, containing no coronary os, is named the *noncoronary cusp* (see Chapter 8).

The aortic valve lies in an oblique plane with the left coronary cusp slightly superior to the right coronary cusp. This explains why during surgery prosthetic valves appear slightly tilted when they are implanted into the aortic root (Titus and Edwards, 1991).

Opening of the valve occurs when left ventricular pressure exceeds aortic pressure. The construction of the valve leaflets is such that the free edge of each cusp approaches the aortic wall, thereby allowing maximum opening of the orifice. This is enhanced by an increase in the diameter of the aortic root during systole. The pressure difference between the ventricle and the aorta disappears by midsystole, and forward blood flow is maintained by the effect of mass acceleration. On reversal of the flow, the cusps fall back and their edges contact each other to close the valve and prevent backflow (Braunwald, 2001).

The skeleton of the aortic valve is in fibrous continuity with the anterior leaflet of the mitral valve (which forms part of the ventricular outflow tract) and with the membranous septum. Conduction tissue lies below the right coronary cusp. It is essential that surgeons and perioperative nurses exercise great caution during operations performed on either valve so that they can avoid

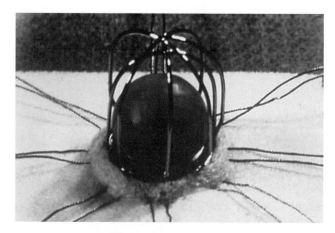

FIGURE 12-1 Original Harkin caged ball valve. The sewing ring could be trimmed to facilitate its insertion into the aortic root. (Courtesy Baxter Healthcare Corp., Edwards CVS Div., Santa Ana, Calif.)

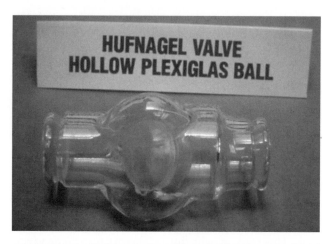

FIGURE 12-2 Hufnagel valve. Although this valve was placed in the descending aorta and did not "replace" the aortic valve, it did show that foreign material could be implanted in the bloodstream without disastrous effects. (Courtesy Baxter Healthcare Corp., Edwards CVS Div., Santa Ana, Calif.)

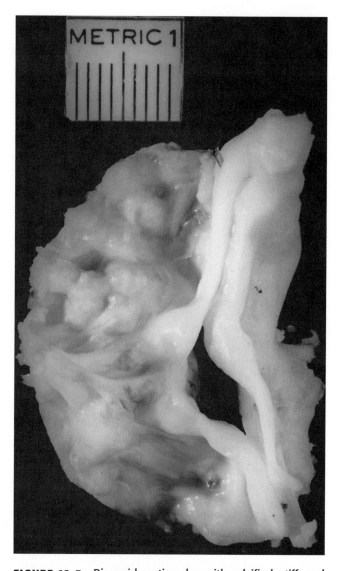

FIGURE 12-3 Bicuspid aortic valve with calcified, stiffened leaflets producing stenosis. Note the greatly reduced orifice area. (Courtesy William C. Roberts, MD; Michael Spencer, photographer.)

injury to the conduction pathways and to the structural components of the adjacent valve.

Aortic Valve Disease

ETIOLOGY AND PATHOLOGY

Aortic valve stenosis or regurgitation may be the result of a number of conditions that affect the valve leaflets and the annulus. Stenotic lesions obstruct left ventricular outflow and may be located at the valve level, below the valve (subvalvular), or above the valve (supravalvular).

Congenital malformations

Congenital malformations are a common cause of aortic stenosis, with the bicuspid aortic valve (Fig. 12-3) being the most common cause of aortic stenosis. Bicuspid valves are rarely symptomatic at birth, but the turbulent flow across the leaflets produces fibrosis, stiffening, and calcification, which leads to symptomatic stenosis generally in the sixth decade. Aortic regurgitation may be associated with a bicuspid valve, but this is less common (Roberts, 1970; Perloff, 1997).

Unicuspid and dome-shaped valves are rare in adults. Occasionally a patient may have a unicuspid valve that goes undetected until calcification and fibrotic degen-

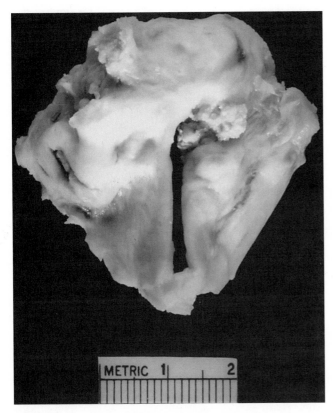

FIGURE 12-4 Stenotic unicuspid aortic valve with fibrosed leaflets. Note the calcium particles. (Courtesy William C. Roberts, MD; Michael Spencer, photographer.)

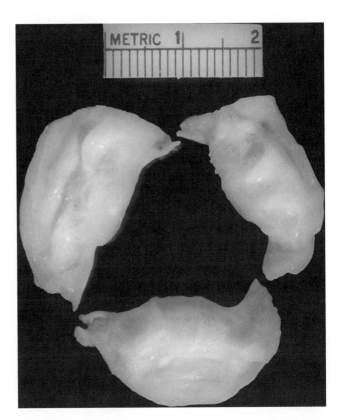

FIGURE 12-5 Rheumatic trileaflet (e.g., morphologically normal) aortic valve. The thickened, glistened, and smooth leaflet are typical of rheumatic changes. (Courtesy William C. Roberts, MD; Michael Spencer, photographer.)

eration produce symptoms (Fig. 12-4). Severe forms usually cause immediate stenotic symptoms in early life; valvotomy is performed to enlarge the orifice.

Rheumatic fever

Rheumatic fever continues to be a significant etiologic factor in aortic valve disease. Inflammatory changes affect the aortic valve in a manner similar to that of the mitral valve, although it occurs less frequently. Granulation tissue and scarring produce contracted leaflets with rolled edges (Fig. 12-5). These changes make the valve more susceptible to degeneration from atherosclerosis and calcium deposition. Eventually there is stiffening of the cusps and fusion of the commissures, producing a stenotic orifice. The rheumatic process also may destroy fibrous tissue within the annulus, which can lead to annular dilation and regurgitation through the incompetent valve. Mixed lesions occur in fibrotic leaflets that both restrict forward flow and fail to prevent backward flow.

Senile calcific aortic stenosis

With the decline of acute rheumatic fever in the United States and a growing geriatric population, the predom-

inant cause of aortic stenosis has shifted from inflammatory lesions to degenerative lesions associated with aging (Rosenhek and others, 2000). These valves are calcified heavily but normally have a tricuspid configuration (Fig. 12-6).

Bacterial endocarditis

Bacterial endocarditis is an increasingly important etiologic factor in the development of aortic valve disease. It may occur on a structurally normal valve but more often affects rheumatically scarred or congenitally malformed aortic valves. *Staphylococcus aureus* is the most common organism. Vegetations and thrombus developing on the leaflets may break off and embolize to the heart, brain, or other organs, and they may cause valvular obstruction. However, the infectious process more often produces valvular incompetence from destruction of the valve and supporting structures. If there is erosion or perforation of the leaflets (Fig. 12-7), acute regurgitation occurs with rapid hemodynamic deterioration. Especially virulent cases of endocarditis are seen among intravenous drug users who use unsterile needles (Glower, 1995).

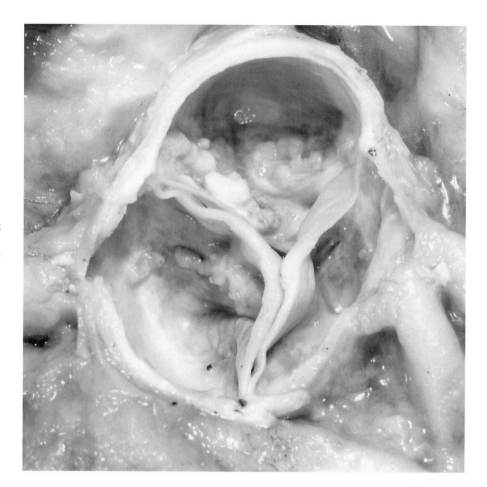

FIGURE 12-6 Degenerative calcific stenosis of a trileaflet aortic valve. (Courtesy William C. Roberts, MD; Michael Spencer, photographer.)

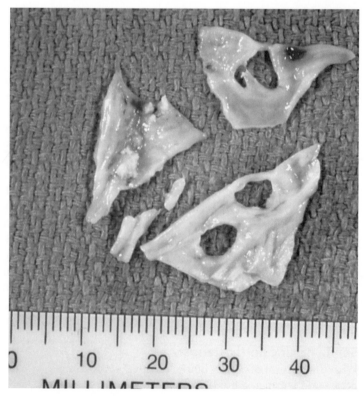

FIGURE 12-7 Perforated aortic valve leaflets resulting from bacterial endocarditis. The patient had acute aortic insufficiency. (Courtesy Edward A. Lefrak, MD.)

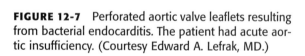

Marfan's syndrome

Chronic or acute regurgitation in an aortic valve with apparently normal leaflets occurs with annular dilation associated with Marfan's syndrome. This is a generalized connective tissue disorder that weakens the wall of the aorta, producing dilation and aneurysmal formation of the annulus, the sinuses of Valsalva, and the ascending aorta (see Chapter 14). Acute intimal tearing and dissection of the aorta stretches the supporting structures of the valve in such a way that the leaflets are unable to coapt.

Similar degenerative changes appear in some patients who do not have Marfan's syndrome. This is termed a *forme fruste* of the syndrome.

Other conditions

Trauma. Aortic insufficiency may be caused by blunt trauma or extreme muscular exertion, which can rupture or perforate the leaflets. Frequently this occurs in a previously diseased valve (Mattox, Estrera, and Wall, 2001).

Tertiary syphilis. Syphilitic aortitis, once a major cause of aortic root and annular dilation, has declined significantly since the introduction of antimicrobial therapy (Westaby, 1997).

PATHOPHYSIOLOGY

Aortic stenosis

Gradual, chronic obstruction to left ventricular outflow resulting from congenital or acquired aortic stenosis creates an increasing pressure load on the left ventricle (Fig. 12-8). The ventricle must work harder to generate

a pressure higher than the aortic pressure in order to propel blood through the narrowed orifice (afterload) into the systemic circulation. Ventricular muscle is able to maintain a relatively normal cardiac output by the compensatory mechanism of concentric hypertrophy.

Hypertrophy develops as a result of the increased energy expenditure demanded of each cardiac cell. Pressure overloading stimulates the myocyte to produce new contractile proteins so that these energy demands can be met. Individual cells enlarge, but the overall number of cells, as well as the capillary network that replenishes their energy resources, remain constant. Although the capillary-to-myocyte ratio is the same, the distances between them is increased in proportion to the degree of cellular hypertrophy. This is most evident in the deeper myocardial layers of the subendocardium and papillary muscles, which are particularly vulnerable to ischemia. Even pharmacologic coronary vasodilation fails to perfuse the subendocardium adequately, further jeopardizing these cells. The situation is aggravated by increased wall stress (a determinant of myocardial oxygen consumption) in the severely hypertrophied heart. Compounding the problem is the reduced diastolic compliance associated with the thickened ventricle. Thus when the ventricle becomes stiff, diastolic filling (preload) is impaired (Rosenhek and others, 2000).

The ventricle cannot compensate indefinitely. Eventually the reduction in energy-producing mitochondria within the cells and the increased distance between capillaries and the interior of the myocyte produce an adverse metabolic environment.

Although cardiac output can be maintained for a considerable period in aortic stenosis, derangements in afterload, preload, and contractility eventually produce heart failure. Left ventricular dilation occurs, which predisposes the heart to left-sided failure and left atrial enlargement. Right-sided heart failure eventually develops as backward volume creates increased pulmonary pressure, which cannot be accommodated by the low-pressure right-sided heart circuit. Contractility of both ventricles decreases, and myocardial cell death can occur without treatment (Berne and Levy, 2001).

The cardinal symptoms of aortic stenosis are syncope, angina pectoris, and dyspnea (Table 12-1). These are related respectively to insufficient blood flow to the brain and the heart and to impaired left ventricular function. Concomitant coronary artery disease exacerbates anginal episodes. Ventricular decompensation results in pulmonary congestion and dyspnea. Exercise-induced fatigue is associated with the reduction in cardiac output. Nonspecific symptoms include dizziness, palpitations, and fatigue. Symptoms usually become apparent when the valve

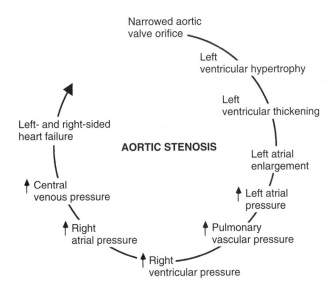

FIGURE 12-8 Pathophysiology of aortic stenosis. (From Kinney MR and others: *Andreoli's comprehensive cardiac care,* ed 8, St Louis, 1996, Mosby.)

TABLE **12-1**
Signs, Symptoms, and Findings of Aortic Valve Disease

AORTIC STENOSIS	AORTIC REGURGITATION (INSUFFICIENCY)
Signs Powerful, heaving PMI to left and below MCL Systolic thrill over aortic area, sternal notch Slowly rising carotid pulse BP normal or systolic BP normal with high diastolic reading Harsh, midsystolic murmur over sternum or apex	**CHRONIC** Hyperdynamic PMI to left and below MCL Forceful apical impulse displaced to left and down Prominent, rapidly rising and collapsing carotid pulse Wide pulse pressure with diastolic BP less than 60 mm Hg Faint diastolic murmur along left sternal border **ACUTE** Weakness Congestive failure Pulmonary edema Tachycardia Short diastolic murmur Hypotension
Symptoms Syncope Angina pectoris Exertional dyspnea Fatigue Paroxysmal nocturnal dyspnea Dizziness Palpitations Sudden death	**CHRONIC** Orthopnea Atypical chest pain Exertional dyspnea Palpitations Paroxysmal nocturnal dyspnea Nocturnal angina with diaphoresis **ACUTE** Dyspnea
Chest X-Ray Film Prominent ascending aorta (poststenotic dilation) Calcification on valve Concentric LV hypertrophy Pulmonary congestion	LV enlargement Pulmonary congestion
Electrocardiogram LV hypertrophy Ventricular tachycardia Sinus bradycardia	LV hypertrophy
Echocardiography Persistent echoes from obstructed flow Poor leaflet movement LV hypertrophy Poststenotic dilation of aorta Increased velocity through valve Pressure gradient between LV and aorta	Diastolic vibrations of anterior leaflet of MV and septum Vegetations on leaflets Regurgitant flow mapped (color Doppler)
Cardiac Catheterization Confirms valve lesion Assesses LV function Detects coronary artery disease, MV problems Measures valve orifice, pressure gradient	Assesses degree of regurgitation, LV and MV function, PA pressures Detects coronary artery disease (less common with AI)

AI, Aortic insufficiency; *BP,* blood pressure, *LA,* left atrium; *LV,* left ventricle; *MCL,* midclavicular line; *MV,* mitral valve; *PA,* pulmonary artery; *PMI,* point of maximal impulse.
Modified from Braunwald E, Zipes DP, Libby P, editors: *Heart disease: a textbook of cardiovascular medicine* ed 6, Philadelphia, 2001, WB Saunders.

orifice area is less than 1 cm², and severe symptoms are seen with an orifice area of less than 0.5 cm². The interval between the discovery of a systolic murmur and the appearance of symptoms can vary from 1 month to 10 years (Glower, 1995).

The appearance of symptoms is an ominous sign, and surgical valve replacement is strongly recommended (Rosenhek and others, 2000); once symptoms occur, the 2-year survival rate is below 50% (Otto, 2000). Appropriate management of *asymptomatic* aortic stenosis is less clear cut. The incidence of sudden death without preceding symptoms and the potential risk of irreversible myocardial damage (Braunwald, 2001) suggest that early elective surgery may be prudent. However, concerns about the risks of valve surgery and the potential complications associated with valve prostheses complicate the decision to operate. Rosenhek and colleagues (2000) attempted to identify predictors of outcome that would facilitate the timing of surgery. Their findings suggest that although surgery in asymptomatic patients may be delayed until symptoms develop, there is great variability among patients.

Asymptomatic patients with very severe gradients (100 mm Hg), moderate to severe valvular calcification (on echocardiogram), and evidence of a rapid increase in the velocity of the jet of blood squirting through the stenosed valve may be at increased risk and should be seriously considered for elective surgery (Rosenhek and others, 2000; Banning and Hall, 1997). Otto (2000) also suggests consideration of surgery for asymptomatic patients who live in areas remote from medical care or who may anticipate a long waiting time for elective surgery.

Other forms of left ventricular outflow tract obstruction

Subvalvular impedance to outflow may also be caused by asymmetric hypertrophy of the ventricular septum, which protrudes into the left ventricular outflow tract (LVOT). The condition, often referred to as *idiopathic hypertrophic subaortic stenosis* (IHSS), is now more commonly known as *hypertrophic cardiomyopathy* (HCM). It is probably an inherited disorder, but it does occur in patients without a family history. Medical therapy initially consists of beta-adrenergic blocking medications to lower ventricular contractility and pharmacologic control of frequently associated dysrhythmias. Surgery is indicated when there is a significant left ventricular-aortic gradient and symptoms persist despite medical treatment (Hazinski, 1999).

Septal hypertrophy often is associated with systolic anterior motion (SAM) of the aortic leaflet of the mitral valve; the leaflet protrudes toward the septal bulge, further obstructing flow (Kirklin and Barratt-Boyes,

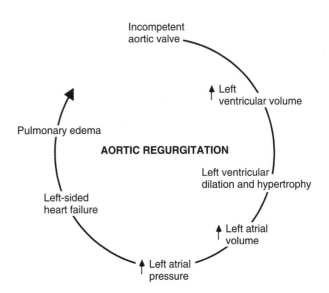

FIGURE 12-9 Pathophysiology of aortic regurgitation/insufficiency. (From Kinney MR and others: *Andreoli's comprehensive cardiac care,* ed 8, St Louis, 1996, Mosby.)

1993; Alpert, Sabik, and Cosgrove, 1998). Surgery for this problem is discussed in this chapter.

Aortic insufficiency

Aortic insufficiency is the result of a primary valve disorder or aortic root disease. The volume overload associated with mild, chronic aortic insufficiency in a majority of cases can be tolerated for almost two decades before the patient becomes symptomatic because the heart gradually dilates to compensate for the additional burden placed on it (Fig. 12-9). Regurgitant aortic volume is added to blood coming from the left atrium during diastole. As end-diastolic volume increases (preload), the left ventricle contracts more forcefully to expel the blood volume. This chronic overload state stimulates the eventual development of left ventricular hypertrophy.

Left ventricular decompensation occurs, and increased chamber pressure is reflected backward to the left atrium, the pulmonary vasculature, and the right side of the heart (Abramczyk and Brown, 1996). Without timely surgical intervention, failure becomes irreversible. Patients with a severely compromised left ventricle preoperatively have a less favorable outcome.

In contrast to chronic aortic insufficiency, acute aortic insufficiency is poorly tolerated for several reasons. The normal-size left ventricle is incapable of accommodating the increased, regurgitant volume and ejecting it with each heartbeat (and increasing the cardiac output). The lowered diastolic pressure that results from volume regurgitating into the ventricle impairs coronary filling by lowering perfusion pressure. Heart failure rapidly ensues.

Diagnostic Evaluation of Aortic Valve Disease

Evaluation of the patient with aortic valve disease begins with the history and physical examination. Diagnosis often is made with the standard electrocardiogram (ECG) and chest x-ray film, although invasive and noninvasive imaging techniques (see Box 12-1) may provide additional detail useful to clinical decision making.

AORTIC STENOSIS

Cardiomegaly is not seen commonly in patients undergoing radiologic and electrocardiographic examinations unless severe valvular stenosis producing dilation is present. Cardiac size may appear normal, although valvular calcification and left ventricular hypertrophy are often apparent on chest x-ray films.

Echocardiography can identify the level of left ventricular outflow tract obstruction: supravalvular, valvular, or subvalvular. Supravalvular and subvalvular lesions are generally congenital in origin; most acquired lesions are at the valvular level. When obstruction is caused by asymmetric hypertrophy of the left ventricular septum, bulging septal tissue can be observed.

In elderly and hypertensive patients, a systolic ejection murmur may be the result of aortic sclerosis rather than significant aortic stenosis. Echocardiography can distinguish between the thickened but mobile leaflets of sclerosis and the relatively immobile cusps of the stenotic valve. Often the structure of the valve (e.g., bicuspid) can be determined, as well as left ventricular chamber and aortic root size, ventricular wall thickness, and other abnormalities. Regional and global left ventricular wall motion can be assessed with two-dimensional imaging.

The addition of color flow Doppler imaging allows quantification of the obstruction and measurement of the gradient, although cardiac catheterization–derived gradients may be more precise (Kern, 1999). The aortic valve area can be calculated with reasonable accuracy.

Cardiac catheterization is not necessary for the diagnosis of aortic stenosis but is mandatory for evaluating the presence and significance of coronary artery disease. There is a high incidence of coronary artery disease in adults, and the need for myocardial revascularization should be considered before valve replacement.

Cardiac catheterization also may be performed to assess left ventricular function and to measure the pressure gradient across the valve. Occasionally a severely obstructed aortic valve orifice does not allow retrograde passage of a catheter into the left ventricle for injection of dye (to visualize ventricular contractility) or measurement of systolic intraventricular pressure. In severe stenosis, pressure gradients may be 50 mm Hg or more between the left ventricle and the ascending aorta. To attain an aortic pressure of 100 mm Hg beyond the valvular obstruction, the ventricle must generate a pressure of 150 mm Hg. Absence of a significant gradient may not be benign, however; it can reflect a weakened left ventricle incapable of generating sufficient pressure.

AORTIC INSUFFICIENCY

Left ventricular enlargement (Fig. 12-10) with the apex displaced downward and to the left is commonly seen with x-ray examination. An enlarged ascending aorta also may be seen. Serial chest x-ray films are examined for increasing cardiac enlargement as an indication of the progression of the disease. The electrocardiogram shows signs of left ventricular hypertrophy. If atrial fibrillation is present (and not related to another disorder), it is usually a sign of elevated left ventricular end-diastolic pressure referred back to the left atrium and an indication of advanced disease.

Echocardiography is used to determine the size of the ventricle, assess left ventricular function, and estimate regurgitant flow. It is particularly valuable as a noninvasive method of serially following the patient's progress.

Cardiac catheterization is used to visualize the degree of reflux and associated pathologic conditions of the aortic root, other valves, and coronary arteries. Elevated pulmonary and ventricular pressures are important prognostic indicators and provide information about optimal timing of surgery. Unfortunately, deciding when to operate is less precise for aortic insufficiency than it is for aortic stenosis. The problem is compounded in the asymptomatic patient with severe aortic regurgitation because the degree of left ventricular impairment (an important predictor of survival) may be difficult to determine. However, surgery rarely

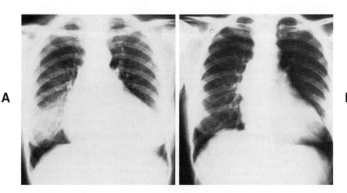

FIGURE 12-10 Aortic insufficiency. **A,** Preoperative chest x-ray film shows dilated left ventricle. **B,** Postoperatively the ventricle has returned to a more normal size and contour. (Courtesy Edward A. Lefrak, MD.)

is contraindicated, because death is virtually a certainty without it. To a great extent, timing of surgery for insufficiency still depends on clinical intuition, as well as quantitative data (Glower, 1995).

Surgery for Aortic Valve Disease

REPARATIVE TECHNIQUES

Techniques to repair the stenotic aortic valve have been more challenging than those for the mitral valve and are performed less commonly. This is caused in part by the more precise closing mechanism of the aortic valve. There is little overlap of the leaflets when the aortic valve is closed, as compared with the mitral leaflets when the mitral valve is closed. Thus imprecise repairs can produce regurgitation that is not well tolerated by the ventricle. Some patients, however, are unable to take anticoagulants or undergo reoperation for bioprosthetic failure or other valve-related complications. These patients may receive temporary benefit from balloon valvuloplasty (performed by the cardiologist in the cardiac catheterization laboratory) or surgical debridement under direct visualization. Allograft valve replacement may be an alternative.

Percutaneous balloon aortic valvuloplasty

With the success of percutaneous balloon aortic valvuloplasty (PBAV) in children with congenital aortic stenosis, attempts were made to employ the technique in adults with calcific aortic stenosis. Although early results showed promise, a restenosis rate approaching 50% has reduced the enthusiasm for this procedure. Currently PBAV is considered a short-term option for palliation in a limited number of adults who are debilitated or at high risk. Indications for PBAV include contraindications to valve surgery (such as very poor left ventricular function) and as a palliative measure for patients scheduled to undergo major noncardiac surgery. Age per se is not a contraindication. The expected outcome is a satisfactory reduction in the pressure gradient (less than 30 mm Hg) and an increase in the valve area (approximately 25% greater than baseline). Restenosis generally occurs within the first 6 to 12 months (Kern, 1999).

Surgical valvuloplasty

Attempting to improve on the results of closed balloon techniques and to avoid prosthetic replacement, surgeons have devised alternative procedures. Valvuloplasty for aortic regurgitation has been described by Cosgrove (Fraser and Cosgrove, 1994), Duran (1997), and David (1999), who have attempted to repair prolapsed aortic leaflets. With these techniques, excess cusp tissue is resected or plicated; annular dilation is repaired by reducing the annular circumference with pledgeted mattress sutures placed through the valve commissures (Fig. 12-11).

Aortic valvotomy

Valvotomy is performed under direct visualization in infants and children with congenital aortic stenosis. The fused leaflets are sharply divided with a knife.

AORTIC VALVE REPLACEMENT

Because reconstruction and repair of acquired lesions of the aortic valve have met with limited success, valve replacement is still considered the treatment of choice for aortic valve disease. Because of the risks associated with prosthetic valves, surgery may be delayed until symptoms warrant intervention but is performed before irreversible failure develops.

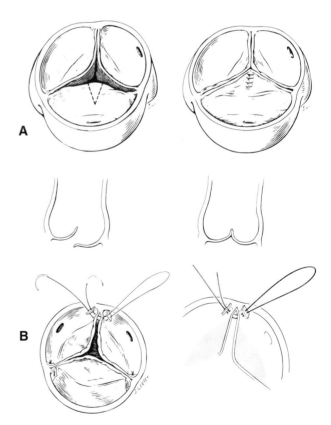

FIGURE 12-11 **A,** Triangular resection of the free edge of the prolapsing cusp results in normal leaflet size and coaptation. **B,** Annuloplasty performed by placement of horizontal mattress sutures buttressed with felt at each commissure. The suture goes through the annulus (but not the leaflet) into the outflow tract and back through the annulus. (From Cosgrove DM and others: Valvuloplasty for aortic insufficiency, *J Thorac Cardiovasc Surg* 102[4]:571, 1991.)

Timing of surgery and results

As noted previously, patients with symptomatic aortic stenosis are recommended for surgery; patients who have aortic stenosis but are asymptomatic are encouraged to have periodic echocardiographic examinations to monitor the degree of valvular calcification. Operative mortality for patients with good left ventricular function is 2% to 8% (Kirklin and Barratt-Boyes, 1993).

Optimal timing of surgery for aortic insufficiency is determined less easily because the severity of the lesion is more difficult to quantify, as compared with aortic stenosis; the effects of volume overloading (regurgitation) are less predictable than those associated with pressure overloading (stenosis). In patients with chronic aortic insufficiency who have minimal impairment of left ventricular (LV) function, mortality may be as low as 1% (Banning and Hall, 1997). If the ventricle is dilated and LV function is more significantly impaired, perioperative risk increases.

Other considerations affect the timing and subsequent success of surgery. A thorough dental assessment is performed, and abscessed or carious teeth are repaired or removed before surgery so that they are not an entry site for bacteria. Infections in other parts of the body are a strict contraindication to surgery and must be resolved before valve surgery is performed. Antiplatelet medications such as aspirin and dipyridamole and anticoagulants such as warfarin (Coumadin) (e.g., for patients with chronic atrial fibrillation) are discontinued preoperatively to reduce the incidence of excessive perioperative bleeding.

Prostheses and their selection

Aortic valve prostheses tend to have a less bulky sewing ring than their mitral prosthetic valve counterparts. They are constructed in this way to reduce as much as possible the amount of material that would take up space within the valve orifice. This provides greater flow through the opening of the prosthesis. Some porcine aortic valve manufacturers (who produce the modified orifice Hancock valve, for example) further modify the valve by removing the leaflet containing a muscle shelf (found in all pig aortic valves) and replacing it with a leaflet from another pig valve that does not have this restrictive leaflet. Thus two pig valves are necessary to produce these bioprostheses.

Unfortunately, all prosthetic valves have inherent disadvantages (see Box 11-6 and Table 11-5). The hemodynamic performance of a prosthesis is critical in aortic valve surgery, and the residual transvalvular gradients associated with prosthetic aortic valves can make selection of a suitable replacement prosthesis difficult. For example, an active lifestyle requires an increased cardiac output during exercise. This is hemodynamically significant, especially in patients with small aortic roots having annular diameters of 19 to 21 mm or less. Although a 19-mm prosthesis generally provides acceptable transvalvular blood flow, in large or very active persons the orifice of a 19-mm prosthesis may not allow sufficient stroke volume and cardiac output to meet tissue demands. (One could expect to see postoperative tachydysrhythmias as a compensatory mechanism for the decreased cardiac output.) With the further narrowing of the orifice from the presence of the prosthetic sewing ring, increasing the cardiac output requires greater ventricular work to overcome the pressure load. In these cases a significant residual pressure gradient restricts the potential effectiveness of valve replacement.

When the annulus is smaller than 19 mm, the surgeon may consider enlargement procedures so that a 19-mm or larger prosthetic valve can be implanted. A mechanical valve usually is selected in order to avoid reoperation, which is more likely with a bioprosthesis that can deteriorate over time.

In general, hemodynamic performance is acceptable for most currently available prostheses with an annular diameter of 25 mm or more. In the smaller annulus (23 mm or less), the excellent flow characteristics of the St. Jude Medical valve make it a popular prosthesis for many patients who can tolerate lifelong anticoagulation. In patients unable to take anticoagulants, a biologic valve is often the prosthesis of choice.

A newer bioprosthesis that combines the hemodynamic advantages of the allograft (see the following) with the universal availability of biologic prostheses is the unstented aortic root porcine tissue valve (Fig. 12-12). The prosthesis is made from an explanted aortic pig valve that is treated with a glutaraldehyde solution to fix the tissue and an antimineralization agent to retard leaflet calcification (Meyers, 1997). Covering the outer surface of the valve is a thin layer of fabric that facilitates suturing and handling of the prosthesis. Because there is

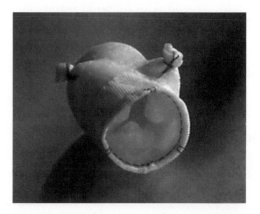

FIGURE 12-12 Stentless aortic porcine bioprosthesis. Note the retained coronary arteries. The prosthesis can be used to replace the aortic root or can be trimmed to replace the aortic valve alone. (Courtesy Medtronic, Inc.)

no stent, the functional opening of the stentless valve is larger than the orifice of a comparably sized stented valve and provides greater flow (David and others, 1998).

An unstented allograft (homograft) is also an option, and it may be preferable in the small aortic root because there is no sewing ring to reduce the size of the orifice. (*Allograft* is now the correct term for tissue from one person's body placed in another person. The term is used preferentially by the Food and Drug Administration to regulate these grafts, which were commonly known as *homografts*.)

Aortic valve allograft (homograft)

Patients requiring valve replacement but who are considered unsuitable candidates for insertion of a mechanical or biologic prosthesis may benefit from an aortic valve allograft (homograft) (Fig. 12-13; Box 12-1). Unstented aortic valve allografts are advantageous in small aortic roots because there is no sewing ring to decrease the size of the orifice. In addition, allografts do not require anticoagulation and are advantageous in patients with active aortic valve endocarditis (McGiffen and Kirklin, 1997).

Ross (1962; Box 12-2), Barratt-Boyes (1964), and O'Brien, McGriffin, and Stafford (1989), who laid the

---

BOX 12-1
Allografts (Homografts): Clinical Considerations

No emboli, turbulence, or hemolysis
Deterioration occurs gradually
Degeneration manifested at about 7 years
Incidence of degeneration uncertain
Slow process of degeneration; valve-related deaths rare
Patient survival better than with prosthestic valves
Satisfactory valve for children
Quality of life is excellent
May be immunologically active

Modified from Ross D: Application of homografts in clinical surgery, *J Cardiac Surg* 1(3 suppl):175, 1987.

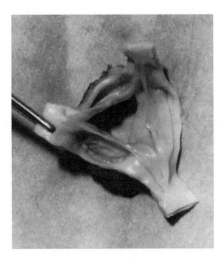

FIGURE 12-13 Unstented aortic valve allograft (homograft). The attached aorta and subvalvular tissue have been removed by the surgeon. Stented allografts are mounted on a frame. (Courtesy CryoLife, Inc., Kennesaw, Ga.)

BOX 12-2
RN First Assistant Considerations During Aortic Valve Surgery

When retracting aorta, be especially cautious to avoid lacerating aortic wall, coronary ostia, and adjacent structures.

If handheld coronary ostial cannulas are used for cardioplegia, ensure that no air is present in tubing before infusion; prepare cannulas for infusion (e.g., flush) when ECG activity is noted or surgeon requests it; left coronary ostial cannula is usually shaped like an L, and right coronary ostial cannula is usually shaped like a J.

When retroplegia cardioplegia is used, anticipate back bleeding from the coronary ostia and the need to suction more frequently (unless there is a pause in suturing while cardioplegia solution is given).

Adjust position of aortic root retractors as stitches are placed into each commissure.

Assist in keeping valve suture pledgets aligned.

Keep sutures from tangling with use of suture holder, suture tags, or other method per protocol.

Keep running count of stitches in each leaflet (or annular segment), as well as total count.

Use moist sponges to clean instruments, suction tips, and so on, of loose calcium particles or other debris.

Use open-tip suction to remove calcium pieces and other debris; suction frequently and whenever loose material is noted in operative field; alert surgeon to presence of material.

Keep bioprostheses moist with frequent saline irrigation (with bulb syringe); prevent drying out.

Watch for calcium particles in crevices of aorta or aortic root (especially where surgeon's view may be obscured) and on tips of instruments and suction catheters. Do not hesitate to wipe tips of instruments used by team members when debris is present (and before instruments are inserted into surgical site).

If heart must be elevated to inspect coronary anastomosis suture lines, do so cautiously to avoid puncturing ventricle with prosthetic struts.

If patch enlargement is performed, maintain alignment of material while surgeon cuts and shapes patch and during insertion into aortic root.

If eye cautery (battery powered) is used to create an opening in prosthetic graft for anastomosis, remove all pieces of excised graft material.

When implanting a Starr-Edwards 1260 aortic ball-and-cage prosthesis, ball poppet can be removed to facilitate insertion of stitches; ball should be stored in safe place until needed; it is easily reinserted into cage after stitches are tied and cut.

When surgeon is tying annular stitches, use Freer or similar instrument to separate sutures.

After the heart resumes beating, monitor the ECG for signs of ischemia, which may be an indication of coronary ostial obstruction by the prosthesis.

groundwork for the use of allografts, stress the excellent long-term results and advocate the use of these grafts in all patients with pathologic conditions of the aortic valve and root. One of the few exceptions is the elderly patient in whom a bioprosthesis would give a comparable result.

Despite its advantages, the aortic valve allograft is not commonly used because of the technical difficulty of insertion (compared with prosthetic valve replacement), less convenient availability (compared with prostheses), and concerns about allograft failure (McGiffin and Kirklin, 1997).

Pulmonary allografts (Fig. 12-14), another graft source, also may be used. Both aortic and pulmonary allografts are procured from cadavers without a history of communicable disease, disseminated malignancy, diabetes, hypertension, hyperlipidemia, or previous sternotomy. The grafts are obtained from cadaver hearts under sterile conditions in an operating room, subjected to microbial testing, treated with nutrient media

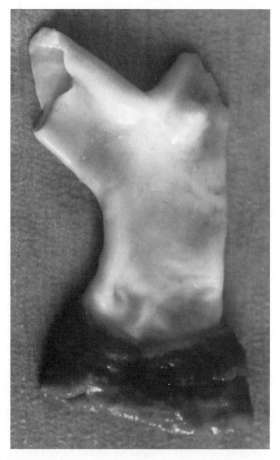

FIGURE 12-14 Pulmonary allograft (homograft) containing the pulmonary valve, main pulmonary artery, and proximal portion of the bifurcation of the right and left pulmonary arteries. (Courtesy CryoLife, Inc., Kennesaw, Ga.)

and antibiotics, and cryopreserved in a special freezer. Before freezing, the leaflets of the valve are assessed for proper function and the diameter of the annulus is measured. The allograft is sealed in a plastic bag and frozen in liquid nitrogen. Long-term storage is maintained at approximately −196° C (O'Brien, McGriffin, and Stafford, 1989). When needed for surgery, an array of grafts in different sizes is transported in a portable freezer. Once the appropriate graft is selected, it is thawed and implanted.

Pulmonary autografts also are being used more often. The patient's pulmonary valve may be used to replace the aortic valve, and a pulmonary allograft is inserted to replace the autograft. Advantages of the allograft include excellent hemodynamics, nonthrombogenicity, and a lower incidence of postoperative infection. They are especially suitable for use in young women and children and may be advantageous for patients with recurrent endocarditis, in whom it is preferable to avoid synthetic foreign material. A disadvantage may be long-term durability, but Chambers and colleagues (1997) describe excellent results 20 years after surgery. Although primary tissue failure does occur, the onset is not sudden, and it does not progress rapidly, as compared with some other bioprosthetic valves (Oury and Maxwell, 1997).

Patient teaching considerations
Teaching considerations for patients undergoing aortic valve surgery are based on the particular lesion, the type of surgery performed, and the impact that the disease and the treatment have on the patient (Table 12-2). As in all patients with valvular heart disease, the perioperative nurse should elicit the patient's understanding of the anticipated procedure and answer questions of the patient and family. Nurses explain that the procedure will be tailored to the patient's needs, with anatomic considerations often playing a decisive role. Assessing the patient's lifestyle and activity level is important because an active 80 year old, for example, may require a more hemodynamically satisfactory prosthesis than a sedentary 60 year old. Various options and reasons provided by the surgeon for the selection of one prosthesis over another can be clarified for the patient.

As with patients undergoing mitral valve replacement, the ability and desire to follow recommended therapeutic regimens must be evaluated. Anticoagulation-related hemorrhage and endocarditis should be discussed and safety measures identified (Abramczyk and Brown, 1996). Bioprosthetic failure, thrombosis of the disk occluder, and dehiscence also can occur. Laboratory follow-up is required to adjust warfarin levels and maintain prothrombin times within an acceptable range.

TABLE **12-2**
Standards of Nursing Care for Aortic Valve Surgery

NURSING DIAGNOSIS	PATIENT OUTCOME	NURSING ACTIONS
Anxiety related to disease, surgery, and postoperative events	Patient demonstrates reduced levels of anxiety that promote therapeutic regimen	Elicit questions and concerns about disease and proposed treatment Identify and reinforce effective coping mechanisms; respect some denial Provide comfort measures; identify perceived needs and expectations
Knowledge deficit related to inadequate knowledge of planned surgery and perioperative events	Patient demonstrates knowledge of physiologic and psychologic responses to aortic valve surgery	Determine patient's understanding of aortic valve disease; possible surgical interventions (aortic valve or root enlargement, valve replacement); types, benefits, and risks of prostheses; and preferences if any Determine patient's understanding of surgical procedure; describe (briefly) immediate preoperative events that will occur while patient is awake; reinforce or clarify what patient (and family) has been told by surgeon; elicit expected outcome of surgery Assess patient's lifestyle (exercise limits, geographic location, proximity to laboratory facilities, community resources, support groups); note age and, if female, ability or desire to have children, possible need for anticoagulation If additional myocardial revascularization procedures are to be performed (coronary artery bypass grafts), assess patient's understanding and clarify as necessary Assess patient's ability to cooperate with possible anticoagulation regimen; assess family support mechanism
Risk for infection related to surgery	Patient is free of infection related to aseptic technique	Culture excised valve and suture as requested Confine and contain instruments and supplies used to excise infected valve tissue Place mechanical prosthesis in antibiotic solution before implantation as requested by surgeon Keep instruments free of debris Document lot and serial numbers of implants
Risk for altered skin integrity	Patient's skin integrity is maintained	In severely thin and malnourished patients (cardiac cachexia), use additional padding to protect skin, joints, and bony prominences
Risk for injury related to use of valve retractor	Patient is free of injury from use of retraction devices	Use handheld valve retractors with caution to avoid injury to aortic wall, coronary ostia
Risk for injury related to: Retained foreign objects	Patient is free of injury related to: Retained foreign objects	Account for valve sizers, holders, handles, and other items Keep instruments free of tissue, suture, and calcium debris Confirm that Starr-Edwards ball poppet is securely replaced in cage (model 1260 prosthesis)
Chemical hazards	Chemical hazards	Label syringes containing antibiotic solutions, heparinized saline, or other solutions; use only physiologically compatible solutions to rinse bioprosthetic valve; do not place bioprosthesis in antibiotic solution (injures valve); follow protocol for removing glutaraldehyde from bioprostheses (rinsing in three baths of saline for at least 2 minutes each); keep bioprostheses moist with saline during implantation

Modified from Seifert PC: Cardiac surgery. In Rothrock JC: *Perioperative nursing care planning,* ed 2, St Louis, 1996, Mosby.

Continued

Procedural considerations

Aortic valve instruments are added to the basic cardiac setup (Box 12-3). Longer knife handles, needle holders, scissors, and forceps may be required, particularly in patients with a deep chest cavity. One or two handheld aortic valve leaflet retractors (Fig. 12-15) are used for exposure (see Box 12-2 for registered nurse [RN] first assistant considerations).

Because of the presence of extensive calcification on many native valves, some surgeons prefer to use a taper cutting needle (rather than a plain taper needle) for easier insertion of the stitches into the calcified annulus. Alternately colored stitches are used (as they are for mitral valve replacement).

Prosthetic valves and accessories for sizing and implanting the prosthesis should be immediately available

TABLE 12-2
Standards of Nursing Care for Aortic Valve Surgery—cont'd

NURSING DIAGNOSIS	PATIENT OUTCOME	NURSING ACTIONS
Physical hazards	Physical hazards	Have available type and sizes of valvular prostheses desired by surgeon; store valves in cool, dry location; have appropriate accessories to size and insert valve; have necessary suture available (pledgeted, nonpledgeted, multicolored)
		Cardioplegia solution may be infused directly into coronary ostia; have handheld cannulas available (L-shaped tip for left coronary os; J-shaped tip for right coronary os); have appropriate tubing for retrograde cardioplegia infusion; determine if initial bolus of cardioplegia solution will be given via aortic root (patients with aortic stenosis and minimal or no insufficiency) and have tubing, connectors, and other items as needed
		If aortic enlargement is planned, have patch material and suture per surgeon's request
		Be prepared with needles and venting catheters to deair left ventricle (superior right pulmonary venous catheter often is inserted); test vents to ensure they are suctioning
Thermal injury	Thermal injury	If aortic valve allograft is used, avoid contact with graft in frozen condition; follow manufacturer's instructions for thawing graft in warm water baths; use insulated gloves when handling cryopreserved valve; if allografts are stored on premises, monitor temperature of storage tank to protect viability of allograft; replace coolant as necessary
		In patients with left ventricular hypertrophy, anticipate need for additional topical cold solutions and more frequent infusion of cardioplegia solution to provide transmural cooling/cardioplegic arrest
Risk for self-care deficit related to inadequate knowledge of rehabilitation period	Patient demonstrates knowledge of rehabilitation period as it relates to self-care abilities	Assess patient's knowledge of signs/symptoms of valve failure
		Assess patient's understanding of medications prescribed; signs/symptoms of anticoagulation-related hemorrhage, thrombosis, emboli; need for antibiotic prophylaxis before invasive procedures; need for follow-up laboratory tests (prothrombin time)
		Identify signs/symptoms of anticoagulation-related hemorrhage (notify physician):
		Nosebleeds, bleeding gums
		Red or brown urine
		Red or black bowel movements
		Bleeding from cuts that cannot be stopped, bruises that get larger
		Severe and persistent headaches
		Abdominal pain
		Faintness, dizziness, or unusual weakness
		Excessive menstrual flow
		Identify signs/symptoms of suboptimal anticoagulation (notify physician):
		Stroke, transient ischemic attacks
		Closing sound of prosthesis no longer audible; absent "click"
		Sudden onset of congestive heart failure
		List precautions for patients receiving anticoagulants:
		Use a soft-bristled toothbrush
		Use electric shavers rather than razors
		Wear gloves when gardening
		Do not go barefoot
		Trim nails with a soft emery board instead of scissors or clippers
		Avoid sports in which skin may be broken or internal injuries may occur
		Provide patient with name of person to contact if questions/problems arise
		Provide information for obtaining and using medical alert bracelet

---

BOX 12-3
Aortic Valve Surgery: Procedural Considerations

Instrumentation
Handheld aortic valve retractors

Valve Prostheses and Accessories
Mechanical heart valves
Bioprostheses (porcine or bovine pericardium)
Sizers (obturators), range of sizes, specific to prosthesis
Sizer (obturator) handles
Prosthetic valve holders and handles (some prostheses are packaged with an attached holder); sterile nurse applies handle into holder

Supplies
Valve suture, single and multipack (multicolored):
  Pledgeted
  Nonpledgeted
Suture organizer (if used)
Preferred patch material (for enlarging aortic root)
Free pledgets, precut or cut to size
18- or 19-gauge needle to deair ventricle
Long (spinal) 18-gauge needle for transseptal deairing of ventricle
Additional basins for bioprosthetic saline rinse, antibiotic solutions, allograft thawing/preparation, or glutaraldehyde preparation of autologous pericardium
Culture tubes (for valve tissue, suture, rinse solutions)
Venting lines for deairing left ventricle
Left superior pulmonary venting catheter (apical vent rare)
Two-stage venous cannula commonly used

Positioning
Supine
If coronary bypass grafts to be performed, patient positioned as for removal of leg vein (see Chapter 10)

Skin Preparation
Midline of chest, inner aspect of both legs shaved
Legs washed at least to knees

Draping
Anterior chest exposed
Legs exposed from groin to knees (can be covered with a towel if access is not required)
Anesthesia screen placed over lower legs to keep drapes off feet

Special Infection Control Measures
Confine and contain tissue and instruments from infected tissue
Culture valve tissue, rinse solutions, and other items as requested by surgeon
Place mechanical prostheses in antibiotic solution before insertion as requested by surgeon
Keep instruments free of debris
Document lot and serial numbers of all implants

Special Safety Measures
Label syringes and containers of solutions, medications:
  Antibiotic solution
  Heparinized saline
  Glutaraldehyde
Account for all sizers, handles, and holders used to size and insert a prosthesis, as well as pledget material, suture needles, hypodermic needles
Monitor presence of ventricular failure and possible need for mechanical ventricular support (intraaortic balloon or ventricular assist device)
Keep prostheses stored in a cool, dry, contamination-free location
If using Starr-Edwards ball-and-cage valve, keep poppet in safe place while suturing valve ring

Documentation/Report to Cardiac Surgical Intensive Care Unit*
Procedure, type of replacement prosthesis
Lot and serial numbers of prosthesis
Preoperative diagnosis (stenosis, regurgitation, or both; congestive heart failure, syncope, angina pectoris; onset)
Epicardial pacemaker lead placement (single, dual), and if being paced
Patient problems, concerns related to valvular heart disease, surgery
Preoperative left ventricular function (e.g., ejection fraction)
Completion of valve implant card (and sent to manufacturer)

*In addition to standard documentation/postoperative report; see Chapter 6.

---

and distinguishable from each other. The nurse should be able to quickly select the appropriate type and size obturator requested. Even if the surgeon plans to use a specific type of prosthesis (e.g., a mechanical or biologic valve), obturators for both should be on the field because anatomic conditions noted during assessment of the native valve may require a change in plan. It is helpful to arrange and label the obturators according to size

and type, especially when multiple valve replacement is planned. Prosthesis handles also differ depending on the manufacturer and should be differentiated as well.

The surgeon may elect to enlarge a small aortic root. Preferred graft material should be available to perform this procedure.

If an aortic (or pulmonary) valve allograft (Box 12-4) is used, additional basins for thawing and reconstitution of

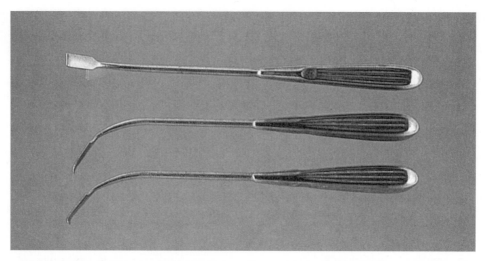

FIGURE 12-15   Aortic valve leaflet retractors. (From Brooks-Tighe SM: *Instrumentation for the operating room: a photographic manual,* ed 4, St Louis, 1994, Mosby.)

BOX 12-4
Comments on Aortic Valve Homografts (Allografts)
Donald Ross
Fellow, Royal College of Surgeons
National Heart Hospital, London

Aortic valve homografts are centrally flowing and are consequently nonobstructive and give rise to neither emboli nor turbulence. They do, however, undergo a slow process of degeneration, giving plenty of time for an elective low-risk second operation. An additional advantage is that they can be used in children.

The quality of life of the homograft patient, who is removed from the dangers of embolism and anticoagulant hemorrhage, the ingestion of pills, regular hematologic checks, restrictions on pregnancy, and the danger of sudden death, is considerably better than that of the mechanical valve patient and very close to normal living.

This quality of life as opposed to quantity is not something that can be evaluated statistically. From the patient's point of view, however, it is a very important feature and is reflected in the fact that most patients ask for a homograft for their second operation.

Long-term results indicate that the unmounted homograft (in contrast to one attached to a stent) in the aortic area gives better results than currently used bioprostheses, and in the right ventricular outflow tract there is no comparable valve.

Since 1982 homografts have remained our preferred method of replacement of the aortic valve, irrespective of age, sex, and the severity of the lesion.

Modified from Ross D: Application of homografts in clinical surgery, *J Cardiac Surg* 1(3 suppl):175, 1987.

---

the graft are needed, along with scissors and clamps or forceps for preparation. Insulated gloves are required to protect the hands of the person retrieving the frozen allograft from the portable freezer. Additional scissors and forceps are needed when the surgeon trims the graft at the field.

Basins are also necessary for rinsing glutaraldehyde-preserved biologic valves; the valve should be rinsed for at least 2 minutes in each of three basins (total time: 6 minutes) containing normal saline. An additional sterile nurse is helpful for procedures that require preparation (thawing, rinsing) of implants. When tissue implants are used, cultures often are taken of the rinse solution, a small piece of the discarded excess allograft, and the needles used for suturing.

Myocardial protection is achieved with retrograde cardioplegia infusion. This method is reliable and easier than the antegrade method, and it reduces the potential injury to the coronary ostia associated with the use of handheld antegrade infusion cannulas. Standard retrograde cardioplegia systems need no special additional preparation for aortic valve surgery.

Occasionally coronary ostial cardioplegia catheters are needed for antegrade cardioplegia infusion if retroplegia cannot be used. The disposable or nondisposable infusion tips are preshaped to facilitate insertion into the left or right coronary os. Generally the left coronary cannula is L-shaped, and the right coronary cannula is J-shaped.

In patients with coronary artery disease (and aortic stenosis with minimal or no insufficiency), both antegrade and retrograde cardioplegia infusion is used, with the initial bolus of cardioplegia solution infused antegradely through the aortic root before the aorta is opened. This is unfeasible in the presence of aortic insufficiency because the incompetent valve leaflets allow the cardioplegia solution to flow preferentially through the valve orifice into the left ventricle rather than into the coronary ostia. This produces ventricular distension and a delay in achieving cardioplegic arrest. If this occurs, the surgeon uses retrograde cardioplegia infusion; bypass grafts are selectively infused antegradely with cardioplegia solution through tubing connected to the retroplegia system.

In left ventricular hypertrophy, transmural cooling may not be achieved sufficiently with retrograde or antegrade cardioplegia alone. The topical application of chilled solutions (saline) to the heart may be required to cool the myocardium thoroughly.

Minimally invasive surgical techniques. Minimally invasive techniques (defined here as a small incision) for aortic valve surgery include total or partial median sternotomy, parasternotomy, thoracotomy, and transverse sternotomy. Concerns about the sacrifice of one or both internal mammary arteries, suboptimal exposure, chest wall instability, and impaired wound healing have led a number of surgeons (Gillinov, Casselman, and Cosgrove, 2000) to favor a partial sternotomy. Advantages of this incision include excellent exposure, relative ease of atrial-aortic cannulation, and the ability to convert to a full median sternotomy when necessary. Standard aortic valve instruments and techniques can be employed with slight modification (e.g., a small Finochietto for chest retraction, smaller chest tubes, and vacuum-assisted venous drainage with a smaller venous cannula).

Port access techniques (see Chapter 9) are employed less frequently for aortic valve procedures than they are for mitral valve surgery because the partial sternotomy approach to the aortic valve allows direct access to the aorta for cross-clamping. External aortic clamping poses fewer risks than endovascular aortic occlusion (Ikonomidis and others, 2000).

Operative procedure: aortic valve replacement

Aortic valve replacement is the excision of the diseased aortic valve and replacement with a biologic or mechanical prosthesis or an aortic valve homograft. Before the procedure begins, the sterile nurse prepares a sterile field on a small table. On this is placed three small round basins, suture scissors, and a pair of forceps. Prosthesis handles specific to the types of prostheses available can be arranged nearby. Culture tubes and syringes are added if a bioprosthesis is selected.

Procedure

1. A median sternotomy is performed, cardiopulmonary bypass is instituted using a two-stage cannula for venous drainage, and the patient is cooled to approximately 22° C (72° F) (Fig. 12-16, *A*). A venting catheter may be passed through the right superior pulmonary vein, past the mitral valve, and into the left ventricle, where it will suction blood and vent air after the valve is implanted.

    The aorta is clamped. Cardioplegia solution is given antegradely through the root or retrogradely through a catheter in the coronary sinus. Direct ostial infusion is accomplished with handheld catheters

(Fig. 12-16, *B*). A cooling pad may be wrapped around the ventricle to enhance cooling.

The valve is exposed through a transverse aortotomy above the coronary ostia (Fig. 12-17).

2. The aortic valve leaflets are excised with a knife or scissors, leaving a rim of tissue at the base of the cusp (Fig. 12-16, *C*). When calcification is present, rongeurs may be used to remove calcified particles. A small round cup with saline is placed in a location where the surgeon can rinse debris from the rongeur tips. The rongeur and other instrument tips are wiped with a moist sponge to remove remaining particles. Care is taken to remove all loose tissue and other debris. (Some surgeons place a small radiopaque sponge into the left ventricular cavity to catch loose material.) Irrigation followed by suction helps to remove debris as well.

3. The surgeon sizes the annulus with obturators specific to the prosthesis desired and requests the appropriate-size valve. Occasionally, anatomic conditions necessitate a different type of valve; because this is a possibility, there should be a table with basins for rinsing a bioprosthesis even if a mechanical valve was the original valve of choice.

4. The valve selected is delivered to the field after the type and size are verified by circulating and sterile nurses. Identification tags attached to the prostheses are cut with scissors, taking care not to injure the valve.

    a. **Mechanical valve:**

    (1) Starr-Edwards—the poppet is removed and placed in a dish with heparinized saline; the valve handle is attached by engaging the top of the cage, and the prosthesis is placed on the back table until needed.

    (2) Medtronic-Hall—the prosthesis and attached handle are taken from the package and placed on the back table until needed.

    (3) St. Jude Medical—the valve within its valve stand is removed from the container; the handle is screwed into the holder preattached to the prosthesis, and the prosthesis is removed from its valve stand. The prosthesis is placed on the back table until needed.

    b. **Biologic valve:**

    (1) Carpentier-Edwards porcine and pericardial aortic valve (model 2700)—the valve is transferred with forceps from the container to the table prepared with basins of saline. The valve handle is screwed into the preattached valve holder. Any packing material is removed, and the bioprosthesis is placed in the first of three basins containing normal saline. The valve is gently agitated (holding the handle) for a minimum of 2 minutes. The valve is placed in the second basin for 2 minutes and in the third

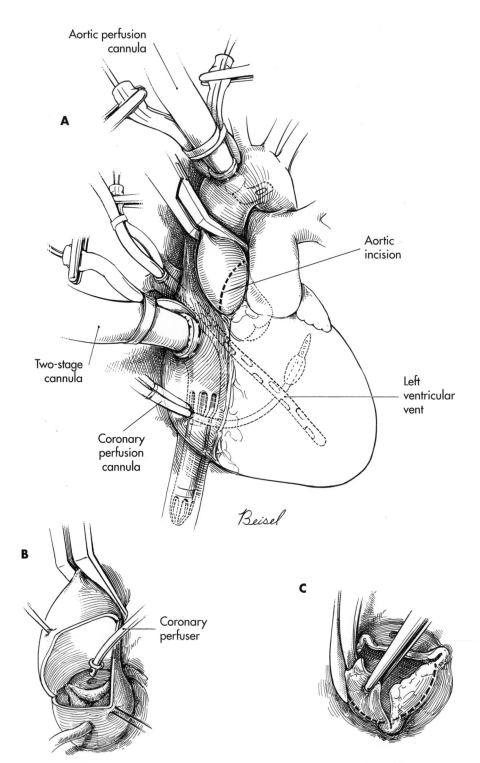

FIGURE 12-16 Aortic valve replacement. **A,** Arterial inflow is established with an aortic perfusion cannula in the ascending aorta distal to the cross-clamp. The two-stage venous cannula is inserted into the right atrium; the distal openings receive blood from the inferior vena cava, and the proximal openings (in the atrium) drain blood returning from the superior vena cava and the coronary sinus. A catheter is inserted through the right superior pulmonary vein and passed into the left ventricle to suction away blood during the valve replacement and to vent air after the valve is implanted and before the cross-clamp is removed. A retrograde cardioplegia infusion catheter can be inserted into the coronary sinus via the right atrium. **B,** The aortotomy is made above the aortic valve, and two retraction sutures are placed in the aorta. If retroplegic arrest cannot be used, handheld coronary ostial perfusers are inserted into the coronary ostia. Shown is the left cannula tip, which is often L-shaped for ease of insertion. The right coronary ostium is below and under the aortic incision; a perfuser with a J-shaped tip makes insertion into the right ostium easier. **C,** Valve leaflets are resected.

Continued

basin for 2 minutes. Cultures may be taken of the last bath solution (or all three basins) with a 10-ml syringe and sent to the laboratory. A separate syringe is used for drawing up a sample from each bath culture. After the valve has been adequately rinsed free of the glutaraldehyde storage solution, it is placed in a saline-

moistened sponge and placed on the back table until needed. The prosthesis should not be allowed to dry.

   (2) Hancock porcine valve—the procedure is similar to that for the Carpentier-Edwards valve.

5. Pledgeted (or nonpledgeted) sutures are passed through the valve annulus and then into the pros-

D

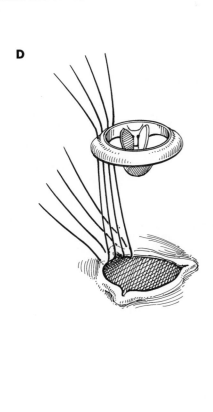

E

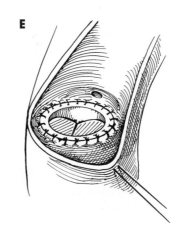

F

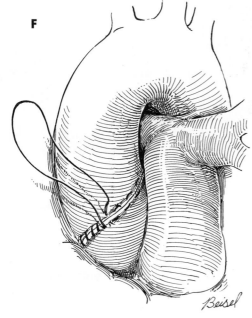

FIGURE 12-16, cont'd   D, Stitches with pledgets in the subannular position are placed in the annulus and then into the sewing ring of a low-profile prosthesis. **E,** Prosthesis in position with the stitches tied and cut. **F,** The aorta is closed with a running suture. (For clarity, the cross-clamp is not shown.) (From Waldhausen JA and others: *Surgery of the chest,* ed 6, St Louis, 1996, Mosby.)

thetic sewing ring (Figs. 12-16, *D,* and 12-18). Some surgeons prefer to place the annular stitches first, followed by insertion of the sewing ring sutures. Felt-pledgeted sutures provide a good seal between the skirt of the prosthesis and the annulus, thereby helping to prevent the development of perivalvular leaks (Waldhausen and others, 1996).

6. The valve is threaded into the annulus, and the stitches are tied and cut (Figs. 12-16, *E,* 12-19, and 12-20.)
7. The aortotomy is closed with a single or double running suture. To close a transverse aortic incision without tension, a folded towel may be placed under the handle of the cross-clamp to tilt it forward

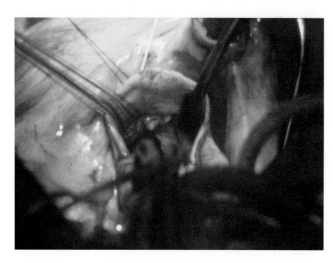

FIGURE 12-17 The aortic root is exposed through a transverse aortotomy. (Courtesy Edward A. Lefrak, MD; Doug Yarnold, CRNA, photographer.)

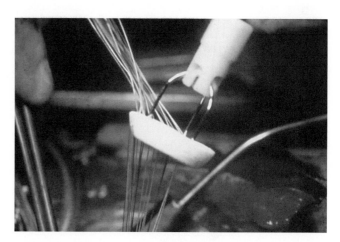

FIGURE 12-18 Nonpledgeted interrupted sutures are passed through the sewing ring of a Starr-Edwards 1260 aortic valve. Note that the poppet has been removed to facilitate insertion of the sutures. (Courtesy Edward A. Lefrak, MD; Doug Yarnold, CRNA, photographer.)

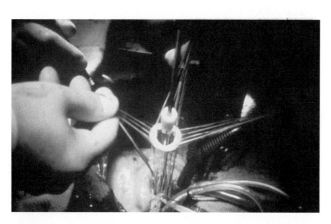

FIGURE 12-19 All the stitches have been inserted into the native annulus and the sewing ring; they are grouped into three sets to correspond with the aortic commissures. (Courtesy Edward A. Lefrak, MD; Doug Yarnold, CRNA, photographer.)

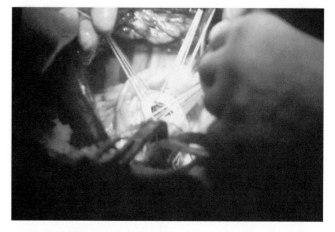

FIGURE 12-20 The prosthesis is seated into the annulus. After the stitches are tied and cut, the poppet is replaced in the cage. (Courtesy Edward A. Lefrak, MD; Doug Yarnold, CRNA, photographer.)

slightly, thereby bringing the edges of the aortotomy into closer approximation. If the aortic tissue is of poor quality, felt buttressing of the suture line may be performed (Waldhausen and others, 1996).

8. The left ventricle is deaired, and the cross-clamp is removed.

Operative procedures: enlargement of the small aortic root

The following procedures are intended to enlarge the diameter of the annulus by 2 to 3 mm, allowing insertion of at least a 19-mm aortic valve prosthesis.

Patch enlargement of the proximal ascending aorta (Fig. 12-21). When narrowing of the aorta is confined to the proximal ascending aorta, patch repair can be performed by making an oblique aortotomy and extending it into the noncoronary cusp. A diamond-shaped patch of preclotted woven Dacron or glutaraldehyde-preserved pericardium is sewn to the edges of the aortotomy. The size of the graft determines by how much the aorta is enlarged (Waldhausen and others, 1996).

Nicks procedure (Fig. 12-22). An oblique incision is made in the aortic root. The valve leaflets are excised, and the annulus is measured. The incision is

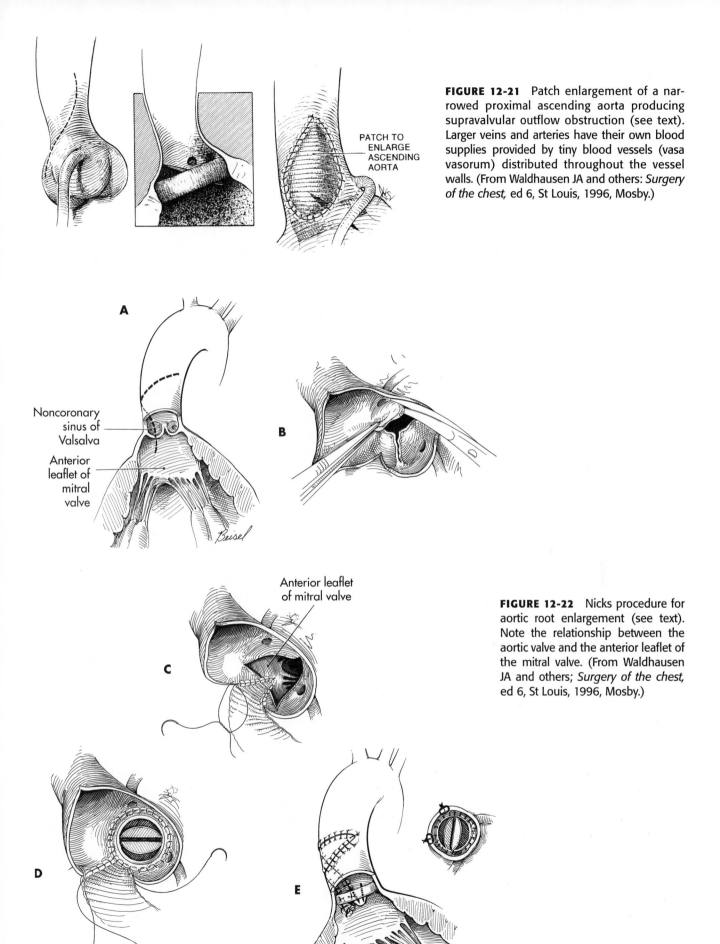

FIGURE 12-21 Patch enlargement of a narrowed proximal ascending aorta producing supravalvular outflow obstruction (see text). Larger veins and arteries have their own blood supplies provided by tiny blood vessels (vasa vasorum) distributed throughout the vessel walls. (From Waldhausen JA and others: *Surgery of the chest,* ed 6, St Louis, 1996, Mosby.)

PATCH TO ENLARGE ASCENDING AORTA

A

Noncoronary sinus of Valsalva

Anterior leaflet of mitral valve

B

Anterior leaflet of mitral valve

C

FIGURE 12-22 Nicks procedure for aortic root enlargement (see text). Note the relationship between the aortic valve and the anterior leaflet of the mitral valve. (From Waldhausen JA and others; *Surgery of the chest,* ed 6, St Louis, 1996, Mosby.)

D

E

continued downward to the noncoronary sinus, dividing the aortic annulus, and extended only to the origin of the anterior mitral leaflet. A wedge-shaped Dacron patch is fashioned and sutured from the apex of the aortotomy to just beyond the annulus with 4-0 polypropylene. Felt pledgets may be needed (Waldhausen and others, 1996).

Manouguian procedure (Fig. 12-23). The incision is more medial than that of the Nicks procedure. The transverse aortotomy is made into the commissure between the left coronary cusp and the noncoronary cusp and extended toward the center of the fibrous origin of the anterior mitral leaflet. A Dacron or pericardial patch is sutured to the V-shaped defect in the anterior mitral leaflet and the aortic root, thereby reestablishing continuity between the two (Manouguian and Seybold-Epting, 1979).

Konno-Rastan procedure (Fig. 12-24). The left ventricular outflow tract is enlarged by opening and enlarging the right ventricular outflow tract through the septum, creating a ventricular septal defect.

The aorta is incised vertically, and the incision is carried down into the right coronary cusp, avoiding the coronary orifice. The right ventricle is incised transversely below the pulmonary valve, and the ventricular septum is then incised.

A Dacron patch is cut to fit the area from the septotomy, across the annulus, to the ascending aorta. At the location of the annulus, the patch needs to be cut large enough to accept a sufficiently large prosthesis.

The patch is sutured to the septum and then to the edges of the annulus. A valve prosthesis is brought to the field and sutured to the native annulus and to the patch graft. Finally, the patch is sutured to the aortotomy. The ventriculotomy is closed with a pericardial patch or Dacron patch. Another method is to use a patch to close just the septal defect and then insert the larger patch to close the aortotomy and ventriculotomy (Waldhausen and others, 1996).

This technique is particularly useful in children requiring an adult-size prosthesis. Complications include injury to the right coronary artery or the pulmonary valve, transection of a major left coronary artery septal perforator, complete heart block, and bleeding.

Left ventricular apicoabdominal aortic conduit (Fig. 12-25). Patients with a congenital, diffusely obstructed left ventricular outflow tract may benefit from this procedure.

The left ventricular apex is exposed through a median sternotomy. The apex is stabbed well to the left of the anterior descending coronary artery with a blade. A plug of myocardium is excised, and a specially made flanged cannula is inserted into the ventriculotomy. Interrupted pledgeted sutures are placed around the cannula to secure it to the myocardium. The cannula tip must penetrate the entire myocardial wall in order to avoid obstruction of the cannula tip.

The proximal end of a valved conduit is anastomosed end-to-end to the ventricular cannula; the distal end of the conduit is attached end-to-side to the descending thoracic or abdominal aorta. The advantage of sewing the conduit to the abdominal aorta is that if the valve within the conduit must be replaced, it is more easily accessible by laparotomy than by sternotomy, which would require dissection of sternal adhesions (Waldhausen and others, 1996).

Operative procedure: allograft (homograft) replacement of the aortic valve, aortic root

Allografts are most commonly used in the aortic position. Because of the more complex structure of the mitral and tricuspid apparatus, allografts are infrequently used to replace these valves. Less commonly, the graft is mounted on a stent and used for tricuspid valve replacement (see Chapter 13).

Unmounted aortic allografts consisting of only the valve, or the valve and a portion of the attached aorta, are used to replace the excised native valve or the aortic root of the patient. Occasionally the graft is mounted onto a stent for aortic valve replacement, but this reduces the orifice area that is gained with the freehand insertion technique (McGiffen and Kirklin, 1997; Karp, 1997).

Supplies for allograft thawing include a sterile field prepared on a separate table, three 300-ml basins, a 50-ml syringe, two pairs of straight suture scissors, a Kelly clamp, vascular forceps, dissecting scissors (Metzenbaum or Cooley My scissors), and a specimen cup containing 10 ml of sterile saline.

A variety of implantation techniques have evolved (Cox, 1997). In the free-standing root replacement, coronary "buttons" are created and sewn to the cylindrical graft. The subcoronary technique in which the aortic sinuses of the graft are excised (scalloped) is described in the next section.

Procedure

1. A supply of cryopreserved grafts is transported to the operating room in a portable liquid nitrogen storage cylinder.

    In some institutions, fresh allografts are procured on the premises. They are measured, immersed in antibiotic solution and a preservative, and implanted. Cryopreservation is more common.

2. After the heart is arrested, a transverse, vertical, or semivertical incision is made in the aorta.

3. The recipient aortic root is sized with standard valve obturators or special cylindric sizers. The appropriate-

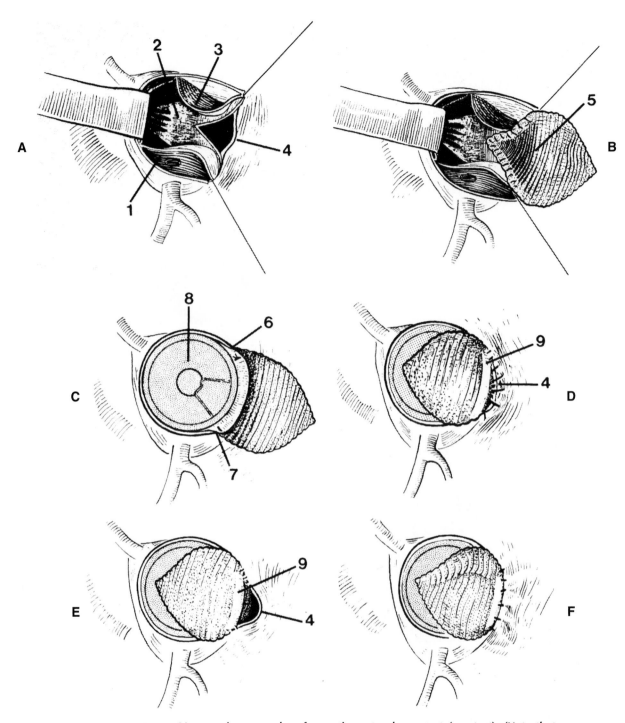

FIGURE 12-23 Manouguian procedure for aortic root enlargement (see text). (Note that the prosthesis—Bjork-Shiley—is no longer available in the United States). *1,* Left semilunar cusp; *2,* anterior mitral leaflet; *3,* noncoronary semilunar cusp; *4,* left atrial wall; *5,* patch; *6-7,* enlargement of the aortic valve ring; *8,* aortic valve prosthesis; *9,* sewing ring of the prosthesis. (From Manouguian S, Seybold-Epting W: Patch enlargement of the aortic valve ring by extending the aortic incision into the anterior mitral leaflet: new operative technique, *J Thorac Cardiovasc Surg* 78[3]:402, 1979.)

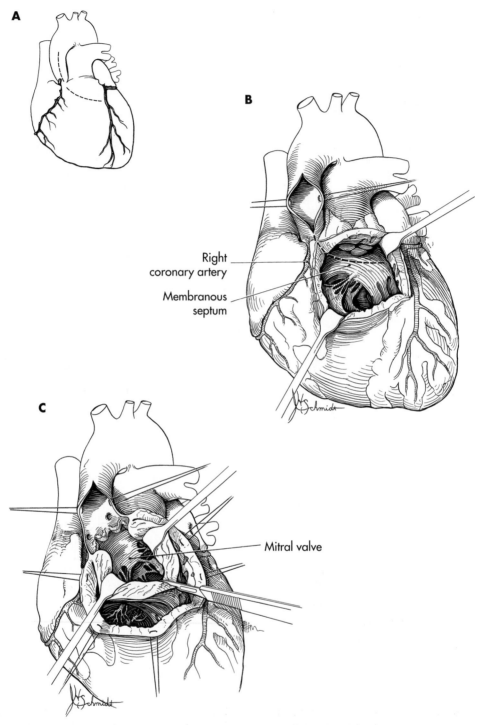

FIGURE 12-24 Konno-Rastan procedure for aortic root enlargement (see text). (From Waldhausen JA and others: *Surgery of the chest,* ed 6, St Louis, 1996, Mosby.)

Continued

size allograft is selected, and if it is cryopreserved, it is taken from the portable freezer.

4. During thawing and reconstitution, concomitant procedures such as coronary artery bypass grafting may be performed.

5. Using insulated gloves, the circulating nurse (or a technician) removes the selected frozen valve from the container and places the bag holding the graft into a basin of warm (about 42° C [108° F]) water. Once the bag is pliable enough to open, it is dried

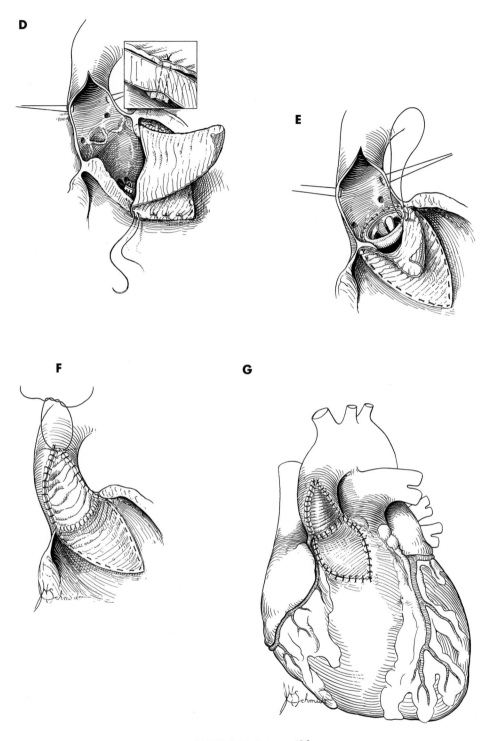

FIGURE 12-24, cont'd

and the top of the bag is cut with sterile scissors, exposing the inner storage bag. The sterile nurse removes the inner bag with the sterile clamp and transfers it to a warm sterile water bath; the transferring forceps are removed from the field.

After a few minutes the inner bag is opened, and the contents are placed in the first of four basins filled with nutrient medium. The graft is rinsed in each basin for 2 minutes (total time: 8 minutes) and delivered to the field. This

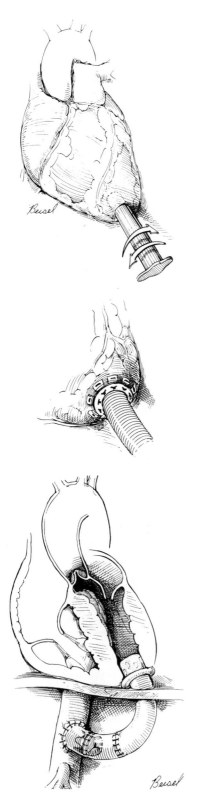

FIGURE 12-25 Left ventricular apicoabdominal conduit (see text). (From Waldhausen JA, and others: *Surgery of the chest,* ed 6, St Louis, 1996, Mosby.)

procedure varies according to the allograft supplier's protocol.

6. The lower muscular margin is trimmed in preparation for implantation. A piece of excess tissue may be sent to the laboratory for aerobic, anaerobic, and fungal cultures.

7. The graft requires both proximal and distal suture lines.

a. Proximal suture line (Fig. 12-26, *A*): Marking sutures helps to align each allograft commissure and the corresponding point below the native valve annulus. The valve is inverted into the left ventricle, and each of these marking sutures is tied. The suture line is then performed with interrupted or continuous sutures (Fig. 12-26, *B*). Special caution is taken in the area of the membranous septum to avoid injury to bundle of His conduction tissue.

b. The graft is everted and brought back up into the aorta.

c. The allograft is then scalloped so that when it is in position it will expose the native coronary ostia (Fig. 12-26, *C*).

d. Distal suture line (Fig. 12-26, *D*): Three double-armed sutures are used for the distal suture line, using the knots of the previous proximal sutures as a guide. Each suture is passed through the graft and the adjacent native sinus using a continuous over-and-over technique. The suture is run along the edge of the graft to the top of the pillar, passed through the pillar and the aortic wall, and then tied outside the aorta. The other two pillars are sutured in the same way.

8. When the suture lines are completed, the surgeon tests the valve for competency. Saline is instilled into the left ventricle, and the valve leaflets are tested for competency.

9. The aorta is closed.

Aortic valve replacement may be performed using the Ross procedure, in which the patient's pulmonary valve (autograft) replaces the aortic valve. The autograft is harvested from the right ventricular outflow tract and implanted into the native aortic root as described previously. The right ventricular outflow tract is reconstructed with a pulmonary allograft (Elkins, 1999; Chambers and others, 1997).

Operative procedure: myomyectomy for hypertrophic subaortic stenosis (Morrow and others, 1975)

A bar or wedge of hypertrophic septal muscle is excised in order to relieve left ventricular outflow obstruction (Fig. 12-27).

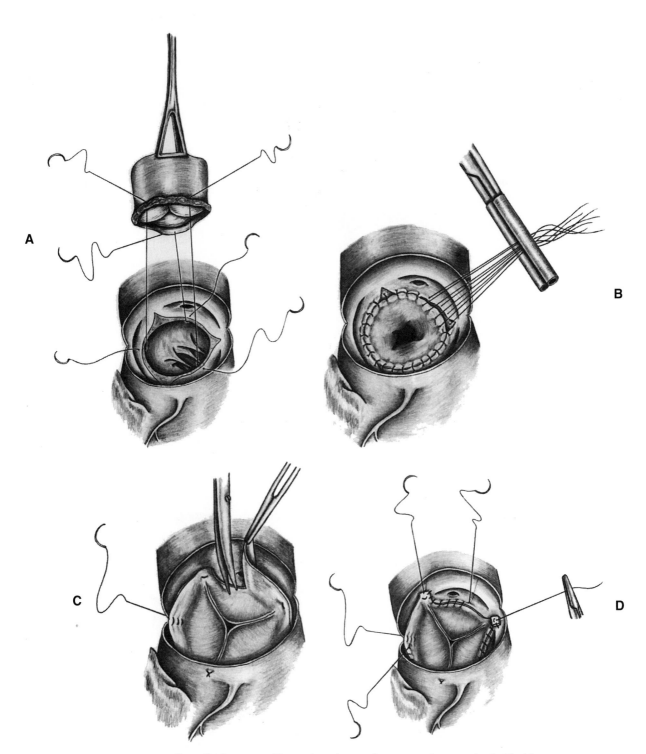

FIGURE 12-26 Allograft (homograft) aortic valve replacement (see text). **A,** Marking sutures are placed from the base of the sinuses of both the aortic root and the allograft. The proximal suture line begins with sutures at the midpoint of each sinus of Valsalva. **B,** The allograft has been inverted and sewn below the native annulus with continuous or interrupted sutures. **C,** The valve is everted, and the commissures are anchored. The sinuses containing the right and left coronary ostia are scalloped to allow blood to enter the coronary circulation. **D,** The noncoronary sinus is left intact, and the distal suture line is a running suture below the coronary orifices. (From Randolph JD and others: Aortic valve and left ventricular outflow tract replacement using allograft and autograft valves, *Ann Thorac Surg* 48:345, 1989; drawing by M. LaWaun Hance, SA, PA-C.)

A

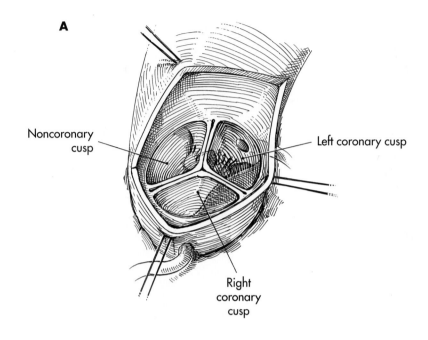

Noncoronary cusp

Left coronary cusp

Right coronary cusp

B

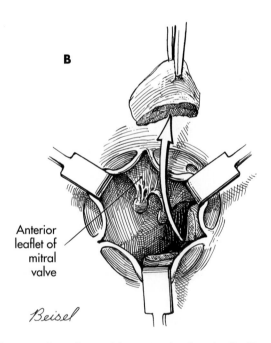

Anterior leaflet of mitral valve

Beisel

FIGURE 12-27   Morrow procedure for resection of septal hypertrophy (see text). (From Waldhausen JA, and others; *Surgery of the chest,* ed 6, St Louis, 1996, Mosby.)

Procedure

1. An incision is made in the ascending aorta and extended down into the noncoronary cusp sinus of Valsalva.
2. The (normal) aortic valve leaflets are retracted and protected from injury.
3. Bulging hypertrophic septal muscle beneath the right coronary leaflet is assessed. The anterior leaflet of the mitral valve may be thickened and opaque.
4. A flat narrow ribbon retractor is passed through the aortic valve annulus to displace and protect the anterior mitral leaflet.
5. A knife with a No. 10 or 12 hook blade is used to shave excess septal tissue. (An angled knife handle facilitates this maneuver.) A second myotomy is

made parallel to the first incision so that a generous wedge can be excised. Cutting too deeply into the hypertrophied septum can cause a ventricular septal defect.

6. Resection of the muscle bar may be completed with scissors, a rectangular knife, or, if necessary, an angled rongeur. Loose myocardial fragments are removed. Care is taken to avoid injury to conduction tissue under the right and noncoronary cusps.

7. The incision is closed. If a ventricular septal defect was created, it is closed and the repair is evaluated by transesophageal echocardiography (TEE).

Associated procedures

Aortic valve endocarditis. Surgery for aortic valve endocarditis is performed when there is evidence of recurrent septic emboli, the appearance of new or more serious dysrhythmias, resistance to antibiotic therapy, or profound hemodynamic deterioration. Valve replacement is performed in the usual manner unless there is extension of the infection onto the annular or subannular structures.

Abscess cavities must be obliterated, and if necessary, the prosthetic valve is translocated above the coronary ostia. In this case bypass grafts are performed to vascularize the heart. Allografts, the Ross procedure, or composite valve grafts with coronary ostial reimplantation (see Chapter 14) are alternative procedures.

Aortic valve replacement with coronary artery bypass grafting. Aortic valve replacement is similar to mitral valve replacement with coronary artery bypass grafting as described in Chapter 11. Distal anastomoses can be accomplished before valve replacement; the proximal grafts usually are attached after the aortotomy is closed and the patient is being rewarmed. The distal anastomoses routinely are done first so that elevation of the heart after valve insertion (with possible injury to the myocardium) can be avoided.

Double valve replacement. Double valve replacement of the aortic and mitral valves is described in Chapter 11. The relationship between the mitral and aortic valves and the relative differences in size can be seen radiologically in Fig. 12-28.

Completion of the Procedure

Once the valve is implanted, measures are taken to evacuate air from the left ventricle. During closure of the aortotomy, the left ventricle is allowed to fill with blood. This is done by clamping (or turning off) the left ventricular vent. Just before the aortotomy suture is tied, the aorta is allowed to fill with blood. The patient is placed in Trendelenburg's position, and the ascending aortic needle vent (which was previously tested to

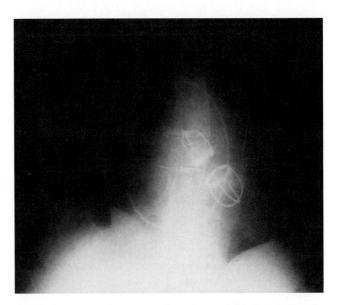

FIGURE 12-28 Chest x-ray film of a patient after a double valve replacement with a Starr-Edwards 1260 aortic valve (smaller cage) and a 6120 mitral valve prosthesis. (Courtesy Edward A. Lefrak, MD.)

be sure it was suctioning and not infusing) is placed in the ascending aorta and turned on to remove air within the left ventricle.

The cross-clamp is then removed, and the ventricular vent is turned on again. It is important that the ventricle not be allowed to eject blood (and possibly a bolus of air) before deairing is accomplished. An additional maneuver is hypodermic needle aspiration of the left ventricular apex (cautiously elevated by the surgeon to avoid endocardial puncture by the prosthesis). A long (spinal) needle may be used for transseptal evacuation of air from the left ventricle if the surgeon wants to avoid elevating the apex.

The pulmonary venous venting catheter is removed, and the entry site is closed with a figure-eight or a purse-string suture. The operating bed is returned to a level position. The ascending aortic vent is left in place until the surgeon is satisfied that deairing has been completed.

After the left ventricle has been deaired and hemostasis of the suture lines has been achieved, cardiopulmonary bypass is terminated and the chest is closed. Temporary atrial and ventricular pacing wires are attached, and drainage tubes are inserted. As in most cardiac procedures, preoperative ventricular function is the strongest predictor of operative risk.

Postoperative Complications

Prosthesis-related complications of thromboembolism, anticoagulation-related hemorrhage, and infection pose a risk for patients with prosthetic valves. Aortic valve

TABLE 12-3
Perioperative Problems and Complications of Aortic Valve Surgery

COMPLICATION/PROBLEM	INTERVENTIONS
Intraoperative	
Aorta and aortotomy	
Calcification of ascending aorta	Cannulation of femoral artery for CPB may be required
	If cross-clamp cannot be safely applied, may need to use deep hypothermia and circulatory arrest (see Chapter 9)
	When closure of aortotomy is difficult, may need to perform endarterectomy and decalcification and use felt-buttressed suture closure
Bleeding from aortic suture line	Close approximation of aortotomy edges may be facilitated by using marking stitches to align aortic edges; when there is a transverse aortotomy, a folded towel placed under handle of cross-clamp will tip upper aortotomy edge forward and closer to lower edge
	If retracting aorta, avoid pulling too hard so that incision line is not torn
	Surgeon may want to use felt buttressing to close a friable aorta or reinforce suture line with an aortic circumferential collar of Dacron (e.g., 8-mm tube graft) or PTFE
	Repairs are best performed when systemic blood pressure against aortic suture line is low; avoid hypertension
Aortic valve annulus	
Detachment of anterior mitral leaflet from annulus	Repair mitral leaflet and annulus with pledgeted sutures
Perforation of annulus	Avoid vigorous removal of calcium deposits; repair with pledgeted sutures
Suture interference with prosthetic function	When pledgeted sutures are used, their position may be subannular or supraannular depending on where they will be less likely to interfere with opening or closing mechanism of prosthesis
Coronary arteries and their origin	
Injury to coronary ostia	Use caution with direct ostial infusion
	Avoid injury caused by instrument manipulation of ostial and periostial tissue
Embolization of surgical debris	Give meticulous attention to removal of calcium and tissue particles, suture fragments, and other debris
	Open-tip suction catheters, copious irrigation, and sponges placed to occlude coronary openings (and also LV cavity) help to avoid this complication
Ostial obstruction	Signs of ischemia may indicate prosthetic obstruction of ostia; may need to reposition valve
	Caged-ball valves should not be placed in small aortas because of potential obstruction
Misorientation of prosthetic valve	Major orifice of disk valve should be oriented so that it opens in such a way that it enhances left coronary artery perfusion in diastole
Conduction pathways: heart block	Injury to AV node or bundle of His near commissure of noncoronary or right cusps may cause heart block; this should be distinguished from the transient block that may occur from edema and mechanical trauma of surgery
	Temporary atrial and ventricular pacing wires are used to pace heart for a few days; if conduction remains blocked, permanent transvenous lead and a generator may be inserted
Postoperative	
Valvular deterioration (allograft, autograft, or bioprosthesis)	Process is usually gradual, not catastrophic; if bioprosthesis is damaged, a new murmur will appear; replacement is indicated
Prosthetic failure; thrombosed occluder (disk or ball)	Cessation of valve noise alerts patient or clinician, sternotomy, assessment of valve, and replacement may be required; can be catastrophic (but less likely than with mitral valve prosthesis); when thrombus obstructs valve opening, debridement may first be attempted; thrombolytic therapy can be tried as well
Prosthetic dehiscence perivalvular leak	A new murmur with decreased hematocrit (from hemolysis) alerts clinician; surgical exploration may result in placement of additional stitches or in prosthetic replacement
Prosthetic valve endocarditis with or without root abscess	Elevated temperature and positive blood cultures alert clinician; surgical debridement and drainage, reconstruction or patch repair of any defects, or valve replacement may be required
	Relatively independent of prosthesis used; high-dose antibiotics instituted
Inefficient hemodynamic performance or prosthesis	Inadequate cardiac output may require reoperation to replace prosthesis or implant an allograft in an effort to improve transvalvular flow
	Patient activity may require modification
Anticoagulation-related hemorrhage	Readjust warfarin (Coumadin) dosage; recommend more frequent laboratory studies until prothrombin time is within acceptable range
	Refer for additional teaching and family support
	Assess dietary, medication, and lifestyle habits for risk
Thromboembolism, embolism related to surgical intervention	Adjust anticoagulation dosage to prolong prothrombin time; report neurologic deficits
	Give meticulous attention to removal of surgical debris and intraoperative cleaning of instruments

AV, Atrioventricular; *CPB,* cardiopulmonary bypass; *LV,* left ventricular; *PTFE,* polytetrafluoroethylene.
Modified from Wisman CB, Waldhausen JA: Aortic valve surgery. In Waldhausen JA, Orringer MB: *Complications in cardiothoracic surgery,* St Louis, 1991, Mosby; Seifert PC: Cardiac surgery. In Meeker MH, Rothrock JC, editors: *Alexander's care of the patient in surgery,* ed 11, St Louis, 1999, Mosby.

surgery is associated particularly with risks of stroke or other neurologic deficit (from particulate or air emboli), persistent bleeding (from coagulation disorders), and myocardial infarction (from coronary atheroembolism). Complete heart block is uncommon unless concomitant procedures involving the conduction pathways within the ventricular septum or the area below the right and noncoronary cusps have been performed.

In patients with aortic valve allografts (or pulmonary autografts), leaflet prolapse may result from misalignment of the graft and the native annulus. The surgeon assesses the repair for signs of aortic regurgitation by palpating the aorta for thrills (vibrations of blood hitting against the aortic wall) and leaflet closure. Intraoperative TEE usually detects the problem early enough for technical repair. Table 12-3 lists problems and complications related to the intraoperative and postoperative periods.

References

Abramczyk EL, Brown MM: Valvular heart disease. In Kinney MR, Packa DR: *Andreoli's comprehensive cardiac care*, ed 8, St Louis, 1996, Mosby.

Alpert JS, Sabik J, Cosgrove DM: Mitral valve disease. In Topol EJ, editor: *Comprehensive cardiovascular medicine*, Philadelphia, 1998, Lippincott-Raven.

Banning AP, Hall RJ: Aortic valve disease: management and indications for surgery. In Piwnica A, Westaby S, editors: *Surgery for acquired aortic valve disease*, Oxford, UK, 1997, Isis Medical Media.

Barratt-Boyes BG: Homograft aortic valve replacement in aortic incompetence and stenosis, *Thorax* 19:131, 1964.

Berne RM, Levy MN: *Cardiovascular physiology*, ed 8, St Louis, 2001, Mosby.

Braunwald E: Valvular heart disease. In Braunwald E, Zipes DP, Libby P, editors: *Heart disease: a textbook of cardiovascular medicine*, ed 6, vol 2, Philadelphia, 2001, WB Saunders.

Brooks-Tighe SM: *Instrumentation for the operating room: a photographic manual*, ed 4, St Louis, 1994, Mosby.

Chambers JC and others: Pulmonary autograft procedure for aortic valve disease: long-term results of the pioneer series, *Circulation* 96(7):2206, 1997.

Cosgrove DM and others: Valvuloplasty for aortic insufficiency, *J Thorac Cardiovasc Surg* 102(4):571, 1991.

Cox JL: Introduction to homograft and autograft valve replacement, *Oper Techniq Cardiac Thorac Surg* 2(4):253, 1997.

David TE: Aortic valve repair for management of aortic insufficiency, *Adv Card Surg* 11:129, 1999.

David TE and others: Aortic valve replacement with stentless porcine aortic valves: a ten-year experience, *J Heart Valve Dis* 7(3):250, 1998.

Duran CM: Reconstructive surgery for acquired aortic valve disease. In Piwnica A, Westaby S, editors: *Surgery for acquired aortic valve disease*, Oxford, UK, 1997, Isis Medical Media.

Elkins RC: The Ross operations in patients with dilatation of the aortic annulus and of the ascending aorta, *Oper Techn Cardiac Thorac Surg* 2(4):331, 1997.

Fraser CD Jr, Cosgrove DM 3rd: Surgical techniques for aortic valvuloplasty, *Tex Heart Inst J* 21(4):305, 1994.

Gibbon JH: Application of a mechanical heart and lung apparatus to cardiac surgery, *Minn Med* 37:371, 1954.

Gillinov AM, Casselman FP, Cosgrove DM: Minimally invasive heart valve surgery: operative technique and results. In Yim APC and others, editors: *Minimal access cardiothoracic surgery*, Philadelphia, 2000, WB Saunders.

Glower DD: Acquired aortic valve disease. In Sabiston DC Jr, Spencer FC, editors: *Surgery of the chest*, ed 6, vol 2, Philadelphia, 1995, WB Saunders.

Harken DE and others: Partial and complete prostheses in aortic insufficiency, *J Thorac Cardiovasc Surg* 40(6):744, 1960.

Hazinski MF: *Manual of pediatric critical care*, St Louis, 1999, Mosby.

Hufnagel CA, Harvey WP: The surgical correction of aortic insufficiency, *Bull Georgetown U Med Center* 6:60, 1953.

Ikonomidis JS and others: Post access heart valve surgery. In Yim PC and others, editors: *Minimal access cardiothoracic surgery*, Philadelphia, 2000, WB Saunders.

Karp RB: Inclusion or mini-root homograft aortic valve replacement, *Oper Techn Cardiac Thorac Surg* 2(4):281, 1997.

Kern MJ: *The cardiac catheterization handbook*, ed 3, St Louis, 1999, Mosby.

Kinney MR and others: *Andreoli's comprehensive cardiac care*, ed 8, St Louis, 1996, Mosby.

Kirklin JW, Barratt-Boyes BG: *Cardiac surgery: morphology, diagnostic criteria, natural history, techniques, results, and indications*, ed 2, vol 2, New York, 1993, Churchill Livingstone.

Manouguian S, Seybold-Epting W: Patch enlargement of the aortic valve ring by extending the aortic incision into the anterior mitral leaflet: new operative technique, *J Thorac Cardiovasc Surg* 78(3):402, 1979.

Mattox KL, Estrera AL, Wall MJ: Traumatic heart disease. In Braunwald E, Zipes DP, Libby P: *Heart disease: a textbook of cardiovascular medicine*, ed 6, Philadelphia, 2001, WB Saunders.

McGiffin DC, Kirklin JK: Homograft aortic valve replacement: the subcoronary and cylindrical techniques, *Oper Techn Cardiac Thorac Surg* 2(4):255, 1997.

Meyers D: Freestyle aortic root bioprostheses. In Piwnica A, Westaby S, editors: *Surgery for acquired aortic valve disease*, Oxford, UK, 1997, Isis Medical Media.

Morrow AG and others: Operative treatment in hypertrophic subaortic stenosis: techniques, and the results of pre and postoperative assessments in 83 patients, *Circulation* 52(1):88, 1975.

O'Brien MF, McGriffin DC, Stafford EG: Allograft aortic valve implantation: techniques for all types of aortic valve and root pathology, *Ann Thorac Surg* 48(4):600, 1989.

Otto CM: Aortic stenosis—listen to the patient, look at the valve, *N Engl J Med* 343(9):652, 2000.

Oury JH, Maxwell M: An appraisal of the Ross Procedure: goals and technical guidelines, *Oper Techn Cardiac Thorac Surg* 2(4):289, 1997.

Perloff JK: Congenital heart disease in adults. In Braunwald E: *Heart disease: a textbook of cardiovascular medicine*, ed 5, vol 2, Philadelphia, 1997, WB Saunders.

Randolph JD and others: Aortic valve and left ventricular outflow tract replacement using allograft and autograft valves, *Ann Thorac Surg* 48:345, 1989.

Roberts WC: Anatomically isolated aortic valvular disease: the case against its being of rheumatic etiology, *Am J Med* 49(2):151, 1970.

Rosenhek R and others: Predictors of outcome in severe, asymptomatic aortic stenosis, *N Engl J Med* 343(9):611, 2000.

Ross DN: Application of homografts in clinical surgery, *J Cardiac Surg* 1(3, Suppl):175, 1987.

Ross DN: Homograft replacement of the aortic valve, *Lancet* 2:487, 1962.

Seifert PC: Cardiac surgery. In Rothrock JC: *Perioperative nursing care planning*, ed 2, St Louis, 1996, Mosby.

Starr A, Edwards ML: Mitral replacement: clinical experience with a ball-valve prosthesis, *Ann Surg* 154:726, 1961.

Titus JL, Edwards JE: The aortic root and valve: development, anatomy, and congenital anomalies. In Emery RW, Arom KV, editors: *The aortic valve*, Philadelphia 1991, Hanley & Belfus.

Waldhausen JA, and others: *Surgery of the chest*, ed 6, St Louis, 1996, Mosby.

Westaby S: The aortic valve. In Piwnica A, Westaby S, editors: *Surgery for acquired aortic valve disease*, Oxford, UK, 1997, Isis Medical Media.

Wisman CB, Waldhausen JA: Aortic valve surgery. In Waldhausen JA, Orringer MD: *Complications in cardiothoracic surgery*, St Louis, 1991, Mosby.

13

Tricuspid and Pulmonary Valve Procedures

The three goals of a valvuloplasty are: to give a predictable result, to preserve normal valve function, and to provide a definitive repair.

Alain Carpentier, MD, 1974 (p. 344)

O f the four cardiac valves, the tricuspid is most likely to undergo surgical repair rather than replacement in order to avoid the risk of valve-related complications such as thromboembolism, thrombosis, and anticoagulation-related problems (Kratz and others, 1985).

Surgery on the pulmonary valve is performed rarely in adults but on occasion may be necessary. It is discussed later in this chapter.

Tricuspid Valve Procedures

Tricuspid Apparatus

The tricuspid valve is the largest of the four cardiac valves and is similar to the mitral valve in form and function (see Chapter 11). It is situated so that it lies in a plane caudad to the mitral valve (Braunwald, 1998). Like the mitral apparatus, the tricuspid apparatus consists of the leaflets, annular tissue, chordae tendineae, papillary muscles, and the ventricular wall.

In addition to the lower pressures within the right side of the heart, there are other differences. One of these is that, unlike the bicuspid mitral valve, the tricuspid valve has three leaflets: the anterior, posterior, and septal (Fig. 13-1). Of surgical significance is that the penetrating portion of the conduction system, the bundle of His, and the atrioventricular node can be found at the base of the septal leaflet.

Another notable difference is that there is no discrete tricuspid annulus; rather, there is a relatively undefined ring of tissue to which the bases of the three leaflets are attached to the heart at the atrioventricular junction. (For ease of discussion, the term *annulus* will be used throughout the chapter.) Surrounding this

ring of tissue is the base of the aortic valve, the membranous septum, the central fibrous body (also known as the right fibrous trigone), the right coronary artery, the coronary sinus, and the bundle of His (Fig. 13-2).

Two-dimensional echocardiographic studies have shown that both mitral and tricuspid annular tissue change dynamically during the cardiac cycle. The tricuspid annulus reaches its maximum size in late diastole and its minimum size in midsystole; the annular area can change in size by as much as 39%. That the tricuspid valve demonstrates a greater reduction in circumference than the mitral valve (up to 31% reduction) is thought to be caused by the fact that tricuspid annular tissue is composed largely of myocardium and thus exhibits greater reduction during ventricular systole when the myocardium contracts (Tei and others, 1982). Evaluating annular size and function is helpful in planning the surgical procedure and provides additional clinical data for the surgeon performing digital palpation of the tricuspid valve before instituting cardiopulmonary bypass.

Tricuspid Valve Disease

Tricuspid valve disease requiring surgery is rarely an isolated lesion except when there is a congenital malformation. More often it is a functional disorder secondary to valve disease in the left side of the heart. In contrast, structural tricuspid valve disease affects the valve itself and produces stenosis or regurgitation. It is most often caused by infective endocarditis, congenital heart disease, or rheumatic fever (Doty, 2000). Other structural factors include diffuse connective tissue disorders, right atrial tumors, carcinoid syndrome (distortion of the valve by endocardial fibrosis created by a metastasizing gastrointestinal carcinoma), congenital lesions such as

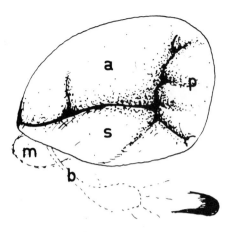

FIGURE 13-1 Normal tricuspid valve. Note the location of the conduction tissue relative to the septal leaflet. *a,* Anterior leaflet; *p,* posterior leaflet; *s,* septal leaflet, *b,* bundle of His; *m,* membranous septum. (From Carpentier A and others: Surgical management of acquired tricuspid valve disease, *J Thorac Cardiovasc Surg* 67[1]:53, 1974.)

Ebstein's anomaly (Hetzer and others, 1998) or atrioventricular canal, and trauma (Braunwald, 1998; McCarthy and Cosgrove, 1997).

TRICUSPID REGURGITATION

Functional tricuspid regurgitation (insufficiency) often is caused by mitral or aortic valve disease producing left ventricular failure, which creates chronically elevated left atrial pressure. This leads to increased pulmonary vascular resistance, pulmonary hypertension, and eventually right ventricular failure, causing right ventricular dilation, tricuspid annular dilation, and subsequent valvular regurgitation (Doty, 2000). In these cases the leaflets themselves may be relatively normal in appearance.

With the development of tricuspid insufficiency, increased right atrial volume raises right atrial pressure, which is reflected backward to the venous system. At the same time forward blood flow is reduced as a result of regurgitation of blood into the right atrium. Eventually, right-sided cardiac output is reduced (Fig. 13-3).

Rheumatic disease

Tricuspid rheumatic inflammatory changes are almost never seen in isolation; they commonly affect the mitral or the aortic valve as well. The process of fibrosis and contraction of the leaflets is similar to that affecting the mitral valve except that calcification is rarer on the tricuspid valve.

Marfan's syndrome

Patients with Marfan's syndrome may demonstrate annular dilation unrelated to pulmonary hypertension (Braunwald, 2001). Marfan's syndrome and other con-

nective tissue disorders (such as those associated with mitral valve prolapse also may affect the leaflets. The mucoid or myxomatous elements of the leaflets proliferate to a greater extent than the sturdier fibrosa element (Roberts, 1987). This produces excessive thinning and stretching of the leaflet tissue, thereby resulting in valvular regurgitation (Fig. 13-4).

Coronary artery disease

Acute thrombosis of the coronary arteries supplying the right ventricle and in particular the inferior wall are an etiologic factor in the development of tricuspid insufficiency (Cohn, 2000). Impaired contractility from right ventricular failure results in a reduction in the narrowing of the annulus during systole. Annular dilation primarily affects the anterior and posterior leaflets; usually only a portion of the septal leaflet annulus becomes dilated (Fig. 13-5). Although pulmonary symptoms are common with left ventricular failure, they are often absent in primary right-sided heart failure, which causes congestion and distension of the venous system (Kinney and others, 1998).

Endocarditis

Although the tricuspid valve is usually an uncommon source of infection, septic endocarditis is being seen with increasing frequency in patients who are intravenous drug users (Relf, 1993).

Ebstein's anomaly

Ebstein's anomaly (Fig. 13-6) is a congenital disorder that may not require surgical intervention until adulthood. The posterior and often the septal leaflets are adherent and tethered to the right ventricular wall. Although the anterior leaflet normally is attached to the annular ring, all three leaflets are usually malformed, being either enlarged or reduced in size, and thickened and distorted. The downward displacement of the posterior and septal leaflets in the right ventricle creates a division of the chamber into a proximal "atrialized" portion with a thin wall and pressures similar to those of the right atrium. The distal ventricular portion consists mainly of apical and infundibular portions of the ventricle. Tricuspid regurgitation is present and may be mild to severe, depending on the degree of leaflet displacement (Hetzer and others, 1998).

Although the anomaly manifests itself during infancy, clinical symptoms may not appear until adolescence or adulthood. Cardiomegaly and hepatomegaly frequently accompany tricuspid regurgitation. Conduction delays, supraventricular tachycardia, and other rhythm disturbances are common and may pose an increased risk during cardiac catheterization. The type of surgery depends on the severity of the lesion and the presence of refractory congestive heart failure or con-

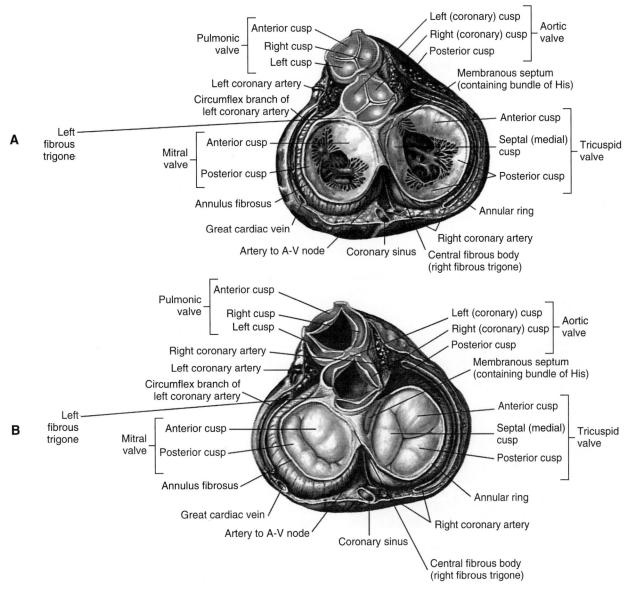

FIGURE 13-2 Superior view of cardiac valves during diastole **(A)**, and systole **(B)**. Note the relationship of the tricuspid valve to the surrounding structures. (From Canobbio M: *Cardiovascular disorders,* St Louis, 1990, Mosby.)

duction disorders. When feasible, valve repair is preferred (Carpentier and others, 1998; Doty, 1997), but replacement may be necessary if the valve is very deformed. Associated atrial septal defects are closed, and conduction disturbances are treated as necessary.

TRICUSPID STENOSIS

Pure tricuspid stenosis is unusual in the adult. When it occurs, it is usually caused by rheumatic disease (which often produces a mixed stenotic and regurgitant lesion), mechanical obstruction by thrombus, bacterial vegetations, tumors (such as atrial myxomas), or meta-static carcinoid lesions (Braunwald, 1998). Congenital absence of the tricuspid valve (tricuspid atresia) is uncommon, but there are reported cases of adults with this malformation (Jordan and Sanders, 1966). Survival depends on the presence of a shunt or a defect to provide an alternative route for blood flow (Roberts, 1987).

The pathologic changes in tricuspid stenosis are similar to those seen in mitral stenosis. The commissures fuse, thereby narrowing the central opening, and right atrial and central venous pressures become elevated (Fig. 13-7), producing symptoms of systemic venous congestion.

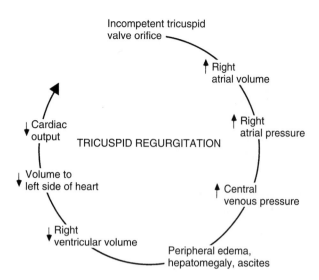

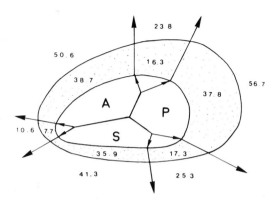

FIGURE 13-5 Tricuspid insufficiency. Dilation primarily affects the posterior *(P)* and anterior *(A)* leaflets. Numbers indicate the average lengths of the attachment of the leaflets in a normal *(central numbers)* and a dilated *(peripheral numbers)* orifice. S, Septal. (From Carpentier A and others: Surgical management of acquired tricuspid valve disease, *J Thorac Cardiovasc Surg* 67[1]:53, 1974.)

FIGURE 13-3 Pathophysiology of tricuspid regurgitation. (From Kinney MR and others: *Comprehensive cardiac care,* ed 8, St Louis, 1996, Mosby.)

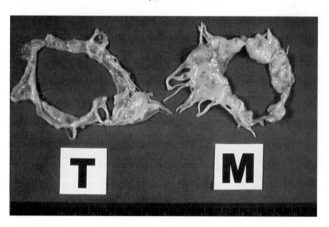

FIGURE 13-4 Myxomatous proliferation of tricuspid *(left)* and mitral *(right)* valves producing valvular insufficiency. (Courtesy Edward A. Lefrak, MD.)

Diagnostic Evaluation of Tricuspid Valve Disease

PHYSICAL EXAMINATION

With both tricuspid valve regurgitation and stenosis, signs and symptoms of right-sided congestion appear (Fig. 13-8). These include hepatomegaly, ascites, right upper abdominal tenderness, increased abdominal girth, and anorexia from liver and intestinal engorgement. Jugular venous distension and edema result from elevated right atrial pressure, and fatigue occurs from low cardiac output. Hepatomegaly may be present; elevated bilirubin levels suggest hepatic congestion from severe right ventricular dysfunction or hepatic ischemia from a low output state (Braunwald, 1998).

Tricuspid regurgitation is more common than stenosis and should be suspected in patients who continue to complain of symptoms despite optimal medical treatment. A moderate degree of tricuspid insufficiency can be tolerated quite easily for many years in some patients; this is in sharp contrast to the more adverse effects of mitral insufficiency.

In addition to the clinical features related to systemic venous congestion and reduced cardiac output, the physical examination generally reveals a systolic (regurgitant) or diastolic (stenotic) murmur along the left lower sternal margin and a prominent jugular venous pulse. The murmur usually is augmented during inspiration and reduced during expiration, particularly during Valsalva's maneuver, which may help to distinguish tricuspid murmurs from mitral murmurs. In patients with tricuspid regurgitation, there may be prominent right ventricular pulsations along the left parasternal region (Braunwald, 1998).

In patients with both stenotic and regurgitant valves, the electrocardiogram usually shows changes associated with enlargement of the right atrium, such as atrial fibrillation. If the right ventricle is enlarged, incomplete right bundle-branch block also may be evident. Chest roentgenograms commonly reveal an enlarged right atrium with tricuspid stenosis or regurgitation; the superior vena cava may be enlarged with tricuspid stenosis.

Clinical findings and hemodynamic data alone are often inadequate to make a diagnosis. The severity of the lesion often requires confirmation at surgery by noting the appearance of the right atrium, digitally palpating the valve before instituting cardiopulmonary bypass, and visually inspecting the valve structure and the size of the annulus (Kirklin and Barratt-Boyes, 1993).

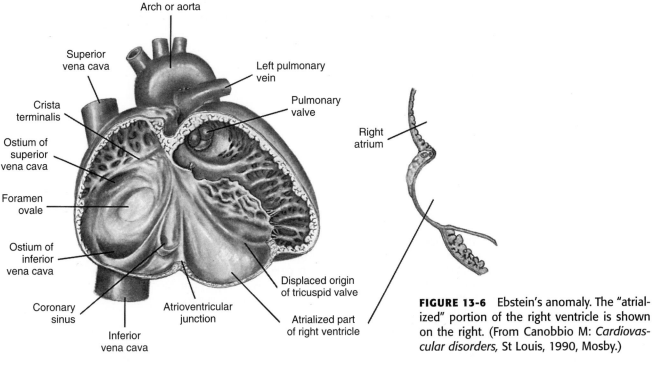

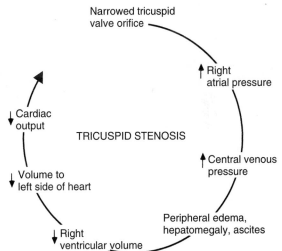

FIGURE 13-6 Ebstein's anomaly. The "atrialized" portion of the right ventricle is shown on the right. (From Canobbio M: *Cardiovascular disorders,* St Louis, 1990, Mosby.)

DIAGNOSTIC STUDIES

Diagnosing tricuspid valve disease presents a number of challenges related to the technique used, right-sided heart hemodynamics, and the left-sided lesions that are often present. Distinguishing tricuspid problems from aortic or mitral valve disease may be difficult because many of the available diagnostic techniques are better at evaluating left-sided rather than right-sided problems.

Echocardiography

Color flow echocardiography often is used to make the diagnosis of tricuspid regurgitation; vegetations may be seen in patients with endocarditis. Doppler methods are used to estimate both the severity of the lesion and the pulmonary artery pressure. Doppler echocardiography has enhanced detection of even minor (and inaudible) amounts of tricuspid regurgitation, but no gold standard exists for measuring the severity of tricuspid regurgitation (Braunwald, 1998).

Doppler methods also can be used to compute the transvalvular pressure gradient with stenotic valves (normally there is no difference in pressure between the atrium and the ventricle during diastole). Usually a mean diastolic gradient exceeding 4 mm Hg will produce symptoms of systemic venous congestion (unless sodium intake has been limited and diuretics have been given). Because the pressures in the right side of the heart are already low, small variations between the right atrium and the ventricle become significant (Braunwald, 2001).

FIGURE 13-7 Pathophysiology of tricuspid stenosis. (From Kinney MR and others: *Comprehensive cardiac care,* ed 8, St Louis, 1996, Mosby.)

Cardiac catheterization

Invasive procedures such as cardiac catheterization may be unreliable, and false-positive results are not uncommon. One reason is that angiographic catheters are inserted into a systemic vein and threaded antegradely into the right atrium, across the tricuspid valve, and into the right ventricle, where dye is injected. Catheter-induced tricuspid regurgitation is easily produced when the catheter crosses the valve (Fig. 13-9). Even though

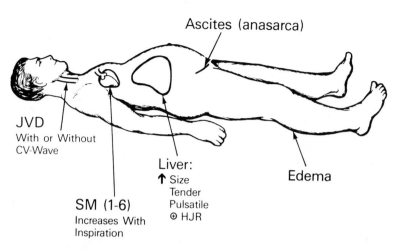

FIGURE 13-8 Clinical signs of tricuspid insufficiency producing systemic venous congestion. *JVD,* Jugular venous distension; *SM,* systolic murmur; *HJR,* hepatojugular reflux. (From Cohen SR and others: Tricuspid regurgitation in patients with acquired, chronic, pure mitral regurgitation. I. Prevalence, diagnosis, and comparison of preoperative clinical and hemodynamic features in patients with and without tricuspid regurgitation, *J Thorac Cardiovasc Surg* 94[4]:481, 1987.)

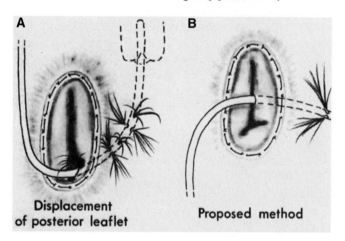

FIGURE 13-9 A, Mechanism of catheter-induced regurgitation in a patient who has had a tricuspid annuloplasty. The same mechanism can cause artifacts during preoperative evaluation. **B,** Alternative method for minimizing catheter-induced regurgitation. (From Grondin P and others: Carpentier's annulus and De Vega's annuloplasty, *J Thorac Cardiovasc Surg* 70[5]:852, 1975.)

such artifacts may produce only a slight increase in the amount of regurgitation detected, in the low-pressure right side of the heart even small increases may be suggestive of a more serious problem than actually exists.

In contrast, mitral valve studies are performed by passing the catheter retrogradely from the aorta into the left ventricle, where dye is injected to detect the presence of mitral valve regurgitation. The catheter does not need to cross the mitral valve, thereby minimizing the possibility of the catheter's interfering with mitral leaflet function. In view of these difficulties, noninvasive techniques such as echocardiography are routine advocated for studying

the tricuspid valve; cardiac catheterization still is used for evaluating other disorders such as coronary artery disease.

Other problems that may be encountered are catheter-induced premature ventricular contractions and catheter dislocation during the injection of contrast dye. Although these problems tend to increase the possibility of false-positive findings, right ventricular angiography probably remains the most objective standard for diagnosing tricuspid regurgitation.

Assessment of tricuspid stenosis is more accurate when right atrial and right ventricular pressures are measured simultaneously rather than sequentially with the pull-back technique (e.g., the catheter is advanced to the right ventricle and pressures are measured, after which the catheter is pulled back into the right atrium and pressures are measured). Left-sided cardiac catheterization is performed routinely to study associated lesions of the mitral or aortic valve, left ventricular function, and the severity and extent of existing obstructive coronary artery disease.

SURGERY FOR TRICUSPID VALVE DISEASE

Because operations for tricuspid valve disease commonly are related to left-sided valvular lesions, surgical outcome is affected by the perioperative status of the left side of the heart. In general, surgical outcome is more successful in patients without severe systemic venous hypertension or right ventricular dysfunction, fixed pulmonary hypertension, or incomplete repairs of left-sided problems (McGrath and others, 1990). In the presence of these derangements, tricuspid regurgitation may actually worsen after surgery.

TABLE **13-1**
Standards of Nursing Care for Tricuspid Valve Surgery*

NURSING DIAGNOSIS	PATIENT OUTCOME	NURSING ACTIONS
Anxiety related to disease, surgery, and perioperative events	Patient demonstrates acceptable levels of anxiety and is able to cooperate with therapeutic regimen	Elicit questions and concerns about tricuspid disease and treatment Identify learning needs; refer if necessary for later follow-up Institute measures to relieve systemic venous congestion: rest, cautious intravenous infusion, avoidance of pressure on abdomen; elevate head of stretcher
Knowledge deficit related to inadequate knowledge of planned surgery and perioperative events	Patient demonstrates knowledge of physiologic and psychologic responses to tricuspid valve surgery	Determine patient's understanding of tricuspid valve disease; possible surgical interventions (annuloplasty, replacement, excision, commissurotomy); types, benefits, and risks of prostheses; and preferences if any Clarify patient's understanding of possible need for permanent pacemaker caused by surgical proximity to conduction tissue If additional procedures are planned, refer to specific standards of care Assess mitral and aortic valve disease in addition to tricuspid valve disease; assess left ventricular and right ventricular function; note presence of pulmonary hypertension, liver dysfunction, other problems related to systemic venous congestion
Risk for injury related to use of valve retractor	Patient is free of injury from use of retraction devices	Use handheld valve retractors with caution to avoid injury to conduction tissue, atrial septum, and surrounding tissue

Risk for injury related to:
 	
  Physical hazards
	The patient is free of injury related to:
	
	  Physical hazards
		
		Have available type and sizes of valvular prostheses desired by surgeon; store valves and annuloplasty rings in cool, dry location; have appropriate accessories to size and insert prostheses; have necessary suture available (pledgeted, nonpledgeted, multicolored); have tricuspid sizers for tricuspid rings; have appropriate bypass and cardioplegia cannulas/catheters
		Have double venous cannulas, right-angle cannulas (per surgeon's request); caval tourniquets or clamps
		Have left atrial line and suture for securing

Electrical hazards	Electrical hazards	Have temporary and permanent epicardial atrial and ventricular pacing leads; have temporary and permanent pacemaker generator per surgeon's request; check for kinks in leads Test pacer leads and generator to ensure they are working properly

Risk for self-care deficit related to inadequate knowledge of rehabilitation period	Patient demonstrates knowledge of rehabilitation period as it relates to self-care abilities	Assess patient's knowledge of signs/symptoms of tricuspid valve failure
		Assess patient's understanding of possible complications of surgery performed and knowledge of reportable signs and symptoms:
		  Heart block: slow pulse, fatigue, syncope
		  Regurgitation/stenosis: edema, jugular venous pulsation, abdominal discomfort, fatigue
		  Endocarditis: fever, anemia, murmur, chills, weight loss, microembolic petechiae
		Know complications of prosthetic valves (see Chapter 11 on mitral valve surgery and Chapter 12 on aortic valve surgery) and reportable signs and symptoms
		Refer for counseling if history of illicit drug use
		Refer for pulmonary and cardiac rehabilitation as needed

Modified from Seifert PC: Cardiac surgery. In Rothrock JC: *Perioperative nursing care planning,* ed 2, St Louis, 1996, Mosby.
*See also Chapter 11 on mitral valve surgery.

Patient teaching considerations

Because tricuspid valve dysfunction often is related to left-sided valvular lesions, patient teaching considerations include learning needs associated with both the tricuspid valve disease and concomitant aortic or mitral valve disease (Table 13-1). The nurse can clarify how left-sided lesions affect the tricuspid valve and produce symptoms of systemic venous congestion. When pulmonary function has been affected by the valvular disorder, the patient can be informed about rehabilitative regimens that enhance both pulmonary and cardiac function.

Psychologic and social responses to the disease and the interventions can be investigated with the patient and family. When the etiology is related to intravenous drug use, referrals to addiction treatment programs should be considered. The risk of recurring endocarditis from continued drug use needs to be stressed.

Patients may undergo valve repair or replacement (or excision). As part of the consent process, the surgeon reviews the risks and benefits of the planned procedure, and the nurse can clarify this information and discuss the functional implications for postoperative activities of daily living.

When valve replacement is planned, patient teaching is directed toward the type of prosthesis (or allograft) to be used and its postoperative implications. Unlike bioprostheses and allografts, mechanical valves require chronic anticoagulation, and attendant risks and precautions should be part of the patient teaching (see Chapter 11 on mitral valve surgery).

Procedural considerations

Instrumentation and supplies (Box 13-1) are similar to those used for mitral valve surgery (see Chapter 11). If surgery on the mitral or aortic valve is planned, specialty items related to those procedures should be included.

Intracardiac hemodynamic monitoring of the right side of the heart is performed with a central venous pressure line inserted before surgery. Because a pulmonary artery balloon catheter interferes with the surgical exposure, pressure monitoring of the left side of the heart may require insertion of a left atrial line after completion of the tricuspid repair. Transesophageal echocardiography (TEE) is used to monitor right- and left-sided cardiac function.

Cardiopulmonary bypass for tricuspid valve surgery is achieved with separate venous cannulas inserted into the superior and inferior venae cavae (Box 13-1). A right-angle cannula in the superior vena cava provides an unobstructed operative site. Umbilical tapes (or caval clamps) are placed around the cavae and tightened with tourniquets. This forces all the systemic venous return to enter the openings in the distal ends of the cannulas and prevents venous return from obscuring the right atrium and tricuspid valve. In the presence of long-standing tricuspid regurgitation and associated liver dysfunction, use of an inferior vena caval tourniquet may produce significant back pressure on the liver, leading to hepatocellular necrosis; some authors (Kay, 1992) suggest avoidance of caval snares. A cardiotomy suction is used to remove coronary sinus drainage.

Often the surgeon performs a digital examination of the tricuspid valve before inserting the superior vena

---

BOX 13-1
Tricuspid Valve Surgery: Procedural Considerations*

Instrumentation

Mitral valve instruments and self-retaining retractors
Handheld tricuspid valve retractors
Caval clamps (see Fig. 13-13)

Valve Prostheses and Accessories

Annuloplasty rings: specific for tricuspid valve (e.g., Carpentier-Edwards) or those that can be used in either atrioventricular valve (e.g., Duran ring)
Mechanical heart valves (mitral prostheses are used)
Bioprostheses (mitral prostheses are used)
Sizers (obturators) (in range of sizes) specific to prosthesis; use tricuspid sizers for tricuspid annuloplasty rings
Sizer handles (Carpentier ring sizers have special handles; Duran ring sizers require a Kelly or tonsil clamp for grasping)
Prosthetic valve holders and handles (some prostheses are packaged with an attached holder); sterile nurse applies handle into holder
Mitral valve supplies and suture (may use 3-0 suture in right side of heart instead of 2-0 commonly used in left side of heart)

Supplies

Individual caval cannulas; may use right-angle cannula (see Fig. 13-12, *B*)
Umbilical (caval) tapes and tourniquets
Retrograde cardioplegia catheter
Left atrial line and supplies for insertion
French-eye needles
Pacemaker supplies: temporary atrial and ventricular (epicardial) leads; temporary pacemaker generator (Have permanent pacer supplies—epicardial leads, generator, and pacing system analyzer [PSA]—available. Need for permanent generator may not be apparent until the postoperative period, at which time permanent leads are placed)

Positioning, Skin Preparation, Draping, Special Safety Measures

Same as for mitral valve

Documentation/Report to the Intensive Care Unit

Same as for mitral or aortic valve plus information related to specific repair (type of prosthesis used, e.g., ring or valve); right-sided problems such as right-sided myocardial infarction, congenital anomalies of tricuspid valve, conduction disturbances related to lesion or surgery; history of pulmonary hypertension; history of liver dysfunction

*See also Chapter 11 on mitral valve surgery. If additional procedures are performed, see appropriate chapter for procedural considerations.

---

caval cannula into the right atriotomy. The purpose of this is to detect the degree of tricuspid insufficiency. Because many factors contribute to the amount of

RN First Assistant Considerations During Tricuspid Valve Surgery

Determine need for and type of pressure monitoring lines in right side of heart (e.g., CVP, pulmonary artery catheter); discuss with anesthesia personnel and surgeon before skin preparation.

Note location of septal leaflet and tricuspid annulus, sinoatrial (SA) node, and atrioventricular (AV) node; avoid injury to structures from instruments or excessive manipulation.

Adjust retractors, surgical lights, and other equipment as necessary to expose surgical site; use caution retracting septum, septal and other leaflets, and membranous septum.

Keep right atrium clear of blood returning via coronary sinus with cardiotomy suction; use care in exposing coronary sinus for retroplegia infusion.

Monitor electrocardiogram, systemic and pulmonary pressures, central venous pressure, and cardiac output; compare with observed cardiac contractions in anticipation of conduction disturbances requiring permanent pacemaker system; assist with insertion of temporary (or permanent) epicardial leads/generator.

Monitor central venous pressure for right-sided heart filling pressures or evidence of tricuspid regurgitation; monitor left-sided heart function by direct inspection of heart or left atrial pressure line or indirectly via systemic blood pressure.

Anticipate use of left atrial pressure line and assist with insertion.

If repairing Ebstein's anomaly, inspect surgical area for atrial septal defect or other congenital anomalies; assist in repair.

CVP, Central venous pressure line.

insufficiency—blood volume, atrial fibrillation, pulmonary hypertension, cardiac insufficiency, and anesthesia—some authors have cautioned that overestimation or underestimation of the degree of insufficiency is possible (Carpentier, 1983). Studies have not demonstrated a statistical correlation between the degree of tricuspid regurgitation palpated at surgery and the severity of regurgitation by the patient history, physical examination, or preoperative hemodynamic data (although longer duration of preoperative symptoms of congestive heart failure does seem to correlate with more severe tricuspid regurgitation). More accurate assessments are likely to result when sodium restriction and diuresis have been instituted preoperatively (Cohen and others, 1987).

Whether the tricuspid valve disease is isolated or occurs in combination with mitral or aortic valve disease, cold cardioplegic arrest is used to protect the entire heart. Retroplegia is valuable in these procedures for protecting the right side of the heart (especially in the presence of a right dominant coronary system) because there is often some degree of right ventricular dysfunction. With the right atrium opened, a retroplegia catheter can be inserted into the coronary sinus under direct vision. Surgeons may use a combined approach with both antegrade and retrograde protection of the right and left sides of the heart; when antegrade cardioplegia is given, coronary venous return exiting the coronary sinus will temporarily obscure the operative field.

One of the most serious complications associated with tricuspid valve procedures is the creation of heart block from injury to the atrioventricular node and the bundle of His located along the annular portion of the septal leaflet. Injury also may be caused by edema from surgical manipulation or to a suture placed in the conduction pathway. Another potential danger is injury to the right coronary artery. Precautions include gentle handling of tissue, avoidance of unnecessary instrument manipulation of conduction tissue, and optimum exposure of the surgical site (Box 13-2).

Associated left-sided lesions are repaired first, followed by the tricuspid valve procedure (Mullany and others, 1987). With respect to myocardial revascularization procedures, if saphenous vein coronary bypass grafts are performed to the right coronary artery (or to the posterior descending branch of the right coronary artery), the proximal anastomosis to the aorta is done after the right atrium is closed.

TRICUSPID VALVE REPAIRS

Procedural considerations

A number of reparative procedures can be performed. The DeVega suture annuloplasty is a simple procedure that requires less operative time than other, more complex reparative techniques (Grondin and others, 1975; Rivera, Duran, and Ajuria, 1985). One of the complications of this technique is suture dehiscence (with resulting insufficiency).

Annuloplasty rings. A variety of annuloplasty rings with specific sizers is available. Rings and sizers should be differentiated from mitral valve devices, as well as from each other. Interrupted sutures commonly are used to insert annuloplasty rings, but a continuous suture technique can be used (Gay, 1990). In general, women require a smaller size than men.

Carpentier tricuspid rings are available in even-numbered sizes (e.g., 30, 32, 34, 36). The rings are similar to their mitral annuloplasty counterparts except that the tricuspid ring has a gap in that portion corresponding to the area adjacent to conduction tissue; the gap prevents the placement of sutures in this critical area. Obturators are made of nondisposable plastic and require sterilization before use; they are also different in shape from those for the mitral annuloplasty ring. The reusable metal obturator handle does fit both tricuspid and mitral rings (see Chapter 3). The ring itself is held

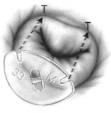

Mitral

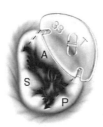
Tricuspid

FIGURE 13-10 One side of the Duran annuloplasty ring sizer is used for tricuspid valve repairs *(right),* and the other side is used for mitral valve repairs *(left).* (Courtesy Medtronic, Inc.)

by the assistant during implantation; no ring holder is available.

Duran annuloplasty rings with disposable sizers are available in odd-numbered sizes (e.g., 31, 33, 35) and can be used in either the tricuspid or mitral position. However, orientation of the ring and the sizers must be appropriate for the valve repaired (Fig. 13-10). When sizing the tricuspid valve, the obturator is held with the side displaying the initial *T* for tricuspid (the reverse side, with the initial *M,* is used to measure a mitral valve). A tonsil or Kelly hemostat is used to grasp the central bar of the obturator, and the sizer is lowered onto the valve. The notches are aligned with the commissures of the septal leaflet, and the anterior leaflet is extended to cover the surface of the selected obturator. The obturator with the surface area most nearly matching the anterior leaflet and commissural notch spacing corresponds to the size ring that should be used.

The Duran ring is supplied with an attached holder; a metal reusable handle is screwed into the plastic holder. The ring/holder assembly needs to be oriented so that the word *tricuspid* is at the upper side (the word *mitral* appears upside down on the assembly). After the sutures have been placed and the prosthesis has been lowered into the annulus, the retaining sutures are cut to remove the holder.

The Cosgrove-Edwards annuloplasty ring (see Fig. 11-24) is attached to a frame with a handle to facilitate insertion of stitches into the prosthetic sewing ring. Carpentier-Edwards tricuspid sizers are used. Once suturing is completed, the holder/handle assembly is removed.

Operative procedure: repair of the tricuspid valve

1. A median sternotomy is performed. Atrial purse-string sutures are placed in the appendage and the atrial wall for bypass cannulas. Before inserting the cannula into the appendage opening, the surgeon

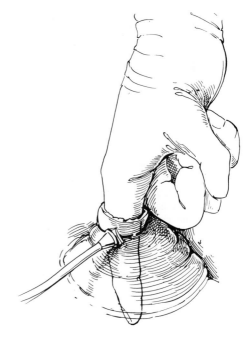

FIGURE 13-11 Before insertion of the venous drainage cannula, the surgeon places a finger through the right atriotomy to palpate the tricuspid valve and to detect the degree of tricuspid regurgitation. (From Waldhausen JA, Pierce WS: *Johnson's surgery of the chest,* ed 5, St Louis, 1985, Mosby.)

may place a finger through the atriotomy to palpate the tricuspid valve (Fig. 13-11) in order to determine the degree of valvular regurgitation.

A minimally invasive right parasternal approach can be employed (Lazzara and Kidwel, 1998). In patients requiring repeat sternotomy, this approach may be preferable because there is less risk of bleeding and graft trauma (e.g., to mammary or saphenous vein grafts in coronary bypass patients) associated with reopening the sternum. Standard surgical instruments can be used. Cardiopulmonary bypass is achieved with femoral vein–femoral artery cannulation. An additional venous cannula can be "Yd" to the superior and inferior venae cavae (Klokocovnik, 2000).

2. Double venous cannulas are inserted so that they do not cross one another in the right atrium. A right-angle cannula (Fig. 13-12) may be used in the superior vena cava. Occluding tapes or caval clamps (Fig. 13-13) are tightened around the cavae and cannulas to prevent venous return from obscuring the surgical site. Cardioplegia solution is infused antegradely through the aortic root.

3. The right atrium is opened longitudinally along the atrioventricular groove to expose the tricuspid valve, and retractors are inserted (see Chapter 11

A

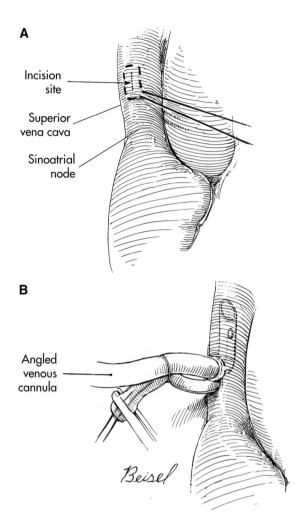

Incision site

Superior vena cava

Sinoatrial node

B

Angled venous cannula

Beisel

FIGURE 13-12 Insertion of a right-angle venous cannula. **A,** Pursestring suture in the superior vena cava. **B,** Right-angle venous cannula with a tourniquet. (From Waldhausen JA, Pierce WS, Campbell DB: *Surgery of the chest,* ed 6, St Louis, 1996, Mosby.)

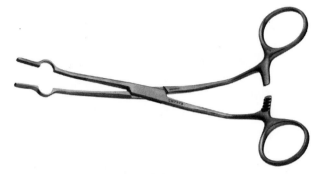

FIGURE 13-13 The caval clamp is placed over the superior vena cava and venous cannula (see text). (Courtesy Baxter Healthcare Corp, V. Mueller Div, Chicago.)

on mitral valve surgery). Cardiotomy suctions are used to remove coronary sinus drainage. Retroplegia may be given under direct vision.

4a. Kay bicuspidization technique (Kay, 1992): This is one of the earliest reparative techniques developed for the tricuspid valve; it is now infrequently performed. The annulus of the posterior leaflet is plicated with sutures, producing a two-leaflet valve.

4b. De Vega suture annuloplasty technique (Rabago and others, 1980): A double-armed, felt-pledgeted suture is placed in or near the tricuspid valve ring, beginning at the anteroseptal commissure and continuing along the anterior and posterior leaflet annulus to the level of the coronary sinus in the area of the septal leaflet (Fig. 13-14, *A*). The suture

is placed into a second pledget. The other arm of the suture is then similarly placed (in reverse), and the two ends of the suture are tied over the pledget at the anteroseptal commissure (Fig. 13-14, *B*). To achieve the correct size for the annulus, a valve obturator may be inserted into the annular opening; the suture is then pulled up against the sizer, and the stitch is tied.

This technique is used less frequently than the Carpentier and Duran annuloplasty repairs.

4c. Carpentier annuloplasty ring technique (Carpentier, 1983): Carpentier's (1974) goals of predictability, preservation of valve function, and definitive repair form the basis for the development of the ring annuloplasty technique that is used widely to repair the tricuspid valve. According to Carpentier (1983), predictability is achieved by precise measurement of the leaflets with sizing obturators and valve function is preserved with restoration of a normal valve orifice using a preformed ring. If these goals are achieved, a definitive repair can be expected.

A prosthetic semirigid ring is inserted in a manner similar to that for a mitral valve ring annuloplasty. The annuloplasty ring itself differs, however, in that there is a gap in the ring corresponding to the annular area containing nodal and bundle conduction tissue. The size of the ring is determined with special tricuspid obturators (Fig. 13-15) that are used to measure the anterior leaflet. Another method is to select the obturator with notches corresponding to the commissures on either side of the septal leaflet (this technique is based on the finding that the septal leaflet is relatively unaffected by annular dilatation and tends to retain its normal size and shape).

Interrupted, alternately colored sutures are placed around the circumference of the annulus

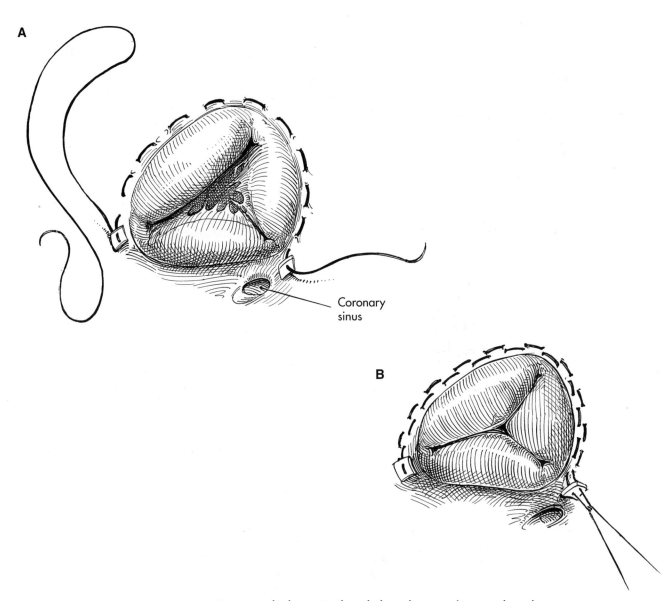

A

B

Coronary
sinus

FIGURE 13-14 De Vega annuloplasty. **A,** The pledgeted suture is started at the posteroseptal commissure and continued counterclockwise to the anteroseptal commissure, where another pledget is attached. **B,** The suture is brought back to the starting point, and the two ends are tied around an obturator to achieve the correct size. (From Waldhausen JA, Pierce WS, Campbell DB: *Surgery of the chest,* ed 6, St Louis, 1996, Mosby.)

(except the conduction tissue portion of the septal leaflet) and then into the corresponding area on the prosthetic ring (Fig. 13-16). When the stitches are tied, the excess annular tissue is evenly drawn up against the prosthesis, thereby reducing the annular size and also remodeling the annulus (Fig. 13-17).

4d. Duran annuloplasty ring technique (Duran, 1989): A flexible circular ring (see Fig. 5-64) is used to reduce and selectively remodel the annulus (see Chapter 11 for illustration of the Duran ring in mitral repair). Obturators are used for sizing, and

stitches are placed into the annulus in a manner similar to that for the Carpentier technique. In the area of the septal leaflet, Duran recommends that sutures be placed superficially at the base of the septal leaflet rather than deep into the annulus in order to avoid creation of heart block.

4e. Cosgrove annuloplasty ring technique (McCarthy and Cosgrove, 1997; Gillinov and Cosgrove, 1998): A flexible semicircular ring (see Fig. 11-24) is used to produce a measured plication of the annulus at the base of the anterior and posterior leaflets,

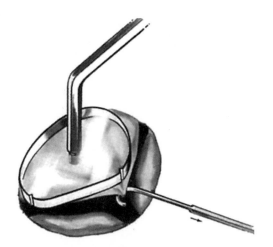

FIGURE 13-15 Sizing is performed by measuring the anterior leaflet with obturators. The two notches in the edge of the obturator correspond with the commissures on either side of the septal leaflet. (From Carpentier A: Cardiac valve surgery—the "French correction," *J Thorac Cardiovasc Surg* 86[3]:323, 1983.)

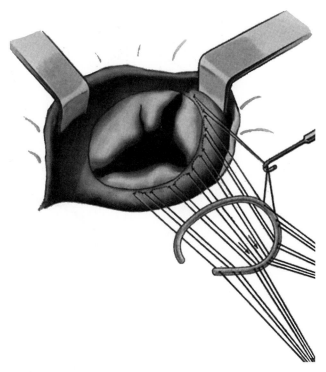

FIGURE 13-16 Suturing of the prosthetic ring using mattress sutures. The interval between sutures is reduced at the commissures *(arrows).* (From Carpentier A: Cardiac valve surgery—the "French correction," *J Thorac Cardiovasc Surg* 86[3]:323, 1983.)

which typically represent the areas of greatest dilation. Avoiding the placement of sutures in the septal leaflet minimizes the risk to conduction tissue. Carpentier-Edwards sizers are used to determine the appropriate Cosgrove ring. Stitches are placed into the annular portions of the anterior and posterior leaflets, then into the semicircular Cosgrove ring. The ring is slid into position and the stitches tied. According to Cosgrove, the procedure produces a universally flexible tricuspid annulus and preserves the physiologic shape and motion.

5. The repairs are tested for residual insufficiency (a bulb syringe often is used), and the right atrium is closed. TEE is used to evaluate the repair.
6. A left atrial pressure monitoring line may be inserted and secured with a fine silk suture (Fig. 13-18).
7. Temporary atrial and ventricular pacing wires are attached, and the patient is weaned from cardiopulmonary bypass. Occasionally, permanent epicardial pacing leads are attached.
8. Hemostasis is achieved, chest tubes are inserted, and all incisions are closed.

Operative procedure: tricuspid valve commissurotomy for tricuspid stenosis

Open commissurotomy (Fig. 13-19) is performed for tricuspid valve stenosis. An annuloplasty ring often is inserted to remodel the annulus to create a more normal configuration and prevent residual insufficiency. When the posterior leaflet is retracted, it may be excluded on insertion of the annuloplasty ring, producing a bicuspid valve (Carpentier, 1983).

Procedure

1. All three commissures are incised sharply to mobilize the leaflets; some secondary chordae tendineae may require resection.
2. An annuloplasty ring is inserted. Occasionally bicuspidization is performed when the posterior leaflet is retracted (Fig. 13-19, *C*).

TRICUSPID VALVE REPLACEMENT

Even when replacement is performed for dysfunctional mitral or aortic valves, implantation of a tricuspid prosthesis is avoided when possible. The exception can occur in the presence of massive tricuspid regurgitation, destruction of the valvular apparatus, fixed pulmonary hypertension, or severe right ventricular dysfunction (Ohata and others, 2000).

When valve replacement is indicated, the lower stresses found in the lower-pressure environment of the right ventricle (as compared with the left ventricle) favor the use of bioprosthetic valves (or aortic valve allografts mounted on a stent), whose leaflets do not seem to degenerate as quickly as they do under the higher pressures generated in the left side of the heart (Nakano and others, 2001; Kawano and others, 2000).

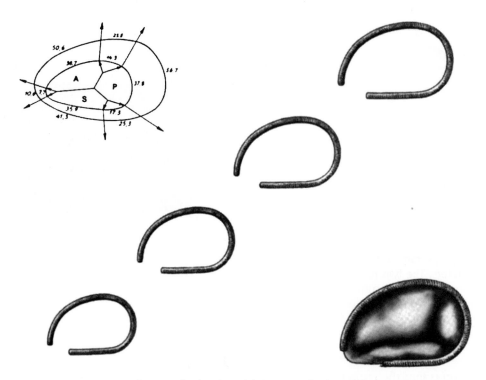

FIGURE 13-17 Carpentier prosthetic tricuspid ring annuloplasty. Shown are dimensions *(left)*, various sizes of rings *(middle)*, and completed annuloplasty *(right)*. (From Carpentier A: Cardiac valve surgery—the "French correction," *J Thorac Cardiovasc Surg* 86[3]:323, 1983.)

Bioprostheses also are favored because they are less thrombogenic than mechanical valves, which have a significant incidence of thrombosis in the right side of the heart. The mechanism of thrombus formation is related to the presence of synthetic materials contacting blood; the process may be accelerated in the right side of the heart because blood flow is slower and more apt to promote venous stasis. Optimum warfarin (Coumadin) anticoagulation is mandatory.

On occasion a bioprosthesis may be considered unsuitable because of a high potential for late calcification, stenosis, or failure. If an allograft is unavailable, a mechanical valve must be used. Although the long-term results with most mechanical valves have been disappointing because of thrombosis, prosthetic endocarditis, and anticoagulation-related hemorrhage, the St. Jude Medical valve has shown good results. The advantages of this valve appear to be related to its central laminar flow pattern, rapid leaflet motion, and low residual gradient (Singh, Feng, and Sanofsky, 1992).

Mechanical prostheses also are often used for patients with Ebstein's anomaly (see Fig. 13-6). Valve replacement can produce long-lasting clinical improvement (Abe and Komatsu, 1983), although reparative techniques (Carpentier and others, 1988) are also used.

Procedural considerations

Mitral valve prostheses are used for tricuspid valve replacement. During excision of the valve leaflets, a portion of the septal leaflet is retained. In this area, sutures are placed into the retained leaflet tissue rather than into the body of the annular ring. This aids in reducing the risk of injury to the conduction pathways.

Operative procedure: tricuspid valve replacement with a biologic or mechanical prosthesis

1. The tricuspid valve is exposed as described in step 3 of the procedure for repair of the tricuspid valve, and the leaflets are excised. A portion of the septal leaflet tissue where it joins the annulus is retained for placement of sutures in this section.
2. The valve ring is sized with obturators, and the appropriate (mitral) prosthesis is delivered to the field. If a bioprosthesis is used, it is rinsed with saline to remove the glutaraldehyde storage solution (see Chapter 11 on mitral valve surgery).
3. Individual, alternately colored sutures are placed in the valve annulus and the prosthetic sewing ring. The valve is seated, and the stitches are tied.
4. The atrium is closed, and the procedure is completed as described in step 8 of the procedure for repair of the tricuspid valve.

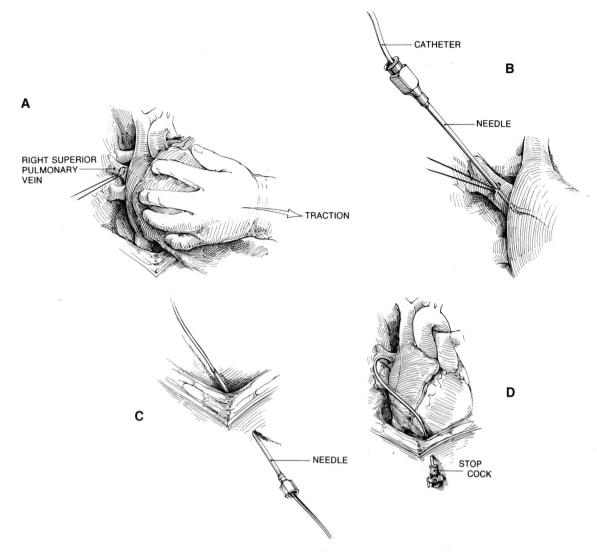

FIGURE 13-18 Left atrial pressure monitoring line. **A,** The right atrium is retracted to expose the right pulmonary vein, and a pursestring suture is inserted. **B,** The monitoring catheter is inserted into the left atrium via a catheter introducer needle (some devices have a peel-away introducer). The introducer is removed, and the pursestring suture is tied. An additional suture may be used to attach the catheter to the pericardium. **C,** The catheter is threaded through a large-bore needle passed through skin and subcutaneous tissue into the pericardium. The catheter is brought out to the skin. **D,** A stopcock can be added, and the catheter is secured to the skin with a suture. Blood is aspirated to ensure proper placement of the catheter, which is then attached to pressure tubing connected to a transducer. (From Waldhausen JA, Pierce WS, Campbell DB: *Surgery of the chest,* ed 6, St Louis, 1996, Mosby.)

Operative procedure: allograft (homograft) replacement of the tricuspid valve

The advantages of central flow and freedom from anticoagulation, hemolysis, and prosthetic noise have made aortic (and pulmonary) allografts attractive for valvular lesions in the left side of the heart and for reconstruction of the right ventricular outflow tract (see Chapter 12 on aortic valve surgery). When tricuspid valve replacement is necessary, these advantages have been cited by those who prefer the allograft to a prosthetic valve. Like tissue valves, allograft durability is enhanced by lower right-sided heart pressures (Kirklin and Barratt-Boyes, 1993; Ross, 1987).

Procedure

1. The aortic valve (or pulmonary valve) allograft is evaluated to confirm the absence of any structural abnormalities and is prepared as described in Chapter 12.

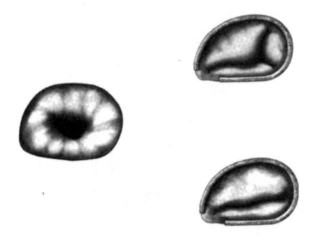

FIGURE 13-19 Tricuspid valve commissurotomy and repair with an annuloplasty ring. (From Carpentier A: Cardiac valve surgery—the "French correction," *J Thorac Cardiovasc Surg* 86[3]:323, 1983.)

2. The allograft is mounted onto a stent or frame (or attached to a segment of Dacron graft) and sewn to the tricuspid annular ring. If the graft is not used immediately, it can be stored in solution at 4° C (39.5° F) or it can be cryopreserved.

TRICUSPID VALVULECTOMY

Special problems may be encountered in patients with intractable bacterial endocarditis (often caused by *Staphylococcus aureus* or *Pseudomonas aeruginosa*) that cannot be controlled with intensive antibiotic therapy (Relf, 1993). In these patients, who are often intravenous drug users, florid vegetations involving all three leaflets may make valve repair by debridement of the vegetations or valvuloplasty unfeasible. Replacement of the valve is associated with thrombotic complications and a significant incidence of reinfection, leading to prosthetic valve endocarditis. In an effort to avoid continued sepsis and recurring infection (generally attributed to resumption of drug use), some researchers have performed initial valvulectomy, followed if necessary by a later second operation for tricuspid valve replacement (Braunwald, 1998). Others (Stern and others, 1986) have questioned the need for excision and prefer initial implantation of a bioprosthesis. Absence of the tricuspid (or pulmonary) valve can be tolerated hemodynamically by some patients, unlike aortic or mitral valve excision without replacement.

Indications for surgery generally include persistent sepsis, recurrent septic pulmonary emboli, and valvular insufficiency leading to acute right-sided heart failure (Braunwald, 1998).

Operative procedure

1. A median sternotomy and bicaval cannulation for cardiopulmonary bypass are performed. Cardioplegic arrest is used to protect the heart.
2. The right atrium is incised longitudinally.
3. The tricuspid valve is excised totally, with care taken to preserve the conduction tissue in the area of the septal leaflet. Portions of infected tissue may be cultured. (It may be advisable to confine and contain the instruments used to excise the infected valve.)
4. If the infectious process extends to the pulmonary valve, excision of that valve may be indicated. A supravalvular incision is made in the pulmonary artery, and the valve is excised.
5. The surgical field is irrigated, debris is removed, and all incisions are closed.

Postoperatively valvulectomy patients require additional volume to maintain an adequate right atrial systolic pressure and right ventricular preload. Intravenous antibiotic therapy is continued for a number of weeks to eradicate the infection. With the valve excised, patients will display a pulsatile liver (from reflux), but in this case it does not necessarily indicate right-sided heart failure (Cohen and others, 1987). A second operation may be undertaken for prosthetic valve replacement subsequent to a cure of the endocarditis or if medical treatment has failed to control hemodynamic derangements associated with right-sided or biventricular failure.

Postoperative Considerations

When tricuspid valve surgery is performed in conjunction with operations for aortic and mitral valve lesions, the results of surgery are dependent on the success of the operation for the left-sided lesions, the degree and reversibility of both left and right ventricular dysfunction, and the amount and reversibility of pulmonary hypertension (Duran, 1989). As with most cardiac operations, better results can be obtained if the operation is performed before the development of congestive heart failure. In addition to the benefits of cardiac rehabilitation, pulmonary rehabilitation may be helpful in these patients. If valve replacement with a mechanical prosthesis has been performed, warfarin anticoagulation is started approximately 48 to 72 hours after surgery (Kirklin and Barratt-Boyes, 1993).

COMPLICATIONS

The clinician is alert to the appearance of complete heart block throughout the postoperative hospital stay (Table 13-2), especially when valve replacement has

TABLE 13-2
Postoperative Complications of Tricuspid Valve Surgery

COMPLICATION	INTERVENTIONS
Rhythm Disturbances (Complete Heart Block)	
Early onset: may be caused by edema; may be iatrogenically related to suture placement in conduction tissue; increased risk with combined tricuspid surgery and mitral valve replacement (compression of firm prosthetic sewing rings)	Permanent pacemaker may be inserted; usually epicardial lead is inserted via thoracotomy to avoid possible injury to valve prosthesis from transvenous insertion; occasionally epicardial leads are placed at time of surgery when heart block has been strongly suspected or confirmed.
Delayed onset: usually related to scar formation around prosthetic annulus; may be idiopathic degeneration of surrounding tissue	Same
Recurrent/Residual Tricuspid Regurgitation	
More likely in patients with irreversible pulmonary hypertension or continued mitral valve problems (prosthetic malfunction, endocarditis)	Repair left-sided lesion Replace mitral prosthesis Repair/replace tricuspid valve
Residual Tricuspid Diastolic Gradient	
May be related to tricuspid prosthetic (valve or ring) annulus being too small; residual stenosis	Replace with larger prosthesis
Persistent Right Ventricular Failure	
Related to dysfunctional right ventricle	Valve replacement may (or may not) improve condition Medical treatment includes diuretics, low-sodium diet, rest, and digitalis
Prosthesis-Related Complications	
Prosthetic valve endocarditis Anticoagulation-related hemorrhage Bioprosthetic degeneration: may occur later than with left-sided bioprosthesis because of lower stresses in right ventricle	See Chapter 11 on mitral valve surgery
Prosthetic dehiscence from torn suture or fractured ring Prosthetic thrombosis: high risk in right side of heart; may occur early or late; is generally caused by inadequate anticoagulation of mechanical valve	Repair annuloplasty Intravenous thrombolysis can be useful when thrombosis first occurs; thrombectomy and valve replacement (with bioprosthesis)

Modified from Grattan MT, Miller DC, Shumway NE: Management of complications of tricuspid valve surgery. In Waldhausen JA, Orringer MB: *Complications in cardiothoracic surgery,* St Louis, 1991, Mosby.

been performed. Heart block may not become apparent until a few days after surgery, especially if temporary pacing has been used in the immediate postoperative period. ECG monitoring should be continued until a stable rhythm is established at an adequate rate (Kirklin and Barratt-Boyes, 1993). If permanent pacing is indicated, transvenous leads may be avoided because of the possibility of injuring the native valve or bioprosthesis or of becoming entrapped in a mechanical prosthesis. When late heart block appears, it can be corrected with an epicardial lead placement through a thoracotomy approach (Grattan, Miller, and Shumway, 1991).

Complications related to annuloplasty techniques include residual regurgitation or stenosis. The former commonly is caused by irreversible pulmonary hypertension, although suture dehiscence may be a cause. The latter may be the result of too small a prosthesis

being inserted. Prosthetic valve replacement is associated with a number of complications described in Chapters 11 and 12 on mitral and aortic valve surgery.

Pulmonary Valve Procedures

Pulmonary Valve Disease

The pulmonary valve, the smallest of the cardiac valves, has three leaflets and is similar to the aortic valve. It is situated between the distal right ventricular outflow tract and the entrance to the main pulmonary artery. When the pericardium is opened during median sternotomy, the bulging outline of the anterior sinuses surrounding the valve leaflets can be seen on the front of the heart at the entrance to the main pulmonary artery.

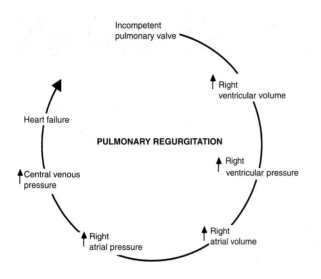

FIGURE 13-20　Pathophysiology of pulmonary regurgitation. (From Kinney MR and others: *Comprehensive cardiac care,* ed 8, St Louis, 1996, Mosby.)

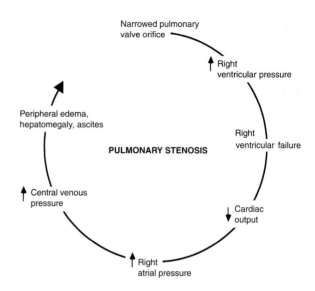

FIGURE 13-21　Pathophysiology of pulmonary valve stenosis. (From Kinney MR and others: *Comprehensive cardiac care,* ed 8, St Louis, 1996, Mosby.)

They are even more apparent when the right ventricular outflow tract is distended.

Acquired lesions of the pulmonary valve are rare, and this is probably related to the conditions within the right side of the heart, such as lower pressures and less turbulent blood flow, which subject the valve to less stress as compared with the valves in the left side of the heart. Rheumatic fever and infective endocarditis are less likely to affect the pulmonary valve than they are the other valves of the heart (Braunwald, 1998). When pulmonary valve disorders do exist, they usually are associated with primary pulmonary hypertension, or they develop secondary to lesions in the left side of the heart (e.g., mitral or aortic valve disease) that produce pulmonary hypertension leading to pulmonary valvular regurgitation (Fig. 13-20). Correction of the left-sided lesion often reduces the degree of regurgitation.

Other causes of pulmonary insufficiency are dilation of the pulmonary valve ring or the pulmonary artery secondary to pulmonary hypertension or connective tissue disorders such as Marfan's syndrome. Infective endocarditis, valvular damage caused by the prolonged use of pulmonary artery monitoring catheters, carcinoid syndrome, direct trauma to the heart, and previous valvulotomy for pulmonary stenosis may also be etiologic factors. Symptoms of pulmonary regurgitation include dyspnea and fatigue, but these are not usually apparent unless there is coexisting pulmonary hypertension (Braunwald, 1998).

Stenotic lesions causing obstruction to flow may result from infectious or inflammatory processes, tumors, carcinoid plaques, or atheromas. Although acute rheumatic fever does involve the pulmonary valve, as well as the other valves of the heart, it rarely causes appreciable chronic fibrosis or dysfunction (Altrichter and others, 1989).

Typically, pulmonary valve stenosis is a congenital lesion. The valve may be bicuspid or tricuspid; it may be accompanied by infundibular muscular stenosis causing right ventricular outflow tract obstruction. Depending on its severity, pulmonary stenosis may not be recognized until childhood or adulthood (Fig. 13-21). Symptoms include dyspnea on exertion, fatigue, and occasionally cyanosis (Braunwald, 1998). These are manifestations of congestive failure as a result of chronic pressure overloading of the right ventricle, reduced cardiac output from obstruction to flow, and an inadequate supply of oxygenated blood to the systemic circulation.

DIAGNOSTIC EVALUATION OF PULMONARY VALVE DISEASE

In addition to a thorough medical history, diagnostic evaluation includes an electrocardiogram to identify the presence right ventricular hypertrophy, right atrial dilation, and conduction disturbances; a chest x-ray film to detect right ventricular enlargement, pulmonary artery dilation, and pulmonary vascular changes; and color flow Doppler echocardiography to visualize and quantify valvular hemodynamic changes. Cardiac catheterization is used for surgical candidates to assess pulmonary artery–right ventricular pressure gradients, the degree of regurgitation, left-to-right shunts, and other possible anomalies or lesions (Braunwald, 1998).

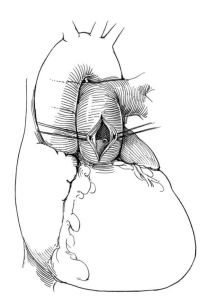

FIGURE 13-22 Incision and retraction of the pulmonary artery for exposure of the pulmonary valve. (From Waldhausen JA, Pierce WS, Campbell DB: *Surgery of the chest,* ed 6, St Louis, 1996, Mosby.)

SURGERY FOR PULMONARY VALVE DISEASE

Percutaneous balloon valvuloplasty commonly is performed for isolated pulmonary valve stenosis (Doty, 1997). The success of balloon dilation procedures is in part the result of the frequent absence of calcification on the pulmonary valve, in contrast to that on valves in the left side of the heart (Altrichter and others, 1989).

When valves are dysplastic or hypoplastic, surgical treatment may be performed to repair or, rarely, to replace the valve. Surgery for acquired pulmonary regurgitation is uncommon. If pulmonary valve replacement is indicated, aortic valve prostheses are used. Increasingly, allografts are being used in preference to mechanical or bioprosthetic valves. They are used widely in children to replace the pulmonary valve or to reconstruct the right ventricular outflow tract (Ross, 1987).

Operative procedure: open commissurotomy for pulmonary valve stenosis

1. A median sternotomy is performed, and cardiopulmonary bypass is established using double-venous cannulation to keep venous return from obscuring the surgical site. The heart is arrested with cardioplegia solution or fibrillated with an alternating-current (AC) fibrillator so that air cannot be ejected into the left side of the heart.
2. The pulmonary artery is opened transversely or longitudinally (Fig. 13-22) to expose the pulmonary valve. Traction sutures may be used to facilitate exposure.

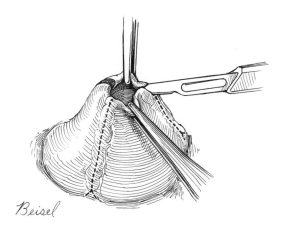

FIGURE 13-23 Commissurotomy for pulmonary stenosis. Incisions are made along the dotted lines. (From Waldhausen JA, Pierce WS, Campbell DB: *Surgery of the chest,* ed 6, St Louis, 1996, Mosby.)

3. The valve is inspected, and the commissures are incised to the annulus with a knife (No. 11 blade) (Fig. 13-23). Hegar dilators may be used to calibrate the valve orifice and the infundibulum.
4. If annular enlargement is indicated, a patch (autologous pericardium or prosthetic patch material) is used to enlarge the annulus and at the same time close the incision.
5. If infundibular hypertrophy restricts right ventricular outflow, part of the muscle can be resected.
6. If a patch has not been used, the incision is closed primarily (Waldhausen, Pierce, and Campbell, 1996).
7. To resume cardiac action in the fibrillating heart, direct-current (DC) countershock is applied to defibrillate the heart.
8. Incision sites are inspected for hemostasis, cardiopulmonary bypass is terminated, chest tubes are inserted, and all incisions are closed.

References

Abe T, Komatsu S: Valve replacement for Ebstein's anomaly of the tricuspid valve: early and long-term results of eight cases, *Chest* 84(4):414, 1983.

Altrichter PM and others: Surgical pathology of the pulmonary valve: a study of 116 cases spanning 15 years, *Mayo Clin Proc* 64(11):1352, 1989.

Braunwald E: Valvular heart disease. In Fauci AS and others: *Harrison's principles of medicine,* ed 14, New York, 1998, McGraw-Hill.

Braunwald E: Valvular heart disease, editor. In Braunwald E, Zipes DP, Libby P, editors: *Heart disease: a textbook of cardiovascular medicine,* ed 6, Philadelphia, 2001, WB Saunders.

Canobbio M: *Cardiovascular disorders,* St Louis, 1990, Mosby.

Carpentier A: Cardiac valve surgery—the "French correction," *J Thorac Cardiovasc Surg* 86(3):323, 1983.

Carpentier A: Discussion of Boyd AD and others: Tricuspid annuloplasty: five and one-half years' experience with 78 patients, *J Thorac Cardiovasc Surg* 68(3):344, 1974.

Carpentier A and others: A new reconstructive operation for Ebstein's anomaly of the tricuspid valve, *J Thorac Cardiovasc Surg* 96(1):92, 1988.

Cohen SR and others: Tricuspid regurgitation in patients with acquired, chronic, pure mitral regurgitation. I. Prevalence, diagnosis, and comparison of preoperative clinical and hemodynamic features in patients with and without tricuspid regurgitation, *J Thorac Cardiovasc Surg* 94(4):481, 1987.

Cohn LH: Surgical treatment of coronary artery disease. In Goldman L, Bennett JC, editors: *Cecil's textbook of medicine*, ed 21, vol 1, Philadelphia, 2000, WB Saunders.

Doty BD: *Cardiac surgery: operative technique*, St Louis, 1997, Mosby.

Doty JR: Tricuspid valve disease, www.ctsnet.org/doc/4471, 2000 (accessed November 27, 2000).

Duran CM: Tricuspid valve repair. In Grillo HC and others, editors: *Current therapy in cardiothoracic surgery*, Philadelphia, 1989, BC Decker.

Gay WA: *Atlas of adult cardiac surgery*, New York, 1990, Churchill Livingstone.

Gillinov AM, Cosgrove DM: Tricuspid valve repair for functional tricuspid regurgitation, *Oper Tech Thorac Cardiovasc Surg* 3(2):134, 1998.

Grattan MT, Miller DC, Shumway NE: Management of complications of tricuspid valve surgery. In Waldhausen JA, Orringer MB: *Complications in cardiothoracic surgery*, St Louis, 1991, Mosby.

Grondin P and others: Carpentier's annulus and De Vega's annuloplasty: the end of the tricuspid challenge, *J Thorac Cardiovasc Surg* 70(5):852, 1975.

Hetzer R and others: A modified repair technique for tricuspid incompetence in Ebstein's anomaly. *J Thorac Cardiovasc Surg* 115(4):857, 1998.

Jordan JC, Sanders CA: Tricuspid atresia with prolonged survival, *Am J Cardiol* 18:112, 1996.

Kawano H and others: Tricuspid valve replacement with the St. Jude Medical valve: 19 years of experience, *Eur J Cardiothorac Surg* 18(5):565, 2000.

Kay JH: Surgical treatment of tricuspid regurgitation, *Ann Thorac Surg* 53:1132, 1992.

Kinney MR and others: *AACN clinical reference for critical care nursing*, ed 4, St Louis, 1998, Mosby.

Kirklin JW, Barratt-Boyes BG: *Cardiac surgery*, ed 2, New York, 1993, Churchill Livingstone.

Klokocovnik T: Minimally invasive parasternal approach to tricuspid valve avoids repeat sternotomy, *Tex Heart Inst J* 27(1):55, 2000.

Kratz JM and others: Trends and results in tricuspid valve surgery, *Chest* 86(6):837, 1985.

Lazzara RR, Kidwel FE: Right parasternal incision: a uniform minimally invasive approach for valve operations, *Ann Thorac Surg* 65(1):271, 1998.

McCarthy JF, Cosgrove DM 3rd: Tricuspid valve repair with the Cosgrove-Edwards annuloplasty system, *Ann Thorac Surg* 64(1):267, 1997.

McGrath LB and others: Tricuspid valve operations in 530 patients: twenty-five-year assessment of early and late phase events, *J Thorac Cardiovasc Surg* 99(1):124, 1990.

Mullany CJ and others: Repair of tricuspid valve insufficiency in patients undergoing double (aortic and mitral) valve replacement. Perioperative mortality and long-term (1 to 20 years) follow-up in 109 patients, *J Thorac Cardiovasc Surg* 94(5):740, 1987.

Nakano K and others: Tricuspid valve replacement with bioprostheses: long-term results and causes of valve dysfunction, *Ann Thorac Surg* 71(1):105, 2001.

Ohata T and others: Surgical strategy for severe tricuspid valve regurgitation complicated by advanced mitral valve disease: long-term outcome of tricuspid valve supra-annular transplantation in eighty-eight cases, *J Thorac Cardiovasc Surg* 120(2):280, 2000.

Rabago G and others: The new De Vega technique in tricuspid annuloplasty (results in 150 patients), *J Cardiovasc Surg* 21(2):231, 1980.

Relf MV: Surgical intervention for tricuspid valve endocarditis: vegetectomy, valve excision, or valve replacement? *J Cardiovasc Nurs* 7(2):71, 1993.

Rivera E, Duran C, Ajuria M: Carpentier's flexible ring versus De Vega's annuloplasty. A prospective randomized study, *J Thorac Cardiovasc Surg* 89(2):196, 1985.

Roberts WC: *Adult congenital heart disease*, Philadelphia, 1987, FA Davis.

Ross D: Application of homografts in clinical surgery, *J Cardiac Surg* 1(3 suppl):175, 1987.

Seifert PC: Cardiac surgery. In Rothrock JC: *Perioperative nursing care planning*, ed 2, St Louis, 1996, Mosby.

Singh AK, Feng WC, Sanofsky SJ: Long-term results of St. Jude Medical valve in the tricuspid position, *Ann Thorac Surg* 54(3):538, 1992.

Stern HJ and others: Immediate tricuspid valve replacement for endocarditis. Indications and results, *J Thorac Cardiovasc Surg* 91(2):163, 1986.

Tei C and others: The tricuspid valve annulus: study of size and motion in normal subjects and in patients with tricuspid regurgitation, *Circulation* 66(3):665, 1982.

Waldhausen JA, Pierce WS: *Johnson's surgery of the chest*, ed 5, St Louis, 1985, Mosby.

Waldhausen JA, Pierce WS, Campbell DB: *Surgery of the chest*, ed 6, St Louis, 1996, Mosby.

14

Surgery on the Thoracic Aorta

The operation now proposed by the writer is applicable to . . . all fusiform and saccular aneurisms, whether traumatic or idiopathic, in which the conditions for securing provisional haemostasis can be obtained . . . These cases offer admirable opportunities for the conservative application of ateriorrhaphy, with the view of preserving the lumen of the injured vessel, and thus maintaining their functional value as blood carriers.

Rudolph Matas, MD, 1903

Matas' treatment of aneurysms was limited to the peripheral vascular system because in the early twentieth century there were no methods to provide circulatory support or prosthetic grafts to replace the diseased aorta. Most aneurysms of the thoracic aorta were inoperable. Occasionally, saccular aneurysms could be treated by clamping the neck of the lesion, excising the aneurysmal sac, and suturing the remaining edges of the aorta. The contributions of Matas were significant nonetheless because he was one of the first to suggest techniques that have become commonplace today: obtaining proximal and distal control of the artery, performing minimal dissection of adjacent structures, and restoring normal, unobstructed flow through the vessel (Cooley, 1989).

The Aorta

The normal aorta is a remarkably strong conduit that can withstand the impact of 2.5 to 3 billion heartbeats in an average lifetime. The aorta is the primary blood conductor and, with its major branches, supplies blood to all the major organs of the body (see Fig. 8-19). When surgery requires temporary occlusion of a portion of the aorta, tissues receiving blood from that segment are deprived of oxygen, nutrients, and the other metabolic requirements. In procedures on the heart, measures are instituted to protect the myocardium and the brain from the effects of ischemia. In procedures on the thoracic aorta, one has to be especially concerned about the neurologic effects of ischemia not only on the brain but also on the spinal cord. In treating lesions of the ascending aorta, and in particular of the aortic arch, which necessitates temporary interruption of cerebral blood flow, there is a risk for stroke.

When disorders of the descending thoracic aorta or thoracoabdominal aneurysms are being treated, interruption of aortic blood flow to the spinal cord can cause paralysis. Prevention of these complications is a major consideration during surgery on the thoracic aorta (Box 14-1).

The Aortic Wall

Like all arteries, the aortic wall consists of three layers (Fig. 14-1). The *tunica intima* is the thin inner layer made up of endothelial cells; the thick middle layer, the *tunica media,* consists of relatively little smooth muscle (as compared with the peripheral arteries) but contains a large amount of laminated and intertwining sheets of elastic tissue arranged in spiral fashion; the outermost layer, the *tunica adventitia,* contains mainly collagen but also the vasa vasorum and lymphatics, which nourish the aortic wall. The structure of the aortic wall facilitates both the forward propulsion of blood and its circulation throughout the body.

When blood is ejected by the left ventricle, the aorta distends and then recoils, propelling the blood distally into the arterial bed. As the patient ages, smooth muscle and elastic tissue in the aorta and its branches tend to stiffen, producing an increase in the systolic blood pressure and a reduction in the distensibility of the aortic wall. The development of arteriosclerosis and hypertension associated with aging, as well as the existence of inherited or acquired disorders such as infection, inflammation, atherosclerosis, or autoimmune diseases, can produce pathologic changes in the aortic wall, leading to the formation of aortic aneurysms and other disorders of the thoracic aorta (Kirklin and Barratt-Boyes, 1993).

Aortic Aneurysms and Aortic Dissections

ANEURYSM

An aneurysm is a localized or diffuse dilation of the arterial wall; it occurs with increasing frequency between the fifth and seventh decades of life (Isselbacher, Eagle, and De Sanctis, 1997). Thoracic (and abdominal) aortic aneurysms are characterized by weakening and degeneration of the medial layer, which leads to progressive enlargement of all layers of the vessel. There is compression of the surrounding structures and, if untreated, eventual rupture with exsanguination. When thoracic aneurysms rupture into the pericardium, death is usually caused by cardiac tamponade. The standard treatment for aneurysms is the surgical restoration of vascular continuity by relining or replacing the diseased aorta with a prosthetic graft.

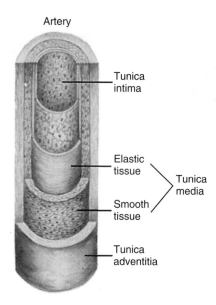

FIGURE 14-1 The aortic wall consists of three layers: the inner tunica intima; the tunica media, composed of elastic and muscular tissue; and the tunica adventitia. (From Canobbio MM: *Cardiovascular disorders,* St Louis, 1990, Mosby.)

AORTIC DISSECTION

Aortic dissection is a unique condition affecting the aortic media. It is the most common catastrophe involving the aorta, occurs more often in men than women, and ruptures acutely more frequently than abdominal aortic aneurysm (David, 1999; Westaby, 1997). Repeated biomechanical stress, often in combination with hypertension and a congenital predisposition, produces an intimal tear (Fig. 14-2) through which blood enters and creates a dissecting hematoma of variable distance within the tunica media. As blood continues to enter the false lumen, it enlarges and impinges on the true lumen. Eventually this causes compression of the arterial branches of the aorta. The torn intima may create a flap of tissue or progress to create a circumferential dissection with intussusception of the intima into the distal portion of the aorta (Borst, Heinemann, and Stone, 1996).

The intimal tear may originate in any portion of the aorta but is most often found in the ascending thoracic aorta just above the coronary ostia and in the descending thoracic aorta just distal to the subclavian artery. It can occur in the presence of an atherosclerotic aorta. Progression of an ascending aortic dissection may be prevented or halted by severe atherosclerosis of the aortic arch, which causes atrophy and fibrosis of the underlying media.

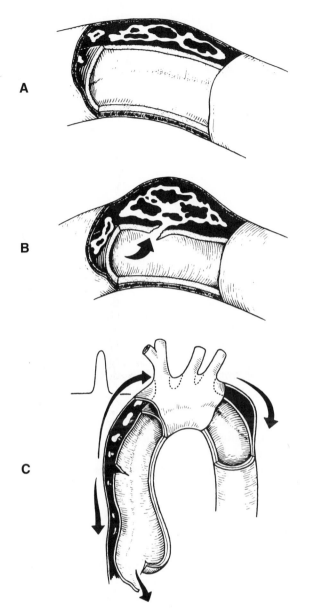

FIGURE 14-2 Pathogenesis of aortic dissection. **A,** Medial and intimal degeneration in the aortic wall predispose the vessel to injury. **B,** Hemodynamic forces acting on the aortic wall produce an intimal tear, directing the bloodstream into diseased media. **C,** The resulting dissecting hematoma is propagated in both directions by a pulse wave produced by each myocardial contraction. (From Wheat MW: Acute dissecting aneurysms of the aorta. In Goldberger E: *Treatment of cardiac emergencies,* ed 5, St Louis, 1990, Mosby).

Although the term *dissecting aortic aneurysm* is often applied to all these lesions, it is appropriate only for those dissections that are superimposed on preexisting fusiform aneurysms. *Aortic dissection* is considered a more accurate designation when the affected aorta was not previously aneurysmal. Dilation of the vessel is

caused mainly by the dissecting hematoma rather than by a transmural dilation of all layers of the aortic wall. The dissection may be classified as acute if it is less than 2 weeks in duration; chronic dissections are those present for more than 2 weeks (Kirklin and Barratt-Boyes, 1993).

Surgery is recommended for all patients with dissections of the ascending aorta and the transverse aortic arch (David, 1999). Dissections of the descending thoracic aorta are treated surgically when there is continuing enlargement of the vessel, danger of imminent rupture, or other complications, usually related to interruption of blood flow through branching blood vessels. Uncomplicated descending thoracic aortic aneurysms not in danger of rupture often are treated medically with antihypertensive and beta-adrenergic blocking medications, analgesics, sedatives, and rest.

Classification of Aortic Aneurysms and Aortic Dissections

Aneurysms and dissections of the thoracic aorta may be classified according to location, morphology, and etiology. Consideration of all three factors is critical to perioperative nurses and surgeons alike for preparing and executing the surgical plan. In particular, this knowledge provides the most meaningful information for determining the indications for operation, the surgical approach (including positioning and instrumentation), and the technique of circulatory support.

LOCATION

For simplicity, aortic disease typically is described according to the principal structural region in which it occurs (i.e., ascending, transverse, or descending aorta) (Fig. 14-3), although the disease process or injury often crosses these anatomic boundaries. Descending aortic aneurysms may be confined to the thoracic section of the aorta (above the diaphragm), or they may occupy both thoracic and abdominal sections of the aorta (thoracoabdominal aneurysms).

Aortic dissection has prompted distinctive classification systems based on the portion of the aorta affected. It is especially important to ascertain whether the dissection involves the ascending aorta because there is a high risk of rupture in this region. DeBakey and colleagues (1965) were the first to place dissections into three categories: types I, II, and III (Fig. 14-4). In type I dissections, the intimal tear originates in the ascending aorta and the dissecting hematoma extends to the descending thoracic aorta or beyond. Type II dissections involve the ascending aorta only. Type III dissections occur in the descending thoracic aorta. The other most

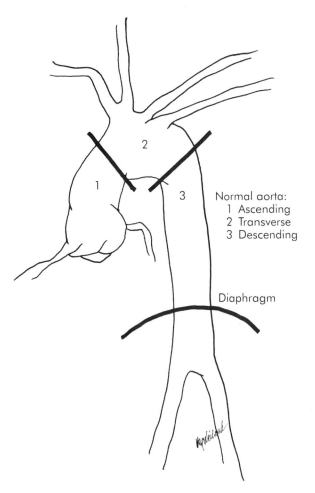

FIGURE 14-3 Structural regions of the thoracic aorta. (Drawing by Anne Weiland, NP.)

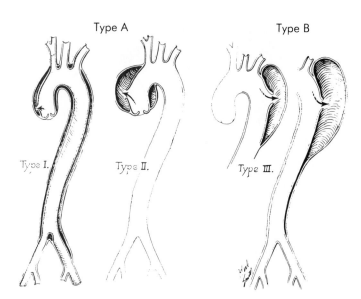

FIGURE 14-4 Location of aortic dissections. The Stanford system classifies aortic dissections based on involvement of the ascending aorta (type A) or noninvolvement (type B). The Debakey system classifies dissections into type I, II, or III. (From DeBakey ME and others: Surgical management of dissecting aneurysms of the aorta, *J Thorac Cardiovasc Surg* 49:130, 1965.)

commonly used classification system is the one devised at Stanford by Daily and his associates (1970) (see Fig. 14-4). It divides dissections into two types: type A, located in the ascending aorta, and type B, involving the descending aorta.

MORPHOLOGY

Morphologically, aneurysms commonly are described as true or false (Fig. 14-5). *True aneurysms* involve all three layers of the arterial wall: intima, media, and adventitia; the full thickness is dilated beyond normal limits. Aneurysms can be subdivided further into saccular or fusiform aneurysms. The former is a localized outpouching from the vessel wall, frequently attached by a neck of tissue. Fusiform aneurysms involve circumferential dilation.

False aneurysm implies a separation of intima from outer layers. The innermost aortic intimal width may be normal in size, with the aneurysm affecting the outermost layers. Also known as *pulsating hematomas*, false an-

eurysms are produced when injury to the inner layers causes extravasation of blood through the intimal and medial layers but the hematoma is contained by the adventitial layer (Cohn, 1995). Aortic dissections are a form of false aneurysm.

ETIOLOGY

Lesions may be either congenital or acquired. Acquired diseases may be complicated by underlying inherited histologic disorders that compromise vascular integrity and accelerate the degenerative process.

Congenital aneurysms

Congenital forms are rare. When they do occur, they often are related to anatomic anomalies or inherited metabolic disorders. Coarctation of the aorta produces hypertension and increased pressure on the aortic wall proximal to the coarctation. A bicuspid aortic valve increases turbulent blood flow and reduces laminar flow, thereby placing greater lateral stress on the aorta and causing local injury (Kirklin and Barratt-Boyes, 1993).

Acquired aneurysms/dissections

Acquired aneurysms and dissections of the thoracic aorta are associated with medial degeneration, arteriosclerosis, atherosclerosis, and trauma. Hypertension is a common finding in these patients and can further weaken an aortic wall already damaged by other causes. Aneurysms tend

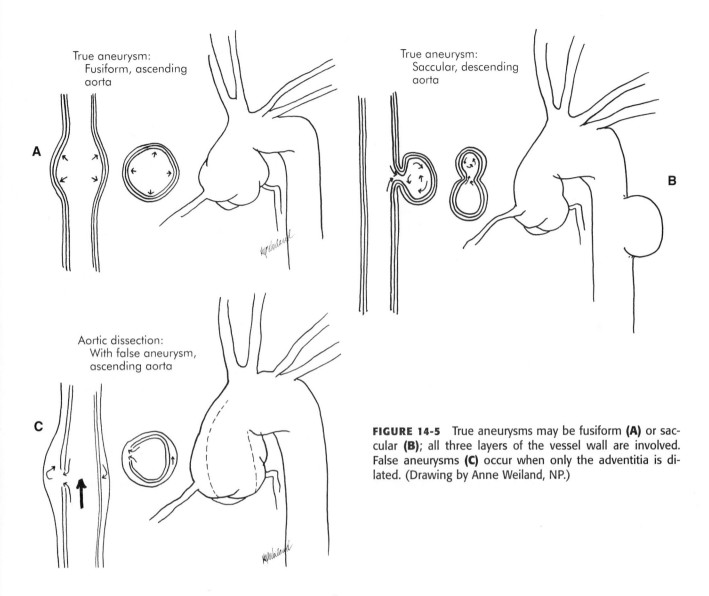

FIGURE 14-5 True aneurysms may be fusiform **(A)** or saccular **(B)**; all three layers of the vessel wall are involved. False aneurysms **(C)** occur when only the adventitia is dilated. (Drawing by Anne Weiland, NP.)

to occur in older patients with atherosclerotic disease, but patients with inherited connective tissue disorders, which can aggravate an existing problem, may acquire an aneurysm or dissection at an earlier age.

Medial degeneration

Most thoracic aortic aneurysms, and in particular aneurysms of the ascending aorta, are caused by medial degeneration. *Cystic medial necrosis* often is used to describe this condition, but the term is a misnomer because true cysts and necrosis of the smooth muscle cells are absent. Rather, there is degeneration and loss of smooth muscle cells and elastic tissue with scarring and fibrotic changes.

The causes of this degenerative process are unknown but are thought to be related to biochemical defects in the synthesis or degradation of collagen, elastin, or mucopolysaccharides within the medial layer of the wall. It is uncertain whether this is a primary medial defect producing dilation (and occasionally dissection) or whether it is an ongoing process of repetitive aortic injury and repair. There is often a history of hypertension, and this is significant because of the additional constant stress it places on the vessel wall. Over time the aortic wall weakens and dilates, and a vicious cycle of further weakening and dilation eventually produces rupture or dissection.

Marfan's syndrome

Patients with Marfan's syndrome demonstrate similar degenerative changes in the elastic fibers of the aortic media and have a characteristic constellation of signs. These are musculoskeletal characteristics that are the result of skeletal overgrowth: excessive height; kyphoscoliosis; slender, spiderlike fingers and toes; chest wall deformities such as pectus excavatum (funnel chest) or pectus carinatum (pigeon chest); weak joint capsules; and elongated facial features. Ocular manifestations include exophthalmos, dislocated lens, shallow anterior chamber, detached retina, cataracts, and myopia.

It is thought that an additional inherited connective tissue disorder produces a deficiency of the microfibrillar fibers forming the scaffolding for elastin, which is one of the primary components of the tunica media. Abnormalities in the development of these fibers cause them to elongate progressively over time and fragment the elastic lamellae of the media, thereby affecting the aorta's ability to withstand the constant stress of pulsatile blood flow and other biomechanical forces.

These changes accelerate the degenerative process, resulting in the appearance of cardiovascular lesions at an early age and often in an emergency setting. The most frequently encountered of these problems are dilation and rupture of the aortic root (complicated by aortic dissection), aortic valve regurgitation, and mitral valve prolapse. These cardiovascular problems form part of a triad of signs and symptoms that also includes musculoskeletal deformities and ocular abnormalities. Patients who do not display the external stigmata associated with Marfan's syndrome but who have a positive family history and display annuloaortic dilation are said to have an incomplete form (*forme fruste*) of the disorder (Pyeritz, 1990).

Annuloaortic ectasia

Annuloaortic ectasia is a pathoanatomic description for a combination of aneurysm of the aortic root, dilation of the aortic annulus, and subsequent aortic valve insufficiency. The lesion, named by Ellis, Cooley, and DeBakey in 1961, is associated with aortic medial degeneration (with or without Marfan's syndrome) that is idiopathic or attributable to the aging process. Aortic dissection and rupture may complicate annuloaortic ectasia.

Usually there is cephalad displacement of the coronary orifices with aneurysms that involve the sinuses of Valsalva. Composite replacement of the aortic valve and the aortic root (with coronary reimplantation) is often required, as it is for most lesions involving the aortic root and valve. Ironically, the upward displacement of the coronary ostia seen in ecstatic lesions makes their reimplantation into the graft somewhat easier because there is more room for the surgeon to perform the ostial anastomoses. Normally placed coronary artery ostia are more difficult to implant directly into a combined valve-graft prosthesis (Cooley, 1991).

Atherosclerosis

Atherosclerotic lesions are found more commonly in the descending thoracic and abdominal aorta but also may affect the ascending aorta or aortic arch. They generally occur in older patients. The media undergoes atrophy and fibrous replacement with avascular connec-

tive tissue. Aortic dilation compromises the ability of the vasa vasorum to nourish the vessel wall. As the wall is exposed to both greater tension and diminishing nutrition, the aneurysm enlarges, resulting in eventual rupture if untreated (Cohn, 1995).

Trauma

Blunt chest trauma from automobile and motorcycle accidents can transect the aorta, resulting in immediate death in approximately 85% of cases (Girardi and Isom, 1999). The most common mechanism of injury is related to the acceleration-deceleration of the body when it contacts an immovable object (e.g., dashboard or steering wheel) and the continued movement of internal organs, specifically the heart and great vessels. As these internal organs continue to move forward, the aorta tears at those points where it is attached within the chest. Most commonly this is the aortic *isthmus,* where the aorta is attached to the ligamentum arteriosum, and the left subclavian artery (see Chapter 19), where the ligamentum arteriosum (the remnant of the fetal ductus arteriosus) connects the aorta and the pulmonary artery. It also can occur before the takeoff of the innominate artery where the right side of the aortic arch is fixed.

Direct trauma, rather than acceleration-deceleration injury, is more likely to injure the ascending aorta and the aortic arch. When all layers of the aortic wall are transected, exsanguination is rapid and survival rates are low.

Survival of traumatic transection of the aorta initially depends on the formation of a false aneurysm whereby the adventitia remains intact and contains the hematoma with support from surrounding mediastinal structures. Without the creation of this false aneurysm, there would be rapid extravasation of the blood volume, allowing insufficient time for prevention or repair of the rupture.

A widened mediastinum or a suspicious shadow may be seen on the chest x-ray film. Early diagnosis and prompt surgical treatment may be delayed, however, because there may be little or no external evidence of chest trauma or because additional injuries may divert attention from the aortic tear. Also, patients may be unable to describe symptoms when head trauma affects their mental status (Girardi and Isom, 1999).

Other causes

Now rare, but at one time the most common cause of thoracic aneurysms, *syphilis* produces inflammatory changes, with scarring and destruction of the aortic wall, leading to fusiform or saccular aneurysms. Also seen with less frequency are aneurysms caused by infection, commonly termed *mycotic aneurysms.* These tend to be saccular and are found mainly in intravenous drug abusers and patients who are immunosuppressed. Surgical excision is often necessary to prevent rupture and to remove the lesion, which tends to be highly resistant to antibiotic treatment.

Ehlers-Danlos syndrome is a connective tissue disorder affecting collagen formation. Aortic dissection is one of the internal complications of the syndrome. *Takayasu's disease* produces an arteritis that affects all layers of the arterial wall and is associated with the formation of fusiform or saccular aneurysms.

The hemodynamic stresses of pregnancy may contribute to acute dissection and rupture of the aorta, but usually there is some underlying predisposition for this to occur. Intraoperative aortic dissections or postoperative false aneurysms (pseudoaneurysms) may occur at aortic cannulation sites, in areas where arterial anastomoses are performed, and at the femoral (or brachial) artery entry site of cardiac angiographic catheters. Dissections of the aorta or the coronary arteries may occur during angiography or angioplasty.

Diagnostic Evaluation of Thoracic Aortic Disease

SIGNS AND SYMPTOMS

Improved survival and reduced morbidity in patients with thoracic aortic lesions are dependent on early diagnosis. The presence of a thoracic aneurysm or dissection often is first suggested by symptoms related to compression or obstruction of surrounding mediastinal structures, dissection, or rupture (Table 14-1).

The pain of dissection is the classic symptom. It is often described as "ripping," "tearing," or "splitting." It is often intense from onset. When the pain persists despite large doses of analgesics, it is thought to indicate progression of the dissection. Abrupt cessation of pain followed by recurrence may signal impending rupture. In patients with proximal aortic dissections, the pain may be located in the anterior part of the chest; descending aortic dissections may produce pain in the posterior part of the thorax, although such specificity is not always present.

Compression of adjacent nerves can produce voice changes; obstruction of the tracheobronchial tree can cause dyspnea or cough. Bloody sputum may be a sign of rupture. If dilation of the aortic root is present, the valve leaflets are unable to coapt, and acute insufficiency with congestive heart failure ensues (Cohn, 1995).

Patients with aortic dissections may present emergently, and signs and symptoms are assessed. Difficulty breathing or swallowing is suggestive, especially when associated with complaints of excruciating pain. If the

false lumen of the dissection obstructs vital branches as a result of the false lumen's compressing the true lumen, symptoms may be apparent. These include mental status changes from cerebral ischemia, reduced urinary output from renal artery compression, and abdominal pain from mesenteric obstruction. Other symptoms include pulse deficits producing unequal bilateral radial, brachial, carotid, or femoral pulses if the artery on one side has been obstructed by the hematoma (Fig. 14-6).

Not infrequently, signs and symptoms may alert the clinician to consider a diagnosis of acute myocardial infarction. Differentiating between dissection and infarction usually focuses on the quality, location, and duration of the pain and on the presence (infarction) or absence (dissection) of electrocardiographic or enzymatic evidence of infarction. Myocardial pain usually builds up more gradually, has a squeezing quality to it, and is located in the anterior part of the chest with or without radiation to the jaw and arms. In the age of thrombolytic therapy for acute myocardial infarction, administration of such agents can have disastrous consequences for patients with aortic dissection (Cigarroa and others, 1993).

DIAGNOSTIC TESTS

Routine laboratory tests may provide little useful information unless massive hemorrhage has reduced the level of hemoglobin. When there is ischemia to major branches of the aorta as a result of a dissection, the clinician may require abnormal liver, kidney, or gastrointestinal function studies.

The electrocardiogram may show hypertrophy of the left ventricle in patients with chronic hypertension and may be used to rule out myocardial infarction. It also may be helpful in the presence of a dissection that extends retrogradely and occludes the entrance to the coronary artery (producing ischemia or infarction) or affects the interatrial septum (producing heart block). A chest roentgenogram usually shows a mediastinal mass associated with the aortic shadow. A widened mediastinum and pleural fluid may be evident.

Transthoracic echocardiography (TTE) and transesophageal echocardiography (TEE) using Doppler color flow mapping have significantly improved prompt diagnosis by displaying the entire aorta and the presence of pericardial fluid and by demonstrating specific lesions, such as aortic valve insufficiency and an aortic flap if dissection is present. The tests are noninvasive, widely available, and easily and quickly performed. TEE may be contraindicated in patients with esophageal disease, but important side effects are rare (Cigarroa and others, 1993).

TABLE 14-1
Signs, Symptoms, and Findings of Thoracic Aortic Disease

ASCENDING AORTA	AORTIC ARCH	DESCENDING AORTA
Signs and Symptoms		
Acute aortic valve insufficiency: new murmurs, pulmonary edema, congestive heart failure	Hoarseness from pressure on recurrent laryngeal nerve	
Angina	Cough, dyspnea, bloody sputum	
Severe, unremitting chest or back pain with dissection	Same	Same
Pain related to pressure on adjacent structures	Same	Same
Unequal peripheral pulses with dissection	Same	Same
Marfan's syndrome stigmata: excessive height; slender, spiderlike fingers and toes	Same	Same
Brachiocephalic venous distension from compression of superior vena cava	Dysphagia from esophageal compromise	Nausea and vomiting from duodenal pressure
Changes in mentation	Same	
Reduction in urinary output	Same	
Chest X-Ray Film		
Dilated ascending aorta	Dilated aortic arch	Dilated descending aorta
Possible hemopericardium	Same	Same
Possible hemothorax	Same	Same
Pulmonary edema	Same	
Widened mediastinum	Same	
	Deviated trachea or esophagus	Same
Electrocardiogram		
Dysrhythmias		
Ischemic changes from impaired coronary perfusion		
Usually not diagnostic	Same	Same
Echocardiography (TTE and TEE)	Same	Same; TEE more useful
Visualize aneurysm		
Aortography	Same	Same
Location of aortic tear in dissection; extent of dissection; true and false lumen	Same	Same
Blood flow to branches of aorta; compression of major branches		
Aortic valve insufficiency		
Computed Tomographic Scanning	Same	Same
Location, size, and extent of aneurysm/dissection		
Cardiac Catheterization		
Coronary artery disease, cardiac or pulmonary shunts, aortic insufficiency		

TEE, Transesophageal echocardiography; *TTE,* transthoracic echocardiography.
Modified from Doty J: Acute aortic dissection [On-line], 2000. Available: www.ctsnet.org/residents/ctsr/archives/75txt.html (accessed November 27, 2000).

Aortography (see Fig. 14-6) confirms the diagnosis and best defines the location and condition of the aortic arch branch vessels and the function of the aortic valve. It is particularly useful for detecting involvement, such as occlusion, of one or more major branches of the aorta and remains one of the definitive methods of diagnosing dissections of the thoracic aorta (Cigarroa and others, 1993; Doty, 2000).

Cardiac catheterization with aortography and left ventriculography may be performed to determine aor-tic valve function and to identify shunts when there is a sinus of Valsalva rupture into a cardiac chamber, but cardiac catheterization may be unnecessary (or unsafe) for diagnosis. In patients with involvement of the ascending aorta, the possibility of catheter-induced injury to the vessel wall may preclude selective coronary angiography or other procedures that pose a risk to the patient.

Computed tomographic (CT) scanning with or without contrast enhancement is useful for diagnosing aor-

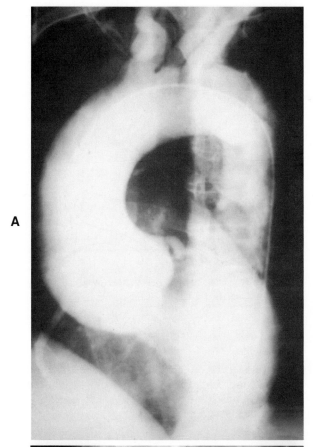

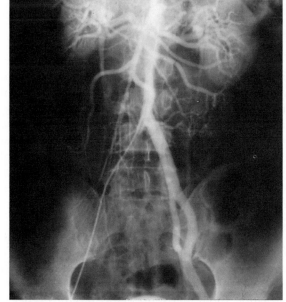

FIGURE 14-6 A, Dissection of the ascending aorta with involvement of the brachiocephalic vessels. **B,** Occlusion of the right iliac artery by false lumen of aortic dissection. (Courtesy Edward A. Lefrak, MD.)

tic dissection and for determining the size of aneurysmal dilation. It is noninvasive (although contrast material must be injected) and is usually available in many hospitals. Disadvantages include its inability to detect the involvement of branch vessels or delineate the coronary arteries. Magnetic resonance imaging (MRI) provides extraordinary accuracy, but there are important disadvantages, including the amount of time required to obtain and compute the images and the relative inaccessibility of patients (who are often hemodynamically unstable) when they are inside the MRI tube. In addition, there is the danger of the effect of the strong magnetic field on metallic implants such as pacemakers, aneurysm clips, and possibly certain metallic prosthetic heart valves (Malarkey and McMorrow, 2000).

Less invasive techniques (e.g., TEE and CT scanning) are recommended to provide a more rapid diagnosis and initiate surgical repair expeditiously, although selective angiography is valuable when noninvasive imaging is inconclusive (Coselli, LeMaire, and Walkes, 1999).

When aortic dissection is diagnosed, the point of origin must be determined in preparation for surgical repair. Dissections originating in the ascending aorta are true surgical emergencies because of the danger of rupture with intrapericardial hemorrhage and death from cardiac tamponade.

Surgery on the Thoracic Aorta

In general, saccular aneurysms with a narrow neck may be tangentially excised using a partial-occlusion clamp. Where there is greater involvement of the vessel, total-occlusion clamps may be required to control the aorta proximally and distally. Occasionally, direct closure of the aorta may be performed when the defect is not too large (and the tissue is relatively sturdy), but patch repair is usually necessary to avoid tension on the suture line, especially with fragile tissue.

Fusiform aneurysms require circumferential replacement to restore vascular continuity. Two techniques can be used. The inclusion technique is one wherein the aorta is incised longitudinally and a prosthetic graft is inserted within the lumen of the vessel and anastomosed proximally and distally to healthy aorta; the remnant aortic wall may then be closed around the graft for hemostasis (Fig. 14-7). The other technique is to excise the diseased portion of the aorta entirely, interpose the synthetic graft, and perform proximal and distal end-to-end anastomoses (Fig. 14-8). Other technical considerations depend on the location and cause of the lesion (Kirklin and Barratt-Boyes, 1993).

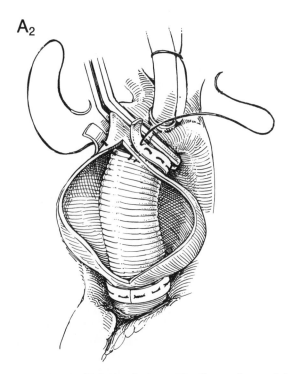

FIGURE 14-7 Inclusion technique. The diseased aorta is incised, a graft is placed within the wall, and the vascular continuity is restored with anastomoses to the proximal and distal portions of the aorta. The remnant wall may be wrapped around the graft. (From Waldhausen JA, Pierce WS: *Johnson's surgery of the chest,* ed 5, St Louis, 1985, Mosby.)

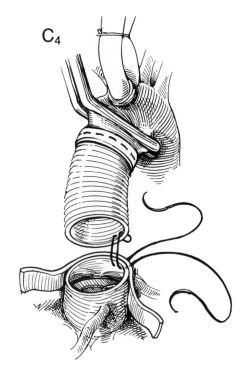

FIGURE 14-8 Excision technique. The diseased aorta is resected and replaced with a graft. (From Waldhausen JA, Pierce WS: *Johnson's surgery of the chest,* ed 5, St Louis, 1985, Mosby.)

INITIAL THERAPY

Whether medical or surgical therapy is planned, initial treatment for dilation of the thoracic aorta, and in particular aortic dissections, consists of lowering intravascular pressures in order to forestall rupture and retard progression of the dissecting hematoma. This includes treating not only the absolute blood pressure in the aorta but also the force with which the aortic pressure rises with left ventricular ejection (dP/dt). This is reflected by the steepness of the pulse wave that is generated by each contraction, and it is this that is especially damaging to the dissecting aorta. Treatment is aimed at modifying the strength of the contractions, decreasing the cardiac impulse, and lowering systemic blood pressure.

Because the increased shearing force can extend the dissection, pharmacologic therapy is instituted promptly. Medications to reduce contractility of the left ventricle and lower blood pressure include beta-adrenergic blockers (e.g., propranolol, a negative inotrope), calcium channel blockers, vasodilators (e.g., sodium nitroprusside), and antihypertensive agents, which decrease left ventricular work and stroke volume. Aggressively managing pain and limiting intravenous fluid administration also are recommended (Coselli, LeMaire, and Walkes, 1999).

PATIENT TEACHING CONSIDERATIONS

The gradual or sudden onset of symptoms related to thoracic aneurysm and the excruciating pain associated with aortic dissection make these lesions particularly stressful to patients both physically and emotionally. Because of the frequent emergent need for surgery, extensive preoperative teaching is usually not possible. The preoperative interview may be limited to a quick assessment of the patient's status, and significant information about the location and type of disorder is communicated to perioperative nurses preparing for surgery (Table 14-2).

If the patient is conscious and is attended by family or friends, the perioperative nurse may provide a brief overview of the planned procedure, the expected length of surgery (this can be highly variable), and information about how (and when) progress reports will be communicated during surgery. Under the circumstances, reassuring the patient and family with a gentle handgrip and calm efficiency may be more beneficial than detailed explanations. The family should be directed to a waiting area where they can be contacted during surgery. More extensive teaching may need to be deferred to the postoperative period.

TABLE 14-2
Standards of Nursing Care for Surgery on the Thoracic Aorta

NURSING DIAGNOSIS	PATIENT OUTCOME	NURSING ACTIONS
Anxiety/fear related to lack of understanding of pathologic lesion and surgery	Patient demonstrates reduced anxiety and fear as a result of sufficient understanding of lesion and surgical treatment	Assess patient's/family's understanding of lesion and proposed surgery Describe events that are taking place in understandable terms Clarify misconceptions, provide reassurance, offer comfort measures Briefly describe proposed surgery and anticipated length of time in operating room (may vary widely) Determine where family will be waiting and where they can receive patient progress reports
Knowledge deficit related to inadequate knowledge of planned surgery and perioperative events	Patient demonstrates knowledge of physiologic and psychologic responses to surgery on thoracic aorta	Determine patient's understanding of aortic lesion, possible surgical interventions (replacement of aortic segment, with or without aortic valve replacement, coronary artery bypass grafts); see standards for aortic valve surgery (Chapter 12) and coronary artery bypass (Chapter 10) Determine patient's understanding of surgery for ascending, arch, descending, or thoracoabdominal aortic lesion; describe immediate preoperative events (while patient is awake); reinforce or clarify what patient (and family) has been told by surgeon; elicit expected outcome of surgery
Risk for infection related to surgery	Patient is free of infection related to aseptic technique	Prepare leg at least to knees to expose leg vein Refer to aortic valve (Chapter 12) and coronary artery bypass (Chapter 10) for procedural considerations Keep instruments free of debris Document lot and serial numbers of grafts, valves, Teflon felt strips and pledgets, and other implants; maintain sterility of graft during preclotting procedures
Risk for altered skin integrity	Patient's skin integrity is maintained	Prepare chest cautiously to avoid traumatizing enlarged aorta Protect lower extremities with anesthesia screen over feet If deep hypothermia is to be used, pad face to prevent frostbite; pad extremities
Risk for injury from positioning	Patient is free of injury from positioning	When using lateral position, avoid nerve/pressure injury by padding extremities, using axillary roll, placing pillows between legs, and supporting head, feet, hands, and arms; stabilize patient anteriorly and posteriorly (tape, vacuum positioning devices) For semilateral position, have rolled towel (or similar device) to elevate left side of chest Follow standard for supine position (see Chapter 5)

Risk for injury related to:
  Retained foreign objects
 	
  Chemical hazards
	Patient is free of injury related to:
	  Retained foreign objects
	
	  Chemical hazards
		Account for all prosthetic material
		Keep instruments free of tissue and suture debris
		Label syringes and basins containing antibiotic solutions, fibrin glue, blood components, and other solutions/fluids
		Follow standard for aortic valve surgery (see Chapter 12) if valve replacement is to be performed

Risk for self-care deficit related to inadequate knowledge of rehabilitation period	Patient demonstrates knowledge of rehabilitation period as it relates to self-care abilities	Assess patient's knowledge of signs/symptoms of recurring aneurysm or dissection If patient has Marfan's syndrome, refer for education and follow-up, including counseling Refer for counseling and education if patient has history of hypertension Provide name of person if there are questions or concerns If aortic valve has been replaced, refer to standards for aortic valve surgery (Chapter 12); if coronary bypass has been performed for coronary artery disease, refer to standards for coronary artery bypass (Chapter 10)

Modified from Seifert PC: Cardiac surgery. In Rothrock JC: *Perioperative nursing care planning,* ed 2, St Louis, 1996, Mosby.

TABLE **14-3**

Surgery on the Thoracic Aorta: Special Considerations

ASCENDING AORTA	AORTIC ARCH	DESCENDING AORTA
Instrumentation		
Sternotomy setup	Sternotomy setup	Thoracotomy setup
Vascular clamps	Vascular clamps	Vascular clamps
Femoral bypass instruments	Femoral bypass instruments	For femoral bypass with thoracoabdominal procedure: abdominal instruments and retractors
Aortic valve instruments		
Coronary bypass instruments		
Prostheses and Accessories		
Woven tube grafts and sizers	Same	Same
Aortic graft-valve prostheses, sizers, and holders		Intraluminal devices
Heart valves (see procedural considerations for aortic valve surgery, Chapter 12)		
Aortic allografts		
Supplies		
Anastomotic suture, long (36 inches) for continuous technique or multipack for interrupted stitches; polypropylene or polyester	Same	Same
Valve suture, single and multipack (multicolored), pledgeted and nonpledgeted		Suture to ligate/anastomose intercostal branches
Suture organizer (if used)		
Free pledgets, precut or cut to size	Same	Same
Felt strips (cut from patch)	Same	Same
Knitted grafts for collars (6, 8, or 10 mm)	Same	Same
Supplies for coronary artery bypass (see Chapter 10) and aortic valve replacement (see Chapter 12)		
Eye cautery to cut opening into graft for anastomosis of bypass grafts, arterial branches, etc.	Same	Same
Circulatory Support		
Single or double venous cannulas for atrial cannulation	Same	Variable; may use left-sided heart bypass (LA or LV* to aorta), Gott shunt, or femoral vein–femoral artery bypass (with oxygenator)
Femoral bypass supplies, extra tubing and connectors to attach atrial cannula to femoral venous line		
Antegrade cardioplegia supplies (handheld coronary ostial perfusers)	Same	Very rarely used
Retrograde cardioplegia supplies	Same	Very rarely used
Supplies for deep hypothermia (topical ice bags for head, padding to protect facial prominences and extremities)	Same	Very rarely used
Venting needles, suction catheters for removing air from heart or aorta	Same	Same as for venting aorta
Cerebral protection catheters, supplies	Same	Rarely used
Positioning		
Supine	Proximal arch	Lateral: may use positioning device (beanbag)
Groin exposed	Supine	
	Distal arch	Groin exposed
	Semilateral	Thoracoabdominal aneurysm: semi-lateral
	Groin exposed	
Skin Preparation		
Midline of chest, inner aspect of both legs shaved	Same	Same, except chest shave not necessary unless hair interferes with incision
Legs washed at least to knees	Same	

*LA, Left atrium; LV, left ventricle.

TABLE 14-3 *Surgery on the Thoracic Aorta: Special Considerations—cont'd*		
ASCENDING AORTA	**AORTIC ARCH**	**DESCENDING AORTA**
Draping		
Anterior chest exposed	Same	Left lateral area of chest and groin exposed
Legs exposed from groin to knees (can be covered with a towel if access is not required)	Same	
Anesthesia screen placed over lower legs to keep drapes off feet	Same	Same
Special Infection Control Measures		
Maintain sterility of graft	Same	Same
Keep instruments free of debris	Same	Same
Document lot and serial numbers of all implants	Same	Same
(See procedural consideration for aortic valve surgery, Chapter 12, coronary artery bypass, Chapter 10)		
Special Safety Measures		
Keep blood bank informed of need for blood/blood products	Same	Same
Have autotransfusion system ready for use	Same	Same
Label syringes and containers of solutions, medications: antibiotic solution, glutaraldehyde, etc.	Same	Same
Account for all sizers, handles, holders used for prostheses; pledget material, suture, needles	Same	Same
Documentation/Report to Cardiac Surgical Intensive Care Unit*		
Preoperative diagnosis	Same	Same
Procedure, location, and type of repair	Same	Same
Renal function, urinary output, neurologic status	Same	Same

*In addition to standard documentation/postoperative report; see Chapter 6.

SURGERY ON THE ASCENDING THORACIC AORTA

Procedural considerations

Knowledge about the type of lesion and its treatment will assist the perioperative nurse in planning care. Of critical importance is an awareness of the aortic region involved. Because of the emergency nature of many of these cases (often at night or on weekends), the time between diagnosis and surgery may be very short. All too often the operating room (OR) team is told that the patient has a "thoracic aneurysm" without being told the location of the aneurysm. Valuable time can be wasted if preparations have been made on the assumption that a patient has an aneurysm in the descending aorta when the aneurysm is in fact in the ascending aorta. Prompt communication to the OR team about the status of the patient and the location of the aneurysm is invaluable when one is trying to prepare for surgery as quickly as possible.

Aneurysms or dissections of the ascending aorta are best approached with the patient in a supine position; sternotomy instruments and supplies are required (Table 14-3). Graft prostheses and sizers should be available so that the correct-size graft can be readily opened when requested. Because the patient is given systemic heparin, woven grafts are used; they demonstrate the least amount of bleeding through the interstices of the fabric, as compared with knitted grafts (see Chapter 3). Currently available grafts rarely require preclotting before use in patients given systemic heparin.

When there is evidence of significant aortic valve insufficiency, valve instruments and supplies (including prostheses) should be immediately accessible. If the patient has concomitant coronary artery disease or if the aortic root containing the coronary ostia must be excised, then coronary bypass instruments should also be available. Aortic valve replacement with graft replacement of the aortic root and reimplantation of the coronary ostia (the Bentall–DeBono procedure, described later in this chapter) requires a special conduit that is composed of a woven graft with an aortic valve prosthesis attached to the proximal end.

The operative procedure may be staged when there is diffuse disease of the aorta involving both proximal and distal segments. The most symptomatic and life-threatening segment is replaced first, and the other segment is repaired weeks or months later (see Borst "elephant trunk" technique, described later in this chapter). If both segments require simultaneous surgery, two incisions may be used to provide access to the lesions (Crawford and others, 1990). Because of the significant morbidity and mortality and the technical complexity associated with staged procedures, they are avoided when possible (Cooley, 1995).

Cardiopulmonary bypass

Cannulation for cardiopulmonary bypass (CPB) usually is performed via the right atrium and the femoral artery because the aorta may be too fragile to cannulate. If the aorta is greatly dilated, posing a high risk of rupture, the femoral artery may be cannulated before the sternum is opened. The subclavian artery also may be cannulated (Sabik and others, 1995) for arterial perfusion in patients with extensive disease.

On rare occasions the femoral vein may be cannulated for venous return of the lower extremities. Long venous drainage cannulas are available that can be inserted into the femoral vein and advanced to the right atrium, but venous return may be inadequate (with disastrous consequences) if it drains by gravity alone (passive drainage). The cannulas work best when venous return is actively drained with a centrifugal pump. Because femoral venous drainage is incomplete, the right atrium is cannulated to receive blood returning from the superior vena cava after the chest is opened. After the aorta is controlled, a cannula is inserted into the right atrium or superior vena cava and connected to tubing that is "Yd" into the femoral venous line. Complete venous drainage can then be achieved.

In aortic dissections, one of the potential dangers of femoral artery (retrograde) cannulation and perfusion of the aortic branches is cannulation of the false lumen rather than the true lumen of a dissected aorta, with a resulting malperfusion. Partially or totally occluding the venous line while gradually initiating femoral arterial inflow is done so that there is not a rapid change from the antegrade flow, produced by the contracting ventricle through the aortic valve, to the retrograde flow, produced by the bypass pump via the cannula in the femoral artery. Venous return is then allowed to drain freely. (If retrograde flow was initiated suddenly, the force of the blood could propel an existing intimal flap up against a major aortic branch or extend the dissection.) Transesophageal or epicardial color flow echocardiography also can be used to ensure that the correct lumen has been entered, that perfusion of the vital organs is occurring, and that the dissection is not being extended.

The perfusionist initiates arterial pump flow slowly, comparing the arterial line pressure with the patient's right and left (radial) arterial blood pressures. If the discrepancy among the pressures is too large, malperfusion is suspected. Renal and cardiac function also are monitored for signs of diminished perfusion.

Sternotomy

The period during which the chest is opened and the aorta is clamped can be characterized as one of controlled tension and anticipation in the OR. Often there is only a thin layer of adventitia confining an aortic dissection, and blood can be seen swirling beneath tissue. Extreme caution must be taken to avoid any injury that could produce a ruptured aorta (Box 14-2).

The quality of the tissue has other implications for surgical repair. In aortic dissections, for example, chronic lesions have tissue that is often sturdier and can be repaired more easily than that in aortas that have dissected acutely. In the latter case the tissue tends to be fragile, delicate, and prone to tearing (described later). This has prompted some researchers to treat aortic tissue with biologic glue (composed of gelatin, resorcin, and formaldehyde) to strengthen the tissue (described later). When tissue is weak, it is more difficult to

---

BOX 14-2

RN First Assistant Considerations During Surgery on the Thoracic Aorta

Assist surgeon as necessary during diagnostic procedure, especially when there is high risk of rupture (may need to perform emergency thoracotomy or sternotomy; have emergency instruments available). Report presence of invasive monitoring lines, urinary drainage catheters, and other lines to operating room staff so that time is not wasted preparing these.

Determine whether aneurysm originates in ascending or descending thoracic aorta; communicate with OR personnel to prepare instrumentation/supplies for sternotomy or thoracotomy, respectively, and for method of circulatory support planned by surgeon.

Anticipate and prepare possible methods of circulatory (cerebral, spinal) support depending on the type of lesion and its location: femoral vein–femoral artery bypass, hypothermic circulatory arrest, retrograde cerebral perfusion, left heart bypass.

Anticipate aortic valve replacement (or repair/resuspension) in patients with aortic root dilation or evidence of aortic insufficiency. If Bentall–DeBono procedure is performed, be prepared for coronary revascularization (bypass grafts, coronary artery ostial reimplantation into graft). Anticipate more extensive procedures in patients with Marfan's syndrome.

Use extreme caution after suture during repairs/anastomoses of dissected aortic tissue, which is fragile and tears easily. Note location of phrenic and vagus nerves, alert surgeon to their location, and avoid injuring nerves.

achieve adequate hemostasis; the perioperative nurse can anticipate the use of buttressing felt strips, reinforcing wraps, and other methods to secure the suture line in these situations.

Operative procedure: repair of an ascending aortic aneurysm

Consideration is given to the extent of the lesion proximally and distally and to involvement of the aortic valve. The following procedure is performed when the aneurysm is limited to a segment of the ascending aorta and there is minimal or no aortic valve insufficiency. Significant aortic valve incompetence and aortic root enlargement are usually indications for replacement of these structures with a composite graft (see discussion of Bentall–DeBono procedure).

Procedure

1. The patient is placed in the supine position, and a median sternotomy is performed.
2. Cardiopulmonary bypass is instituted.
   a. If the distal portion of the ascending aorta is normal, it may be cannulated for arterial inflow; the proximal transverse aortic arch also may be used. The right atrium is cannulated with single or double cannulas for venous drainage.
   b. If there is no suitable place to cannulate the ascending aorta for arterial inflow or the right atrium for venous return or if there is a high risk of injury to the aorta during sternal opening, femoral vein–femoral artery cannulation may be performed before opening the chest. Following administration of systemic heparin, the cannulas are inserted into the exposed vein and artery. Bypass is initiated after the chest is opened to perfuse the body and achieve systemic hypothermia.

      When feasible, a cannula is inserted into the superior vena cava and connected by tubing to the femoral venous line after the sternum is opened.
3. After the aorta is clamped across healthy tissue, the aneurysm is incised longitudinally to a point above the entrance to the coronary ostia; the aortic wall may be preserved for later wrapping, or it is excised. Minimal dissection of surrounding tissue is performed.
4. Retrograde cardioplegia is infused. The left ventricular venting catheter is inserted into the right superior pulmonary vein and threaded through the mitral valve into the left ventricle; a pulmonary artery vent may be used.
5. The aneurysmal aortic wall and the aortic valve are inspected.
   a. If there is minimal aortic valve incompetence and the valve is morphologically normal (and there is no underlying connective tissue disorder), it may

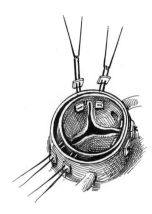

FIGURE 14-9 Resuspension of the aortic valve commissures with pledged sutures to restore aortic valve competence. (From Waldhausen JA, Pierce WS, Campbell DB: *Surgery of the chest,* ed 6, St Louis, 1996, Mosby.)

be resuspended (Fig. 14-9) with pledgeted mattress sutures placed at the level of the commissures and passed through the layers of the aortic wall. Aortic root reconstruction with felt reinforcement is another, less common technique to salvage the native valve (Coselli, LeMaire, and Walkes, 1999).
   b. If the valve requires replacement, this is done in the standard fashion (see Chapter 12). A collar of aorta is retained for anastomosis of the graft.
6. The aorta is sized, and the appropriate graft is delivered to the field.
7. The proximal and distal anastomoses are made to the healthy aorta with a running 2-0 or 3-0 polypropylene or polyester suture. The suture line may be reinforced with strips of felt (Fig. 14-10).
8. The remaining aorta (if not excised) is trimmed and wrapped around the completed repair, and the edges are oversewn with a continuous suture. Some authors suggest an additional strip of felt around the aorta at the location of the proximal and distal anastomoses (Waldhausen, Pierce, and Campbell, 1996; Fig. 14-11).
9. Air is removed from the left side of the heart through the right superior pulmonary venous venting catheter, needle aspiration of the left ventricular apex, or needle venting of the ascending aorta with the patient in the deep Trendelenburg position. The cross-clamp is removed, the patient is rewarmed, and cardiopulmonary bypass is discontinued.

Bentall–DeBono procedure

Annuloaortic ectasia or aortic dissection involving the aortic root and aortic valve generally requires their replacement, especially in patients with Marfan's syndrome or other degenerative disorders.

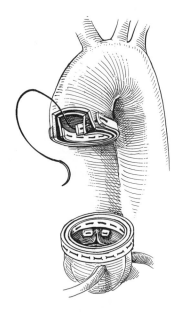

FIGURE 14-10 Proximal and distal sections of aorta are sandwiched between felt strips to obliterate false lumen. (From Waldhausen JA, Pierce WS, Campbell DB: *Surgery of the chest,* ed 6, St Louis, 1996, Mosby.)

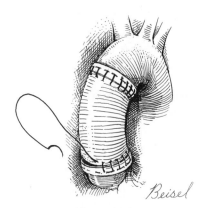

FIGURE 14-11 Proximal and distal anastomoses. (From Waldhausen JA, Pierce WS, Campbell DB: *Surgery of the chest,* ed 6, St Louis, 1996, Mosby.)

The procedure, described by Bentall and DeBono (1968), involves the use of a valved conduit to replace the aortic valve and ascending aorta (see Chapter 3). The coronary ostia are reimplanted into openings made in the graft, and the remnant aortic wall is then wrapped around the graft.

A number of modifications have been made to the operation to reflect technical improvements. Problems include hemorrhage from anastomotic suture lines, disruption of the coronary ostia, pseudoaneurysm formation at the coronary ostial or aortic suture lines, and injury from clamping the fragile aortic wall (Kirklin and Barratt-Boyes, 1993).

Conduit size. An important consideration in these procedures is proper sizing of both the proximal end of the conduit (containing the prosthetic valve) and the distal graft portion of the conduit. The distal end can be sized with graft sizers; the graft may be beveled to better fit the aorta.

In sizing the proximal end, the surgeon considers the graft and the valve contained within it. In commercially manufactured conduits the process of sewing the graft to the valve adds 2 mm to the diameter of the valve contained within the conduit. Thus when the surgeon sizes the annulus, the size obturator that fits best (rather than the size of the valve within the conduit) determines the size of the conduit. A 23-mm annulus will have a 23-mm conduit (containing a 21-mm valve prosthesis) implanted. If the surgeon determines that a 25-mm obturator fits best into the annulus, the surgeon

should be given a 25-mm conduit, which contains a 23-mm valve. The obturators should correspond to the type of conduit used (e.g., St. Jude Medical obturators to determine the appropriate St. Jude Medical conduit).

Another consideration related to conduits is that a low-profile valve commonly is used because it is technically easier to reimplant the coronary ostia, as compared with a higher-profile valve (e.g., a ball-and-cage valve). Also, mechanical valves tend to be favored because of their greater durability as compared with bioprostheses, which could require difficult reoperation (Coselli, LeMaire, and Walkes, 1999). Aortic allografts and pulmonic autografts (with pulmonary allografts to replace the pulmonic valve and pulmonary artery) have been used as alternatives to the composite graft (Kouchoukos, 1991).

Cannulation and sternotomy are similar to the procedure just described for an ascending aortic aneurysm.

Operative procedure: annuloaortic ectasia or aortic dissection—modified Bentall–DeBono technique (Fig. 14-12)

1. The sternum is divided, and the pericardium is opened. The aneurysm is inspected. The femoral artery is cannulated for arterial inflow; a two-stage venous cannula is inserted for venous drainage.
2. The distal ascending aorta is clamped (Fig. 14-13). If there is a dissection involving the proximal aortic arch, hypothermic circulatory arrest may be used (see later section) in order to avoid clamping (and possibly further injuring) the dissected aorta.
3. The aorta is incised transversely or longitudinally. If dissection is present, the location of the intimal tear is noted. Cardioplegia solution is infused retrogradely. Rarely, the coronary ostia are infused with cardioplegia solution. Stitches may be placed into each side of the aneurysmal aortic wall for retraction.

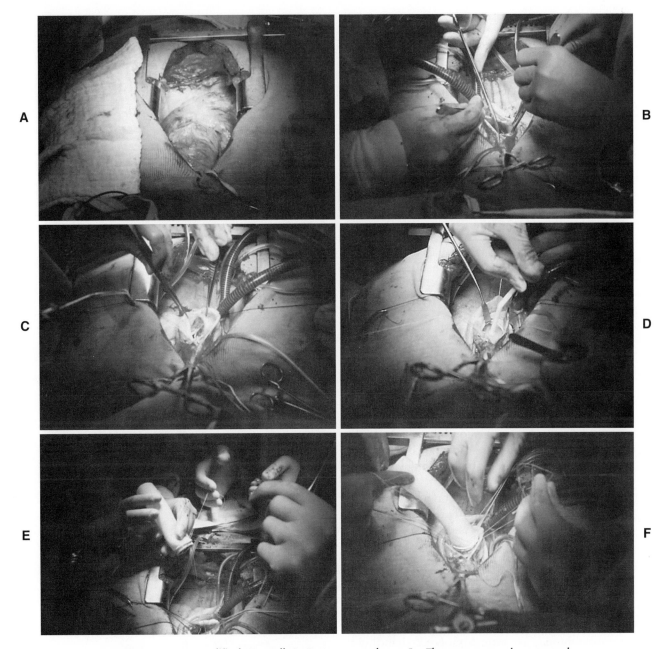

FIGURE 14-12 Modified Bentall–DeBono procedure. **A,** The aneurysm is exposed through a median sternotomy (head is at bottom of picture). **B,** The aneurysm is incised. **C,** The aortic valve is inspected. **D,** The aortic annulus is sized with an obturator. Note the aortic leaflet retractor. **E,** After stitches have been inserted into the aortic annulus, stitches are placed in the sewing ring of the valve end of the conduit. Another technique is to place stitches into the annulus and prosthesis sewing ring at the same time. **F,** After all the stitches have been inserted, the prosthesis is seated and the stitches are tied. (Courtesy Edward A. Lefrak, MD; Doug Yarnold, CRNA, photographer.)

Continued

4. The aortic valve and the sinuses of Valsalva are inspected. The openings to the coronary arteries are identified, and their position relative to the annulus is noted (elevated or in the normal position).

5. The aortic valve leaflets are excised, and the annulus is measured with obturators of the type of prosthetic valve contained in the valved conduit.
   a. Conduit: The appropriate-size conduit is delivered to the field. When the conduit is being

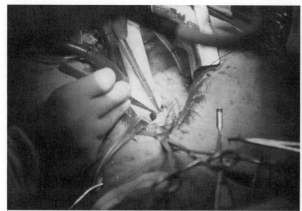
G

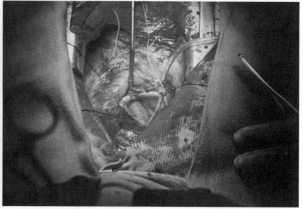
H

FIGURE 14-12, cont'd Modified Bentall–DeBono procedure. **G,** The left coronary ostium is reimplanted into the graft. **H,** The completed repair. The aortic wall will be closed around the graft after protamine has been infused to reverse the heparin and hemostasis has been achieved. Note that the patient is off bypass and that the venous cannulas have been removed. (Courtesy Edward A. Lefrak, MD; Doug Yarnold, CRNA, photographer.)

preclotted, the valve portion should not be immersed in the preclotting medium; the valve occluder mechanism should be checked to ensure that it is moving freely. If a prosthesis handle is available and the surgeon elects to use it, it should be attached to the conduit (Fig. 14-14).

   b. Allograft: An aortic allograft (e.g., homograft) may be inserted as described in Chapter 12 on aortic valve surgery.

6. The proximal (valve) end of the conduit is inserted into the annulus (Fig. 14-15). The interrupted or continuous suture technique is used (see Chapter 12). Pledgets may be used to buttress the annulus. Cardioplegia solution is infused before entry to the coronary arteries is reestablished.

7. Coronary circulation is restored. No matter which of the following techniques is used for a synthetic graft, an opening must be made into the graft for the anastomosis. A battery-powered, handheld (eye) cautery is helpful for making the opening and simultaneously heat-sealing the graft edges to prevent fraying.

   a. A button of aorta surrounding both the left and the right coronary ostia is retained and anastomosed to the respective openings made in the graft using a continuous 4-0 polypropylene suture. Cephalad displacement of the coronary ostia, commonly found in annuloaortic ectasia, facilitates this method of reimplanting the coronary ostia. The anastomosis can incorporate the remnant aortic wall as well (Fig. 14-16). A "washer" of Teflon felt may be placed around each ostial anastomosis to buttress the tissue.

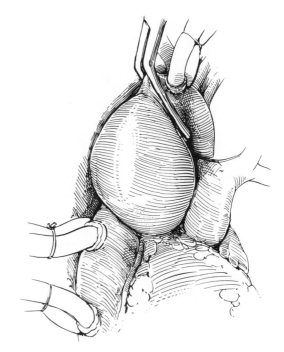

FIGURE 14-13 The distal aorta is clamped. (From Waldhausen JA, Pierce WS, Campbell DB: *Surgery of the chest,* ed 6, St Louis, 1996, Mosby.)

   b. Cabrol, Pavie, and Mesnildrey (1986) devised a reimplantation technique (Fig. 14-17) aimed at reducing tension on the coronary ostial suture line. One end of an 8- or 10-mm woven tube graft is anastomosed end-to-end to the origin of the left coronary artery. The graft is brought across the anterior aspect of (or behind) the aor-

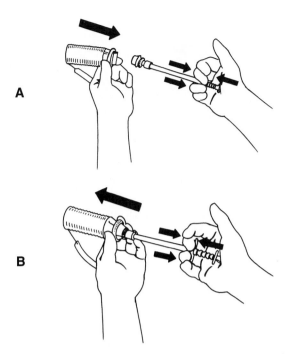

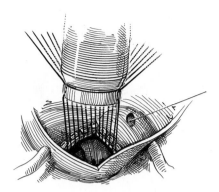

FIGURE 14-15 The valve end of the graft-valve conduit is sewn into the aortic annulus. (From Waldhausen JA, Pierce WS, Campbell DB: *Surgery of the chest,* ed 6, St Louis, 1996, Mosby.)

FIGURE 14-14 **A,** The conduit handle (specific to the prosthesis) is inserted. The handle jaws are aligned with the lateral openings in the St. Jude Medical valve; the end of the handle is depressed, and the jaws are inserted into the prosthesis. **B,** Removal of the handle from the prosthesis. (Courtesy St. Jude Medical Center, Inc., Minneapolis, Minn.)

tic graft to the right coronary ostium, where it is cut and anastomosed end-to-end to the right ostium. An opening is cut into the coronary graft and into the aortic graft at a level above the prosthetic valve, and a side-to-side anastomosis is performed. Arterial blood flows into the aortic graft opening and then into both coronary ostia.

c. Saphenous vein or a 6- to 8-mm prosthetic (Dacron or PTFE) graft is interposed between the coronary ostia and the aortic graft (Kouchoukos, 1991).

d. In patients with obstructive coronary artery disease, saphenous vein bypass grafts are anastomosed distally to the heart and proximally to the aortic graft.

8. After coronary continuity is reestablished, cardioplegia solution may be infused through the graft and into the coronary openings (this may be technically difficult) or given retrogradely.

The graft is brought up to the location of the distal anastomosis, and excess graft is cut. If the aorta is dissected, the location of the intimal tear must be excluded from the remaining aorta, or redissection will occur (Fig. 14-18). In addition, circumferential strips of Teflon felt may be used to sandwich the

distal edges of the transected aorta to obliterate the false lumen. (When available, biologic glue may be used to seal the edges together before suturing the aorta.

9. The distal anastomosis is performed with a running 2-0 or 3-0 polypropylene or polyester suture incorporating all layers of the felt (see Fig. 14-11).

10. The patient is placed in Trendelenburg's position, and a venting needle is placed in the most anterior portion of the aorta (Waldhausen, Pierce, and Campbell, 1996). Air is removed from the left ventricle with a needle or with a venting catheter in the right superior pulmonary vein.

11. The cross-clamp is removed, and the anastomoses and graft are inspected for bleeding. Pledgeted or nonpledgeted sutures are used to reinforce suture lines as necessary.

12. If oozing from the graft or suture line persists, a variety of techniques are available:

a. The inclusion wrap technique involves wrapping the prosthetic graft with the remaining aortic wall and oversewing the approximated aortic edges. Additional felt strips or graft wraps may be used. (The wrap technique also has been suggested for protection from infection [Borst, Heinemann, and Stone, 1996].)

This technique is currently less popular because tight wrapping may place stress on the suture lines and possibly disrupt the coronary ostial-graft anastomoses or occlude coronary blood flow.

b. Tissue glue (variously made from fibrin sealant, gelatin-resorcin-formalin [GRF], or other biologic adhesives) is used for hemostasis of the suture lines. In some instances the glue is used to seal dissected aortic wall layers (Borst and others,

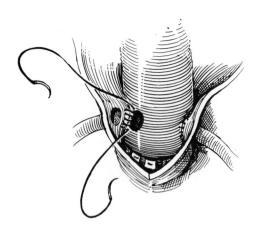

FIGURE 14-16 Anastomosis of the right coronary ostium to the prosthetic graft. The left coronary ostial reimplantation has been completed. (From Waldhausen JA, Pierce WS: *Johnson's surgery of the chest,* ed 5, St Louis, 1985, Mosby.)

1996). (At the time of this writing, GRF has not been approved for use in the United States by the Food and Drug Administration.)

  c. The Cabrol technique (Cabrol, Pavie, and Mesnildrey, 1986) is used to decompress the perigraft space when the inclusion-wrap technique is being used. A fistula is created between the aortic wrap and the right atrium (Fig. 14-19). This allows collected blood to drain into the right side of the heart. If the fistula does not close spontaneously and bleeding persists, re-operation may be necessary.

13. After removal of air from the left side of the heart and the aorta, the OR bed is brought to a level position. While rewarming is completed, temporary pacing wires and chest tubes are inserted.

14. Cardiopulmonary bypass is discontinued, and the chest is closed.

Surgery on the Aortic Arch

PROCEDURAL CONSIDERATIONS

Cerebral protection

In aneurysms involving the ascending aorta when there is (relatively) normal distal ascending aortic tissue, cerebral perfusion is achieved by cross-clamping the aorta proximal to the origin of the branches of the aortic arch and allowing femoral artery retrograde perfusion of the head and upper body. In aneurysms involving the transverse aortic arch, unless each branch vessel is selectively cannulated (as performed in the past with generally unsatisfactory results), cerebral perfusion must be temporarily interrupted while the arch is repaired. This period of circulatory arrest necessitates

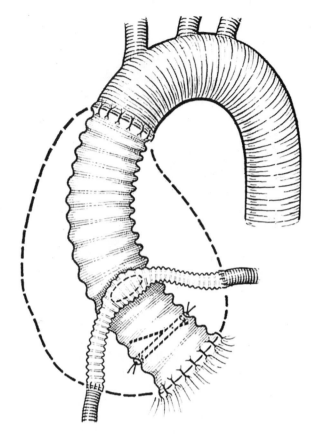

FIGURE 14-17 Cabrol technique for reestablishing coronary circulation. The ends of the graft are anastomosed to each coronary ostium, and a side-to-side anastomosis of the transverse graft is made to the graft-valve conduit. (From Cabrol C, Pavie A, Mesnildrey P: Long-term results with total replacement of the ascending aorta and reimplantation of the coronary arteries, *J Thorac Cardiovasc Surg* 91[1]:17, 1986.)

protective measures to protect the brain (and the rest of the body). Techniques that can be employed include hypothermia, circulatory arrest, and retrograde cerebral perfusion (RCP); they are intended to minimize the effects of oxygen deprivation, create a bloodless field, and reduce the incidence of embolism (Safi and others, 1993; Svensson and Crawford, 1997).

Hypothermia and *circulatory arrest* commonly are combined for cerebral protection during surgery on arch aneurysms or dissections and complex ascending aortic lesions. Hypothermia reduces the metabolic rate, thereby allowing longer intervals of cerebral oxygen deprivation without significant sequelae. Patients may be cooled to 12° to 18° C (53.6° to 64.4° F). At 18° C the metabolic rate is approximately 40% of normal, thus providing a relatively safe period in which to perform the distal repairs (Moon and Miller, 1999). Circulatory arrest avoids the use of aortic cross-clamps during the arch repair and reduces the risks associated with retro-

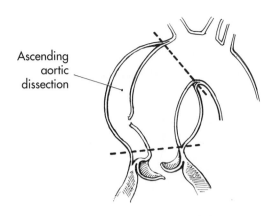

Ascending
aortic
dissection

FIGURE 14-18 The dissected portion of the aorta must be identified and excluded during the repair to avoid redissection. (From Waldhausen JA, Pierce WS, Campbell DB: *Surgery of the chest,* ed 6, St Louis, 1996, Mosby.)

grade arterial perfusion through the femoral CPB line, which could cause additional intimal tears, dislodgment of atheromatous material, and possible cerebral malperfusion (David, 1999).

The patient is cooled internally with CPB (at a rate of approximately 1° C per minute), with the arterial line inserted into the femoral artery (or in some cases the subclavian artery). External cooling can be achieved with a cooling blanket and ice packs to the head (and on occasion to the entire body surface area). Because of the increased risk of lethal dysrhythmias with hypothermia, members of the cardiac team should monitor closely the electrocardiogram for signs of ventricular irritability or fibrillation and be ready to institute appropriate measures if this occurs. Continuous TEE can be used to monitor the development—and avoidance—of left ventricular distension. It is also important to avoid manipulation of the aorta, especially in older patients who may have a clot or atheroma in the aortic lumen that can be dislodged. Debris also can be dislodged by altered CPB flow (especially near the tip of the perfusion cannula).

Once the desired temperature is reached (by monitoring esophageal, nasopharyngeal, rectal, bladder, or jugular venous temperature), the bypass pump is turned off and the distal arch anastomoses are performed (McCullough and others, 1999). Determination of a safe interval of arrest is difficult but arrest periods of 40 minutes (Svensson and others, 1993) and 60 minutes (Griepp and others, 2000) with minimal or no neurologic injury have been reported.

Inadvertent rewarming should be avoided. Internal cooling is achieved by the circulation of blood cooled with the heat exchanger within the bypass circuit. When the patient is under circulatory arrest and the bypass pump is turned off, internal cooling cannot be

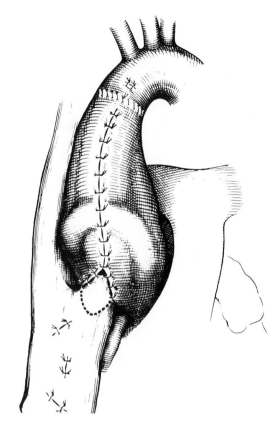

FIGURE 14-19 Cabrol technique to close the aneurysmal wall over the prosthesis. A fistula is created between the perioprosthetic space and the right atrial appendage. (From Cabrol C, Pavie A, Mesnildrey P: Long-term results with total replacement of the ascending aorta and reimplantation of the coronary arteries, *J Thorac Cardiovasc Surg* 91[1]:17, 1986.)

maintained with perfusion of cold blood. Cooling must be maintained by other methods. The room temperature setting should remain low (13° to 15° C [55° to 60° F]), and the cooling blanket should be set appropriately. If bags of ice are applied around the patient's head, they should be checked by the circulating nurse and replenished with additional ice as necessary. All needed equipment and supplies should be readily available to avoid prolonging the period of circulatory arrest unnecessarily. The procedure should be performed as efficiently as possible to minimize delays, which could increase the risk of cerebral injury.

Additional measures that have been used to protect the brain include avoidance of hyperglycemia (which can generate increased amounts of lactate and lower intracellular pH, leading to increased acidosis), the use of pharmacologic agents such as corticosteroids and barbiturates, and hemodilution (to reduce blood viscosity). The electroencephalogram (EEG) and cortical somatosensory evoked potentials (Oliver, Nuttall, and Murray,

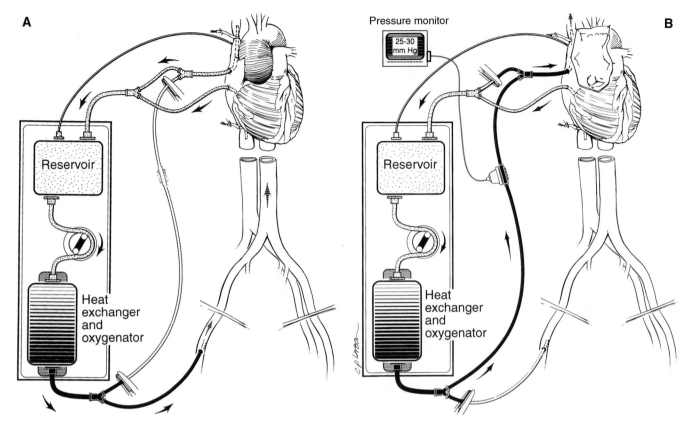

A

B

Pressure monitor

25-30 mm Hg

Reservoir

Heat exchanger and oxygenator

Reservoir

Heat exchanger and oxygenator

FIGURE 14-20 CPB circuit modified for retrograde cerebral perfusion. **A,** A Y connection between the arterial line and the superior vena cava line; a clamp on this connecting line allows CPB with progressive cooling. **B,** After initiating hypothermic circulatory arrest, the clamps are repositioned to allow RCP via the SVC cannula. (From Coselli JS, LeMaire SA, Walkes J-C: Surgery for acute Type A dissection, *Oper Techn Thorac Cardiovasc Surg* 4[1]:13, 1999.)

1999) can be used to monitor brain activity, which is considered to be minimal with adequate hypothermia.

After the distal and arch anastomoses are completed, the graft is clamped proximal to the arch branches, air and debris are removed, and retrograde cerebral perfusion (discussed in the following) is discontinued. CPB is reestablished. TEE may be used to confirm that the true lumen is being perfused and to look for residual air. The proximal anastomosis is then performed while the patient rewarms. Rewarming is performed slowly at a rate of 1° C (1.8° F) every 2 to 3 minutes; differences between the temperature of the circulating blood and the core body temperature (as measured by the esophageal temperature) should not be greater than approximately 10° C (18° F). A larger temperature gradient could injure blood cells and tissue (Griepp and others, 2000).

Retrograde cerebral perfusion (RCP) (Fig. 14-20) via the superior vena cava (SVC), or antegrade cerebral perfusion via the subclavian artery, can be employed, especially when a prolonged (more than 60 minutes) pe-

riod of circulatory arrest is anticipated (Safi, Petrika, Miller, 2001; Svensson, 2001).

RCP is instituted after the circulation has been arrested and during the period of arrest. In one method of implementing RCP, the CPB circuit is adapted by inserting a Y connection into the arterial line and another Y into the venous drainage line (Fig. 14-20). The venous drainage tubing is clamped (see Fig. 14-20, *A*). To initiate RCP, the femoral arterial line is clamped, and the previously inserted Y connection off the arterial line is opened (see Fig. 14-20, *B*), thereby perfusing the cerebral circulation with arterialized blood. A tourniquet is tightened around the cannula. According to the method used by David (1999), the initial flow rate should be approximately 300 ml per minute and is increased to maintain a venous pressure 25 to 30 mm Hg in the SVC. RCP may be employed for the duration of circulatory arrest.

Before bypass is restarted, the SVC retrograde cerebral perfusion line can be used to flush particulate matter or air from the vessels (Griepp and others, 2000). To

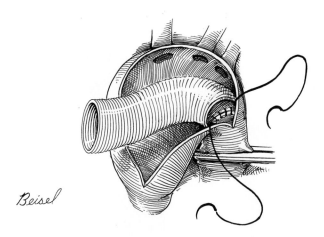

FIGURE 14-21 Distal anastomosis for an aortic arch aneurysm. (From Waldhausen JA, Pierce WS, Campbell DB: *Surgery of the chest,* ed 6, St Louis, Mosby.)

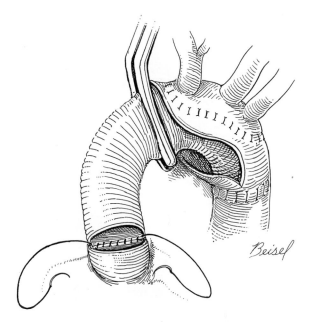

FIGURE 14-23 The graft is clamped, cardiopulmonary bypass is resumed, and the proximal anastomosis is performed. (From Waldhausen JA, Pierce WS, Campbell DB: *Surgery of the chest,* ed 6, St Louis, 1996, Mosby.)

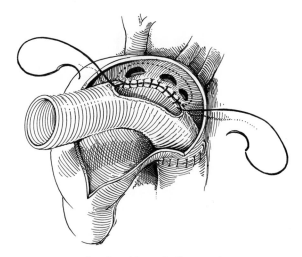

FIGURE 14-22 The brachiocephalic arteries are anastomosed as an island to the prosthetic graft. (From Waldhausen JA, Pierce WS, Campbell DB: *Surgery of the chest,* ed 6, St Louis, 1996, Mosby.)

terminate RCP, the retrograde line is clamped and the venous return line is opened, allowing the resumption of venous drainage into the venous reservoir.

Operative procedure: repair of a transverse aortic arch

Two anastomotic techniques for arch aneurysms are described in the following: total arch replacement (Figs. 14-21 to 14-23) and hemiarch replacement (Fig. 14-24). According to Moon and Miller (1999), the hemiarch replacement technique is more advantageous than the total replacement because only 15 to 30 minutes of circulatory arrest at 20° to 22° C (68° to 71.6° F) may be required, versus a substantially longer period of circu-

latory arrest at lower core temperatures, both of which prolong CPB and impair coagulation processes.

Total arch replacement (Coselli, LeMaire, and Walkes, 1999; David, 1999) (see Figs. 14-21 to 14-23)

1. The patient is placed in the supine position, and median sternotomy is performed. External and internal cooling to the desired temperature is achieved with topical cold applications and right atrial–femoral artery CPB.

2. Once the patient is cooled, the aorta may be clamped (less favored) or the pump turned off to create circulatory arrest and a bloodless field. The heart is likely to fibrillate, and manual massage may be employed to decompress the heart before a left ventricular vent is inserted. The left ventricular (LV) vent is frequently inserted via the right superior pulmonary vein in order to decompress the heart. In some cases an LV apical vent may be inserted (Moon and Miller, 1999).

3. Retrograde cardioplegia is infused to arrest and protect the myocardium. Intermittent retroplegia reinfusion washes out metabolic wastes.

4. The patient is placed in Trendelenberg's position and RCP instituted.

5. The aneurysm is incised, and a tube graft is selected. Atherosclerotic material, formed thrombus, and other debris are removed from the aorta and arch vessels.

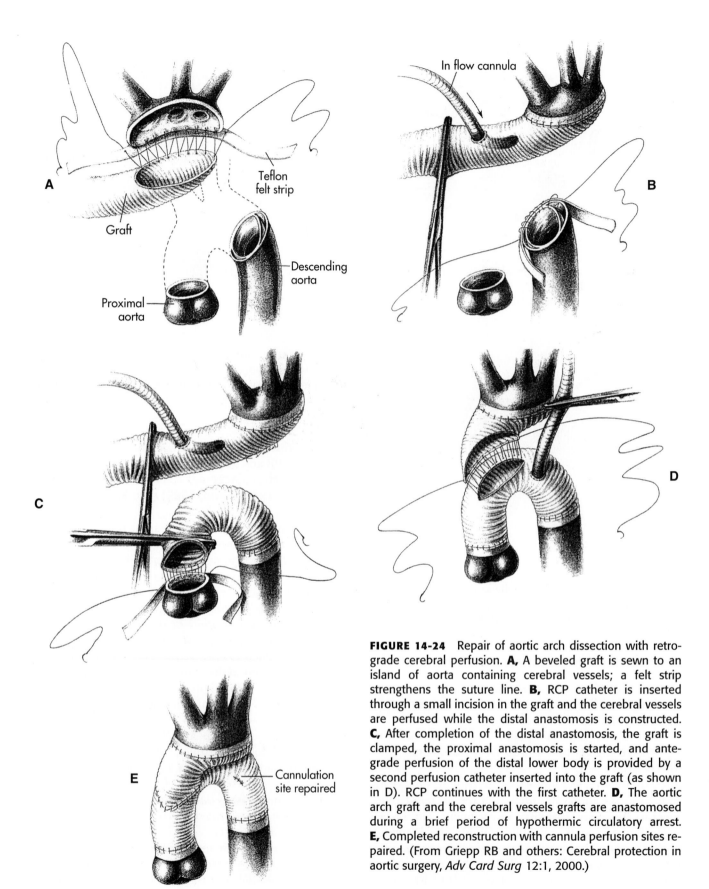

FIGURE 14-24 Repair of aortic arch dissection with retrograde cerebral perfusion. **A,** A beveled graft is sewn to an island of aorta containing cerebral vessels; a felt strip strengthens the suture line. **B,** RCP catheter is inserted through a small incision in the graft and the cerebral vessels are perfused while the distal anastomosis is constructed. **C,** After completion of the distal anastomosis, the graft is clamped, the proximal anastomosis is started, and antegrade perfusion of the distal lower body is provided by a second perfusion catheter inserted into the graft (as shown in D). RCP continues with the first catheter. **D,** The aortic arch graft and the cerebral vessels grafts are anastomosed during a brief period of hypothermic circulatory arrest. **E,** Completed reconstruction with cannula perfusion sites repaired. (From Griepp RB and others: Cerebral protection in aortic surgery, *Adv Card Surg* 12:1, 2000.)

6. The phrenic nerve and the recurrent laryngeal branch of the vagus nerve, which cross the aortic arch, are identified. Injury to the former can affect diaphragmatic movement, and injury to the latter can produce vocal cord paralysis on the side of the affected nerve.

7. The distal anastomosis (see Fig. 14-21) to the descending thoracic aorta is performed with a continuous 2-0 or 3-0 polypropylene or polyester suture.

8. Implantation of the brachiocephalic arteries (see Fig. 14-22) is done by making an oval opening (with an eye cautery) in the convex portion of the graft. The graft is anastomosed to the common origin of the branch vessels (rather than to each individual artery).

9. After the distal anastomoses are completed, an occlusion clamp is placed on the graft proximal to the arch vessels (See Fig. 14-24). With the patient in deep Trendelenburg's position, air is evacuated from the arch and its branches, and blood is allowed to fill the aortic arch and branch vessels. Cardiopulmonary bypass is slowly resumed, the perfusion flow rate is gradually increased, and rewarming is initiated.

10. The proximal anastomosis is performed with a continuous 2-0 or 3-0 polypropylene or polyester suture. Retroplegia is infused as necessary.

11. The suture lines are inspected for hemostasis, and air is removed from the left side of the heart and aorta. Rewarming is completed, and bypass is terminated. Temporary pacing wires and chest tubes are inserted, and all incisions are closed.

Hemiarch replacement (Griepp and others, 2000; Moon and Miller, 1999)

1. The patient is positioned, cooled, and arrested as described for the total arch replacement technique described in steps 1 to 4 for total arch replacement.

2. The aorta is transected just proximal to the innominate artery.

3. An island containing the arch vessels is created and anastomosed to a beveled graft (see Fig. 14-24, A). Antegrade cerebral perfusion is given through the graft after completion of the anastomosis (see Fig. 14-24, B).

4. A second graft is selected, anastomosed to the distal portion of the aorta, and clamped; then the proximal anastomosis is sewn (see Fig. 14-24, C).

5. Antegrade perfusion of the lower body is instituted with a second perfusion catheter (see Fig. 14-24, D).

6. Another brief period of circulatory arrest is initiated, during which time the aortic arch graft is connected to the second graft with an end-to-side anastomosis.

7. The cannulation site for the antegrade perfusion cannula is repaired (see Fig. 14-24, E).

8. Hemostasis is achieved, and the procedure completed as described for total arch replacement.

Extension into the descending aorta

When the arch lesion extends into the descending thoracic aorta, the procedure may have to be modified. The patient can be placed in a semilateral position and a transverse bilateral thoracotomy incision made. The femoral artery is cannulated for arterial infusion; venous drainage may be obtained from the right atrium. The surgeon may stand to the left of the patient for the distal anastomosis and then move to the right side to perform the arch and proximal anastomoses.

The "elephant trunk" technique devised by Borst, Frank, and Schaps (1988) can be used to repair extensive aortic aneurysms and dissections, especially those requiring staged operations. The aortic arch is replaced, but instead of a conventional anastomosis being done between the distal end of the arch graft and the origin of the descending aorta, an appropriate length of the terminal graft is first invaginated. The circular reflection fold thus created is then sutured end-to-end to the descending aorta. Before the anastomotic suture is tied, the invaginated portion of the graft is advanced into the downstream portion of the aorta (where it is suspended freely like an elephant trunk). Air is removed from the aorta and the space between the graft and the aneurysm by retrograde perfusion. If another operation is needed to repair the aorta downstream from the first repair, the distal end of the elephant trunk can be exposed through a left thoracotomy and anastomosed to another graft to replace the descending thoracic aorta. This technique allows graft-to-graft anastomoses for subsequent repairs on the descending (and abdominal) aorta and obviates the need for proximal graft-to-aorta anastomoses (thus avoiding having to sew on aneurysmal or chronically dissected aortic tissue, which may not hold sutures securely (Moon and Miller, 1999).

SURGERY ON THE DESCENDING THORACIC AORTA

Although surgery is the standard treatment for dissections and aneurysms of the ascending aorta and the transverse aortic arch, there is no single standard treatment for lesions of the descending thoracic aorta. In particular, surgery for dissections of the descending aorta may not always be indicated.

Reports (Daily and others, 1970; Wheat and others, 1969) of improved survival with medical versus surgical therapy in uncomplicated descending thoracic aortic dissections prompted clinicians to reserve surgery for patients whose aorta had ruptured or who demonstrated expansion of the dissection, continuing pain, and ischemia of visceral organs. These findings have been reconfirmed by Glower and colleagues (1990). As with other dissections, initial therapy is directed toward lowering blood pressure and myocardial contractility to retard progression of the intimal tear.

Minimally invasive techniques

Although minimally invasive techniques have not been widely applied to thoracic aortic disease, endoluminal grafting technology, originally developed to treat abdominal aortic aneurysms (May and others, 1997), has been applied by Dake and colleagues (1998) to patients with aneurysms of the descending thoracic aorta. Problems encountered include thromboembolism, stroke, paraplegia (possibly caused by sudden occlusion of a large number of intercostal artery branches), endoleaks, and poor flexibility. Others (Terai and others, 2000) have investigated the use of balloon catheters to treat Stanford type B dissections. Although in its early stages, vascular stenting of the thoracic aorta is likely to have a greater future role in the treatment of aortic disease.

Procedural considerations

When surgery is being planned, the need for circulatory support must be considered. The heart is not arrested except in very complex lesions, when circulatory arrest may be used; it continues beating to perfuse the upper body. Thus myocardial protection techniques, such as systemic hypothermia and cardioplegia, are not used. Surgery is performed under normothermic conditions. Circulatory support may be used, however, to perfuse the kidneys, spinal cord, and lower extremities while the descending thoracic aorta is occluded.

Spinal cord injury

Of major concern during the period of aortic clamping is ischemic injury to the spinal cord, resulting in paraparesis or paraplegia, which can occur in as many as 40% of cases (Gharagozloo, Neville, and Cox, 1998). The risk of injury is increased in the presence of dissection and other complex aortic lesions, perioperative hypotension, prolonged aortic cross-clamping and reperfusion injury, increased cerebrospinal fluid (CSF) pressure, and the sacrifice of critical intercostal or lumbar (in thorocoabdominal aneurysms—see p. 423) arteries.

Techniques proposed to reduce the risk of injury include use of oxygen free radical scavengers, drainage of cerebrospinal fluid, induction of hypothermia, admin-istration of pharmacologic agents, expeditious surgery, distal aortic perfusion, identification of vascular supply, and preservation of intercostal arteries.

When most or all of the descending thoracic aorta is involved, the incidence of spinal cord injury increases, especially when the aorta is dissected. Distal hypotension of the aorta, which can occur when the aorta is cross-clamped, causes a decrease in the perfusion pressure of the spinal cord. If there is a prolonged period of cross-clamping, during which time spinal perfusion pressure is significantly reduced, neural ischemia occurs. As a result, energy stores (e.g., adenosine triphosphate [ATP]) are depleted and neurotoxic enzymes are released. Additionally, the production of destructive oxygen free radicals that occurs after the restoration of the circulation (reperfusion) is increased. Free radicals cause a loss of cellular membrane integrity and increase the amount of substances that produce vasospasm and microvascular thrombosis. Free radical scavenger enzymes (superoxide dismutase and catalase) have been employed to control free radicals, but their effectiveness has not been clearly demonstrated (Gharagozloo, Neville, and Cox, 1998).

When the aorta is occluded, blood pressure increases in the aorta proximal to the cross-clamp. This proximal aortic hypertension not only increases cardiac afterload but also increases cerebrospinal fluid (CSF) pressure. As CSF pressure increases, blood pressure in the spine decreases, resulting in a reduction in spinal blood flow. Spinal cord perfusion pressure can be increased with drainage of the CSF (Acher and Wynn, 1998). One technique for draining CSF is to place an intrathecal catheter in the second lumbar space. CSF pressure can be continuously monitored, and CSF can be drained through the catheter. The CSF drainage catheter should not be placed in a patient receiving heparin because of the increased risk for bleeding (Gharagozloo, Neville, and Cox, 1998).

Another protective technique is to infuse cold (4° C [39.2° F]) normal saline through the CSF catheter to produce regional hypothermia. This lowers the metabolic rate of the spinal tissue and has been shown to reduce the incidence of paraplegia (Cambria and Davison, 1998). Core cooling with cardiopulmonary bypass and circulatory arrest also has been used. In patients without aortic insufficiency or coronary artery disease, this technique is generally contraindicated because the retrograde flow employed can regurgitate through an incompetent valve to cause LV distension; in addition, the reduced coronary perfusion pressure associated with retrograde CPB can aggravate coronary ischemia (Rokkas and Kouchoukos, 1998).

Pharmacologic agents, such as barbiturates (which reduce neuronal metabolism) and corticosteroids (which are membrane stabilizers and free radical scavengers) also have been employed to reduce spinal cord ischemic injury. Other drugs have been used to combat the ischemic effects of endogenous opiates (endorphins). Opiates appear to decrease cerebral blood low and increase vascular resistance; opium antagonists (e.g., naloxone) have been shown to reduce neurologic deficits in patients undergoing thoracic and thoracoabdominal aneurysms (Acher and others, 1994).

Because there are numerous factors related to spinal cord injury and no one protective technique has demonstrated consistent avoidance of injury, many surgeons perform surgery expeditiously, using the clamp-and-go technique with few or no additional supportive procedures. When cross-clamp times are less than 25 minutes, the probability of lower extremity neurologic deficit is almost nonexistent (Gharagozloo, Neville, and Cox, 1998). When there is a complex lesion and the anticipated cross-clamp time is expected to be longer than 25 to 30 minutes, additional protective measures are likely to be employed.

One of these additional protective techniques is distal aortic perfusion. The most commonly used methods include roller pumps, passive shunts, and centrifugal pumps. The earliest form of perfusion was accomplished with roller pumps and the institution of cardiopulmonary bypass. With *left atrial–distal aorta bypass,* a form of left-sided heart bypass, a cannula is placed in the left atrium to receive oxygenated blood, which travels through tubing to a cannula in the distal aorta. The roller pump is interposed in the tubing to propel the blood into the distal vascular bed. An oxygenator in the circuit is not required because blood from the left atrium is freshly oxygenated. The need for systemic heparinization, and the associated increased risk of hemorrhage, makes this method less popular than others. *Femoral vein–femoral artery bypass* also has been used for distal perfusion. An oxygenator is required to oxygenate the femoral venous return before it is pumped into the femoral artery.

Heparinized shunts (e.g., the Gott shunt), placed between the proximal portion of the descending thoracic aorta (or the left ventricular apex) and the aorta (or femoral artery) distal to the distal cross-clamp, do not require systemic heparin administration (Fig. 14-25). However, because these are passive shunts, the blood flow cannot be regulated. Thus if the native perfusion pressure is less than 60 mm Hg (considered the lower end required for perfusion pressure), the shunt is unable to provide adequate perfusion.

Centrifugal pumps can overcome some of the difficulties associated with roller pumps and passive shunts and are considered by some to be the best method of maintaining distal aortic perfusion (Gharagozloo,

Neville, and Cox, 1998). Flow can be regulated, there is less damage to blood components compared with roller pumps, shed blood can be collected and reinfused, and minimal heparin is required. However, in some cases bypass techniques have been shown to result in high morbidity and mortality compared with the clamp-and-go technique. This may be related to atheroemboli or air emboli resulting from the cannulation of the diseased aorta (Svensson and Loop, 1988). Also, although perfusion techniques may provide blood flow to the distal aorta, they may not protect the spinal cord. If the arteries supplying the spinal cord arise from the excluded (clamped) aorta, the spinal cord will remain ischemic. Methods to identify the blood supply to the spinal cord can help clinicians to predict the relative degree of risk for spinal cord injury after surgery on the descending thoracic aorta.

Anterior and posterior spinal arteries perfuse the spinal cord. The anterior spinal artery is supplied by a variable number of radicular arteries that supply the thoracic and upper abdominal region. The major radicular artery, the *arteria radicularis magna* (ARM), also referred to as the *artery of Adamkiewicz,* arises between T7 and L1 and joins the anterior spinal artery in a variety of locations (Svensson, 1998). Even with excellent distal perfusion, the spinal cord may remain relatively ischemic if the ARM flow cannot reach the excluded segment of aorta. Efforts to identify the location of the ARM preoperatively have been attempted, but this technique has not been implemented widely for fear that the injection of angiographic contrast material could itself cause paralysis (Kieffer and others, 1989). Monitoring somatosensory evoked potentials (SEP) is another method to test the function of the spinal cord (and, indirectly, spinal cord ischemia). A drawback of SEP is that it tests the more ischemia-resistent axons and not necessarily the more ischemia-sensitive cells (Svensson, 1998).

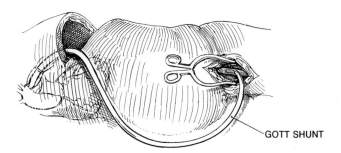

GOTT SHUNT

FIGURE 14-25 Gott shunt. The proximal end is in the descending aorta just beyond the takeoff of the subclavian artery. The distal end is in the left common femoral artery. (From Waldhausen JA, Pierce WS: *Johnson's surgery of the chest,* ed 5, St Louis, 1985, Mosby.)

A technique to enhance blood flow to the affected aortic tissue is to incorporate portions of the intercostal arteries between T9 and T12 into the prosthetic graft. Disappointing results may be related to the prolongation of cross-clamp time required for the anastomoses and to reimplantation of the "wrong" (e.g., not containing the ARM) cluster of intercostal arteries. Newer methods to identify the critical arteries have been described by Svensson (1998), who has studied spinal motor responses with the use of an electrode alongside the spinal cord. In cases involving the upper thoracic aorta, reimplantation may not be critical. In cases involving a short segment of the lower thoracic aorta and those involving a longer segment of thoracic aorta or the thoracoabdominal aorta, implantation of critical intercostals and lumbar arteries is recommended (Gharagozloo, Neville, and Cox, 1998).

Nursing considerations

The aneurysm is approached via a left posterolateral thoracotomy through the fourth or fifth intercostal space. If the lesion is extensive, a proximal incision and a distal incision may be required. Equipment and supplies for placing the patient in a lateral position need to be available, as well as thoracotomy instruments and vascular clamps. Instruments and supplies for distal perfusion (e.g., CPB, shunts) are available and ready, depending on surgeon preference.

Operative procedure: repair of a descending thoracic aortic aneurysm/dissection

1. The patient is positioned for lateral thoracotomy and the skin prepared from the shoulder to the knees. Access to the groin must be maintained for possible cannulation or blood pressure monitoring lines.
2. An incision is made in the left fourth intercostal space, and a rib retractor is inserted. The location of the incision may be altered, and a second incision may be required for better exposure.
3. If requested, circulatory support/distal perfusion is instituted.
   a. Left atrial–distal aorta bypass: A pursestring suture with a tourniquet is placed in the left atrium, and a cannula is inserted through a stab wound. The cannula is connected to tubing attached to a centrifugal pump or threaded through a roller pump. The distal end of the tubing is connected to a cannula that has been inserted through a pursestring suture into the femoral artery.

   A modification of this technique provides distal hypothermia via a heat exchanger incorporated into the circuit in an effort to improve protection of the spinal cord (Cooley and Jones, 2000).

   b. Femoral vein–femoral artery bypass: Institution of bypass is performed as described in Chapter 9.
   c. Gott shunt: Double pursestring sutures (3-0 polyester) with tourniquets are placed in the proximal portion of the descending aorta and the distal aorta or common femoral artery. The proximal and distal ends of the shunt (7 mm or 9 mm) are inserted through stab wounds into the aorta and/or femoral artery (see Fig. 14-25).
4. The aortic lesion is assessed and isolated between vascular clamps. A tube graft is selected and delivered to the field.
5. The aneurysm is opened longitudinally. Intercostal artery orifices are oversewn with suture ligatures for hemostasis; larger, critical intercostals may be anastomosed end-to-side to the graft (Fig. 14-26).
6. The graft is anastomosed end-to-end to the aorta proximally with a 3-0 polypropylene double-armed suture and distally with a 3-0 or 4-0 suture. A longer, 36-inch suture may be used to reduce the need for additional sutures to complete the anastomosis. If the aorta is dissected, felt strips may be used to obliterate the false lumen and strengthen the anastomotic site (see Fig. 14-26; Fig. 14-27).
7. After the anastomoses are completed and the graft is deaired, the distal clamp is removed. The proximal

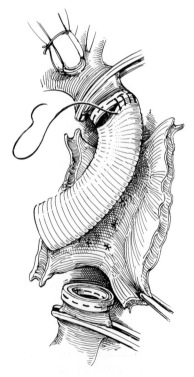

FIGURE 14-26 Proximal anastomosis for repair of the descending thoracic aorta. (From Waldhausen JA, Pierce WS: *Johnson's surgery of the chest*, ed 5, St Louis, 1985, Mosby.)

clamp then is removed slowly (to avoid sudden hypotension), and the graft is inspected for hemostasis. The remnant aortic wall may be wrapped around the completed repair.

8. Cannulas or shunts are removed and insertion sites repaired.

Use of intraluminal prostheses

In the presence of acute aortic dissection, conventional suture anastomoses can be problematic because aortic tissue is often friable and easily torn and often is associated with a prolonged cross-clamp time. This challenge was addressed by Dureau and his colleagues (1978) with the introduction of a sutureless graft prosthesis that could be quickly inserted into the ascending aorta with tape ligatures.

The prosthesis is constructed by attaching rigid, velour-covered rings at each end of a Dacron tube graft. An array of diameter widths and lengths is available. Tapered versions can be used in locations where there is a significant disparity between the proximal and distal vessel lumen. A variable-length prosthesis also is made that uses a movable fixation ring. In cases in which the surgeon prefers to construct a conventional anastomosis at the distal or proximal end, the ring at that end can be removed. Concerns about prosthetic migration of

grafts (originally positioned in the ascending or transverse arch) occluding the coronary and cerebral vessels have limited the use of these devices. Occasionally they are used in the descending aorta (Fig. 14-28).

SURGERY FOR THORACOABDOMINAL ANEURYSMS

Lesions involving both the thoracic and abdominal aorta pose a significantly increased risk of morbidity and mortality. They usually occur in older patients with atherosclerotic disease and may attain considerable size before they are discovered. Of major importance during surgery is revascularization of the major visceral organs supplied by the celiac artery and the superior and inferior mesenteric arteries, restoration of renal blood flow, and preservation of the spinal cord. Spinal cord and renal injury are the most frequent complications of surgery. Circulatory support such as that described for repairs of descending thoracic lesions may be used. Generally, cardiopulmonary bypass is not used, but some authors have suggested that the use of hypothermic circulatory arrest may be beneficial in preserving spinal cord function (Rokkas and Kouchoukos, 1998).

Determining the patency of the major visceral arteries helps in planning the operation. Vessels occluded by the aneurysmal process (often the inferior mesenteric artery) are not reimplanted.

Procedural considerations

To provide access to both the descending thoracic and abdominal aortic segments, the patient is placed in the supine position with a roll or pillow under the left side of the chest to achieve a 45-degree modified lateral position. Both thoracotomy and laparotomy instrumentation are added to the vascular clamps and other instruments required for the repair.

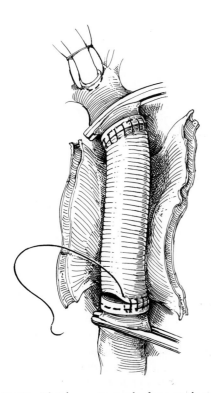

FIGURE 14-27 Distal anastomosis for repair of the descending thoracic aorta. (From Waldhausen JA, Pierce WS: *Johnson's surgery of the chest,* ed 5, St Louis, 1985, Mosby.)

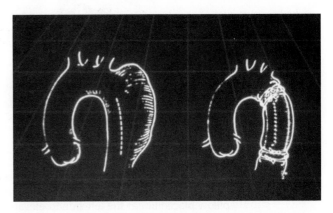

FIGURE 14-28 Intraluminal prosthesis positioned in the descending thoracic aorta. (Courtesy Bard Vascular Systems Div., Billerica, Mass.)

Operative procedure: repair of a thoracoabdominal aortic aneurysm

1. The patient is positioned, and the initial thoracic incision is made through the intercostal space, allowing the best access to the proximal portion of the thoracic aortic lesion. (This may be between the sixth or seventh intercostal space or lower [Fig. 14-29].) The incision is continued to the midline of the abdomen and down the linea alba to a point below the umbilicus.
2. If circulatory support is being used, it is instituted (as described previously).
3. A thoracotomy retractor is inserted into the thoracic incision; rib cutters may be needed.
4. The diaphragm is opened a few centimeters to expose the proximal abdominal aorta. Care is taken to avoid injury to the phrenic nerve, the lung, the liver, and other organs. An abdominal retractor is inserted.
5. The aneurysm is inspected, and the extent of the lesion proximally and distally is determined. If separate proximal and distal lesions are present, the operation can be performed in two stages (Fig. 14-30).
6. For aneurysms involving one segment the thoracoabdominal aorta only, repair is done in one operation. The abdominal viscera are mobilized and retracted to the right. The distal aorta or iliac arteries are dissected.

7. Before cross-clamping the aorta, heparin may be given (1 mg/kg of body weight [1000 units]) to prevent thrombosis or microemboli.

   Pharmacologic agents are used to control blood pressure and maintain hemodynamic stability. The aorta is cross-clamped proximally. The distal aorta or iliac arteries may be occluded or may be allowed to back bleed (Cooley, 1998). Occasionally, balloon occlusion catheters, gauze packing, or clamps are used to control profuse back bleeding.
8. The aorta is incised longitudinally, the lumen is measured, and the desired graft is delivered to the field. The proximal anastomosis is performed with a continuous 3-0 or 4-0 suture. Large intercostal and lumbar arteries may be reattached to the graft to help preserve spinal cord integrity (see Fig. 14-30, *B*).
9a. When the visceral vessels and renal arteries are involved, the celiac and superior mesenteric arteries are anastomosed to openings made in the graft with a battery-powered, handheld cautery. If possible, they are reimplanted as a unit along with the right renal artery (Fig. 14-30).

   If the inferior mesenteric artery is patent, it is anastomosed to the graft. The left renal artery is reattached directly or with a short segment of 6 or 8 mm Dacron graft (or splenic artery if the spleen has been removed) (see Fig. 14-30, *B*).

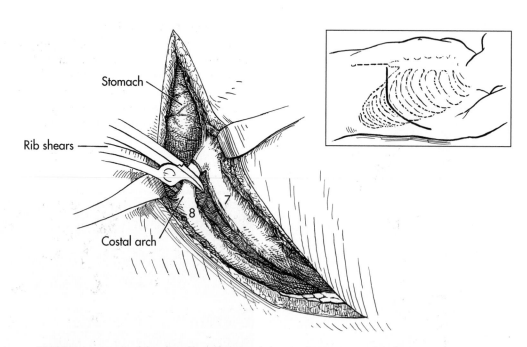

FIGURE 14-29 Incision line for a thoracoabdominal aneurysm. The thoracotomy incision is carried to the midline and extended to beyond the umbilicus. Not shown is the roll or pillow placed under the left side to elevate the chest for exposure of the descending thoracic aorta. (From Waldhausen JA, Pierce WS, Campbell DB: *Surgery of the chest,* ed 6, St Louis, 1996, Mosby.)

9b. If the visceral vessels and renal arteries are not involved, they can be excluded from the repair. The graft is beveled to repair the posterior portion of the abdominal aorta (Fig. 14-31).

10. The distal anastomosis is made to the distal abdominal aorta. If the aneurysm extends to the iliac arteries, a bifurcated graft is used. (A bifurcated segment of graft may need to be anastomosed end-to-end to the distal portion of the tube graft.)

11. Air is evacuated, and each anastomosis is tested for hemostasis after completion. The aneurysmal sac is closed around the graft, and the viscera are replaced in the peritoneum. If circulatory support has been used, it is discontinued and incision sites are repaired.

12. A chest tube is inserted into the thorax, and an abdominal drain is inserted if excessive bleeding is anticipated.

13. Thoracic and abdominal incisions are closed.

Completion of the Procedure

After completion of the surgery, patients are transported to the surgical intensive care unit. In procedures involving extensive dissection (e.g., thoracoabdominal aneurysms), bleeding may be greater than that anticipated with other types of surgery. In addition to monitoring cardiac performance, attention also is focused on renal and neurologic function, especially when blood flow to the brain and the spinal cord has been interrupted.

Postoperative Complications

Complications associated with repairing the thoracic aorta are listed in Table 14-4. Complications and patient teaching considerations for aortic valve prostheses are discussed in Chapter 12.

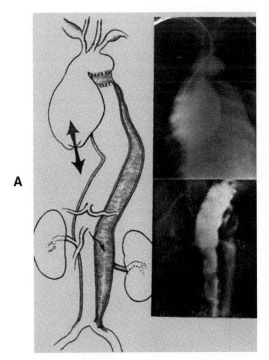
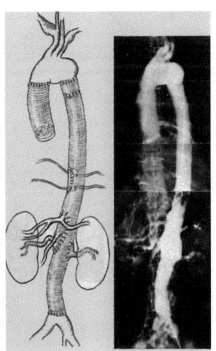

FIGURE 14-30 A, Fusiform aneurysm of the ascending aorta and separate chronic dissecting aneurysm involving the entire descending thoracic and abdominal aorta (the patient had already undergone a graft replacement for a descending thoracic aneurysm). **B,** Drawing of staged operations showing graft replacement of the ascending aorta. Note reimplantation of intercostal arteries, visceral vessels, and both renal arteries. (From Crawford ES and others: Thoracoabdominal aortic aneurysms: preoperative and intraoperative factors determining immediate and long-term results of operations in 605 patients, *J Vasc Surg* 3:389, 1986.)

TABLE 14-4

Perioperative Problems and Complications of Surgery on the Thoracic Aorta

COMPLICATION/PROBLEM	PREVENTION/INTERVENTIONS
Hemorrhage	
Excessive bleeding may be caused by technical problems, excessive blood transfusions, prolonged cardiopulmonary bypass runs, excessive hemodilution, and coagulation defects related to hypothermia or intrinsic bleeding disorders	Intervention depends on cause of bleeding
	Hemorrhage at suture lines:
	Use felt strips to bolster suture line
	Use fibrin glue and other topical hemostatic agents
	Use preclotted grafts (or those manufactured to minimize interstitial bleeding)
	Wrap suture line with Dacron graft (8 or 10 mm)
	Excessive blood transfusions:
	Avoid unnecessary connections or kinks in bypass circuit (damages blood cells)
	Use cardiotomy suction gently, in pooled blood
	Use fresh bank blood
	Use autotransfusion system
	Prolonged bypass runs/excessive hemodilution:
	Avoid unnecessary delays during procedure
	May require clotting factors
	Membrane oxygenators and centrifugal pumps have been shown to preserve cell integrity
	Administer desmopressin (DDAVP) to enhance activation of clotting factors
	Coagulation defects caused by hypothermia; when rewarming:
	Do not allow OR to become too cold
	Restart warming mattress
	Use warm irrigation
	Cover exposed skin when access not required
	Coagulation defects caused by intrinsic bleeding disorder:
	Provide appropriate replacement therapy
	Platelets may be required if there is history of aspirin

Modified from Kouchoukos NT, Wareing TH: Management of complications of aortic surgery. In Waldhausen JA, Orringer MB: *Complications in cardiothoracic surgery,* St Louis, 1991, Mosby; Moon MR, Miller DC: Aortic arch replacement for dissection, *Oper Techn Thorac Cardiovasc Surg* 4(1):33, 1999.

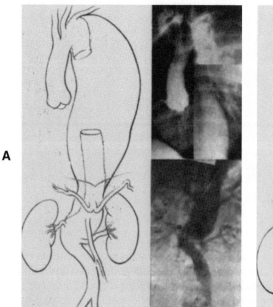 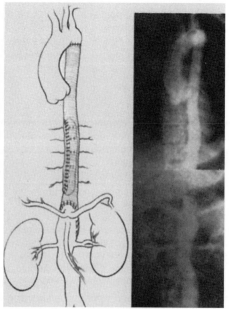

FIGURE 14-31 **A,** Aneurysm of the descending thoracic aorta and upper abdominal aorta. **B,** Intercostal arteries have been reimplanted into the graft. The visceral vessels and renal arteries are excluded from the repair. (From Crawford ES and others: Thoracoabdominal aortic aneurysms: preoperative and intraoperative factors determining immediate and long-term results of operations in 605 patients, *J Vasc Surg* 3:389, 1986.)

TABLE **14-4**
Perioperative Problems and Complications of Surgery on the Thoracic Aorta—cont'd

COMPLICATION/PROBLEM	PREVENTION/INTERVENTIONS

Central Nervous System Injury

Embolization of particulate matter or air can cause neurologic injury; spinal cord paralysis is a complication of operations on descending thoracic and thoracoabdominal aorta; phrenic and vagus nerve injury can cause, respectively, paralysis of left diaphragm and left vocal cord; perfusion of false lumen in dissections can cause brain damage

Intervention depends on the type of injury
  Embolization:
    Remove all atheromatous and other debris from instruments and surgical site
    Evacuate air completely from heart, aorta, and arch vessels
    Gently manipulate vessels and perform careful debridement
    Place in deep Trendelenburg's position before reestablishing arterial flow
    Use hypothermic circulatory arrest; occasionally, selective perfusion of arch vessels may be used in repair of aortic arch
    Monitor EEG, temperature, and evoked potentials
  Spinal cord paralysis:
    Minimize ischemic time; avoid delay
    Maintain adequate distal flow and perfusion pressure with shunt or bypass; avoid hypotension
    Monitor spinal cord function with evoked potentials
    Limit amount of aorta resected
  Phrenic and vagus nerve injury:
    Avoid stretching or severing nerves during surgery of aortic arch or proximal descending aorta
    Note location of retractors
    Brain injury from perfusion of false lumen (as well as injury to viscera):
    May need to use circulatory arrest and open technique
    May need to cannulate graft for antegrade flow after completion of first anastomosis
    Monitor EEG, evoked potentials
    Simultaneously monitor femoral and both radial pulses
  (See text for additional details)

Infection of Prosthetic Grafts

1% to 2% of all patients develop infection of prosthetic graft; mortality can be 25% to 75%; most infections are result of Intraoperative contamination; risk is increased when operative time is prolonged, reoperation is performed, or there is excessive infusion of blood products

Prompt reoperation may be needed with replacement of infected prosthesis; a pedicle flap of omentum may be placed over graft
Use strict operative sterile technique
Provide antibiotic treatment (may require lifetime maintenance)
Perform preoperative antibiotic prophylaxis
Chlorhexidine gluconate may be preferred to povidone-iodine as operative cleansing agent

Pulmonary Complications

Diffuse interstitial edema with reduced pulmonary compliance and acute respiratory failure may occur postoperatively; possible causes include anaphylatoxins generated during cardiopulmonary bypass, injury to lungs during retraction, or infusion of drugs or blood products

Provide mechanical ventilation at low inspiratory pressures in combination with positive end-expiratory pressure (PEEP); maintain 90% or greater arterial oxygen saturation
Use caution during surgery to avoid injury to lungs from retraction and manipulation
Use ultrafiltration to avoid excessive hemodilution during bypass; use membrane oxygenation
Provide judicious infusion of blood products during surgery; antihistamines

Formation of Pseudoaneurysm at Anastomosis, Recurrent Dissection

Associated with composite graft replacement of ascending aorta and aortic valve, or supracoronary graft replacement of ascending aorta for aortic dissection; may be greater risk in patients with connective tissue disorders (e.g., Marfan's syndrome); attributed to tension on suture line, persistent bleeding at anastomoses or between graft and aortic remnant closed over graft, and pathologic condition of aorta; may be caused by infection

Avoid tension on suture lines (e.g., use interposition of vein or synthetic graft between aortic graft and coronary ostia; use Cabrol technique) (see text)
Use measures to reduce bleeding
Use measures to prevent or treat infection (see previous)
May need to avoid inclusion technique of wrapping remnant aneurysmal sac around graft
In patients with dissections and Marfan's syndrome, composite graft replacement may be preferable to supracoronary graft replacement (so that weakened tissue is excluded from repair)
Reoperation to repair or replace graft and pseudoaneurysm should be done before it becomes too enlarged

References

Acher CW and others: Combined use of cerebral spinal fluid drainage and naloxone reduces the risk of paraplegia in thoracoabdominal aneurysm repair, *J Vasc Surg* 19(2):236, 1994.

Acher CW, Wynn MM: Multifactoral nature of spinal cord circulation, *Semin Thorac Cardiovasc Surg* 10(1):7, 1998.

Bentall H, De Bono A: A technique for complete replacement of the ascending aorta, *Thorax* 23(4):338, 1968.

Borst HG, Frank G, Schaps D: Treatment of extensive aortic aneurysms by a new multiple-stage approach, *J Thorac Cardiovasc Surg* 95(1):11, 1988.

Borst HG, Heinemann MK, Stone CD: *Surgical treatment of aortic dissection*, New York, 1996, Churchill Livingstone.

Cabrol C, Pavie A, Mesnildrey P: Long-term results with total replacement of the ascending aorta and reimplantation of the coronary arteries, *J Thorac Cardiovasc Surg* 91(1):17, 1986.

Cambria RP, Davison JK: Regional hypothermia for prevention of spinal cord ischemic complications after thoracoabdominal surgery: experience with epidural cooling, *Semin Thorac Cardiovasc Surg* 10(1):61, 1998.

Canobbio MM: *Cardiovascular disorders*, St. Louis, 1990, Mosby.

Cigarroa JE and others: Diagnostic imaging in the evaluation of suspected aortic dissection: old standards and new directions, *N Engl J Med* 328(1):35, 1993.

Cohn LH: Thoracic aortic aneurysms and aortic dissection. In Sabiston DC, Spencer FC, editors: *Surgery of the chest*, ed 6, vol 2, Philadelphia, 1995, WB Saunders.

Cooley DA, Jones BA: Use of selective hypothermia to protect the spinal cord, during resection of thoracoabdominal aneurysms, *Tex Heart Inst J* 27(1):29, 2000.

Cooley DA: Single-clamp repair of aneurysms of the descending thoracic aorta, *Semin Thorac Cardiovasc Surg* 10(1):87, 1998.

Cooley DA: Retrograde replacement of the thoracic aorta, *Tex Heart Inst J* 22(2):162, 1995.

Cooley DA: Experience with hypothermic circulatory arrest and the treatment of aneurysms of the ascending aorta, *Semin Thorac Cardiovasc Surg* 3(3):166, 1991.

Cooley DA: Evolution of surgical treatment of thoracic aortic aneurysms, *Ann Thorac Surg* 48(1):137, 1989.

Coselli JS, LeMaire SA, Walkes J-C: Surgery for acute Type A dissection, *Oper Techn Thorac Cardiovasc Surg* 4(1):13, 1999.

Crawford ES and others: Diffuse aneurysmal disease (chronic aortic dissection, Marfan, and mega aorta syndromes) and multiple aneurysm: treatment by subtotal and total aortic replacement emphasizing the elephant trunk operation, *Ann Surg* 211(5):521, 1990.

Crawford ES and others: Thoracoabdominal aortic aneurysms: preoperative and intraoperative factors determining immediate and long-term results of operations in 605 patients, *J Vasc Surg* 3:389, 1986.

Daily PO and others: Management of acute aortic dissections, *Ann Thorac Surg* 10(3):237, 1970.

Dake MD and others: The "first generation" of endovascular stent-grafts for patients with aneurysms of the descending thoracic aorta, *J Thorac Cardiovasc Surg* 116(5):689, 1998.

David TE: Surgery for acute Type A aortic dissection, *Oper Techn Thorac Cardiovasc Surg* 4(1):2, 1999.

DeBakey ME and others: Surgical management of dissecting aneurysms of the aorta, *J Thorac Cardiovasc Surg* 49:130, 1965.

Doty J: Acute aortic dissection [On-line], 2000. Available: www.ctsnet.org/residents/ctsn/archives/75txt.html (accessed November 27, 2000).

Dureau G and others: New surgical technique for the operative management of acute dissections of the ascending aorta: report of two cases, *J Thorac Cardiovasc Surg* 76(3):385, 1978.

Ellis PR, Cooley DA, DeBakey ME: Clinical considerations and surgical treatment of annuloaortic ectasia, *J Thorac Cardiovasc Surg* 42:363, 1961.

Gharagozloo F, Neville RF Jr, Cox JL: Spinal cord protection during surgical procedures on the descending thoracic and thoracoabdominal aorta: a critical overview, *Semin Thorac Cardiovasc Surg* 10(1):73, 1998.

Girardi LN, Isom OW: Surgery for acute aortic transection, *Oper Techn Thorac Cardiovasc Surg* 4(1):77, 1999.

Griepp RB and others: Cerebral protection in aortic surgery, *Adv Card Surg* 12:1, 2000.

Isselbacher EM, Eagle KA, DeSanctis RW: Diseases of the aorta. In Braunwald E, editor: *Heart disease: a textbook of cardiovascular medicine*, ed 5, vol 2, 1997, Philadelphia, WB Saunders.

Kieffer E and others: Preoperative spinal cord arteriography in aneurysmal disease of the descending thoracic and thoracoabdominal aorta: preliminary results in 45 patients, *Ann Vasc Surg* 3(1):34, 1989.

Kirklin JW, Barratt-Boyes BG: *Cardiac surgery*, ed 2, New York, 1993, Churchill Livingstone.

Kouchoukos NT: Composite graft replacement of the ascending aorta and aortic valve with the inclusion-wrap and open techniques, *Semin Thorac Cardiovasc Surg* 3(3):171, 1991.

Kouchoukos NT, Wareing TH: Management of complications of aortic surgery. In Waldhausen JA, Orringer MB: *Complications in cardiothoracic surgery*, St Louis, 1991, Mosby.

Malarkey LM, McMorrow ME: *Laboratory tests and diagnostic procedures*, ed 2, Philadelphia, 2000, WB Saunders.

Matas R: An operation for the radical cure of aneurism based on arteriorrhaphy, *Ann Surg* 53:38, 1903.

May J and others: Concurrent comparison of endoluminal repair versus no treatment for small abdominal aortic aneurysms, *Eur J Vasc Endovasc Surg* 13:472, 1997.

McCullough JN and others: Central nervous system monitoring during operations on the thoracic aorta, *Oper Techn Thorac Cardiovasc Surg* 4(1):87, 1999.

Moon MR, Miller DC: Aortic arch replacement for dissection, *Oper Techn Thorac Cardiovasc Surg* 4(1):33, 1999.

Oliver WC, Nuttall G, Murray MJ: Thoracic aortic disease. In Kaplan JA, editor: *Cardiac anesthesia*, ed 4, Philadelphia, 1999, WB Saunders.

Pyeritz RE: Marfan syndrome, *N Engl J Med* 323(14):987, 1990.

Rokkas CK, Kouchoukos NT: Profound hypothermia for spinal cord protection in operations on the descending thoracic and thoracoabdominal aorta, *Semin Thorac Cardiovasc Surg* 10(1):57, 1998.

Sabik JF and others: Axillary artery: an alternative site of arterial cannulation for patients with extensive aortic and peripheral vascular disease, *J Thorac Cardiovasc Surg* 109(5):885, 1995.

Safi HJ, Petrik PV, Miller CC 3rd: Brain protection via cerebral retrograde perfusion during aortic arch aneurysm repair: updated in 2001, *Ann Thorac Surg* 71(3):1062, 2001.

Safi HJ and others: Brain protection via cerebral retrograde perfusion during aortic arch aneurysm repair, *Ann Thorac Surg* 56(2):270, 1993.

Seifert PC: Cardiac surgery. In Rothrock JC, *Perioperative nursing care planning,* ed 2, St Louis, 1996, Mosby.

Svensson LG: Invited commentary on Safi and others (2001), *Ann Thorac Surg* 71:1064, 2001.

Svensson LG: Management of segmental intercostal and lumbar arteries during descending and thoracoabdominal aneurysm repairs, *Semin Thorac Cardiovasc Surg* 10(1):45, 1998.

Svensson LG, Crawford ES: *Cardiovascular and vascular disease of the aorta,* Philadelphia, 1997, WB Saunders.

Svensson LG, Kaushik SD, Marinko E: Elephant trunk anastomosis between left carotid and subclavian arteries for aneurysmal distal aortic arch, *Ann Thorac Surg* 71(3):1050, 2001.

Svensson LG, Loop FD: Prevention of spinal cord ischemia in aortic surgery. In Bergan JJ, Yao JST, editors: *Arterial surgery: new diagnostic and operative techniques,* Orlando, 1988, Grune & Stratton.

Svensson LG and others: Deep hypothermia with circulatory arrest: determinants of stroke and early mortality in 656 patients, *J Thorac Cardiovasc Surg* 106(1):19, 1993.

Terai H and others: Treatment of acute stanford type B aortic dissection with a novel cylindrical balloon catheter in dogs, *Circulation* 102(19 suppl 3): III259, 2000.

Waldhausen JA, Pierce WS, Campbell DB: *Surgery of the chest,* ed 6, St Louis, 1996, Mosby.

Waldhausen JA, Pierce WS: *Johnson's surgery of the chest,* ed 5, St Louis, 1985, Mosby.

Westaby S: Acute type A dissection. In Piwnica A, Westaby S, editors: *Surgery for acquired aortic valve disease,* Oxford, UK, 1997, Isis Medical Media.

Wheat MW: Acute dissecting aneurysms of the aorta. In Goldberger E: *Treatment of cardiac emergencies,* ed 5, St Louis, 1990, Mosby.

Wheat MW Jr and others: Acute dissecting aneurysms of the aorta: treatment of results in 64 patients, *J Thorac Cardiovasc Surg* 58(3):344, 1969.

15 Mechanical and Biologic Circulatory Assistance

Inside the body, the pump faces a very hostile environment. It's a hot saltwater solution with enzymes whose job it is to dissolve matter . . . . Then you have the problem of size constraints. There are no voids in the body, so there's a big challenge when you try to insert anything. And finally, you have to interface with blood, whose reaction to a foreign object is to encapsulate it and try to exteriorize it . . . . That's why it has taken us so long. We've had to develop new materials, figure out how to deal with blood, and design systems that are compatible with the anatomy.

Victor Poirier, 1992 (p. 26)

What patients and families want more than anything else from you is honesty and straightforwardness, even in the worst of situations.

Daniel James Waters, 1995 (Instruction 17)

The insertion of a temporary total artificial heart (TAH) by Cooley and his associates in 1969 and the implantation of the Jarvik-7 permanent TAH (Fig. 15-1) in 1982 by DeVries (1988) were major landmarks in the search for a mechanical cardiac pump. Although these early devices were fraught with problems, they stimulated the growth of an array of circulatory support systems.

These mechanical circulatory support (MCS) devices have become an increasingly important addition to the cardiac surgical armamentarium for the treatment of heart failure and cardiogenic shock (Hunt and Frazier, 1998). The evolution of these devices has enabled cardiac specialists to support patients' hemodynamics during surgery, as a bridge to transplant, a bridge to recovery, or end-destination (e.g., final therapy) (Stevenson and Kormos, 2001).

In 1953 the era of mechanical circulatory support was ushered in by Gibbon (1954) with the introduction of the heart-lung machine (Cooley, 1999). Several factors have propelled the development of these devices. Orthotopic heart transplantation currently is recognized as the most widely accepted treatment for end-stage congestive heart failure (Arabia and others, 1999). The introduction of effective immunosuppressive medications has improved survival after transplant. A shortage of donor hearts often means that the condition of many patients with heart failure deteriorates during the wait for a donor organ. Bridging patients' waiting time to transplant with mechanical devices has fueled the evolution of these assist devices

(Wieselthaler and others, 2000). The development of blood-contacting surfaces that promote neoendothelialization within the mechanical pumps (resulting in a reduction in the incidence of thrombus formation and embolization) also has helped to reduce complications and make these devices more attractive treatment options.

After nearly half a century of mechanical circulatory support, researchers and cardiac specialists continue to develop next-generation devices that are smaller, more easily portable, and completely implantable. In addition to the design of these devices, a wider application

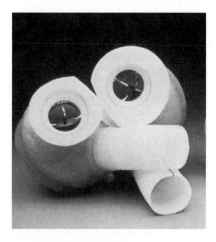

FIGURE 15-1 Symbion Jarvik-7 total artificial heart. (From Quaal SJ: *Cardiac mechanical assistance beyond balloon pumping,* St Louis, 1993, Mosby.)

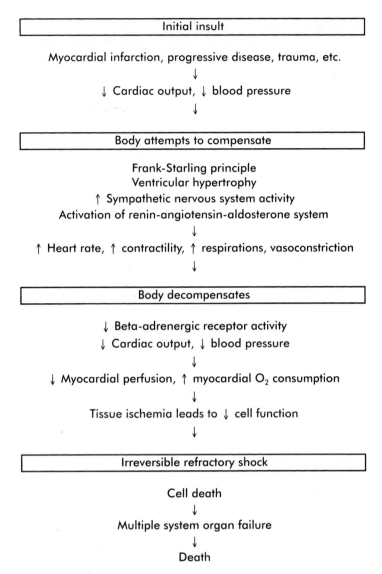

FIGURE 15-2 Sequence of events resulting in heart failure and cardiogenic shock. (From Quaal SJ: *Cardiac mechanical assistance: beyond balloon pumping*, St Louis, 1993, Mosby.)

of the technology may hold hope for patients with heart failure who are not transplant candidates.

Heart Failure

In healthy patients the heart muscle contracts to generate a cardiac output that is adequate to perfuse the entire body. *Heart failure* is the inability of this pump to adequately circulate blood, and remains a leading cause of illness in the United States, affecting approximately 4.7 million people total, and approximately 500,000 individuals per year (Albert, 1999). Understanding the causes of heart failure and its sequelae (structural, functional, and cellular) is important when the surgical team is identifying treatment goals and selecting a particular device.

There are several ways to conceptualize heart failure. One way is to describe the failure as *acute* or *chronic*. Acute severe myocardial injury may result in sudden impairment of cardiac output and cardiogenic shock (Fig. 15-2; Albert, 1999). This acute injury is seen in the cardiovascular operating room in the form of post-cardiotomy cardiogenic shock in approximately 2% to 6% of adult cardiac surgery procedures (Helman and others, 1999). Chronic congestive heart failure now is described as a syndrome that results from impaired ventricular function (Cohn, 1997). Four interacting hemodynamic forces determine ventricular function: contractility, preload, afterload, and heart rate (Albert, 1999). Box 15-1 identifies conditions that can affect one or more of these determinants of cardiac performance.

BOX 15-1
Selected Causes of Heart Failure

1. Mechanical Abnormalities
Increased afterload
  Aortic stenosis
  Systemic arterial hypertension
  Coarctation of the aorta
Increased preload
  Valvular regurgitation
  Shunts
  Increased venous return
Altered contractility
  Myocardial infarction
  Ventricular aneurysm
Obstruction of or impairment to cardiac chamber filling
  Mitral stenosis
  Tricuspid stenosis
  Pericardial constriction
  Cardiac tamponade
  Massive pulmonary embolus
  Intracardiac tumor
Traumatic injury
  Myocardial contusion
  Penetrating cardiac injury

2. Myocardial Abnormalities
Idiopathic cardiomyopathies
  Dilated
  Hypertrophic
  Restrictive
Neurovascular cardiomyopathy
  Duchenne's muscular dystrophy
Myocarditis
  Bacterial
  Viral
  Mycotic
  Protozoal
Metabolic deficiencies
  Diabetes mellitus
  Beriberi
  Acid-base imbalance
  Electrolyte imbalance
  Malnutrition
Cardiotoxic/cardiodepressant effect
  Alcohol
  Cocaine
  Radiation exposure
  Electrical shock
  Tricyclic antidepressants

Chemotherapeutic agents
  Adriamycin
  Vincristine
Theophylline
Poison
  Plant
  Animal, insect
  Environmental
Effects of aging
Ischemia
  Acute
  Chronic
Infarction
Metabolic disorders
  Acromegaly
  Hypoparathyroidism
  Pheochromocytoma
  Hyperthyroidism
  Cardiac glycogenesis
Other disease
  Amyloidosis
  Carcinoid heart disease
  Sarcoidosis
  Endocarditis
  Acute cardiac allograft rejection
  Crohn's disease
  Chronic obstructive pulmonary disease
  Connective tissue disorders
  AIDS-related cardiomyopathy
  Cocaine-induced heart disease
  Anaphylactic shock
  Septic shock

3. Conduction System Abnormalities
Bradydysrhythmias
  Extreme sinus bradycardia
  Junctional rhythm
Tachydysrhythmias
  Prolonged supraventricular tachycardia
  Ventricular tachycardia
Conduction disturbance
  High-grade heart block
  Atrioventricular dissociation
  Complete heart block
Fibrillation
  Atrial
  Ventricular

AIDS, Acquired immunodeficiency syndrome.
Modified from Colucci WS, Braunwald E: Pathophysiology of heart failure. In Braunwald E, Libby P, Zipes DP, editors: *Heart disease: a textbook of cardiovascular medicine,* ed 6, Philadelphia, 2001, WB Saunders.

Compensatory Mechanisms in Heart Failure

When the hemodynamic status deteriorates, compensatory mechanisms are triggered to improve blood flow. If ventricular function does not improve and hemo-dynamics continue to be compromised, the need for compensatory mechanisms persists and can contribute to ventricular dilation, which creates a change in the ventricular geometry that is referred to as *remodeling* (Cohn, 1997).

FRANK-STARLING MECHANISM

One of the first compensatory mechanisms to be activated by the heart when the body attempts to improve cardiac output is the Frank-Starling mechanism. Increased diastolic filling pressures (preload) stretch the myocardial muscle fibers. This allows the ventricle to eject more forcefully and thereby produce a correspondingly larger stroke volume. In the presence of progressive heart failure, the effectiveness of the mechanism is limited because the elevated pressures of failure increase ventricular wall tension (Quaal, 1993).

VENTRICULAR HYPERTROPHY

Chronic overloading and increased pressure stimulates ventricular hypertrophy. Initially the increased muscle mass is capable of generating higher ejection volumes to maintain cardiac output. Worsening cardiac failure and increased myocardial oxygen consumption eventually result in refractory failure.

INCREASED SYMPATHETIC ACTIVITY

The sympathetic nervous system is activated as the body attempts to improve cardiac output. Increased sympathetic tone is modulated by the baroreceptors in the aorta and carotid sinus (Albert, 1999). When the sympathetic system is triggered, norepinephrine and epinephrine are released into the body. Stimulation of the sympathetic system accelerates the heart rate and increases the strength of the myocardial contraction. An increase in sympathetic tone also causes vasoconstriction. In heart failure there is a prolonged activity of sympathetic stimulation. High plasma levels of norepinephrine are associated with structural changes in the ventricle (remodeling) (Cohn, 1997). The remodeled ventricle has expanded chamber size, increased wall stress, greater oxygen consumption, impaired function, and higher risk for dysrhythmias (Acker, 1999). This mechanical distension of the ventricles results in myocyte death by producing a downregulation of cellular biologic and genetic function such that the cells are programmed to die (Bartling and others, 1999).

RENIN-ANGIOTENSIN-ALDOSTERONE SYSTEM

Other organ systems respond to insufficient blood flow with compensatory mechanisms. The kidneys release renin when subjected to decreased blood flow. This initiates a biofeedback loop, which stimulates the renin-angiotensin-aldosterone system. Renin stimulates angiotensin, which in turn activates a potent vasoconstricting substance called *angiotensin II* by angiotensin-converting enzyme. Angiotensin II stimulates the release of aldosterone, which causes sodium retention. This increases the circulating volume within the vascular system, thereby increasing flow through the kidneys. Treatment may include the use of angiotensin-converting enzyme (ACE) inhibitors and atrial natriuretic peptides (ANP) to induce diuresis and suppress the renin-angiotensin axis (Massin, 1998).

ADDITIONAL VASOCONSTRICTORS

Vasopressin and endothelin also are released into the bloodstream in the presence of decreased blood flow. These substances cause fluid retention and vasoconstriction (Albert, 1999).

CARDIOMYOPATHY

The result of prolonged failure is structural changes in the shape and size of the ventricle, called *cardiomyopathy* (Fig. 15-3), which can be classified as *dilated*, *restrictive*, or *hypertrophic* cardiomyopathy. An *unclassified* cardiomyopathy also exists. An example of unclassified cardiomyopathy is *noncompaction* syndrome, which is a congenital abnormality. Isolated ventricular noncompaction (IVNC) results from the arrest of the compaction of the myocardial layers, producing thick, spongy ventricular walls. Patients with this rare form of cardiomyopathy are predisposed to thromboembolic events, dysrhythmias, and heart failure (Oechslin and others, 1999). The diagnosis of IVNC is best accomplished with echocardiography. Idiopathic cardiomyopathy remains the most common reason for heart transplantation.

Initial Medical Management

The goal of medical management is to reduce the symptoms of failure by manipulating preload and afterload (Cohn, 1997). In the operating room, management of poor ventricular function may include inotropic agents such as phosphodiesterase inhibitors (e.g., amrinone), dopamine, or dobutamine; diuretics; and vasoconstrictors or vasodilators, depending on the need to affect preload or afterload, respectively.

For patients with pulmonary hypertension contributing to right ventricular failure, prostacycline may be used for pulmonary vasodilation. Additionally, inhaled nitric oxide (NO) may be introduced into the ventilatory circuit to decrease pulmonary pressures (Hare and others, 1997; Richenbacher, 1999). Nitric oxide is produced in the body as a gas;

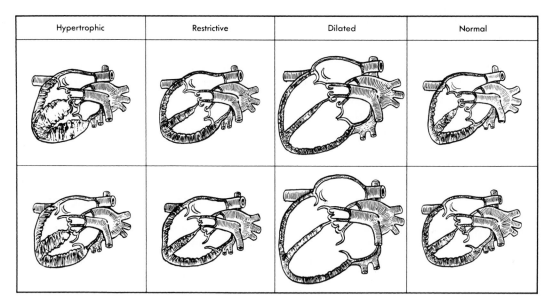

FIGURE 15-3 Types of cardiomyopathies compared with a normal heart. (From Thelan LA, Davie JK, Urden LD: *Textbook of critical care nursing: diagnosis and management,* St Louis, 1990, Mosby.)

TABLE 15-1
Circulatory Assist Devices

NAME OF DEVICE	LENGTH OF INTENDED USE	RIGHT, LEFT, BIVENTRICULAR SUPPORT	FLOW PATTERN	INDICATIONS AND DISTINGUISHING FEATURES
ECMO	Short term		Nonpulsatile	Usually pediatric; pulmonary support
IABP	Short term	Right or left	Augment	Cardiogenic shock
Hemopump	Short term		Augment	Cardiogenic shock; no longer manufactured in the United States
External centrifugal pumps: Sarns 3M St. Jude Medical Lifestream BioMedicus BioPump BioActive BioPump	Short term	Right, left, biventricular		Cardiogenic shock Support during arch or thoracic aorta surgery Widely available, simple, inexpensive
Abiomed BVS 5000	Intermediate	Right, left, biventricular	Pulsatile	Cardiogenic shock, bridge to recovery bridge to transplant
Thoratec	Long term	Right, left, biventricular	Pulsatile	Postcardiotomy shock, bridge to transplant
HeartMate	Long term	Left	Pulsatile	Bridge to transplant
Novacor	Long term	Left	Pulsatile	Bridge to transplant
Axial-flow impeller pumps: Jarvik 2000 DeBakey HeartMate II Sun Medical				Investigational
Non–blood contacting: Abiomed Heart Booster				Investigational
TAH: CardioWest Sarns 3M Abiomed				Investigational

ECMO, Extracorporeal membrane oxygenation; *IABP,* intraaortic balloon pump; *TAH,* total artificial heart.
Modified from Willman VL: *Expert panel review of the NHLBI [National Heart, Lung, and Blood Institute] total artificial heart program, June 1998–November 1999* [Online], 2001. Available: http://www.nhlbi.nih.gov/resources/docs/tah-rpt.htm (accessed May 2, 2001).

it is the active component of endothelium-derived relaxing factor and is released by the endothelial lining of the vascular walls. When released, NO causes local vasodilating effects. Inhaled NO, administered via the ventilatory circuit, assists in the management of patients with right ventricular failure, especially during implantation of a ventricular assist device (Nathan and Kraus, 2000).

Circulatory Assist Devices

When maximum medical management has not satisfactorily improved the patient's hemodynamic status, mechanical assist devices must be considered in order to support the heart and the circulation, reduce cardiac work, enhance myocardial oxygenation, and increase organ perfusion. Depending on the degree of cardiac dysfunction, devices are available that can

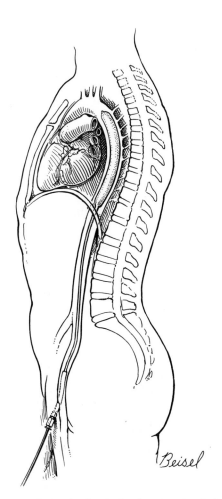

FIGURE 15-4 Lateral view of placement of intraaortic balloon in descending thoracic aorta. (From Waldhausen JA, Pierce WS, Campbell DB: *Surgery of the chest,* ed 6, St Louis, 1996, Mosby.)

partially or totally support ventricular stroke volume and cardiac output. Patients in acute decompensation may need to be rescued with immediate circulatory support (see Stevenson and Kormos, 2001, and the March 2001 supplement of the *Annals of Thoracic Surgery,* which are devoted to circulatory assistance in heart failure).

Multiple classification schemes have been used to describe assist devices in relation to their availability, position, intended use, source of energy, flow pattern, and reliance on native cardiac function. Because there does not currently exist one device that is indicated for all causes and conditions of heart failure and ventricular support, it is important to examine each device for its use, benefits, and limitations (Table 15-1; Hunt and Frazier, 1998).

INTRAAORTIC BALLOON PUMP

The intraaortic balloon pump (IABP) provides counterpulsation that supports a failing heart by decreasing myocardial oxygen demand and improving coronary artery perfusion (Bojar and Warner, 1999). The device works on the principle of internal counterpulsation (Figs. 15-4 and 15-5). Balloon inflation with helium or carbon dioxide during diastole propels blood both antegradely to perfuse the distal organs and retrogradely to perfuse the brain and coronary arteries. By propelling aortic blood flow both in the antegrade and retrograde directions during diastole, systemic organ perfusion and coronary perfusion, respectively, are enhanced, and cardiac output is augmented. By deflating just before systole, the device reduces the work of the heart and the myocardial oxygen demand by lowering afterload.

History

In 1962 Moulopoulos and colleagues developed the concept of diastolic augmentation using a balloon placed over a catheter introduced into the descending thoracic aorta (Bolooki, 1998). Jacobey (Kantrowitz, 1990) further modified the concept by suggesting counterpulsation; Kantrowitz and his colleagues (1968; 1990) applied improved balloon pumping techniques in the clinical setting for patients suffering from cardiogenic shock. In the late 1970s and early 1980s, percutaneous balloon catheter insertion widened the application of counterpulsation to patients outside the operating room.

Indications

Currently IABP systems are used to treat patients with cardiogenic shock after myocardial infarction (MI), patients with deteriorating hemodynamics in the cardiac

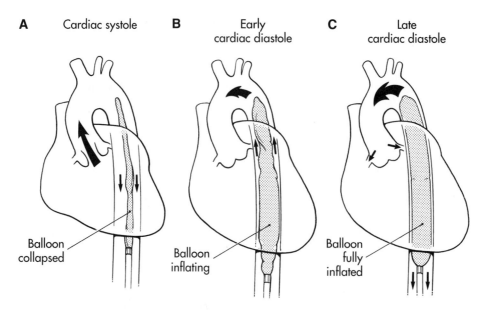

A Cardiac systole   **B** Early cardiac diastole   **C** Late cardiac diastole

Balloon collapsed   Balloon inflating   Balloon fully inflated

FIGURE 15-5   **A,** Balloon collapsed during systole. **B,** Balloon inflating during early diastole. **C,** Balloon fully inflated during late diastole (see text). (From Waldhausen JA, Pierce WS, Campbell DB: *Surgery of the chest,* ed 6, St Louis, 1996, Mosby.)

catheterization laboratory and in the operating room (OR), and as a bridge to transplant. IABPs also are used in conjunction with other assist devices (Bolooki, 1998).

Contraindications

Contraindications to IABP include aortic insufficiency, aortic dissection, and aortic and peripheral vascular atherosclerosis (Bojar and Warner, 1999). Aortic insufficiency would allow blood to preferentially enter the left ventricle rather than the coronary arteries, resulting in decreased coronary perfusion and increased ventricular distension. Aortic dissection or aneurysm is considered a contraindication because of the risk of aortic rupture.

Operative considerations

The balloon catheter is commonly inserted percutaneously via the femoral artery (Fig. 15-6, *A*), threaded up the aorta in a retrograde manner, and positioned in the descending thoracic aorta distal to the left subclavian artery and proximal to the renal arteries (see Fig. 15-4) (Bolooki, 1998).

Operative procedure

1. The groin is prepped and draped in the usual fashion.
2. The femoral pulse is located, and an 18-gauge needle attached to a 10-ml syringe is introduced into the femoral artery using Seldinger technique (Fig. 15-6, *B*).

3. On entering the artery, a guidewire is threaded into the femoral artery, and the needle is removed. If there is extensive aortoiliac disease, passage of the guidewire may be difficult, requiring a silicone-coated or J-tipped guidewire to facilitate insertion (Fig. 15-7).
4. An incision is made at the site of the guidewire to allow for the dilator that will be used to dilate the artery.
5. The dilator is inserted over the guidewire; the dilator is removed (and may be replaced with a larger dilator to enlarge the vessel). The balloon catheter size is selected (based on the patient's weight and age). Excess air from the balloon is removed. The surgeon may place the balloon over the patient's chest to measure the distance from the left subclavian artery to the femoral artery entry site; a heavy silk tie may be used to mark the proximal end of the balloon where it will exit the femoral artery.
6. After the artery has been dilated, the balloon is inserted over the guidewire (Fig. 15-6, *C*) and advanced gradually until the guidewire is seen protruding from the proximal end of the balloon. The guidewire is removed.
7. The balloon is connected to the pump. The pressure line coming off the balloon is connected to a transducer for blood pressure monitoring.

    Both electrocardiogram (ECG) electrodes and a pressure monitoring line are connected to the pump console to facilitate timing of inflation and deflation of the balloon. Synchronization of balloon

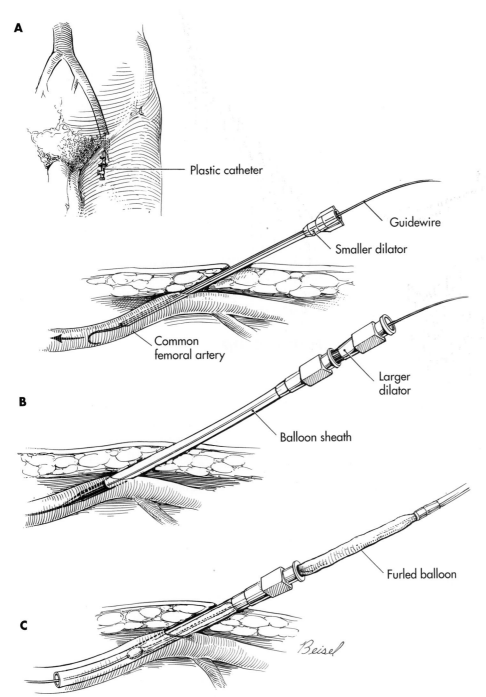

A

Plastic catheter

Guidewire

Smaller dilator

Common
femoral artery

B

Larger
dilator

Balloon sheath

Furled balloon

C

Beisel

FIGURE 15-6 A, Catheter inserted in left groin for later insertion of intraaortic balloon. **B,** A Seldinger needle is inserted into the femoral artery, and a guidewire is threaded into the aorta. The needle is removed, and a small dilator is inserted. Increasingly larger dilators are used to enlarge the tissue track. **C,** The balloon is inserted into the femoral artery. (From Waldhausen JA, Pierce WS, Campbell DB: *Surgery of the chest,* ed 6, St Louis, 1996, Mosby.)

inflation and deflation usually is based on the arterial waveform and the echocardiogram (Bolooki, 1998). Electrocautery can interfere with the ECG, as can dysrhythmias, artifact, and pacemaker spikes. When cautery is in use, pressure monitoring (arterial waveform) is used to time the balloon.

Direct ascending aorta insertion

When bilateral aortoiliac atherosclerotic disease prevents retrograde IABP insertion via the femoral artery,

direct ascending aorta (or transverse arch) insertion may be considered (Fig. 15-8; Bonchek and Olinger, 1981). The procedure is done via sternotomy incision with transesophageal echocardiogram (TEE) guidance. The aorta is partially occluded with a clamp, and a small portion of the aortic wall is excised. A Dacron graft is anastomosed to the aortotomy, and the balloon is inserted in the antegrade direction through the graft into the artery. Because the prosthetic graft first must be anastomosed to the aorta, there is a time delay that

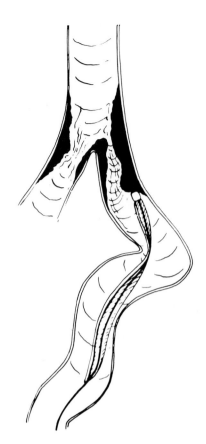

FIGURE 15-7 Tortuous artherosclerotic artery impedes advancement of balloon catheter. Use of a Teflon-coated guidewire may help to direct balloon past the obstruction. (From Quaal SJ: *Comprehensive intra-aortic balloon pumping,* St Louis, 1984, Mosby.)

may be tolerated poorly in a deteriorating patient. Placement of the graft may be technically difficult if the aorta is crowded with bypass grafts and the arterial infusion cannula. To discontinue the IABP, it is removed through the graft, which is then trimmed and oversewn (Waldhausen, Pierce, and Campbell, 1996).

Complications of IABP

The inability to balloon properly can occur with atrial pacing, rapid heart rates, dysrhythmias, volume loss from the balloon, and balloon rupture. Vascular complications related to IABP include aortic (or iliac or femoral) dissection or rupture, embolization, distal ischemia, and thrombocytopenia (Bojar, 1999).

INTRAPULMONARY BALLOON PUMP

Although rarely used because of the availability of right ventricular assist devices, it is possible to support right ventricular function with a balloon pump (Bolooki, 1998). Direct insertion into the pulmonary artery for

right ventricular support has been used to promote pulmonary blood flow and decrease right ventricular workload (Fig. 15-9). An intrapulmonary balloon pump (IPBP) may be best suited for patients with pure right-sided failure, such as those with pulmonary hypertension.

A pulmonary artery catheter designed to be threaded directly from the femoral vein into the pulmonary artery is under development. Currently the procedure for IPBP placement is similar to that for direct aortic insertion. A graft is anastomosed to the pulmonary artery, and the balloon is threaded through the graft and the artery. Removal is achieved by reopening the sternotomy incision, removing the catheter, and oversewing the graft (Bolooki, 1998).

Complications of IPBP include difficulty with placement related to exposure of the pulmonary artery, difficulty closing the sternum (Bolooki, 1998), vascular injury, air embolism or thromboembolism, hemorrhage, and infection.

Hemopump

HISTORY

The Hemopump was designed originally by Richard Wampler in 1972 (Sweeney, 1999). The device has been under investigation in the United States since 1988 but has not been approved by the federal Food and Drug Administration (FDA) and is no longer manufactured in the United States. It has enjoyed a wider clinical experience in Europe.

Ventricular Assist Devices

Ongoing research and development of ventricular support devices have prompted an expansion of indications for ventricular assist devices (VADs), including postcardiotomy shock, reversible ventricular failure and myocardial recovery, failed transplanted heart (Couper, Dekkers, and Adams, 1999), and end-destination therapy (Maloney, 2000). Unlike the IABP and the Hemopump, which provide pressure assistance to the failing heart by reducing afterload and augmenting existing coronary and systemic circulation, VADs provide volume assistance to the heart by greater decompression of the ventricle and diversion of blood flow from the native ventricle to the artificial pump. VAD systems can function independently of the heart, whereas the IABP and the Hemopump can only augment (not replace) existing ventricular function.

The two primary objectives of mechanical assistance are to decrease the workload of the right and/or left ventricle and restore adequate organ perfusion. Deter-

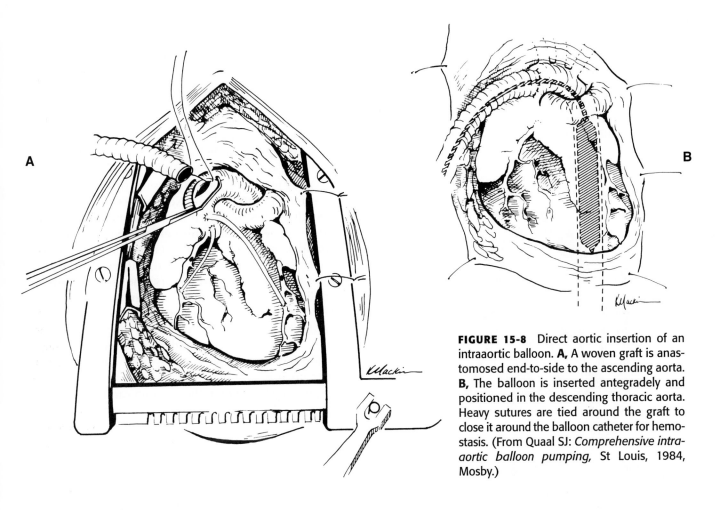

FIGURE 15-8 Direct aortic insertion of an intraaortic balloon. **A,** A woven graft is anastomosed end-to-side to the ascending aorta. **B,** The balloon is inserted antegradely and positioned in the descending thoracic aorta. Heavy sutures are tied around the graft to close it around the balloon catheter for hemostasis. (From Quaal SJ: *Comprehensive intraaortic balloon pumping,* St Louis, 1984, Mosby.)

mination of VAD placement depends on which side of the heart is affected. Most often VADs are used to support the left ventricle (LVAD), but they may be used for the right ventricle (RVAD) or for both chambers (biventricular [BiVAD]); (see Table 15-1).

By taking over cardiac function, VADs enable the heart to rest and recover from reversible injuries. When end-stage cardiomyopathy or irreversible injury preclude recovery, VADs can maintain adequate body perfusion and forestall multisystem organ failure until a donor heart becomes available for patients who are appropriate candidates for transplantation. Patients with end-organ dysfunction may not be suitable candidates; Box 15-2 list contraindications to VAD insertion.

Although a VAD can support the circulation independently of ventricular function, it cannot replace pulmonary function. Patients with chronic cardiac and pulmonary failure may eventually require heart-lung transplantation (see Chapter 16). Extracorporeal membrane oxygenation (ECMO; see Chapter 9) has been used when there is a need for rapid institution of cardiac and pulmonary support (Segesser, 1999).

EXTERNAL CENTRIFUGAL AND ROLLER PUMPS

Roller and centrifugal pumps are components of the cardiopulmonary bypass (CPB) machines that circulate the blood through the device for support during cardiac surgery. The pumps themselves can be used alone, without the oxygenator, to support a failing heart. These devices were part of the original armament for mechanical assistance and have enjoyed widespread use.

Centrifugal pumps

The Medtronic BioMedicus (Fig. 15-10) pump has been available for more than 15 years and has been used clinically more than 1.5 million times (Noon, 1999). In addition to their use for postcardiotomy cardiogenic shock, centrifugal pumps can be used for support during surgery on the heart and the thoracic aorta, during cardiac transplantation, and (rarely) for ECMO.

Centrifugal pumps are constructed from three smooth, rotating blades mounted in a cone-shaped housing that is sealed at the bottom with a magnet. The magnet on the cone is connected to a magnet on the console motor. When the motor is activated, the motor magnet and the attached cone magnet revolve, rotating the blades and creating centrifugal force inside the cone. This centrifugal force creates a vortex and supplies kinetic energy to the spinning blood within the lower portion of the cone. The number of blade revolutions per minute regulates cardiac output. Cannula size and site selection vary depending on indications such as

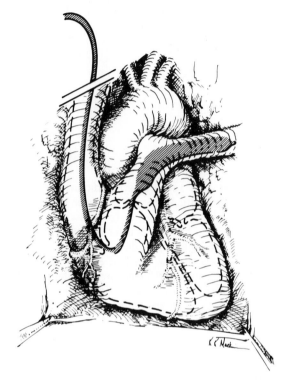

FIGURE 15-9 Transvenous insertion of pulmonary artery balloon. The balloon may also be inserted directly into the PA via a graft anastomosed to the artery. (From Quaal SJ: *Comprehensive intra-aortic balloon pumping*, St Louis, 1984, Mosby.)

failure to wean from bypass versus cardiac failure unrelated to surgical procedure (Curtis and others, 1999).

Advantages of the centrifugal pump include widespread availability, relatively low cost, and ease of insertion (Katz, 1999). Additional advantages include the transference of high volumes of energy at low pressures, thus decreasing red blood cell trauma; reduction of the possibility of air embolus (because air rises to the top of the cone, where it is trapped); and minimal risk of creating excessive outflow pressure, which could lead to disruption of the circuit (Noon, 1999).

Disadvantages include the need for moderate levels of systemic heparin administration when the pump is running at low flow rates and an appreciable degree of hemolysis, although it is less than that seen with roller pumps. Given these two factors, the most common complication is bleeding (Curtis and others, 1999). Like roller pumps, centrifugal devices produce nonpulsatile flow, which is nonphysiologic (although there is some controversy about the advantage or disadvantage of short-term nonpulsatile flow). IABP has been used in conjunction with these devices in an attempt to provide pulsatile flow. Often the sternum cannot be closed in these situations and may require temporary closure with Silastic sheeting (Fig. 15-11). To decrease bleeding from the sternal edges, bone wax may be applied (Curtis and others, 1999).

Another common complication of centrifugal pump therapy is renal failure. A three-way connector may be placed between the cardiac cannula and the centrifugal pump bypass tubing. This allows for a connection to an ultrafiltration system or hemodialysis catheter (Curtis and others, 1999). Other factors related to maintaining patients on centrifugal pumps include immobility and its sequelae (e.g., pulmonary and musculoskeletal complications) and the risk of infection related to the open chest.

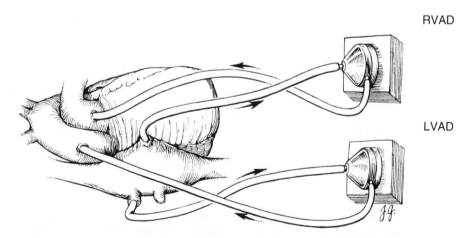

FIGURE 15-10 Left and right ventricular support with a Biomedicus centrifugal pump. (From Katz N: Left and right ventricular assist with the Bio-Medicus centrifugal pump, *Op Tech Thorac Cardiovasc Surg* 4[4]:268, 1999.)

Roller pumps

Roller pumps were initially used for mechanical support for postcardiotomy failure because it was easy to convert from bypass to roller pump (Litwak and others, 1976). Currently the use of roller pumps is limited to CPB support during surgery and ECMO (Scherr, Jensen, and Koshal, 1999) because of increased bleeding secondary to anticoagulation, blood cell injury secondary to trauma from the bypass circuit, and the problems associated with centrifugal pumps. Heparin-coated circuits (see Chapter 9) reduce cellular injury. Air embolus presents a constant danger, and disconnection between sections of the bypass circuit pose additional risk because of the high pressures that can be generated.

Cannulation techniques for centrifugal and roller pumps are similar. CPB is not necessary, but a sternotomy (or thoracotomy) is required for insertion. Portable roller pumps are used. Before cannulation the surgeon determines whether a patent foramen ovale exists. Because such a defect could produce interatrial shunting, with the possibility of arterial blood desatura-

tion, air embolus, and right-side overloading, the defect is closed primarily or repaired with a patch.

For left ventricular support, a drainage cannula is placed in the left atrium, and the inflow cannula is positioned in the femoral artery or the ascending aorta. Right ventricular support is achieved by cannulating the femoral vein or the right atrium (outflow) and the pulmonary artery (inflow). When biventricular support is indicated, both right and left ventricular circuits are established.

Pulsatile Devices

Pulsatile VADs have incorporated biocompatible blood-contacting surfaces to allow for extended use with minimal anticoagulation. Pulsatile blood flow also may be more physiologic and reduce the degree of hemolysis (Scherr, Jensen, and Koshal, 1999). Although each device described in this section has unique characteristics (Goldstein and Oz, 2000), there are many procedural similarities in the implantation of these devices. Basic standards of nursing care (Table 15-2) are broadly

---

BOX 15-2
Contraindications and Considerations Related to VAD Insertion

Technical
Body surface area less than 1.5 m² or greater than 2.5 m²
Weight greater than 150% of ideal
Highly calcified aorta (particularly at proposed site of outflow conduit ananstomosis)
Substantive aortic insufficiency
Prosthetic aortic valve
Pacemaker dependence or presence of an implantable defibrillating device

Anticoagulation
Primary coagulopathy
Prothrombin time with INR greater than 1.8 or activated partial thromboplastin time greater than twice the control value in patients not on anticoagulant therapy

Hemodynamic
Right atrial pressure greater than 22 mm Hg despite aggressive diuresis or vasodilator therapy
Pulmonary capillary wedge pressure generally less than 15 mm Hg when treated
Cardiac index generally greater than 2 liters per minute per m² without parenteral inotropes

Pulmonary
Patient chronically ventilator dependent
Recent pulmonary embolism
Substantively impaired pulmonary function (FEV₁ less than 50% predicted)

Fixed pulmonary hypertension (systolic pulmonary artery pressure greater than 60 mm Hg, transpulmonary gradient greater than 17 mm Hg, pulmonary vascular resistance greater than 5 Woods units while on intensive pulmonary vasodilator therapy

Peripheral Vascular
Significant abdominal aortic aneurysm (greater than 4.5)
Cerebrovascular disease (perioperative stroke or TIA in the presence of internal carotid artery plaque or lesion)

Active Systemic Infection
Fever greater than 38° C

Irreversible End-organ Dysfunction
Hepatic cirrhosis
Liver enzymes greater than 3 times upper normal or bilirubin greater than 3 ml per dl
Platelet count less than 50,000
Serum creatinine greater than 3 mg per dl or creatinine clearance less than 30 ml per hour

Psychosocial (Might Impair Compliance)
Alcohol dependence or abuse
Major psychiatric illness
Inadequate social support systems

FEV₁, Forced expiratory volume in 1 second; *INR,* international normalized ratio; *TIA,* transient ischemic attack.
Modified from Richenbacher WE, editor: *Mechanical circulatory support,* Austin, Tex, 1999, Landes Bioscience.

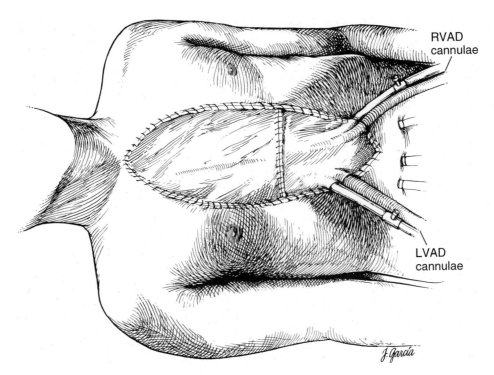

RVAD
cannulae

LVAD
cannulae

FIGURE 15-11 Silastic sheeting may be used to cover the pericardial cavity when the sternal edges cannot be approximated. The sheeting is sewn to the sternal edges. (From Katz N: Left and right ventricular assist with the Bio-Medicus centrifugal pump, *Op Tech Thorac Cardiovasc Surg* 4[4]:268, 1999.)

applicable to each device. Meeting specific requirements before VAD insertion necessitates a cohesive, well-informed team, according to Frazier (Box 15-3), whose comments (Seifert, 1994) remain as pertinent today as they were in 1994.

ABIOMED

History and indications

The Abiomed BVS 5000 Bi-Ventricular Support System (Abiomed, Danvers, Mass.) is an external, automatic, pneumatically driven, pulsatile biventricular support device intended for short-term right, left, or biventricular support after cardiotomy (Fig. 15-12). It is connected to the patient via a transthoracic cannulation technique.

The Abiomed was the first device to receive FDA approval for biventricular support of postcardiotomy heart failure patients. The two-chambered device is also FDA approved for right ventricular failure after implantation of a left ventricular assist device, after a failed heart transplant, and for other causes of reversible ventricular failure (Couper, Dekkers, and Adams, 1999).

Design

The system uses a microprocessor-based drive console to supply pneumatic power to a disposable blood pump

(DiCorte and Van Meter, 1999). Heart rate and pump intervals are determined automatically by sensing driveline air flow at the console, which drives the blood pumps independently.

Operative considerations

Right atrial–to–pulmonary artery cannulation and left atrial–to–ascending aorta cannulation are used for RVADs and LVADs, respectively. Cannulas and insertion techniques are similar to Thoratec (see p. 444). Femoral vein–femoral artery bypass may be used during device insertion. The distal end of the outflow cannulas have an attached Dacron graft that is anastomosed to the pulmonary artery (for right-side support) or the aorta (for left-side support). The Dacron graft has an thin external coating to eliminate the need for preclotting (the graft should *not* be preclotted).

Trileaflet polyurethane valves are used to maintain unidirectional blood flow. The pump is composed of two seamless chambers made of polyurethane. The upper chamber is a reservoir that fills passively like the native atrium; the lower chamber contains inflow and outflow valves. When the lower chamber is full, the console collapses it with a pulse of positive-pressure air (DiCorte and Van Meter, 1999).

TABLE 15-2

Standards of Nursing Care for Ventricular Assist Devices

NURSING DIAGNOSIS	PATIENT OUTCOME	NURSING ACTIONS
Powerlessness related to dependence on mechanical device, uncertainty about prognosis, and outcome of treatment	Patient and family understand purpose of treatment and expected outcome so that sense of powerlessness is reduced and coping abilities are enhanced	Discuss questions and concerns about disease and need for cardiac support Identify fears and address specific concerns Allow family interaction with patient to degree possible Address patient/family concerns about critical nature of patient's status/prognosis Keep family informed about patient's status; report changes in condition Support feelings of partnership with health care team
Knowledge deficit about disease, use of VAD, planned surgery, and perioperative events	Patient demonstrates knowledge about physiologic and psychologic responses to disease and VAD	Determine the patient's understanding of cardiac disease, need for and purpose of VAD (e.g., bridge to transplantation) Encourage patient and family to ask questions about VAD; explain/teach to patient's and family's level of understanding Determine understanding of VAD complications: stroke, infection, hemorrhage; clarify misconceptions
Risk for infection related to multiple wounds, compromised cardiac function	Patient is free of infection	Prepare VAD components with strict aseptic technique; maintain a wide sterile barrier Report deviations in laboratory values (e.g., white blood cell count) Control room traffic, have necessary supplies and equipment collected in one area Dress all wounds; if sternum is left open, cover incision with sterile covering; skin and subcutaneous tissue only may be closed
Risk for injury related to:	Patient is free from injury related to:	
Positioning	Positioning	When moving patient, use caution to avoid disrupting lines, cables, cannulas Avoid bending the leg in patients with femoral artery cannulas (e.g., IABP)
Physical hazards	Physical hazards	Have available VADs, lines, cannulas, connectors, graft material, wrenches, extra vascular clamps, and other implantation supplies; have backup supplies and equipment; avoid scratching or otherwise injuring VAD and VAD components Have TEE setup prepared Be familiar with type of VAD (e.g., centrifugal, electric, roller pump, pneumatic and how inserted) Have VAD drive system in OR; ensure it is functioning properly; have backup power source immediately available Ensure that all connections are tight; avoid kinking of lines Have defibrillator immediately available in anticipation of cardiac arrest Have cannulation supplies appropriate for inflow and outflow sites (e.g., LV apex, aorta, PA, left or right atrium) Prepare prosthetic valve components per manufacturer's instructions (if applicable) Do not apply any liquids, gels, or other products to device components unless specifically indicated Assist with deairing measures to reduce risk of air embolus Ensure that cannulas are connected to drive system/power source appropriately Anticipate insertion of hemodialysis catheter, left atrial line; have necessary supplies available Anticipate heparin reversal (in VADs not needing heparinization at standard flow rates); patient may be placed on antiplatelet or heparin therapy, depending on type of VAD and physician preference Plan postoperative transport route to minimize delay; ensure transport power source is working (if battery used, ensure they are fully charged before transport)

LV, Left ventricle; *PA,* pulmonary artery.
Modified from Seifert PC: Cardiac surgery. In Rothrock JC, *Perioperative nursing care planning,* ed 2, St Louis, 1996, Mosby.

Continued

TABLE 15-2
Standards of Nursing Care for Ventricular Assist Devices—cont'd

NURSING DIAGNOSIS	PATIENT OUTCOME	NURSING ACTIONS
Electrical hazards	Electrical hazards	Confirm that drive system is working; have backup
		Avoid contact between VAD and defibrillator paddles, cautery, and pacing wires
Foreign objects	Foreign objects	Account for additional instruments and supplies associated with VAD insertion: wrenches, connectors, etc.; if covers placed over VAD pump openings to prevent air entering the pump, account for these as well
Risk for altered fluid and electrolyte imbalance	Fluid and electrolyte balance is maintained	Prepare for insertion of hemodialysis catheter (patient may have high potassium levels)
		Ensure that inotropic drugs are available (per medical order)
		Check connections and rest of VAD system for bleeding; have hemostatic agents available; avoid puncturing graft components or injuring prosthetic valves
		Observe chest tubes for excessive drainage; be prepared for mediastinal exploration for excess bleeding

BOX 15-3
Comments on Implantation of a Ventricular Assist Device
O.H. Frazier, MD
Texas Heart Institute
Houston, Texas

For an optimal surgical implant of a ventricular assist device, a knowledgeable team is of the utmost importance. All team members need to be thoroughly informed about the many aspects of the device that is going to be used, such as:
  Indications for use
  Method of insertion
  Proper setup and initiation
  Any time a ventricular assist device is required, it is of an emergent nature, whether the device is approved for general use or is investigational. The physician, OR nurses, and circulatory support team must be able to work quickly and expertly together. Frequently there is little time to "run" for needed supplies.
  A checklist has proved to be beneficial to our team and is used during most implants. From a prepared list, a variety of sutures and equipment are maintained in the operating room to help eliminate any guesswork. For investigational devices, a preimplant checklist is available to ensure adherence to the investigative protocol. The foremost concern to the surgeon is having a well-educated team, working together, to achieve one goal—a good implant— in order to ensure the best possible outcome for the LVAD patient.

Drainage cannulas must be inserted in a manner that avoids impedance to device filling or obstruction of blood drainage. Blood drains by gravity from either atrium into the external pumps, which are positioned below the level of the patient's atria (see Fig. 15-12). This passive filling prevents the atria from collapsing around the cannulas and minimizes hemolysis from blood trauma. It also prevents air from being suctioned into the system (DiCorte and Van Meter, 1999).

Advantages

The Abiomed system has the capability to provide biventricular support. The system also has wide application both for postcardiotomy patients and as a bridge to transplantation in patients with small to large body surface areas.

Disadvantages

Patients require anticoagulation, have limited mobility, and commonly experience bleeding. Proper function is dependent not only on proper cannula insertion intraoperatively but also on adequate volume status and appropriate pump height (e.g., below the atria to facilitate passive drainage). If the pump is too high, atrial drainage will be inadequate; if it is too low, there will be prolonged filling of the pump and the heart can become distended.

THORATEC

The Thoratec (Berkeley, Calif.; formerly called the Pierce-Donachy) VAD is a paracorporeal system that is driven pneumatically to provide mechanical assistance to the left, right, or both ventricles (Arabia and others, 1998). This system is indicated for both bridge to transplant and bridge to recovery. The pumps (Fig. 15-13) are powered by compressed air from the console, which alternately compresses and empties the blood sacs to achieve pulsatile flow. Prosthetic valves are incorporated into the inflow and outflow portions of the pump to maintain unidirectional blood flow. During the filling phase, blood flows from the heart, through the inflow cannula and valve, and into the inner compartment. This compartment is lined with a very smooth biocompatible proprietary polymer (developed by Thoratec) that is intended to reduce the formation of

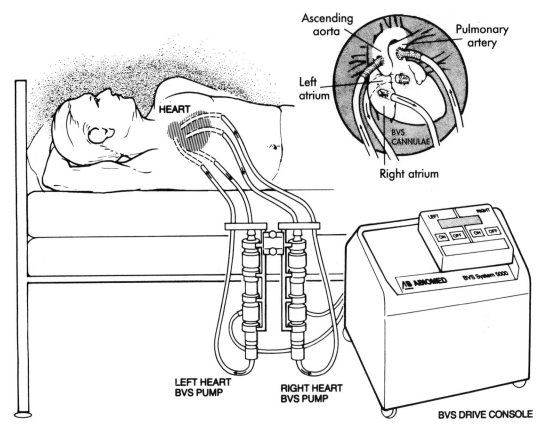

FIGURE 15-12 Abiomed BVS 5000 console and blood pumps at the patient's bedside. (Courtesy Abiomed, Inc., Danvers, Mass.)

thrombus. Pressurized air between the inner and outer compartments causes the diaphragm to push against the inner compartment, ejecting blood in pulse waves through the outflow valve and cannula and into the aorta (LVAD) or pulmonary artery (RVAD).

The use of povidone-iodone (Betadine) ointment or acetone on the Thoratec device is contraindicated because these products can cause the polyurethane to crack.

Operative considerations

Preclotting of the graft material is performed on a separate sterile table. Care is taken not to allow clot to enter the inside of the cannula. In preparation for the placement of the inflow and outflow cannulas, tunnels are created from the pericardial space to the skin, just below the costal margin. It is important to verify proper VAD pump alignment with the arrows marked on the inlet and outlet valve housing; these components are secured with the proper-colored housing nut using the appropriate wrench.

LVAD: atrial cannulation. The atrial cannula should not be cut.

1. The left ventricular apex is lifted and retracted to the patient's right side to expose the left atrial appendage.

2. Double concentric pursestring sutures are placed at the base of the appendage; pledgets or buttons may be placed at the beginning and end of each pursestring.

3. The pursestring needles are cut, and tourniquets are applied to each suture.

4. The left atrial appendage is incised, and the atrial cannula is inserted (Fig. 15-14). The tourniquet is tightened around the cannula and secured. In addition, a ligature is tied around each tourniquet and cannula. The cannula is filled with saline and clamped to prevent loss of fluid and the introduction of air into the atrium. In patients with a large left atrium or with a surgically absent left atrial appendage, an alternative insertion site for the left atrial cannula may be the roof of the left atrium, called the *atrial dome* (Fig. 15-15).

5. The cannula is passed through the tunnel and brought out through the subcostal incision (Fig. 15-16). The cannula is allowed to fill with atrial blood and is reclamped where it exits the skin. Alternatively, the cannula may be attached to the suction line of the bypass circuit.

Aortic Cannulation

6. A partial-occlusion clamp is placed on the ascending aorta, and a small segment of aorta is excised. The

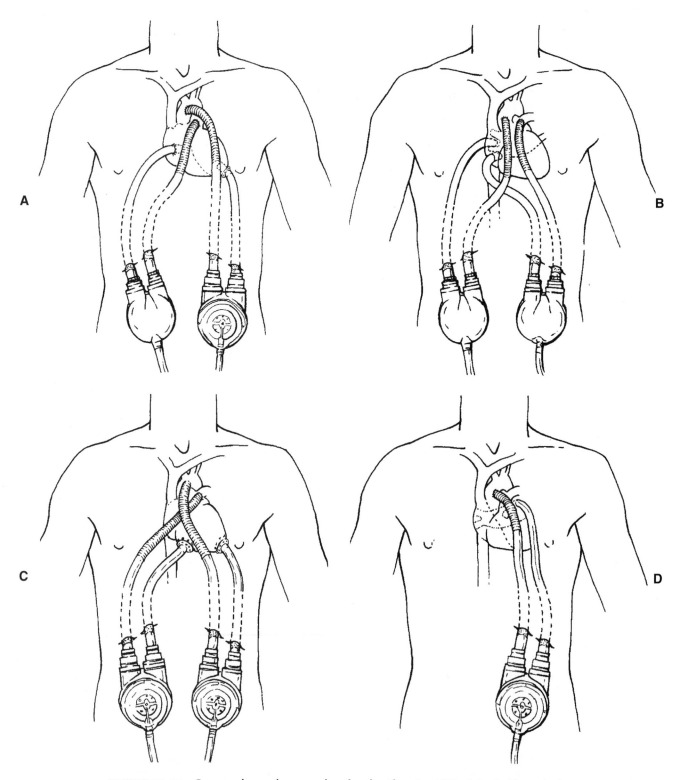

FIGURE 15-13 Commonly used approaches for the Thoratec VAD. **A** to **C,** Biventricular support methods used for bridge to transplantation, postcardiotomy support, and higher flow rates, respectively. **D,** Left ventricular support. (From Pae WE, Lundblad O: Thoratec paracorporeal pneumatic ventricular assist device, *Op Tech Thorac Cardiovasc Surg* 4[4]:352, 1999.)

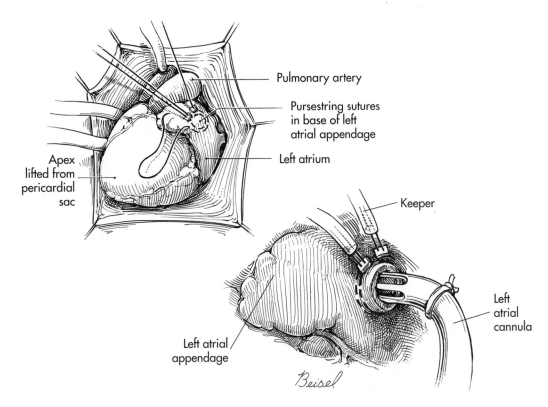

FIGURE 15-14 After double pursestring sutures are placed at the base of the left atrial appendage, the cannulas are inserted. (From Waldhausen JA, Pierce WS, Campbell DB: *Surgery of the chest,* ed 6, St Louis, 1996, Mosby.)

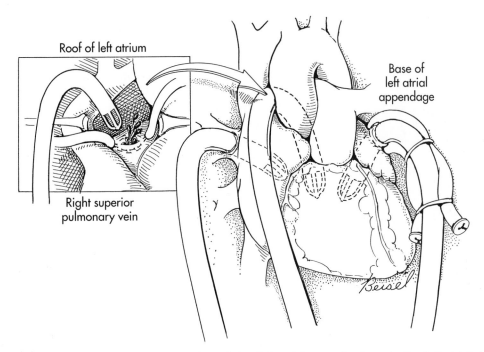

FIGURE 15-15 Insertion of the left atrial cannula through the left atrial dome. (From Waldhausen JA, Pierce WS, Campbell DB: *Surgery of the chest,* ed 6, St Louis, 1996, Mosby.)

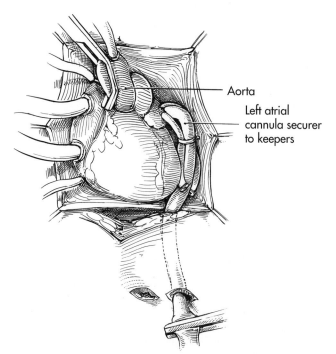

FIGURE 15-16 The left atrial cannula is brought out through the subcostal skin incision. (From Waldhausen JA, Pierce WS, Campbell DB: *Surgery of the chest,* ed 6, St Louis, 1996, Mosby.)

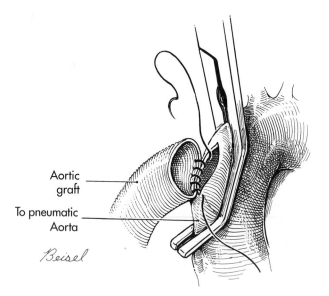

FIGURE 15-17 Anastomosis of the graft to the aorta. (From Waldhausen JA, Pierce WS, Campbell DB: *Surgery of the chest,* ed 6, St Louis, Mosby.)

Dacron graft end of the arterial cannula is anastomosed to the aortotomy (Fig. 15-17).

7. The cannula is filled with saline, clamped, and tunneled to the medial subcostal incision.
8. The cannulas are attached to the pump after deairing has been completed (Fig. 15-18). The system is checked and pumping is initiated.

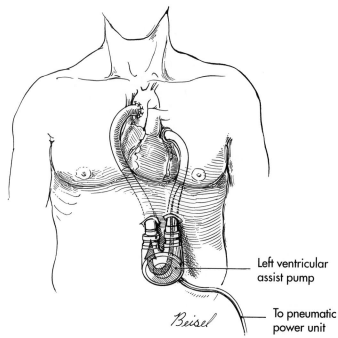

FIGURE 15-18 Pump attached to cannulas for left ventricular support. The chest has been closed. (From Waldhausen JA, Pierce WS, Campbell DB: *Surgery of the chest,* ed 6, St Louis, 1996, Mosby.)

RVAD. The tunnels and cannula are placed in the right atrial appendage and the pulmonary artery (see Fig. 15-13) in a manner similar to the technique described for the LVAD.

Advantages. The paracorporeal approach allows the device to be implanted in a range of body sizes (Waldhausen, Pierce, and Campbell, 1996).

Disadvantages. The need for anticoagulation is a limiting factor for some patients and a source of complications for others. The current drive console requires the patient to remain hospitalized. To address this issue the manufacturer has nearly completed development and testing of a portable driver (Farrar and others, 1997).

Implantable Systems

The two best known implantable devices are the Novacor N100PC left ventricular assist system (LVAS; Baxter, Oakland, Calif.) and the HeartMate TCI (formerly Thermo Cardiosystems, Inc., Woburn, Mass., currently Thoratec, Berkeley, Calif.; Table 15-3). They are both left ventricular assist devices that have implantable pumps, external controllers, and external power sources (McCarthy, 1999). The internal pumps are connected to the controllers and power supply via a cable that exits the patient's abdominal wall through a stab site. These are long-term devices capable of supporting patients for many months and in some cases 2 or more years.

	NOVACOR	TCI VE DEVICE
TABLE 15-3 ***Comparison of the Novacor and TCI Systems***		
Anticoagulation	Low-molecular-weight dextran, then heparin, then warfarin (Coumadin)	Aspirin; additionally, some centers use persantine
Pump housing material	Seamless polyurethane	Sintered titanium microspheres
Pump capacity	65 ml	83 ml
Valves	Porcine	Porcine

NOVACOR

Development of the Novacor system (Fig. 15-19) was initiated in 1969 and first implanted in 1984 at Stanford. The device was FDA approved for use as a bridge to transplant in September 1998 (on the same day as the HeartMate TCI device.) In 1999 Robbins and Oyer reported their longest device implant to be 860 days. The application of this device for end-destination therapy in nontransplantable patients is currently under investigation in a study called INTrEPID (Investigation of Non–Transplant-Eligible Patients who are Inotrope Dependent).

HEARTMATE I

The HeartMate I system was first developed with a pneumatic drive console implantable pneumatic [IP] that had to remain plugged into the wall; a battery with 30 minutes of energy storage enabled patients to take short walks within the hospital. These constraints prevented patients from being discharged with the device.

The next version of the HeartMate LVAD (Fig. 15-20) has an electrically driven pump (vented electric [VE]) with batteries that allow it to be carried by the patient in a harness and provide the patient with approximately 6 hours of untethered time. At night the patient must be tethered to a power base unit (Petty, 1999).

Surgical implantation

Surgical implantation for the Thoractec, Novacor, and HeartMate pumps is similar; the following description reflects both the Novacor (McCarthy, 1999) and the HeartMate (Sun, 1999) devices. It is important to stress that for VAD insertion, the *inflow* cannula refers to that through which blood flows away *from* the heart to the pump; the *outflow* cannula is that which pumps blood from the pump *into* the systemic (LVAD) or pulmonary (RVAD) circulation.

1. An incision is made from the sternal notch to the umbilicus.
2. Before heparin administration a pocket for the pump is created within the peritoneal or preperitoneal cavity (Poirier, 2000).

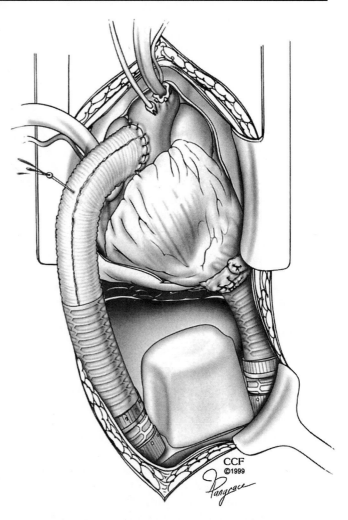

FIGURE 15-19 The Novacor left ventricular assist device. The device inflow graft allows blood to flow from the left ventricle to the pump; the outflow graft pumps blood from the device to the aorta. A needle vent is shown in the outflow portion of the graft; active venting may also be employed with an aortic venting catheter *(shown).* (From McCarthy PM: Implantable left ventricular assist device insertion techniques, *Op Tech Thorac Cardiovasc Surg* 4[4]:277, 1999.)

3. Drive lines are tunneled to an exit point to provide stability for the drive line, to ensure proper positioning intraoperatively, and to decrease drive line movement postoperatively. Drive line movement

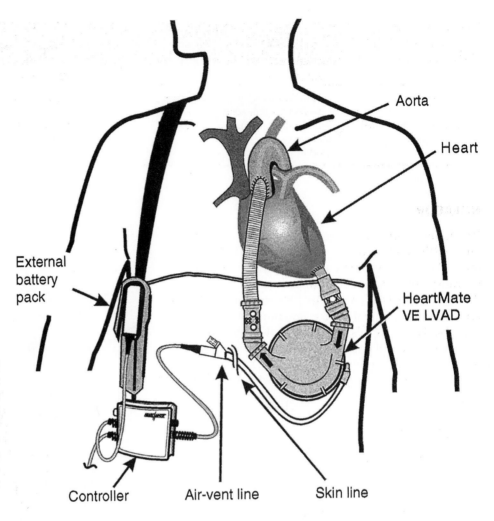

Aorta

Heart

HeartMate
VE LVAD

External
battery
pack

FIGURE 15-20 An implanted HeartMate TCI vented electric (VE) left ventricular system. The external battery pack allows the patient to ambulate. (From Slater JP, Williams M, Oz MC: Implantation techniques for the TCI HeartMate left ventricular assist system, *Op Tech Thorac Cardiovasc Surg* 4(4):330, 1999.)

Controller   Air-vent line   Skin line

causes local damage to the skin at the exit site and increases the risk for infection.

4. CPB is instituted.
5. The left ventricular apex is opened with a coring device (Fig. 15-21).
6. The inflow cannula traverses the diaphragm and is secured to a Teflon cuff that has been sutured to the ventricular apex with horizontal mattress, Teflon-pledgeted Dacron sutures (Figs. 15-22 and 15-23).
7. The inflow graft is attached to the pump (Fig. 15-24). Tightening of the graft-conduit attachment is first performed manually; then it is further tightened with a wrench (shown for the Novacor system) or other device.
8. The outflow graft is stretched to approximate its length after it is distended with blood; then it is cut at an angle to facilitate the subsequent end-to-side anastomosis to the aorta (Fig. 15-25).
9. The outflow graft is anastomosed to the ascending aorta (see Figs. 15-19 and 15-20). Autologous peri-

cardium may be used to buttress the 4-0 polypropylene suture for the graft.

10. The patient is then placed in Trendelenburg's position during deairing and device activation in order to decrease the risk of air embolization to the brain.

Advantages. The advantage of the Novacor and HeartMate systems is that they can be implanted for long-term support (McCarthy and others, 1998; Savage and others, 1999). Both these systems permit the patient to ambulate (Fig. 15-26). Once instructed how to interact with the system, the patient can be discharged from the hospital with the system in place.

Disadvantages. These devices depend on well preserved right ventricular function. Because they require that the patient have a sufficiently large body habitus to accept the device components, patient selection is limited. This limitation has prompted a number of studies to investigate the possibility of using these devices, not only as a bridge to transplantation but as an end destination itself.

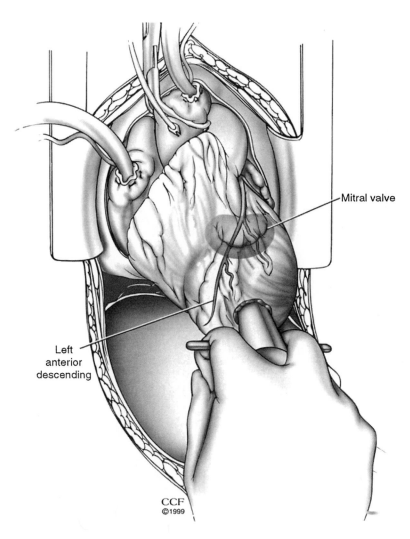

Mitral valve

Left
anterior
descending

CCF
©1999

FIGURE 15-21 After institution of cardiopulmonary bypass and aortic cross-clamping, the left ventricular apex is opened with a coring device; the direction of the coring knife is along the ventricular septum (not toward the septum) and is directed at the mitral valve. (From McCarthy PM: Implantable left ventricular assist device insertion techniques, *Op Tech Thorac Cardiovasc Surg* 4[4]:277, 1999.)

Total Artificial Heart

The CardioWest (CWT) C-70 total artificial heart (CardioWest Technologies, Inc., Tucson, Ariz.) is the direct descendant of the Jarvik-7 (see Fig. 15-1) TAH. Based on the pioneering work of Kolff (1993) and others, the CardioWest C-70 heart is an orthotopically placed mechanical assist device that was first implanted in 1993 (Arabia and others, 1999; Copeland and others, 1999).

The device has not yet been FDA approved, but it is being investigated as a bridge to transplantation. The device is a pneumatically driven pump with polyurethane ventricles and mechanical heart valves and connects to an external console. A diaphragm separates the blood from air. This diaphragm is displaced by compressed air during systole. The CardioWest has a maximum flow of 10 liters per minute (LPM), but 6 to 8 LPM is a more common flow rate. Before heparin administration the arterial grafts are preclotted, the atrial cuffs are trimmed, and the drive lines are tunneled. The patient is then given heparin and placed on CPB.

The native ventricles are removed, and the prosthetic ventricles are sutured to the atria, the aorta, and the pulmonary artery.

An advantage of the device is that the need for inotropes is eliminated because the ventricles have been replaced. A disadvantage of the system is the large size of the console, which prevents the patient from being discharged. A portable console is being developed.

HeartSaver VAD (Mussivand and others, 1999)

Among the newer devices being developed is the HeartSaver VAD (Worldheart Corp., Ottawa, Canada), an intrathoracic, completely implantable VAD. The system contains a pump with hydraulic fluid that pushes blood during systole (an electrohydraulic actuating mechanism), a direct current (DC) motor, an impeller blade, and pump housing. The pump is attached to an implanted battery that is recharged transcutaneously by a process called transcutaneous energy transfer (TET).

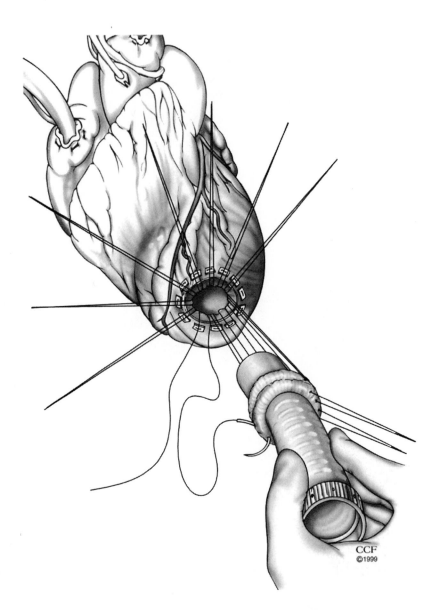

FIGURE 15-22 Pledgeted sutures are inserted around the ventriculotomy and then are passed through the apical sewing ring of the inflow cuff. The cannula is advanced into the LV apex, and the sutures are tied and cut. (From McCarthy PM: Implantable left ventricular assist device insertion techniques, *Op Tech Thorac Cardiovasc Surg* 4[4]:277, 1999.)

The system also eliminates the need for percutaneous venting through a mechanism that allows the diaphragm portion of the fluid pump to be in contact with the lungs, through which air can be expelled. Additionally, the controller system uses infrared communications to obtain and send information with the unit; biotelemetry capability makes it possible for an external controller to connect to a public telephone line.

Implantable Axial Flow Systems

Four continuous axial-flow systems are in development: the Jarvik 2000 heart, the DeBakey/NASA VAD, the HeartMate II (formerly the Nimbus/Pittsburgh axial-flow blood pump), and the Sun Medical/HIJ/Waseda/Pittsburgh (Wieselthaler and others, 2000; DeBakey, 1999). The advantage of continuous flow devices is that they are smaller, so the systems may become completely implantable. This gives the devices wider application and makes them vibration free and possibly less expensive. This has fueled investigational studies by Nose and others (1999) of a miniaturized implanted centrifugal pump in animal models.

General Considerations to Prepare for Mechanical Circulatory Support Implants

TRAINING

Extensive preparation is required before implementing a mechanical circulatory support program (Van Meter, Hollenbach Ordoyne, and Kateiva, 1999; Richenbacher,

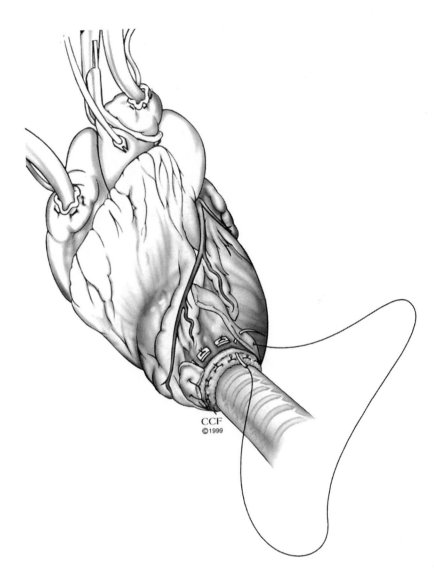

FIGURE 15-23 In order to avoid air entrainment through the inflow graft, a strip of felt is sewn around the ventricular insertion site. (From McCarthy PM: Implantable left ventricular assist device insertion techniques, *Op Tech Thorac Cardiovasc Surg* 4[4]:277, 1999.)

1999; Jones and others, 1999). Thorough training of operating room staff, perfusionists, anesthesia care providers, critical care staff, transplant coordinators, clinical specialists, and post–open-heart surgery ward staff is mandatory. Consultants in cardiology, neurology, nephrology, infectious medicine, hematology, cardiac rehabilitation, and psychiatry or psychology are integral members of the team, as are members of the accounting, dietary, and pastoral care departments.

Policies and procedures developed in accordance with manufacturers' guidelines are essential for a successful program. If the device being used has not yet been FDA approved, clinicians must follow strict protocols and federal guidelines to achieve good clinical practice. Questions or concerns about implementing the investigational protocol and ensuring proper documentation should be directed to the institutional review board (IRB) of the hospital, the research department, or the principal investigator. Guidelines set by the investigating institution, the manufacturer, and the FDA must be followed. Special considerations are listed in Box 15-4.

PATIENT CONSIDERATIONS

When a patient candidate for mechanical circulatory support is assessed, both physiologic and psychosocial factors should be considered. Understanding the patient's current living situation, adjustment to illness, financial capability, legal factors, and mental status enables the nurse to work with the individual to optimize the experience (Jones and others, 1999). Of special importance to the perioperative nurse is the mental status of the patient just before surgery.

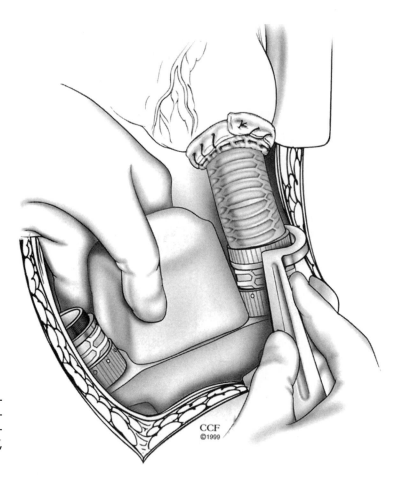

FIGURE 15-24 Tightening the inflow cannula (Novacor device shown). (From McCarthy PM: Implantable left ventricular assist device insertion techniques, *Op Tech Thorac Cardiovasc Surg* 4[4]:277, 1999.)

Patients with a bridge-to-transplantation VAD may experience a variety of emotions. These feelings can focus on uncompleted tasks, a loved one who is ill or injured, increased anxiety over the cost of hospitalization, conflicting feelings about the need for someone to die in order to receive a donor heart, or a sense of powerlessness associated with the need for circulatory assistance. Savage and Canody (1999) studied the adaptive behaviors of patients coping with prolonged hospitalization; the researchers found that the use of humor, the creation of supportive relationships, and participation in diversional activities are all considered effective by patients. Nurses can apply these findings to assist patients in coping during the perioperative period by allowing family interaction with the patient before surgery, clarifying questions and concerns, identifying (and addressing) fears, and using humor to reduce strong emotions (see Table 15-2).

Complications of Mechanical Circulatory Systems

Complications may occur during the intraoperative and postoperative periods and after discharge in pa-

tients with ambulatory systems (Morales and others, 2000).

BLEEDING

Bleeding from cardiac and vascular suture lines can result in cardiac tamponade and affect filling of the device (Barker and Devries, 1993; Pavie and others, 1999). Devices that require systemic heparin administration increase the risk of hemorrhage. The ability to avoid full heparin administration during the period of support has reduced bleeding complications significantly; many devices require only dextran, aspirin, dipyridamole, or low-dose heparin. Bleeding is of additional concern with internal devices because of the extensive soft tissue dissection required to create a pocket for the pump. Reoperation may be necessary for control of persistent bleeding.

THROMBOEMBOLISM

Thromboembolism (TE) has been a persistent, albeit less frequent, complication. Cerebral vascular accidents have been associated with mechanical circulatory sup-

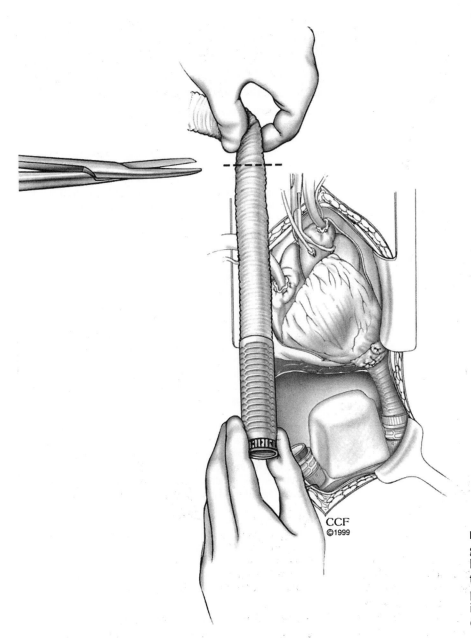

CCF
©1999

FIGURE 15-25 Measuring the outflow graft before cutting; the cut edge is beveled to facilitate the anastomosis to the aorta. (From McCarthy PM: Implantable left ventricular assist device insertion techniques, *Op Tech Thorac Cardiovasc Surg* 4[4]:277, 1999.)

port (MCS). The risk of thrombus formation is greatest during periods of reduced pump flow, such as occurs during weaning; blood stasis increases the risk of thrombogenesis. Before weaning from a device, the patient's anticoagulation levels are increased.

The risk of TE has been lowered as a result of improvements in the blood sac linings and modifications in the connections between components of the VAD circuit. These modifications cause less trauma to the blood, thereby reducing stimulation of the clotting mechanism.

INFECTION

Infection is another common complication of circulatory support devices, often related to preoperative debil-

itation, invasive lines, and duration of support (Helman and others, 1999). Postoperative drive line infections have been linked to movement of the line and skin breakdown at the incision and exit sites; careful selection of the exit site is essential. Immobilization of the drive line is important for reducing the incidence of infection. VAD surfaces may also affect the immune system by reducing CD4 T-cell counts, thus increasing the patient's susceptibility to infection (Ankersmit and others, 1999; Richenbacher, 1999).

HEMOLYSIS

Hemolysis is encountered less frequently because of improvements in the interior portion of the VAD

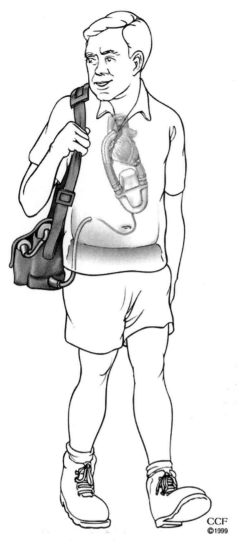

FIGURE 15-26 Ambulation with an implantable LVAD. The drive line exits far to the right and above the patient's beltline. The drive line is connected to the external controller and batteries. A shoulder bag or vest system makes the power system portable. (From McCarthy PM: Implantable left ventricular assist device insertion techniques, *Op Tech Thorac Cardiovasc Surg* 4[4]:277, 1999.)

circuit. Seams and connections have been made less traumatic, thereby decreasing the mechanical injury to the blood cells (Dasse and others, 1987; Houel and others, 1999).

RIGHT VENTRICULAR FAILURE

In patients with LVAD systems there is a risk of right ventricular failure caused by dilation of the right ventricle when the left ventricle is unloaded. In other words, when the volume preload of the native left ventricle is reduced as a result of the VAD pump's receiving blood from the LV, that volume is shifted to the native

RV, with the result that the RV preload is increased significantly. If there is inadequate right ventricular function, which is necessary to provide an adequate left ventricular preload, LV preload (which is necessary to fill the VAD pump) is impaired. Inotropic drugs, volume infusion and replacement, and nitric oxide may be required to maintain filling and emptying of the right ventricle (Argenziano and others, 1998). Thus if the right side of the heart cannot propel blood forward or if venous return to the right side of the heart is reduced, then LV filling and VAD pump filling are impaired. This results in reduced cardiac output.

DEVICE-RELATED COMPLICATIONS

Device complications may be related to the specific design of the system. Prevention of power failure (or the activation of the backup system should a power failure occur) becomes paramount in supporting the patient. Abdominal placement of the pumps for implantable devices has been associated with wound dehiscence, diaphragmatic hernia, bowel adhesions, and colon perforation (Frazier and others, 1992; Phillips and others, 1992). Internal pumps may lead to early satiety (a sense of having eaten sufficiently) as a result of physical pressure on the stomach; this may place postoperative patients at risk for nutritional deficiencies (el-Amir and others, 1996). If a portion of the VAD cannula or the pump is in contact with the costal margin, the patient may experience chronic pain; if the cannula or the pump cannot be positioned to avoid pain, intercostal nerve blocks may provide some relief (Richenbacher, 1999).

These complications illustrate some of the physical limitations (e.g., size, shape, and weight) of devices that are positioned internally. Additionally, the implantation of these devices may necessitate immobility, and the complications associated with immobility (e.g., skin breakdown) may be observed in this patient population.

HUMAN LEUKOCYTE ANTIGEN SENSITIZATION

Stimulation of antibodies in VAD patients during support has been documented (Massad, 1997; DeNofrio and others, 2000). This increased sensitivity, leading to antibody activation, is directly associated with cardiac allograft rejection after transplant. The panel of reactive antibodies (PRA) test is used to measure the patient's antibody levels. Patients shown to have clinically significant positive PRA levels who return to the OR for VAD explant or orthotopic heart transplant may require plasmapheresis during surgery to remove the leukocytes in order to prevent subsequent acute allograft rejection.

Other Surgical Interventions for Heart Failure

DYNAMIC CARDIOMYOPLASTY

The use of skeletal muscle to replace or repair a damaged ventricle has been studied experimentally since the 1930s. Salmons and Sreter (1976) demonstrated that skeletal muscle can be transformed with low-frequency electrical stimulation to a highly fatigue-resistant muscle; conditioning for 4 to 6 weeks provides sufficient fatigue resistance to allow indefinite pacing at normal heart rates (Chiu, 1991). Carpentier and Chachques (1985; 1991) performed the first successful clinical dynamic cardiomyoplasty, during which they applied a left latissimus dorsi muscle (LDM) pedicle graft to the ventricular surface. They then stimulated the muscle with a cardiac pacemaker so that it would contract in synchrony with the heart. The use of long-term repetitive stimulation with an electrical stimulator that discharges an electrical impulse (not unlike a pacer generator) transforms the muscle from skeletal and fatigue-prone to fatigue-resistant cardiac muscle (Jatene and others, 1991; Acker, 1999).

Patient selection

Cardiomyoplasty (Fig. 15-27) has been performed in patients with severe, chronic, and medically intractable myocardial failure. These patients may not be suitable candidates for transplantation because of associated medical problems, psychosocial contraindications, age, or other exclusion criteria (Magovern and Magovern, 1998; Stewart and others, 1993). Additionally, donor organs are scarce, and patients themselves may refuse transplantation; mechanical assist devices may be unsuitable or unavailable to some patients in heart failure, although cardiomyoplasty does not necessarily preclude eventual insertion of a mechanical assist device or cardiac transplantation. These considerations prompted interest in skeletal muscle as a biologic ventricular assist device.

The principal indications for cardiomyoplasty are dilated and ischemic cardiomyopathy (Magovern and Magovern, 1998). Hypertrophic cardiomyopathy is usually contraindicated because the latissimus dorsi muscle (LDM) is unable to compress the thickened ventricular wall. Patients with end-stage cardiac disease who may be candidates for transplantation or bridge devices are not candidates for myoplasty because there is little hemodynamic benefit from the procedure during the first few postoperative weeks, during which time the muscle pedicle is recuperating and is not yet conditioned to resist fatigue. Thus patients undergoing the procedure must be able to withstand the stress of the surgery and

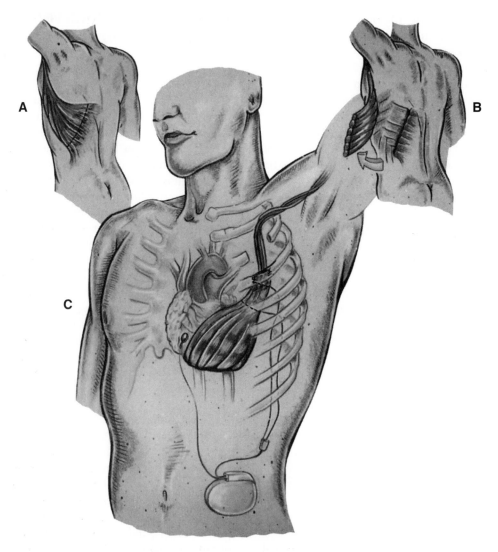

FIGURE 15-27   A, The left dorsi latissimus is dissected free. **B,** The wrap is swung around to the mediastinum (see text). **C,** Completed LDM muscle wrap with cardiomyostimulator implanted in the abdominal pocket (see text). (Courtesy Medtronic, Inc.)

the immediate postoperative period. Contraindications include significant pulmonary dysfunction, renal failure, complex ventricular dysrhythmias, degenerative muscle disease, previous left thoracotomy incision, and preoperative need for inotropic agents and IABP (Frazier and Myers, 1999). Postoperatively, inotropes and IABP may be required to support the patient until the muscle wrap begins to function.

Procedural considerations
The left LDM is commonly used because of its proximity to the heart, its large bulk, and the presence of a single main blood supply and a single motor nerve that is suitable for electrode placement and stimulation. The

LDM dissection produces little residual functional impairment for the patient (Chiu, 1991; Koroteyev and others, 1991). Other muscles that have been used as pedicle grafts to cover the heart include the right LDM, the pectoralis muscle, and the rectus abdominis muscle. The psoas muscle and the diaphragm have also been used. Concomitant coronary artery bypass grafting or left ventricular aneurysmectomy may be performed (see Chapter 10).

The procedure is performed in two parts: LDM muscle dissection and cardiac wrap. With the patient lying on the right side for a left LDM and on the left side for a right LDM, a longitudinal incision is made from the axilla to the iliac crest over the lateral border of the

LDM; the muscle is dissected free from its insertions in the vertebrae, ribs, and iliac crest. Care is taken to retain the thoracodorsal neurovascular bundle. Stimulating electrodes are implanted in the muscle and tested to obtain a response from the skeletal muscle. Curariform muscle-paralyzing drugs are omitted. The pedicle is placed in the pleural cavity via a transected second or third rib. A drain is placed, and the wound is closed.

After the muscle dissection is completed, the patient is placed in the supine position and a median sternotomy incision is made. The LDM is retrieved from the left pleural cavity, and the stimulating electrodes are tested. The muscle is then wrapped around the heart and sutured to the myocardium or pericardium. Sensing electrodes are placed on the ventricle and tested to ensure that the electrodes sense the R wave, which will trigger the stimulator. A pocket is formed beneath the rectus abdominis muscle in the upper abdomen, and the cardiac sensing and muscle-stimulating electrodes are tunneled to the pocket and connected to the stimulator or generator.

Unless concomitant procedures requiring CPB are performed, CPB is not required, although it is available. Patients who are at increased risk and cannot tolerate long procedures may require a two-stage operation: The first stage involves the LDM dissection, and the second stage creates the muscle wrap. A progressive electrical stimulation protocol for the LDM to produce fatigue resistance is started approximately 2 weeks after the cardiac wrap is created. This delay allows healing and restoration of the collateral blood supply to the pedicle. Electric stimuli are delivered as systolic bursts during each cardiac cycle and continue at an increasing rate over the following few weeks.

A report issued by the National Heart, Lung, and Blood Institute (Willman, 2001) cited no clear benefit from cardiomyoplasty, and the procedure is no longer under active clinical investigation. However, the contributions of Magovern and others (1991), Carpentier and Chachques (1991), Chiu (1991), and others have certainly had an impact on using skeletal muscle in new ways for treating heart failure.

SKELETAL MUSCLE–POWERED ASSIST DEVICES

The genetic modification of skeletal cells also is being studied. Unlike cardiac muscle, skeletal muscle can regenerate and proliferate to restore injured muscle cells, and the potential exists for transplanting a patient's own skeletal cells for myocardial repair (El Oakley and others, 2001).

Skeletal muscle ventricles (SMV), described by Lu and others (1993) and Thomas and Stephenson (2001), have been constructed experimentally from conditioned

latissimus dorsi muscle to provide arterial augmentation in a manner similar to that with the IABP. Mechanical ventricular assist devices powered by conditioned skeletal muscles not requiring an external power source also are being investigated (Whalen and others, 1999; Willman, 2001). Animal studies have been conducted to test the Thoratec system (Farrar, Reichenbach, Hill, 1994) to determine if it can be powered by skeletal muscle. These investigations demonstrate the evolution of mechanical assistance and the ingenuity with which ventricular assistance is being pursued.

Pericardial Devices

Pericardial devices that are conceptually similar to cardiomyoplasty have been developed using synthetic wraps. In 1965 the use of the pericardial cup was introduced by Anstadt and colleagues (Anstadt, Blakemore, and Baue, 1965). The Anstadt cup provides direct mechanical ventricular actuation (DMVA) and has had demonstrable success (Kung and Rosenberg, 1999; Lowe, Hughes, and Biswas, 1999). Abiomed (Danvers, Mass.) is developing an assist device that provides pericardial support (Kung and Rosenberg, 1999). This device has three components: a synthetic wrap, a hydraulic pump, and a reservoir.

Devices that wrap the heart are technically challenging because they make coronary artery bypass grafting difficult once the heart is wrapped. Techniques to connect the wrap to the heart represent additional challenges (Kung and Rosenberg, 1999).

Future Challenges

Historically the shortage of donor cardiac organs to treat end-stage cardiac disease has fueled the search for mechanical adjunctive or replacement therapy. Current investigations into the use of nonhuman (xenograft) hearts, skeletal or myocellular transplantation, and organogenesis through tissue engineering may result in a reduction in the demand for allograft donor organs and possibly provide a definitive cure for cardiac disease. Until these innovative potential treatments become a reality, cardiac assistive techniques and devices will continue to be developed and refined (El Oakley and others, 2001; Willman, 2001).

Among these refinements is a circulatory assist device to treat the pediatric population. This need has prompted design modifications to adapt to the smaller body habitus of children. The return of continuous flow devices may make smaller models clinically feasible.

Cost containment and reimbursement issues are significant concerns in the provision of health care in the new millennium. In order to tailor the intervention to the patient, adjunctive therapy combining assist device implantation, coronary revascularization, angiogenesis, and myocyte transplantation can be anticipated in the future.

Circulatory assist devices are undergoing intense scrutiny in comparison with maximal medical therapy for heart failure in order to compare the cost effectiveness of each intervention. Heart failure remains a leading cause of illness and death, and the determination of which treatment to choose will continue to be a pressing issue in the health care arena.

Access to circulatory assistance technology has increasingly become a cost issue. Because not every hospital has the fiscal, technical, or professional resources to support a circulatory assistance program, there are inherent inequities in the ability to care for individuals with heart failure. This situation poses a challenge for facilities with and without an MCS program. In health care institutions without this technology, patients must be transported to another facility; this can delay treatment for a critically ill patient. For those institutions receiving the patient, the MCS team must provide intense intervention in a patient who is not well known to the team.

Cost considerations represent only some of the concerns facing both patients and caregivers. Questions of how, when, where, and with whom these devices and techniques should be used require careful and compassionate inquiry by patients and families, physicians, nurses, technologists, administrators, and legislators. Increasingly patients and their loved ones are becoming actively involved in decisions about their treatment. The questions and dilemmas facing clinicians and consumers can only become more complicated; their resolution can be achieved with inclusive and open deliberation.

References

Acker MA: Dynamic cardiomyoplasty: at the crossroads, *Ann Thorac Surg* 68(2):750, 1999.

Albert N: Heart failure: the physiologic basis for current therapeutic concepts, *Crit Care Nurse* 19(3 suppl):2, 1999.

Ankersmit HJ and others: Quantitative changes in T-cell populations after left ventricular assist device implantation: relationship to T-cell apoptosis and soluble CD95, *Circulation* 100(19 suppl):II211, 1999.

Ann Thorac Surg 71(suppl 3), 2001. (Supplement devoted to mechanical circulatory support for heart failure.)

Anstadt GL, Blakemore WS, Baue AE: A new instrument for prolonged mechanical massage, *Circulation* 31:43, 1965 (abstract).

Arabia FA and others: Implantation technique for the CardioWest total artificial heart, *Ann Thorac Surg* 68(2):698, 1999.

Arabia FA and others: Biventricular cannulation for the Thoratec ventricular assist device, *Ann Thorac Surg* 66(6):2119, 1998.

Argenziano M and others: Randomized, double-blind trial of inhaled nitric oxide in LVAD recipients with pulmonary hypertension, *Ann Thorac Surg* 65(2):340, 1998.

Barker LE and DeVries WC: Total artificial heart. In Quaal SJ, editor: *Cardiac mechanical assistance beyond balloon pumping,* St Louis, 1993, Mosby.

Bartling B, and others: Myocardial gene expression of regulators of myocyte apoptosis and myocyte calcium homeostasis during hemodynamic unloading by ventricular assist devices in patients with end-stage heart failure, *Circulation* 100 [19 Supp II]:II-216, 1999.

Bojar RM, Warner KG: *Manual of perioperative care in cardiac and thoracic surgery,* ed 3, Malden, Mass, 1998, Blackwell Science.

Bolooki H: *Clinical application of the intra-aortic balloon pump,* ed 3, Armonk, NY, 1998, Futura.

Bonchek LI, Olinger GN: Direct ascending aortic insertion of the "percutaneous" intraaortic balloon catheter in the open chest: advantages and precautions, *Ann Thorac Surg* 32(5):512, 1981.

Carpentier A, Chachques JC: Clinical dynamic cardiomyoplasty: method and outcome, *Semin Thorac Cardiovasc Surg* 3(2):136, 1991.

Carpentier A, Chachques JC: Myocardial substitution with a stimulated skeletal muscle: first successful clinical case, *Lancet* 1(8440):1267, 1985.

Chiu RC: Dynamic cardiomyoplasty: an overview, *Pacing Clin Electrophysiol* 14(4 Pt 1):577, 1991.

Cohn JN: Overview of the treatment of heart failure, *Am J Cardiol* 80(11 A):2L, 1997.

Colucci WS, Braunwald E: Pathophysiology of heart failure. In Braunwald E, Libby P, Zipes DP, editors: *Heart disease: a textbook of cardiovascular medicines,* ed 6, Philadelphia, 2001, WB Saunders.

Cooley DA: Mechanical circulatory support systems: past, present and future, *Ann Thorac Surg* 68(2):641, 1999.

Cooley DA and others: First human implantation of cardiac prosthesis for staged total replacement of the heart, *Trans Am Soc Artif Intern Org* 15:252, 1969.

Copeland JG and others: Arizona experience with CardioWest Total Artificial Heart bridge to transplantation, *Ann Thorac Surg* 68(2):756, 1999.

Couper GS, Dekkers RJ, Adams DH: The logistics and cost-effectiveness of circulatory support: advantages of the ABIOMED BVS 5000, *Ann Thorac Surg* 68(2):646, 1999.

Curtis JJ and others: Centrifugal pumps: description of devices and surgical techniques, *Ann Thorac Surg* 68(2):666, 1999.

Dasse KA and others: Clinical experience with textured blood contacting surfaces in ventricular assist devices, *ASAIO Trans* 33(3):418, 1987.

DeBakey ME: A miniature implantable axial flow ventricular assist device, *Ann Thorac Surg* 68(2):637, 1999.

DeNofrio D and others: Detection of anti-HLA antibody by flow cytometry in patients with a left ventricular assist device is associated with early rejection following heart transplantation, *Transplantation* 69(5):814, 2000.

De Vries WC: The permanent artificial heart: four case reports, *JAMA* 259(6):849, 1988.

DiCorte CJ, Van Meter CH: Abiomed RVAD and LVAD implantation, *Op Tech Thorac Cardiovasc Surg* 4(4):301, 1999.

el-Amir NG and others: Gastrointestinal consequences of left ventricular assist device placement, *ASAIO J* 42(3):150, 1996.

El Oakley RM and others: Myocyte transplantation for myocardial repair: a few good cells can mend a broken heart, *Ann Thorac Surg* 71(5):1724, 2001.

Farrar DJ and others: Portable pneumatic biventricular driver for the Thoratec ventricular assist device, *ASAIO J* 43(5):M631, 1997.

Farrar DJ, Reichenbach SH, Hill JD: In vivo measurements of skeletal muscle in a linear configuration powering a hydraulically actuated VAD, *ASAIO J* 40(3):M309, 1994.

Frazier OH, Myers TJ: Left ventricular assist system as a bridge to myocardial recovery, *Ann Thorac Surg* 68(2):734, 1999.

Frazier OH and others: Multicenter clinical evaluation of the Heart Mate 1000 IP left ventricular assist device, *Ann Thorac Surg* 53(6):1080, 1992.

Gibbon JH: Application of a mechanical heart and lung apparatus to cardiac surgery, *Minn Med* 37:171, 1954.

Goldstein DJ, Oz M, editors: *Cardiac assist devices,* Armonk, NY, 2000, Futura Publishing.

Hare JM and others: Influence of inhaled nitric oxide on systemic flow and ventricular filling pressure in patients receiving mechanical circulatory assistance, *Circulation* 95(9):2250, 1997.

Helman DN and others: Left ventricular assist device bridge-to-transplant network improves survival after failed cardiotomy, *Ann Thorac Surg* 68(4):1187, 1999.

Holman WL and others: Ventricular assist device infections, *Ann Thorac Surg* 68:711, 1999.

Houel R and others: Pseudointima in inflow conduits of left ventricular assist devices, *Ann Thorac Surg* 68(2):717, 1999.

Hunt SA, Frazier OH: Mechanical circulatory support and cardiac transplantation, *Circulation* 97(20):2079, 1998.

Jatene AD and others: Left ventricular function changes after cardiomyoplasty in patients with dilated cardiomyopathy, *J Thorac Cardiovasc Surg* 102(1):132, 1991.

Jones KL and others: Nursing care of the patient requiring mechanical circulatory support. In Richenbacher WE, editor: *Mechanical circulatory support,* Austin, Tex, 1999, Landes Bioscience.

Kantrowitz A: Origins of intraaortic balloon pumping, *Ann Thorac Surg* 50(4):672, 1990.

Kantrowitz A and others: Initial clinical experience with intraaortic balloon pumping in cardiogenic shock, *JAMA* 203(2):113, 1968.

Katz N: Left and right ventricular assist with the Bio-medicus centrifugal pump, *Op Tech Thorac Cardiovasc Surg* 4(4):268, 1999.

Kolff WJ: Total artificial hearts, ventricular assist devices, or nothing? In Quaal SJ, editor: *Cardiac mechanical assistance beyond balloon pumping,* St Louis, 1993, Mosby.

Koroteyev A and others: Skeletal muscle: new techniques for treating heart failure, *AORN J* 53(4):1005, 1991.

Kung RT, Rosenberg M: Heart booster: a pericardial support device, *Ann Thorac Surg* 68(2):764, 1999.

Litwak RS and others: Use of a left heart assist device after intracardiac surgery: technique and clinical experience, *Ann Thorac Surg* 21(3):191, 1976.

Lowe JE, Hughes GC, Biswas SS: Non-blood contacting biventricular support: direct mechanical ventricular actuation, *Op Tech Thorac Cardiovasc Surg* 4(4):345, 1999.

Lu H and others: Skeletal muscle ventricles: left ventricular apex to aorta configuration, *Ann Thorac Surg* 55:78, 1993.

Magovern JA, Magovern GJ: Cardiomyoplasty. In Baue AE and others, editors: *Glenn's thoracic and cardiovascular surgery,* ed 6, vol 2, Stamford, Conn, 1996, Appleton & Lange.

Magovern JA and others: Indications and risk analysis for clinical cardiomyoplasty, *Semin Thorac Cardiovasc Surg* 3(2):145, 1991.

Maloney LD: An engineer for the long haul, *Design News* (Feb 10):66, 1992.

Massad MG and others: Factors influencing HLA sensitization in implantable LVAD recipients, *Ann Thorac Surg* 64(4):1120, 1997.

Massin EK: Outpatient management of congestive heart failure, *Tex Heart Inst J* 25(4):238, 1998.

McCarthy PM: Implantable left ventricular assist device insertion techniques, *Op Tech Thorac Cardiovasc Surg* 4(4):277, 1999.

McCarthy PM and others: One hundred patients with the HeartMate left ventricular assist device: evolving concepts and technology, *J Thorac Cardiovasc Surg* 115(4):904, 1998.

Morales DL and others: Six-year experience of caring for forty-four patients with a left ventricular assist device at home: safe, economical, necessary, *J Thorac Cardiovasc Surg* 119(2):251, 2000.

Moulopoulos SC and others: Diastolic balloon pumping (with carbon dioxide) in the aorta: A mechanical assistance to the failing circulation, *Am Heart J* 63:669, 1962.

Mussivand T and others: Progress with the HeartSaver ventricular assist device, *Ann Thorac Surg* 68(2):785, 1999.

Nathan SD, Kraus T: Inhaled nitric oxide use in cardiac surgery, *Kardia* 11(1):6, 2000.

Noon GP and others: Acute and temporary ventricular support with Bio Medicus centrifugal pump, *Ann Thorac Surg* 68(2):650, 1999.

Nose Y and others: Development of a totally implantable biventricular bypass centrifugal blood pump system, *Ann Thorac Surg* 68(2):775, 1999.

Oechslin EN and others: Long-term follow-up of 34 adults with isolated left ventricular noncompaction: a distinct cardiomyopathy with poor prognosis, *J Am Coll Cardiol* 36(2):493, 1999.

Pae WE, Lundblad O: Thoratec paracorporeal pneumatic ventricular assist device, *OR Tech Thorac Cardiovasc Surg* 4(4):352, 1999.

Pavie A and others: Preventing, minimizing, and managing postoperative bleeding, *Ann Thorac Surg* 68(2):705, 1999.

Petty M: Left ventricular assist systems, *Med Electron* (April):34, 1999.

Phillips WS and others: Surgical complications in bridging to transplantation: the Thermo Cardiosystems LVAD, *Ann Thorac Surg* 53(3):482, 1992.

Poirier VL: LVADs—a new era in patient care, *J Cardiovasc Manage* 11(2):26, 2000.

Quaal SJ: *Comprehensive intra-aortic balloon pumping,* St Louis, 1984, Mosby.

Quaal SJ, editor: *Cardiac mechanical assistance beyond balloon pumping,* St Louis, 1993, Mosby.

Richenbacher WE, editor: *Mechanical circulatory support,* Austin, Tex, 1999, Landes Bioscience.

Robbins RC, Oyer PE: Bridge to transplant with the Novacor left ventricular assist system, *Ann Thorac Surg* 68(2):695, 1999.

Salmons S, Sreter FA: Significance of impulse activity in the transformation of skeletal muscle type, *Nature* 263(5572):30, 1976.

Savage EB and others: The AB-180 circulatory support system: summary of development and plans for phase I clinical trial, *Ann Thorac Surg* 68(2):768, 1999.

Savage LS, Canody C: Life with a left ventricular assist device: the patient's perspective, *Am J Crit Care* 8(5):340, 1999.

Scherr K, Jensen L, Koshal A: Mechanical circulatory support as a bridge to cardiac transplantation: toward the 21st century, *Am J Crit Care* 8(5):324, 1999.

Segesser LK: Cardiopulmonary support and extracorporeal membrane oxygenation for cardiac assist, *Ann Thorac Surg* 68:672, 1999.

Seifert PC: *Cardiac surgery,* St Louis, 1994, Mosby.

Slater JP, Williams M, Oz MC: Implantation techniques for the TC1 HeartMate left ventricular assist system, *Op Tech Thorac Cardiovasc Surg* 4(4);330, 1999.

Stevenson LW, Kormos RL: Mechanical Cardiac Support 2000: current applications and future trial design, *J Thorac Cardiovasc Surg* 121(3):418, 2001.

Stewart JV and others: Cardiomyoplasty: treatment of the failing heart using the skeletal muscle wrap, *J Cardiovasc Nurs* 7(2):23, 1993.

Sun BC and others: 100 long-term implantable left ventricular assist devices: the Columbia Presbyterian interim experience, *Ann Thorac Surg* 68(2):688, 1999.

Sweeney MS: The Hemopump in 1997: a clinical, political, and marketing evolution, *Ann Thorac Surg* 68(2):761, 1999.

Thelan LA, Davie JK, Urden LD: *Textbook of critical care nursing: diagnosis and management,* St Louis, 1990, Mosby.

Thomas GA, Stephenson LW: As originally published in 1993, skeletal muscle ventricles: left ventricular apex to aorta configuration: updated in 2001, *Ann Thorac Surg* 71(5):1736, 2001.

Van Meter CH Jr, Hollenbach Ordoyne SK, Kateiva JE: Ventricular assist device programs: design and function, *Ann Thorac Surg* 68(2):643, 1999.

Waldhausen JA, Pierce WS, Campbell DB: *Surgery of the chest,* ed 6, St Louis, Mosby.

Waters DJ: *A heart surgeon's little instruction book,* St Louis, 1995, Quality Medical Publishing.

Whalen RL and others: A ventricular assist device powered by conditioned skeletal muscle, *Ann Thorac Surg* 68(2):780, 1999.

Wieselthaler GM and others: First clinical experience with the DeBakey VAD continuous-axial-flow pump for bridge to transplantation, *Circulation* 101(4):356, 2000.

Willman VL: *Expert panel review of the NHLBI [National Heart, Lung, and Blood Institute] total artificial heart program, June 1998–November 1999* [On-line], 2001. Available: http://www.nhlbi.nih.gov/resources/docs/tah-rpt.htm (accessed May 2, 2001).

16 *Transplantation for Heart and Lung Disease*

A new heart will I give you,
A new spirit put within you.
I will remove the heart of stone from your flesh,
And give you a heart that feels.

From the Yom Kippur Morning Service, "Gates of Repentance"

General Considerations

Transplantation has become a clinical reality. In 1999, there were 304 centers worldwide providing cardiac transplantation. Acceptance of this treatment by Medicare has been demonstrated by the decision in 1986 to reimburse institutions meeting federal criteria for cardiac transplantation; most private insurers cover heart transplantation (Miniati, Robbins, Reitz, 2001).

Other forms of thoracic organ replacement (e.g., heart-lung and lung transplantation) are increasingly being reimbursed by government and third party payers. Refinements in donor and recipient selection, immunosuppression, methods to diagnose rejection, and infection control, as well as improvements in preservation and implantation technique have improved survival and enhanced the quality of life for transplant recipients. Ongoing investigations involving cardiac myocyte transplantation, xenotransplantation, genetically engineered drugs, ABO-incompatible heart transplantation in infants, and the total artificial heart offer a widening array of treatment options for heart failure.

HEART TRANSPLANTATION

In 1937, Vladimir Demikhov transplanted a heterotopic heart in a dog. In 1947 he performed the first isolated lung transplantation. Demikhov's work in the Soviet Union went largely unnoticed in the United States until the past decade, although a number of transplant surgeons, especially those living outside the United States, were aware of his contributions (Krau, 2000; Konstantinov, 1998; Cooper, 1969).

In 1960, the feasibility of performing a human cardiac transplantation was described by Richard Lower (Lower and Shumway, 1960). The only other physician in attendance was Lower's mentor, Norman Shumway, from Stanford University (Cabrol, 1992b). Just more than 30 years later, almost 1000 participants attended a 1992 meeting of the International Society for Heart and Lung Transplantation (Cabrol, 1992a). The tremendous growth in the popularity of cardiac transplantation during that interval was not only because of Christiaan Barnard's (1967) first human transplant, but because of the sustained investigations of Lower (who was to continue his work in Richmond, Virginia) and Shumway. Lower and Shumway, their colleagues, and the early investigators such as Alexis Carrel (see Chapter 1), Demikhov, and Peter Medawar (1944) (whose research demonstrated that organ rejection is an immune process) made transplantation a viable intervention for end-stage heart disease (Westaby, 1997; Reitz, 2002).

Although the anastomotic techniques developed by Lower and Shumway gave clinicians a rapid and effective surgical method for performing orthotopic cardiac replacement (e.g., exchanging one person's heart for that of another), rejection of the allograft forced most investigators to abandon transplantation. The problem continued to be studied by Shumway in California and Lower in Virginia, who were able to improve survival with azathioprine and corticosteroids (e.g., prednisone) for immunosuppression. The addition of cyclosporine in the 1980s led to a triple-drug regimen that reduced the severity of rejection episodes, and newer medications have further reduced episodes of organ rejection and the side effects associated with many of the drugs (Shumway, 2000).

HEART-LUNG TRANSPLANTATION

The development of heart-lung transplantation was stimulated by the studies performed on cardiac replacement. Pulmonary problems such as hypertension and interstitial fibrosis could complicate otherwise successful heart transplants because the right ventricle would be unable to overcome the increased afterload associated with these lung alterations. Thus two organ systems—the heart and the lungs—would fail, necessitating heart-lung transplantation. The first long-term survivor of this combined procedure was a patient of Bruce A. Reitz, Shumway, and their associates at Stanford University in 1981 (Reitz, Pennock, and Shumway, 1981).

LUNG TRANSPLANTATION

Lung transplantation—single and double—became clinically feasible as a result of the efforts of Joel D. Cooper and the Toronto Lung Transplant Group (1986). Although numerous lung transplantations had been attempted before the first successful experience in Toronto in 1983, respiratory failure, rejection, infection, and dehiscence of the tracheal or bronchial anastomoses made these attempts unsuccessful. Use of cyclosporine, avoidance of steroids in the early postoperative period, and methods to protect and revascularize the airway anastomoses demonstrated improved results (Meyers and Patterson, 2000).

AVAILABILITY OF DONOR ORGANS

An inadequate supply of donor organs for the growing number of transplant candidates remains a continuing problem. It is estimated that there are between 12,000 and 27,000 potential organ donors; of those only 12% to 20% actually become donors (Van Bakel, 1997). This shortage of donor organs has stimulated liberalization of donor criteria (e.g., increasing the age limit) and prompted federal regulatory mandates (e.g., that imminent deaths be reported to organ procurement organizations) in order to meet the demand (Bogan, Rosson, and Petersen, 2000). While there is greater awareness of the need for organs and more frequent family-initiated discussions about organ donation, delays in potential donor identification and insufficient understanding of selection criteria and the recovery process remain problems. In addition, personnel may be hesitant to approach a grieving family, even with required laws that mandate such requests.

Significant increases in organ donation have been demonstrated when the discussion of death and the discussion of donation occur at distinctly separate times—a process known as *decoupling* (Bogan, Rosson, and Petersen, 2000).

Emotional Aspects of Transplantation

Transplantation places great emotional stress on the recipient awaiting transplantation and on the family of the organ donor. It also generates many feelings, sometimes conflicting, among the personnel who participate in the care of brain-dead patients before removal of organs and among those who are involved in the recovery and implantation procedures.

TRANSPLANT CANDIDATE

Patients accepted for organ transplantation worry that they may not survive the waiting period—not an unwarranted fear considering that in 1998, of 4185 people waiting for a donor heart, 1078 died while on the waiting list (Bogan, Rosson, and Petersen, 2000). Candidates also may be concerned that the new organ, once implanted, will not function. In addition, there may be deep-seated fears about the insertion of another person's body parts into their own.

Although it is important to educate the patient about the technical and immunologic aspects of organ transplantation, it is also important to provide emotional support. Patients not only must understand the necessity of complying with lifelong immunosuppression therapy, frequent checkups, and endomyocardial biopsies but also must accept these lifestyle changes if they are to have a successful outcome. Family support is important to help the candidate cope with the stress of waiting. Often the family's home and social commitments are interrupted so that members can devote their attention to the transplant candidate (Augustine, 2000).

DONOR FAMILY

Families who are considering organ donation or who have already consented to donate undergo a range of emotions. Nurses, transplant coordinators, surgeons, and others involved with the care of donors can provide support during the period when the family is making or accepting the decision to donate. Emotional assistance before, during, and after donor retrieval is important (Thelan and others, 1998).

Feelings of guilt related to the death of the loved one may compound the array of emotions felt by family members. Although family members at first may deny the diagnosis of brain death and detach themselves emotionally and physically, this does not necessarily imply that they do not wish to talk to someone about the death at a later time. Nurses who are aware of this can be prepared to interact with the family when appropriate; usually the family initiates this interaction. Nurses and organ recovery coordinators can be especially helpful to families during this period by clarifying the concept of brain death in relation to the artificial maintenance of cardiac and respiratory function. Confusion over inconsistent terminology, too much information at one time, and too little clarification of brain death contribute to families' concerns (Bogan, Rosson, and Petersen, 2000).

Sensitivity to the family's feelings, empathy, and acceptance of the emotions of being felt reflect compassionate understanding of this painful experience. This is a critical component in assisting families in viewing organ donation as a humane and honorable act and as a way of attaching meaning to the loss of their loved one. Important needs of families also include receiving information and support, frequent visiting of the loved one, and, for many, consenting to organ donation (Riley and Coolican, 1999).

CAREGIVERS

Transplantation also has an emotional impact on nurses and other caregivers involved in the selection and care of donors, organ recovery, and the transplant procedure.

Kiberd and Kiberd (1992) studied nurses' attitudes toward organ donation, procurement, and transplantation. Operating room (OR) nurses were less likely to consent to donate than were nurses in other units. The authors suggest that this may be related to environmental factors (e.g., participating in the surgery, which was perceived by some respondents to be "mutilating" and "disrespectful"). With respect to organ procurement, the authors found that only 10% of the operating room nurses in the study felt that they had been supported in their efforts. Complaints from these OR nurses included not enough nursing staff provided; no feedback on the outcome of transplantation; short notice; time consumption; lack of education, psychologic support, and respect from surgeons and physicians; and feelings of discomfort after being left alone with a dead patient after organ retrieval.

Plante and Bouchard (1995) studied critical care nurses' attitudes toward organ recovery and found that nurses with greater experience in donor care and support from peers and administrators tended to have more positive attitudes. Both studies indicate that positive experiences influence attitudes. In addition, the need for support and counsel should be considered for caregivers, transplant candidates, and families of donors.

Organ Recovery

Initial identification of potential donors usually is made by health care providers, who may talk to the family about donation. According to a 1998 referral policy from the Health Care Financing Administration (now called the *Center for Medicare and Medicaid Services*), members of an organ procurement organization (OPO) should be con-

tacted before pronouncement of death to determine suitability for donation. After the individual's death is pronounced, donation can be discussed with the family by an OPO representative with special training in organ donation procedures (Medicare and Medicaid Programs, 1998; Lilly and Langley, 1999; Sullivan, Seem, and Chabalewski, 1999). A patient is not considered a candidate until pronunciation of brain death: total and irreversible absence of all brain and brainstem function according to the Uniform Determination of Death Act (1997). Because ventilators and other mechanical means of life support can maintain vital functions even after the brain has ceased to function and clinical signs (e.g., neuroreflexive spontaneous movements) can suggest retention of some basic brain function, there is persistent debate and confusion about the concept of *brain death* (Sullivan, Seem, and Chabalewski, 1999; Capron, 2001). Confirmatory tests such as cerebral angiography, electroencephalography, and transcranial Doppler ultrasonography are employed to confirm the diagnosis of death (Wijdicks, 2001; Capron, 2001).

Although brain death is the usual stated reason for death, the Uniform Determination of Death Act identifies two ways to declare death: (1) brain death or (2) irreversible cessation of circulatory and respiratory function. In the past two decades organ donors traditionally have been in the first group. Donor organs from the second group, *non–beating heart donors* (NBHDs), are being used increasingly to reduce the organ shortage, especially for kidney transplants. Admittedly rare, both hearts and lungs have come from NBHDs (usually from donors who retain just enough mainstem brain function to prevent their meeting the criteria for a diagnosis of brain death). Experimental research on the use of NBHD lungs (Egan, 2000; Takashima and others, 2000; Steen and others, 2001) has demonstrated improved outcomes after lung transplantation. Further research may promote more widespread clinical use of NBHDs for thoracic organs.

Inclusion and exclusion criteria for organ donation are used to ensure that the donor's organs will provide optimal function when transplanted. After a donor is identified and accepted, permission is sought from the next-of-kin, and the retrieval process is begun.

Recovery coordinators assist with the donor's medical management, arrange for the arrival of transplant recovery teams (and granting of temporary surgical privileges), collect necessary legal and administrative forms and documents, assist with the procurement procedure, and coordinate donor and recipient teams. Because of the limited supply of donor organs, recovery of a single organ (rather than multiple organ retrieval) is now less common. In a multiple organ donation the organs generally are removed in the following order: heart, lungs (or heart and lungs en bloc), liver, pancreas, kidneys, and small intestine. After solid organs are removed, tissue recovery (e.g., skin) is performed in the OR, the morgue, or the coroner's office (Bogan, Rosson, and Petersen, 2000). Coordinators provide an important communication link between the multiple organ recovery teams, which facilitates efficient procurement.

To ensure fair distribution of suitable organs, the United Network of Organ Sharing (UNOS, www.unos. org), in collaboration with local organ procurement organizations (see Association of Organ Procurements Organizations at www.aopo.org), allocates the organs based on a nationwide, computerized waiting list. The UNOS policy on allocation was revised in 1999 to make donor hearts available to the sickest *local* patient first, and then to patients progressively more geographically distant from the donor hospital. Allocation status is designated 1A, 1B, 2, or 7 (Box 16-1), with each level further defined by location; local status 1A patients (those with a life expectancy of less than 7 days) have the highest priority (Hobson, 2000). Most patients in status 1 remain hospitalized awaiting a donor heart and transplantation (Greer and Webb, 2000). Availability of these items should be confirmed, however. The team will have cold cardioplegia for donor hearts and cold pulmonary flush solutions for donor lungs. The transplant coordinator assists this process by discussing requirements with the staff of the donor hospital and providing a list of needed instruments and supplies. The staff can collect these before arrival of the retrieval team. Often extra tables and round basins are needed as well for preparation and packaging of the organs before their transport back to the waiting recipient.

Ideally heart and lung organs have an ischemic time of less than 4 hours, although there are reports that lungs may remain undamaged for a few hours longer (Meyers and Patterson, 2000). To avoid unnecessary delay, which could produce ischemic injury, preparation for implantation of the organs should be completed before the arrival of the donor organ.

Recipient Preparation

When the recovery team has been notified that a donor is available, the recipient is notified to prepare for surgery. Patients who have been discharged to their homes often carry a beeper so that they can be paged to come to the hospital; on arrival they are admitted and readied for the operation. Patients within the hospital are prepared for transport to the OR suite.

Once the procurement team has reviewed the chart on the donor patient and confirmed the compatibility of the donor lymphocyte and ABO status with the recipient, the organ is visually inspected. The recipient team is notified, and the recipient patient is transported to the OR. The circulating nurse greets the patient and family and provides reassurance. The family is directed to a waiting area, where the surgeon will speak with them after the

procedure. Usually patients and family members have mixed feelings of excitement and apprehension.

Venous and arterial lines may have been inserted before transport to the OR. Once in the OR the patient is positioned comfortably and covered with warm blankets. The OR staff completes the setup for the procedure while additional monitoring lines are inserted into the patient.

Patients with ventricular assist devices (VADs, see Chapter 15) are transported to the OR with the functioning VAD. The VAD is removed only after confirma-

---

BOX 16-1

Criteria for Status Adult Classification (Based on UNOS Policy 3.7, Effective January 1999)

Status 1A

Patient is admitted to the transplant center and has at least one of the following in place:
1. Mechanical circulatory support for acute hemodynamic compromise that includes at least one of the following:
   a. Left or right ventricular assist device transplanted for 30 days or less.
   b. Total artificial heart.
   c. Intra-aortic balloon pump.
   d. Extracorporeal membrane oxygenator.
2. Mechanical circulatory support for more than 30 days with documented evidence of significant device related complications such as thromboembolism, mechanical failure, device infection, or life-threatening ventricular arrhythmias.
3. Mechanical ventilation.
4. Continuous infusion of a single high-dose inotrope, or multiple intravenous inotropes along with continuous hemodynamic monitoring or filling pressures. (Currently, qualification for Status 1A with this criterion is valid for 7 days with one-time, 7-day renewal for each occurrence of a Status 1A listing of same patient.)
5. A patient who does not meet the criteria specified in 1, 2, 3, or 4 may be listed as Status 1A if the patient is admitted to the listed transplant center hospital and has a life expectancy of less than 7 days without a transplant.

Status 1B

Patient can be in or out of hospital and has at least one of these devices or therapies in place:
1. Left or right ventricular assist device for more than 30 days.
2. Continuous infusion of intravenous inotropes.

Status 2

Patient at home or outside the hospital in need of a transplant but does not meet the criteria for Status 1A or 1B.

Status 7

Patient considered temporarily unsuitable to receive a transplant because he or she is too ill to proceed or because the patient's condition is improving without a transplant.

tion that the donor organ is acceptable and after initiation of cardiopulmonary bypass (CPB). The patient often is placed on femoral vein–femoral artery bypass to reduce the risk of lacerating the Dacron graft component of the left ventricular device or the biventricular device, which can occur when opening the chest for CPB (Lefrak, 2001).

Heart Transplantation

Cardiac homotransplantations may be orthotopic or, less commonly, heterotopic. In the former the recipient heart is excised and replaced with a donor human heart. Heterotopic transplantation, the so-called piggyback procedure, is the insertion of a donor heart into the right pleural cavity; the donor acts as an auxiliary pump for the remaining native heart (see p. 477). Other forms of cardiac replacement are also being studied.

Xenotransplantation, replacing a human heart with the heart of another species (e.g., a baboon) has been performed and caused a sensation when Bailey and associates (1985) implanted a baboon heart into a neonate. Bailey and colleagues did demonstrate the technical feasibility of such an operation and stimulated continuing research into the mechanisms of rejection. The baboon, which is not an endangered species, provides anatomy and physiology similar to a human but tends to be small. This limits the use of baboon organs to pediatric patients or small adults. Other limitations include the infrequency of blood type O and a concern that infectious baboon diseases may be transmitted to human recipients.

Studies have also included pigs (whose hearts are similar to human heart and whose heart valves as used as bioprostheses in humans) in an effort to increase the donor supply. Genetic manipulation to reduce the pig-human antigen-antibody response (which, between species, causes a catastrophic, hyperacute form of rejection) and to prevent transmission of genetically encoded porcine viruses is being researched (Derenge and Bartucci, 1999; Michler and Itescu, 2000). The use of xenotransplants as a bridge to an allograft (e.g., human) transplant also is being studied.

Another area of research involves tissue engineering to construct and manufacture replacement cardiac cells, which has the potential to repair damaged heart muscle. Myocytes have been altered to differentiate into cardiac cells, which are then implanted into the myocardium, creating a form of cellular cardiomyoplasty, or cardiac cell transplantation (Chiu, 1999).

ETIOLOGY

Approximately 46% of the patients undergoing cardiac transplantation have nonischemic cardiomyopathy (see Chapter 15), with generalized left ventricular dysfunc-

tion commonly of idiopathic or viral origin. About 45% have end-stage ischemic heart disease; the remainder have valvular heart disease, congenital disease, or myocarditis (Cupples and Spruill, 2000).

Patients often have signs of low cardiac output (forward failure), as well as pulmonary and hepatic congestion (backward failure). The ventricles become dilated and unable to eject an adequate right or left cardiac output. Although compensatory mechanisms may be adequate to provide a sufficient cardiac output during rest, cardiac output is inadequate during physical exertion or emotional stress. Reduced systemic perfusion can lead eventually to multisystem organ failure and death. Mechanical support devices (see Chapter 15) may be used in these patients to avert irreversible organ failure.

SELECTION CRITERIA

Selection criteria are becoming more flexible in experienced transplant programs with long-term success rates. The UNOS (2000) Status Classification System (see Box 16-1) reflects hemodynamic variables; additional considerations include functional status (New York Heart Association Functional Status III or IV), end-stage heart disease (less than 50% 1-year survival) not amenable to therapy, absence of irreversible systemic illness, willingness to comply with medical advice and resume an active lifestyle, and psychosocial support and stability (Cupples and Spruill, 2000). Although age limits are generally regarded to be 60 years of age or less, age criteria is flexible and is based on physiologic age rather than on a strictly chronologic age. On occasion the age limits have been extended, and candidates who are 60 years of age or older are not unknown. Contraindications to heart transplantation are listed in Box 16-2.

Two significant issues are addressed during the candidate evaluation process: (1) the capability of the patient to resume a relatively normal lifestyle after

---

BOX 16-2
Contraindications to Heart Transplantation

Advanced age (older than 70 years)
Irreversible hepatic, renal, or pulmonary dysfunction
Severe peripheral vascular or cerebrovascular disease
Insulin-requiring diabetes mellitus with end-organ damage
Active infection
Recent cancer with uncertain status
Psychiatric illness, poor medical compliance
Systemic disease that would significantly limit survival or rehabilitation
Pulmonary hypertension with pulmonary vascular resistance greater than 6 Wood units, or 3 Wood units after treatment with vasodilators

transplantation and (2) the ability to follow a strict postoperative regimen that includes daily medications, unpleasant drug side effects, and frequent follow-up tests. Because there is some subjectivity in evaluating the criteria, the evaluation usually is performed by a multidisciplinary team consisting of physicians (e.g., cardiologist, surgeon, infectious disease specialist), nurses, social workers, dieticians, and psychologists or psychiatrists. Other consultants are included as necessary. These individuals also form the posttransplant care team (Cupples and Spruill, 2000). The patient who has been accepted for transplantation also should be considered a member of the team.

Contraindications to transplantation are those that would place the donor organ recipient at excessive risk of morbidity and mortality. Among the factors are active infection, coexisting malignancy, systemic illness with poor prognosis, severe obesity or cachexia, irreversible pulmonary disease, acquired immunodeficiency disorder (AIDS), advanced age (typically more than 60 to 65 years old, although this may be modified), and psychosocial instability (Greer and Webb, 2000).

Transplant criteria also apply to patients who have had a VAD inserted as a bridge to transplantation. Although these patients may demonstrate significant improvement in their clinical status, their underlying disease remains an indication for transplantation.

PATIENT TEACHING

Patient teaching (Box 16-3) for heart transplant candidates is critical if the chronic immunosuppression and frequent follow-up care regimens are to be successfully integrated into the patient's lifestyle. Patients may focus on the transplant procedure alone and may not consider their life after transplantation. The ability to concentrate and remember what has been taught may be affected by low cardiac output. These factors make family involvement an important aspect of teaching (Greer and Webb, 2000).

PROCEDURAL CONSIDERATIONS

Organ retrieval teams bring sterile containers for organ transport and any special instruments that may not be available at the organ recovery site. Cold cardioplegia and infusion tubing, along with any other solutions needed, also are transported. To save time, especially after the donor heart has been removed, the recovery team should bring only a minimum number of nondisposable items; this reduces the time needed for cleaning these items before departure (see Fig. 16-1).

> ### BOX 16-3
> ### *Teaching Considerations for Heart Transplant Patients*
>
> **Pretransplant**
> - Clinical condition requiring surgery
> - Planned surgery
> - Average waiting time
> - UNOS status listing
> - Notification of donor and family when donor available
> - Preoperative protocol
> - Survival statistics
> - Postoperative quality of life
> - Financial considerations
> - Physiologic and psychologic evaluation
> - Possibility of surgery cancellation during donor evaluation
>
> **Posttransplant**
> - Intensive care unit, equipment, monitors
> - Rejection process
>   - Signs and symptoms
>   - Basic pathology
>   - Detection by endomyocardial biopsy
>   - Laboratory tests
>   - Prevention of rejection through immunosuppression
>   - Basic action and side effects of prescribed drugs and alternative drugs
> - Infection
>   - Signs and symptoms
>   - Basic precautions by patient, family, and staff
>   - Wound care
>   - Hospital procedure
>   - Antibiotic prophylaxis
> - Late complications (graft atherosclerosis, hypertension)
> - Schedule for biopsies and clinic visits
> - Emotional sequelae: anxiety, depression, stress disorders
> - Stress management
> - Lifestyle recommendations after transplant
>   - No smoking
>   - Diet (e.g., low cholesterol)
>   - Exercise regimen; cardiac rehabilitation
>   - Lifelong medication
>   - Vital signs and weight records
>   - Close medical supervision
>
> Modified from Augustine SM: Heart transplantation: long-term management related to immunosuppression, complications, and psychological adjustments, *Crit Care Nurse Clin NA* 12(1):69, 2000; De Geest SD: Psychosocial and behavioral issues in transplantation [On-line], 2000.
> Available: http://surgery.medscape.com/Medscape/CNO/2000/ISHLT/Story.cfm_id=1155 (accessed April 30, 2001).

The traditional technique for orthotopic transplantation, as described by Lower and Shumway in 1960 (Fig. 16-2), has been widely employed. In this method a large portion of the posterior walls of the right and left atria are retained in the recipient; the donor heart is implanted with relatively long atrial suture lines and direct end-to-end anastomoses of the aorta and the pulmonary artery. The technique has been modified (see the following) by placing the

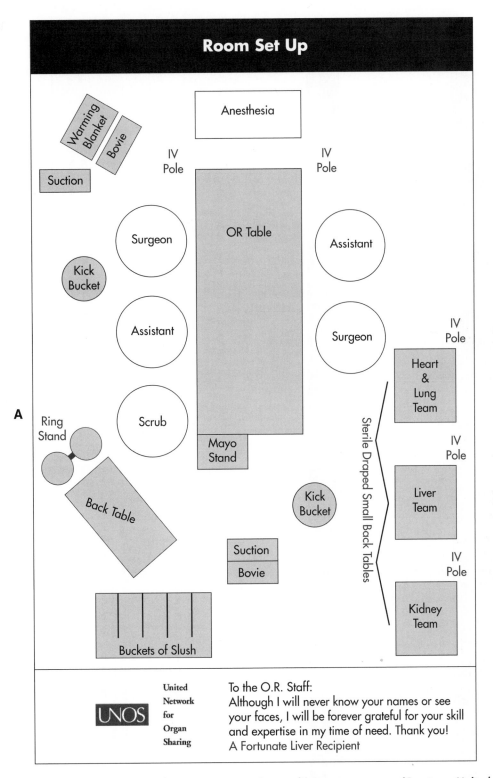

FIGURE 16-1 A, Operating room setup for multi-organ recovery. (Courtesy United Network for Organ Sharing, Richmond, Virginia) *Continued*

Procedure: Organ Recovery—Single or Multi-Organ

Position of Patient:	Supine with arms out or tucked, depending on organs to be recovered and surgeon preference. Place warming blanket under patient or use a lower-body Bear Hugger.
Skin Prep:	Solution varies according to surgeon preference. Prep from clavicle to mid-thigh.
Drapes:	Laparotomy drapes are acceptable with a wider area of exposure. Free draping is also acceptable and may be preferred.

Grounding pads, EKG electrodes and other devices should be placed on the posterior side of the body away from the sterile field.

Suture and Needles
Depends upon surgeon preference—examples

Ties:	0, 2-0, 3-0, and 4-0 silk ties* #1 and #4 silk ties*
Suture:	2-0 silk on cutting or taper needle* 4-0 & 5-0 prolene on taper needle* 1 or 2 nylon on cutting needle for closure*
Other:	ligaloops/endoloops, umbilical tapes* vessel paws, bone wax*
Hold:	large and small hemaclips skin stapler with rotating head
Dressing:	sterile 4x4s* shroud kit*

Instruments and Equipment
Specific tray names will vary according to institution

Basic:	skin prep tray* gowns X 5-10* electrocautery units X 2 lap tapes* blades - #10 X 3, #15 X 2, #11 X 2* suction sets X 2-3 (for large fluid volumes) suction tips X 2ea. yankaur, poole or octopus major laparotomy tray	razors towels X 5 grounding pad X 2* raytec sponges
Special:	vascular tray sternal saw extra long balfour vascular stapler (hold) gallbladder dilators (hold)	assorted vascular clamps sternal retractor mallet GIA, LDS (hold) large basins X 2-3 (hold)
Extras:	sterile ice defibrillator with sterile internal paddles available headlight available ice machine available or several bags of unsterile ice I.V. poles (one for each organ to be recovered)	slush (or capabilities)**

Some organ recovery agencies' customized packs will contain these items. Check with your recovery agency to prevent duplication.

**If no slush machine, contact your recovery agency for the formula for making slush. This procedure needs to be initiated at least one hour prior to the recovery case.*

Visiting recovery teams may bring additional items, which you may need to autoclave.

B

FIGURE 16-1, cont'd B, Procedure and equipment and supply recommendations for single-organ or multi-organ recovery. (Courtesy United Network for Organ Sharing, Richmond, Virginia)

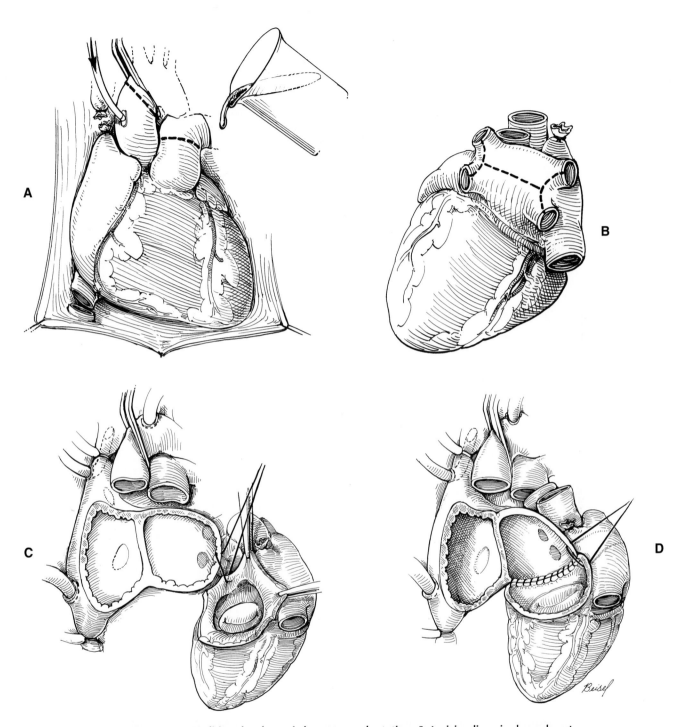

FIGURE 16-2 Traditional orthotopic heart transplantation. **A,** Incision lines in donor heart. Cold saline is poured over heart. **B,** Posterior portion of the heart showing incision lines connecting pulmonary veins. **C** and **D,** Left atrial anastomosis. (From Waldhausen JA, Pierce WS, Campbell DB: *Surgery of the chest,* ed 6, St Louis, 1996, Mosby.)

Continued

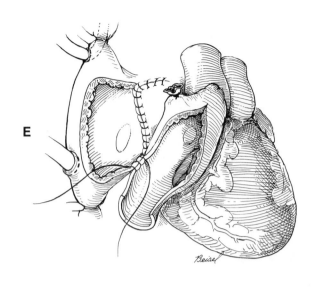

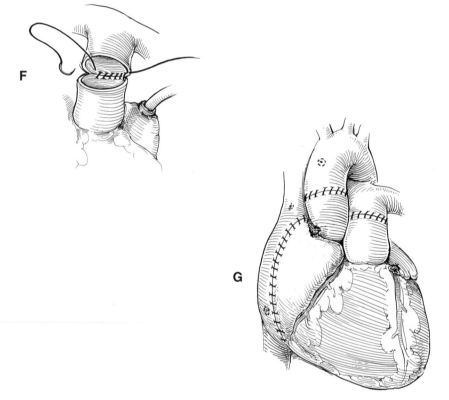

FIGURE 16-2, cont'd   Traditional orthotopic heart transplantation. **E,** Right atrial anastomosis. **F,** Pulmonary artery anastomosis. **G,** Completed transplant. (From Waldhausen JA, Pierce WS, Campbell DB: *Surgery of the chest,* ed 6, St Louis, 1996, Mosby.)

anastomoses at the level of the superior and inferior vena cavae and the pulmonary veins (Fig. 16-3; described in the following); aortic and pulmonary anastomoses are similar to the traditional technique. The caval-caval technique has nearly replaced the traditional Lower-Shumway method (Lefrak, 2001).

Implantation procedures are relatively straightforward, but certain considerations are important. Different set-ups are required for donor organ retrieval and recipient transplantation. The sterile setup should be ready in advance of the arrival of the donor organ. The period of ischemia includes implantation time and

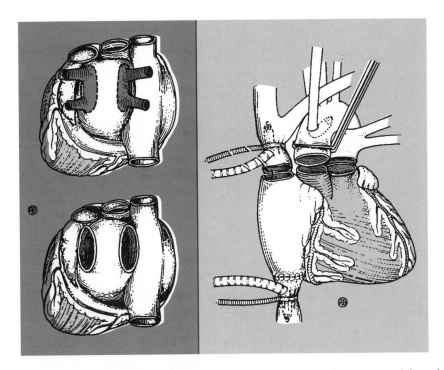

FIGURE 16-3   Total heart replacement by pulmonary venous anastomoses on right or left and caval anastomosis at the superior and inferior vena cava (bicaval technique). Aorta and pulmonary artery attached as in the conventional technique. (From Braunwald E, Zipes DP, Libby P, editors: *Heart disease: a textbook of cardiovascular medicine,* ed 6, Philadelphia, 2001, WB Saunders.)

ends only after the cross-clamp has been removed and the new heart receives systemic blood flow. Any delay in preparing for surgery can jeopardize the myocardium. Extra-long suture (54 inches) and longer instruments may be useful for deep anastomoses of the left atrium or pulmonary veins. Immunosuppressive medications given in the OR should be available, along with blood and blood products (Table 16-1).

OPERATIVE PROCEDURE: TRADITIONAL ORTHOTOPIC CARDIAC TRANSPLANTATION (WALDHAUSEN, PIERCE, AND CAMPBELL, 1996; LOWER AND SHUMWAY, 1960)

Retrieval of the donor heart

1. A median sternotomy is made to expose the heart and great vessels. Palpable thrills over the great vessels, obvious atherosclerotic coronary lesions, or obvious myocardial contusion may contraindicate the use of the heart.
2. The aorta, pulmonary artery, and venae cavae are dissected in a manner that maximizes the length of each vessel. The cavae are occluded and divided; the aorta is cross-clamped and proximally injected with cold antegrade cardioplegia (see Fig. 16-2, *A*).
3. The left atrium (LA) is vented by incising the right superior pulmonary vein or by amputating the tip of

the LA appendage (when simultaneous lung harvest is performed). Topical cold saline is applied to the heart.

4. The heart is removed by dividing the pulmonary veins and severing the aorta and pulmonary artery (see Fig. 16-2, *B*).
5. The donor heart is placed in a basin of cold saline and inspected for atrial septal defect, patent foramen ovale, and valve disease. The LA is opened by connecting the orifices of the pulmonary veins (see Fig. 16-2, *B*).
6. The donor heart is placed into two or more sterile bags containing cold saline (or other preservation solution); the bags are placed in a cooler with ice and are immediately transported to the site where the heart will be inserted into the recipient.

Recipient preparation

1. A median sternotomy is performed to expose the heart and great vessels.
2. Bicaval cannulation for cardiopulmonary bypass is performed, and a caval tape is placed around each cava. The suitability of the donor organ is confirmed before the procedure is continued.
3. The patient is cooled to the desired temperature, the recipient aorta is cross-clamped, and the caval tapes are tightened.

TABLE **16-1**
Standards of Nursing Care for Heart and Lung Transplantation

NURSING DIAGNOSIS	PATIENT OUTCOME	NURSING ACTIONS
Anxiety/fear related to waiting for donor organ, uncertainty about prognosis, function of organ, and outcome of transplant	Recipient and family understand purpose of transplant and expected outcome so that anxiety/fear is reduced and coping abilities are enhanced	Discuss questions and concerns about disease and need for transplant Identify fears and address specific concerns Allow family interaction with patient to provide emotional support Address patient's/family's concerns about critical nature of patient's status/prognosis Keep patient/family informed about patient's status and organ availability
Knowledge deficit about disease, planned transplant surgery/retrieval, and perioperative events	Recipient demonstrates knowledge about physiologic and psychologic responses to disease and transplant	**Recipient** Determine patient's understanding of cardiac/pulmonary disease, need for, and purpose of transplantation Encourage patient and family to ask questions about transplantation, anticipated lifestyle changes, need for immunosuppression, need for biopsy/endoscopy, infection, need for close medical supervision; explain/teach to patient's and family's level of understanding Verify recipient's understanding of need to be readily available if a donor is found; devise system to contact recipient at all times (e.g., beeper) Determine understanding of transplant complications: signs/symptoms of infection, rejection, organ failure, related diseases (e.g., CMV, CAD, pulmonary changes)
Risk for infection related to immunosuppression, compromised cardiac function	Donor family demonstrates understanding of brain death and process of organ recovery Patient is free of infection	**Donor Family** Clarify "brain death" Explain organ retrieval procedure (as requested) If possible, describe disposition of donor organs Prepare donor organs with strict aseptic technique; have sterile containers to pack and transport organs Have separate sterile fields for organs Clean outside of transport case before entering recipient OR Have recovery team change into clean scrub clothes before entering recipient OR Control room traffic; have necessary supplies and equipment prepared before implantation procedure
Risk for injury related to: Positioning	Patient is free of injury related to: Positioning	Provide comfort measures (e.g., warm blanket, pillow, head of bed elevated) while awaiting verification from recovery team about organ Determine patient position before surgery (e.g., lateral or supine position for single lung transplant, supine position for heart, heart-lung, double lung transplants); have positioning supplies/equipment available When moving patient with a VAD, use caution to avoid disrupting lines, cables, cannulas, etc.
Physical hazards	Physical hazards	**Care by Donor Recovery Team** Be prepared to respond immediately if contacted to retrieve organ; have necessary supplies collected and ready to go; collect additional items (such as those requiring refrigeration) Bring only supplies/instruments needed; keep cleaning requirements to minimum to avoid prolonging ischemic time

BiVAD, Biventricular assist device; *CAD,* coronary artery disease, *CMV,* cytomegalovirus; *CVP,* central venous pressure; *ETA,* estimated time of arrival; *ICU,* intensive care unit; *IV,* intravenous; *IJ,* internal jugular; *PA,* pulmonary artery
Modified from Seifert PC: Cardiac surgery. In Rothrock JC: *Perioperative nursing care planning,* ed 2, St Louis, 1996, Mosby.

TABLE 16-1

Standards of Nursing Care for Heart and Lung Transplantation—cont'd

NURSING DIAGNOSIS	PATIENT OUTCOME	NURSING ACTIONS
		Provide direction and guidance to staff from recovery hospital
		Provide list of instruments/supplies needed; bring special items unlikely to be found at recovery hospital (e.g., solutions, special staplers for pulmonary procedures)
		Assist with infusion of cardioplegia solution (heart) and/or pulmoplegia (lung) perfusion, as requested
		If multiple organ recovery is planned, be aware that most other organs are dissected free and the heart is excised first
		Avoid placing donor organs in direct contact with ice
		Be prepared to depart donor hospital as soon as possible after donor organ(s) have been excised; notify recipient hospital of ETA
		If donor and recipient are at same hospital, follow same procedures as for excision and protection of heart, sterile setups, etc.; transport of organ from OR to OR may be similar to care by donor recovery team at different hospital (per surgeon's request)
		Care of Donor—Staff of Recovery Hospital
		Prepare OR in advance of recovery team arrival; confirm that consents and other donor documents are in order
		Place warming blanket on OR bed (to avert cardiac irregularity or standstill from hypothermia)
		Collect instruments/ supplies requested by recovery team; confirm with transplant coordinator or designate
		Have extra IV poles, portable overhead lights, small tables, basinware, ice, extra suction and cautery, and backup sternal saw and power source
		Provide brief orientation to recovery team: location of rooms, bathrooms, donor OR, scrub sinks, flash sterilizers, refrigerator (and coffee); familiarize with donor OR—tables, instruments, supplies, etc.
		Provide assistance with organ recovery
		Care of Recipient—Recipient Team
		Prepare patient/OR in advance of arrival of donor organ; coordinate with surgeon, anesthesiologist, and recovery team
		Place warming blanket on bed and activate
		Anticipate use of CVP (PA line may interfere with surgical site); plan for insertion of PA line after skin closure (as requested)
		Patient's sternum or chest may be opened before arrival of donor organs (especially if recipient has had previous sternotomy)
		Cannulation for CPB may or may not be performed, depending on surgeon's preference; be prepared for double atrial cannulation (venous) and ascending aortic cannulation (arterial) for heart transplant; groin cannulation may be used for lung procedures requiring CPB
		Have long suture for deep anastomoses as requested (e.g., 54-inch suture)
		Anticipate extensive venting procedures; have necessary venting catheters, tubing, etc.
		Anticipate meticulous hemostasis after each anastomosis; once areas of posterior dissection and anastomosis (e.g., LA) become obscured by anterior anastomoses, hemostasis is more difficult to achieve

Continued

TABLE **16-1** *Standards of Nursing Care for Heart and Lung Transplantation—cont'd*		
NURSING DIAGNOSIS	PATIENT OUTCOME	NURSING ACTIONS
Risk for injury related to—cont'd:	Patient is free of injury related to—cont'd:	**Care of Recipient—Recipient Team—cont'd** For lung procedures, have staplers and fiberoptic bronchoscope to inspect lungs, suture lines Notify ICU when donor organ is functioning Be alert for hyperacute rejection in OR; donor heart may have to be removed and replaced by biVAD until new heart donor can be found
Foreign objects	Foreign objects	Inspect donor organs for tissue residue from preparation of donor organ (trimmings, etc.)
Risk for altered fluid and electrolyte imbalance	Fluid and electrolyte balance is maintained	**Donor** Have appropriate storage solution/perfusates (donors often have high potassium levels) **Recipient** Have blood available; communicate with surgeon/blood bank about special orders (e.g., irradiated blood to decrease risk of disease transmission) Ensure that immunosuppressive drugs are available (per order) Be aware that chest drainage may not accurately reflect amount of blood in pericardium (caused by enlarged pericardial cavity of recipient and donor heart smaller than excised native heart)
Risk for ineffective participation in rehabilitation resulting from not understanding or following prescribed regimens	Patient understands prescribed regimens and verbalizes effects on activities of daily living	Assess patient's/family's understanding of heart biopsy/bronchoscopy to assess organ function, signs of rejection; explain biopsy procedure: right internal jugular approach, local anesthesia (or anesthesia standby), small specimen excised from right ventricle Explain need for frequent cultures (throat, urine, blood, sputum, bronchial) and blood studies (white blood cell count, platelet count) Describe antibiotic prophylaxis before invasive procedures, dental work; need to avoid sick family members and friends; signs and symptoms of infection or rejection Elicit patient's/family's understanding of medications, diet, weight control, exercise, cessation of smoking, and other prescribed regimens; refer for cardiopulmonary rehabilitation Provide name of contact persons for follow-up, questions, concerns

4. The pulmonary trunk and aorta are transected above their respective semilunar valves. The atria are incised to leave intact posterior portions of the right and left atrial walls, as well as the interatrial septum of the recipient.

5. The recipient heart is then excised.

Implantation of the donor heart

1. The donor heart is removed from the transport container and placed on the back table. The surgeon evaluates the heart and trims the atrial walls and great vessels in preparation for the anastomoses.

2. The donor heart is placed in the pericardial cavity and aligned with the interatrial septum and the right and left atrial wall remnants of the recipient heart.

3. The donor LA wall (see Fig. 16-2, *C* and *D*) is anastomosed with a 54-inch running polypropylene suture. After completion of the anastomosis, a left-sided heart vent may be placed through the LA appendage to decompress the left ventricle (LV) and remove air.

4. The right atrial (RA) wall is anastomosed (see Fig. 16-2, *D* and *E*) with a long, running polypropylene suture.

5. The pulmonary artery anastomosis is completed (see Fig. 16-2, *F*).

6. While the patient's temperature is warmed to normal, the aortic anastomosis is completed (see Fig. 16-2, *G*). Air is removed from the heart with the LV vent.

7. An aortic venting needle is inserted into the ascending aorta. The patient is placed in Trendelenburg's position, and the cross-clamp is removed with continuous venting of the aorta.
8. If the heart does not start to beat spontaneously, it is defibrillated.
9. A recuperation period is provided by maintaining CPB and allowing the heart to rest (particularly if ischemic time has been prolonged).
10. When the patient has been rewarmed, CPB is discontinued. Chest drainage tubes and temporary epicardial pacing wires are inserted, and the chest incision is closed. A pulmonary artery pressure catheter may be inserted for postoperative monitoring.

Modification of orthotopic transplantation

Modifications to the procedure by Blanche and Colleagues (1997) have reduced some of the dysrhythmias and valvular dysfunction associated with the traditional atrial anastomoses (see Fig. 16-3). By creating end-to-end anastomoses between the superior vena cava and the inferior vena cava (instead of atrial-to-atrial anastomoses), there is a more physiologic atrial contribution to ventricular filling and less distortion of the mitral and tricuspid annuli. This results in less atrioventricular valve regurgitation and fewer rhythm disturbances (Miniati, Robbins, and Reitz, 2001). A cuff of recipient LA is sewn to the donor LA. Pulmonary artery and aortic anastomoses are performed as described in the traditional procedure (see p. 476).

HETEROTOPIC CARDIAC TRANSPLANTATION

Heterotopic (piggyback) transplantation is the insertion of a second heart into the right pleural cavity. The donor heart works in tandem with the recipient's native heart. It was originally performed by Carrel and Guthrie (1905), who transplanted a dog heart into the neck of a recipient dog with anastomoses to the recipient's carotid artery and jugular vein.

This type of transplantation has a limited role because the recipient's native heart function continues to deteriorate, producing symptomatic deterioration in the patient. Moreover, chronic anticoagulation, in addition to chronic immunosuppression, is required to prevent thromboembolism from originating in the dysfunctional native heart.

Possible indications for heterotopic transplantation include a size mismatch between a small donor and a large recipient and as a biologic assist device. Another indication is the presence of severe pulmonary hypertension. In patients with pulmonary hypertension and right ventricular hypertrophy, pulmonary vasodilator treatment may be initiated before transplant to reduce the afterload that initially would be faced by the transplanted organ. The procedure is technically more difficult, the extra heart can compress lung tissue, and monitoring rejection is complicated by the position and angle of the donor organ (Emery and Arom, 1996).

Another procedure may be preferable to the heterotopic operation: the domino donor procedure, whereby a heart-lung donor's organs are given to a patient with pulmonary disease and mild right ventricular hypertrophy (with no other abnormalities) secondary to the pulmonary hypertension. The excised heart from the heart-lung recipient in turn is implanted into a patient with elevated pulmonary vascular resistance requiring a cardiac transplant. The rationale is that implanting a heart with a normal right ventricular wall into a patient with elevated pulmonary pressures will cause the transplanted heart to fail before it can compensate by hypertrophy (Winkel, Kao, and Costanzo, 1996).

Procedure (Emery and Arom, 1996)

Donor recovery is similar to that for orthotopic transplantation, except that more caval tissue is taken during recovery. A prosthetic graft may be required to bridge the gap between one or both great vessels of the donor and recipient. Nursing considerations are similar to those for orthotopic transplantation.

1. The pericardium on the recipient's right side is freed and allowed to fall into the right chest, thereby exposing the right atrium.
2. CPB is instituted and an incision made into the LA anterior to the pulmonary veins; this incision in the recipient is sewn to the single left pulmonary vein orifice (made by connecting the orifices of the left pulmonary veins) or the donor (Fig. 16-4, *A* and *B*). The right pulmonary veins will have been ligated previously.
3. The superior vena cava of the donor is sewn to that of the recipient (Fig. 16-4, *C*).
4. The aortas are joined with an end-to-side anastomosis; the pulmonary arteries are similarly joined end to side, often using graft material (see Fig. 16-4, *C*).

POSTOPERATIVE CARE

Postoperatively the patient is taken to a private room in the surgical intensive care unit (ICU). Isolation practices vary, but strict isolation procedures have not been shown to be more beneficial than modified protective isolation procedures consisting of gowns, masks, and careful hand washing. Immediate postoperative care

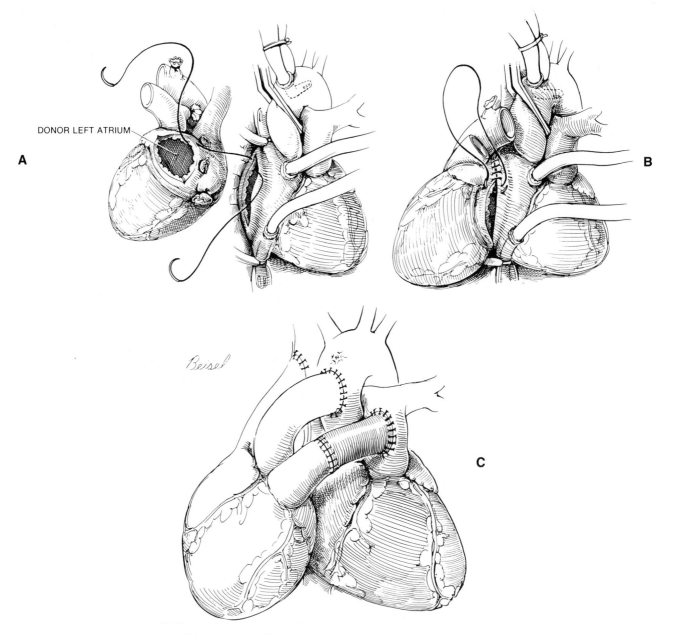

FIGURE 16-4 Heterotopic cardiac transplantation. **A** and **B,** Left atrial anastomoses. **C,** A remnant of the donor SVC is anastomosed to the side of the recipient SVC. The donor ascending aorta and pulmonary artery are anastomosed end-to-side to their respective counterparts (see text.) (From Waldhausen JA, Pierce WS: *Johnson's surgery of the chest,* ed 5, St Louis, 1985, Mosby.)

differs little from that after more routine heart surgery, except for the use of immunosuppression (Hunt, Schroeder, and Berry, 2001).

Although a healthy donor heart is tolerant of ischemia, postoperative cardiac dysfunction is a common occurrence. Patients often require a combination of inotropic drugs and vasodilators for a few hours or days after surgery. Isoproterenol may be used to support the right ventricle of the donor heart. Heart failure may be aggravated by pulmonary hypertension caused by pretransplant pulmonary dysfunction in the recipient, increased cardiac output ejected by the donor, reperfusion injury, or the adverse effects of CPB (see Chapter 9) during the transplant procedure. Drug therapy, adequate ventilation, and monitoring of blood gases are all important considerations during postoperative care.

TABLE 16-2
Effects of Denervation on the Heart

NORMAL	DENERVATION
Loss of Sympathetic Innervation	
Sympathetic fibers release norepinephrine and acetylcholine, leading to:	Without direct stimulation, response to stress and exercise depends on other mechanisms
Increased conduction through sinoatrial and atrioventricular nodes	Muscle activity increases venous return to heart, increasing cardiac output
Increased heart rate	Later, heart rate and cardiac output increase from circulating catecholamines
Increased stroke volume	There is delayed response to exercise
Immediate response to exercise	When preload is decreased, orthostatic hypotension occurs, resulting from a lack of compensatory increase in heart rate
Loss of Parasympathetic Innervation	
Parasympathetic fibers (including vagus nerve) inhibit conduction through atrioventricular node	Faster resting heart rate (usually 90 to 100 beats per minute) occurs
	Valsalva maneuver, carotid massage, and atropine have no effect on heart rate
Loss of Pain Receptors	
Angina is present during cardiac ischemia	There is no angina

From Dressler DK: The patient undergoing cardiac transplant surgery. In Guzzetta CE, Dossey BM: *Cardiovascular nursing: holistic practice,* St Louis, 1992, Mosby.

Another factor is the effect of severing the neural connections to the heart. Because sympathetic (e.g., adrenergic) and parasympathetic (e.g., vagus) nerves are interrupted, the denervated heart (Table 16-2) must rely on noncardiac mediators to augment heart rate and contractility in order to increase the cardiac output. Manipulation of volume (preload) and inotropic medications, as well as atrial pacing, may be necessary to maintain adequate stroke volume. Circulating noncardiac catecholamines provide another means of increasing heart rate and contractility. Bengel and others (2001) have shown that sympathetic reinnervation occurs in heart transplant recipients and has a positive impact on both myocardial contractility and heart rate. However, reinnervation is not complete, and patients are usually unable to return to a normal level of exercise (Hunt, 2001).

Chest pain receptors are also cut, resulting in an inability to feel angina pectoris. Sensory afferent reinnervation of the donor heart can occur months after transplantation and is thought to be related to the reestablishment of sympathetic fibers and myocardial norepinephrine stores. These findings are significant because patients are at risk for accelerated coronary atherosclerosis, and anginal symptoms are an important warning signal.

Because right atrial tissue from both donor and recipient is present after the traditional transplant procedure, the electrocardiogram (ECG) shows two P waves. Only the P wave of the donor heart is conducted to the rest of the heart because the impulse from the recipient's native atrial tissue is unable to cross the suture line. (This inability of impulses to cross suture lines is the basis for the Maze procedure to treat atrial fibrillation; see Chapter 17.) Bradycardia is not unusual after surgery, but in general dysrhythmias are uncommon. However, the appearance of atrial flutter may signal rejection. Occasionally patients require a pacemaker, but this complication is seen less frequently with the modified, bicaval anastomostic technique (Miniati, Robbins, and Reitz, 2001).

Bleeding may be another problem encountered postoperatively. Because the recipient pericardium is often enlarged secondary to cardiomegaly, there is additional space between the pericardium and the smaller donor heart in which blood can accumulate without detection. Moreover, many patients are taking anticoagulants (e.g., warfarin) preoperatively to protect them from thromboembolism related to left ventricular dilation and atrial fibrillation. Adhesions from previous surgery may cause increased bleeding, and liver dysfunction (from preoperative right-sided congestion) may impair coagulation processes. Homologous blood transfusions are avoided when possible to reduce the risk of disease transmission; autotransfusion is used whenever possible. A number of chronic complications occur in the transplant patient (Box 16-4).

REJECTION

Rejection of the transplanted heart remains a major threat to long-term survival. The basic problem is the

BOX 16-4
Major Chronic Complications After Cardiac Transplantation

Related to chronic immunosuppression
  General
    Infections
    Malignancy
  Cyclosporine
    Arterial hypertension
    Renal dysfunction
    Hyperlipidemia
    Gingival hypertrophy
    Hypertrichosis
    Neurologic: tremor, headache
  Azathioprine
    Neutropenia
    Hepatic dysfunction
    Pancreatitis
  Steroids
    Osteoporosis
    Hypertension
    Obesity
    Hyperlipidemia
    Glucose intolerance
    Sodium retention
    Myopathy
    Skin changes
    Cholelithiasis
Not directly related to immunosuppression
  Rejection
  Transplant coronary artery disease
  Nonspecific graft failure
  Tricuspid regurgitation

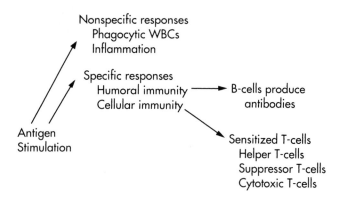

FIGURE 16-5 Overview of the immune system. When confronted with a foreign substance, the immune system may respond through specific or nonspecific responses. Cellular immunity with the stimulation of small sensitized T-cells is thought to be the most important response in relation to transplant rejection. (From Dressler DK: The patient undergoing cardiac transplant surgery. In Guzzetta CE, Dossey BM: *Cardiovascular nursing: holistic practice,* St Louis, 1992, Mosby.)

TABLE 16-3
Phagocytes and Their Functions

PHAGOCYTE	FUNCTION
Monocytes	Migrate from blood tissues to become macrophages
Macrophages	Scavenger cells in tissues
	Present antigen to T cells
	Secrete enzymes, complement proteins, and immune regulatory factors (cytokines)
	Activated by lymphokines
Neutrophils	Contain granules capable of destroying alien organisms
	Key role in inflammatory reactions
Eosinophils	Contain granules capable of destroying alien organisms
	Weaker phagocyte
Basophils	Contain granules capable of destroying alien organisms
	Key role in allergic reaction

specific and nonspecific responses of the recipient's immune system to foreign antigens (Fig. 16-5, Table 16-3). The immunologic process that affects the donor heart can be hyperacute, acute, or chronic, and severe or mild.

Hyperacute rejection occurs immediately after transplantation and becomes apparent in the OR. It is caused by a humoral response related to ABO incompatibility and a reactive lymphocyte cross-match between recipient and donor. Platelet thrombi are deposited throughout the coronary arteries, and endothelial damage and interstitial hemorrhage are manifested. This produces global myocardial ischemia and cardiac failure. When hyperacute rejection occurs, the donor heart must be removed and replaced with a biventricular assist device (BiVAD) until another cardiac organ becomes available for transplantation.

Acute rejection (Fig. 16-6) commonly occurs within the first 3 months after transplant. It is activated by T-lymphocytes producing interstitial and perivascular mononuclear cell infiltration. If untreated, it progresses to cellular death.

Transvenous endomyocardial biopsy (Fig. 16-7) is performed to study the histologic changes characteristic of acute rejection. Results should be correlated to the clinical picture because sampling errors can occur (e.g., tissue from scarred regions, tissue taken from an area free of rejection but surrounded or adjacent to an area of rejection).

Rejection is categorized as mild, moderate, severe, resolving, or resolved. During the first few months postoperatively, biopsies are performed frequently (Table 16-4). Clinical signs and symptoms of rejection warrant prompt

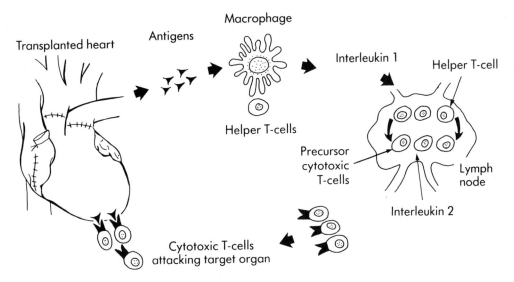

FIGURE 16-6 Acute rejection process. Antigens on the transplanted cells are recognized as foreign by macrophages and precursors of helper T-cells. The interaction between these cells results in the release of IL-1, which causes helper T-cells to mature. The helper T-cells then interact with precursors of cytotoxic T-cells. Another hormone, IL-2, is released and promotes proliferation and maturation of the cytotoxic T-cells. These cells then circulate to the transplanted heart, combine with the antigens on the transplanted cells, and attempt to destroy the transplanted cells. (From Dressler DK: The patient undergoing cardiac transplant surgery. In Guzzetta CE, Dossey BM: *Cardiovascular nursing: holistic practice,* St Louis, 1992, Mosby.)

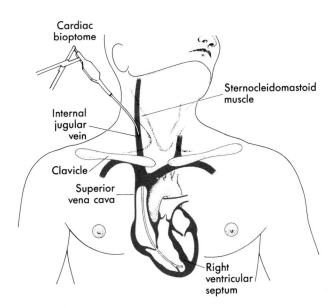

FIGURE 16-7 Technique of endomyocardial biopsy. The bioptome is inserted through the right internal jugular vein. (From Macdonald SN, Naucke NA: Heart transplantation. In Smith SL: *Tissue and organ transplantation: implications for professional nursing practice,* St Louis, 1990, Mosby.)

biopsy. Noninvasive methods such as radionuclide testing, transesophageal and transsternal echocardiography, and blood tests (including immunosuppression drug levels) are among the routine tests performed in patients.

TABLE 16-4
Recommended Frequency of Endomyocardial Biopsy for Routine Monitoring of Heart Transplant Rejection*

TIME AFTER TRANSPLANT	INTERVAL	NUMBER OF BIOPSIES
Day 14	First biopsy	1
1-4 wk	Every week	3
5-12 wk	Every 2 wk	4
3-6 mo	Every mo	3
6 mo to indefinite	Every 3 mo	

*Rebiopsy if indeterminate and 10 d after conclusion of rejection treatment. From Braunwald E, Zipes DP, Libby P, editors: *Heart disease: a textbook of cardiovascular medicine,* ed 6, Philadelphia, 2001, WB Saunders.

IMMUNOSUPPRESSION

Immunosuppression for minimizing or preventing rejection has become more patient specific with the ongoing development of newer agents. The availability of these newer agents also has reduced the reliance of steroids, which produce cushingoid (i.e., moon-faced) features and other complications (see Table 16-3). Current immunosuppression regimens often involve a triple drug therapy that includes cyclosporine or tacrolimus, azathioprine or mycophenolate mofetil

(MMF), and prednisone. Tacrolimus (originally called FK-506 [Szeto and Rosengard, 2002]) is comparable to cyclosporine in survival rate and incidence of rejection but may have less severe side effects, such as nephrotoxicity and hyperglycemia. MMF inhibits the proliferation of B- and T-lymphocytes and has demonstrated excellent survival rates in comparison with azathioprine. Other immunosuppression drugs include OKT3, a monoclonal antibody that causes T-lymphocyte cell lysis and may be used as induction therapy for heart transplant recipients and for treating severe rejection. Interleukin-2 receptor antagonists also can be used in the early postoperative period to reduce the frequency and severity of rejection (Miniati, Robbins, and Reitz, 2001).

INFECTION

Because immune therapy lowers the body's defense against infection, opportunistic pathogens (normally controlled by the body's immune system) can cause infection. Infection can occur anywhere, but the most common site is the lungs. Bacterial, viral, fungal, or parasitic organisms may be responsible (Table 16-5).

Prevention is the best protection. Donors are screened preoperatively for transmissible diseases. Recipients are extubated within the first 24 hours if possible, and invasive lines and catheters are discontinued as soon as permissible. Patients also are encouraged to ambulate soon after surgery to prevent pulmonary complications. Strict infection control practices, especially frequent hand washing, are important. Perioperative antibiotic treatment is standard; long-term prophylaxis may be used, but generally organism-specific drugs are preferred.

CORONARY ARTERY DISEASE

The development of coronary artery disease (CAD) in the transplanted heart has become a major long-term problem. The disease tends to be diffuse and concentric; the use of intravascular ultrasound (see Chapter 4) can demonstrate the degree of disease with greater precision than coronary angiography alone. The warning symptom of angina pectoris is rare because the allograft heart is essentially denervated.

The cause of allograft vasculopathy is thought to be related to a complex immune mechanism producing intimal proliferation and hyperplasia (Miniati, Robbins, and Reitz, 2000). The prognosis for survival is generally poor, but preventive strategies such as lipid-lowering drugs show some promise in retarding the proliferation of CAD. New immunosuppression agents that can retard the development of allograft coronary disease are under

TABLE 16-5 *Peak Incidence of Common Infections After Cardiac Transplantation*	
ORGANISM	SOURCE
Month 1 Posttransplant	
Staphylococci	Lung, wound, urine, blood
Gram-negative bacteria	Lung, wound, urine, blood
Herpes simplex virus	Mucocutaneous
Candida	Mucocutaneous
Aspergillus	Lung
Months 2 to 5 Posttransplant	
Cytomegalovirus	Lung, gastrointestinal tract, heart, eye
Herpes zoster virus	Dermatomes
Pneumocystis carinii	Lung
Toxoplasmosis gondii	Central nervous system, lung, heart
Listeria monocytogenes	Central nervous system
Legionella pneumophila	Lung
Nocardia asteroides	Lung, soft tissues
Later than 6 Months Posttransplant	
Community-acquired bacteria	Variable

study. Patients with established disease may undergo balloon angioplasty or coronary artery bypass surgery, but results have not demonstrated long-term success. In selected patients, *retransplantation* may be performed (Hunt, Schroeder, and Berry, 2001).

Patient Discharge Teaching

Discharge planning (see Box 16-3) focuses on assisting patients and families in coping with the short- and long-term effects of transplantation. A large amount of information is provided that requires repetition and reinforcement. New information should build on what is already known and should take into consideration the psychologic makeup of the patient. It is especially important that patients know about rejection, infection, drug complications, expected quality of life, and lifestyle recommendations; this can be facilitated by making them part of an OR transplant care team (Lefrak, 2001).

AUTOTRANSPLANTATION

Another form of transplantation has been employed for malignant cardiac tumors. When conventional surgical excision of the tumor is not successful, the patient may undergo explantation and replacement (i.e., *autotransplantation*) of the heart. Wagner,

Hutchisson, and Baird (1999) describe autotransplantation for removal of a tumor encroaching on the mitral valve.

The heart was removed by dividing the right atrial junction from the superior and inferior venae cavae, transecting the ascending aorta and the pulmonary artery, and incising the left atrium so that a left atrial cuff was retained. The heart was placed in cold saline, and cardioplegic solution was infused directly into the left main coronary artery. The tumor was removed and the valve replaced with a prosthesis. (A bioprosthesis usually is implanted so that anticoagulation is not necessary should future surgery be required.) The heart was reimplanted by anastomosing the inferior and superior venae cavae, aorta, pulmonary artery, and left atrial cuff.

When resection of an extensive tumor is not possible (and metastases have not been detected), orthotopic transplantation may be performed (Grandmougin and others, 2001).

Heart-Lung Transplantation

Patients with end-stage lung disease associated with severe right ventricular failure may be candidates for heart-lung procedures. The most common indications in the past were primary pulmonary hypertension or Eisenmenger's syndrome. The latter is a condition in patients with atrial or ventricular septal defects who have pulmonary overloading, which leads to hypertension; eventually this causes reversal of the shunt from one that is left-to-right to one that is right-to-left, producing cyanosis. Closure of the defect does not result in improvement when a severely elevated pulmonary vascular resistance poses too high an afterload for the right ventricle to overcome; heart-lung replacement may be the only therapeutic option, although complex congenital heart disease is the main indication (Miniati, Robbins, and Reitz, 2001; Griffith and Magliato, 1999).

With the development of improved lung transplantation techniques, a number of these patients may benefit from single- or double-lung sequential transplantation (see the following section), especially if it is performed before irreversible right ventricular decompensation occurs. Given the shortage of donor organs, this technique allows distribution of organs to more candidates because the donor heart can be used in another patient requiring cardiac transplantation.

The *domino procedure* may be performed, whereby the recipient patient with end-stage lung disease receives a donor heart and lungs and donates his or her normal heart to an isolated heart transplant candidate. Changes in the UNOS policy 3.7 (see Box 16-1) to require heart-lung candidates to be listed separately on both lung and heart waiting lists has made the domino procedure more rare in the United States (Griffith and Magliato, 1999).

Other limiting factors for heart-lung transplantation include the requirement that both the donor heart and lungs are normal or at least satisfactory and that the donor and recipient be similar in weight, height, and chest size. Size matching is especially important between the donor lungs and recipient thorax because lungs that are too large could produce cardiac tamponade when the sternum is closed; when this occurs, sternal closure may have to be delayed for a few days to allow reduction in the amount of pulmonary edema. Careful fluid management helps to prevent pulmonary overload and possible damage to the lungs.

Avoiding pulmonary infection related to endotracheal intubation preoperatively in the donor or to spillage from the trachea during either retrieval or transplantation procedures is another consideration in heart-lung (and lung) procedures. Trachial or bronchial stumps are closed with disposable stapling devices to prevent cross-contamination.

Recipient preparation varies from cardiac transplantation in that in addition to removal of the heart, removal of the diseased native lungs and insertion of the donor lungs must be done in such a way that the phrenic, vagus, and recurrent laryngeal nerves are not injured during dissection. Transection of the right or left phrenic nerves can cause unilateral or bilateral paralysis of the diaphragm; recurrent laryngeal nerve injury affects laryngeal motor function; and vagal interruption can cause, among other problems, severe gastrointestinal dysfunction and persistent diarrhea. Meticulous hemostasis is mandatory (Griffith and Magliato, 1999).

Two modifications to the traditional three anastomotic techniques (i.e., trachea, right atrium, and aorta) have helped to reduce the incidence of certain complications. Bicaval right-sided anastomoses, described under othotopic heart transplantation (see Fig. 16-3), have reduced torsion and tricuspid valvular regurgitation that may be seen with the traditional right atrium–to–right atrium method. The second change, which is seen more often in lung transplantation, is the performing of *bibronchial* anastomoses (each donor mainstem bronchus is anastomosed to its respective recipient bronchus) to reconnect the airway (rather than the traditional tracheal anastomosis). This modification reduces bleeding that often occurs after dissection of the bronchial vessels in and around the carina and has enhanced the integrity of the airway connection (Griffith and Magliato, 1999).

OPERATIVE PROCEDURE: HEART-LUNG TRANSPLANTATION (GRIFFITH AND MAGLIATO, 1999)

Organ retrieval

Excision of the donor organ is done only after broncho-scopic inspection of the lungs and visual assessment of the heart. Aerosolized antibiotics are instilled into the lungs. The heart and lungs may be removed en bloc (as one unit) or separately. Median sternotomy is the stan-dard incision for donor organ removal; often a bilateral, intercostal transsternal ("clamshell") incision is employed for the transplantation into the recipient (Fig. 16-8, *A*).

Procedure

1. Abdominal organs (to be removed at the same time as the heart and lungs) are prepared; Prostaglan-din E_1 (a pulmonary vasodilator) is then infused into the donor lungs.

2. The superior vena cava (SVC) is stapled.
3. The inferior vena cava (IVC) is divided at the di-aphragm. If concomitant liver removal is per-formed, the length of the heart portion of the IVC may be shortened to give more IVC length to the liver allograft.
4. The aorta is cross-clamped, and cardioplegia is in-fused into the aortic root. The left atrial appendage is amputated to allow decompression of the left ventricle and the pulmonary veins.
5. Pulmoplegic solution is infused into the lungs while the lungs are gently inflated.
6. After the aortic cardioplegia is infused, the aorta is transected (which also allows the pulmonary flush [pulmoplegia] to escape).
7. The inferior right and left pulmonary ligaments are divided, and the pericardium abutting the di-aphragm is divided.

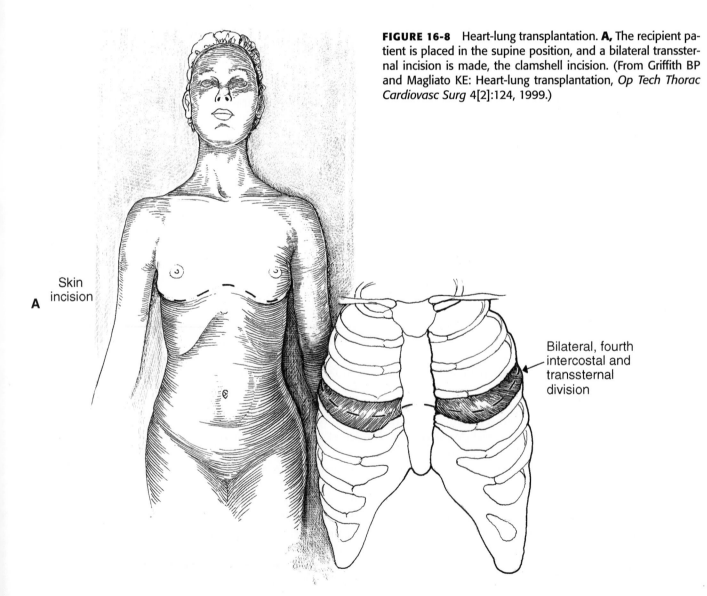

Skin incision

A

Bilateral, fourth intercostal and transsternal division

FIGURE 16-8   Heart-lung transplantation. **A,** The recipient pa-tient is placed in the supine position, and a bilateral transster-nal incision is made, the clamshell incision. (From Griffith BP and Magliato KE: Heart-lung transplantation, *Op Tech Thorac Cardiovasc Surg* 4[2]:124, 1999.)

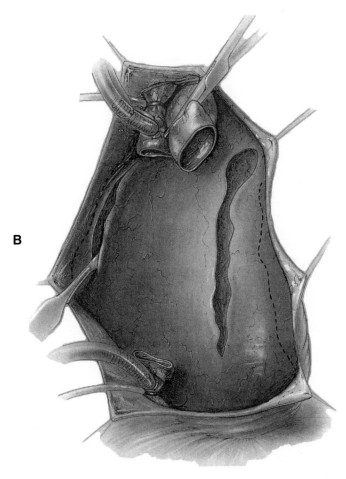

B

FIGURE 16-8, cont'd   Heart-lung transplantation. **B,** Right and left pericardial windows are made, avoiding the phrenic nerves *(dotted lines)*.

Continued

8. The bronchial arteries are closed with hemoclips (cautery may not be reliable).
9. The endotracheal (ET) tube is withdrawn, and the trachea is stapled and divided.
10. The heart-lung block is removed, packaged, and stored for transport to the recipient.

Recipient preparation
1. The patient is placed in the supine position with the arms tucked at the side (or elevated above the head in large patients). An arterial line and pulmonary artery catheter are inserted, as well as a transesophageal echocardiography (TEE) probe to monitor cardiac function.
2. Although median sternotomy has been the traditional incision, a bilateral, intercostal (fourth interspace) transsternal incision (see Fig. 16-8, A) is preferred by some authors (Griffith and Magliato, 1999).

3. The pericardium and both pleura are inspected for adhesions and other potential problems. (Adhesions may produce excessive bleeding and contraindicate transplantation.)
4. CPB is initiated with arterial inflow infused into the innominate artery and venous return draining from cannulas in the IVC and SVC.
5. The ascending aorta is occluded just below the aortic infusion cannula.
6. The right pulmonary artery and all pulmonary veins are divided at their pericardial junction.
7. The LA is removed from the RA, with the atrial septum left intact (for later anastomotic attachment).
8. At this point the pericardial well contains an RA cuff and a portion of the left pulmonary artery (PA). When bicaval (e.g., IVC and SVC) anastomoses are planned (versus right atrial anastomoses), a greater portion of the RA is excised.
9. Pulmonary ligaments are divided, hilar structures are isolated, and the pulmonary arteries and veins are divided.
10. The bronchial vessels are clipped, the mainstem bronchi are stapled, and the lungs are amputated. Meticulous hemostasis of the posterior mediastinum and peribronchial areas is critical because these areas are not easily accessible once the donor organs are implanted.

Implantation
1. After the incision is made, the pleural cavities are entered by incising each pleura anterior (Fig. 16-8, B) to the pericardium (incising the pleura lateral could injure the phrenic nerves running along the lateral borders of the pericardium.)
2. The donor heart and lungs are brought to the field, and the organs are positioned by passing the (larger) right lung (Fig. 16-8, C) behind the right atrial cuff (or directly through the right pericardial window when the atrium has been removed to perform bicaval anastomoses), and the heart is positioned within the pericardium.
3. Bibronchial anastomoses are performed (Fig. 16-8, D). The inner, membranous portion of each bronchus is anastomosed with a running absorbable suture (Fig. 16-8, D1). The cartilaginous portion is joined by interrupted absorbable sutures (Fig. 16-8, D2), and the anastomoses are completed (Fig. 16-8, D3).
4. Air is vented from the ascending aorta, and a left ventricular apical vent is introduced via the left atrial appendage.
5. Bicaval anastomoses are performed (Fig. 16-8, E). After the IVC portion is completed, the SVC anastomosis is achieved by connecting the recipient SVC to the SVC and some atrial tissue of the donor. The aorta is anastomosed with a running suture.

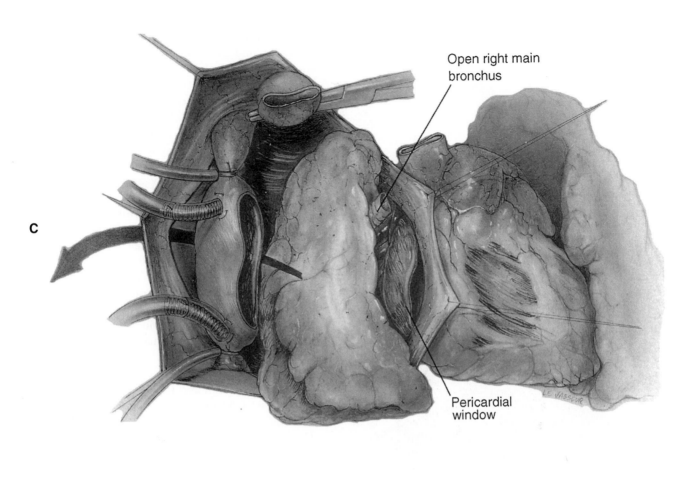

C

Open right main bronchus

Pericardial window

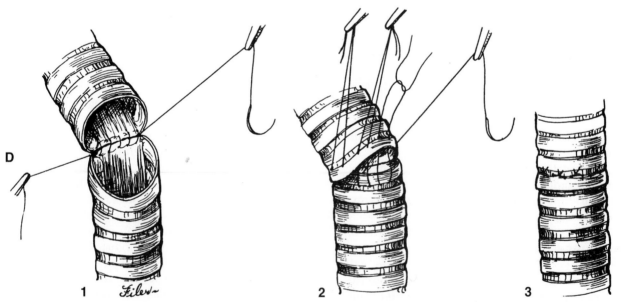

D   1   2   3

FIGURE 16-8, cont'd   Heart-lung transplantation. **C,** The heart and lungs are brought into the field and the right lung is swung behind the right atrium, through the right pericardial window, and into the right pleural space. **D,** Bibronchial anastomoses are performed. *1,* The membranous portion of one bronchus is anastomosed with a running suture; *2,* The cartilaginous portion of the bronchus is anastomosed with interrupted sutures; *3,* The completed bronchial anastomosis. (From Griffith BP and Magliato KE: Heart-lung transplantation, *Op Tech Thorac Cardiovasc Surg* 4(2):124, 1999.)

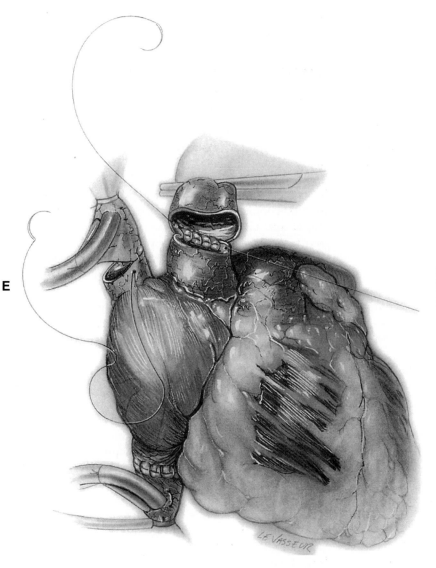

E

FIGURE 16-8, cont'd   E, The IVC anastomosis is completed and the aorta and SV are connected with running sutures.

6. The donor and recipient aortas (see Fig. 16-8, *E*) are anastomosed end to end with a continuous 4-0 polypropylene suture. Topical lavage is discontinued, and rewarming is begun. Air is removed from the aorta and left side of the heart, and the cross-clamp is removed.
7. Caval tourniquets are removed, and ventilation is started. Venting catheters are taken out of the heart, and the entry sites are oversewn. CPB is terminated.
8. Temporary pacing wires and chest tubes are placed; hemostasis is achieved, and the sternum is closed.

Postoperative period

In addition to the problems associated with cardiac transplantation discussed previously, heart-lung recipients are also at risk for developing complications relating to the lung transplant (see the following section). Perioperative complications include injury to major

nerves, pulmonary edema, and tracheal or bronchial anastomotic dehiscence.

Early death (e.g., within 30 days) is caused primarily by graft failure and hemorrhage. Infection (often bacterial) is the most common cause of death within the first year; cytomegalovirus infection also occurs in more than half the patients. Beyond 1 year the leading cause of death is bronchiolitis obliterans, a syndrome producing small airway obstruction, thought to be caused by episodes of acute reaction of the lung (but not necessarily the heart). Transbronchial biopsy is performed routinely to monitor for rejection (Griffith and Magliato, 1999).

Lung Transplantation

Experimental lung transplants were performed in the 1940s and 1950s, and the first human lung transplant was accomplished in 1963 by James Hardy in Mississippi

(Hardy, 1964; 1986). Early poor results were attributed not only to poor patient selection but also to ischemia and deterioration of the bronchial airway, rejection, and sepsis. Bronchovascular or bronchopleural fistulas developed, and the use of immunosuppressive therapy with prednisone and azathioprine was found to further retard healing of the bronchial anastomoses (Lochyna, 1999).

With the substitution of cyclosporine for the steroids and the use of a circumferential omental pedicle flap to revascularize the bronchial anastomosis and prevent the formation of fistulas, survival improved significantly for investigators from the University of Toronto. They performed the first successful long-term single-lung transplant in 1983 on a patient with end-stage pulmonary fibrosis (Toronto Lung Transplant Group, 1986).

Bilateral, en bloc lung transplantation was performed a few years later in a patient with end-stage emphysema.

Bilateral sequential lung transplantation with one lung from one donor and a second lung from another donor currently is performed more commonly than en bloc double-lung transplantation. In some patients with bilateral lung disease, single-lung transplantation can be performed. The choice of which side to transplant is based not only on donor organ availability but also on pathologic features (replacing the lung with the worst function), anatomic features (no adhesions or anomalies), and physiologic features (the side with greater chest capacity). Important advantages of single-lung transplantation are that the use of one lung provides another organ for another patient requiring transplantation and that the procedure can be performed without the use of CPB (Lonchyna, 1999). Additional advantages are listed in Box 16-5. Occasionally the domino procedure (described previously) may be performed.

Candidates generally have obstructive and interstitial lung diseases and are not expected to live longer than 1 to 2 years. Patients demonstrate diminished exercise capacity, oxygen dependence, and worsening pulmonary function tests. Contraindications include chronic infectious lung disease, end-organ failure, malnourishment, sepsis, ventilator dependence, malignancy, or other life-threatening disease.

PROCEDURAL CONSIDERATIONS

For both single and bilateral sequential lung transplants, the retrieval team reviews the chest-x-ray films to determine the size and condition of the lungs. Evidence of infiltrates, aspiration, or consolidation would make a donor unacceptable. Adequate gas exchange is confirmed by arterial blood gas analysis. If the arterial oxygen saturation declines over time, the donor lung may not be suitable. A bronchoscopy is performed, and specimens are taken for culture and Gram's stain. (Gram's stain results can be used to guide antibiotic therapy in the recipient.) The final assessment of the donor lungs is direct inspection after both pleural spaces have been opened.

Patients with head injuries resulting from motor vehicle trauma provide a significant number of potential donors, but associated blunt chest trauma causing pulmonary contusion can contraindicate use of the lungs (Perreas, Milano, and Wallwork, 2000). Ideally retrieval time is no more than 4 hours; when multiple organ procurement is performed or retrieval sites are a great distance, close coordination is mandatory to maintain an ischemic time of less than 4 hours. Flying time (one way) may be limited to less than $2\frac{1}{2}$ hours.

For single-lung transplant recipients, CPB is available on a standby basis (but is rarely needed); the groin is prepared and draped for cannulation if needed. If CPB is not used, heparinization can be avoided. In certain patient populations (e.g., those with pulmonary fibrosis) receiving a single lung, 25% of the recipients required CPB. Strict aseptic technique is used for endotracheal intubation and nasogastric tube insertion. For bilateral lung transplants, CPB often can be avoided (Meyers and Patterson, 1999).

OPERATIVE PROCEDURE: LUNG ORGAN RETRIEVAL (LONCHYNA, 1999; MEYERS AND PATTERSON, 1999)

If the donor heart is to be used for transplantation, cardiectomy is performed before the lung is removed.

Procedure
1. A left atrial incision is made, leaving an adequate cuff for both the heart and the lung.
2. Prostaglandin E_1 is injected intravenously, and cold electrolyte solution (pulmoplegia) is flushed through the inflated lungs via the pulmonary artery. Cold lavage may be used in the pleural spaces.
3. The left atrial appendage is amputated or cannulated to allow returning flush solution to exit the heart (the

---

BOX 16-5
Advantages of Single-Lung Transplantation

- One lung donor provides organs for two lung recipients
- Increased donor availability
- Decreased recipient waiting time
- Decreased need for intraoperative cardiopulmonary bypass
- Potential shorter recovery and hospital stay
- Preservation of native heart
- Heart rejection avoided
- Accelerated graft atherosclerosis not as prevalent

From Thelan LA and others: *Critical care nursing: diagnosis and management*, ed 3, St Louis, 1998, Mosby.

rationale for this is the same as it is for heart-lung procedures, described previously). The right side of the heart is vented by transecting the IVC. The aorta is then clamped (and cardioplegia solution is infused).

4. After flushing has been completed, the pulmonary artery is divided at the bifurcation.

5. The lungs are inflated, and the bronchus is dissected and divided between staple lines. (Inflating and stapling the lungs prevents flooding of the lungs by the transport solution and reduces the risk of infectious matter spilling into the lungs.)

6. One lung (or both lungs) is removed; it remains connected to the left atrial cuff and the pulmonary artery. If a single-lung transplant is to be performed on two patients at the same center, the lungs are taken en bloc and divided at the recipient hospital.

7. The organ is immersed in cold solution and placed in a sterile bag, packed into one or two additional sterile bags, and placed in a cooler for transport. The lung can be used either for single-lung, bilateral lung, or sequential lung procedures.

OPERATIVE PROCEDURE: SINGLE-LUNG TRANSPLANTATION

1. Approximately 1 hour before the arrival of the donor lung, arterial and pulmonary pressure lines are inserted, and the patient is anesthetized and intubated with a double-lumen tube. TEE is performed to monitor heart function.

2. For single-lung transplants the patient may be positioned laterally with the affected side up and the position maintained for the entire procedure.

   An anterolateral incision also can be used. For double-lung procedures, two disconnected anterolateral incisions may be employed (Fig. 16-9, *A*).

3. The chest, abdomen, and both groins are prepared and draped. (Usually the contralateral groin is used if CPB is necessary.)

4. After the incision is made, Finochietto chest retractor (shown in Fig. 16-9, *B*, inserted into the patient's right chest) is used to spread the ribs vertically, while a Balfour is used to spread the chest laterally. (Other retractors may be preferred by the surgeon.) Note that the sternum is not divided.

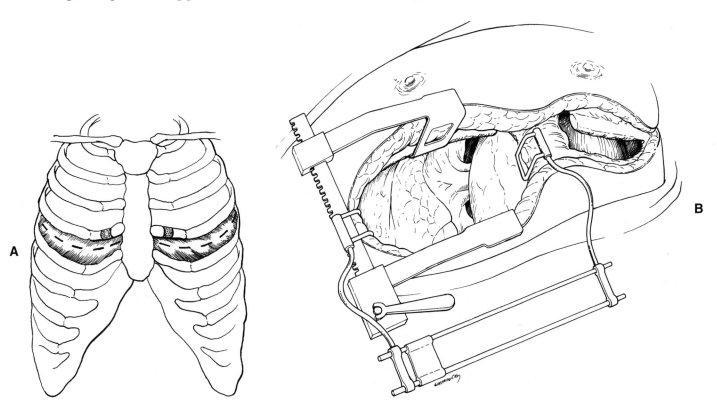

FIGURE 16-9 Lung transplantation. **A,** Two disconnected anterolateral incisions are made. **B,** A Finochietto chest retractor spreads the (right) ribs vertically, and a Balfour retractor spreads the incision laterally (different retractors can be used depending on surgeon preference). (**A** from Meyers BF, Patterson GA: Bi-lateral lung transplantation, *Op Tech Thorac Cardiovasc Surg* 4[2]:162, 1999; **B-F** from Meyers BF, Patterson GA: Technical aspects of adult lung transplantation, *Semin Thorac Cardiovasc Surg* 10[3]:213, 1998.)

Continued

5. The recipient pulmonary artery, veins, and right (or left) bronchus are prepared for their eventual anastomosis to the corresponding donor vessels and structures. The pericardium is opened around the pulmonary veins.

6. To determine if the patient can withstand lung transplantation without CPB, the pulmonary artery is occluded for about 5 minutes to test the patient's response. If CPB is deemed necessary, it is instituted after arrival of the donor organ.

7. Once the donor lung has arrived and is found to be acceptable, the recipient lung is excised.

8. The recipient pulmonary artery is occluded and transected just beyond the first bifurcation.

9. The bronchus is transected just before its bifurcation. The endotracheal tube to the affected bronchus is used to occlude the bronchial orifice.

Implantation of the donor lung

10. The donor lung is brought to the field and oriented into the chest.

11. The bronchial anastomosis of the right lung is depicted in Fig. 16-9, *C*. Duval lung retractors are placed on the recipient's (stapled) right pulmonary artery and pulmonary veins (the clamped double vessels).

The bronchial anastomosis of the left lung is shown in Fig. 16-9, *D*. Duval lung retractors are applied to the stapled lung pulmonary artery and pulmonary veins.

12. The right pulmonary artery anastomosis is performed with a partial occlusion clamp on the artery (Fig. 16-9, *E*), taking caution to avoid including the PA catheter in the jaws of the clamp. Some surgeons may sew the clamp to the wound edge to avoid slipping or premature opening of the clamp.

13. The arterial anastomosis is performed (Fig. 16-9, *F*). Retraction with a sponge stick enhances visualization.

14. TEE is used to assess right ventricular function during the significant pulmonary changes occurring with pulmonary artery clamping and unclamping, to monitor left ventricular function, and to look for retained air (Meyers and Patterson, 1999). Chest tubes are inserted.

15. The double-lumen endotracheal tube is exchanged for the single-lumen tube. Fiberoptic bronchoscopy is performed to assess the patency of the anastomoses and the donor airway. Retained secretions

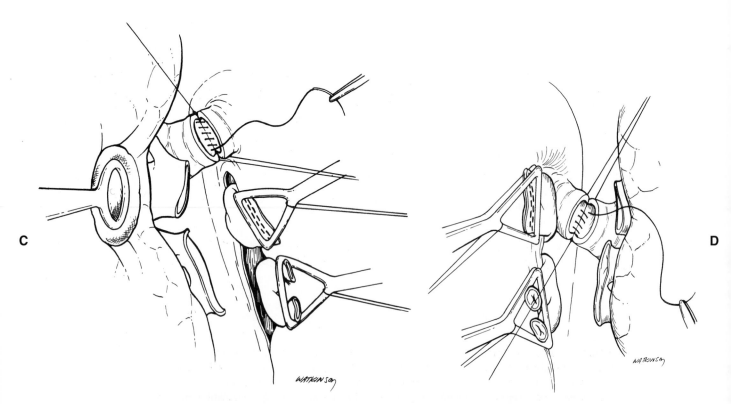

C   D

FIGURE 16-9, cont'd   Lung transplantation. **C,** Right lung bronchial anastomosis; note use of Duval lung clamps and the use of sponge stick for retraction. **D,** Left lung bronchial anastomosis. (**B-F** from Meyers BF, Patterson GA: Technical aspects of adult lung transplantation, *Semin Thorac Cardiovasc Surg* 10[3]:213, 1998.)

are suctioned. The patient is transported to the ICU. Most patients are extubated the first or second postoperative day.

BILATERAL LUNG TRANSPLANTATION

Donor retrieval is similar to that for single-lung recovery. Each lung is removed from the donor after left atrial incision and transection of the pulmonary arteries and the bronchi. The en bloc procedure is performed infrequently; bilateral single-lung transplants or sequential single-lung transplants are more common.

The least functional lung is resected and replaced first. The order is significant in that CPB may be avoided because the remaining (more healthy) lung can provide sufficient oxygenation while the less healthy lung is replaced. CPB is likely to be employed when there is hemodynamic instability, inadequate oxygenation, deterioration of RV function, or dramatic increases in pulmonary artery pressure (Meyers and Patterson, 1998).

The bilateral anterolateral incision (see Fig. 16-9, *A*) usually provides sufficient exposure. If a larger incision is required, the sternum can be transected (with ligation of the right and left internal mammary arteries)

and the incision converted to a full clamshell. A sternal saw or Lebsche knife (a large knife that is hit with a mallet to cut bone) is used for emergency bone splitting when an electric or pneumatic saw is unavailable.

Radial or femoral arterial lines are inserted for blood pressure monitoring, and TEE is standard for assessing ventricular function and the presence of intracavity air.

The donor lungs are removed as described earlier and inserted into their respective pleural cavity through the right and left pericardial windows that have been created (see Fig. 16-8, *C*). Bibronchial, pulmonary artery, and atrial anastomoses are performed as described earlier, chest tubes are inserted, and the procedure is completed. If the sternum has been transected, it is reapproximated with heavy wire; some authors (e.g., Meyers and Patterson, 1998) also may place a Steinmann pin to secure the closure and prevent the migration of the sternal wires.

After the skin incisions are closed, the double-lumen ET tube (if used) is replaced with a single-lumen tube. The patient is transferred to the intensive care unit.

Transplantation of living donor lobes

Bilateral implantation of lower pulmonary lobes from two blood group–compatible living donors is a newer

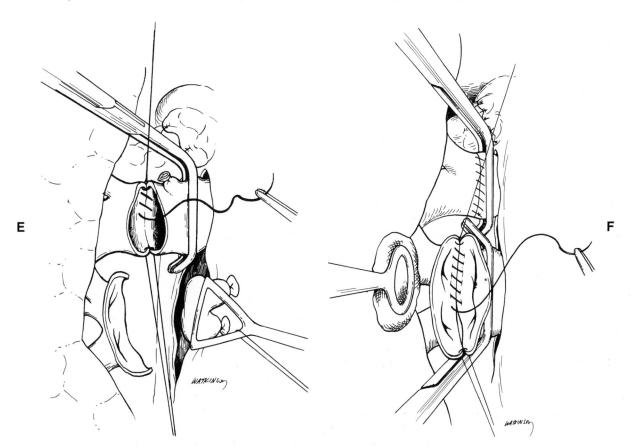

E F

FIGURE 16-9, cont'd Lung transplantation. **E,** Pulmonary artery anastomosis. **F,** Atrial anastomosis. (**B-F** from Meyers BF, Patterson GA: Technical aspects of adult lung transplantation, *Semin Thorac Cardiovasc Surg* 10[3]:213, 1998.)

technique that has been performed mainly on patients with cystic fibrosis, although patients with primary pulmonary hypertension, postchemotherapy pulmonary fibrosis, and obliterative bronchiolitis can also benefit (Barr and others, 1998). It is recommended that the donor lobes should be larger than the recipient so that the donor lobes fill each hemithorax, thereby avoiding persistent unfilled pleural space. Results have been similar to cadaver whole-lung transplantation, and there are few serious complications in donors. This technique has the potential to expand the donor base (Watson and Starnes, 1996; Arcasoy and Kotloff, 1999).

Other (e.g., upper, middle) lobes have been transplanted, but the right and left lower lobes seem most suitable for the recipient's right and left sides, respectively. Both these lobes can be excised with an adequate bronchus, pulmonary artery, and pulmonary vein to allow for functional anastomoses to the corresponding recipient structures (Watson and Starnes, 1996).

Potential donors are evaluated from each patient's extended family and from unrelated friends. Donors are tested for blood type compatibility and size matching, and they receive a chest x-ray examination. Detailed psychological and social evaluations are also performed. After the initial screening, potential donors undergo pulmonary function testing, ventilation/perfusion scanning, exercise stress testing (in older patients), echocardiogram, and chest computed tomography scanning. The final decision is made based on which donor is considered more appropriate for the right versus the left lower lobe (Barr and others, 1998).

Postoperative management includes an immunosuppression regimen, antibiotic therapy, and pulmonary function measurements. Fewer severe episodes of rejection have been seen in the living-related lung transplant group compared to the standard cadaver lung transplant patients. A unique pattern of unilateral rejection in a bilateral lung transplant recipient has been noted in some patients (Barr and others, 1995).

POSTOPERATIVE PERIOD

The transplanted lung is susceptible to fluid overload. This may be the result of a number of causes. Reperfusion edema may be the result of hypothermia and CPB (if used), as well as intraoperative ischemia; it may be affected by the disruption of pulmonary lymphatics and increased extravascular water accompanying implantation. In patients who have undergone CPB, bleeding may be a problem; and suboptimal myocardial preservation may cause postoperative left ventricular dysfunction. Oximetry, arterial, and pulmonary pressures; cardiac output; and mixed venous saturation are measured.

Patients are extubated when the lung is working well. Patients may have a prolonged ileus, necessitating nasogastric tube suctioning and intravenous total parenteral nutrition. Chest physiotherapy is started while the patient is intubated. Ambulation is started as early as possible.

Immunosuppression is initiated in the immediate postoperative period and consists of cyclosporine or tacrolimus, azathioprine or MMF, and prednisone. Bacterial infections are common but not generally lethal.

Acute rejection is common, with two or three episodes often occurring within the first month. Rejection is manifested by temperature elevation (which may be slight), deterioration of gas exchange as evidenced by decreased exercise tolerance, and infiltrates (seen on x-ray films). Bronchoscopic lung biopsy is the procedure of choice for diagnosing acute rejection, which is treated with methylprednisone.

Chronic rejection is a persistent problem and often appears as bronchiolitis obliterans (itself considered an immunologic, acute form of rejection). Currently there is no effective treatment for this complication (which is also seen in heart-lung recipients), so preventive strategies (e.g., lung biopsy, prompt treatment for acute rejection) are critical (Arcasoy and Kotloff, 1999). Infectious complications, especially those related to CMV, continue to be a problem.

Follow-up care includes frequent blood tests to monitor immunosuppression levels and blood counts. Exercise testing, bronchoscopy, pulmonary function studies, and arterial blood gases also are used, especially in anticipation of the onset of bronchiolitis obliterans. Colds or other illnesses persisting for more than a few days warrant prompt investigation. Cardiac and pulmonary function are evaluated every 3 months (or more) the first year and every 6 months after that.

Conclusion

Despite the advances made in all forms of transplantation, donor organ shortages have limited the widespread use of transplantation techniques. Methods to optimize the efficient use of available organs is reflected in the variety of combinations used for heart-lung, single-lung, and bilateral sequential lung replacement procedures. Nurses and other health care professionals can help these efforts by engaging in educational activities for the community and professional colleagues and by participating in the identification of potential donors. Future efforts will be aimed at overcoming problems associated with xenotransplantation, refining immunosuppression therapy, and gaining greater insights into the mechanisms of rejection.

References

Arcasoy SM, Kotloff RM: Lung transplantation, *N Engl J Med* 340(14):1081, 1999.

Augustine SM: Heart transplantation: long-term management related to immunosuppression, complications, and psychosocial adjustments, *Crit Care Nurs Clin North Am* 12(1):69, 2000.

Bailey LL and others: Baboon-to-human cardiac xenotransplantation in a neonate, *JAMA* 254(23):3321, 1985.

Barnard CN: A human cardiac transplant: an interim report of a successful operation performed at Groote Schuur Hospital, Cape Town, *S Afr Med J* 41:1271, 1967.

Barr ML and others: Living-related lobar transplantation: recipient outcome and early rejection patterns, *Transplant Proc* 27(3):1995, 1995.

Barr ML and others: Recipient and donor outcomes in living related and unrelated lobar transplantation, *Transplant Proc* 30:2261, 1998.

Bengel FM and others. Effect of sympathetic reinnervation on cardiac performance after heart transplantation, *N Engl J Med* 345(10):731, 2001.

Blanche C and others: Heart transplantation with bicaval and pulmonary venous anastomoses: a hemodynamic analysis of the first 117 patients, *J Cardiovasc Surg (Torino),* 38(6):561, 1997.

Bogan LM, Rosson MW, Petersen FF: Organ procurement and the donor family, *Crit Care Nurs Clin North Am* 12(1):23, 2000.

Braunwald E, Zipes DP, Libby P, editors: *Heart disease: a textbook of cardiovascular medicine,* ed 6, Philadelphia, 2001, WB Saunders.

Cabrol C: Presidential address, *J Heart Lung Transplant* 11(4, pt 1):595, 1992a.

Cabrol C: Special recognition award to Richard Lower, *J Heart Lung Transplant* 11(4, pt 1):597, 1992b.

Capron AM: Brain death—well settled yet still unresolved, *N Engl J Med* 344(16):1244, 2001.

Carrel A. Guthrie CC: The transplantation of veins and organs, *Am Med* 10:1101, 1905.

Chiu RC: Cardiac cell transplantation: the autologous skeletal myoblast implantation for myocardial regeneration, *Adv Card Surg* 11:69, 1999.

Cooper DK: Transplantation of the heart and both lungs. I:historical review, *Thorax* 24(4):383, 1969.

Cupples SA, Spruill LC: Evaluation criteria for the pretransplant patient, *Crit Care Nurs Clin North Am* 12(1):35, 2000.

De Geest SD: Psychological and behavioral issues in transplantation. http://surgery.medscape.com/medscape/cno/2000/ISHLT/story.cmf_id=1155 (accessed April 30, 2001).

Derenge S, Bartucci MR: Issues surrounding xenotransplantation, *AORN J* 70(3):428, 1999.

Dressler DK: The patient undergoing cardiac transplant surgery. In Guzzetta CE, Dossey BM: *Cardiovascular nursing: holistic practice,* St Louis, 1992, Mosby.

Egan TM: Non-heart-beating lung donors: yes or no? *Ann Thorac Surg* 70(5):1451, 2000.

Emery RW, Arom KV: Techniques in cardiac transplantation. In Emery RW, Miller LW, editors: *Handbook of cardiac transplantation,* St Louis, 1996, Mosby.

Grandmougin D and others: Total orthotopic heart transplantation for primary cardiac rhabdomyosarcoma: factors influencing long-term survival, *Ann Thorac Surg* 71(5):1438, 2001.

Greer ME, Webb JP: For those who wait: care of the status 1 patient awaiting cardiac transplantation, *Crit Care Nurs Clin North Am* 12(1):49, 2000.

Griffith BP, Magliato KE: Heart-lung transplantation, *Op Tech Thorac Cardiovasc Surg* 4(2):124, 1999.

Hardy JD: *The world of surgery 1945-1985: memoirs of one participant,* Philadelphia, 1986, University of Pennsylvania Press.

Hardy JD: The transplantation of organs, *Surgery* 56:685, 1964.

Hobson JE: How the system functions: the roles of the United Network of Organ Sharing, the organ procurement and transplantation network, and the organ procurement organization in heart transplantation, *Crit Care Nurs Clin North Am* 12(1):11, 2000.

Hunt S: Reinnervation of the transplanted heart—why is it important? *N Engl J Med* 345(10):762, 2001.

Hunt SA, Schroeder JS, Berry GJ: Cardiac transplantation, mechanical ventricular support, and endomyocardial biopsy. In Fuster V, Alexander RW, O'Rourke RA, editors: *Hurst's the heart,* ed 10, vol 2, New York, 2001, McGraw-Hill.

Kiberd MC, Kiberd BA: Nursing attitudes towards organ donation, procurement, and transplantation, *Heart Lung* 21(2):106, 1992.

Konstantinov IE: A mystery of Vladimir P. Demikhov: the 50th anniversary of the first intrathoracic transplantation, *Ann Thorac Surg* 65(4):1171, 1998.

Krau SD: The evolution of heart transplantation, *Crit Care Nurs Clin North Am* 12(1):1, 2000.

Lefrak EA: Personal communication, 2001.

Lilly KT, Langley VL: The perioperative nurse and the organ donation experience, *AORN J* 69(4):779, 1999.

Lonchyna VA: Single lung transplantation, *Op Tech Thorac Cardiovasc Surg* 4(2):142, 1999.

Lower RR, Shumway NE: Studies on orthotopic homotransplantations of the canine heart, *Surg Forum* 11:18, 1960.

Macdonald SN, Naucke NA: Heart transplantation. In Smith SL: *Tissue and organ transplantation,* St Louis, 1990, Mosby.

Medawar PB: The behavior and fate of skin autografts and skin homografts in rabbits, *J Anat* 78:176, 1944.

Medicare and Medicaid Programs: Hospital conditions of participation; identification of potential organ, tissue, and eye donors and transplant hospitals' provision of transplant-related data, *Federal Register,* 63:33856, 1998.

Meyers BF, Patterson GA: Current status of lung transplantation, *Adv Surg* 34:301, 2000.

Meyers BF, Patterson GA: Bilateral lung transplantation, *Op Tech Thorac Cardiovasc Surg* 4(2):162, 1999.

Meyers, BF, Patterson GA: Technical aspects of adult lung transplantation, *Semin Thorac Cardiovasc Surg* 10(3):213, 1998.

Michler RE, Itescu S: Xenotransplantation: are we making any progress? Report on the 20th Annual Meeting and Scientific Sessions of the International Society for Heart and Lung Transplantation, 2000, http://www.medscape.com/medscape/cno/2000/ISHLT/Story.cfm?story_id=1157 (accessed April 30, 2000).

Miniati DN, Robbins RC, Reitz BA: Heart and heart-lung transplantation. In Braunwald E, Zipes DP, Libby P, editors: *Heart disease: a textbook of cardiovascular medicine,* ed 6, vol 2, Philadelphia, 2001, WB Saunders.

Perreas KG, Milano C, Wallwork J: Donor management tactics for cardiothoracic transplantation, *Transplant Rev* 14(2): 127, 2000.

Plante A, Bouchard L: Occupational stress, burnout and professional support in nurses working with dying patients, *Omega* 32(2):93, 1995.

Reitz BA: History of heart and heart-lung transplantation. In Baumgartner WA and others, editors: *Heart and lung transplantation*, Philadelphia, 2002, WB Saunders.

Reitz BA, Pennock JL, Shumway NE: Simplified operative method for heart and lung transplantation, *J Surg Res* 31(1):3, 1981.

Rickenbacher PR, Hunt SA: Long-term complications of transplantation. In Emery RW, Miller LW: *Handbook of cardiac transplantation*, St Louis, 1996, Mosby.

Riley LP, Coolican MB: Needs of families of organ donors: facing death and life, *Crit Care Nurs* 19(2):53, 1999.

Seifert PC: Cardiac surgery. In Rothrock JC: *Perioperative nursing care planning*, ed 2, St Louis, 1996, Mosby.

Shumway NE: Thoracic transplantation, *World J Surg* 24(7): 811, 2000.

Steen S and others: Transplantation of lungs from a non-heart beating donor, *Lancet* 357(9259)825, 2001.

Sullivan J, Seem DL, Chabalewski F: Determining brain death, *Crit Care Nurse* 19(2):37, 1999.

Szeto WY, Rosengard BR: Basic concepts in transplantation immunology and pharmacologic immunosuppression. In Baumgartner WA and others: *Heart and lung transplantation*, Philadelphia, 2002, WB Saunders.

Takashima S and others: Short-term inhaled nitric oxide in canine lung transplantation from non-heart-beating donor, *Ann Thorac Surg* 70(5):1679, 2000.

Thelan LA and others: *Critical care nursing: diagnosis and management*, ed 3, St Louis, 1998, Mosby.

Toronto Lung Transplant Group: Unilateral lung transplantation for pulmonary fibrosis, *N Engl J Med* 314:1140, 1986.

Uniform Determination of Death Act, 12 Uniform Laws Annotated (U.L.A.) 589, 1997.

United Network for Organ Sharing (UNOS): Critical data for 2000: U.S. facts about transplantation, 2000, http://www.unos.org (accessed August 25, 2001).

Van Bakel AB: The cardiac transplant donor: identification, assessment, and management, *Am J Med Sci* 314(3):153, 1997.

Wagner S, Hutchisson B, Baird MG: Cardiac explantation and autotransplantation, *AORN J* 70(1):99, 1999.

Waldhausen JA, Pierce WS: *Johnson's surgery of the chest*, ed 5, St Louis, 1985, Mosby.

Waldhausen JA, Pierce WS, Campbell DB: *Surgery of the chest*, ed 6, St Louis, 1996, Mosby.

Watson TJ, Starnes VA: Pediatric lobar lung transplantation, *Sem Thorac Cardiovasc Surg* 8(3):313, 1996.

Westaby S: *Landmarks in cardiac surgery*, Oxford, 1997, Isis Medical Media.

Wijdicks EFM: The diagnosis of brain death, *N Engl J Med* 344(16):1215, 2001.

Winkel E, Kao W, Costanzo MR: Pulmonary hypertension and cardiac transplantation. In Emery RW, Miller LW, editors: *Handbook of cardiac transplantation*, St Louis, 1996, Mosby.

17 Surgery for Cardiac Dysrhythmias

The heart is always marching, unless it misses signals from its conductor.

John Stone, MD, 1990 (p. 127)

Treat each day as if it were your last, and each patient as if he or she were your first.

Douglas P. Zipes, MD, 2001 (p. 1469)

Disorders affecting the electrical activity of the heart produce changes in the rate or rhythm of cardiac impulses. These disorders commonly are divided into those affecting impulse formation, those affecting impulse conduction, and a combination of the two (Rubart and Zipes, 2001). Historically patients with symptomatic, excessively slow heart rates (bradycardia) were first treated with pacemaker electrodes placed directly on the epicardial surface of the heart. Epicardial electrodes are still widely used for temporary pacing during the perioperative period, but transvenous pacemaker leads have largely supplanted epicardial pacemaker leads for permanent pacing (Samuels and Samuels, 2000).

Excessively fast heart rates (tachycardia) and those disorders that degenerate into ventricular fibrillation were first treated by Beck and his colleagues (Beck, Pritchard, and Fell, 1947), who used direct (internal) defibrillation of the heart. Within the next decade, Zoll and his associates (1956) successfully applied transthoracic direct current to defibrillate a patient. The clinical implantation of a permanent automatic defibrillator was first described by Mirowski and others (1980).

Corrective surgery on the heart itself for underlying dysrhythmias was introduced in 1968 when Sealy (Cobb and others, 1968) surgically divided an abnormal conduction pathway that was producing tachycardia in a patient with Wolff-Parkinson-White (WPW) syndrome. Early attempts to treat atrial fibrillation employed cryoablation techniques to control the irregular rhythm by creating a preferred pathway to the atrioventricular node for the electrical impulses. The concept of interrupting abnormal electrical circuits while permitting conduction of the normal sinus impulse was further developed by Cox and his colleagues (1991a; 1991b; 1991c) and led to the creation of a surgical cure called

the Maze procedure. Subsequent developments and refinements have been aided by a greater understanding of the anatomic and electrophysiologic principles of the conduction system. Advances in electrophysiologic diagnostic and therapeutic capabilities have expanded the use of both surgical procedures and percutaneous catheter interventions. In particular, pacemakers and internal defibrillators increasingly are inserted in the cardiac catheterization or electrophysiology (EP) laboratory. Whether in the EP or cardiac catheterization laboratory (or the operating room), patients have universal needs for safety, education, and the effective use of the array of sophisticated equipment and devices to treat dysrhythmias. Pacemakers and internal defibrillators are included in this chapter because an increasing number of perioperative nurses are caring for patients in the catheterization and EP laboratories.

Conduction System

The action of contraction and relaxation reflects the heart's conversion of electrical stimulation into mechanical work. The resulting pumping activity is performed in a regular pattern and at a sufficient rate to optimize cardiac output for the individual's hemodynamic needs. Disturbances in the initiation, rate, rhythm, or conduction of the electrical impulses that stimulate the myocardium can alter contractility, making the pumping action of the heart less efficient and tissue perfusion inadequate. Ventricular fibrillation, for example, is considered a lethal dysrhythmia because the uncoordinated impulses being discharged in the ventricle produce an unorganized ventricular contraction that is ineffectual in ejecting blood (Berne and Levy, 2001). However, minor rhythm disturbances are common, and those that do not interfere with cardiac output and are not life threatening may not require treatment. The severity of the dysrhythmia is determined by its effect on cardiac output and the clinical status of the patient.

Automatic and rhythmic beating of the heart begins early in embryonic life. During cardiogenesis two types of cardiac tissue develop: contractile cells of the myocardium that can respond to a stimulus and pacemaker cells capable of spontaneously initiating an electrical impulse that stimulates myocardial cells to contract. Al-

though all normal cardiac tissue is excitable (able to respond to an electrical stimulus), only pacemaker cells are capable normally of initiating the impulse without an outside stimulus (automaticity). When a cardiac impulse (also known as action potential) is generated, the heart's inherent conductivity allows it to be transmitted to other areas of the heart (Marriott and Conover, 1998; Box 17-1).

To understand why and how surgery and other invasive techniques are used to treat dysrhythmias, it is help-

---

BOX 17-1
Glossary of Terms

Aberrancy   Temporary, abnormal intraventricular conduction of a supraventricular impulse (e.g., a premature atrial beat conducted to the ventricle).

Accessory pathway   Extramuscular tract between the atrium and the ventricle, outside the normal conduction tract, that is capable of conducting an impulse, either antegrade or retrograde; seen in Wolff-Parkinson-White syndrome.

Action potential   Generation and transmission of an electrical impulse through the cell. It is a precise and rapid sequence of changes in the movement of transmembrane ionic currents (mainly sodium, calcium, and potassium) that represents the electrical cardiac cycle. It consists of five phases: phases 0 to 3 make up electrical systole, and phase 4 makes up electrical diastole.

   Phase 0   Rapid depolarization; the electrical gradient changes rapidly from approximately -65 mV to $+20$ mV as sodium rapidly enters the cell (fast sodium channels). Because it is a significant change, it appears on the electrocardiogram (ECG). Class I antidysrhythmic drugs (e.g., lidocaine, procainamide) are sodium channel blockers.

   Phase 1   Initial rapid repolarization of the cell caused by inactivation of sodium and calcium.

   Phase 2   Plateau of the action potential; results from the influx of calcium and sodium (slow channels). Class IV antidysrhythmic drugs (e.g., verapamil) block calcium influx.

   Phase 3   Terminal rapid repolarization phase that begins with closing of slow channels. It is completed by the passive movement of potassium out of the cell and the active transport of sodium out of the cell by the sodium pump. During this phase the electrical gradient (transmembrane potential) is returned to -65 mV. Because this is a major electrical change, it appears on the ECG. Activation can be initiated during this phase with a lessor stimulus than is required at maximum repolarization. Class III antidysrhythmic drugs (e.g., amiodarone) delay phases 2 and 3; these agents slow repolarization and prolong refractoriness, thereby making the myocardium less irritable.

   Phase 4   Slow depolarization of pacemaker cells produced by slow influx of sodium and potassium and calcium currents.

Anistropy   Propagation of an impulse along the axis of the fibers; much faster than across the axis of the fibers.

Automaticity   Capability of a cell to depolarize spontaneously, reach threshold potential, and initiate an action potential. Characteristic of pacemaker cells.

Altered automaticity   Ability of cells, not normally possessing the property of automaticity, to depolarize automatically.

Enhanced normal automaticity   Rapid automatic activity caused by steepening of phase 4 depolarization in pacemaker cells; can occur with excess catecholamines, especially in the presence of ischemia.

Circus movement tachycardia   Any reentry tachycardia; generally reserved for atrioventricular (AV) reentry using an accessory pathway and the AV node.

Conductivity   Ability of cardiac cells to receive an electrical stimulus and transmit it to other cells.

Depolarization   Reduction of a membrane potential to a less negative value.

Ectopy   Cardiac dysrhythmia caused by initiation of an excitation impulse at a site other than the sinus node; may occur in healthy and diseased hearts at a site of irritated myocardium.

Excitability   Ability of a cardiac cell to respond to an electrical stimulus; irritability.

Preexcitation   Activation of part of the ventricular myocardium earlier than would be expected if the activating impulses traveled only down the normal routes.

Reentry   Reactivation of a tissue for the second or subsequent time by the same impulse.

Refractory period   Period during which the cell (or fiber) is unable to respond normally to a stimulus because it has been activated too recently by a previous stimulus. During the *effective* refractory period, no stimulus can evoke a response; during the *relative* refractory period, a strong stimulus can evoke a response, but conduction velocity may be reduced through the AV node.

Repolarization   Restoration of the cell's resting membrane potential; occurs between phase 1 and the end of phase 3 of the action potential.

Resting membrane potential   Electrical gradient that exists between the inside and the outside of a myocardial cell at rest.

Rhythmicity   Ability of the heart to contract with regularity.

Threshold potential   Transmembrane potential (electrical gradient) that must be achieved before an action potential can be initiated.

Triggered activity   Rhythmic activity that results when a series of after-depolarizations reach threshold potential; can be induced by digitalis.

Modified from Marriott HJL, Conover MB: *Advanced concepts in arrhythmias,* ed 3, St Louis, 1998, Mosby; Doty JR: Cardiac arrhythmia—bradycardia [On-line], 2000a. Available: http://ctsnet.org/doc/4457 (accessed November 27, 2000); Doty JR: Cardiac arrhythmia—tachycardia [On-line], 2000b. Available: http://ctsnet.org/doc/4457 (accessed November 27, 2000).

ful to review how electrical impulses are normally generated and transmitted from the atria to the ventricles through the network of cells and fibers that make up the conduction system.

Conduction of Electrical Impulses

The conduction system comprises the sinoatrial (SA) node, the internodal pathways, the atrioventricular (AV) junction, the bundle of His and its right and left branches, and the Purkinje fibers. In the healthy heart these impulses travel from right to left and from head to toe. The electrocardiogram (ECG) provides a pictorial record of this electrical activity by registering potential changes in the electrical field of the heart (Fig. 17-1). The ECG does not record this electrical activity directly (that would require the placement of an electrode into the cell itself), nor does it represent the mechanical activity of the heart.

SINOATRIAL NODE

Impulses originate in the SA node, a mass of neuromuscular tissue lying between the entrance of the superior vena cava and the right atrium in the sulcus terminalis.

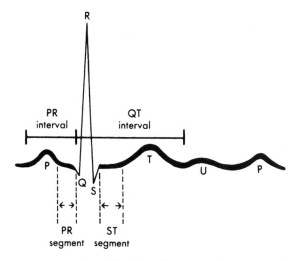

FIGURE 17-1 The deflections in a normal ECG are the P wave (atrial depolarization), QRS complex (ventricular depolarization), and T wave (ventricular repolarization). The U wave is sometimes present and follows the T wave. The PR segment is the interval between the end of the P wave and the beginning of the QRS complex. The ST segment is the interval between the end of the QRS complex and the beginning of the T wave. The PR interval is from the onset of the P wave to the onset of the QRS complex. The QT interval is from the onset of the QRS complex to the end of the T wave. (From Kinney MR, Packa DR, editors: *Andreoli's comprehensive cardiac care,* ed 8, St Louis, 1996, Mosby.)

The SA node receives its blood supply from the sinus node artery, which runs lengthwise through the center of the node. The nodal artery arises from the right coronary artery or, less commonly, from the left coronary artery. (Ischemic injury caused by obstructive lesions in the coronary artery supplying the SA node can cause nodal dysfunction.)

Electrophysiologic mapping of the right atrium has demonstrated a number of sites within the area of the SA node that can initiate impulses spontaneously. No single cell in the sinus node is thought to serve as the sole pacemaker. A number of cells probably discharge impulses that merge to form a single wavefront. Different types of cells have been identified. Pacemaker (P) cells (also called nodal cells) within the center of a pacemaker site initiate the action potential; surrounding transitional (T) cells conduct the impulse to the atrial tissue and atrial muscle cells, which extend as peninsulas into the nodal boundaries. Collectively these sites serve as an *atrial pacemaker complex* (Berne and Levy, 2001). Because the SA node generates impulses at a faster rate (approximately 60 to 100 beats per minute) than other neuromuscular tissues of the heart, it excites other potential pacemakers before they can reach the threshold necessary to spontaneously depolarize themselves and initiate an impulse (Rubart and Zipes, 2001). As a result, the SA node suppresses the automatic generation of impulses by other (potential) pacemaker sites, such as the AV junction (which has an intrinsic rate of approximately 40 to 60 impulses per minute) and the ventricular fibers (approximately 20 to 40 impulses per minute). Because of the higher rate of impulse formation, the normal SA node acts as the primary pacemaker of the heart and the main controller of the heart rate. Conversely, when the sinus node does not generate impulses at a sufficiently rapid rate, it does not suppress latent pacemakers. One or more of these may reach threshold and depolarize to take over the function of the primary pacemaker.

From the atrial pacemaker complex the impulse is conducted radially throughout the right atrium. The anterior internodal myocardial band enters the interatrial band (Bachmann's bundle), which conducts the impulse from the SA node directly to the left atrium. Conduction of the impulse from the SA node to the AV node is thought to occur over three groups of internodal tissue: the anterior, middle, and posterior internodal pathways, collectively referred to as internodal atrial myocardium. These pathways do not appear to be histologically discreet tracts like those that make up the bundle branches. Preferential nodal conduction is thought to be related more to fiber orientation (anistropy) and size rather than to specialized tracts (Rubart and Zipes, 2001).

ATRIOVENTRICULAR JUNCTION

The AV node, situated between the atria and the ventricles, is composed of three regions. (1) The atrionodal (AN) region is located between the atrium and the anatomic AV node; this also is referred to as the transitional zone. (2) The nodal (N) region, also known as the compact portion, corresponds to the AV node and is located posteriorly on the right side of the interatrial septum near the coronary sinus and directly above the insertion of the septal leaflet of the tricuspid valve. (3) The nodal-His (NH) region is situated between the N region and the bundle of His (Paul, 2001). Collectively these three regions, along with the bundle of His, are called the AV junction (Fig. 17-2). Cardiac rhythms formerly classified as *nodal* are now more appropriately considered *junctional*. Blood flow to the AV junction is received from a branch of the right coronary artery in most individuals (Marriott and Conover, 1998).

What is physiologically and clinically significant about the AV node itself is the reduction in velocity of the impulse that occurs in this area. This is because of the fibrotic nature of the tissue, which, unlike faster conducting myocardial cells, impedes the speed of the impulse. This delay (seen on the ECG between the P wave and the QRS complex) allows the atria to contract and the ventricles to fill. This delay also protects the ventricle when there are excessively rapid atrial impulses. Without the delay, too many of these impulse would be conducted to the ventricles, producing excessive contractions and limiting ventricular filling (Paul, 2001). Another mechanism occurring in the normal heart that protects the ventricle from excessive contractions is that the AV node allows only a fraction of the atrial impulses to traverse the junctional region (Berne and Levy, 2001).

Of surgical significance is the location of the AV junction, which is contained within the triangle of

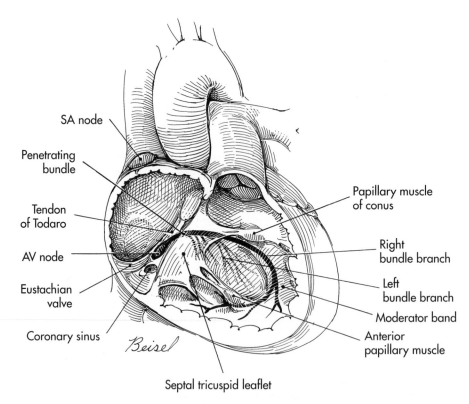

FIGURE 17-2 Anatomic landmarks used during surgery on the conduction system. The AV node lies at the apex of the triangle of Koch, which is formed by the tendon of Todaro, the tricuspid valve annulus, and the coronary sinus (the base of the triangle). The penetrating bundle of His passes through the central fibrous body into the septum, staying at the inferior border of the membranous septum on the left side. The branching portion gives off the fasciculi of the posterior radiation of the left bundle branch. At its bifurcation it then divides into the right bundle and the anterior radiation of the left bundle branch. The right bundle branch passes to the right side of the septum and goes to the anterolateral papillary muscle (moderator band). Conduction tissue does not extend beyond the papillary muscle of the conus (medial papillary muscle). (From Waldhausen JA, Pierce WS, Campbell DB: *Surgery of the chest,* ed 6, St Louis, 1996, Mosby.)

Koch, an anatomically discreet region bordered by the tricuspid valve annulus, the tendon of Todaro, and the thebesian valve of the coronary sinus (Fig. 17-3; see Fig. 17-2). This triangular area is carefully avoided during cardiac procedures to prevent iatrogenic injury to the conduction system (Skubas and others, 1999).

Accessory pathways

In most persons AV junctional tissue and the bundle of His provide the only pathway for impulses traveling from the atrium to the ventricles. In some persons alternative routes (accessory pathways) exist between the atria and the ventricles that can allow impulses to travel not only in a forward normal (antegrade) fashion but also in a backward (retrograde) or circular direction. These accessory pathways are thought to be the result of a developmental failure to interrupt the AV myocardial continuity present in the primitive heart and are related to gestational development.

During the early stages of development there is a discrete ring of muscle fibers surrounding the AV junction. This ring becomes fibrotic, thereby slowing conduction velocity between the upper and lower cardiac chambers. When the continuity of some fibers fails to be divided, one or more pathways remain, in addition to the AV node and bundle of His, through which an impulse can pass from atria to ventricles. Often these conduct faster than the AV node because they are made up of working myocardium, which offers less resistance to the impulse than AV nodal tissue. These accessory pathways may be responsible for conducting impulses that can prematurely excite the ventricles (preexcitation) and produce lethal dysrhythmias. Some impulses may be delayed in one of the pathways and reenter the circuit, thereby self-perpetuating the impulse (see subsequent section on reentry). Catheter ablation using radiofrequency waves, cryosurgery, or direct severing of these accessory pathways can be performed. Patients with WPW syndrome, the most common form of preexcitation, often benefit from ablation therapy.

VENTRICULAR CONDUCTION

Cells in the NH region gradually merge with the bundle of His, which forms the upper portion of the ventricular conduction system. The bundle is situated along the right side and the top of the ventricular septum (near the septal leaflet of the tricuspid valve). It

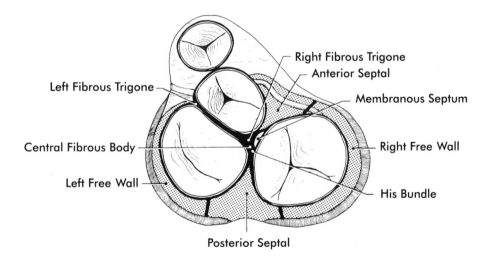

FIGURE 17-3 Diagram of the superior view of heart with the atria cut away, demonstrating the boundaries of each of the four anatomic areas where accessory pathways can occur in Wolff-Parkinson-White syndrome. The boundaries of the left free wall space are the mitral valve annulus and the ventricular endocardial reflection extending from the left fibrous trigone to the posterior septum. The boundaries of the posterior septal space are the tricuspid valve annulus, the mitral valve annulus, the posterior superior process of the left ventricle, and the ventricular epicardial reflection. The boundaries of the right free wall space are the tricuspid valve annulus and the epicardial reflection extending from the posterior septum to the anterior septum. The boundaries of the anterior septal space are the tricuspid valve annulus, the membranous portion of the interatrial septum, and the ventricular epicardial reflection. All accessory connections must insert into the ventricle somewhere within these anatomic boundaries. (From Cox JL, Gallagher JJ, Cain, ME: Experience with 118 consecutive patients undergoing operation for the Wolff-Parkinson-White syndrome, *J Thorac Cardiovasc Surg* 90[4]:490, 1985.)

then divides into a right bundle and a left bundle. The right bundle follows the right side of the septum. The left bundle penetrates the septum and further divides into an anterior and a posterior division, or fascicle (Mirvis and Goldberger, 2001). Right or left bundle-branch block occurs when transmission is delayed or interrupted in the respective main bundle branch; left anterior or left posterior hemiblock refers to conduction blocks within the respective left bundle branches (fascicles).

The right and left bundle branches subdivide into the Purkinje fibers, which penetrate the subendocardium of each ventricle. Conduction is most rapid through the Purkinje system, allowing rapid activation of the ventricles. The Purkinje system also plays a protective role in limiting the number of atrial impulses that can stimulate ventricular contraction. It can accomplish this because the Purkinje fibers have a long refractory period during which they will not respond to further excitation. Consequently they will not normally allow premature contractions of the ventricles. When there are accessory pathways or other AV connections that bypass the AV node, rapidly firing impulses can be transmitted to the ventricles, producing ventricular tachycardia. Transmission of the impulses over the ventricles begins with the left and then the right endocardial surface of the interventricular septum (except the basal portion) and the papillary muscles. (Early papillary muscle contraction helps to tether the mitral and tricuspid valve leaflets so that they do not evert into their respective atria during ventricular systole.)

The impulse rapidly spreads along the endocardial surface of both ventricles. It spreads less rapidly from endocardium to epicardium, especially in a hypertrophied left ventricular wall. The basal epicardial and septal regions are activated last (Mirvis and Goldberger, 2001).

Atrial repolarization follows a path similar to atrial depolarization. Ventricular repolarization occurs in the opposite direction, beginning at the epicardium (where ventricular depolarization ended) and finishing at the endocardium (Mirvis and Goldberger, 2001).

FACTORS INFLUENCING THE INITIATION OR CONDUCTION OF IMPULSES

In addition to intrinsic disturbances of cardiac tissue, electrical events can be modified by chamber geometry (such as left ventricular hypertrophy or atrial septal defect), autonomic nervous system influences, hemodynamics, blood flow, wall motion changes, electrolyte abnormalities, drugs, surgical trauma and edema, and ischemic heart disease.

Both sympathetic (adrenergic) and parasympathetic fibers of the autonomic system can modify the generation and transmission of impulses. The sympathetic system directly affects both atria and ventricles by stimulating an increase in the rate and conduction of impulse and augmenting the force of atrial and ventricular contractions. It also increases the excitability of the heart. The parasympathetic system has less control over the ventricles, but the vagus branches do influence the sinus node and the AV junction by causing a reduction in the rate of discharge from the SA node, decreasing the excitability of the AV junctional fibers and further slowing conduction through the AV node. Increased heart rates are usually the result of decreased vagus tone (e.g., as can be produced pharmacologically with atropine) rather than increased sympathetic activity (Rubart and Zipes, 2001).

It is likely that the autonomic nervous system may have competitive effects on cardiac rhythm. For example, sympathetic stimuli may be antidysrhythmic by improving contractility and coronary blood flow in a failing heart; however, the increase in myocardial oxygen demand accompanying increased contractility in a heart with ischemic coronary artery disease may promote the development of cardiac dysrhythmias. The effects of sympathetic stimulation may explain why anxiety and psychologic stress can be significant factors in the onset of ventricular fibrillation (Zipes, 1997a). An awareness of this interaction offers an important rationale for providing emotional support and comfort measures in the anxious patient.

The electrophysiologic effects of coronary ischemia can be especially deleterious because inadequate blood flow alters regional myocardial pH, potassium, calcium, and other electrolyte levels and the concentration of metabolic end-products. Infarction or ischemic injury to conducting tissue alters the ability to generate or conduct impulses and is responsible for a number of supraventricular and ventricular dysrhythmias. Surgical interruption or pharmacologic blockade of efferent sympathetic responses can be used to control the dysrhythmias; catheter ablation is under investigation.

Surgery can produce direct trauma or tissue injury (such as edema) leading to temporary (or permanent) conduction blocks. Surgery on the tricuspid valve, repairs of congenital anomalies involving the atrial septum, and other operations in areas containing conduction tissue pose a risk of injury. The surgical division of accessory pathways may also produce conduction blocks (requiring permanent pacemaker).

Although the nervous system does affect heart rate and contractility, intact nervous pathways are not required for the heart to function, as cardiac transplant patients with denervated hearts have demonstrated. This is because the heart is capable of initiating its own impulse, responding to that impulse, and doing so with regularity. These reflect, respectively, the characteristics of automaticity, excitability, and rhythmicity (see Box 17-1).

Categorizing Dysrhythmias

Rhythm disturbances may be classified as major dysrhythmias (which require treatment) and minor dysrhythmias (which may not); supraventricular dysrhythmias (above the ventricle, specifically above the bundle of His) and ventricular dysrhythmias; and bradydysrhythmias (slow heart rates) and tachydysrhythmias (fast heart rates). The pathogenesis of these disturbances is attributed to disorders of *impulse formation,* such as abnormal automaticity and triggered activity, and disorders of *impulse conduction,* such as block and reentry mechanisms (see Box 17-1; Rubart and Zipes, 2001).

ABNORMAL AUTOMATICITY

Abnormal automaticity is caused either by enhancement of normal automaticity or by the development of abnormal automaticity in both pacemaker cells and nonpacemaker cells as a result of certain disease states. Enhanced automaticity may develop in the sinus node or His-Purkinje fibers. For example, sympathetic nervous system activity with increased catecholamine release can alter sinus node automaticity to produce sinus tachycardia. Such stimulation can be related to strong emotions, such as fear or anxiety, or to emotional tension. Additional factors include exercise, fever, anemia, hyperthyroidism, myocardial disease, or anoxia. Medications such as atropine, isoproterenol, or epinephrine also may enhance automaticity. Excessive vagal tone may depress automaticity and produce sinus bradycardia. Depressed sinus function also can allow lower centers, such as the bundle of His, to fire impulses faster and thereby usurp the sinus node as the primary pacemaker.

Abnormal automaticity producing dysrhythmias occurs in working atrial or ventricular myocardium cells and pacemaker cells. A declining membrane potential enables the cell membrane to reach threshold prematurely, resulting in a spontaneous depolarization. Often this is related to disease or metabolic derangements such as ischemia, infarction, cardiomyopathy, hypokalemia, or hypocalcemia (Rubart and Zipes, 2001).

TRIGGERED ACTIVITY

Triggered activity is another disorder of impulse formation producing dysrhythmias. Triggered impulses are those that are repetitively fired during or after the repolarization phase of an ectopic cell. If the cell reaches threshold potential during the period when the calcium or sodium channels are activated, it can be "triggered" to depolarize (again) spontaneously. Excess digitalis or catecholamines are often the cause of this mechanism; other factors include ischemia, increased ventricular wall tension (e.g., from the pressure overload of aortic stenosis), and heart failure (Marriott and Conover, 1998).

BLOCK

Conduction delay and block can produce either bradydysrhythmia or tachydysrhythmia (Rubart and Zipes, 2001). Slow rates can result when the impulse is stopped and is followed by a slow escape rhythm (e.g., an intrinsically slower ventricular beat.) Impulses can be slowed or blocked when cellular membranes impede the velocity of conduction or when the strength of the impulse itself is not strong enough to propagate the impulse. Fast heart rates can result when the blocked impulse allows reentry to occur (see the following).

REENTRY

The reentry mechanism (Fig. 17-4) is responsible for sustaining the majority of ventricular dysrhythmias, such as ventricular tachycardia, and supraventricular dysrhythmias, such as supraventricular tachycardia,

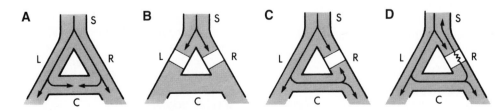

FIGURE 17-4 Reentry and the role of unidirectional block. **A,** An excitation wave traveling down a single bundle *(S)* of fibers continues down the left *(L)* and right *(R)* branches. The depolarization wave enters the connecting branch *(c)* from both ends and is extinguished at the zone of collision. **B,** The wave is blocked in branches *L* and *R*. **C,** Bidirectional blocks exists in branch *R*. **D,** Unidirectional block exists in branch *R*. The antegrade impulse is blocked, but the retrograde impulse is conducted through and reenters bundle *S* (see text). (From Berne RM, Levy MN: *Cardiovascular physiology,* ed 8, St Louis, 2001, Mosby.)

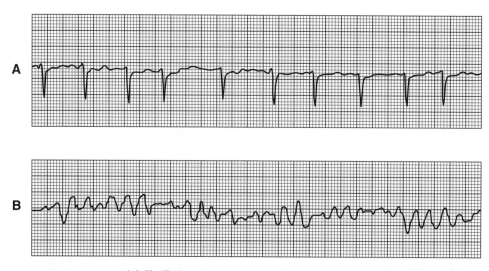

FIGURE 17-5 **A,** Atrial fibrillation. **B,** Ventricular fibrillation. (From Berne RM, Levy MN: *Cardiovascular physiology,* ed 8, St Louis, 2001, Mosby.)

atrial flutter, and atrial fibrillation. Reentry occurs when a cardiac impulse restimulates a portion of the heart that has already been stimulated. Three conditions are necessary: an additional circuit (e.g., an accessory pathway), unequal responsiveness in the limbs of the circuit, and slow conduction (Berne and Levy, 2001). For example, a descending impulse enters two limbs of a circuit: the normal AV route and an accessory pathway. When one limb has recovered while the other remains refractory, the refractory limb prevents passage of the impulse when it first approaches; the wave front travels only down the responsive limb. (If both limbs were still refractory, the impulse would be arrested; if both limbs had recovered, the impulse would have continued. In either case, reentry could not occur.)

When the wave front reaches the distal end of the refractory limb and that region has had time to recover, the impulse is transmitted backward through the previously refractory portion and arrives at the original forking point. The two pathways available to the impulse also have recovered by now and accept the impulse. It is as though a new impulse has originated from the forking point, but actually it is still the sinus impulse starting a second wave front. This mechanism creates a reciprocal rhythm that produces a circulating wave, or *circus movement.*

PROCEDURAL CONSIDERATIONS

A practical way to categorize disturbances of rhythm and conduction is to divide them into bradydysrhythmias and tachydysrhythmias that are supraventricular or ventricular. Determination of their origin is important because prognosis and treatment differ. Supraventricular dysrhythmias, such as sinus tachycardia, atrial fibrillation (Fig. 17-5), or premature atrial complexes, originate in

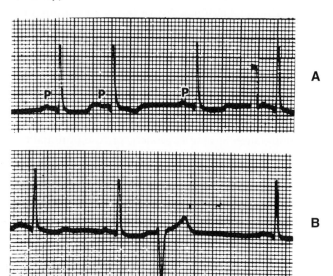

FIGURE 17-6 **A,** Premature atrial depolarization. **B,** Premature ventricular depolarization. The premature atrial depolarization (the second beat in the *top tracing*) is characterized by an inverted P wave and normal QRS and T waves. The interval following the premature depolarization is not much longer than the usual interval between beats. The brief rectangular deflection just before the last depolarization is a standardization signal. The premature ventricular depolarization **(B)** is characterized by bizarre QRS and T waves and is followed by a compensatory pause. (From Berne RM, Levy MN: *Cardiovascular physiology,* ed 8, St Louis, 2001, Mosby.)

the atrium or AV junction. Electrophysiologically these are generally characterized by normal (narrow) QRS complexes. Ventricular dysrhythmias, such as ventricular tachycardia or fibrillation, or premature ventricular complexes, commonly produce a bizarre (wide) QRST

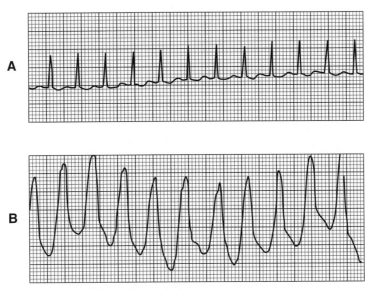

FIGURE 17-7 **A,** Supraventricular tachycardia. **B,** Ventricular tachycardia. (From Berne RM, Levy MN: *Cardiovascular physiology,* ed 8, St Louis, 2001, Mosby.)

complex that has a prolonged QRS interval (Rubart and Zipes, 2001). Fig. 17-6 illustrates this difference by comparing premature atrial complexes and premature ventricular complexes; Fig. 17-7 demonstrates differences between supraventricular tachycardia and ventricular tachycardia. The tachydysrhythmias are of special concern because they can result in life-threatening symptoms such as hypotension, syncope, or pulmonary edema. Persistent ventricular tachycardia can degenerate into ventricular fibrillation (see Fig. 17-5), causing sudden death. These dysrhythmias, usually caused by abnormal mechanisms (e.g., altered automaticity, triggered activity, and reentry), may be evaluated with a number of diagnostic tests.

Diagnostic Evaluation of Dysrhythmias

After taking a careful history of the patient, the physician orders noninvasive diagnostic tests. The most common is the 12-lead resting ECG; an exercise ECG and ambulatory (Holter) monitoring also may be performed (Table 17-1). These tests are used to detect significant episodes of ectopic activity, ventricular tachycardia, and asystole. Rhythm disturbances are fairly uncommon in healthy young persons, but certain dysrhythmias, such as premature ventricular contractions (PVCs), are not necessarily abnormal. Recent studies have even raised the possibility that PVCs may be a *marker* for patients at risk of sudden death, rather than being causally related to sudden death—the PVC may be unrelated to the tachydysrhythmia producing sudden death (Rubart and Zipes, 2001).

Other noninvasive electrocardiographic techniques are available, although they may be employed less frequently. They may be used to identify the risk for sudden death, to distinguish supraventricular from ventricular tachycardias, to localize the site of the rhythm disturbance, and to identify the causes of syncope.

Esophageal electrocardiography is performed by placing an electrode into the esophagus, which is adjacent to the posterior atria. Atrial recordings with this technique can point to the origin of the dysrhythmias. Atrial (and occasionally ventricular) pacing also can be achieved with a catheter electrode in the esophagus.

Atrial ECGs can be performed with the temporary epicardial pacing wires implanted in cardiac surgery patients. Disturbances of rate and rhythm (especially atrial fibrillation) are common postoperatively, and atrial ECGs can be used to diagnose and plan treatment for sinus abnormalities, atrial fibrillation or flutter, and sinus or junctional tachycardias. For differentiating the origin of rapid heart rates, atrial ECGs are especially valuable because they enable the clinician to select the most appropriate therapy.

SIGNAL-AVERAGED ELECTROCARDIOGRAPHY

Signal-averaged ECG is used for patients at risk for sudden cardiac death from ventricular dysrhythmias. Signal averaging enables detection of low-amplitude waveforms in the ECG that are normally masked by muscle movement and electronic "noise" from amplifiers and electrodes. These low-amplitude signals are called *late potentials,* occurring at the end of or just after the QRS complex. They are thought to originate from

TABLE 17-1
Evaluation Before Electrophysiologic Testing*

PROCEDURE	PURPOSE
History and physical	Identify signs/symptoms of cardiac or neurologic disease
	Identify factors known to exacerbate arrhythmias
	Details of syncopal events
Neurologic evaluation (if history and physical suggest)	
EEG	Rule out seizure disorder
CT/MRI	Identify focal lesion
Carotid ultrasound	Identify significant cerebrovascular disease
12-lead ECG	Previous myocardial infarction
	Intraventricular conduction delays
	Prolonged QT interval
	Preexcitation syndromes
24- to 48-hr ambulatory electrocardiography	Correlation of symptoms with electrocardiographic events
	Quantitation of ambient ectopy
	Diurnal variation in arrhythmia
Event recorder	Correlation of symptoms with electrocardiographic events
Head-up tilt table testing	Diagnose vasovagal/vasodepressor syncope
Echocardiogram/radionucleotide ventriculography	Assessment of left ventricular and right ventricular size and function
	Detect valvular pathology
Stress test (with or without perfusion scanning)	Detect reversible ischemia
	Assess effects of catecholamines on arrhythmia induction
Cardiac catheterization	Define coronary anatomy

ECG, Electrocardiogram; *EEG*, electroencephalogram; *CT*, computed tomography; *MRI*, magnetic resonance imaging.
*Selected procedures may vary depending on the clinical presentation.
From Kern MJ: *The cardiac catheterization handbook*, ed 3, St Louis, 1999, Mosby.

damaged (e.g., infarcted) areas of myocardium, which conduct more slowly than normal tissue. The resulting delayed conduction provides one of the requirements for reentry ventricular tachycardia, which can lead to sudden death.

A computer-based technique is used to combine hundreds of QRS complexes. Noise is canceled, and a high-resolution signal is created and amplified to detect late potentials.

Electrophysiologic studies

EP testing is an invasive procedure performed with multipolar catheter electrodes introduced into the venous or arterial system and threaded into the heart. The catheter electrodes can be positioned in the atria or ventricles to test the regions of the His bundle, bundle branches, accessory pathways, and other structures (Chambers, Skeehan, and Hensley, 1999). EP catheter interventions to treat dysrhythmias have become the first-line management for many rhythm disorders. Increasingly, pharmacologic therapy can be avoided when correction of the dysrhythmia by EP intervention can be accomplished.

In addition to diagnostic and therapeutic interventions (Box 17-2), EP testing also can be employed to evaluate therapy and to identify patients at risk for sudden cardiac death (Chambers, Skeehan, and Hensley,

1999). The interpretation of EP tests (as with many other tests) may be complicated by false-negative responses (not finding a specific abnormality known to be present) or false positive responses (inducing a dysrhythmia with little or no clinical significance).

Less common is the use of the upright tilt-table test. When the test is used, it is performed with the patient in the supine position on a tilt table. The patient is tilted upright to a maximum of 60 to 80 degrees for 20 to 45 minutes in order to stimulate syncope and to differentiate between cardioinhibitory and vasopressor causes of the syncope. In many centers, EP testing has largely replaced the tilt-table test.

EP testing commonly is performed in the EP laboratory or in the cardiac catheterization laboratory if there is not a dedicated EP laboratory (Fig. 17-8). It also can be performed in the operating room (OR) in conjunction with surgical procedures affecting the conduction system (e.g., internal defibrillator insertion or ablation procedures); the initial diagnosis is frequently made in the EP laboratory.

Although bradydysrhythmias and tachydysrhythmias can be diagnosed initially with an ECG, EP studies are valuable for distinguishing between, for example, an intrinsic conduction abnormality of the sinus node and an autonomic nervous system dysfunction (such as excessive vagal tone) producing bradycardia. In addition to

---

BOX **17-2**
Clinical Applications of Electrophysiologic Studies

Diagnostic

Diagnose sinus node dysfunction
Determine site of AV nodal block
Define cause of syncope of unclear etiology
Differentiate VT from SVT in cases of wide complex tachycardia
Define mechanism of SVT or VT and map site of origin of tachycardia

Therapeutic

Guide drug therapy for sustained VT, aborted sudden death or SVT
Select appropriate candidates for cardioverter-defibrillator and antitachycardic pacing therapy
Test efficacy or device therapy for ventricular tachyarrhythmias
Select appropriate candidates for catheter ablative and surgical therapy
Test efficacy of ablative and surgical therapies

Interventional

AV nodal ablation or modification for atrial fibrillation
Ablation for atrial tachycardia and atrial flutter
AV nodal modification (slow-pathway or fast-pathway ablation)
Accessory pathway ablation in WPW
Ablation of ventricular tachycardia

Prognostic

Risk stratification in asymptomatic WPW
Risk stratification in patients post–myocardial infarction
Risk stratification in patients with nonsustained VT

VT, Ventricular tachycardia; *SVT,* supraventricular tachycardia; *WPW,* Wolff-Parkinson-White syndrome.
From Kern MJ: *The cardiac catheterization handbook,* ed 3, St Louis, 1999, Mosby.

---

obtaining intracardiac electrograms, electrophysiologists attempt to reproduce the clinical dysrhythmia in order to uncover the causes of the disturbance and to institute treatment. This is accomplished with programmed electrical stimulation (PES) to initiate and terminate dysrhythmias.

Often potentially dangerous dysrhythmias, such as ventricular tachycardia, are induced. As a precaution in the event the EP catheters are unable to revert to a slower, normal heart rate, external defibrillator patches are applied to patients undergoing PES. Defibrillation capability must be verified before the start of the EP test. When applying patches (or paddles), the nurse should ensure that they are applied in such a way that the defibrillation current can cross the left ventricle. Patch placement may be the right shoulder–left ventricular apex (near the left midclavicular line), anteroposterior to the left ventricle, or some other configuration that allows current to reach the left ventricle. (In the OR, external paddles may be indicated when adhesive pads interfere with the sterile field.) Backup equipment should be available, and personnel directly involved with patient care should be thoroughly familiar with the use of both external defibrillator adhesive pads and external defibrillator paddles.

Patient safety considerations mandate that all equipment for emergency resuscitation be available (Miller and Zipes, 2001). Emergency drugs and supplies for assisted ventilation also should be present, along with oxygen and suction.

PES is a sterile procedure with the patient prepped and draped to expose the catheter entry sites. Usually both femoral veins and arteries are used; internal jugular and subclavian sites also may be used. Arterial pressure is measured with a catheter in the femoral artery; the femoral veins are used most commonly for the electrode

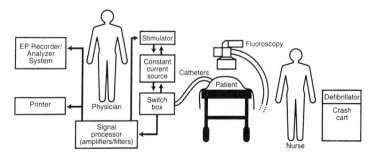

FIGURE 17-8 General setup of the equipment used for electrophysiologic studies. (From Kern MJ: *The cardiac catheterization handbook,* ed 3, St Louis, 1999, Mosby.)

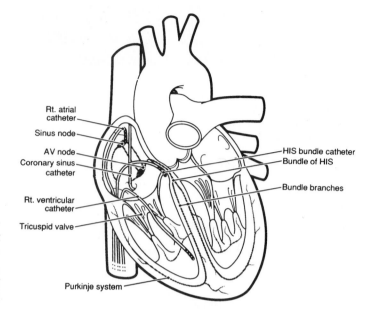

FIGURE 17-9 The catheter positions for routine electrophysiologic study are shown positioned in the high right atrium near the sinus node, in the area of the atrioventricular node and His bundle, in the right ventricular apex, and in the coronary sinus. (From Kern MJ: *The cardiac catheterization handbook,* ed 3, St Louis, 1999, Mosby.)

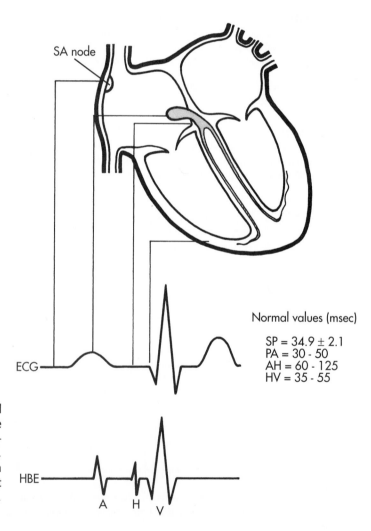

FIGURE 17-10 Electrical events in the heart as related to surface ECG and His bundle electrogram *(HBE).* The approximate relationship of SA node discharge is also related to surface ECG. *SP,* SA conduction time. *PA,* Intraatrial conduction time; *AH,* AV nodal conduction time; *HV,* His-Purkinje conduction time. (From Marriott HJL, Conover MB: *Advanced concepts in arrhythmias,* ed 3, St Louis, 1998, Mosby.)

catheters. Baseline measurements are taken of the conduction times between sections of the conduction pathway. Multipolar electrode catheters are inserted to permit stimulation and recording from each catheter (Fig. 17-9). Each electrode is connected to monitors or recorders and to the stimulator. Catheter electrodes commonly are positioned in the high right atrium, low right atrium, coronary sinus, and right ventricular apex and along the bundle of His. The electrodes can simultaneously stimulate, pace, and record activities at these various sites to produce an EP map of the heart. Programmed stimulation is used to induce or reproduce the clinical dysrhythmias and to define its underlying electrical basis. Pacing capability is used to suppress or overdrive the dysrhythmia.

Bundle of His recordings (Fig. 17-10) provide valuable information in differentiating supraventricular causes of ventricular disturbances from ventricular ones. Impulses originating in the atrium are reflected in recordings of bundle of His activity, whereas ectopic ventricular foci do not produce bundle of His activation.

EP testing in general (and PES in particular) tends to take longer than a diagnostic cardiac catheterization with or without angioplasty and stent insertion. Physical and emotional comfort measures, interventions to protect skin integrity, and patient education promote a successful result.

Intraoperative electrophysiologic studies. When surgical repair for dysrhythmias is indicated, intraoperative electrophysiologic mapping is employed to locate, for example, accessory pathways that may not have been identified during preoperative EP studies. Computerized intraoperative mapping systems can record multiple electrograms simultaneously. Often this technique obviates the need for cardiopulmonary bypass (CPB), thus eliminating its potentially deleterious sequelae; allows rapid and accurate identification of dysrhythmias; and minimizes cardiac manipulation during mapping. Cardiac mapping is performed after cannulation for CPB (but before CPB is initiated) with a nylon mesh band containing multiple electrodes. The band is placed on the atrium or the ventricle and electrograms are taken of the heart. The information is put through a computer, and a graphic display is created to guide the surgeon (Skubas and others, 1999). When the endocardial surfaces (such as the inside of the right atrium) are studied, a handheld probe electrode can be used.

THERAPY FOR DYSRHYTHMIAS

Pharmacologic therapy

Antidysrhythmia drugs are selected according to their mechanism of action (Table 17-2) and may be used for either ventricular or supraventricular rhythm disturbances. Because all have side effects of varying severity, their use has decreased as the number (and success) of percutaneous procedures has increased.

Amiodarone has been employed frequently to treat refractory supraventricular and ventricular dysrhythmias (Gonzalez, Kannewurk, and Ornato, 1998). The drug slows SA nodal firing and AV nodal conduction time and prolongs the refractory period in the AV node, the atria, and the ventricles. However, it has a number of serious side effects and a long half-life. Consequently the drug is not used in patients with asymptomatic ventricular tachycardia of short duration. Side effects

TABLE 17-2
Classification of Antidysrhythmic Drugs

GENERIC NAME	CLASS	COMMENTS
		Class I drugs change the sodium ion influx that allows the cells to depolarize
Quinidine	IA	Class IA drugs slow conduction and prolong refractoriness
Procainamide	IA	
Disopyramide	IA	
Lignocaine	IB	Class IB drugs shorten the refractory period
Mexiletine	IB	
Flecainide	IC	Class IC drugs slow conduction without changing refractoriness
Encainide	IC	
Propafenone	IC	
Propranolol	II	Class II drugs are adrenergic blockers
Acebutolol	II	
Atenolol	II	
Amiodarone	III	Class III drugs prolong refractoriness
Sotalol	III	
Verapamil	IV	Class IV drugs block calcium influx
Diltiazem	IV	

Modified from Doty JR: Cardiac arrhythmia—tachycardia [On-line], 2000b. Available: http://ctsnet.org/doc/4458 (accessed November 27, 2000).

include SA node blockade, bradycardia, myocardial depression, pulmonary toxicity, and hypotension.

Recently the use of intravenous amiodarone has been shown to be more effective than lidocaine in improving survival in patients with out-of-hospital cardiac arrest because of shock refractory (e.g., the failure of three or more defibrillation attempts) ventricular fibrillation or tachycardia (Kudenchuk and others, 1999). Amiodarone is now recommended as a first-line therapy for the management of ventricular fibrillation and pulseless ventricular tachycardia (Guidelines, 2000; Eisenberg and Mengert, 2001).

Amiodarone (in combination with beta blocker medications) also has been studied for prophylaxis against atrial fibrillation after cardiac surgery (Giri and others, 2001). Patients receiving oral amiodarone for a few days before surgery demonstrated a lower incidence of AF postoperatively (compared with those receiving a placebo), but the potential disadvantages of preoperative amiodarone (e.g., risk of pulmonary toxicity, bradycardia) necessitate further investigation (Bharucha and Kowey, 2000).

NONPHARMACOLOGIC THERAPY

Because of the serious complications and suboptimal efficacy associated with many dysrhythmia drugs, nonpharmacologic therapy has become the treatment of choice for an increasing number of conduction disorders (Finkelmeier, 2000). Among the various forms of treatment are ablative therapy; surgical interruption, isolation, or excision of dysrhythmogenic myocardial tissue; and pacemaker and implantable defibrillator insertion.

Ablation therapy

Endocardial catheter ablation is performed most commonly with radiofrequency (RF) energy; lasers and cryogenic devices are less frequently used. RF energy produces thermal injury to the targeted tissue. One of the advantages of RF energy is that it creates small, discrete lesions that reduce the risk of injury to tangential normal tissue (Fig. 17-11; Morady, 1999; Miller and Zipes, 2001).

Ablation techniques often are performed in patients with AV reentry tachycardias (e.g., WPW syndrome). The precise location of the dysrhythmic focus is identified and ablated percutaneously in the EP laboratory. The ablation catheter is maneuvered into position, and the energy source is activated to destroy the selected tissue. When AV junctional ablation is performed, complete AV block may develop, necessitating permanent pacemaker insertion. Other complications include ventricular tachycardia and fibrillation, thromboembolism,

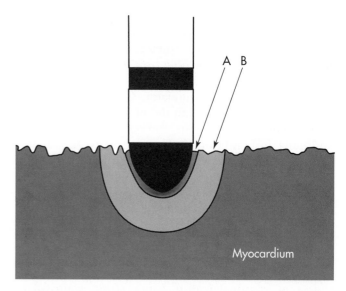

FIGURE 17-11 Mechanism of heating during radiofrequency catheter ablation. Because current density drops off rapidly as a function of distance from the electrode surface, only a small shell of myocardium adjacent to the distal electrode (*A*) is heated directly. The major portion of the lesion (*B*) is produced by conduction of heat away from the electrode-tissue interface into surrounding tissue. (From Langberg JJ, Leon A: Energy sources for catheter ablation. In Zipes DP, Jalife J, editors: *Cardiac electrophysiology: from cell to bedside,* ed 2, Philadelphia, 1994, WB Saunders.)

hemopericardium with tamponade, and transient hypotension. Surgical ablation is now infrequently performed.

Supraventricular Dysrhythmias

BRADYDYSRHYTHMIAS

Pacemakers

Traditionally, temporary and permanent pacemakers have been used for patients with compromised cardiac output caused by profound bradycardia. Early pacemakers fired at a fixed rate; they did not have the ability to sense the patient's native heartbeat. With the introduction of sensing capabilities, pacemakers could determine the intrinsic heart rate and generate an electrical impulse whenever the heart did not initiate a beat on its own within a preset period. With an adequate underlying rate, the pacemaker impulse is inhibited. This shift from continuous pacing to continuous sensing eliminated the hazard of the pacemaker competing with the intrinsic heartbeat (and potentially creating a ventricular dysrhythmia) and prolonged the battery life of the generator.

Pacemakers have evolved from devices that were capable of stimulating a single chamber to those able to sense and stimulate both atrial and ventricular chambers; adjust rates to physiologic demands; provide telemetric information and autoprogram and reprogram functions; and provide antitachycardia functions (Fig. 17-12). The ability to program pacemakers has led to greater flexibility in adapting to changing metabolic requirements and underlying rhythm derangements. Pacemaker systems are capable of modulating the rate of impulse generation (the rate-responsive mode), as well as modifying the amount of energy (the output) required to stimulate an impulse. Dysrhythmia detection is also available in the latest systems. Pacemakers can be used in combination with antidysrhythmic drugs to control reentrant tachydysrhythmias. They can also be used to treat tachycardias by sensing a rapid ventricular rate and instituting a faster (overdrive) pacing stimulus to terminate the tachydysrhythmia. These functions have been included in the descriptive code established by the Inter-Society Commission on Heart Disease Resources (Box 17-3). Patients likely to benefit from these newer devices are those with a clinical tachycardia that can be reliably initiated and terminated in the EP laboratory. Patients at risk for ventricular fibrillation because of ventricular tachydysrhythmias originating from multiple sites may be treated more appropriately with an internal defibrillator (Bernstein and others, 1987).

Temporary pacemakers. Temporary pacing may be used as an emergency measure to stabilize a patient with deteriorating hemodynamic function as a result of sudden heart block. A permanent pacemaker can be implanted after the patient is stabilized. Temporary pacemaker leads (contained within a pacing Swan-Ganz catheter) may be inserted transvenously with a percutaneous method, or leads can be applied externally in the form of adhesive patches. Temporary epicardial leads commonly are used in postoperative cardiac surgery patients to control transient postoperative rhythm disturbances (Atlee, 1999).

Permanent pacemakers. Permanent pacing systems are indicated for patients with chronic or recurrent severe bradycardia caused by AV block or sinus node malfunction (Doty, 2000a). They also may be used for overdrive pacing in patients with ventricular tachycardia or tachycardia-bradycardia syndromes. Historically, pacemaker insertion was performed only in the OR, but currently many pacemakers are inserted in the cardiac catheterization (or EP) laboratory. Patient needs for safety, education, anxiety reduction, and infection control are similar in the OR and the interventional laboratory (Table 17-3).

Although permanent epicardial leads were common in the past, they are used rarely (even when concomitant cardiac surgery is performed) because of the high thresholds created by the scar tissue that forms at the lead insertion site. However, epicardial leads (Fig. 17-13) may be necessary in cases in which an endovascular (Fig. 17-14) lead cannot be inserted. This situation can occur in patients with congenital or acquired stenosis of the superior vena cava or other central veins or when other catheters are present (such as a dialysis or Hickmann catheter).

Pacemaker system

A cardiac pacemaker can be thought of as a system consisting of a power supply, housing, leads, and an electronic circuit. These components are necessary for both temporary and permanent pacemakers.

Power supply. Implantable (permanent) pacemaker generators most often contain lithium batteries, whose longevity is determined by battery size and capacity, current settings, rate and mode of stimulation, and lead design. Single-chamber leads and generators pace one chamber (usually the ventricle). Dual-chamber pulse generators have two sensing and stimulating channels to pace the atrium and the ventricle.

TABLE **17-3**
Standards of Nursing Care for Pacemakers and Implantable Cardioverter Defibrillators

NURSING DIAGNOSIS	PATIENT OUTCOME	NURSING ACTIONS
Anxiety related to dysrhythmia surgery/pacemaker insertion, postoperative effects	Patient demonstrates acceptable level of anxiety that promotes effectiveness of pacemaker/ICD treatment	Elicit questions and concerns about dysrhythmia and proposed treatment Identify and reinforce effective coping mechanisms; respect some denial; expect concern about relying on a "machine" Provide comfort measures; identify perceived needs and expectations

Knowledge deficit related to inadequate knowledge of planned surgery and function of devices	Patient demonstrates knowledge of physiologic and psychologic responses to device insertion	Determine patient's understanding of dysrhythmia, conduction disturbance
		Determine patient's/family's understanding of surgical procedure; briefly describe perioperative events; if local anesthesia is used, tell patient what to expect; reinforce or clarify what patient (and family) has been told by surgeon; elicit expected outcome of surgery
		Pacer:
		    Elicit patient's preference (if any) for location of generator pocket
		    Allow patient to keep hearing aid if local anesthesia is used; provide comfort measures (e.g., pillow, drapes off face)
		ICD:
		    If generator placement is to be performed with patient under local anesthesia, prepare for sensation of fibrillation/defibrillation (usually sedation used); provide emotional support and comfort measures

Risk for infection related to surgery	Patient is free of infection related to aseptic technique	Protect sterility of test cables, guidewires, etc; use sterile covers for wands and other devices that cannot be sterilized Confine and contain instruments and supplies used to excise infected tissue Keep instruments and guidewires free of blood and debris Document lot and serial numbers of implants
Risk for altered skin integrity	Patient's skin integrity is maintained	In thin, malnourished, or very elderly patients with poor skin turgor, use additional padding to protect skin, joints, and bony prominences
Risk for injury related to:	Patient is free of injury related to:	
Retained foreign objects	Retained foreign objects	Account for screwdrivers, electrode caps, and other small accessory items Check generator pockets for retained sponges
Physical hazards	Physical hazards	Have available appropriate equipment/supplies such as leads, generators, testing devices, and accessory items; confer with technical representative and surgeon to ensure that all necessary items are available If fluoroscopy is used, provide lead shields, aprons for personnel and patient Monitor ECG for severe bradycardia or ventricular ectopy, tachycardia, and fibrillation When transvenous leads are inserted (pacer or ICD), be alert for signs of pneumothorax or hemothorax: SOB, absent or diminished breath sounds, cyanosis, restlessness, tachypnea, decreased oxygen saturation, hypotension For ICD insertion, be prepared to open chest; institute CPB if patient does not defibrillate Use magnets with caution and in consultation with physician when activating/deactivating devices Keep instruments, device components clean; wash powder off gloves
Electrical hazards	Electrical hazards	Minimize use of electrocautery; avoid near generator or leads, and with active ICD Confirm defibrillator settings with surgeon when testing ICD (e.g., 10-20 J for internal defibrillation; 350 J or more for external shock) Apply appropriate conducting gel with external defibrillator paddles Defibrillate on verbal command of surgeon
Thermal injury	Thermal injury	Avoid placing external defibrillator paddles/pads over generator When testing (fibrillating) patient, have defibrillator charged and ready to shock

APR, Cardiopulmonary resuscitation; *ICD,* implantable cardioverter defibrillator; *J,* joule; *MRI,* magnetic resonance imaging; *SOB,* shortness of breath.
Modified from Seifert PC: Cardiac surgery. In Rothrock JC: *Perioperative nursing care planning,* ed 2, St Louis, 1996, Mosby.

TABLE 17-3
Standards of Nursing Care for Pacemakers and Implantable Cardioverter Defibrillators—cont'd

NURSING DIAGNOSIS	PATIENT OUTCOME	NURSING ACTIONS
Thermal injury—cont'd	Thermal injury—cont'd	Avoid pouring ice slush or ice chips directly on phrenic nerve (in lateral pericardium)

Risk for self-care deficit related to inadequate knowledge of device function	Patient demonstrates knowledge of device as it relates to self-care abilities	Assess patient's knowledge of signs/symptoms of pacer/ICD function
		Assess patient's understanding of signs/symptoms of infection: redness, swelling, warmth, pain, fever
		Use patient education material provided by manufacturer
		Complete documentation and submit forms as indicated for follow-up and patient ID card; stress importance of keeping ID card on person at all times (may be required for security clearance at airport because devices can set off security alarms)
		Provide information for obtaining medical alert ID bracelet/necklace; provide name of person to contact in emergencies (or dial 911)
		Pacer:
		  Discuss safety issues:
		    Limit use of electric razors, hairdryers, and other electrical devices over generator site
		    Do not lean directly over running engines
		    Inform physician before undergoing diagnostic procedures that use magnetic fields or intense radiation
		  Provide instruction related to:
		    Taking own pulse and maintaining record
		    Reporting prolonged hiccoughing or chest twitching
		    Battery failure; note change in heart rate (5 beats more or less than set rate), dizziness or fainting, weakness or fatigue, chest pain, swelling in extremities; failure is gradual
		    Telephonic testing procedure
		ICD:
		  Discuss possible personal concerns:
		    Driving restrictions
		    Appearance of generator pocket
		    Dependence on ICD, fear of shocks or malfunction, sensation of shock
		  Instruct patient to report:
		    ICD shocks; keep diary
		    Rapid heart rate, dizziness, fainting
		  Instruct patient that precautions are required for the following:
		    Arc welders, large transformers
		    Security systems (e.g., airport)
		    MRI, diathermy, lithotripsy, nerve stimulators, electrocautery, radiation therapy
		  Instruct patient that precautions are not required for the following:
		    Small hand tools
		    Microwave ovens, satellite dish
		    Ultrasound, lasers, diagnostic radiation
		  Address family concerns:
		    ICD discharge, notification of physician
		    Activities of daily living, travel, driving
		    Signs and symptoms of malfunction
		    Need for CPR if device fails or has already delivered full sequence of shocks
		    Making contact with person receiving a shock (produces buzzing or tingling)

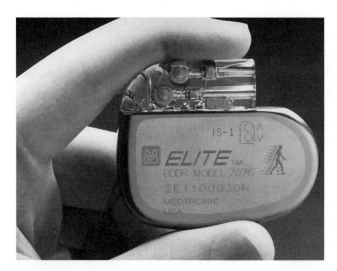

FIGURE 17-12 Dual-chamber cardiac pacemaker generator, capable of synchronized rate-responsive pacing in both chambers of the heart and counting and recording electrical events. Information stored in the generator can be retrieved and monitored to ensure proper function. (Courtesy Medtronic, Inc.)

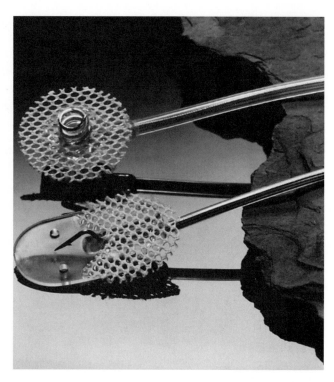

FIGURE 17-13 Permanent epicardial screw-in *(top)* and stab *(bottom)* pacemaker leads. (Courtesy Medtronic, Inc.)

Temporary generators are powered by alkaline batteries. They are never line powered (attached to a wall outlet) because of the danger of current leaks into the myocardium.

Housing. The power supply and the electronic circuitry of the generator are enclosed separately within an inert metal container (see Fig. 17-12). The box is hermetically sealed to prevent moisture and tissue from injuring the internal components of the device and to prevent the surrounding tissue from being injured.

Lead. The lead acts as the conductor of the pacing stimulus to the myocardium and as the sensor of P waves or QRS complexes (depending on whether the atrium or the ventricle, respectively, is sensed). Rubber or plastic is used to insulate all but the distal tip of the lead that directly contacts the myocardium. The contacting portion of the lead is known as the *electrode.* Transvenous atrial leads typically have a screw configuration; the tip is rotated into the atrial appendage (unless the appendage has been resected during prior cardiac surgery) or the atrial wall. Transvenous ventricular lead tips often have a tined tip that is passively placed into the trabecular tissue of the ventricle (see Fig. 17-14).

Epicardial atrial leads (see Fig. 17-13) commonly have a fish-hook tip that is affixed by "stabbing" the atrial tissue. Ventricular epicardial leads have a pigtail design that screws into the ventricular muscle (see Fig. 17-13). Fixation sutures may be used to anchor the leads. The leads are tunneled to a subcutaneous pocket for the generator in a manner similar to that described for transvenous insertion in the following.

Electronic circuit. The electronic circuit modifies the energy available in the power supply in order to create the appropriate duration and amplitude of an impulse. A timing element within the circuit determines the frequency of stimulation. The stimulus is applied to the atrium or to the ventricle or to both chambers sequentially, depending on the type of pacemaker device inserted. When two chambers are paced, two output and timing circuits are required, along with two sensing components; a separate timing mechanism is used to create an AV delay. Additional circuitry provides other pacing/antitachycardia functions.

Patient teaching considerations

Pacemaker insertion is a commonplace procedure and may be perceived as "routine" by clinicians. Assumptions about the relative simplicity of insertion and the positive effects that these devices have on the clinical status of the patient should not be generalized to patients' psychologic perceptions about the impact that a pacemaker has on their lives. Dependence on a machine that the patient cannot control may have a profound emotional effect. Patients' acceptance levels vary depending on demographic variables such as support systems, environment, and socioeconomic status. These considerations should be integrated into the educational programs designed for patients and families (Kinney and Packa, 1996).

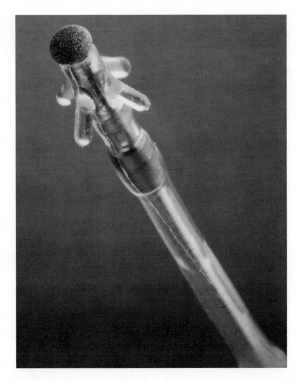

FIGURE 17-14 Steroid-eluting transvenous cardiac pacing lead with tined tip. Treating the lead with a steroid reduces inflammation of the myocardium and can extend the battery life by allowing effective stimulation with electrical impulses of less intensity. (Courtesy Medtronic, Inc, Minneapolis, Minn.)

Patient teaching addresses the reason for pacemaker insertion, the system components, the surgical procedure (with conscious sedation), and postoperative considerations related to the pacemaker and to functional activities (Table 17-3). The nurse can show the patient a pacemaker similar to the one being implanted. Many patients may not be aware that pacemaker generators are relatively small ($1\frac{3}{4} \times 1\frac{1}{2} \times \frac{1}{4}$ inches or smaller) and lightweight (a little more than 1 ounce). The patient can be shown the pacing leads and how they are implanted into the heart distally and attached to the generator proximally. Photographs of the small scar and the slight skin pocket bulge can help patients to prepare for their postoperative appearance. These teaching sessions also provide the patient with an opportunity to ask questions and clarify misconceptions.

Patient preparation for transvenous insertion in the operating room or cardiac catheterization laboratory focuses on what can be expected during the procedure. Including sensory stimuli (e.g., color, temperature, size or room; sounds, conversations; number and roles of personnel) enables the patient to anticipate and mentally plan for the experience. If the patient wears a hearing aid, it is helpful to allow the patient to keep it in place so that questions asked of the patient during surgery will be heard. The patient should be aware that local anesthesia will reduce the discomfort from the incision, that sedation is available, and that a drape will separate his or her face from the periclavicular incision site. The procedure lasts approximately 1 hour, and that information can be relayed to the patient and waiting family; efforts to make the patient as comfortable as possible will enhance the smoothness of the procedure. Additional teaching is performed after the completed procedure.

Procedural considerations

The transvenous route is the most common insertion method and is performed with fluoroscopy. Location of the generator pocket is important. A unit that is too close to the axilla may be painful and interfere with arm movement. It also may lead to skin breakdown and infection. A generator that is too close to the clavicle may be painful during arm motion and when the patient is supine (Waldhausen, Pierce, and Campbell, 1996). (Excessive arm movement during the early postoperative period also may cause the leads to become dislodged.)

When the procedure is performed in the OR, the nurse coordinates efforts with the OR control desk and the radiology department to have the appropriate x-ray equipment ready and tested before the start of the procedure. Pacing leads, generators, testing devices, and other necessary supplies to insert and test the system should be available (Box 17-4).

In patients with existing pacemaker generators, special precautions should be taken with the use of electrosurgical units. Excessive currents near the vicinity of the generator may cause dysrhythmias or myocardial burns from transmission of the current down the electrode. Reprogramming of the pacer generator may be required if electrocautery energy disrupts generator function. Patients with exteriorized wires are also susceptible to electrical shock hazards; exposed wires should be covered.

OPERATIVE PROCEDURE: INSERTION OF A TRANSVENOUS PACEMAKER SYSTEM

1. The patient is in the supine position with both subclavian vein areas of the upper chest and shoulders exposed.
2. Local anesthetic (1% lidocaine) is infiltrated into the skin over the area where the subclavian vein is to be punctured; this may be the same site as the pocket for the generator (Fig. 17-15).

   The patient is placed in Trendelenburg's position (to engorge the vein). The patient's head is turned to the opposite side.
3. A cutdown is performed to isolate the right or left subclavian vein, and the vessel is encircled with heavy sutures or umbilical tapes.

BOX **17-4**
Procedures for Dysrhythmias: Considerations

Instrumentation

Basic sternotomy setup for open chest procedure
Mitral valve retractors if mitral valve exposure is necessary for dysrhythmia surgery
Minor set for transvenous insertion of pacemaker or ICD leads

Supplies*

Sterile drapes for fluoroscopy unit
Sterile sleeves for "wands" and other testing devices that cannot be sterilized
Sterile magnet
Leads and patches (subcutaneous)
Generators
Guidewires, introducers, stylets
Alligator test cables, probes, ECG cables
Device programmers/analyzers
EP "socks," belts for intraoperative EP testing
Service kits (e.g., screwdrivers, sterile caps, etc.)
Adaptor kits and connectors
Culture tubes (e.g., if revising pacer or ICD pocket)

Equipment

Defibrillator (and backups); internal and external defibrillation capability; external defibrillation patch system may also be requested
Fibrillator (for induction of dysrhythmia during testing)
Testing equipment appropriate for device inserted (EP machines, computer programmers, analyzers)
Fluoroscopy machine for transvenous route

Positioning

Supine
Modified thoracotomy may be used for some ICD procedures

Skin Preparation

Chin to groin, side to side; prep over both subclavian veins

Draping

Anterior and lateral chest and abdomen, right and left sternoclavicular areas (over subclavian vein) exposed
Anesthesia screen placed over head to keep drapes off face

Special Infection Control Measures

Confine and contain tissue and instruments from infected tissue
Secure leads, testing devices, etc., that are passed off field
Culture tissue and other items as requested by surgeon/electrophysiologist
Keep guidewires, leads, etc., free of blood and debris

Special Safety Measures

Label syringes and containers holding medications and solutions:
  Antibiotic solution
  Heparinized saline
  Lidocaine topical anesthetic

Documentation/Report to Postprocedure Care Unit†

Procedure: type of device, manufacturer, lot and serial numbers of all implanted components
Preoperative diagnosis (e.g., complete heart block, ventricular tachycardia, sudden death)
Pacemaker; rate settings; type and location of leads, generator; pacer function (e.g., DDD—both atrium and ventricle paced and sensed, and capable of either triggering or inhibiting a response)
ICD: location of transvenous electrode, generator; ICD function (e.g., defibrillation with bradycardia pacing; status—active, inactive)
Patient problems, concerns related to dysrhythmia, procedure, function of device
Documentation required for investigational devices
Documentation of all personnel

ICD, Implantable cardioverter defibrillator.
* As applicable to procedure.
† In addition to standard documentation/postoperative report; see Chapter 6.

4. The vein is punctured with a needle through which a guidewire is introduced (Fig. 17-16).
5. A dilator sheath is advanced over the guidewire to enlarge surrounding tissue; the dilator is removed. The lead is introduced over the guidewire, and the sheath is peeled away (Fig. 17-17). The guidewire is removed.
6a. If a single ventricular lead (e.g., VVI) is to be inserted, it is threaded through the right atrium and tricuspid valve and into the right ventricle under fluoroscopy. Stylets inserted through the electrode can be used to manipulate the lead into position within the right ventricle.

   Alligator cables are attached: one prong of each cable is connected to the lead, and the second prong is clipped to the subcutaneous tissue as a ground. The proximal ends of the cables are passed off the field and inserted into the pacing analyzer system. Thresholds and other conduction parameters are tested to confirm that the lead will function appropriately.
6b. If dual-chamber pacing is used, a second electrode is placed in the right atrium and the position is checked by fluoroscopy. Leads may have a tined tip or a screw-in tip to foster a secure attachment in the right atrium; a stylet may be used to position the lead within the atrial trabeculations. Testing is performed (see step 6A).
7. The incision site is enlarged, if necessary, to become a pocket for the pacer generator, or a pocket

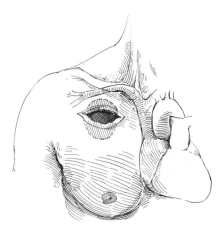

FIGURE 17-15   A skin incision is made where the pocket is to be formed; the pocket may be made just under the right *(shown)* or left subclavian vein. (From Waldhausen JA, Pierce WS, Campbell DB: *Surgery of the chest,* ed 6, St Louis, 1996, Mosby.)

FIGURE 17-16   With the patient in Trendelenberg's position and the head turned to the opposite side, the subclavian vein is punctured through the upper margin of the wound. The guidewire is introduced. (From Waldhausen JA, Pierce WS, Campbell DB: *Surgery of the chest,* ed 6, St Louis, 1996, Mosby.)

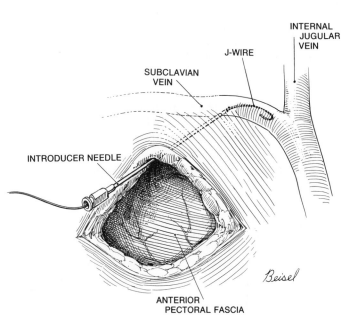

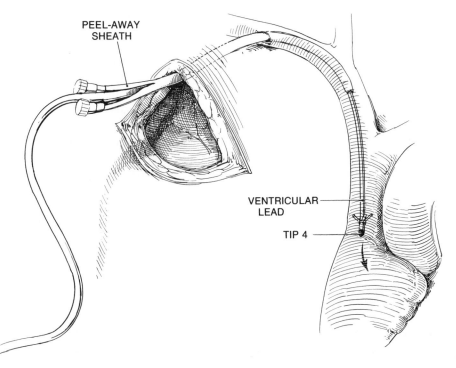

FIGURE 17-17   The dilator sheath is advanced over the guidewire; the wire and dilator are then removed, and the pacer lead is introduced into the sheath. The electrode lead is advanced into the right atrium. (From Waldhausen JA, Pierce WS, Campbell DB: *Surgery of the chest,* ed 6, St Louis, 1996, Mosby.)

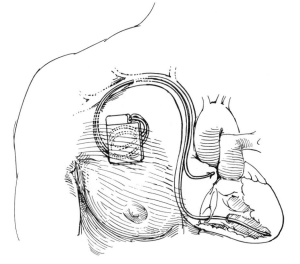

FIGURE 17-18 Both atrial and ventricular leads have been inserted and tunneled to the pacer pocket, where they are connected to the generator. (A single pocket may be used for the leads and the generator.) Excess electrode is coiled and placed behind the generator, which is placed into the pocket. (From Waldhausen JA, Pierce WS, Campbell DB: *Surgery of the chest,* ed 6, St Louis, 1996, Mosby.)

is formed near the venous insertion site, and the leads are tunneled to the pocket.

8. The leads are connected to the generator, which is placed into the pocket. Excess lead is coiled and placed behind the generator (Fig. 17-18). Incisions may be irrigated with antibiotic solution.

9. Subcutaneous tissue and skin are closed with absorbable suture, and dressings are applied.

The generator may be sutured to the pectoral fascia in patients who may be considered at risk for migration of the generator (e.g., those with poor wound healing).

Postoperative period

In the immediate postoperative period, pacemaker function is assessed and additional teaching is performed. The patient is taught to take an apical pulse and to inspect the incisional area for signs of infection. Signs of pacemaker malfunction are reviewed, and the telephone number of a person to contact should be available for reporting occurrences. An identification card is given to the patient, who should carry it at all times. The card includes information such as the name of the pacemaker manufacturer; model, lot, and serial numbers; implantation date; and name and telephone number of the physician. If problems arise, this information is vital for troubleshooting and, if necessary, for reprogramming the generator.

Transtelephonic monitoring is used for periodic assessment of pacemaker function. ECG rhythm strips are transmitted to the physician's office and reviewed. These rhythm strips can also detect when a generator battery change is needed.

Battery and lead changes. When the power source or a transvenous lead must be replaced (or reprogrammed), the procedure can be performed on an outpatient basis. The skin pocket is reopened, and the generator is exposed and removed along with the attached leads. The leads are disconnected, and a new generator is connected to the leads and tested. It is then replaced in the skin pocket, and the incision is closed.

Transvenous lead replacement requiring lead extraction may be performed by the electrophysiologist in the EP laboratory. Usually the existing leads become embedded in the atrial or ventricular endocardium. If the leads cannot be dislodged and removed, they may be left in place and new leads inserted on the contralateral side. The remaining leads are disconnected from the generator and capped so that there are no exposed wires remaining. When malfunctioning leads must be removed, surgical standby may be requested; if cardiac tamponade occurs, emergency surgery is performed.

Biventricular pacing for heart failure

Although pacemaker therapy commonly is used for bradydysrhythmias, dual-site pacing of both the right and the left ventricles has emerged as a treatment for patients with dilated cardiomyopathy and congestive heart failure. This cardiac resynchronization therapy (CRT) is under investigation in the United States; CRT is approved in Europe for the treatment of heart failure (Saxon, Kumar, and De Marco, 2000).

When the left ventricle and the right ventricle are paced simultaneously, a more physiologic depolarization sequence occurs. By improving the sequence of electrical activation (resynchronization), and creating a more coordinated and efficient left ventricular contraction, hemodynamic function can improve (Barold, 2000).

Insertion of the leads is similar to that for a dual-chamber (AV) pacemaker; the electrodes are inserted transvenously into the right atrium and the right ventricle. Additionally, a third lead is placed in the coronary sinus and extended into the cardiac vein (or a tributary) to a position in the left side of the heart; this lead functions as the second ventricular pacing lead. The procedure is performed in the EP laboratory.

TACHYDYSRHYTHMIAS

The goals of treatment for supraventricular tachydysrhythmias are to localize the initiating focus or abnormal conduction pathway and to ablate, excise, or otherwise destroy the dysrhythmogenic site. EP studies are performed to locate and identify the lesion; often percutaneous catheter ablation can be performed at the same time.

Occasionally, surgical treatment is performed on patients who have failed attempted RF ablation or who have concomitant cardiac disease requiring surgery. Additional EP testing is then performed in the OR.

Catheter ablation for Wolff-Parkinson-White syndrome

WPW syndrome is commonly treated with percutaneous catheter ablation using radiofrequency currency to destroy the abnormal conduction tract. The WPW dysrhythmia is related to the existence of one or more accessory pathways (also known as Kent bundles) producing early activation (preexcitation) of part or all of the ventricle by an impulse originating in the sinus node or the atrium. The most common rhythm disturbance is *circus movement* reentry tachycardia. During circus movement tachycardia, the impulse travels in a circuit: atrium–AV node–bundle of His–bundle branch–ventricle–accessory pathway–atrium. In this situation the impulse travels antegradely (slow pathway) from the atrium to the ventricle (AV) through the normal pathway (AV node–bundle of His) and then reenters the atrium retrogradely (fast pathway) from the ventricle through the accessory pathway. Retrograde conduction through the accessory pathway does not produce ventricular preexcitation.

Alternatively, antegrade AV conduction can occur over the accessory pathway (causing preexcitation of the ventricle), and retrograde ventricular–atrial (VA) conduction can occur through the bundle of His–AV node pathway. For circus movement to occur, the cardiac impulse travels a loop of cardiac fibers and reenters previously excited tissue (see Fig. 17-4). To achieve this the impulse must be conducted slowly around the loop, and one of the two AV pathways must be blocked in one direction in order to allow the impulse to reenter the circuit (Berne and Levy, 2001). When atrial fibrillation occurs in patients with WPW syndrome, the accessory pathways may provide a relatively unimpeded route for the rapid atrial impulses to reach the ventricle and thereby stimulate ventricular fibrillation.

The success of RF ablation in treating these accessory pathways has all but eliminated the need for surgical ablation. When surgery is indicated, intraoperative EP mapping is used to identify the pathways, which can be located in one or more locations in the left free wall, right free wall, and posterior and anterior septal positions (see Fig. 17-3). Surgical approaches include the endocardial approach (dissecting the AV groove) and the epicardial approach (dissecting tissue from the AV groove to the mitral valve annulus). After dissection, EP mapping evaluates the results. If abnormal conduction persists, cryoablation (to $-60°$ C/$-76°$ F) may be performed.

Treatment for paroxysmal supraventricular tachycardia

Paroxysmal supraventricular tachycardia may be caused by an accessory pathway or by atrioventricular nodal reentrant tachycardia (AVNRT). Early treatment for AVNRT consisted of catheter ablation of the bundle of His with insertion of a permanent pacemaker. RF ablation of the slow pathway (compared with the fast pathway) is associated with less inadvertent heart block and has demonstrated long-term success (Tracy and others, 2000; Clague and others, 2001).

Surgical treatment can be performed with selective cryoablation of the reentrant pathway (avoiding the normal AV conduction tract and thereby preventing heart block). Other supraventricular tachycardias caused by the reentry mechanism also can be surgically treated with multiple incisions that interrupt abnormal connections; cryoablation also can be employed. These procedures are advantageous because they often preserve the continuity of the atrial pacemaker complex with the atrial septum and the ventricles (Skubas and others, 1999; Morady, 1999).

Surgery for atrial fibrillation

Atrial fibrillation (AF) is the most common sustained tachydysrhythmia occurring in humans. Its incidence increases with age and the presence of heart disease (Prystowsky and others, 1996; Narayan, Cain, and Smith, 1997). The primary mechanism causing AF is a reentry phenomenon during which impulses arising in the atria form multiple irregular circuits. A second distinct mechanism causing AF is a rapidly firing focus (or foci), usually located in or near a superior pulmonary vein (Falk, 2001). Interestingly, the Maze III procedure for atrial fibrillation (see p. 519), which includes (in part) encircling the pulmonary veins with incisions, can convert AF to sinus rhythm.

The detrimental sequelae of atrial fibrillation include (1) an irregularly irregular ventricular response to the chaotic atrial impulses, (2) hemodynamic compromise resulting from loss of an atrial kick and decreased ventricular filling time, and (3) increased vulnerability to thromboembolism (TE) caused by loss of effective atrial contraction and stasis of blood in the atrium (Cox and others, 1991a; 1991c). The thromboembolic risk is one of the major reasons that AF is associated with increased morbidity and mortality (Ozcan and others, 2001; Ad and Cox, 2000).

Types of atrial fibrillation. *New-onset* AF (within 24 hours) may spontaneously convert to sinus rhythm. *Recurrent paroxysmal* AF refers to episodic periods of the dysrhythmia, which has a sudden onset and sudden termination, reverting to sinus rhythm before resumption of another period of fibrillation. If AF is longer than 24 hours, it is considered *persistent;* the likelihood of spontaneous conversion decreases and is rare when AF lasts longer than 1 week. *Lone atrial fibrillation* refers to AF occurring in the absence of documented underlying cardiac disease or a history of hypertension (Falk, 2001).

Often atrial fibrillation is precipitated by underlying cardiac disease such as atrial fibrosis or localized atrial myocarditis. Additionally a trigger may be required to initiate the dysrhythmia. Increased susceptibility to autonomic nervous stimulation and cardiac surgery are two significant triggers of AF (Falk, 2001).

Treatment. In highly symptomatic patients (e.g., those with pulmonary edema), patients with a previous embolic event, and patients at high risk for thromboembolism, antidysrhythmic therapy or anticoagulant therapy may be prescribed. In patients with unstable angina or acute myocardial infarction, electrical cardioversion may be the most appropriate initial therapy because drug therapy is often unpredictable. Patients should receive warfarin therapy for approximately 3 weeks before elective cardioversion; anticoagulation should be maintained for 4 weeks after the procedure (Tracy and others, 2000).

Percutaneous catheter ablation of the AV node with insertion of a permanent pacemaker has been performed in patients with atrial fibrillation to alleviate symptoms, improve exercise tolerance, and control the ventricular rate. However, ablation does not eliminate atrial fibrillation (Ozcan and others, 2001).

In patients with atrial fibrillation triggered by a rapidly firing focus originating in the pulmonary veins, RF energy has been applied to the ectopic foci in the pulmonary veins. A modification of this technique involves using RF energy to isolate the pulmonary veins from the atrium, with a resulting reduction in spontaneous atrial ectopy and abolition of atrial fibrillation (Falk, 2001).

Implantable atrial defibrillators were developed after the demonstrated success of ventricular defibrillators. Current models combine both atrial and ventricular

defibrillation capability. Some devices allow the patient to activate the atrial defibrillation component, thereby enabling the patient to avoid unexpected, painful shocks (Falk, 2001).

Surgery for AF. Early surgical procedures attempted to blunt the sequelae of atrial fibrillation by ablating the bundle of His or by creating an isolated strip of muscle to direct impulses from the SA node to the AV node/bundle of His and from there to the ventricles (the *corridor procedure*). Unfortunately, the first procedure could not reestablish sinus rhythm and therefore could not provide an atrial kick; the risk of TE also remained. The corridor procedure could correct the irregular ventricular rhythm produced by atrial fibrillation, but right and left atrial synchrony could not be reestablished, and the atrial kick remained absent (Cox and others, 1991a).

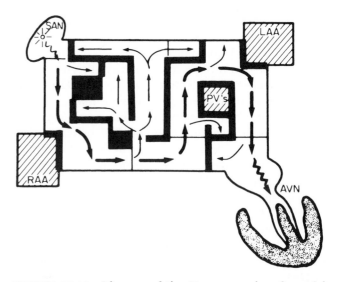

FIGURE 17-19 Diagram of the Maze procedure for atrial fibrillation. Because atrial fibrillation is characterized by the presence of multiple macroreentrant circuits that are fleeting in nature and can occur anywhere in the atria, a surgical procedure based on the principle of the maze was developed. Both atrial appendages are excised, and the pulmonary veins (also considered a source of abnormal circuits) are isolated. Appropriately placed atrial incisions not only interrupt the conduction routes of the most common reentrant circuits but also direct the sinus impulse from the SA node to the AV node along a specified route. The myocardium is electrically activated by providing for multiple blind alleys off the main conduction route between the SA node and the AV node, thereby preserving atrial transport function postoperatively. *SAN,* Sinoatrial node; *RAA,* right atrial appendage; *LAA,* left atrial appendage; *PV's,* pulmonary veins; *AVN,* atrioventricular node. (From Cox JL and others: The surgical treatment of atrial fibrillation: III. Development of a definitive surgical procedure, *J Thorac Cardiovasc Surg* 101[4]:569, 1991c.)

In 1991 Cox and his associates (1991a, 1991b, 1991c; Cox, 1991) introduced the Maze procedure in an attempt to reroute the multiple wave fronts, nonuniform conduction, bidirectional block, and large reentrant circuits occurring during atrial fibrillation. These results were achieved by making multiple incisions so that the impulses (which are unable to cross sutured incisions) were routed from the SA node to the AV node (Fig. 17-19).

According to Cox (2000b), the original Maze procedure resulted in two unexpected problems: (1) Many patients were unable to increase their heart rate sufficiently to meet the cardiac output required for physical exertion because one or more of the Maze incisions interrupted the sinus-tachycardia region of the SA node; and (2) prolonged intraatrial conduction resulted in a delayed and ineffective left atrial contraction.

These problems led to the development of the Maze II procedure, but this modification was technically difficult and required transection of the superior vena cava (SVC) for exposure (Cox, Schuessler, and Boineau, 2000). Further modification led to the Maze III (described in the following; Fig. 17-20), which corrected the problems encountered with the Maze I and reduced the difficulties associated with the Maze II (Cox, 2000b). Modifications continue to be made by other surgeons (Ad and others, 2000; McCarthy, 2000; Kim and others, 2001; Kosakai, 2000), and Cox himself (2000a; Cox and Ad, 2000) has developed a minimally invasive approach.

Operative procedure: the Maze III procedure (Cox, 2000b)

Excellent surgical exposure is critical. The patient is placed in the supine position.

Procedure

1. A median sternotomy is performed.
2. The superior vena cava is mobilized from the azygos vein to the right atrium. The anatomic groove between the right pulmonary artery and the right superior pulmonary vein is developed, and the posterior left atrium is freed from the pericardium.
3. The aorta and pulmonary artery are retracted to the left.
4. The interatrial groove is developed as for mitral valve surgery (see Chapter 11), except that the dissection is completed as much as possible inferiorly and superiorly.
5. The aorta is dissected from the pulmonary artery and encircled with an umbilical tape.
6. The SVC and inferior vena cava (IVC) are encircled with caval tapes and cannulated; the SVC is cannulated high and the IVC cannulated low to enhance exposure. The aorta is cannulated, and a cardioplegia vent needle is inserted into the ascending aorta.
7. A pulmonary artery vent is placed just beyond the pulmonary valve and connected to the aortic vent line.
8. CPB is instituted, the caval tapes are tightened, and the patient is systemically cooled.

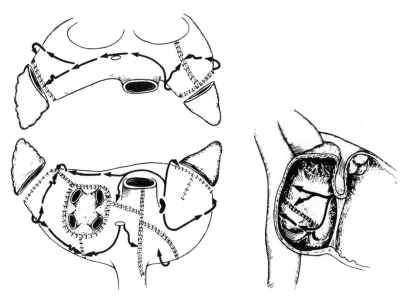

FIGURE 17-20 Maze III procedure. Two-dimensional depiction of incisions for Maze III procedure. Note encircling incisions of the four pulmonary veins *(left;* see text.) (From Cox JL, Schuessler RB, Boineau JP: The development of the Maze procedure for the treatment of atrial fibrillation, *Semin Thorac Cardiovasc Surg* 12[1]:2, 2000.)

9. The aorta is cross-clamped, and the heart is arrested with hyperkalemic cardioplegia infused into the aortic root.

10. The right atrial appendage is excised.

11. The first incision is made from the right side of the base of the excised atrial appendage toward the IVC.

12. A second incision is made from the SVC to the IVC; the incisional area close to the IVC is sutured closed immediately (to prevent inadvertent tearing during later retraction).

13. A cardiotomy suction catheter is inserted into the coronary sinus via the atrial appendage keeps the field free of blood exiting the coronary sinus.

14. A third incision is made in the right atrium superior to the IVC cannula, toward the tricuspid valve annulus, taking care not to injure the right coronary artery that runs along the atrioventricular groove.

15. The right atrial free wall is retracted anteriorly and superiorly.

16. Cryolesions are produced close to the tricuspid valve annulus, and the tricuspid end of the incision made in step 14 is closed partially.

17. A fourth incision is made across the first incision at the border of the excised atrial appendage and extended to the anteromedial tricuspid valve annulus; the nearby AV node–His bundle complex is avoided. A cryolesion is made at the tricuspid end of the incision. This fourth incision is closed to the base of the atrial appendage. The remaining tight atrial incisions are left unclosed until the left atrial procedure is completed.

18. A left atriotomy is made along the interatrial groove, and the atrial septum is divided. The atrial septum is retracted to expose the left atrium (LA).

19. The LA appendage is inverted and excised (avoiding the circumflex coronary artery), and the left superior pulmonary vein is isolated with incisions. Additional cryolesions are made near the pulmonary vein, and the LA appendage excision site is closed.

20. Cryolesions are made close to the coronary sinus.

21. Another cryolesion is placed near the mitral valve annulus; the posterior left atriotomy is closed.

22. The lower portion of the pulmonary vein isolation (step 19) is closed; the incision now resembles a standard atriotomy in the interatrial groove.

23. The septal incision is closed, and then the right atrial incisions are closed.

24. Atrial and ventricular pacing wires are attached; CPB is discontinued.

25. Hemostasis is obtained, and chest tubes are inserted. The incisions are closed.

Within the first 3 months after surgery, patients may experience periods of atrial fibrillation. After 3 months, only 1.2% of patients in Cox's (2000b) series continued

to have AF. Overall, 15% of patients required a new pacemaker after surgery. More than 90% of patients had right and left atrial contractions producing forward cardiac output.

Postoperative complications. Complications specifically related to surgery for dysrhythmias include heart block and injury to cardiac structures within the surgical field (e.g., coronary sinus, SVC, IVC, pulmonary veins, tricuspid and mitral valves). Other complications include stroke, coagulopathy, hemorrhage, infection, pulmonary embolism, ventricular dysfunction, and chylopericardium (abnormal lymphatic drainage into the pericardium).

Minimally invasive Maze III procedure

Objectives of the minimally invasive approach include shortened length of stay in the intensive care unit and the hospital, less perioperative morbidity, faster recuperation, decreased costs, and improved cosmesis (Cox, 2000a). The right atrial portion of the procedure is performed off bypass with the heart beating. CPB bypass is started, the aorta is clamped, the heart is arrested, and then the left atrial portion of the procedure is performed.

Procedure

1. The patient is in the supine position with a small rolled towel placed lengthwise under the right chest.

2. Three small incisions are made in the right chest: (1) a submammary incision below the nipple at the fourth intercostal space, (2) a more lateral fourth intercostal space incision, and (3) an intercostal incision one or two interspaces below the submammary incision.

3. A thoracotomy retractor is inserted into the submammary incision, and the patient is cannulated for femoral vein–femoral artery bypass. A Y connection off the venous line enables an SVC cannula to be inserted through the lateral (second) incision into the SVC after exposure of the cava. CPB is not initiated at this time.

4. A double-action clamp is inserted through this incision and will be used later to occlude the aorta; a cardioplegia catheter is inserted into the aortic root.

5. Cryolesions are made in the right atrium.

6. After the right atrial cryolesions are completed, CPB is instituted and a left ventricular venting catheter is inserted through the right superior pulmonary vein.

7. The aorta is cross-clamped, and antegrade cardioplegia is infused.

8. The left atrium is opened and cryolesions are made in the left atrium and around the pulmonary vein orifices and the left atrial appendage. The appendage is closed from the inside with a running suture (to prevent embolization of any clot within the appendage).

9. Mitral or tricuspid valve repair or replacement can be performed at the same time.
10. The incisions are closed and the procedure completed as described previously.

Postoperative complications

Complications specifically related to the surgical treatment for dysrhythmias include heart block and injury to cardiac structures within the surgical field (e.g., coronary sinus, coronary arteries, tricuspid and mitral valves). Other complications that are associated with most open heart procedures include stroke, coagulopathy, hemorrhage, infection, pulmonary embolism, ventricular dysfunction, and chylopericardium.

Ventricular Dysrhythmias

BRADYDYSRHYTHMIAS

Ventricular bradycardias may be seen in patients with chronic conduction delay caused by bundle-branch or fascicular block. Complete trifascicular block is rare, and the rate of progression is slow when there are no intervening causes (such as ischemia, drugs, or electrolyte imbalances). EP studies may be indicated in symptomatic patients whose bundle-branch block is suspected of causing symptoms (e.g., syncope or near-syncope) or in whom knowledge of the site of the block, the severity of the conduction delay, or the response to drug therapy requires further EP studies. Pacemaker implantation (discussed earlier) is the therapy of choice.

TACHYDYSRHYTHMIAS

The most serious of the ventricular rhythm disturbances are the tachydysrhythmias that may deteriorate into ventricular fibrillation because of a primary electrical instability or hemodynamic compromise associated with the rapid heart rate.

Ablation therapy may be palliative in patients with hemodynamically stable ventricular tachycardia that has a discreet focus. Ablation currently is not indicated for ventricular tachycardia or ventricular fibrillation arising from multiple foci, although some investigational studies are underway (Morady, 1999).

Unlike many patients with supraventricular dysrhythmias, patients undergoing surgical therapy for ventricular rhythm disturbances often have left ventricular dysfunction related to ischemic heart disease. Ischemic ventricular tachycardias are commonly caused by reentrant circuits located in the border region between a myocardial infarction or left ventricular aneurysm and the surrounding normal myocardium (Cox, 1991b).

Direct and indirect surgical techniques have been employed. An association between left ventricular aneurysm (post–myocardial infarction) and ventricular tachycardia was made in the late 1950s, and it was suggested that left ventricular aneurysmectomy might eradicate the dysrhythmia (Samuels and Samuels, 2000). These *indirect techniques* performed without electrophysiologic mapping (termed *blind aneurysmectomies*) demonstrated variable success rates because the origin of the tachycardia often was outside the visible scar and landmarks of the dysrhythmic locus were not always visible. A *direct technique* guided by EP mapping was developed to guide the surgery. Although superior results were shown when EP mapping was used, the increased morbidity and mortality associated with the surgery have made implantation of an internal defibrillator the treatment of choice (Doty, 2000b).

Nonischemic forms of ventricular tachydysrhythmias exist, but these occur less often and are most often caused by cardiomyopathy or congenital ventricular dysplasia. Occasionally the tachydysrhythmia is idiopathic, without macroscopic or microscopic evidence of primary cardiac disease (Cox, 1991a; 1991b). A cardioverter defibrillator is commonly implanted to reduce the risk of sudden death in these patients (Miller and Zipes, 2001).

Implantable cardioverter defibrillator

Sudden cardiac death (SCD) affects more than 350,000 people per year in the United States and represents a major health problem (Josephson and others, 2000). SCD is thought to result from ventricular fibrillation (VF) or some sustained ventricular tachycardia (VT) that deteriorates into VF (Hayes and Zipes, 2001).

Automatic external defibrillator. Increased awareness of the causes of SCD and its treatment have raised the national interest in cardiopulmonary resuscitation and early defibrillation for cardiac arrest. Efforts to simplify cardiac resuscitation and improve survival have prompted the growing use of external defibrillators by the lay public, as well as emergency personnel (Kern and Paraskos, 2000). Automatic external defibrillators (AEDs) can be used by firefighters, law enforcement personnel, emergency medical technicians, and others with relatively minimal training to defibrillate victims of cardiac arrest outside of a hospital. AEDs are available in many shopping malls, commercial airplanes, gaming establishments, and other public places.

The AED system consists of sensing electrodes that are applied to the victim and connected to the defibrillator. (The system also contains a razor to shave excess chest hair so that the electrode paddles make proper contact with the skin.) The device analyzes the rhythm, and if a defibrillating shock is indicated, the machine gives a loud verbal command to charge the device. When charged,

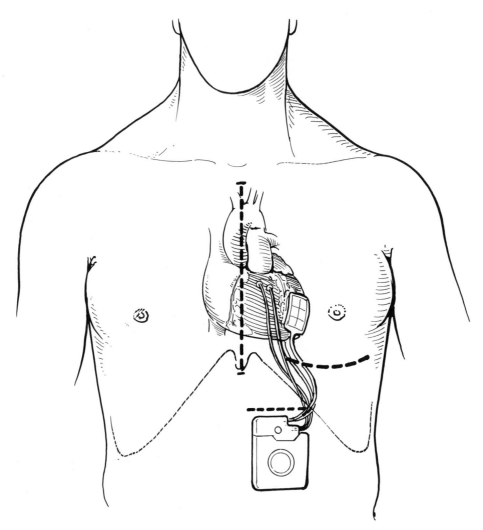

FIGURE 17-21 Thoracotomy ICD insertion. Early ICD insertions were performed via median sternotomy, subxiphoid, or submammary incisions *(dotted lines).* Two sensing leads are positioned on the right ventricle; defibrillator patches are placed on the anterior apical and posterior portions of the left ventricle. The size and weight of the early generators necessitated abdominal insertion; newer generators are smaller and lighter and can be placed in the upper chest. Currently most ICDs are inserted transvenously. (From Waldhausen JA, Pierce WS, Campbell DB: *Surgery of the chest,* ed 6, St Louis, 1996, Mosby.)

the machine gives the command to stand back and then discharges the electric shock.

Implantable cardioverter defibrillators. In patients with a known risk for SCD (e.g., those who have had spontaneous VF unresponsive to pharmacologic therapy), implantable defibrillators have had the greatest impact on preventing SCD (Gregoratos and others, 1998; Josephson and others, 2000). In patients at high risk for SCD, antidysrhythmic drugs and surgery have had mixed success in reducing the chance for SCD; implantable cardioverter defibrillators (ICDs) have had the greatest impact on preventing SCD (Josephson and others, 2000).

The difficulties of managing ventricular tachydysrhythmias are related to the fact that electrical countershock is the only treatment for ventricular fibrillation.

Realizing that patients often died of ventricular tachycardia/fibrillation because the necessary equipment and personnel to defibrillate patients were unavailable, Mirowski and his associates (1980) conceived of an implantable device that could sense the dysrhythmia and deliver a countershock to terminate the life-threatening disorder. The first device of this kind was implanted clinically at Johns Hopkins Hospital in Baltimore in 1980. The first defibrillators were used to treat ventricular fibrillation; by 1982 modifications allowed the Mirowski defibrillator to treat both ventricular fibrillation and ventricular tachycardia.

Early defibrillators consisted of defibrillating patches placed via thoracotomy on the ventricular epicardium and connected to an internal defibrillator that dis-

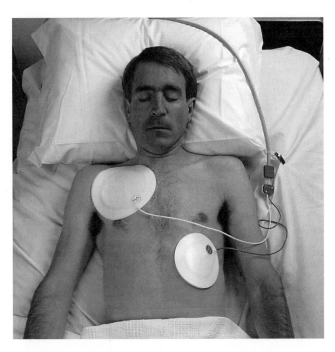

FIGURE 17-22 External defibrillation pads. (Courtesy Medtronic, Inc.)

charged when it sensed ventricular tachycardia or fibrillation (Fig. 17-21). Up to four or five shocks could be delivered per episode of dysrhythmia. The development of nonthoracotomy lead systems inserted transvenously have made epicardial patch systems rare, although in some situations they may be required if the transvenous electrodes fail to defibrillate effectively (Lowe and Wharton, 1995). The first manufactured internal defibrillator bore the proprietary name automatic implantable cardioverter defibrillator (AICD) and was made by Cardiac Pacemakers, Inc.; *ICD* is the generic name for these devices, which are currently manufactured by a number of different manufacturers.

ICD insertion usually is performed in the cardiac catheterization or EP laboratory. Electrophysiologic testing is performed to induce the dysrhythmia and to identify its characteristics. Because testing requires induction of VT or VF, external adhesive defibrillator patches are applied (Fig. 17-22). After diagnosing the characteristics of the problem, the device is inserted.

The transvenous system has a variety of configurations (Fig. 17-23). There may be a single lead containing a sensing component and two shocking coils (one at the distal tip and the other in a proximal portion of the lead). Often this single lead can be used alone. A second electrode may be required; this can be another transvenous lead, or it can be an electrode patch that is placed subcutaneously on the left chest wall. Current devices are not much larger than pacemaker generators and are considerably smaller and weigh less than the early devices. Additionally, defibrillator generators can provide backup pacing for patients who have bradycardia immediately after the defibrillator discharges. Rapid pacing capabilities can terminate VT in selected patients. This antitachycardia pacing (ATP) feature can both prevent the discomfort of a shock and reduce the number of shocks required, thereby enhancing quality of life and prolonging battery life, respectively (Hayes and Zipes, 2001). Multiprogrammable capabilities also include synchronization of the shock, diagnostic and telemetry functions, escalating shocking ranges (0.1 to 35 or 40 joules, depending on patient need), and the ability to take a second look (e.g., if the defibrillator charges for a shock and then the dysrhythmia ceases, the device can sense this and dump the energy; thus the patient is spared an unnecessary and painful shock).

With greater miniaturization of defibrillator devices, improvements in the power sources, better tachycardia recognition, and backup bradycardia pacing, ICDs became the treatment of choice in certain subgroups instead of the treatment of last resort (Waldhausen, Pierce, and Campbell, 1996). Current defibrillator electrodes are designed for transvenous insertion; a subcutaneous patch may be placed in the left side of the chest to expand the number of possible configurations in order to lower the defibrillation threshold (see Fig. 17-23).

Procedure: Transvenous insertion of an ICD

1. With the patient under local anesthesia with sedation, the ICD lead is inserted percutaneously (transvenously) as described for insertion of a permanent pacemaker. The lead position is confirmed fluoroscopically. A pocket for the generator is made in the upper chest or, less commonly, in the abdomen (see Fig. 17-23).

2. If needed, a subcutaneous (SQ) pocket is made in the left side of the chest and the SQ patch is attached. The lead is tunneled to the generator and inserted into the device.

3. Defibrillation testing is performed to sense the rhythm, measure the shocking and pacing thresholds, and determine the lowest energy that consistently defibrillates. When suitable defibrillation thresholds are achieved, the lead is attached to the pectoralis fascia and tunneled to the generator. The lead is inserted into the generator, which is placed in the incisional pocket. The incision is closed.

Complications and follow-up

Fewer complications occur with transvenous insertion (compared with thoracotomy); those that do occur are often associated with venous access and pocket formation. Lead problems (e.g., fracture, cracking, migration) and component or battery failure may occur and are similar to pacemaker problems. ICD-specific complications may include SQ patch migration and inappropriate discharges

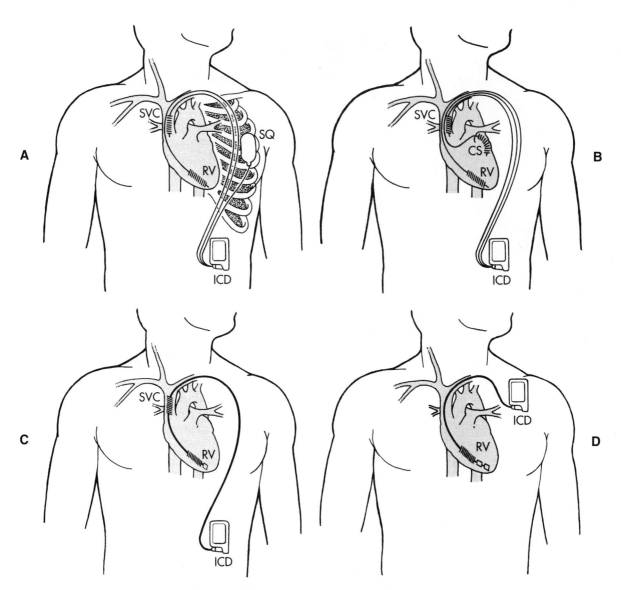

FIGURE 17-23   Nonthoracotomy ICD lead configurations and generator insertion sites (see text). **A,** A three-lead system with shocks delivered from the *RV* electrode to the *SVC* electrode and also to the *SQ* patch electrode. **B,** A three-lead system with shocks delivered from the RV to SVC electrodes and also to the coronary sinus *(CS)* electrode. **C,** A single-lead system with shocks delivered from the RV to SVC electrodes. **D,** A single-lead system with shocks delivered from the RV electrode to the defibrillator. Generators are commonly placed in the left upper chest **(D).** (From Kinney MR, Packa DR, editors: *Andreoli's comprehensive cardiac care,* ed 8, St Louis, 1996, Mosby.)

for short-term VT or supraventricular tachycardias. The fear of painful shocks, anxiety, and depression should be evaluated and may require counseling or, rarely, device removal (Kinney and Packa, 1996).

The device is tested before the patient's discharge from the hospital. Antidysrhythmic drugs may be added or restarted (although usually in lower doses). Stored electrograms are reviewed periodically to monitor de-

vice function. Follow-up is recommended every 2 to 3 months depending on individual need. Periodic chest x-ray films in the first year are used to assess generator, lead, and patch location. Multiple ICD discharges warrant investigation (Hayes and Zipes, 2001). Generator changes can be done with the patient under local anesthesia. Additional teaching considerations are listed in Table 17-3.

References

Ad N, Cox JL: Stroke prevention as an indication for the Maze procedure in the treatment of atrial fibrillation, *Semin Thorac Cardiovasc Surg* 12(1):56, 2000.

Ad N and others: Observations on the perioperative management of patients undergoing the Maze procedure, *Semin Thorac Cardiovasc Surg* 12(1):63, 2000.

Atlee JL: Cardiac pacing and electroversion. In Kaplan JA, editor: *Cardiac anesthesia*, ed 4, Philadelphia, 1999, WB Saunders.

Barold SS: Biventricular cardiac pacing: promising new therapy for congestive heart failure, *Chest* 118(6):1819, 2000.

Beck CS, Pritchard WH, Fell HS: Ventricular fibrillation of long duration abolished by electric shock, *JAMA* 135:985, 1947.

Berne RM, Levy MN: *Cardiovascular physiology*, ed 8, St Louis, 2001, Mosby.

Bernstein AD and others: The NASPE/BPEG generic pacemaker code for antibradyarrhythmia and adaptive-rate pacing and antitachyarrhythmia devices, *Pacing Clin Electrophysiol* 10(4 Pt 1):794, 1987.

Bharucha DB, Kowey PR: Management and prevention of atrial fibrillation after cardiovascular surgery, *Am J Cardiol* 85(10 suppl 1):20, 2000.

Chambers CE, Skeehan TM, Hensley FA: The cardiac catheterization laboratory: diagnostic and therapeutic procedures in the adult patient. In Kaplan JA, editor: *Cardiac anesthesia*, ed 4, Philadelphia, 1999, WB Saunders.

Clague JR and others: Slow pathway ablation and modification successful for long-term treatment of SVT, *Eur Heart J* 22:82, 2001.

Cobb FR and others: Successful surgical interruption of the bundle of Kent in a patient with Wolff-Parkinson-White syndrome, *Circulation* 38(6):1018, 1968.

Cox JL: The minimally invasive Maze-III procedure, *Oper Techn Thorac Cardiovasc Surg* 5(1):79, 2000a.

Cox JL: The standard Maze-III procedure, *Oper Tech Thorac Cardiovasc Surg* 5(1):2, 2000b.

Cox JL: The surgical treatment of atrial fibrillation: IV. Surgical technique, *J Thorac Cardiovasc Surg* 101(4):584, 1991.

Cox JL, Ad N: New surgical and catheter-based modifications of the Maze procedure, *Semin Thorac Cardiovasc Surg* 12(1):68, 2000.

Cox JL, Schuessler RB, Boineau JP: The development of the Maze procedure for the treatment of atrial fibrillation, *Semin Thorac Cardiovasc Surg* 12(1):2, 2000.

Cox JL and others: The surgical treatment of atrial fibrillation: I. Summary of the current concepts of the mechanisms of atrial flutter and atrial fibrillation, *J Thorac Cardiovasc Surg* 101(3):402, 1991a.

Cox JL and others: The surgical treatment of atrial fibrillation: II. Intraoperative electrophysiologic mapping and description of the electrophysiologic basis of atrial flutter and atrial fibrillation, *J Thorac Cardiovasc Surg* 101(3):406, 1991b.

Cox JL and others: The surgical treatment of atrial fibrillation: III. Development of a definitive surgical procedure, *J Thorac Cardiovasc Surg* 101(4):569, 1991c.

Doty JR: Cardiac arrhythmia—bradycardia [On-line], 2000a. Available: http://ctsnet.org/doc/4457 (accessed November 27, 2000).

Doty JR: Cardiac arrhythmia—tachycardia [On-line], 2000b. Available: http://ctsnet.org/doc/4458 (accessed November 27, 2000).

Eisenberg MS, Mengert TJ: Cardiac resuscitation, *N Engl J Med* 344(17):1304, 2001.

Falk RH: Atrial fibrillation, *N Engl J Med* 344(14):1067, 2001.

Finkelmeier BA: *Cardiothoracic surgical nursing*, ed 2, Philadelphia, 2000, JB Lippincott.

Giri S and others: Oral amiodarone for prevention of atrial fibrillation after open heart surgery, the Atrial Fibrillation Suppression Trial (AFIST): a randomized placebo-controlled trial, *Lancet* 357(9259:830, 2001.

Gonzalez ER, Kannewurk BS, Ornato JP: Intravenous amiodarone for ventricular arrhythmias: overview and clinical use, *Resuscitation* 39(1-2):33, 1998.

Gregoratos G and others: ACC/AHA guidelines for implantation of cardiac pacemakers and antiarrhythmia devices: executive summary—a report of the American College of Cardiology/American Heart Association Task Force on Practice Guidelines (Committee on Pacemaker Implantation), *J Am Coll Cardiol* 31(5):1175, 1998.

Guidelines 2000 for cardiopulmonary resuscitation and emergency cardiovascular care: international consensus on science, *Circulation* 102(Suppl I):I-1, 2000.

Hayes DL, Zipes DP: Cardiac pacemakers and cardioverter-defibrillators. In Braunwald E, Zipes DP, Libby P, editors. *Heart disease*, ed 6, vol 2, Philadelphia, 2001, WB Saunders.

Josephson ME, Callans DJ, Buxton AE: The role of the implantable cardioverter-defibrillator for prevention of sudden cardiac death, *Ann Intern Med* 133(11):901, 2000.

Kern KB, Paraskos JA: Task Force I: cardiac arrest, *J Am Coll Cardiol* 35(4):825, 2000.

Kim KB and others: Modifications of the Cox-Maze III procedure, *Ann Thorac Surg* 71(3):816, 2001.

Kinney MR, Packa DR, editors: *Andreoli's comprehensive cardiac care*, ed 8, St. Louis, 1996, Mosby.

Kosakai Y: How I perform the Maze procedure, *Oper Tech Thorac Cardiovasc Surg* 5(1):23, 2000.

Kudenchuk PJ and others: Amiodarone for resuscitation after out-of-hospital cardiac arrest due to ventricular fibrillation, *N Engl J Med* 341(12):871, 1999.

Lowe JE, Wharton JM: Cardiac pacemakers and implantable cardioverter-defibrillators. In Sabiston DC, Spencer FC, editors: *Surgery of the chest*, ed 6, vol 2, Philadelphia, 1995, WB Saunders.

Marriott HJL, Conover MB: *Advanced concepts in arrhythmias*, ed 3, St Louis, 1998, Mosby.

McCarthy PM: Cox-Maze III procedure with mitral valve repair, *Oper Techn Thorac Cardiovasc Surg* 5(1):58, 2000.

Miller JM, Zipes DP: Management of the patient with cardiac arrhythmias. In Braunwald E, Zipes DP, Libby P editors: *Heart disease: a textbook of cardiovascular medicine* ed 6, vol 2, Philadelphia, 2001, WB Saunders.

Mirowski M and others: Termination of malignant ventricular arrhythmias with an implanted automatic defibrillator in human beings, *N Engl J Med* 303(6):322, 1980.

Mirvis DM, Goldberger AL: Electrocardiography. In Braunwald E, Zipes DP, Libby P, editors: *Heart disease: a textbook of cardiovascular medicine* ed 6, vol 2, Philadelphia, 2001, WB Saunders.

Morady F: Radio-frequency ablation as treatment for cardiac arrhythmias, *N Engl J Med* 340(7):534, 1999.

Narayan SM, Cain ME, Smith JM: Atrial fibrillation, *Lancet* 350(9082):943, 1997.

Ozcan C and others: Long-term survival after ablation of the atrioventricular node and implantation of a permanent pacemaker in patients with atrial fibrillation, *N Engl J Med* 344(14):1043, 2001.

Paul S: ECGs and pacemakers, *Crit Care Nurse* 21(1):56, 2001.

Prystowsky EN and others: Management of patients with atrial fibrillation, *Circulation* 93(6):1262, 1996.

Rubart M, Zipes DP: Genesis of cardiac arrhythmias: electrophysiological considerations. In Braunwald E, Zipes DP, Libby P, editors: *Heart disease: a textbook of cardiovascular medicine* ed 6, vol 2, Philadelphia, 2001, WB Saunders.

Samuels LE, Samuels FL: The electrophysiologist and the cardiac surgeon, *Adv Card Surg* 12:97, 2000.

Saxon LA, Kumar UN, De Marco T: Heart failure and cardiac resynchronization therapies: U.S. experience in the year 2000, *Ann Noninvasive Electrocardiol* 5(2):188, 2000.

Seifert PC: Cardiac surgery. In Rothrock JC: *Perioperative nursing care planning*, ed 2, St Louis, 1998, Mosby.

Skubas NJ and others: Anesthesia for electrophysiologic procedures. In Kaplan JA, editor: *Cardiac anesthesia,* ed 4, Philadelphia, 1999, WB Saunders.

Stone J: *In the country of hearts: journeys in the art of medicine,* New York, 1990, Delacourt Press.

Tracy CM and others: American College of Cardiology/American Heart Association clinical competence statement on invasive electrophysiology studies, catheter ablation, and cardioversion, *J Am Coll Cardiol* 36(5):1725, 2000.

Waldhausen JA, Pierce WS, Campbell DB: *Surgery of the chest,* ed 6, St Louis, 1996, Mosby.

Zipes DP: President's page: convocation address: "treat each day as your last and each patient as your first: a personal promise to the profession," *J Am Coll Cardiol* 37(5):1469, 2001.

Zoll PM and others: Termination of ventricular fibrillation in man by externally applied electric shock, *N Engl J Med* 254:727, 1956.

18 Surgery for Adult Congenital Heart Disease

The complications arising from the persistence of a patent ductus arteriosus would seem to make surgical ligation of this anomalous vessel a rational procedure, if such a procedure could be completed with promise of a low operative mortality.

Robert E. Gross, MD, and John P. Hubbard, MD, 1939

The successful ligation in 1939 by Gross (Gross and Hubbard, 1939) of a persistent ductal shunt between the aorta and the pulmonary artery in a 7-year-old girl often is considered the beginning of surgical treatment for congenital malformations of the heart (Taussig, 1982). This achievement also focused on the importance of collaborative efforts between surgeons and their pediatric cardiologic associates and stimulated the development of procedures to palliate or repair a number of congenital deformities (Rashkind, 1982).

Catheter therapy has greatly expanded the treatment options for congenital anomalies. Balloon angioplasty techniques can be used to dilate stenotic valves or vascular strictures. Transcatheter closure of some secundum atrial septal defects (with umbrella-shaped and other similar functioning devices) is becoming the best approach for some patients (Friedman and Silverman, 2001), and percutaneous interventions for other anomalous intracardiac or extracardiac communications are under investigation. Radiofrequency ablation for dysrhythmias is another percutaneous method of treating congenital conduction disturbances. It is anticipated that dysrhythmias also will increase as a greater number of individuals survive into adulthood after complex congenital cardiac repairs, which, in addition to the underlying anatomic abnormalities, can create rhythm problems in adulthood (Warnes and others, 2001).

Before the introduction of extracorporeal circulatory support, surgical treatment of congenital anomalies was limited primarily to extracardiac lesions (such as patent ductus arteriosus [PDA] and coarctation of the aorta) that could be operated on without the necessity of arresting the heart. Surgery for intracardiac malformations, such as the tetralogy of Fallot, consisted of the creation of palliative extracardiac shunts (e.g., the Blalock-Taussig subclavian artery–to–pulmonary artery shunt). Total repair of this and other complex intracardiac lesions had to await cardiopulmonary bypass (CPB) capability and the development of diagnostic methods that were more sophisticated than the stethoscope, three-lead electrocardiogram (ECG), and chest radiograph, which were the only tools available to Gross in 1939 (Gross and Hubbard, 1939).

In the past the frequency of congenital lesions seen in the adult (Box 18-1) was a reflection not only of their

---

BOX 18-1
Most Frequent Congenital Malformations Seen at Surgery in Adults*

Ostium secundum atrial septal defect
Coarctation of aorta
Ventricular septal defect
Pulmonary stenosis
Ostium primum atrial septal defect
Patent ductus arteriosus
Tetralogy of Fallot
Aortic stenosis
Vascular ring
Total anomalous pulmonary venous drainage

*This is one of the earliest tabulations of congenital anomalies seen in the adult; other listings tabulated more recently show a comparable incidence of congenital heart disease in the adult. Exceptions may be the incidence of mitral valve prolapse and the bicuspid aortic valve, which, according to Roberts (1987), are the most common congenital anomalies in the adult.
Modified from Cooley DA, Hallman GL, Hammam S: Congenital cardiovascular anomalies in adults. Results of surgical treatment in 167 patients over age 35, *Am J Cardiol* 17(3):303, 1966.

rate of occurrence but also of their mortality in childhood. The more serious lesions were not seen in later life because they were more likely to cause death in infancy (Cooley, Hallman, and Hammom, 1966). With extraordinary advances in diagnostic and treatment modalities over the past 40 years, approximately 85% of babies born with cardiovascular anomalies can expect to reach adulthood (Warnes and others, 2001). In the United States the number of adults with congenital heart defects (Table 18-1) is approximately 800,000 (Summary of Recommendations, 2001).

The number of older patients with congenital heart disease is increasing steadily and includes patients who have never undergone palliative or reparative procedures in childhood but who require surgical correction in adulthood, those who have had palliation with or without anticipation of repair, those who have had

surgery and require no further operation, and those whose condition is inoperable apart from organ transplantation (Perloff, 1997). Patients who have never had palliative or corrective surgery, as well as those who have undergone surgery, also are susceptible to acquired cardiac disease and valvular dysfunction. Thus perioperative nurses specializing in acquired cardiac disorders are increasingly likely to see both patients with corrected or uncorrected congenital heart disease.

Although this chapter is limited to the congenital deformities most likely to await repair in adulthood, it is helpful to be familiar with the congenital anomalies commonly requiring correction in childhood because the perioperative nurse may encounter these patients when they require surgery for acquired disorders. Nurses can plan care better knowing that there may be sternal (or thoracic) adhesions from prior surgery, altered

---

TABLE 18-1
Description of Selected Congenital Cardiac Lesions Seen in Adulthood

LESION	DESCRIPTION
Anomalous pulmonary venous return	Pulmonary venous return enters systemic venous system rather than left atrium; usually partial rather than total return of pulmonary venous blood flow; usually produces increased pulmonary blood flow; variable cyanosis
Atrial septal defect (ASD)	Communication between right and left atria; three common types of ASD: **Sinus venosus:** Area of entry is superior vena cava into atrium; commonly associated with partial anomalous pulmonary venous return **Ostium secundum:** Area of fossa ovalis (formerly fetal foramen ovale); midportion of septum; most common **Ostium primum:** Area inferior to fossa ovalis; associated with cleft anterior leaflet of mitral valve; least common
Bicuspid aortic valve	Fusion of two of the three cusps, producing a two-cusp valve; prone to eventual calcification and stenosis; one of the most frequent anomalies of the heart
Coarctation of aorta	Aortic constriction caused by both external narrowing and intraluminal membrane **Postductal** (adult): Coarctation located distal to left subclavian artery and PDA, near or at aortic isthmus; produces systolic and diastolic hypertension in proximal aorta, increases left ventricular workload, and stimulates fetal and postnatal development of large collateral vessels to perfuse organs distal to coarctation **Preductal** (infant): Coarctation located proximal to PDA; lower body perfusion dependent on patent ductus; may produce cyanosis of lower extremities; collateral circulation not formed; less common than adult form
Coronary artery fistula	Communication (fistula) between one or more coronary arteries and a cardiac chamber, vena cava, coronary sinus, pulmonary vein, or pulmonary trunk; produces ischemia when the fistula "steals" blood from the myocardium; common malformation
Patent ductus arteriosus	Persistent fetal shunt between aorta and pulmonary artery; produces increased pulmonary blood flow
Pulmonary valve stenosis	Thickened valve leaflets impede blood flow to lungs; increases right ventricular (RV) afterload, producing RV hypertrophy and failure if untreated; balloon dilation commonly used in young patients
Sinus of Valsalva aneurysm	Weakening, dilation of (usually) one of the aortic valve sinuses; may contain small perforations producing murmur; prone to rupture
Tetralogy of Fallot (TOF)	Consists of four anatomic abnormalities: VSD, pulmonary stenosis, aorta that overrides VSD, and RV hypertrophy; results in decreased pulmonary blood flow, causing hypoxia and cyanosis; rare instances exist of untreated TOF in adulthood
Ventricular septal defect (VSD)	Communication between right and left ventricles; may occur beneath aortic valve in membranous septum, in infundibular (perimembranous) septum, beneath septal leaflet of tricuspid valve, or in muscular septum; produces volume and pressure overloading of RV and volume overloading of the pulmonary circulation; small defects often close before adulthood

Modified from Therrien J, Webb GD: Congenital heart disease in adults. In Braunwald E, Zipes DP, Libby P editors: *Heart disease: a textbook of cardiovascular medicine,* ed 6, Philadelphia, 2001, WB Saunders.

anatomy without the familiar landmarks, prostheses (e.g., conduits, occlusive devices, intracardiac or extracardiac patches) that should not be disturbed, and other alterations that affect the performance of surgery.

Among the congenital disorders discussed in this chapter are PDA, atrial septal defect (ASD), and coarctation of the aorta. This chapter also includes a discussion of closure of a PDA in the infant. PDA, a frequently occurring extracardiac congenital disorder, does not require CPB in the infant (unless it is associated with other complex malformations) and is relatively easy to repair. Perioperative cardiac nurses may be presented with such a patient, especially when there are no pediatric centers in the vicinity.

Other congenital deformities and syndromes already discussed in previous chapters include the following:

Mitral valve prolapse	Chapter 11
Bicuspid aortic valve	Chapter 12
Idiopathic hypertrophic subaortic stenosis	Chapter 12
Ebstein's anomaly	Chapter 13
Pulmonary stenosis	Chapter 13
Marfan's syndrome and Ehlers-Danlos syndrome	Chapter 14
Wolff-Parkinson-White syndrome	Chapter 17

When adult patients appear with a congenital lesion more commonly seen in the pediatric population, perioperative nurses can apply principles of surgical management for acquired disorders to these congenital malformations. Although the etiology is different, there are similarities that the perioperative nurse can consider in preparing for these unusual cases. (It is also helpful if a nurse in this situation consults a colleague familiar with congenital cardiac disorders.) For example, patients with tetralogy of Fallot (see Table 18-1) require closure of the ventricular septal defect (VSD), relief of the pulmonary stenosis, and enlargement of the right ventricular outflow tract (often with a synthetic patch). Repair of a congenital VSD would include techniques similar to those used for repair of a postmyocardial infarction VSD (see Chapter 10). Pulmonary stenosis at the valvular level could be repaired by incision of the stenotic pulmonary valve (see Chapter 13) or insertion of a pulmonary allograft (see Chapter 12); subvalvular stenosis may require excision of a portion of the hypertrophied right ventricular outflow tract. Patch closure of the right ventriculotomy may be required: the patch material, suture, and felt pledgets and the surgical technique may be similar to those used for a standard repair of a left ventricular apical aneurysm (see Chapter 10).

Intrauterine Circulation

The fetal lungs do not oxygenate blood; the lungs are nonaerated and filled with fluid, which produces a high pulmonary vascular resistance. Both oxygen and nutrients are provided by the mother, whose blood is circulated to the placenta, where oxygen and other metabolic substrates are exchanged for the metabolic waste products of the fetus. Enriched blood is carried to the fetus through the umbilical vein, passes through the liver, and enters the inferior vena cava (IVC) and right atrium. Most of this blood passes preferentially across the patent foramen ovale (bypassing the high-pressure pulmonary vascular bed) into the left atrium, left ventricle, and ascending aorta to perfuse the brain and coronary circulation (Fig. 18-1).

Blood returning to the superior vena cava (SVC) enters the right atrium and passes through the tricuspid valve into the right ventricle and the pulmonary artery. Much of this blood passes across the nonrestrictive, wide patent ductus arteriosus into the descending aorta rather than into the high-pressure pulmonary system.

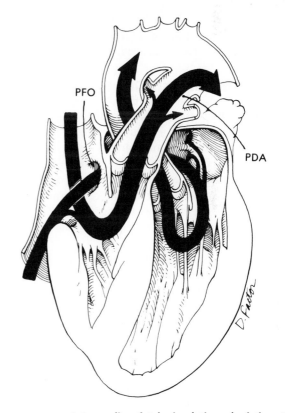

FIGURE 18-1 Intracardiac fetal circulation depicting the normal fetal shunts: the patent foramen ovale *(PFO)* and the *PDA.* Most IVC blood passes across the PFO into the left atrium. The superior vena cava (SVC) return is directed predominantly across the PDA, which is large and nonrestrictive. Note that relatively little blood enters or exits the lungs. Persistent postnatal shunting of blood through the PFO and PDA creates hemodynamic disturbances that may require surgical correction. (From Bove EL: Congenital heart lesions. In Miller TA, editor: *Physiologic basis of modern surgical care,* St Louis, 1988, Mosby.)

TABLE **18-2**
Congenital Malformations Seen in the Adult

MALFORMATION	EXAMPLE
Defects: Absent tissue in cardiac septa (walls), causing shunts	Atrial septal defect
Obstructions: Excess tissue at or near level of cardiac valves or major arteries	Coarctation of aorta; idiopathic hypertrophic subaortic stenosis
Anomalous connections: Abnormal communications between arteries and veins or between vessels and cardiac chambers	Anomalous pulmonary venous return (e.g., into right atrium)
Improperly formed tissue: Having normal function at birth and during adolescence but later causing cardiac dysfunction	Bicuspid aortic valve
Combinations of the above	Tetralogy of Fallot

Modified from Roberts WC: Congenital cardiovascular abnormalities usually "silent" until adulthood. In Roberts WC: *Adult congenital heart disease,* Philadelphia, 1987, FA Davis.

Ductal patency in utero is maintained by prostaglandins and other vasodilator substances (Clyman, 2000). (Prostaglandins may be used *after* birth to keep the ductus open.) Because the right and left ventricles face similar resistances, both ventricles function essentially as one unit. Blood in the aorta returns to the placenta via the umbilical arteries (Hazinski, 1999).

Postnatal Circulatory Changes

At birth, closure of the normal fetal shunts—the foramen ovale and the ductus arteriosus—is necessary to achieve separation of the pulmonary and systemic circulations. Elimination of the placenta (which in utero creates a low systemic vascular resistance) results in an abrupt increase in systemic vascular resistance. Aeration of the lungs gradually decreases pulmonary vascular resistance, promoting greater blood flow to the lungs (Rudolph and Nadas, 1962).

Increased pulmonary venous return to the left atrium elevates left atrial pressure. This causes the septum primum (a flap of tissue on the left atrial wall) to seal closed the foramen ovale (which becomes the fossa ovalis). Increased arterial oxygen tension, a drop in circulating prostaglandins (fetal vasodilators), and a reduction of prostaglandin receptor sites in the ductal wall cause constriction of the smooth muscle in the ductus (which becomes the ligamentum arteriosum). Closure of the ductus results from functional and anatomic mechanisms. Functional closure occurs within hours after birth, when ductal smooth muscle constricts. Anatomic occlusion occurs over the next few days in response to the loss of ductal blood flow (because blood bypasses the ductus and then preferentially enters the lungs); this hypoperfusion creates a zone of hypoxia in the ductal muscle media, which stimulates endothelial proliferation. The neointima thickens, and the smooth muscle cells disappear (Clyman, 2000; Lake, 1999). When either the ductus arteriosus or the foramen ovale fails to close, mixing of oxygenated and unoxygenated blood persists. The higher pressure in the systemic circulation (as compared with the pulmonary circulation) leads to shunting of blood into the pulmonary system, which, if severe enough, may result in congestive heart failure.

Congenital Malformations

Unlike acquired cardiac disease, which imposes pathologic anatomic and physiologic changes in previously normal structures, the major problems associated with congenital disorders of the heart and great vessels are the disturbed hemodynamics and in some lesions the hypoxemia that result from abnormal morphology, intracardiac shunting, and altered pulmonary blood flow (Lake, 1999).

Why some congenital malformations do not require intervention until later childhood or adulthood is related to the nature of the lesion (Table 18-2), the altered volume and pressure loads affecting cardiac function in the neonatal period, and the degree of oxygen saturation of the blood supplying the tissues. Lesions are often categorized as *acyanotic* (those that do not produce systemic arterial desaturation) or *cyanotic* (those that produce a bluish discoloration from venous blood entering the arterial circulation and causing arterial oxygen desaturation). Cyanotic lesions can be the result of right-to-left shunts within the heart or aorta or to transposition of the pulmonary artery and the aorta (Hazinski, 1999).

Also important are the status of the lungs, which can be affected by increased pulmonary blood flow; the type and size of the malformation or defect; the resistance to flow through the abnormal and the normal vascular pathways; and the direction and magnitude of the shunts. For example, an abnormal opening in the ventricular septum produces shunting of blood from the area of higher pressure (usually the left ventricle) to the area of lower pressure (e.g., the right ventricle). An isolated, small VSD will have fewer adverse hemodynamic consequences than a large VSD or multiple VSDs, both of which would sub-

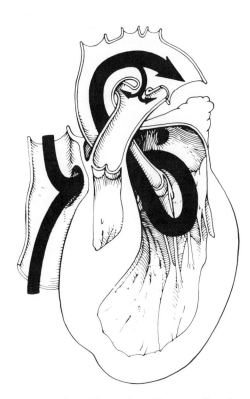

FIGURE 18-2 Tricuspid atresia with normally related great vessels and without a ventricular septal defect. Pulmonary blood flow depends on an atrial septal defect to shunt blood to the left atrium, from where it enters the left ventricle. From there, blood enters the aorta and enters the lungs via a patent ductus arteriosus. When a VSD is also present, blood can cross to the right ventricle and enter the lungs. (From Bove EL: Congenital heart lesions. In Miller TA, editor: *Physiologic basis of modern surgical care,* St Louis, 1988, Mosby.)

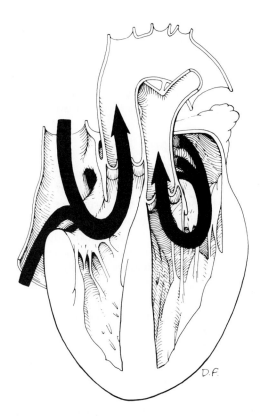

FIGURE 18-3 Transposition of the great arteries. The aorta arises from the right ventricle, and the pulmonary artery arises from the left ventricle, producing severe hypoxemia. For survival, an intracardiac shunt is needed to allow oxygen-saturated blood to enter the aorta and the systemic circulation. (From Bove EL: Congenital heart lesions. In Miller TA, editor: *Physiologic basis of modern surgical care,* St Louis, 1988, Mosby.)

stantially increase the left-to-right shunting of blood into the pulmonary vasculature, eventually resulting in increased pulmonary vascular resistance. If, however, the VSD is associated with a severe obstruction to right ventricular outflow (such as a tightly stenotic pulmonary valve), then there is likely to be higher pressure in the right ventricle as it tries to overcome the resistance to ejection, and this can cause blood to be shunted to the (relatively lower pressure) left ventricle.

Other developmental cardiac abnormalities may be present. Valves may be absent (e.g., tricuspid atresia; Fig. 18-2); chambers may be underdeveloped (e.g., hypoplastic left heart syndrome); systemic and pulmonary arteries may be attached to the "wrong" ventricle (e.g., transposition of the great arteries; Fig. 18-3). Combinations of malformations (e.g., in tetralogy of Fallot) are not uncommon and may not be evident during the initial diagnostic workup. Because of the possibility of finding additional anomalies at operation, a surgeon will explore cardiac and related anatomy meticulously during surgery.

Diagnostic Evaluation of Congenital Heart Disease

A complete history and physical examination incorporates the extent of the cardiopulmonary impairment and other, extracardiac congenital anomalies that are frequently associated with congenital heart disease. Pulmonary infections are common in lungs that are chronically volume overloaded, and the presence, severity, and duration of hypoxemia should be investigated. Bacterial endocarditis also is seen in these patients and is related to the endothelial trauma that can occur from altered circulatory patterns (Lake, 1999).

ELECTROCARDIOGRAM

The ECG provides information about cardiac rhythm, the adverse effects of volume and pressure overload on the ventricles, conduction abnormalities such as bundle-branch blocks, and signs of ventricular hypertrophy.

Interpretation of the ECG should take into consideration the effects of diuresis on electrolyte levels. The classic histologic studies of the conduction system by Lev (1958; 1959; 1960) have been valuable in interpreting ECG patterns and in guiding the surgeon during intraoperative repairs of congenital cardiac anomalies.

CHEST RADIOGRAPHY

Posteroanterior and lateral chest radiographs illustrate cardiac size and configuration, the pattern of pulmonary blood flow, the position of the aortic arch, and skeletal abnormalities (such as rib notching, often seen in patients with coarctation of the aorta). In adults who have had previous surgery for palliation of congenital malformations, the chest x-ray film may show rib deformity from thoracotomy or the extent of adhesions from sternotomy, conduits or shunts, or postoperative complications. Contrast imaging is used for complicated lesions.

ECHOCARDIOGRAPHY

Two-dimensional echocardiography with color flow Doppler is indispensable for the diagnosis of congenital (and acquired) cardiac disorders. Its use may obviate the need for cardiac catheterization, which can be risky in the neonate. Uncomplicated ASD, PDA, and coarctation of the aorta may be diagnosed with precision in many cases. For more complex defects of the atrial or ventricular septum or for small-lumen PDAs, echocardiography has limitations, and diagnosis may require more invasive techniques. Doppler technology provides information about the movement of blood (direction and velocity), pressure gradients across valves and obstructions, and the valve area. In addition to its noninvasiveness, echocardiography avoids ionizing radiation and is relatively inexpensive (Kahn and others, 1999).

CARDIAC CATHETERIZATION

Cardiac catheterization with cineangiocardiography remains an important diagnostic technique for assessing congenital malformations, although echocardiography is becoming increasingly useful for initial diagnosis. Because adults with congenital lesions are also at risk for developing acquired heart disease, cardiac catheterization is done routinely to determine the existence and extent of obstructive atherosclerotic lesions and other acquired disorders and to assess left ventricular function. It also is used to study the direction, magnitude, and approximate location of intracardiac shunts. Intracardiac and intravascular pressures, pressure gradients, and blood oxygen saturations can be measured. For example, the patient whose arterial blood is fully saturated in the aorta can be safely assumed to have no significant right-to-left shunt, whereas documentation of hypoxemia in the aorta indicates shunting of desaturated blood into the systemic circulation (Kern, 1999).

OTHER DIAGNOSTIC TECHNIQUES

Computed tomography (CT) is helpful for diagnosing a number of congenital disorders. CT scans may be especially useful in anomalies associated with the great vessels.

Magnetic resonance imaging (MRI) and positron emission tomography (PET) can provide information about morphology and altered hemodynamics; they also are being used to study cardiac metabolism noninvasively by measuring the phosphorus found in high-energy phosphates (e.g., adenosine triphosphate [ATP]) and other biologically important atomic nuclei used in metabolic processes. MRI is useful for visualizing coarctation of the aorta and is especially valuable in the older patient whose aortic isthmus may not be easily assessed with ultrasonic techniques. (Echocardiography is superior, however, for evaluating flow velocity through shunts and defects [Kahn and others, 1999]).

Radionuclide techniques can be used to quantify left-to-right shunting and systolic ventricular performance, and there is great potential for measuring ventricular volumes and diastolic function (Taylor, 2000).

Patent Ductus Arteriosus

PDA is the most common cause of left-to-right shunting at the level of the great arteries (see Fig. 18-1). Because aortic pressure is higher than pulmonary artery pressure throughout the cardiac cycle, shunting occurs in both systole and diastole. This produces a continuous murmur, often described as "machinery-like." In addition, the low-resistance pulmonary circulation allows a significant amount of aortic diastolic runoff, resulting in a wide pulse pressure and a bounding arterial pulse. A large PDA produces a substantial increase in pulmonary blood flow, leading to pulmonary overloading and eventual heart failure (Lake, 1999). A smaller PDA, producing less left-to-right shunting, may not be clinically significant for many years unless pulmonary hypertension develops.

INFANT PATENT DUCTUS ARTERIOSUS

In preterm infants with a physiologically significant shunt, pharmacologic closure of a PDA has been performed with indomethacin (a prostaglandin inhibitor), although ibuprofen has been shown to be as effective, but with fewer side effects than indomethacin (Van Overmeire and others, 2000). (Conversely, in babies with congenital lesions that severely limit pulmonary blood flow, such as a stenotic or absent tricuspid valve, a PDA may be necessary for survival until surgery can be performed. In such cases prostaglandin may be used to maintain the patency of the ductus.) Nonsurgical methods to close the ductus have included the insertion of occlusive devices under fluoroscopy in the cardiac catheterization laboratory. Minimally invasive techniques, such as video-assisted thoracoscopic surgery (VATS), are also being used to close PDAs, and it can be anticipated that the use of VATS will continue to grow (Burke and Wernovsky, 1997; Maldonado and Nygren, 1999).

Procedural considerations

Surgical closure of a PDA is indicated when the patient is at risk for or has congestive heart failure. The procedure can be performed in the operating room (OR) or in the neonatal intensive care unit (NICU). Where surgery is performed is based on the ability of the infant to withstand the stress of transport to and from the nursery, the availability of infant carrier systems, the creation of a suitable operative environment, the availability and skill of personnel, and surgeon preference (Huddleston, 1991). For infants who are critically unstable and require high-frequency ventilation or extracorporeal membrane oxygenation (ECMO) (see Chapter 9), PDA ligation in the NICU may be preferred in order to avoid the risks of transport (Austin, 2000).

When PDA ligation is performed in the NICU, the primary concern is maintenance of sterility (Huddleston, 1991) to protect the infant from infection. Sterile instruments and supplies required for surgery often are brought to the unit. Other items may be present in the unit or may be transported from the OR as needed (Box 18-2).

Closure of the ductus can be performed in a number of ways. Gross (Gross and Hubbard, 1939) originally ligated the ductus of a 7-year-old girl with No. 8 braided silk. Current ligation techniques may use double ligature of heavy silk (e.g., No. 1) or a pursestring ligature of polypropylene. The ligated ductus may or may not be divided.

Division and oversewing of the cut ductal ends and double application of metal vascular clips with or without division are other methods of ligation. The use of vascular clips has gained some popularity; its proponents maintain that the technique minimizes the risk of tearing friable ductal tissue (especially in the posterior wall of the ductus) in infants, as well as in adults. Before application of the clips, the applier must be checked for easy release of the clip and for correct apposition of the clip applier jaws.

In neonates an important consideration is distinguishing between the various vascular structures: the PDA, aorta, pulmonary artery, and left subclavian artery (Box 18-3). A careful evaluation is necessary to avoid ligating the wrong vessel because in neonates the PDA

BOX 18-2

Instruments and Supplies for Ligation of a Patent Ductus Arteriosus Outside the Operating Room

Instruments*

Knife handles
Vascular forceps
Adson tissue forceps with teeth
Fine dissecting scissors
Suture scissors
Towel clips
Mosquito clamps
Hemostats
Kelly clamps
Right-angle clamps
Vascular clip appliers (assorted sizes)
Needle holders
Vascular clamps (straight and angled)
Suction tip(s)
Sponge sticks
Ribbon retractors
Brain retractors
Vein retractors
Army-Navy retractors
Senn retractors
Eyelid retractors
Rib spreader

Sterile Supplies

Gowns, gloves, drapes
Peanut (Kittner) sponges
Suture (heavy silk ties, vascular suture, closing suture)
Mineral oil
Electrocautery pencil
Suction tubing
Chest catheter (standard chest tube for older patient or red rubber catheter for infant)
Vascular ligating clips (assorted sizes)
Skin preparation materials
Hand scrub brushes

Nonsterile Supplies and Equipment

Electrosurgical unit
Electrosurgical dispersive pad
Spotlight
Radiant warmer (infants)
Surgeon headlights and magnifying loupes
Privacy screens
Surgical hats and masks
Positioning supplies
Physiologic monitoring devices
(Blood and blood products should be available at the start of surgery)

*Size of instruments is dependent on size and weight of patient; type of instruments is dependent on surgeon's preference.
Modified from Huddleston KR: Patent ductus arteriosus ligation: performing surgery outside the operating room, *AORN J* 53(1):69, 1991.

may be quite large and resemble the aorta. The PDA may seem to be in continuity with the descending aorta, whereas the aortic isthmus and aortic arch are smaller (Waldhausen, Pierce, and Campbell, 1996).

Operative procedure: ligation of a patent ductus arteriosus in the infant

The patient is placed in the lateral position with the left side up. Positioning supplies (e.g., axillary rolls, padding between the knees) are the same as those used for any lateral position (see Chapter 9). Small axillary rolls can be made from a rolled cloth diaper, Webril, or a washcloth. Pressure areas are padded, and a dipersive electrode pad is placed around the buttocks. Adhesive tape across the hips may be used to stabilize the patient, although in neonates this may be unnecessary.

Routine monitoring includes ECG, pulse oximetry, and monitoring of blood pressure, temperature, and end-tidal carbon dioxide. Head coverings are used to reduce heat loss from the head; radiant warmers may be used to provide additional warmth. Very small infants present special needs. Finding sufficient space for ECG electrodes and dispersive pads may be a challenge. However, dispersive pads should not be trimmed down because this could cause inadequate dispersion of electrical currents and result in skin burns.

Procedure

1. A thoracotomy incision is made in the third or fourth intercostal space (Fig. 18-4).
2. The ribs are spread with handheld retractors for initial dissection. A Finochietto rib spreader is then inserted. The lungs are carefully retracted downward and forward, taking care to protect the phrenic, recurrent laryngeal, and main vagus nerves (Fig. 18-5).
3. The mediastinal pleura is opened over the aortic isthmus (the portion of the aorta over the PDA, be-

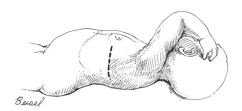

FIGURE 18-4 Incision for repair of a PDA. (From Waldhausen JA, Pierce WS, Campbell DB: *Surgery of the chest*, ed 6, St Louis, 1996, Mosby.)

BOX 18-3
Special Considerations for Patients with Congenital Heart Disease

General Considerations

Review the diagnostic study results in preparation for surgery.
Always expect a more complex lesion than anticipated; other cardiac anomalies may be present.
Ensure that the jaws of vascular clamps, clip appliers, and hemostatic clamps are in proper working order.
Have available array of total- and partial-occluding vascular clamps.

Patient Ductus Arteriosus Repair

Lung compression may be poorly tolerated; use caution when retracting.
Assume that the *aorta* has been clamped until it is confirmed that the PDA has been clamped.
Beware of injuring the vagus and recurrent laryngeal nerves.

Atrial Septal Defect

Plan for bicaval venous cannulation; have a right-angle SVC cannula available.
Anticipate insertion of atrial pressure monitoring lines.
Prepare for insertion of pulmonary monitoring lines at the conclusion of surgery.

Coarctation of the Aorta

Anticipate and be prepared for subclavian flap or graft interposition, patch, or bypass repair.
Maintain cool ambient temperature (an increased incidence of spinal cord paralysis is associated with *hyperthermia*).
Anticipate right and left (radial) arterial blood pressure monitoring lines.

Modified from Maldonado SS, Nygren C: Pediatric surgery. In Meeker MH, Rothrock JC, editors: *Alexander's care of the patient in surgery*, ed 11, St Louis, 1999, Mosby; Lake CL: Anesthesia for patients with congenital heart disease. In Kaplan JA, editor: *Cardiac anesthesia*, ed 4, Philadelphia, 1999, WB Saunders.

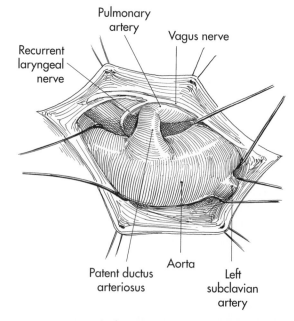

FIGURE 18-5 Surgical exposure for a closure of a PDA. Note the relationships between the PDA, aorta, left subclavian artery, and pulmonary artery, and the location of the vagus nerve and its branch, the recurrent laryngeal nerve. (From Waldhausen JA, Pierce WS, Campbell DB: *Surgery of the chest*, ed 6, St Louis, 1996, Mosby.)

tween the left subclavian artery and the descending aorta); the incision is extended to expose the subclavian artery, the ductus, and the pulmonary artery.

4. The vascular structures are inspected and identified, and the determination is made as to which occlusion technique to use. Retraction sutures may be placed around the aorta proximally and distally, and around the subclavian artery with a clamp (Fig. 18-6, *A*).

5A. Suture ligation: A heavy (No. 1) silk suture may be placed around the ductus and tied (Fig. 18-6, *B*); a second ligature may be placed around the ductus (Fig. 18-6, *C*). Coating the ligature with sterile mineral oil may facilitate its passage around the ductus.

In some neonates the ductus may be very large, and it must be distinguished from the aorta (Fig. 18-7).

5B. Vascular clip: A medium to medium-large vascular clip may be placed across the ductus. This technique minimizes the risk of hemorrhage associated with dissection of the posterior wall of the ductus. (Retraction sutures may not be required.)

5C. Division and oversewing: The ductus may be clamped proximally and distally and divided, and the ends may be oversewn (Fig. 18-8).

5D. Pursestring ligation: A pursestring ligature may be sewn on the aortic side, and another one may be sewn on the pulmonary side; these are tied, occluding the PDA.

6. If the pleura has been entered, air can be removed with the chest tube. In neonates a red rubber catheter can be placed into the pleura through the partially closed incision and then gradually withdrawn while the lungs are inflated and the pneumothorax is evacuated. Once the catheter is removed, the incision is closed completely.

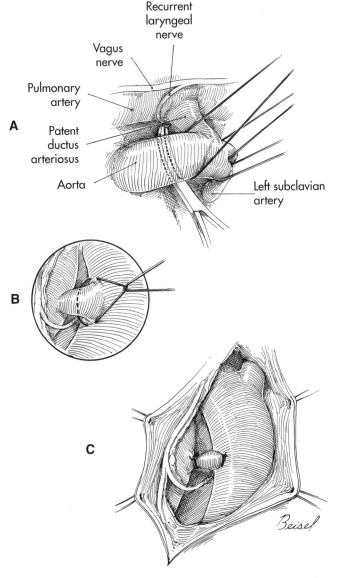

FIGURE 18-6 **A,** Dissection of the posterior wall with a clamp; tissue behind the ductus may be quite dense. **B,** A pursestring ligature of a PDA may be preferred to passing a ligature, or a clamp, around the ductus with a ligature carrier, which requires more extensive dissection and increases the risk of hemorrhage from the posterior wall of the ductus. **C,** Completed double-suture ligation. (From Waldhausen JA, Pierce WS, Campbell DB: *Surgery of the chest,* ed 6, St Louis, 1996, Mosby.)

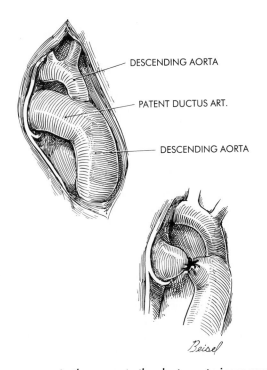

FIGURE 18-7 In the neonate the ductus arteriosus may be quite large and difficult to distinguish from the aorta. (From Waldhausen JA, Pierce WS, Campbell DB: *Surgery of the chest,* ed 6, St Louis, 1996, Mosby.)

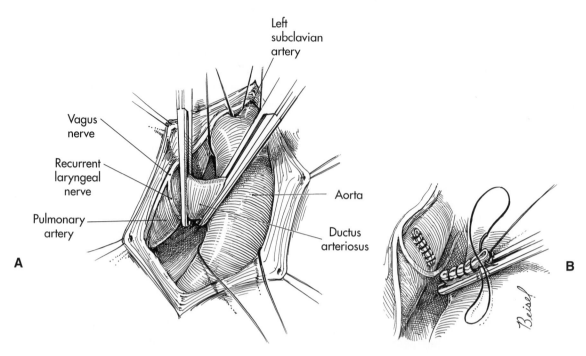

FIGURE 18-8 **A,** Clamps are applied to the aortic and pulmonary sides of the ductus arteriosus. **B,** Division of the ductus is completed, and an over-and-over technique is used to close each end of the ductus. (From Waldhausen JA, Pierce WS, Campbell DB: *Surgery of the chest,* ed 6, St Louis, 1996, Mosby.)

7. The skin closure is completed, and dressings are applied.

Postoperative period

In the absence of other problems, the postoperative course after PDA closure is usually uneventful. Occasionally a ligated ductus becomes patent again; if the re-opened ductus is hemodynamically significant, reoperation is performed to divide and oversew the vessel. Even when a reopened ductus has little clinical impact, closure is advised to reduce the susceptibility to endarteritis.

ADULT PATENT DUCTUS ARTERIOSUS

A ductus that does not close spontaneously within 2 months of birth usually remains persistently patent. It is also more commonly an isolated anomaly. Dyspnea and recurrent respiratory infections are typical presenting symptoms. The presence and severity of symptoms in adults is determined by the size of the PDA, the presence of pulmonary hypertension, and the direction of the shunt. Congestive heart failure is a cause of death in adults patients with PDA. With improved diagnostic techniques and selective antibiotic prophylaxis, the incidence of infective endarteritis has been greatly decreased. Because progressive pulmonary vascular disease may lead to rapid and irreversible cardiac failure, it is recommended that adults with PDA undergo surgical closure.

In adults the ductus may be calcified, sclerotic, and aneurysmal, increasing the risk of rupture. Double ligation (similar to that used in infants) is effective in the uncomplicated adult ductus. In more complicated cases where the ductus is broad and fragile, felt-buttressed sutures or patch closure of the ductal opening inside the aorta may be performed. Left atrial–left femoral artery (left-sided heart bypass) or CPB (occasionally with hypothermia) may be used for the difficult ductus (Waldhausen, Pierce, and Campbell, 1996). In patients with marked elevation of pulmonary vascular resistance, operative closure may not significantly reduce pulmonary hypertension and outcomes may be less favorable (Perloff, 1997).

Atrial Septal Defect

ASDs are among the most common of the congenital malformations seen in adulthood. The defect can occur in three forms (Fig. 18-9): the ostium secundum (the most common), the sinus venosus, and the ostium primum (least common). A common associated lesion in the sinus venosus ASD is partial anomalous pulmonary venous return into the right atrium.

Although blood being shunted from the left atrium to the right atrium increases pulmonary blood flow, the right atrium and the lungs are generally able to tolerate this increased volume for many years. This is because of

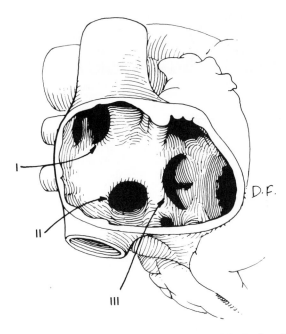

FIGURE 18-9 Location of the three types of ASD. The sinus venosus defect *(I)* is shown with anomalous drainage of the right upper pulmonary vein. The ostium secundum defect *(II)* is in the midportion of the septum in the area of the fossa ovalis. The ostium primum defect *(III)* is located in the base of the septum, with its inferior edge formed by the continuity of the tricuspid and mitral valves. There is often a cleftlike anomaly in the anterior leaflet of the mitral valve visible through the defect. (From Bove EL: Congenital heart lesions. In Miller TA, editor: *Physiologic basis of modern surgical care,* St Louis, 1988, Mosby.)

the distensibility of the atrial wall and the pulmonary vasculature, as well as to the low pressures found within the right side of the heart. Eventually, pulmonary overloading can produce pulmonary hypertension and elevated pulmonary vascular resistance. Pulmonary arterial pressure may begin to approximate systemic arterial pressure, which in turn can lead to a balanced (bidirectional) shunt or to reversal of the shunt whereby higher right-sided pressures create a right-to-left shunt, producing systemic arterial desaturation (e.g., cyanosis). With advancing age, patients also can develop cardiomegaly, atrial dysrhythmias, right ventricular hypertrophy, and right ventricular failure (cor pulmonale) (Perloff, 1997).

The ECG usually demonstrates incomplete right bundle-branch block and a clockwise shift of the heart. Posteroanterior and lateral chest radiographs demonstrate an enlarged right atrium and right ventricle, reflecting the increased ratio of pulmonary blood flow to systemic blood flow (see later discussion). The pulmonary artery shadow is enlarged also. Echocardiography is almost always diagnostic, with transesophageal echocardiography (TEE) widely used to differentiate between the forms of ASD. Atrioventricular valve regurgitation can be demonstrated as well.

Although bacterial endocarditis is often a risk in patients with congenital heart disease, it is unusual in a patient with an ASD because the relatively large septal defect does not produce a "jet" lesion (the forceful squirting of blood against endocardium or endothelium, as occurs with PDA), which would traumatize the inside of the heart and create a potential site for infection.

Symptoms are usually exertional dyspnea and fatigue. Initially these complaints may be attributed to coronary artery disease or rheumatic valvular problems rather than to an ASD. Incomplete right bundle-branch block or atrial fibrillation also may be present, particularly in adults.

Diagnosis usually can be made with modern echocardiographic techniques, but cardiac catheterization may be performed in adults to determine the presence of coronary or valvular heart disease. Cardiac catheterization techniques also have been used extensively to measure pulmonary and systemic pressures, to determine the oxygen saturation of the cardiac chambers and major vessels, and to compute the ratio of pulmonary blood flow to systemic blood flow (Qp/Qs). In the normal heart the stroke volume of the right ventricle equals that of the left ventricle. In the presence of an ASD, which shunts some of the left ventricular preload into the right side of the heart, the pulmonary circulation receives more blood than the systemic circulation. Thus the ratio of pulmonary blood flow to systemic blood flow is higher than the normal Qp/Qs of 1:1. The patient also has an increased oxygen saturation of the right atrial blood (normal is 75%). This is caused by the shunting of freshly oxygenated blood to the right atrium (the increase in venous oxygen saturation is referred to as a *step-up*). Blood samples can be taken from a number of locations between the SVC and the IVC in order to determine the site of the defect and whether there is anomalous pulmonary venous return to the right atrium (which would be reflected in higher oxygen saturation of the blood near the SVC as compared with that near the IVC). Table 18-3 lists cardiac catheterization data of a patient with a secundum ASD.

TRANSCATHETER CLOSURE OF ASD

A variety of percutaneously inserted occlusion devices (variously shaped like buttons, wings, clamshells, or umbrellas) have been introduced for ASD closure and have become an alternative to surgical repair. The devices are most appropriate for secundum defects that are not too large; sinus venous defects; large, complex secundum defects are best repaired with surgery in which the defect and surrounding tissue can be inspected visually (Austin, 2000).

TABLE 18-3

Cardiac Catheterization Laboratory Results of a Patient with Ostium Secundum Atrial Septal Defect

MEASUREMENT	DEFECT	NORMAL
Pressures:		
Right atrium	Mean = 1 mm Hg	Less than 5 mm Hg
Right ventricle	46/0–3 mm Hg	25/0–5 mm Hg
Pulmonary artery	46/18 (mean 26) mm Hg	25/12 (mean 16) mm Hg
Pulmonary artery wedge pressure	Mean = 4	4–12 mean
Left atrium	Mean = 4	8–12 mean
Left ventricle	140/0–6	100–140/0–5
Aorta	140/68	100–140/60-80
Oxygen saturations:		
Superior vena cava	76%	75%
Inferior vena cava	81%	75%
High right atrium	82%	75%
Mid right atrium	84%	75%
Low right atrium	85%	75%
Right ventricle inflow	85%	75%
Right ventricle outflow/pulmonary artery	85%	75%
Left atrium	98%	95%
Left-to-right shunt (ratio of pulmonary blood flow to systemic blood flow)	1.9:1	1:1
Systemic vascular resistance	25 Wood units	Less than 20 Wood units
Total pulmonary resistance	3.4 Wood units	Less than 3.5 Wood units
Pulmonary vascular resistance	2.9 Wood units	Less than 2 Wood units
Angiography: Normal contraction of left ventricle without evidence of mitral regurgitation or mitral valve prolapse		
Coronary angiography: Normal coronary arteries		

Modified from Seifert PC, Lefrak EA: Atrial septal defect: the adult patient, *AORN J* 39(4):617, 1984.

Occasionally, emergent surgical intervention is required after failed transcatheter repair or in situations where cardiac perforation has occurred. Residual shunt, dislocation of the device, or cardiovascular complications are the most frequent complications requiring surgical intervention (Berdat and others, 2000).

Procedural considerations

Monitoring lines consist of arterial and central venous pressure lines; a pulmonary artery pressure catheter hampers exposure of the right atrial surgical site (insertion also may be complicated by the presence of large defects through which the catheter could travel). If left ventricular function requires monitoring, a left atrial line can be inserted during surgery or a pulmonary artery catheter can be introduced after completion of the operation. Nurses should be aware that air in venous lines can pass through the defect and embolize into the systemic circulation. Therefore great caution should be taken to remove any air from peripheral or central venous lines. TEE is commonly used during surgery for ASD in the adult.

Bicaval cannulation is used for venous return so that systemic blood does not obscure the field. A right-angle SVC cannula may be needed if the ASD is high in the right atrium (e.g., sinus venosus ASD). Mild hypother-

mia (32° C [90° F]) is usually sufficient for simple defects. Cardioplegia solution is given antegradely; cardioplegia solution given retrogradely through the coronary sinus is cumbersome with the right atrium opened, but some surgeons do give intermittent retroplegia infusions with a handheld catheter.

A median sternotomy is performed routinely, but a modified right thoracotomy approach also can be used if there are no other suspected anomalies. The cosmetic results of such an anterolateral (submammary) incision have been excellent.

Instrumentation that is used for mitral valve surgery (Chapter 11) also can be used for ASD repair. Autologous pericardium is often used; it heals well and is resistant to infection (Waldhausen, Pierce, and Campbell, 1996). If pericardium is unavailable, knitted patch material may be employed; it is easier to handle and frays less than woven material. Primary closure generally is avoided in adults with large defects in order to prevent distortion of the atrium or excessive tension on the suture line.

Surgery is associated with some risk to the atrioventricular node, which is situated near the coronary sinus and the septal leaflet of the tricuspid valve (Bharati, Lev, and Kirklin, 1983) (Fig. 18-10). Transvenous pacemaker leads can be inserted in the event that heart block is created (see Box 18-3).

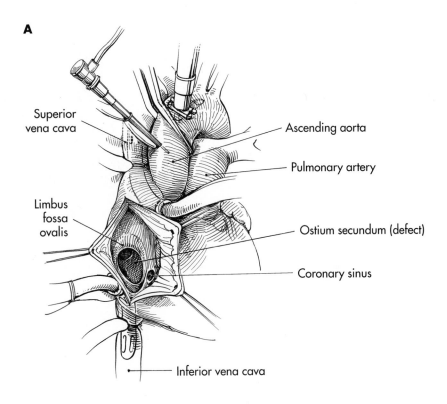

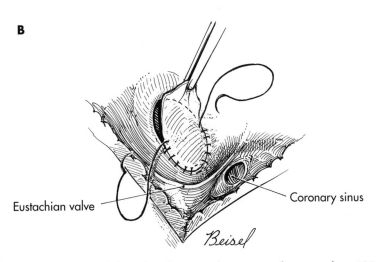

FIGURE 18-10 A, The right atrium is opened to expose the secundum ASD. Occasionally a very small defect may be closed primarily. **B,** Patch repair. (From Waldhausen JA, Pierce WS, Campbell DB: *Surgery of the chest,* ed 6, St Louis, 1996, Mosby.)

Operative procedure: repair of an atrial septal defect

1. A median (or mini-) sternotomy is made, and bicaval cannulation for CPB is performed. A cardioplegia infusion line/venting catheter is placed in the anterior aorta. If pericardium is to be used for closure of the defect, a piece of sufficient size is excised and kept moist and pliable in normal saline until it is needed.

2. After bypass is initiated, the heart is arrested and the right atrium is opened (see Fig. 18-10). Retractors are inserted to expose the atrial septum.

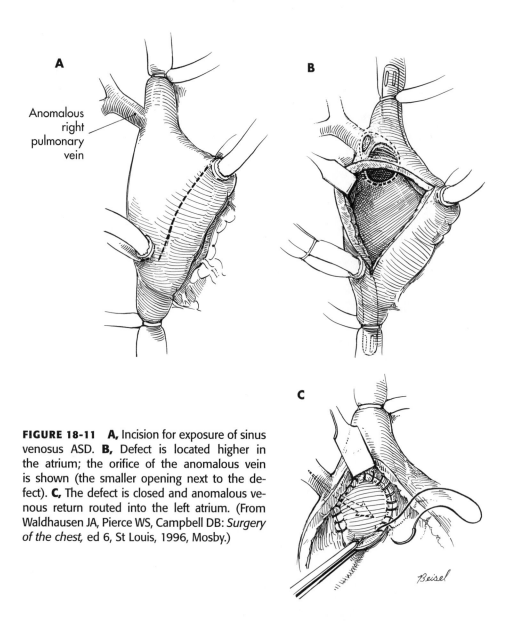

FIGURE 18-11   A, Incision for exposure of sinus venosus ASD. **B,** Defect is located higher in the atrium; the orifice of the anomalous vein is shown (the smaller opening next to the defect). **C,** The defect is closed and anomalous venous return routed into the left atrium. (From Waldhausen JA, Pierce WS, Campbell DB: *Surgery of the chest,* ed 6, St Louis, 1996, Mosby.)

3. The right atrium is carefully inspected to locate the defect and to determine its size and configuration. Surrounding tissue is inspected for other anomalies. If a prosthetic patch is to be used, sterile patch material is delivered to the field and cut to the appropriate size and shape.

4A. Repair of secundum ASD: Suturing of the patch to the edges of the defect is started at the inferior margin (see Fig. 18-10) and proceeds along one side and then the other. Excess material may be trimmed further and the superior repair is then completed. Just before patch closure is completed, air within the left atrium and left ventricle is allowed to escape through the opened portion of the patch.

4B. Repair of sinus venosus ASD: The atrial incision may be modified (Fig. 18-11, **A.**) to facilitate exposure to the defect and to coexisting anomalous pulmonary veins entering the right atrium. Patch repair is performed as in step 4A, but higher in the atrium where the defect occurs (Fig. 18-11, **B** and **C**). If there are one or more anomalous pulmonary veins, the patch is placed in such a way that it redirects pulmonary venous drainage into the left atrium through the defect but does not impede systemic venous return from the SVC into the right atrium (Fig. 18-11, **C**).

If there is a single large vein that drains into the SVC, another technique (Fig. 18-12) is to divide the SVC proximally and distally in relation to the

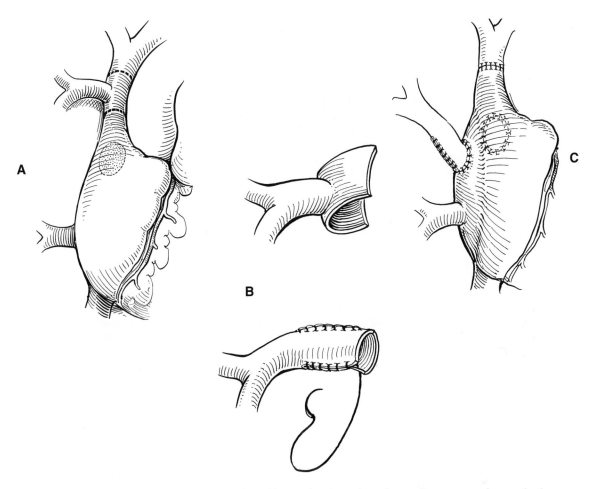

FIGURE 18-12   A-C, Procedure for repair when there is one large anomalous vein (see text). (From Waldhausen JA, Pierce WS, Campbell DB: *Surgery of the chest,* ed 6, St Louis, 1996, Mosby.)

anomalous vein, sew the flaps of the caval tissue together (to provide additional length), and anastomose the vein directly to the left atrium. The SVC is then reapproximated.

5. Closure of the right atrium is performed so that narrowing of the SVC is avoided. The right atrium is partially closed with 4-0 polypropylene. Air is removed from the right atrium and the pulmonary artery, and closure of the atrium is completed. The aortic vent needle is turned on to remove residual air from the left side of the heart.

6. The cross-clamp is removed, and the heart is defibrillated if it does not resume contraction spontaneously. The ECG is monitored for signs of conduction blocks or dysrhythmias. TEE is used to test the repair and to detect the presence of intracardiac air.

7. Temporary atrial and ventricular pacing wires are inserted. A left atrial pressure line may be inserted to monitor left ventricular response to the increased volume and pressure load resulting from closure of the defect.

8. Chest tubes are placed, and the patient is weaned from bypass.

9. After hemostasis has been achieved, the chest and skin are closed.

Postoperative period

Closure of ASDs in adults increases longevity and provides significant improvement in clinical symptoms. The operative risk is low; increased risk is caused primarily by associated problems (e.g., coronary artery disease, valvular dysfunction, dysrhythmias). Although it may require a number of months, there is often a decrease in the size of the heart and a reduction in elevated pulmonary pressures. Cardiac rhythm and atrioventricular conduction often remain unchanged (Stewart and Bender, 1991).

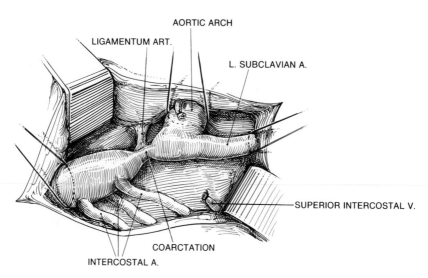

AORTIC ARCH

LIGAMENTUM ART.

L. SUBCLAVIAN A.

SUPERIOR INTERCOSTAL V.

COARCTATION

INTERCOSTAL A.

FIGURE 18-13   Exposure of coarctation of the aorta. Note the relationships between the various structures. The superior intercostal vein has been ligated and divided to facilitate exposure. It is common to find greatly enlarged intercostal arteries, which provide collateral circulation to the distal aorta. The ligamentum arteriosum is the former PDA. (From Waldhausen JA, Pierce WS, Campbell DB: *Surgery of the chest,* ed 6, St Louis, 1996, Mosby.)

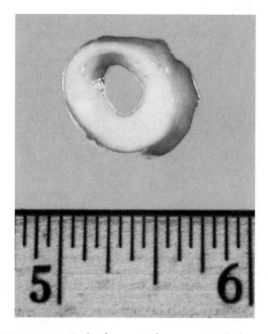

FIGURE 18-14   Excised coarcted segment of the aorta. (Courtesy Nevin M. Katz, MD.)

Coarctation of the Aorta

Coarctation of the aorta is characterized by a localized narrowing of the aortic wall (Fig. 18-13; see also Table 18-1). Abnormally thick medial tissue (Fig. 18-14) projects into the lumen of the aorta, forming a shelf, which creates an obstruction to left ventricular outflow. Blood pressure proximal to the coarctation is elevated (pro-

moting left ventricular hypertrophy), whereas blood pressure distal to the lesion is decreased. Upper-body hypertension and absent or diminished femoral or pedal pulses may be detected during physical examination. There may be a murmur at the left sternal border caused by blood flow through the narrowed aorta. Left-sided rib notching from the extensive collateral circulation and enlarged intercostal vessels pressing against the thorax may be seen on the chest radiograph. These clinical findings suggest coarctation, which often is confirmed by MRI. Cardiac catheterization is usually necessary only if MRI cannot demonstrate the lesion (Oliver, Nuttall, and Murray, 1999). The most common associated congenital malformation is a bicuspid aortic valve (see Chapter 12). Other anomalies include VSD, PDA, and mitral valve abnormalities.

In adults (Fig. 18-14, *A*) the coarctation often is found at the junction of the aortic arch and the descending aorta distal to the left subclavian artery and the ligamentum arteriosum (formerly the PDA). This postductal form of coarctation, in contrast to the preductal (infant) type of constriction (Fig. 18-14, *B*), is the more common form of coarctation and is also more likely to allow survival into adulthood. This is because of the extensive collateral circulation, which provides blood flow to the kidneys and lower extremities. Collaterals develop in utero and continue after birth in response to the resistance to blood flow through the PDA (and the heart) that is created by the aortic constriction. A coarctation located proximal to the ductus does not stimulate collateral development because fetal

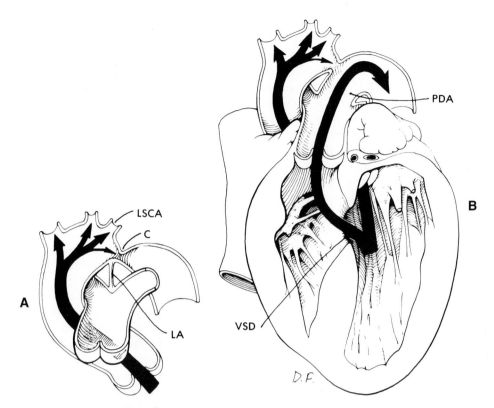

FIGURE 18-15 Hemodynamic abnormalities in coarctation of the aorta. **A,** Pathophysiology in the older child or adult. The coarctation *(C)* is distal to the former patent ductus arteriosus (PDA)—the ligamentum arteriosum *(LA)*—and the left subclavian artery *(LSCA)*. With this postductal form of coarctation, because there is resistance to flow even in utero, the development of collateral circulation is stimulated and provides a means of perfusing the lower body. **B,** In preductal coarctation there is little stimulus to develop collateral circulation, because in the fetus blood flow through the ductus is unimpeded. It is only at birth, when the heart must eject against a greatly increased afterload and perfusion to the lower body is severely compromised, that the effects of the coarctation manifest themselves. Without a *VSD* to allow blood to pass through into the pulmonary artery and cross the *PDA* into the distal aorta, severe hypoxemia develops. (From Bove EL: Congenital heart lesions. In Miller TA, editor: *Physiologic basis of modern surgical care*, St Louis, 1988, Mosby.)

blood flows preferentially through the PDA into the descending aorta (with little blood flow traveling through the aorta proximal to the ductus). Although blood flow in utero is relatively unimpeded with preductal coarctations, at birth this changes dramatically as the ductus closes and the heart must eject the full cardiac output into the constricted aorta. Without collateral circulation a PDA becomes an important conduit for distal blood flow. As the ductus begins to close, heart failure occurs if the coarctation is severe (Hazinski, 1999).

Procedural considerations

In the adult, long-standing collateral circulation to the distal aorta will have enlarged the left subclavian artery and the arteries in the muscles and intercostal spaces.

These arterial walls tend to be very thin, and hemorrhage from them may be troublesome (Waldhausen, Pierce, and Campbell, 1996). A PDA may be found near the most constricted portion of the coarctation; the PDA may be ligated or clipped as previously described.

Positioning, skin preparation, draping, and instrumentation are similar to those used for descending thoracic aortic aneurysms (see Chapter 14). Different sizes of tube grafts should be available. Preparations for surgery should be made sufficiently in advance; unnecessary prolongation of aortic cross-clamp time creates a risk for spinal ischemia and paralysis (see Box 18-3).

Resection of a short coarctation with end-to-end anastomosis of the aorta can be performed in infants, whose tissue may be reapproximated easily. Because recoarctation can occur after the initial operation, a subclavian flap procedure has been devised whereby the left subclavian artery is divided, brought down, and anastomosed to the aorta to create an adequately enlarged lumen. A reverse subclavian flap may be used to enlarge a coarcted aortic arch; the artery is divided, swung around to the proximal portion of the aorta, and anastomosed to the aortic arch. Because ligation of the subclavian artery restricts blood flow to the affected arm, this technique usually is reserved for very young patients who may be able to develop collateral circulation to perfuse the arm. In children with longer coarctations, or in older patients with less elastic tissue or a sclerotic aorta, patch repair or resection with interposition of a tube graft may be necessary to prevent excessive tension on the suture line. Occasionally the coarctation is left in place, and a bypass graft (tube graft) is anastomosed to the aorta proximal and distal to the coarctation.

Percutaneous balloon dilation of the native obstruction has not shown good results, although it has shown a benefit in recoarctation. One reason for these results may be that histologically the aorta distal to the coarctation is similar to that found in Marfan's syndrome (see Chapter 14). Dilation injures this vulnerable segment and may promote the redevelopment of the coarctation. Surgical resection removes the vulnerable aortic section and thus may minimize the possibility of recoarctation (Perloff, 1997). Stents have been successfully used in adults.

Operative procedure: resection of a coarctation of the aorta (Waldhausen, Pierce, and Campbell, 1996)

1. The patient is placed in the lateral position with the left side up, and a thoracotomy incision is made in the fourth intercostal space.
2. The pleura is opened over the coarctation and aortic isthmus, and the lungs are retracted anteriorly and inferiorly.
3. The area of the coarctation, including the transverse aortic arch, the distal aorta, and the left subclavian artery, is dissected as much as possible, using caution to avoid injury to the recurrent laryngeal, vagus, and phrenic nerves. Distally the aorta may be freed almost to the diaphragm.
4. Heavy silk ligatures or umbilical tapes may be placed around the left subclavian artery, the vertebral artery, and the aorta.
5. Vascular occluding clamps are placed on the aorta above and below the coarctation. Intercostal arteries may be occluded temporarily to control bleeding during the repair.
6. The aorta is opened, and the coarctation shelf is excised (Fig. 18-16).

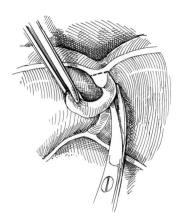

FIGURE 18-16 Excision of the coarctation shelf. (From Waldhausen JA, Pierce WS, Campbell DB: *Johnson's surgery of the chest,* ed 5, St Louis, 1985, Mosby.)

7A. Resection with graft replacement: The appropriate-size graft is delivered to the field and anastomosed end-to-end proximally and distally to the aorta. Because the distal aorta tends to be larger than the proximal aorta (related to poststenotic dilation), the graft can be beveled to approximate the proper lumen size. This technique is similar to that used for resection of a descending thoracic aortic aneurysm (see Chapter 14).
7B. Subclavian flap repair: The left subclavian artery is ligated at the origin of the vertebral artery, which is ligated also. The subclavian artery is divided and swung down onto the aorta, where it is sutured (Fig. 18-17).
8. After completion of the anastomoses, the distal clamp is removed first. The proximal clamp is then removed slowly to prevent a sudden increase in the arterial pressure.
9. Hemostasis is achieved, a chest tube is inserted, and the pleura is closed with absorbable suture. The chest is closed, and dressings are applied. Percutaneous insertion of an intraluminal stent (Fig. 18-18) is another treatment option that can be used to repair coarctation of the aorta.

Postoperative period

Complications that may require reoperation in the early postoperative period include hemothorax (usually from a branch of an intercostal artery) and chylothorax (from injury to the thoracic duct, which allows lymph to drain into the chest). Patients may complain of abdominal pain after surgery; this is thought to be related to the sudden and unaccustomed strong blood flow to the mesentery after repair. In severe cases, bowel infarction may result. Recurrent coarctation is a late complication that may require surgery, balloon angioplasty, or stent insertion.

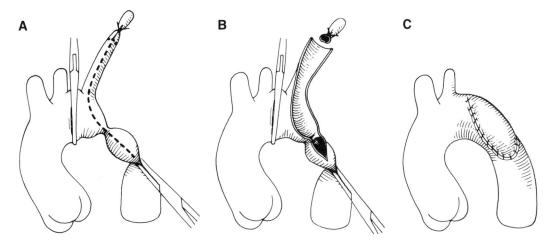

FIGURE 18-17 Repair of coarctation using the subclavian flap procedure. **A,** The left subclavian artery is mobilized and divided distally. **B,** A longitudinal incision is made through the artery and the adjacent aorta; the incision must extend distally beyond the coarctation to normal aorta. **C,** The subclavian flap is brought down onto the aorta and anastomosed. (From Bove EL: Congenital heart lesions. In Miller TA, editor: *Physiologic basis of modern surgical care,* St Louis, 1988, Mosby.)

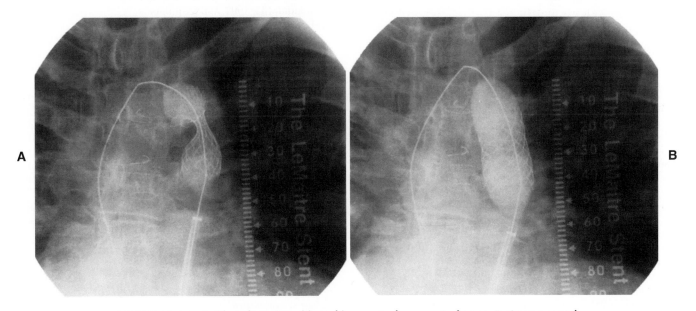

FIGURE 18-18 **A,** Closed stent positioned in coarcted segment of aorta. **B,** Stent opened, expanding lumen of aorta. (Courtesy Michael H. Goldman, MD.)

Although resection of an aortic coarctation results in significant reduction in systemic blood pressure in most adults, persistent and unexplained systemic hypertension can be seen in up to 50% of patients. Although it is unclear why there is continuing hypertension (in the absence of a residual coarctation), it has been suggested that it is related to the time that hypertension existed preoperatively. Thus resection performed in young patients is less likely to result in persistent hypertension; however, the incidence of recoarctation is higher in this group. Other possible factors are reduced distensibility of the proximal aorta, renovascular abnormalities involving the renin-angiotensin system, and essential hypertension (Perloff, 1997).

Unfortunately, other cardiovascular complications are not uncommon and may shorten life expectancy. These include unexplained congestive heart failure, aortic or cerebral vascular rupture, and problems associated with the aortic or mitral valve. Because of the high incidence of abnormal valves associated with coarctation, antibiotic prophylaxis is recommended before invasive procedures are done (Perloff, 1997).

Conclusion

Congenital malformations are not uncommon in the adult. Future trends in congenital heart diseases will depend not only on the number of infants born with malformations (often reported as 6 to 8 in 1000 live births [Lake, 1999]) but also on the impact of early surgical repair and the effects of survivors having children of their own. Although there is variance in the reported incidence of survivors of congenital heart disease having children with cardiac deformities, the American College of Cardiology (Summary of Recommendations, 2001) has predicted a definite increase. Perioperative nurses are likely to encounter an increasing number of adult patients with lesions ranging from the simple secundum ASD to the more complex tetralogy of Fallot.

References

Berdat PA and others: Surgical management of complications after transcatheter closure of an atrial septal defect or patent foramen ovale, *J Thorac Cardiovasc Surg* 120(6):1034, 2000.

Bharati S, Lev M, Kirklin JW: *Cardiac surgery and the conduction system*, New York, 1983, John Wiley & Sons.

Bove EL: Congenital heart lesions. In Miller TA, editor: *Physiologic basis of modern surgical care*, St Louis, 1988, Mosby.

Burke RP, Wernovsky G: Images in clinical medicine. Thoracoscopic clipping of patent ductus arteriosus, *N Engl J Med* 336(3):185, 1997.

Clyman RI: Ibuprofen and patent ductus arteriosus, *N Engl J Med* 343(10):728, 2000.

Cooley DA, Hallman GL, Hammam AS: Congenital cardiovascular anomalies in adults. Results of surgical treatment in 167 patients over age 35, *Am J Cardiol* 17(3):303, 1966.

Friedman WF, Silverman N: Congenital heart disease in infancy and childhood. In Braunwald E, Zipes DP, Libby P, editors: *Heart disease: a textbook of cardiovascular medicine*, ed 6, Philadelphia, 2001, WB Saunders.

Gross RE, Hubbard JP: Surgical ligation of a patent ductus arteriosus: report of first successful case, *J Am Med Assoc* 112(8):729, 1939.

Hazinski MF: *Manual of pediatric critical care*, St Louis, 1999, Mosby.

Huddleston KR: Patent ductus arteriosus ligation: performing surgery outside the operating room, *AORN J* 53(1):69, 1991.

Kahn RA and others: Intraoperative echocardiography. In Kaplan JA, editor: *Cardiac anesthesia*, ed 4, Philadelphia, 1999, WB Saunders.

Kern MJ, editor: *The cardiac catheterization handbook*, ed 3, St Louis, 1999, Mosby.

Lake CL: Anesthesia for patients with congenital heart disease. In Kaplan JA, editors: *Cardiac anesthesia*, ed 4, Philadelphia, 1999, WB Saunders.

Lev M: The architecture of the conduction system in congenital heart disease. III. Ventricular septal defect, *AMA Arch Pathol* 70:529, 1960.

Lev M: The architecture of the conduction system in congenital heart disease. II. Tetralogy of Fallot, *AMA Arch Pathol* 67:572, 1959.

Lev M: The architecture of the conduction system in congenital heart disease. I. Common atrioventricular orifice, *AMA Arch Pathol* 65:174, 1958.

Maldonado SS, Nygren C: Pediatric surgery. In Meeker MH, Rothrock JC, editors: *Alexander's care of the patient in surgery*, ed 11, St Louis, 1999, Mosby.

Oliver WC, Nuttall G, Murray MJ: Thoracic aortic disease. In Kaplan JA, editor: *Cardiac anesthesia*, ed 4, Philadelphia, 1999, WB Saunders.

Perloff JK: Congenital heart disease in adults. In Braunwald E, editor: *Heart disease: a textbook of cardiovascular medicine*, ed 5, Philadelphia, 1997, WB Saunders.

Rashkind WJ: Historical aspects of surgery for congenital heart disease, *J Thorac Cardiovasc Surg* 84(4):619, 1982.

Roberts WC: Congenital cardiovascular malformations usually silent until adulthood. In Roberts WC: *Adult congenital heart disease*, Philadelphia, 1987, FA Davis.

Rudolph AM, Nadas AS: The pulmonary circulation and congenital heart disease, *N Engl J Med* 267:968, 1962.

Stewart JR, Bender HW: Management of complications of surgery for septal defects. In Waldhausen JA, Orringer MB: *Complications in cardiothoracic surgery*, St Louis, 1991, Mosby.

Summary of Recommendations—care of adult with congenital heart disease, 32nd Bethesda Conference, American College of Cardiology, *J Am Coll Cardiol* 37(5):1167, 2001.

Taussig HB: World survey of the common cardiac malformations: developmental error or genetic variant? *Am J Cardiol* 50(3):544, 1982.

Taylor GJ: *Primary care management of heart disease*, St Louis, 2000, Mosby.

Therrien J, Webb GD: Congenital heart disease in adults. In Braunwald E, Zipes DP, Libby P, editors: *Heart disease: a textbook of cardiovascular medicine*, ed 6, Philadelphia, 2001, WB Saunders.

Van Overmeire B and others: A comparison of ibuprofen and indomethacin for closure of patent ductus arteriosus, *N Engl J Med* 343(10):674, 2000.

Waldhausen JA, Pierce WS, Campbell DB: *Surgery of the chest*, ed 6, St Louis, 1996, Mosby.

Warnes CA and others: Task force I: the changing profile of congenital heart disease in adult life, *J Am Coll Cardiol* 37(5):1170, 2001.

19 Cardiac Trauma and Emergency Surgery

Changes do not simply "happen"—they are caused.

Kenneth L. Mattox, 2000 (p. 25)

Chance favors the prepared mind.

Louis Pasteur, as quoted in Vallery-Radot R, *The life of Pasteur*, 1927

Emergency situations are not unusual for perioperative cardiac nurses, many of whom have a disaster mentality that enables them to anticipate and prepare for unusual or unexpected events. Nurses are aware that routine cardiac procedures have the potential for turning into emergencies, given the underlying instability of many patients. When the patient's clinical status deteriorates suddenly outside the operating room (OR), as can occur with acute rupture of an ischemic mitral papillary muscle or postmyocardial infarction ventricular septal defects, prompt surgical intervention is required. Efficient and experienced cardiac perioperative nurses are able to respond quickly and implement the most appropriate treatment. Predetermined protocols, jointly developed by nurses and physician members of the surgical team and confirmed or reviewed as warranted by the patient's clinical status, can facilitate the expeditious transfer of the patient to the OR, opening of the chest, instituting of cardiopulmonary bypass (CPB), and repairing of the injury.

Occasionally patients are too unstable to transport to the OR, and surgery must be performed wherever the patient is located (e.g., the cardiac catheterization laboratory, emergency/trauma department, or critical care unit). The availability of portable systems incorporating CPB capability, instruments, and supplies enables the surgical team to perform emergency procedures in these non-OR settings.

Factors that promote prompt intervention include an awareness of the pathophysiology and the goal of therapy, familiarity with the roles and responsibilities of various team members, and coordination of efforts. Emergency situations, whether caused by trauma, complications of surgery, or accidents, depend on close cooperation and communication.

This chapter describes some of these emergency situations. Many of the principles of trauma care are similar to those applied when life-threatening alterations occur during any cardiac procedure.

Trauma

EPIDEMIOLOGY

Traumatic injuries account for more than 150,000 deaths a year in the United States (Schroen, 1999). Trauma is the leading cause of death between the ages of 1 and 44 years of age. Forty-seven percent of all trauma injury deaths are caused by motor vehicle crashes (MVC), including motorcycle crashes. Alcohol, particularly in adolescents (Spain and others, 1997), is often a contributing factor. Firearm injuries are the second greatest cause of death in trauma patients. Homicide is the second leading cause of death in ages 15 to 24 and the primary cause of death in black males in ages 15 to 34 (Schroen, 1999). Falls far exceed MVCs as the most common cause of nonfatal injury in elderly persons over the age of 75, with the greatest risk of death being falls (Jacobs and Jacobs, 1996). Thoracic injuries contribute significantly to the morbidity and mortality of trauma patients, particularly in the elderly (Keough, 1998).

Military surgeons operating during war have been instrumental in developing not only methods of vascular and myocardial repair but also endotracheal intubation, mechanical ventilation, management of pulmonary injuries, and chest drainage systems. Especially notable is Harkin's (1946) accomplishment during World War II (see Chapter 1) when he operated on 134 soldiers with shell fragments and other missiles in or near the heart; there were no deaths in this series of patients (Westaby, 1997; Symbas and Justicz, 1993).

In addition to improved surgical techniques and interdisciplinary teamwork, rapid transport systems, early resuscitation and stabilization, and prompt surgical intervention have contributed to the success of civilian trauma systems (Mullins and others, 1996; *Resources for Optimal Care of the Injured Patient,* 1999; 1998).

Mechanism of Injury

Cardiac injuries are caused when kinetic energy is absorbed and dissipated by the chest. Kinetic injuries are generally divided into two categories: blunt or penetrating. A detailed description of the crash scene from the first responders can assist in anticipating and diagnosing injuries to the chest. Useful information includes the amount of damage done to the vehicle, condition of the steering wheel and column, approximate rate of speed at impact (highway speed versus residential street speed), direct frontal impact versus side impact, restrained versus unrestrained passengers, ejection of passengers, and deployment of an air bag (Vaden, 1999).

The biomechanics of blunt force injuries, especially for MVCs, has been studied recently. In an MVC, three types of collisions produce crush or compression injuries to the chest and thorax (Feliciano, 1996; Fig. 19-1). The first is when a moving object strikes a stationary object

(e.g., when a motor vehicle impacts a stationary object, such as a tree or another vehicle). Major extrusion into the passenger compartment of the vehicle from front or side impact can cause direct injuries to the occupants. The second is when the victim is thrown against the internal parts of the vehicle, such as the windshield, steering wheel and column, or dashboard. The third collision involves movable and nonmoveable internal organs colliding with each other. An example is when the sternum (moving object) hits the steering column (stationary object); the heart is crushed between the sternum and vertebral column. A second pattern of injury is the deceleration injury. For example, tearing movable internal structures, such as the thoracic aorta, from their nonmoving components, such as the ligamentum arteriosum (Fig. 19-2). The collisions described here may produce not only crush but deceleration injuries as well. Injuries produced by blunt force trauma can range from asymptomatic cardiac contusions to immediate fatal cardiac rupture (May and others, 1999).

The most common penetrating injuries to the heart include stab wounds, gunshot wounds, and impalements. Battle injuries are commonly caused by high-velocity gunshot wounds and missile fragments that produce severe hemorrhage, with death at the scene. Unfortunately, firearm deaths in the civilian population have increased at an alarming rate (Jacobs and Jacobs, 1996). In most civilian shootings the assailant and victim are, on average, about 7 meters apart (Barach,

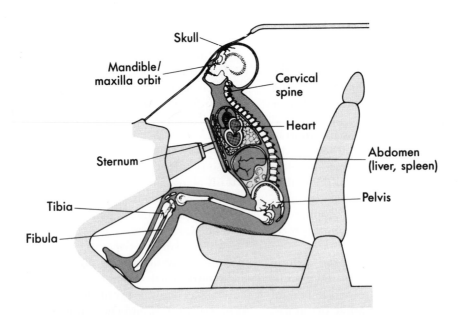

FIGURE 19-1 Potential sites of injury in the unrestrained driver. (From Kidd PS: Assessment of the trauma patient. In Neff JA, Kidd PS: *Trauma nursing: the art and science,* St Louis, 1993, Mosby.)

Tomlanovich, and Nowak, 1986). Tissue damage is caused by direct and indirect mechanisms (Feliciano, 1996). Direct mechanisms cut or lacerate tissue from the missile or fragment and transfer of heat caused by friction. Indirect mechanisms include tissue compression from shock waves that precede and spread out behind the projectile in the wound. Research into the science of wound ballistics has increased significantly. A comprehensive discussion of this controversial and poorly understood science is beyond the scope of this chapter. Wound ballistics, the interaction of both the missile and fragments with the target tissue, are determined by various factors, making accurate prediction of the extent of injury difficult (Feliciano, 1996).

Nursing Considerations

Nursing care focuses on the identification and treatment of the patient's response to injury (Box 19-1). Factors that affect a patient's response include the type of injury, age and developmental level, previous and current health problems, family and social support systems, economic status, level of education, and psychosocial impact of the injury on the victim and family. Appropriate material resources should be selected without duplication. Inadequate or inappropriate instrumentation delays prompt intervention and can foster confusion, increase the level of stress, and possibly incur litigation (Trauma Nursing Coalition, 1992; Kidd, Sturt, and Fultz, 2000).

The perioperative nurse's role as a patient advocate is especially critical in a setting where the patient enters the system severely wounded, often unconscious and intubated, and incapable of communication and self-protection. The legal rights of patients must be protected; advance directives such as those relating to organ donation should be honored, and safety considerations outlined in institutional policies and procedures should be followed. Minimum standards relating to basic aseptic technique, counts, and documentation are adhered to in all but the most critical situations; exceptions should be covered by written policies (e.g., taking an x-ray film postoperatively when sponge or needle counts cannot be performed).

Families and significant others also must cope with the stress that traumatic injuries impose. Because of the suddenness with which such injuries occur, families often are unprepared and may feel helpless to cope with the situation. Nurses can have a positive impact by engendering a sense of hope and providing information about the patient's condition and the care being received (Reeder, 1991).

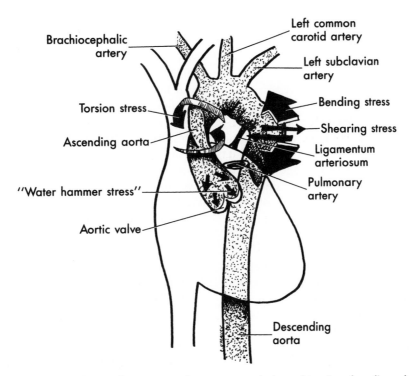

FIGURE 19-2 Cardiac and great vessel anatomy and sites of torsion, bending, shearing, and water hammer stress. (From Kidd PS: Assessment of the trauma patient. In Neff JA, Kidd PS: *Trauma nursing: the art and science,* St Louis, 1993, Mosby.)

BOX 19-1
Preparing for Thoracic Trauma

When a patient with thoracic trauma is admitted to the emergency department, the OR is alerted. The following are questions to ask in preparing for the patient with thoracic injuries.

1. Is this patient hemodynamically stable? What does *unstable* mean? The levels of hypovolemic shock are as follows:

	ESTIMATED BLOOD LOSS	MENTAL STATUS	SKIN	URINE OUTPUT	RESPIRATORY RATE	BLOOD PRESSURE	PULSE
Class I: Compensated	<750 ml (15% of volume)	Slightly anxious, thirsty	Pale	30 ml	14-20	Normal	80-120
Class II: Moderately unstable	750-1500 ml (15%-30% volume)	Mildly anxious, restless	Pale/diaphoretic	20-30 ml	20-30	Normal	>120
Class III: Progressive instability	1500-2000 ml (30%-40% volume)	Anxious, confused	Pale/diaphoretic	5-15 ml	30-40	Low	>120
Class IV: Severe instability	>2000 ml (≥40% volume)	Lethargic, obtunded	Pale/diaphoretic	Low/none	>35	Systolic <90	Falling

2. Is the injury blunt or penetrating? If it is penetrating, is the injury within the cardiac box?
3. Who is the operating surgeon?
4. When will the patient come—immediately or after arteriography?
5. Will the surgeon use the cell saver? Has blood been ordered? How much? Where is it? Has the trauma surgeon initiated the mass transfusion protocol?
6. Is the room warm enough? Anything under 80° F (26.7° C) is too cold. (Why? See Research Highlight 2.)
7. Has the patient been properly and quickly prepped? Prep fast: neck-to-knees and bedside-to-bedside with a single-step prep solution.
8. To count or not to count (e.g., sponges, instruments)? If there is time, yes; if not, no. A written policy should address emergencies when there is no time to count.
9. Is there confirmation that the neck has been cleared? (Always assume the neck has *not* been cleared.)
10. Has the respiratory therapist been called well before the patient is ready to be moved? Generally all patients on ventilators should be moved on the transport ventilator.

Blunt Thoracic Injuries

DIAGNOSTIC EVALUATION

History

Diagnostic evaluation begins with a history (Vaden, 1999). For blunt thoracic trauma, accurate information from the first responders is extremely helpful. Useful information includes the amount of damage done to the vehicle, extrication time, other injuries or deaths at the scene, condition of the steering wheel and column, approximate time of injury, rate of speed at impact (highway speed versus residential street speed), direct frontal impact versus side impact, whether patient was restrained versus unrestrained or ejected, whether an air bag was deployed, level of consciousness, and hemodynamic status during rescue and transport. If the patient is conscious, symptoms may include chest pain, shortness of breath, hemoptysis, stridor, or hoarseness. History of cardiorespiratory diseases or thoracic diseases is useful if it can be obtained.

Physical examination

Physical examination may reveal abrasions, contusions, lacerations, or obvious fractures of the sternum or ribs (Vaden, 1999). Seat belt marks diagonally across the sternum may suggest thoracic injury. Beck's triad (Beck, 1937)—jugular vein distension, muffled heart sounds, and hypotension—are classic physical signs of cardiac tamponade. Other signs include narrow pulse pressure. Pulse pressure is the difference between systolic blood pressure and diastolic blood pressure (systolic minus diastolic) (Roberts, 1996). Changes in pulse pressure reflect changes in cardiac output more accurately than the systolic pressure alone as shock is developing (Wilson, 1992). Pulse pressure less than 30 mm Hg indicates decreased stroke volume. *Pulsus paradoxus* is when the systolic pressure falls by 15 mm Hg or more during inspiration; this occurs in patients with pericardial tamponade. A bulging pseudoaneurysm of a ruptured thoracic aorta, hemothorax, or pneumothorax may shift the trachea from the midline. Diminished or absent breath sounds may indicate hemothorax or pneumothorax. Paradoxic motions of segments of the chest on respiration indicate flail chest segments. Point tenderness of the sternum, rib fractures, or crepitus may occur.

Diagnostic evaluation

Diagnostic evaluation is based on a suggestive mechanism of injury and findings on the initial chest x-ray

Indications for video-assisted thoracic surgery have increased in recent years, but its role in the surgical treatment of blunt and penetrating thoracic injuries is unclear. Recent studies indicate VATS may be useful in the diagnosis and treatment of hemodynamically stable patients with thoracic injuries. Morales and colleagues (1997) successfully used a diagnostic thorascopic pericardial window on normotensive patients with penetrating chest injuries who responded favorably to fluid resuscitation to diagnose hemopericardium. Bar and colleagues (1998) describe a case of a video-assisted extraction of a kitchen knife embedded in the back. The scope was inserted below the tip of the right scapula. The blade had penetrated the pleura but had not injured the lung, mediastinum, or diaphragm. The knife was removed uneventfully and a thoracotomy avoided. Dah-Wei and colleagues (1997) successfully used VATS to treat 56 patients with hemothorax or posthemothorax complications resulting from chest trauma. Researchers agree that VATS applications will increase for hemodynamically stable patients with chest trauma.

Modified from: Bar I and others: Thorascopically guided extraction of an embedded knife from the chest, *J Trauma* 44(1):222, 1998; Dah-Wei L and others: Video-assisted thoracic surgery in treatment of chest trauma, *J Trauma* 42(4):670, 1997; Morales CH and others: Thoracoscopic pericardial window and penetrating cardiac trauma, *J Trauma* 42(2):273, 1997.

film (Vaden, 1999). ECG screening should be done on all patients with blunt thoracic trauma (Pasquale and Fabian, 1998). The diagnostic algorithm used to evaluate blunt thoracic injuries varies depending on regional practice patterns and the relative hemodynamic stability of the patient. A widened mediastinum in the hemodynamically stable patient requires further investigation, such as a diagnostic peritoneal lavage or focused abdominal sonogram. If these are negative, the aorta should be evaluated with an arteriogram of the aortic arch. In the hemodynamically unstable patient, the aorta should be evaluated after a celiotomy for rapid control of intraabdominal hemorrhage. Recent advances in technology include surgeon-performed pericardial and pleural ultrasound, transthoracic (Pasquale, 1998) or transesophageal echocardiogram (Feliciano and Rozychki, 1999), CT scan, and aortic arch angiography (Vaden, 1999; Ahrar and others, 1997). Laboratory tests specific for myocardial contusions may include serial cardiac enzymes. Indications for this test have increased significantly in recent years. Video-assisted thoracoscopy may be used as a diagnostic tool for selected thoracic injuries (Dah-Wei and others, 1997) in hemodynamically stable patients (Research Highlight 19-1). It may be used to diagnose diaphragmatic injuries or suspected cardiac injury or to determine the cause of continued bleeding from a chest tube (Villavicencio, Aucar, and Wall, 1999). It has limited usefulness in the unstable patient. Other structures

contained in the chest may be injured, such as the trachea and esophagus. This discussion is limited to cardiac and great vessel injuries.

SURGICAL MANAGEMENT

The most common blunt injury to the heart is a myocardial contusion, which is treated nonoperatively. Surgical injuries may include injury or rupture of the pericardium; injuries to the septal wall, valves, and coronary vessels; and injuries to the great vessel of the chest, such as the thoracic aorta (Tsikaderis, Dardas, and Hristofordis, 2000). Video-assisted thoracoscopy has been used effectively in evacuating clotted hemothorax (Mattox, Wall, and Pickford, 1996). Recent case reports include the following cardiac injuries caused by blunt force trauma to the chest: rupture of both ventricles (Duba and others, 1999), rupture of the mitral chordae tendineae (Grinberg and others, 1998), rupture of the right atrium (Song, Shimomura, and Suenaga, 1998), and coronary artery occlusive dissection (Ginzburg and others, 1998).

Rupture of the interventricular septum produces an acute left-to-right shunt that is poorly tolerated and requires prompt surgical therapy to close the defect (see Chapter 10 for technique of patch repair). Valvular injuries, such as ruptured chordae tendineae or papillary muscles, often require valve replacement, although reparative techniques are preferred when feasible (see previous chapters for discussion of valve surgery). Repair of the thoracic aorta is described in the following.

Surgery for injury to the thoracic aorta

Although the aortic arch and heart are relatively freely suspended in the mediastinum, the descending aorta is attached at the ligamentum arteriosum (the remnant fetal ductus arteriosus). If the posterior thoracic wall and the vertebral column stop, so does the descending aorta (see Fig. 19-2). The aortic arch and heart, however, continue to swing forward. This action can result in shear forces sufficiently strong enough to partially or completely lacerate the aorta circumferentially. Such deceleration injuries may tear the aorta at the isthmus, which is just distal to the subclavian artery. If all three layers of the aortic wall (intima, media, and adventitia) are torn, exsanguination is almost immediate. If only the intima and media are torn, the adventitia may encapsulate the hematoma and tamponade the bleeding. The resulting pseudoaneurysm (Fig. 19-3) may remain intact long enough for the victim to receive emergency treatment. The mechanism of injury and radiographic evidence provide information about the extent of the injury. Superior mediastinal widening, depression of the left main bronchus, and deviation of the esophagus to the right are significant and warrant aortography or

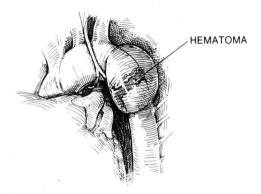

FIGURE 19-3 Hematoma contained within the adventitial layer of a descending thoracic aorta, creating a pseudo-aneurysm. (From Waldhausen JA, Pierce WS: *Johnson's surgery of the chest,* ed 5, St Louis, 1985, Mosby.)

scanning in hemodynamically stable patients (Vaden, 1999).

If the hematoma (e.g., surrounding the lacerated descending thoracic aorta) is not massive or expanding rapidly (and the patient is stable), preoperative diagnostic imaging of the aorta is beneficial because it documents the presence or absence of other vascular injuries and localizes the site of the tear. This information is especially useful for coordinating surgery to repair other injuries, planning the most appropriate surgical procedures, and selecting the best location for the incision (Vaden, 1999).

In preparation for surgery, perioperative nurses have instruments, supplies, and positioning equipment for a left thoracotomy. The procedure is similar to that for a descending thoracic aneurysm (see Chapter 14). Synthetic tube grafts should be available for resection and repair of the aorta. Autotransfusion capability and an adequate supply of banked blood are necessary. CPB may be avoided because of the risk of hemorrhage from systemic heparin administration. Intubation with a double-lumen endobronchial tube allows deflation of the lung on the affected side, thereby enhancing surgical visualization.

Operative procedure: repair of a transected aorta

1. After skin preparation and draping for a left lateral thoracotomy, an incision is made in the fifth intercostal space. The lungs are retracted anteriorly and inferiorly.
2. The hematoma is located, and the aorta above and below is dissected partially to allow placement of occlusive clamps (Fig. 19-4, *A*).
3. The hematoma is incised. If there is a small tear in the aorta, it can be repaired primarily with a running suture (Fig. 19-4, *D*).

4. If the extent of the injury makes primary closure unfeasible, the edges of the aortic wall are trimmed in preparation for insertion of a prosthetic graft.
5. An appropriately sized tube graft is delivered to the field, and the proximal anastomosis is performed (Fig. 19-4, *B*).
6. The distal anastomosis is then performed (Fig. 19-4, *C*).
7. The distal clamp is removed first, and the anastomoses are checked for bleeding. Additional sutures are placed as necessary. The surgical site is assessed for other injuries or areas of bleeding; these are repaired.
8. After hemostasis is achieved, the proximal clamp is slowly removed.
9. Free blood and clotted blood are removed, and the pleural space is irrigated.
10. Two chest tubes are inserted, and the incision is closed.

Pharmacologic control of the aortic blood pressure (e.g., with nitroprusside), expeditious surgery, and early reexpansion of the lung promote successful outcomes. Postoperatively, pulmonary impairment, empyema, and sepsis may complicate recovery. Ischemic injury to the spinal cord or kidneys is less likely to occur with cross-clamping times of less than 30 minutes (Mattox and Wall, 1996).

Penetrating Thoracic Injuries

Penetrating cardiac injuries are caused by bullets, knives, ice picks, and other objects that can pierce the skin and underlying structures. The extent of injury is related to the velocity, size, and internal movement of the object and the tissue being penetrated. Gunshot wounds are generally more lethal than stab wounds because of the higher velocity and the larger area of tissue destroyed. Because of its accessibility, the anterior surface of the heart (primarily the right ventricle) is the most frequent site of injury. Acute hemorrhage or tamponade severely compromises hemodynamic status, leading to shock and acidosis, and the victim often dies before reaching a health care facility.

DIAGNOSTIC EVALUATION

History
When patients do survive long enough to reach a facility, diagnostic evaluation for penetrating thoracic trauma should begin with a history (Vaden, 1999). A history is less useful in anticipating penetrating thoracic injuries than with blunt thoracic injuries. The most useful information from first responders is the approximate time of the incident, response time from the scene to the facility,

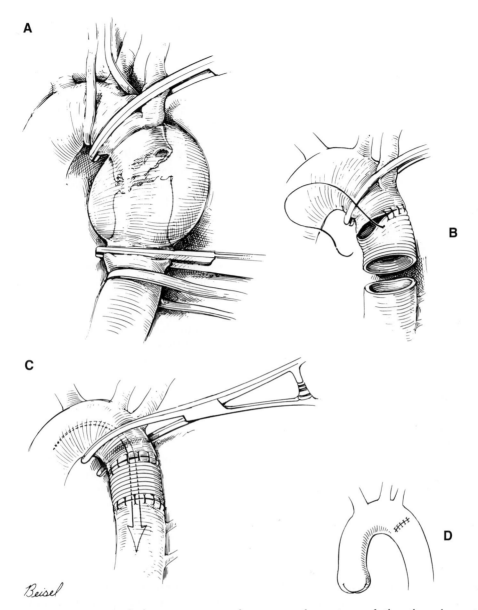

FIGURE 19-4 Surgical management of a traumatic rupture of the thoracic aorta. **A,** Control of the aorta is achieved by placing occlusive clamps above and below the lacerated aorta. Occasionally the proximal clamp is placed across the aorta between the left carotid and the left subclavian arteries, and a separate clamp is applied to the subclavian artery. **B,** The proximal anastomosis is performed with a continuous suture technique (the distal aortic clamp is not shown). **C,** The completed repair. After the distal clamp is removed, the proximal clamp is released slowly. **D,** Primary closure of a small aortic tear. (From Waldhausen JA, Pierce WS: *Johnson's surgery of the chest,* ed 5, St Louis, 1985, Mosby.)

the patient's hemodynamic history during rescue and transport, and the mechanism of injury (Tyburski, 2000). History of cardiorespiratory or thoracic diseases is useful in treating penetrating thoracic injuries as well, but it is often unobtainable.

Physical examination

Physical examination should reveal the entry wounds and perhaps the exit wounds if the projectile passed through the body. Any injury between the midclavicular lines is considered an injury to the heart until proven

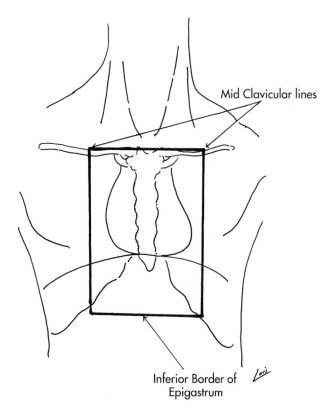

FIGURE 19-5 The cardiac box. Any penetrating injury between the midclavicular lines is considered a heart injury until proven otherwise. (Courtesy L Fernandez, MD.)

otherwise (Fig. 19-5). Beck's triad (Beck, 1937), consisting of hypotension, distended neck veins, and distant (muffled) hearts sounds, may be present with the cardiac tamponade associated with penetrating thoracic trauma. Other signs are similar to those for blunt thoracic injuries: narrow pulse pressure, pulsus paradoxus, shift of the trachea from the midline, diminished or absent breath sounds, and paradoxic chest motions.

Diagnostic evaluation

Specific diagnostic evaluations are often limited by the fact that many of these patients are hemodynamically unstable on admission. Generally, however, a chest x-ray examination and surgeon-performed ultrasound of the heart are obtained.

Iatrogenic injuries

Iatrogenic injury constitutes another category of penetrating trauma. Cardiopulmonary resuscitation (CPR) may fracture ribs and puncture the heart and abdominal organs. Cardiac catheterization, angiographic studies, pacemaker insertions, and percutaneous minimally invasive procedures can be complicated by laceration or dissection of the heart or major blood vessels from

guidewires and catheters (Ivantury, 1996). Prompt recognition of and intervention to repair iatrogenic injury are similar to the diagnosis and treatment of other forms of unexpected injury.

SURGICAL MANAGEMENT OF OPEN CARDIAC WOUNDS

Operative procedure: suture of a heart wound

1. An anterolateral (or midsternal) incision is made.
2. The pericardium is opened, and blood clots are removed. Brisk hemorrhage may be evident; autotransfusion suctions should be available to salvage and reinfuse the blood.
3. The wound is located after a careful search. Occasionally a discreet wound can be covered with a finger (Fig. 19-6, *A*). If digital control cannot be achieved, a urinary drainage catheter with a 5-ml inflatable balloon can be inserted through the wound; the balloon can then be inflated and gently pulled against the inside of the heart (the catheter lumen is occluded to prevent back bleeding).

     Lifting the hypovolemic heart may kink the vena cava, reducing venous return (preload). Ventricular fibrillation may occur, especially if the patient is hypothermic and acidotic and has electrolyte imbalances (Mattox and Wall, 1996). Cardiac massage is performed, and underlying metabolic alterations are corrected. Defibrillation is attempted but may be unsuccessful in the presence of severely altered blood values.
4. Deep traction sutures are placed on either side of the wound, avoiding coronary arteries if possible. Crossing the sutures may close the wound sufficiently to permit removal of the finger and allow suture repair under direct vision (Fig. 19-6, *B*). Polypropylene (4-0, 5-0) may be used with or without pledgets to bolster the suture line; pledgets may be required, especially if coexisting myocardial contusion has weakened the tissue. More extensive lacerations require multiple sutures. Studies indicate that using a skin-stapling device commonly found in most emergency departments may take significantly less time and have essentially the same tissue strength as sutures. Stapling during emergency resuscitation may be considered (Mayrose and others, 1999). If a major coronary artery has been lacerated or ligated, bypass grafting (see Chapter 10) with CPB may be necessary.
5. After hemostasis has been achieved, the traction sutures are removed. Chest tubes are inserted and the incision is closed.

Factors affecting the prognosis of a patient with penetrating heart injuries are related to the physiologic state of the patient when presenting in the emergency department;

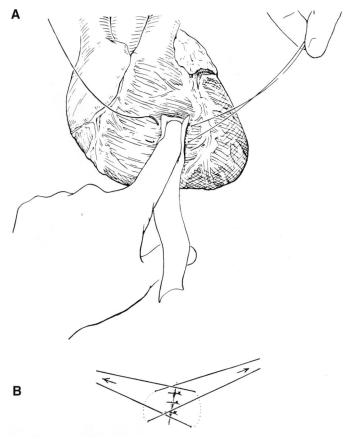

FIGURE 19-6 Suturing of open cardiac wound. **A,** Digital pressure is applied to the wound to control bleeding. **B,** Stay sutures are inserted (avoiding major coronary arteries) for traction and closure of the wound while the repair is performed. (From Waldhausen JA, Pierce WS: *Johnson's surgery of the chest,* ed 5, St Louis, 1985, Mosby.)

the mechanism of injury; and the presence of cardiac tamponade (Tyburski and others, 2000). In a population-based review of 212 penetrating cardiac injuries (Rhee and others, 1998), overall survival was 19.3%, 9.7% for gunshot wounds, and 32.6% stab wounds. The survival rate of patients with penetrating heart wounds who suffered cardiac arrest in the field or during transport is negligible. The use of the emergency room thoracotomy is questionable on pulseless patients with absent blood pressure. Patients presenting in profound shock with a systolic blood pressure below 80 mm Hg should be managed with fluid resuscitation. If fluid resuscitation fails to stabilize the patient, prompt emergency thoracotomy is indicated (Ivantury, 1996).

SURGICAL MANAGEMENT OF PENETRATING WOUNDS TO MAJOR VESSELS

Stab and bullet wounds to the thoracic aorta and its major branches or to veins within the chest may cause rapid exsanguinating hemorrhage unless occlusive vas-

cular clamps can be quickly placed across the proximal and distal segments of the injured vessel. This maneuver allows the surgeon to control the bleeding while the repair is being made. The incision depends on the location of the injury. Generally a median sternotomy affords the best exposure to the pulmonary artery, the ascending aorta, and the proximal arch vessels. The incision can be angled at either side of the neck, if necessary, for access to vessels in that area. A thoracotomy may be indicated for subclavian injuries. Repair depends on the site and extent of the injury (Waldhausen, Pierce, and Campbell, 1996; Vaden, 1999). Either primary suture repair or interposition of a tube graft to bridge the defect may be performed (Mattox, Estrera, and Wall, 2001).

CARDIAC TAMPONADE

Acute tamponade is the most common cardiac emergency seen in patients with penetrating injuries to the heart and pericardium (Fig. 19-7); the condition is seen

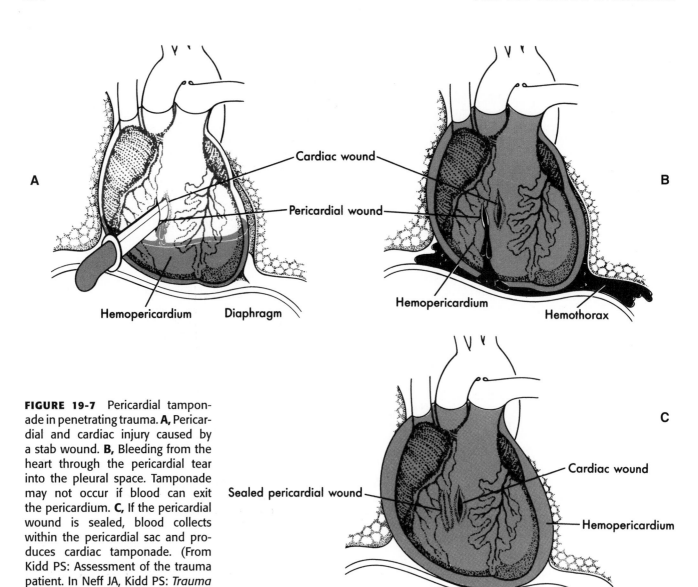

FIGURE 19-7 Pericardial tamponade in penetrating trauma. **A,** Pericardial and cardiac injury caused by a stab wound. **B,** Bleeding from the heart through the pericardial tear into the pleural space. Tamponade may not occur if blood can exit the pericardium. **C,** If the pericardial wound is sealed, blood collects within the pericardial sac and produces cardiac tamponade. (From Kidd PS: Assessment of the trauma patient. In Neff JA, Kidd PS: *Trauma nursing: the art and science,* St Louis, 1993, Mosby.)

less often in patients with blunt trauma to the chest. Because the pericardium is a relatively nondistensible sac encasing the heart, accumulated blood from the injured heart muscle or coronary arteries can cause compression of the myocardium. If the pericardial opening is obliterated by blood clot, lung tissue, or a flap of pericardial tissue, blood within the pericardial sac cannot escape. This prevents adequate filling of the ventricles, resulting in a reduction of cardiac output (Roberts, 1996). The classic signs of tamponade (Beck's triad, described previously) may be difficult to demonstrate clinically, especially during major resuscitation efforts, when heart sounds are difficult to hear, or when patients are uncooperative or combative. The most reliable signs include elevated central venous pressure (CVP)—unless

there is hypovolemia, in which case there would be a low CVP—in association with systemic hypotension, tachycardia, and hemothorax (Roberts, 1996).

Surgical management of cardiac tamponade for either blunt or penetrating injuries may be minimally invasive pericardiocentesis, aspirating fluid from the pericardial sac with a needle. Pericardiocentesis to diagnose or relieve cardiac tamponade caused by trauma is done rarely since the introduction of surgeon-preformed ultrasound (Thourani and others, 1999). More invasive surgical management is the pericardial window (Roberts, 1996). An incision is made just inferior to the xiphoid process, which is lifted; the pericardium is then visualized and incised. A chest tube may be inserted, or a portion of the pericardium may be excised (pericardectomy).

Perioperative Nursing Considerations

Institutions with trauma centers often have perioperative nurse team members functioning within the trauma unit or on call from the OR. Roles vary from institution to institution. Some perioperative nurses function in a separate trauma OR, some act as a liaison between the OR and the emergency/trauma department, and others participate in transporting and treating patients in a designated OR within the surgical suite. The degree of interdepartmental interaction may differ, but a system of communication and planning for rapid intervention is essential to avoid a chaotic situation that can adversely affect patient outcomes (*Resources for Optimal Care of the Injured Patient,* 1999).

Case carts prepared in advance can be especially helpful in avoiding delays. Carts (or other portable units) containing items specific to the type of injury (e.g., thoracic, abdominal, extremity) include instruments and supplies likely to be required. Separate carts also can facilitate performing simultaneous procedures for two or more life-threatening injuries. And because they are portable, these carts can be taken to the emergency department (or other area) if the patient is too unstable to transport to the OR.

When the patient arrives in the OR, positioning, application of dispersive pads, and skin preparation are performed expeditiously. Prior communication with the liaison in the emergency department will assist the perioperative staff in having ready the most appropriate supplies and equipment for the intended procedure. If pneumatic antishock garments (PASG) or military antishock trousers (MASTs) are in place, they should not be removed unless specifically requested by the surgeon or anesthesiologist. It should be noted that the use of MASTs may be declining; studies have demonstrated that pneumatic counterpressure and shock garments used on patients with thoracic trauma have *no* effect on survival when compared with patients not receiving these garments (Mattox and Wall, 1996). A perioperative plan of care for the trauma patient based on nursing intervention classifications (McClosky and Bulechek, 1996) is shown in Table 19-1.

The location of traumatic injury determines the type of incision. Anterolateral thoracotomy through the fourth or fifth interspace provides excellent cardiac exposure and can be extended across the sternum if necessary. This incision has the advantage of keeping the abdominal cavity separate from the thorax and is an important consideration when there are concomitant enteric injuries. A median sternotomy and lateral thoracotomy also may be performed when the injury has been localized, but often it is difficult to determine the precise location of injuries, and the exposure is not as good as it is with the anterolateral approach (Box 19-2). Subxiphoid pericardiotomy is used less often since the advent of ultrasonography; however, it may be useful to assess the pericardium when a concomitant laparotomy is performed (Mattox, Wall, and Pickard, 1996; Ivantury, 1996). Pericardiocentesis (insertion of a large-bore needle into the pericardium to drain blood) may provide emergency relief until surgery can be performed, but it should not delay opening of the chest and performance of a definitive repair.

In addition to release of tamponade and control of the site of bleeding, internal cardiac massage (Fig. 19-8) may be necessary to decompress an arrested or fibrillating heart that has become distended and to perfuse distal organs until cardiac activity can be resumed. In markedly hypovolemic patients, cross-clamping the descending thoracic aorta (Fig. 19-9) may be done to enhance coronary and cerebral blood flow (Mattox and Wall, 1996). Vascular clamps should not be placed on ventricular walls; doing so could cause injury to the myocardium. Partial-occlusion clamps may be used on atrial tissue and on blood vessels with small, discreet injuries that can be repaired primarily.

Internal defibrillation paddles should be available on the surgical field. CPB is usually available on a standby basis, although it can be contraindicated in patients with head or other injuries in whom increased bleeding would result from systemic anticoagulation. Nurses should be prepared to institute CPB quickly.

Inadvertent Hypothermia

Prolonged exposure to cold temperatures from trauma (Research Highlight 19-2) or submersion in cold water can produce hypothermia (core temperatures less than 32° C [90° F]). Hypothermia caused by submersion can occur as a consequence of falling through the ice into water or being in a motor vehicle accident wherein the car veers into a body of cold water. Patients become apneic and pulseless with fixed and dilated pupils.

Conventional warming techniques, such as heating blankets, radiant warmers, body cavity lavage, and airway rewarming, are usually not capable of increasing the body temperature by more than 1° C (1.8° F) per hour. Children are more likely to recover than adults. Institution of CPB has been an effective method in the absence of associated traumatic injuries that would preclude the use of systemic heparin (Letsou and others, 1992). The patient may be placed on bypass with a portable system in the emergency department or brought to the OR.

When there is a risk of bleeding from heparin, an alternative method (devised by Gentilello and Rifley,

TABLE **19-1**

Intraoperative Care Plan of the Patient with Thoracic Trauma Using Nursing Intervention Classifications (1996)

NURSING DIAGNOSIS	NURSING INTERVENTION	EVALUATION CRITERIA
Fluid volume deficit related to third space fluids and preoperative and intraoperative blood loss	Electrolyte monitoring and management: 　Check preoperative lab results 　Monitor ECG for signs of electrolyte deficits 　Monitor blood pressure and vital signs Fluid management and monitoring: 　Assist with starting large-bore central lines 　Insert indwelling urinary catheter and nasogastric tube 　Measure accurate I&O, including blood loss and returned blood 　Administer fluids, blood, and blood products 　Anticipate use of rapid fluid warmer/infuser	Pulse pressure >30 mm Hg Systolic blood pressure >100 mm Hg Diastolic blood pressure >50 Urinary output >30 cc/hr
Decreased cardiac output related penetrating or blunt injury to heart muscle or blood supply	Circulatory care—mechanical assist devices: 　Assist with setup and insertion of device Shock management: 　Monitor ECG for signs of inadequate coronary perfusion 　Anticipate appropriate instrumentation, suture, and supplies for intraoperative control of hemorrhage	Mean arterial pressure >60 Heart rate <110
Impaired gas exchange related to concomitant injury to lung, hemothorax, or pneumothorax	Airway management: 　Assist with intubation, suctioning, cricoid pressure as needed 　Anticipate use of double-lumen endobronchial tube 　Anticipate difficult intubation 　Monitor oxygenation (Sao_2) 　Confirm endotracheal tube location 　Assist with insertion of arterial line and transducer setup	Successful endotracheal intubation Oxygen saturation ≥92% Acceptable arterial blood gases
Hypothermia related to prehospital environment and iatrogentic conditions	Hypothermia treatment: 　Warm the room to 85° F (29° C) 　Insert core temperature monitoring device 　Use warmed fluid, blood, and blood products 　Use warming blanket 　Warm inhalation gases and air 　Cover/wrap head	Core temperature ≥97° F (36.1° C)
Risk for infection related to penetrating projectile and severe immunosuppression of massive trauma	Infection control and protection: 　Apply strict surgical asepsis	Control and contain inherent contamination of penetrating wounds
Altered tissue perfusion: renal related to preoperative and intraoperative blood loss and/or clamping of the aorta superior to the renal arteries	Fluid management and monitoring: 　Assist with starting large bore central lines 　Insert indwelling urinary catheter and nasogastric tube 　Measure accurate I&O, including blood loss and returned blood 　Administer fluids, blood, and blood products 　Anticipate use of rapid fluid warmer/infuser Shock management: 　Monitor ECG for signs of inadequate coronary perfusion 　Anticipate appropriate instrumentation, suture, and supplies for intraoperative control of hemorrhage	Mean arterial pressure >60 Heart rate <110 Cross-clamp <30 minutes Pulse pressure >30 mm Hg Systolic blood pressure >100 mm Hg Diastolic blood pressure >50 Urinary output >30 ml/hr

I&O, Intake and output.

BOX **19-2**
Comments on the Operative Management of Patients with Cardiac Injuries
Kenneth L. Mattox, MD
Baylor College of Medicine
Houston, Texas

The successful operative management of patients with cardiac injuries is dependent on (1) rapid transport to a regional trauma center and (2) immediate care by a surgeon. The injury determines the surgical approach. Injuries from iatrogenic, penetrating, and blunt trauma requiring operation are each approached in a different manner. The objectives, however, are the same: (1) control free hemorrhage from the heart surface, (2) repair any significant valvular or (ventricular) septal damage, and (3) do *no* harm by ligating a coronary artery or creating a shunt or heart block.

Anterolateral incisions are preferred for gunshot wound victims, whereas patients with stab wounds between the nipples are best approached via a median sternotomy. Subxiphoid pericardiotomies should *not* be used by emergency physicians or by general or thoracic surgeons for any suspected cardiac injury. If thoracic injury is suspected, an appropriately large thoracic incision should be used. Simple techniques, virtually always without the use of cardiopulmonary bypass, are preferable to complex reconstructions. Simple sutures, usually using 4-0 polypropylene on a large needle, or mattress suturing is satisfactory. Pledgets are rarely indicated, except in the right ventricle. Fluid overload should be avoided. Adjunctive maneuvers of (vena caval) inflow occlusion, autotransfusion, and deliberate fibrillation are occasionally necessary.

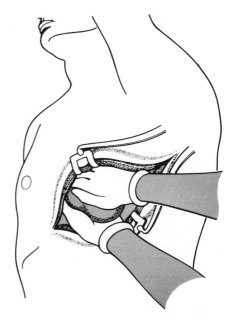

FIGURE 19-8 Left anterolateral thoracotomy provides excellent exposure to the heart, left lung, and descending thoracic aorta. Bimanual massage of the heart is illustrated here. (From Kidd PS: Assessment of the trauma patient. In Neff JA, Kidd PS: *Trauma nursing: the art and science,* St Louis, 1993, Mosby.)

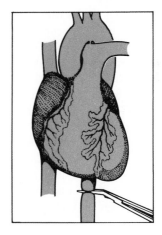

FIGURE 19-9 Clamping the descending thoracic aorta in severely hypovolemic patients can improve blood flow to the coronary arteries and the brain. (From Kidd PS: Assessment of the trauma patient. In Neff JA, Kidd PS: *Trauma nursing: the art and science,* St Louis, 1993, Mosby.)

1991) is continuous arteriovenous rewarming. The system uses a rapid fluid warmer to increase the temperature of the endogenous blood volume 1° C (1.8° F) approximately every 15 minutes.

PROCEDURE FOR REWARMING

The femoral artery and contralateral femoral vein are percutaneously cannulated with a standard renal arteriovenous hemofiltration catheter. Venous access also can be achieved by cannulating the ipsilateral femoral, internal jugular, or subclavian vein. The catheters are connected to a fluid warmer with an inline filter to create a circulatory fistula through the heating mechanism. A blood pump, membrane oxygenator, or systemic heparin administration is not required. The core temperature can be monitored with a pulmonary artery catheter or urinary bladder thermistor. After rewarming, the catheters are withdrawn, and digital pressure is applied for at least 20 minutes. Full neurologic recovery has been demonstrated with this technique (Gentilello and Rifley, 1991).

Pulmonary Embolus

Pulmonary embolus is not a distinct disease but a complication of many medical and surgical disorders (Rutledge and Sheldon, 1996). Deep venous thrombosis (DVT) of the lower extremities is often a precursor to acute pulmonary thromboembolism in trauma

RESEARCH **HIGHLIGHT 19-2**

Research indicates a core body temperature less than 32° C (89.6° F) is associated with 100% mortality in trauma patients. Furthermore, the longer temperatures are sustained at or below 36° C (97° F), the higher the morbidity and mortality rates. Normothermic patients have fewer cardiac arrhythmias, are weaned faster from ventilators, and have fewer postoperative complications in general, including a superior survival rate. Metabolic indicators of acidosis, such as serum bicarbonate levels, adjust more quickly in normothermic patients. Infection rates also are lower in patients kept at normal temperature.

Modified from Gentilello LM and others: Is hypothermia in the victim of major trauma protective or harmful? A randomized, prospective study, *Ann Surg* 226(4):439, 1997; Insler SR and others: Association between postoperative hypothermia and adverse outcomes after coronary artery bypass surgery, *Ann Thorac Surg* 70(1):175, 2000.

patients and in patients who have been on prolonged bed rest or who have indwelling femoral intravenous catheters. In patients at risk for pulmonary embolus, prophylactic measures include administration of low-dose heparin or low-molecular-weight heparin and insertion under fluoroscopy of a filter in the inferior vena cava (IVC) to trap emboli migrating from the IVC to the heart and thereby prevent their entry into the pulmonary circulation. The device may be especially useful in the patient with bleeding complications from anticoagulation therapy or a history of recurrent thromboembolism (Rutledge and Sheldon, 1996).

Studies by Shackford and colleagues (1990) have shown that high-risk factors in trauma patients related to venous thrombosis include stasis, local venous injury, hypercoagulability, and age greater than 45 years. Diagnosis relies on the clinical signs and symptoms of calf swelling, tenderness, warmth, and pedal edema. Doppler echocardiography has replaced venography for assessing pelvic and thigh DVT (Rutledge and Sheldon, 1996).

Acute pulmonary embolus (APE) occurs when a portion of thrombus in a systemic vein, right atrial appendage, or right ventricle dislodges and migrates to the pulmonary artery (PA) or one of its major branches. When approximately 60% or more of the pulmonary circulation is occluded, the right ventricle is unable to eject the blood returning from the systemic circulation. The obstruction causes acute right ventricular dilation with right-sided congestive failure if the obstruction is unrelieved. Clinical signs of APE often include distended neck veins, engorgement of the liver, tachypnea, dyspnea, cough, and wheezing. Massive air emboli or fat emboli (associated with large bone fractures) can produce a similar clinical picture.

In addition to clinical signs and symptoms, the ECG, chest x-ray film, perfusion lung scanning, and pulmonary arteriography may be performed to determine the diagnosis. The ECG may show signs of right ventricular strain, anatomic rotation, axis shifts of the heart, acute myocardial infarction of the inferior portion of the heart, right bundle-branch block, and dysrhythmias such as sinus tachycardia and atrial flutter. Chest radiographs may show nonspecific changes or elevated diaphragm on the affected side. Pleural effusion, PA dilation, and infiltrates may be apparent (Wisner, 1995).

Perfusion scans using radioisotopes are performed to detect changes in the areas supplied by the occluded PA. With APE, defects appear in the scan. Normal perfusion scans exclude the possibility of massive APE. However, other conditions (e.g., pneumonia, emphysema) also can produce abnormal findings. The most accurate test for diagnosis of APE is right-sided heart catheterization with pulmonary arteriography. A positive study shows and intraluminal defect. A sharp reduction in flow also may be seen, although this should be distinguished from concomitant pulmonary or cardiac disease (Rutledge and Sheldon, 1996).

Arterial blood gases (ABGs) are used to monitor ventilation-perfusion defects. Arterial oxygen saturation is decreased as expected; compensatory hyperventilation produces a decreased level of carbon dioxide.

INITIAL TREATMENT

Initial therapy for APE in trauma patients consists of oxygen administration, intravenous thrombolytic therapy (except in the presence of head injury), and pharmacologic treatment for shock. Monitoring is achieved with a central venous or pulmonary artery blood pressure catheter. If the patient does not respond to medical therapy and remains in critical condition (e.g., right-sided heart failure, significant pulmonary obstruction of the pulmonary vasculature), pulmonary embolectomy may be necessary. This is often the case with a massive *saddle* embolus, named for the characteristic shape of a clot that sits at the bifurcation of the main PA.

Perioperative considerations

Surgical mortality is high; in one series of 96 patients mortality was almost 38% (Meyer and others, 1991). Cardiac arrest and associated cardiopulmonary disease and massive pulmonary hemorrhage increase mortality.

Pulmonary embolectomy may be performed on one or both PA branches. Primarily unilateral involvement may be an indication for anterior thoracotomy on the affected side. In patients with bilateral emboli, or emboli within the main PA, median sternotomy and CPB are generally indicated. The risk of bleeding may be increased with systemic heparin administration. Intrabronchial bleeding may occur, and in anticipation of this complication a double-lumen endotracheal tube is inserted so that the unaffected side may continue to be ventilated (Wisner, 1995).

Operative procedure: pulmonary embolectomy with cardiopulmonary bypass

1. A median sternotomy is performed.
2. A venous cannula can be placed in either the right atrium or the right ventricular outflow tract; an arterial cannula is placed in the ascending aorta. CPB is instituted.

   In some cases the aorta is not clamped and the procedure is performed under normothermic conditions. In more complex cases aortic occlusion and cardioplegic arrest with hypothermia may be used. Occasionally, circulatory arrest is required.
3. The PA is dissected medially from the aorta.
4. An incision is made in the main PA, and the thrombus is removed.
5. If the thrombus is in the left or right PA, a second incision may be made, and the branches of the main embolus are removed. Peripheral emboli may be extracted with common bile duct forceps and standard suction tips (Meyer and others, 1991). When the thrombus has been removed, back bleeding of bright red blood will be seen (Wisner, 1995).
6. The arteriotomies are closed; a pericardial or synthetic patch may be inserted to avoid constriction of the PA lumen during closure.

   Ligation or clipping of the IVC or insertion of a vena caval filter may be performed in patients at risk for recurrent DVT or APE.
7. CPB is discontinued, chest tubes are inserted, and the incision is closed after hemostasis has been achieved.

Before heparin reversal with protamine, intrabronchial hemorrhage may occur; a balloon-tipped occlusion catheter can be inserted into the affected mainstem bronchus to tamponade the bleeding until coagulation and hemostasis can be achieved (Wisner, 1995).

Postoperative complications include right ventricular failure in patients with pulmonary hypertension and pulmonary hemorrhage. A few patients may have recurrent pulmonary emboli. Anticoagulation may be administered and a vena caval filter may be inserted prophylactically in patients predisposed to DVT.

Postoperative Complications of Cardiac Surgery

In addition to APE, there are several postoperative complications of cardiac surgery, including hemorrhage with or without tamponade, low cardiac output syndrome, and lethal dysrhythmias that may require emergency management. When there is excessive bleeding from the chest tubes, correction of existing coagulopathies, volume replacement, and pharmacologic manipulation of cardiac output are first attempted. If the patient continues to deteriorate rapidly and becomes profoundly hypotensive or shows signs of tamponade, the chest may have to be reopened in the postoperative intensive care unit (ICU) (Roberts, 1996). If the patient has fibrillated, direct cardiac massage (see Fig. 19-8) can help to decompress the heart and perfuse peripheral organs. Internal defibrillation may be necessary.

When possible, mediastinal exploration is performed within the controlled environment of the OR. However, some patients are unable to tolerate transfer, and exploration in the ICU may be necessary. With some preplanning, these procedures can be performed in the ICU in a manner that is safe, effective, convenient, and less costly, without increasing morbidity and mortality (Kaiser and others, 1990). Important advantages of performing surgery in the ICU are that it saves time, reduces the possibility of further hemodynamic deterioration, and obviates the necessity of disconnecting then reattaching monitors and intravenous infusion lines.

PROCEDURAL CONSIDERATIONS

Having sterile instrumentation and supplies in the ICU is critical in order to avoid delays and enhance preparedness for such emergencies. Communication and coordination among hospital staff members in the OR and ICU are important for establishing protocols, developing instrument and supply inventories, and outlining roles and responsibilities during emergencies (Resources for Optimal Care of the Injured Patient, 1998). Perioperative and critical care nursing responsibilities should be outlined, but there must be flexibility built into any policy or protocol.

A number of questions can arise, and these should be discussed and clarified:

- Are perioperative nurses routinely expected to assist with ICU emergency sternotomy? If they are, how will they be notified?
- What are the critical care nurse's responsibilities? Monitoring? Documenting? Volume/medication infusion?
- What constraints exist in the number of personnel, availability of supplies and equipment, and knowledge of procedures?

A system to alert perioperative cardiac nurses when there is a need for sternal exploration in the ICU (or the OR) should be available at all times. Late-night emergencies may mean a delay in arrival of the perioperative nurses. In this case the critical care nurse may have to assist the surgeon temporarily in opening the chest. Perioperative nurses can provide inservices to critical care personnel about the indications for emergency sternotomy and the goal of exploration. Emphasis should be placed on the basic steps necessary for reopening the chest and the minimum requirements: a knife (or scissors), wire cutters, a sternal retractor, and suction.

The following items may be needed for ICU emergencies and are often found in the unit: privacy screens, sterile gowns and gloves, skin antiseptics, hats and masks, sterile suction tubing the tips, and internal defibrillator paddles. Internal defibrillator cords and paddles must be appropriate for the ICU defibrillator, which may be different from the one used in the OR. Cables from one unit may not be interchangeable with those of another unit; different models from the same manufacturer may not be interchangeable. Occasionally the defibrillator and the cords and cables from the OR may have to be brought to the ICU for internal defibrillation.

Other items that may have to be added to the ICU inventory (or brought to the unit) include a headlight and light source, suture material, and temporary pacing wires. Some units keep an electrosurgical unit (and dispersive pads), but more often a unit is brought from the OR (or an eye cautery is used) along with the surgeon's headlight and light source. Additional lighting is especially useful if it is difficult to achieve adequate illumination of the pericardial cavity.

When the chest must be opened, the chest instrument set can be placed on an overbed table and opened. The ICU nurses may be requested to assist the surgeon until the OR staff arrives. Responsibilities should be jointly delineated by nursing staff from the ICU and the OR, surgeons, and other personnel likely to be involved in resuscitative efforts.

Operative procedure: sternal exploration in the intensive care unit

Ideally there are two perioperative nurses available: one to perform the duties of the sterile nurse and one to act as a circulator. If only one perioperative nurse is available, she or he may perform sterile duties and direct a critical care nurse in preparing the skin and providing sterile supplies. Personnel should wear head coverings and masks.

Procedure

1. The emergency sternotomy tray is placed on a table (or counter) and opened; sterile gowns and gloves are opened. The patient's chest dressings are removed.

2. A sterile drape is opened on another surface (if available), and required sterile supplies (e.g., sponges, suture) are placed on the drape. If another table or counter is unavailable, supplies may have to be opened onto the set of instruments.

3. While a nurse expeditiously prepares the patient's chest with antimicrobial solution (using a spray bottle is the fastest method), the sterile nurse and surgeon wash their hands and then gown and glove.

4. The sterile nurse and the surgeon drape the patient.

5. While draping is performed, the nurse gathers a knife or scissors to open the skin incision and passes sterile suction tubing off the field; this is connected to the wall suction outlet and turned to "high." Sterile internal paddles are prepared, and the cords are passed off to be connected to the defibrillator. (These may have to be done while the surgeon is opening the chest.)

6. The skin incision is opened with the knife or scissors. If staples have been used for chest closure, a staple remover is necessary. Any patient whose chest is closed with staples must have a staple remover accompany him or her to the ICU, and the staple remover must be placed where it can be made available immediately (e.g., taped to the wall near the patient).

7. After the skin is opened, the nurse hands the wire cutters and a wire needle holder (or heavy clamp such as a Kocher clamp) to the surgeon, who cuts and removes the wires.

8. A chest retractor is inserted, and a suction is handed to the surgeon.

9. The surgeon performs cardiac massage if the heart is asystolic. If the heart is fibrillating, internal defibrillation may be attempted first, and the heart is then massaged if cardiac rhythm is not restored. While performing these maneuvers, the surgeon assesses the heart and surrounding structures for areas of bleeding. The sterile nurse or surgical assistant can suction the field and also look for bleeding sites.

10. When cardiac rhythm is restored and the site of bleeding is determined, the repair is performed. This may be application of a vascular ligating clip or use of a suture ligature, or a more complex repair may be required.

Sternal and retrosternal (e.g., from an internal mammary artery pedicle) bleeding can be repaired without the need for CPB. Leaking from coronary artery bypass grafts on the anterior surface of the heart may not require CPB, but suturing a moving heart is difficult. In such a situation the patient may require transport to the OR, where the repair can be performed under more controlled conditions.

Lacerations of the ventricle, posterior coronary artery bypass anastomotic leaks, and other injuries may necessitate the use of extracorporeal circulation to decompress the heart and perfuse the body. Induced cardiac arrest (fibrillation or cardioplegic arrest) may be required.

11. After the repair has been completed, blood clots within the chest tubes are removed, and the drainage tube is repositioned in the chest. The epicardial pacing wires may have been detached; these are reattached to the heart.

The surgical site is reassessed for hemostasis, and the sternum is rewired. Fascia, subcutaneous tissue, and skin are closed, and dressings are applied. (The patient may be transported to the OR for closure, but this is often unnecessary.)

Postoperative course

Standard postoperative monitoring and management are performed after completion of the ICU procedure. Special attention is focused on detecting the recurrence of problems that required ICU sternotomy and signs of infection. Contrary to expectation, there is a low incidence of infection after such procedures (Kaiser and others, 1990).

COMPLICATIONS ASSOCIATED WITH PACEMAKER WIRE REMOVAL

The risk of sudden hemorrhage is also present a few days after surgery when temporary pacemaker wires are discontinued. Removal of the pacing wires (commonly attached to the right atrial and ventricular epicardium during surgery) can produce bleeding secondary to laceration of the myocardium, nearby blood vessels, or an adjacent bypass graft (Johnson, Brown, and Alligood, 1993).

If chest tubes are still in place, a sudden increase in drainage is evident (and tamponade is less likely to develop). However, pacing wire removal is often done after the mediastinal drainage tubes have been removed, and rapid tamponade can develop because blood remains confined to the pericardium. Pericardial tamponade can occur, often within 60 minutes after pacing wire removal, and demonstrate symptoms described earlier in the chapter. Pericardiocentesis may be attempted, but mediastinal exploration in the patient unit or in the OR may be necessary to repair the site of injury and release the tamponade.

References

Ahrar K and others: Angiography in blunt thoracic aorta injury, *J Trauma* 42(4):665, 1997.

Barach E, Tomlanovich M, Nowak R: Ballistics: a pathophysiologic examination of wounding mechanisms of firearms, *J Trauma* 26(3):225, 1986.

Beck CS: Acute and chronic compression of the heart, *Am Heart J* 14:515, 1937.

Duda AM and others: Successful repair of blunt cardiac rupture involving both ventricles, *Cardiovasc Surg* 7(2):263, 1999.

Feliciano DV: Patterns of injury. In Feliciano DV, Moore EE, Mattox KL, editors: *Trauma*, ed 3, Stamford, Conn, 1996, Appleton & Lange.

Feliciano DV, Rozycki GS: Advances in the diagnosis and treatment of thoracic trauma, *Surg Clin North Am* 79(6):1417, 1999.

Gentilello LM and others: Is hypothermia in the victim of major trauma protective or harmful? A randomized, prospective study, *Ann Thorac Surg* 226(4):439, 1997.

Gentilello LM, Rifley WJ: Continuous arteriovenous rewarming: report of a new technique for treating hypothermia, *J Trauma* 31(8):1151, 1991.

Ginzburg E and others: Coronary artery stenting for occlusive dissection after blunt chest trauma, *J Trauma* 45(1):157, 1998.

Grinberg AR and others: Rupture of mitral chorda tendinea following blunt chest trauma, *Clin Cardiol* 21(4):300, 1998.

Harkin DE: Foreign bodies in, and in relation to, the thoracic blood vessels and heart. I. Techniques for approaching and removing foreign bodies from the chambers of the heart, *Surg Gynecol Obstet* 83:117, 1946.

Insler SR and others: Association between postoperative hypothermia and adverse outcomes after coronary artery bypass surgery, *Ann Thorac Surg* 70(1):175, 2000.

Ivantury RR: Injury to the heart. In Feliciano DV, Moore EE, Mattox KL, editors: *Trauma*, ed 3, Stamford, Conn, 1996, Appleton & Lange.

Jacobs BB, Jacobs LM: Epidemiology of trauma. In Feliciano DV, Moore EE, Mattox KL, editors: *Trauma*, ed 3, Stamford, Conn, 1996, Appleton & Lange.

Johnson LG, Brown OF, Alligood MR: Complications of epicardial pacing wire removal, *J Cardiovasc Nurs* 7(2):32, 1993.

Kaiser GC and others: Reoperation in the intensive care unit, *Ann Thorac Surg* 49(6):903, 1990.

Kidd PS, Sturt P, Fultz JH: *Mosby's emergency nursing reference*, ed 2, St Louis, 2000, Mosby.

Keough V and Letizia M: Blunt cardiac injury in the elderly patient, *Int J Nurs* 4(2):38, 1998.

Kidd PS: Assessment of the trauma patient. In Neff JA, Kidd PS: *Trauma nursing: the art and science*, St Louis, 1993, Mosby.

Letsou GV and others: Is cardiopulmonary bypass effective for treatment of hypothermic arrest due to drowning or exposure? *Arch Surg* 127(5):525, 1992.

Liu DW and others: Video-assisted thoracic surgery in treatment of chest trauma, *J Trauma* 42(4):670, 1997.

Mattox KL: TraumaLine 2000: a history of change and a vision for the future, *Bull Am Coll Surg* 85(11):24, 2000.

Mattox KL, Estrera AL, Wall MJ: Traumatic heart disease. In Braunwald E, editor: *Heart disease: a textbook of cardiovascular medicine* ed 6, vol 2, Philadelphia, 2001, WB Saunders.

Mattox KL, Wall MJ: Injury to the thoracic great vessels. Injury to the heart. In Feliciano DV, Moore EE, Mattox KL, editors: *Trauma*, ed 3, Stamford, Conn, 1996, Appleton & Lange.

Mattox KL, Wall MJ, Pickard LR: Thoracic trauma: general considerations and indications for thoracotomy. In Feliciano DV, Moore EE, Mattox KL, editors: *Trauma,* ed 3, Stamford, Conn, 1996, Appleton & Lange.

May AK and others: Combined blunt cardiac and pericardial rupture: review of the literature and report of a new diagnostic algorithm, *Am Surg,* 65(6):568, 1999.

Mayrose MS and others: Comparison of staples versus sutures in the repair of penetrating cardiac wounds, *J Trauma* 46(3):441, 1999.

McClosky JC, Bulechek GM: *Nursing interventions classifications* ed 2, St Louis, 1996, Mosby.

Meyer G and others: Pulmonary embolectomy: a 20-year experience at one center, *Ann Thorac Surg* 51(2):232, 1991.

Mullins RJ and others: Influence of a statewide trauma system on location of hospitalization and outcome of injured patients, *J Trauma* 40(4):536, 1996.

Morales CH and others: Thoracoscopic pericardial window and penetrating cardiac trauma, *J Trauma* 42(4):670, 1997.

Neff JA, Kidd PS: *Trauma nursing: the art and science,* St Louis, 1993, Mosby.

Pasquale M, Fabian TC: Practice management guidelines for trauma from the Eastern Association for the Surgery of Trauma, *J Trauma* 44(6):941, 1998.

Reeder JM: Family perception: a key to intervention, *AACN Clin Issues Crit Care Nurs* 2(2):188, 1991.

Resources for optimal care of the injured patient: 1999, Chicago, 1998, American College of Surgeons' Committee on Trauma.

Rhee PM and others: Penetrating cardiac injuries: a population-based study, *J Trauma* 45(2):366, 1998.

Roberts SL: *Critical care nursing: assessment and intervention,* Stamford, Conn, 1996, Appleton & Lange.

Rutledge R, Sheldon GF: Bleeding and coagulation problems. In Feliciano DV, Moore EE, Mattox KL, editors: *Trauma,* ed 3, Stamford, Conn, 1996, Appleton & Lange.

Schroen A: Epidemiology of trauma. In Nwariaku F, Thal E, editors: *Parkland Memorial Hospital: Parkland trauma handbook,* ed 2, London, 1999, Mosby.

Shackford SR and others: Venous thromboembolism in patients with major trauma, *Am J Surg* 159:365, 1990.

Song MH, Shimomura T, Suenaga Y: Blunt cardiac trauma: successful repair of right atrium rupture, *J Cardiovasc Surg* 39(4):473, 1998.

Spain DA and others: Risk-taking behavior among adolescent trauma patients, *J Trauma,* 43(3):423, 1997.

Symbas PN, Justicz AG: Quantum leap forward in the management of cardiac trauma: the pioneering work of Dwight E Harkin, *Ann Thorac Surg* 55:789, 1993.

Thourani VH and others: Penetrating cardiac trauma at an urban trauma center: 22 year perspective, *Am J Surg* 65(9):811, 1999.

Trauma Nursing Coalition: *Resource document for nursing care of the trauma patient,* Chicago, 1992, Emergency Nurses Association.

Tsikaderis D, Dardas P, Hristofordis H: Incomplete ventral septal rupture following blunt chest trauma, *Clin Cardiol* 23(2):131, 2000.

Tyburski JG and others: Factors affecting prognosis with penetrating wounds of the heart, *J Trauma* 48(4):587, 2000.

Vaden R: Thoracic trauma. In Nwariaku F, Thal E, editors: *Parkland Memorial Hospital: Parkland trauma handbook,* ed 2, London, 1999, Mosby.

Villavicencio RT, Aucar JA, Wall MJ: Analysis of thoracoscopy in trauma, *Surg Endoscopy* 13(1):3, 1999.

Waldhausen JA, Pierce WS: *Johnson's surgery of the chest,* ed 5, St Louis, 1985, Mosby.

Waldhausen JA, Pierce WS, Campbell DB: *Surgery of the chest,* ed 6, St Louis, 1996, Mosby.

Westaby S: *Landmarks in cardiac surgery,* Oxford, UK, 1997, Isis Medical Media.

Wilson RF: *Critical care manual: applied physiology and principles of therapy,* ed 2, Philadelphia, 1992, FA Davis.

Wisner DH: Trauma to the chest. In Sabiston DC, Spencer FC: *Surgery of the chest,* ed 6, vol 1, Philadelphia, 1995, WB Saunders.

20 *Miscellaneous Procedures*

It's great to be alive—and to help others.

Motto of The Mended Hearts, Inc.*

Cardiac Tumors

Primary tumors, benign or malignant, originating in the heart and pericardium are rare and occur less frequently than metastatic neoplasms involving the heart (Salm, 2000). The most common cardiac tumor is the myxoma (Fig. 20-1), which is usually benign and was first resected under direct vision with cardiopulmonary bypass (CPB) by Craoford in 1954 (Schaff and Mullany, 2000; Crafoord, 1955).

To illustrate the rarity of cardiac tumors, in one series of more than 52,500 patients undergoing surgery between 1961 and 1983, only 20 primary cardiac tumors (excluding cardiac myxomas) were found—an incidence of less than 1 in every 2500 cases. Five of the 20 tumors were malignant. In the same series, 51 benign myxomas were found (Reece and others, 1984). Types of benign and malignant cardiac tumors (Box 20-1) occurring in the heart are typical of those that develop in any mass of striated muscle and connective tissue. Approximately 70% of cardiac tumors (mostly myxomas) are benign histologically, and the remainder (mostly sarcomas) are malignant (McAllister and Fenoglio, 1978; Doty, 2000). It has been observed that malignant tumors are more often found in the right side of the heart, whereas those in the left side tend to be benign (McAllister, Hall, and Cooley, 1999).

The causes of most tumors are unclear, but radiation, trauma, and chemotherapy are among the exogenous sources that have been implicated. Of significance to cardiac transplant recipients, long-term immunosuppression regimens have been associated with an increased incidence of malignant neoplasms, such as Kaposi's sarcoma (Kirklin and Barrett-Boyes, 1993a).

*The Mended Hearts, Inc., 7320 Greenville Ave., Dallas, TX, 75231

CLINICAL PRESENTATION

Clinical manifestations of cardiac tumors result from their degree of local invasion, mass effect, embolization, or systemic alterations (Salm, 2000; Silverman, 1980). As the tumor enlarges, it may interfere with valve function, producing regurgitation or stenosis. Blood flow may be obstructed, leading to signs and symptoms of congestive heart failure: dyspnea, orthopnea, elevated venous pressure, and peripheral edema (Colucci and Schoen, 2001). Systemic or pulmonary embolism may occur as a result of fragments breaking off from the main tumor mass, respectively located in the left or right side of the heart. Often there are nonspecific findings that include fever, cachexia (severe weight loss and muscle wasting), malaise, weakness, fatigue, anemia, and arthralgia. Dysrhythmias may be present, but the site of origin may not correlate with the site of the lesion.

DIAGNOSTIC EVALUATION

Laboratory tests may show an elevated erythrocyte sedimentation rate, anemia, and elevated serum gamma globulins (Colucci and Schoen, 2001). The electrocardiogram (ECG) may demonstrate atrial dysrhythmias and various degrees of heart block. Chest radiographs are often nonspecific and may have limited applicability unless the tumor is calcified (Salm, 2000).

The echocardiogram is the most useful diagnostic tool; two-dimensional transthoracic and transesophageal echocardiograms with color flow Doppler techniques often provide precise information about the lesion. Computed tomography (CT) and magnetic resonance imaging (MRI) are also valuable for their ability to distinguish among the various types of tumor tissue (Hupp, Shoaf, and Riggs, 1986; Araoz and others, 2000).

565

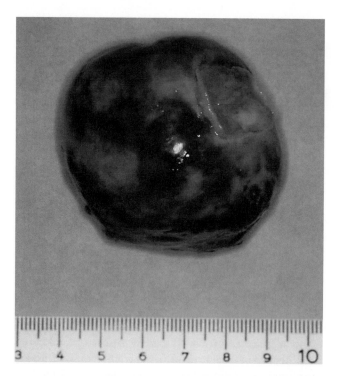

FIGURE 20-1   Benign left atrial myxoma. The tumor is primarily composed of acid mucopolysaccharides and has a soft, smooth, glistening capsule. Myxomas may be small nodules or large masses that fill the atrium and are often attached by a stalk or pedicle to the atrial septum. Myxomas are often pale or, as shown, stained by bleeding into the tumor. (Courtesy Edward A. Lefrak, MD.)

BOX 20-1
*Primary Tumors of the Heart**

Benign Tumors
Atrial myxoma
Lipoma
Papillary (valvular) fibroelastoma
Rhabdomyoma
Fibroma
Hemangioma
Teratoma
Atrioventricular nodal mesothelioma
Bronchogenic cyst

Malignant Tumors†
Angiosarcoma
Rhabdomyosarcoma
Mesothelioma
Fibrosarcoma
Malignant lymphoma
Osteosarcoma (arising in heart)

*Relative incidence; may involve the pericardium.
†Often involve both the heart and the pericardium.
Modified from McAllister HA, Fenoglio JJ: Tumors of the cardiovascular system. In *Atlas of tumor pathology,* fasc 15, ser 2, Washington, DC, 1978, Armed Forces Institute of Pathology.

If all four cardiac chambers cannot be visualized with noninvasive methods, cardiac catheterization and angiography may be indicated. Because of the danger of dislodging fragments from the tumor and subsequent embolization of the tumor pieces, cardiac catheterization is performed with great caution and often only in patients with suspected obstructive coronary artery disease.

Endomyocardial biopsy, first used to monitor the status of a transplanted heart, has been employed to diagnose cardiac tumors. Direct histologic examination of the biopsy specimen can confirm a diagnosis of cardiac malignancy (Salm, 2000).

TREATMENT

Cardiac tumors often can be detected early and excised surgically. Excision of an atrial myxoma (see later discussion) is the most common of the surgical procedures for cardiac tumors. Tumors located within the ventricle or the atrioventricular conduction system or attached to the papillary muscles, chordae tendineae, and cardiac valves also may be excised.

Unfortunately, surgery for most malignant tumors may not be effective because of the large mass of cardiac tissue that is often involved or because of the presence of metastases. Surgery may be performed to establish a diagnosis and to exclude the possibility of a benign tumor that can be cured. Palliation of hemodynamic derangements and physical symptoms can be achieved with aggressive therapy, such as partial resection of a tumor, chemotherapy, immunotherapy, and radiation therapy, alone or in combination. In some cases the heart is explanted, the tumor removed, and the native heart reimplanted (autotransplantation). If the tumor has widely invaded the heart, transplantation with a donor heart may be necessary (Wagner, Hutchisson, and Baird, 1999).

NURSING CONSIDERATIONS

Resection of tumors often requires that a portion of normal tissue be sacrificed. For example, when valve structures are involved, the perioperative nurse anticipates and prepares for the possibility of repair or replacement of the valve. Similarly, surgery in the area of conduction warrants consideration of the potential for a pacemaker. Potential complications and treatments should be discussed by the nurse and the surgeon.

Because the prognosis for primary malignant tumors of the heart and pericardium is often poor, nursing interventions are aimed at maximizing the quality of life. This can be achieved by helping patients and family to cope with the fear of death, reduce emotional distress, retain some degree of control over their life, and maintain as much physical, emotional, and physical comfort as possible.

An early case study by Motock (1966) focused on a patient with sarcoma of the pericardium. Motock's conclusions in the study remain pertinent today, and they reflect the importance of the nurse's behavior and attitude toward a patient (Box 20-2).

ATRIAL MYXOMA

Atrial myxoma, the most common primary cardiac tumor, appearing at almost any age, is gelatinous or mucoid, often with areas of hemorrhage (Kirklin and Barratt-Boyes, 1993a). Unlike intracavitary thrombi, myxomas are covered by endothelium. Myxomas occur predominantly in women; they are usually benign, but malignant myxomas have been reported (Salm, 2000). An echocardiogram usually identifies the tumor; an ECG may show atrial dysrhythmias and various degrees of heart block, but often the rhythm is normal sinus (Reynen, 1995). A heart murmur may be present if a left atrial myxoma prolapses through the mitral valve; this murmur often is referred to as a tumor *plop* and may be audible in the early diastolic phase of the cardiac cycle when the tumor falls into the ventricle.

Myxomas arise from the endocardium and are usually located in the left atrium; right atrial myxomas account for approximately 15% to 20% of all cardiac myxomas (Guhathakurta and Riordan, 2000). Ventricular or mitral valve myxomas are less common. They are solitary tumors that attach by a stalk or pedicle to the atrial septum, often in the area of the fossa ovalis. Surgical removal is indicated soon after the diagnosis is made because of the danger of embolization and risk of sudden death in these patients (Colucci and Schoen, 2001).

Myxomas tend to be sporadic, but there may be a familial pattern. Patients with the familial type are more likely to have recurrence of the lesion after surgery; family members also may have myxomas. *Syndrome myxoma*, also known as *Carney syndrome* (Carney, 1985), is associated with the familial pattern. Patients tend to be younger and may demonstrate extensive facial freckling. They may have noncardiac myxomas and endocrine neoplasms (Schaff and Mullany, 2000).

Operative procedure: excision of a left atrial myxoma

Although a minimally invasive approach has been used, Schaff and Mullany (2000) recommend a median sternotomy incision for men and older women. An anterolateral thoracotomy through a submammary incision can be used for patients seeking a more cosmetic result. Cardiopulmonary bypass (CPB) with cold-blood cardioplegia provides a quiet operative field and facilitates the en bloc removal of these tumors, which tend to be friable and prone to breaking apart. Right or left thoracotomy can be used for difficult reoperations.

To the basic chest set are added atrial retractors. Because complete removal of the tumor pedicle requires excision of the attached portion of the atrial septum, closure of the remaining atrial septal defect is necessary. This may be achieved by primary suture closure or, more commonly, with a patch of autologous pericardium or synthetic patch material.

Procedure (Schaff and Mullany, 2000)

1. A median sternotomy is performed. If the surgeon plans to close the septum with pericardium, a piece is removed for later use. The tissue should be kept moist with saline to retain its pliability.

2. CPB is instituted with bicaval cannulation for venous drainage. Caval tapes or clamps are used to divert all systemic venous return away from the right atrium and into the venous line. The aorta is cross-clamped and the heart arrested with cardioplegia.

Minimal manipulation of the heart before cross-clamping lessens the risk of dislodging tumor fragments.

3. The approach to the tumor can be individualized. For a small left atrial myxoma, the right atrial wall can be incised and a right atrial transseptal incision made to access the tumor. Larger or multi-sited tumors may require a biatrial approach or an incision in the posterior portion of the inter-atrial groove.

4. An atrial retractor is inserted, and the atrium is inspected. The tumor may bulge out of the atrium.

5. The tumor pedicle attached to the atrial septum is located. The pedicle and the full thickness of the atrial septum to which the pedicle is attached are excised.

    Occasionally, proximate conduction tracts must be sacrificed in order to completely remove the tumor. The entire tumor and pedicle are removed.

6. The atria, atrioventricular valves, and ventricles are inspected. Remaining tumor fragments (and other particulate matter) are removed.

7. The septal patch is cut into the desired shape; closure of the interatrial septal defect with peri-cardium or a synthetic patch is often performed with a running (3-0) polypropylene suture. Just before completion of the patch closure, the left atrium is irrigated or allowed to fill with blood to remove as much air as possible.

8. Patch closure is completed, followed by closure of the right atrial wall. Air is evacuated from the left side of the heart.

9. Temporary atrial and ventricular pacing wires are attached, and chest tubes are inserted for drainage.

10. The sternum and chest incision are closed.

Postoperative course

Temporary atrial dysrhythmias (caused by the atriotomies and cardiac manipulation) are common postoperatively. If permanent heart block develops, a transvenous pacemaker system can be inserted. Antibiotic prophylaxis before invasive procedures is recommended in patients with synthetic patch material (Hupp, Shoaf, and Riggs, 1986).

Occasionally there is recurrence of an excised myxoma, usually within 1 to 5 years after surgery. This may result from incomplete initial tumor excision or seeding of tumor cells during surgery, regrowth from the same cells of origin, or multifocal sites of origin unrecognized during the initial procedure. It is often related to the familial form of myxoma. Follow-up with annual echocardiograms for 5 years has been recommended. Family members of patients with the familial form also should be screened by echocardiography (Schaff and Mullany, 2000).

Pericardial Disease

The pericardial sac encloses the heart and consists of parietal and visceral layers between which is approximately 50 ml (although this can vary) of lubricating fluid. It is thought that the function of the pericardium is to stabilize the position of the heart within the chest, reduce friction between the surface of the heart and surrounding tissues, protect the heart against the spread of infection from adjacent structures, prevent cardiac overdilation, and maintain the normal pressure-volume relationships of the cardiac chambers (Spodick, 2001). Thus when disease affects either the pericardial sac itself or the fluid within it, the heart may be unable to function properly.

Surgical indications for pericardial disease include two main categories of patients: those with effusive pericarditis and those with chronic constrictive pericarditis (Liu, 2000). Excess fluid within the limited pericardial cavity can lead to cardiac tamponade; pericardial constriction can limit cardiac filling, leading to reduced cardiac output.

PERICARDIAL EFFUSION

Studies have demonstrated that pericardial fluid is an ultrafiltrate of plasma. When venous or lymphatic drainage of the heart is obstructed (as can occur with trauma or tumors), abnormal amounts of pericardial fluid can accumulate as a result of the altered balance of hydrostatic and osmotic forces. This leads to increased filtration of plasma across the visceral pericardium, producing pericardial effusion. Production of excess pericardial fluid also can be stimulated by inflammation of the pericardium (Gibson and Segal, 1978; Kirklin and Barratt-Boyes, 1993b). Two-dimensional echocardiography is the most useful diagnostic technique and can be used to guide needle aspiration.

PERICARDIOCENTESIS

Aspiration of excess pericardial fluid with a large-bore needle (Fig. 20-2) may be performed for emergency release of a tamponade. Pericardiocentesis also can be performed diagnostically in cancer patients with chronic pericardial effusion to differentiate malignant effusion from postirradiation pericarditis. For chronic effusion, a pericardial window via anterior thoracotomy or video-assisted thoracoscopic surgery (VATS) offers more effective long-term results.

CREATION OF A PERICARDIAL WINDOW

Pericardial drainage may be performed through a right or left anterior thoracotomy, a subxiphoid approach, or

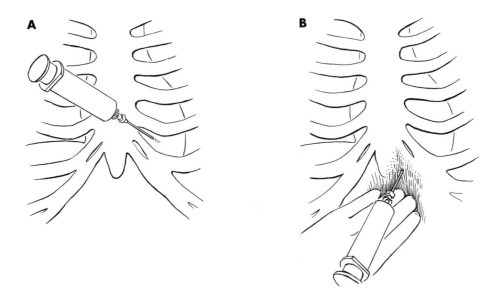

FIGURE 20-2 Pericardiocentesis. Insertion through either **A** or **B** may be used. Advancement of the needle is halted when either intrapericardial blood appears or the motion of the heart is felt by the fingers. An ECG lead may be attached to the needle; a significant change in the ECG tracing alerts the surgeon that contact has been made with the myocardium. (From Waldhausen JA, Pierce WS, Campbell DB: *Surgery of the chest,* ed 6, St Louis, 1996, Mosby.)

thoracoscopically (VATS). With the release of the fluid, a dramatic improvement in systemic blood pressure can be expected. The pericardial drainage should be measured; culture tubes also should be available for bacteriologic and histologic evaluation. Elevating the head of the transport stretcher or the operating room bed may reduce some of the discomfort felt by the patient in the supine position before surgery.

Because there is a risk of sudden cardiac decompensation with positive-pressure ventilation and general anesthesia in these patients, it is recommended that patients be prepared and draped before anesthetic induction to minimize the time interval between ventilation and release of the tamponade. Initially local anesthesia may be used to enhance the patient's hemodynamic status; once the patient has been stabilized, general anesthesia and ventilation may be initiated. In some cases, pericardiocentesis is performed before anesthesia induction; a topical anesthetic is injected to lessen discomfort. Application of external defibrillation pads is recommended (Waldhausen, Pierce, and Campbell, 1996).

Operative procedure: creation of a pericardial window via an anterior thoracoscopy

Thoracoscopy instruments and VATS equipment are prepared. The patient is placed in a semilateral position or supine with the left side slightly elevated by a small roll (Dawes, 1999). The right chest cavity may be entered if the pericardial fluid takes up a significant portion of the left pleural space (Liu, 2000). External defibrillation pads should be applied.

Procedure (Liu, 2000)

1. The first incision is often made in the sixth intercostal space along the midaxillary line.
2. The pleural cavity is entered by blunt dissection, and the space is palpated to determine the presence of adhesions.
3. An 11-mm trocar and a 10-mm, 0-degree, telescope are inserted, and the chest cavity is explored.
4. Two more intercostal incisions are made along the anterior axillary line at approximately the fourth and seventh intercostal spaces. Adjustments may be necessary depending on the patient's anatomy and the location of the lesion.
5. The phrenic nerve is identified and kept in view throughout the entire procedure.
6. An incision is made in the distended pericardium, and the hole is enlarged with a clamp of the surgeon's choice (or with a cautery pencil). The fluid draining into the pleural space is suctioned away.
7. A patch of pericardium is excised to create a window (approximately 3×4 cm).
8. A chest tube is inserted through the previously made inferior incision; remaining decisions are closed.

Operative procedure: creation of a pericardial window via an anterior thoracotomy

Thoracotomy instruments are used. Positioning is similar to thoracoscopy; external defibrillator pads are recommended.

Procedure

1. An incision is made over the anterior left fifth rib; a segment of rib may need to be excised.
2. The pericardium and anterior surface of the heart are exposed by incising the posterior periosteum and parietal pleura.
3. As large a portion of pericardium as possible is removed from the right ventricle and left ventricle (anterior to the left phrenic nerve) with scissors and cautery to create a window. Caution is taken to avoid burn injuries to the heart or the phrenic nerve, and to reduce the risk of causing ventricular fibrillation. Additionally, the heart should be gently retracted to avoid injury during excision of the pericardium.
4. Pericardial fluid and tissue are sent for laboratory study.
5. Posterolateral and anterior chest tubes are brought out from the left pleural space through lower intercostal stab wounds, and the incision is closed.

Operative procedure: creation of a pericardial window via a subxiphoid approach

When only pericardial drainage is required (and a portion of pericardium does not need to be resected), a subxiphoid approach may be employed. This approach also may be useful if the patient is unable to tolerate single-lung ventilation for thoracotomy or thoracoscopy (Liu, 2000).

Procedure

1. The patient is placed in the supine position and sternal instruments are used.
2. An incision is made over the xiphoid process and upper abdomen; the xiphoid process is cut with bone cutters or retracted upwardly.
3. The pericardium is opened, fluid suctioned away, and a drain inserted. The incision is closed.

CONSTRICTIVE PERICARDITIS

Constrictive pericarditis is produced when chronically inflamed pericardium becomes fibrotic, often calcified, and noncompliant. The pericardial space becomes obliterated, and the heart is encased in an adherent layer of scar (measuring 0.5 to 1 cm in thickness) that restricts diastolic ventricular filling. The etiology may be related to chronic effusive pericarditis; it is often viral, although tuberculosis is once again becoming an important etiologic factor. Among patients with chronic renal disease, uremic pericardial disease also is seen (Schoen, 1999; Kirklin and Barratt-Boyes, 1993b).

Clinically the patient demonstrates signs and symptoms similar to those of congestive heart failure. The absence of a history of myocardial disease is important in the differential diagnosis. Dyspnea, fatigue, and weight gain are common complaints, and jugular venous distension, peripheral edema, hepatomegaly, or ascites may be evident. A striking abnormality of constrictive pericarditis, in contrast to the situation with cardiac tamponade (or in healthy persons), is the failure of intrathoracic pressure changes during respiration to be transmitted to the pericardium and cardiac chambers. Thus with constrictive pericarditis, central venous pressure does not fall during inspiration, and venous return to the right atrium does not increase. In some patients systemic venous pressure may increase with respiration (e.g., *Kussmaul's sign*). Kussmaul's sign does not occur in acute cardiac tamponade (Spodick, 2001).

Radiographically the heart may be small; calcification of the pericardium may be seen. The ECG may show nonspecific ST-T wave changes, atrial dysrhythmias, and low QRS voltage. CT scanning may be used to distinguish between thickened pericardium and underlying myocardium; it is often more useful than echocardiography, which may not be able to make the distinction. Cardiac catheterization (and endomyocardial biopsy) may be necessary to differentiate constrictive pericarditis from other cardiac disease, such as restrictive cardiomyopathy, and to asses the status of the coronary arteries.

TREATMENT

Because the disease is progressive and not reversible, the treatment of choice is pericardiectomy. Decortication of the visceral (epicardial) and parietal pericardium adhering to the cardiac chambers often produces dramatic improvement.

A median sternotomy provides excellent exposure and facilitates the repair of lacerations that may occur during removal of the fibrous layer (Waldhausen, Pierce, and Campbell, 1996). This incision also allows rapid institution of CPB if there is sudden cardiac decompensation; CPB should be available on a standby basis (Oliver, De Castro, and Strickland, 1999).

Basic sternotomy instruments are used; lung retractors are required. Ultrasonic debridement may be a useful adjunct when there is dense calcification. Suture ligatures (4-0, 5-0 polypropylene, silk, or other material, depending on the surgeon's preference) and pledgets can be used to repair lacerations. External defibrillator pads should be readily available because manipulation of the heart may cause ventricular fibrillation.

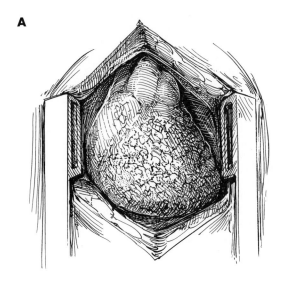

A

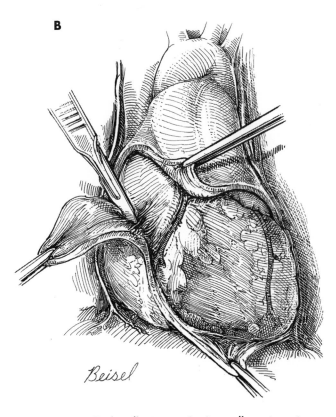

B

Beisel

FIGURE 20-3 Pericardiectomy. **A,** A median sternotomy exposes the fibrous pericardium. **B,** Sharp dissection of the fibrous peel; the right and left phrenic nerves (running along the lateral pericardium) and the epicardial blood vessels are protected during dissection. (From Waldhausen JA, Pierce WS, Campbell DB: *Surgery of the chest,* ed 6, St. Louis, 1996, Mosby.)

Operative procedure: pericardiectomy (Waldhausen, Pierce, and Campbell, 1996)

1. A median sternotomy is performed to expose the heart and great vessels (Fig. 20-3, *A*). The pleurae are opened, and the lungs are displaced laterally. The phrenic nerves are identified and protected.
2. A knife or scissors is used to incise the pericardium (Fig. 20-3, *B*).
3. Pericardial flaps are created and meticulously dissected. Inflation of the lungs is performed intermittently throughout the procedure.
4. Small lacerations of the myocardium can be repaired with pledgeted or nonpledgeted suture ligatures.
5. If pericardial and epicardial adhesions in the region of the right coronary artery pose too great a risk of laceration of the artery, a strip of scar tissue may be retained in the area of the right atrioventricular groove.
6. Dissection is carried laterally over the left ventricle to beyond the left phrenic nerve, which is preserved as a pedicle.
7. The right atrium is freed to the right phrenic nerve, which is preserved as in step 6.
8. Drainage catheters are placed in the pericardium and each pleura, and the chest incision is closed.

Postoperative course

Postoperatively, low cardiac output syndrome may occur, especially in patients with more severe preoperative disability (e.g., functional class III or IV; marked elevation of right ventricular end-diastolic pressure). Preoperative functional status also influences long-term survival, and it is recommended that pericardial resection be performed early in the course of constrictive pericarditis. When performed early, patients can expect definite symptomatic improvement. However, some patients require weeks or months before relief is obtained and elevated venous filling pressures are reduced (Lorell, 1997).

References

Araoz PA and others: CT and MR imaging of benign cardiac neoplasms with echocardiographic correlation, *Radiographics* 20(5):1303, 2000.

Carney JA: Differences between nonfamilial and familial cardiac myxoma, *Am J Surg Pathol* 9(1):53, 1985.

Colucci WS, Schoen FJ: Primary tumors of the heart. In Braunwald E, Zipes DP, Libby P, editors: *Heart disease: a textbook of cardiovascular medicine,* ed 6, vol 2, Philadelphia, 2001, WB Saunders.

Crafoord CL: Discussion of late results of mitral commissurotomy. In Lam CR, editor: *Proceedings: International Symposium on Cardiovascular Surgery,* Philadelphia, 1955, WB Saunders.

Dawes BG: Thoracic surgery. In Alexander EL, Meeker MH, Rothrock JC, editors: *Alexander's care of the patient in surgery,* ed 11, St Louis, 1999, Mosby.

Doty DB: Cardiac tumors, 2000, http://www.ctsnet.org/residents/ctsn/archives/31txt.html (accessed Nov 27, 2000).

Gibson AT, Segal MB: A study of the composition of pericardial fluid, with special reference to the probable mechanism of fluid formation, *J Physiology* 277:367, 1978.

Guhathakurta S, Riordan JP: Surgical treatment of right atrial myxoma, *Tex Heart Inst J* 27(1):61, 2000.

Hupp E, Shoaf B, Riggs TR: Cardiac myxomas: diagnosis, surgical excision, and nursing care, *AORN J* 44(6):928, 1986.

Kirklin JW, Barratt-Boyes BG: Cardiac tumor. In Kirklin JW, Barratt-Boyes BG, *Cardiac surgery: morphology, diagnostic criteria, natural history, techniques, results and indications,* ed 2, vol 2, New York, 1993a, Churchill Livingstone.

Kirklin JW, Barratt-Boyes BG: Pericardial disease. In Kirklin JW, Barratt-Boyes BG, *Cardiac surgery: morphology, diagnostic criteria, natural history, techniques, results, and indications,* ed 2, vol 2, New York, 1993b, Churchill Livingstone.

Liu HP: Minimally invasive surgery for pericardial diseases. In Yim APC, and others: *Minimal access cardiothoracic surgery,* Philadelphia, 2000, WB Saunders.

McAllister HA, Fenoglio JJ: Tumors of the cardiovascular system. In *Atlas of tumor pathology,* facs 15, ser 2, Washington, DC, Armed Forces Institute of Pathology.

McAllister HA, Hall RA, Cooley DA: Tumors of the heart and pericardium: Primary cardiac tumors, *Curr Probl Cardiol* 24:63, 1999.

Motock EC: A patient with sarcoma of the pericardium: a case study, *Nurs Clin North Am* 1(1):15, 1966.

Oliver WC, De Castro MA, Strickland RA: Uncommon diseases and cardiac anesthesia. In Kaplan JA, editor: *Cardiac anesthesia,* ed 4, Philadelphia, 1999, WB Saunders.

Reece IJ and others: Cardiac tumors: clinical spectrum and prognosis of lesions other than classical benign myxoma in 20 patients, *J Thorac Cardiovasc Surg* 88(3):439, 1984.

Reynen K: Cardiac myxomas, *N Engl J Med* 333(24):1610, 1995.

Salm TJ: Unusual primary tumors of the heart, *Semin Thorac Cardiovasc Surg* 12(2):89, 2000.

Schaff HV, Mullany CJ: Surgery for cardiac myxomas, *Semin Thorac Cardiovasc Surg* 12(2):77, 2000.

Schoen FJ: The heart. In Cotran RS, Kumar V, Collins T, editors: *Robbins' pathologic basis of disease,* ed 6, Philadelphia, 1999, WB Saunders.

Silverman NA: Primary cardiac tumors, *Ann Surg* 191(2):127, 1980.

Spodick DH: Pericardial diseases. In Braunwald E, Zipes DP, Libby P, editors: *Heart disease: a textbook of cardiovascular medicine,* ed 6, vol 2, Philadelphia, 2001, WB Saunders.

Wagner S, Hutchisson B, Baird MG: Cardiac explantation and autotransplantation, *AORN J* 70(1):99, 1999.

Waldhausen JA, Pierce WS, Campbell DB: *Surgery of the chest,* ed 6, St Louis, 1996, Mosby.

Index

A

AATS, 25
Abbott, Maude, 11
Abciximab, 114t, 263
Abdominal aorta, 208f
Aberrancy, 496b
Abiomed BVS 5000 Bi-Ventricular
    Support System, 442
Abiomed VAD, 442-444
Ablation therapy, 508
Abnormal automaticity, 501
ACC database, 51
Accessory items, 79b, 80b
Accessory pathways, 496b, 499
Accidents, 38
Acetylsalicylic acid, 114t
Acquired aneurysms/dissections, 398
Action potential, 496b
Activated PTT, 113t, 115f
Active failures, 38
Acute aortic insufficiency, 349
Acute pulmonary embolus (APE), 560
Acute rejection, 480
Acute respiratory failure (ARF), 247
Acute severe myocardial injury, 431
Acute tamponade, 555
Adenosine, 101, 157t
Admission to cardiac ICU, 171b
Admission to cardiac service, 146, 149b
Adrenalin, 156t
Advance directives, 151
Advanced beginner, 28-29
Advanced beginner circulating
    nurse, 29
AEDs, 62, 521
AF, 181, 502f, 517-521
Afterload, 206t, 207
Aging workforce, 24
AICD, 523
Air embolism, 234t, 235
Akinesis, 263b
Alcohol injection, 13
Alexander, Edythe Louise, 17
Alexander's Care of the Patient in Surgery,
    15, 17
Alfenta, 156t
Alfentanil, 156t
A-line, 155

Allen's test, 124b, 274
Allocation status, 466
Allograft, 353
Allograft replacement of aortic valve,
    364-368
Altered automaticity, 496b
Ambient temperature levels, 34
American Association for Thoracic
    Surgery (AATS), 25
American Heart Association, 185
Amiodarone, 507-508
Amrinone, 156t
AN region, 498
Anatomic factors, 96b
Anatomic gifts, 151
Anatomy and physiology, 187-212
    aortic valve, 196
    arterial circulation, 208f
    cardiac chambers, 191-194
    cardiac cycle, 204-205
    cardiac myocyte, 202-203
    cardiac output, 205-207
    cardiac valves, 194-196
    cardiac veins, 199
    cellular contraction, 204
    circulatory system, 207-212
    conduction system, 199-200
    coronary arteries, 196-199
    coronary blood flow, 198
    excitation-contraction of cardiac
        cell, 202-204
    external features of heart, 190
    fetal circulation, 209-212
    innervation of heart, 200-201
    left atrium, 192-193
    left ventricle, 193-194
    location of heart, 187-189
    mitral valve, 194-196
    pericardium, 187-189
    pulmonary circulation, 209
    pulmonary valve, 196
    right atrium, 191-192
    right ventricle, 192
    size/position of heart, 189
    systemic circulation, 207-209
    tricuspid valve, 196
    venous circulation, 210f
Ancef, 157t

Anesthesia provider, 32
Aneurysm, 396-401
ANF, 202
Angina pectoris, 261
Angiotensin II, 433
Angle of Louis, 188f
Angular vein, 210f
Anistropy, 496b
Ankeney sternal retractor, 72f
Annular dilation, 314
Annular ring, 377f
Annuloaortic ectasia, 400
Annuloplasty rings, 92-93, 327-328,
    383-384
Annulus fibrosus, 377f
Anomalous pulmonary venous return,
    528t
ANS, 200
Anstadt cup, 459
Antegrade/retrograde blood
    cardioplegia infusion, 253-256
Anterior commissural leaflet, 311f
Anterior facial vein, 210f
Anterior interventricular sulcus, 190f
Anterior leaflet, 192f, 196
Anterior papillary muscle, 193f, 194f,
    196, 498f
Anterior scallop, 311f
Anterior septal, 499f
Anterior tibial artery, 208f
Anterior tibial vein, 210f
Anterolateral papillary muscle, 310f
Anterolateral thoracotomy, 214t, 226f,
    227f
Anteromedial leaflet, 196
Antibody immunosuppression, 15
Antidysrhythmic drugs, 507t
Anxiety, 132, 176
AORN, 17, 23
AORN Journal, 17
AORN patient outcome standards,
    131b
AORN perioperative patient-focused
    model, 132f
Aorta, 208f, 395. *See also* Thoracic
    aortic disease.
Aortic anastomoses, 291
Aortic aneurysms, 396-401

Page numbers followed by f indicate figures; t, tables; b, boxes.

Aortic arch, 190f
Aortic arch replacement, 417-419
Aortic graft valve prostheses, 91-92
Aortic insufficiency, 349
Aortic leaflet, 196, 311f
Aortic and pulmonary allografts, 91
Aortic root, 196
Aortic stenosis, 347-349, 350
Aortic valve, 343, 377f
Aortic valve allograft, 353-354, 358
Aortic valve endocarditis, 371
Aortic valve leaflet retractors, 358f
Aortic valve replacement, 351-371
Aortic valve replacement with
     coronary artery bypass grafting,
     371
Aortic valve surgery, 343-374
  allograft replacement, 364-368
  aortic insufficiency, 349, 350
  aortic stenosis, 347-349, 350
  aortic valve allograft, 353-354, 358
  aortic valve endocarditis, 371
  aortic valve replacement with
     CABG, 371
  aortic valvotomy, 351
  bacterial endocarditis, 345
  completion of procedure, 371
  congenital malformations, 344
  diagnostic evaluation, 350
  documentation, 357b
  double valve replacement, 371
  enlargement of small aortic root,
     362-364
  equipment, 357b
  Kanno-Rastan procedure, 364, 366f,
     367f
  left ventricular apicoabdominal aor-
     tic conduit, 364, 368f
  LVOT obstruction, 349
  Manouguian procedure, 364, 365f
  Marfan's syndrome, 347
  minimally invasive surgical tech-
     niques, 359
  Morrow procedure, 368-371
  myomyectomy for hypertrophic
     subaortic stenosis, 368-371
  Nicks procedure, 362-364
  nursing care, 355t, 356t
  operative procedure (replacement),
     359-362
  patch enlargement of proximal
     ascending aorta, 362, 363f
  patient teaching, 354
  PBAV, 351
  postoperative complications, 371-
     373
  procedural considerations, 355-359
  pulmonary allografts, 354
  reparative techniques, 351
  replacement, 351-371
  rheumatic fever, 345
  RNFA considerations, 353b
  safety measures, 357b
  senile calcific aortic stenosis, 345
  signs/symptoms of disease, 348t

Aortic valve surgery—cont'd
  special considerations, 357b
  surgical valvuloplasty, 351
  tertiary syphilis, 347
  valve prostheses, 343, 344f, 352-353
Aortic valvotomy, 351
Aortic wall, 395
Aortocaval cannulation, 239
Aortography, 402, 403f
APE, 560
Apex, 189, 190f, 192f
Apical ventricular aneurysm patch
     repair, 296
Apoptosis, 204t, 261
Aprotinin, 166, 169t
Arch of aorta, 208f
Arcuate artery, 208f
ARF, 247
Arterial blood gases, 113t
Arterial catheters, 65, 66f
Arterial circulation, 208f
Arteria radicularis magna (ARM), 421
Arterioles, 209
Artery of Adamkiewicz, 421
Artery to A-V node, 377f
Ascending aorta, 190f
Aspinall, Mary Jo, 18
Aspirin, 114t
Assessment. *See* Evaluation,
     Preoperative assessment.
Association of periOperative
     Registered Nurses (AORN),
     17, 23
Asymptomatic aortic stenosis, 349
Asynergy, 263b
Asynersis, 263b
Atheroemboli, 181
Atherosclerosis, 259, 400
Atlas of Congenital Heart Disease
     (Abbott), 11
Atrial appendage, 190f
Atrial fibrillation (AF), 181, 502f, 517-
     521
Atrial myxoma, 312, 567
Atrial natriuretic factor (ANF), 202
Atrial pacemaker complex, 497
Atrial septal defect (ASD), 536-541
Atrionodal (AN) region, 498
Atrioventricular (AV) junction, 199-
     200, 498
Atrioventricular (AV) node, 191
Atrioventricular groove, 191
Atrioventricular nodal reentrant
     tachycardia (AVNRT), 517
Atrioventricular valves, 309
Atropine, 156t
Autologous blood salvaging methods,
     160
Automatic external defibrillators
     (AEDs), 62, 521
Automatic implantable cardioverter
     defibrillator (AICD), 523
Automaticity, 199, 496b
Autonomic nervous system (ANS),
     200

Autotransfusion suction, 235
Autotransfusion system, 63-64
Autotransplantation, 482-483
AV junction, 199-200, 498
Avitan, 156t
Avitene, 167t
AV node, 191, 200
AVNRT, 517
Axillary artery, 208f
Axillary vein, 210f
AXIS 360-degree coronary stabilizer,
     75f
Azathioprine, 480b, 481
Azygos (low) flow principle, 7

B

Baby boomers, 24t
Bachmann's bundle, 497
Bacitracin, 157t
Backup instruments, 34
Bacterial endocarditis, 312, 345
Bailey, Charles, 13
Balanced, 197
Balloon angioplasty, 265f
Barnard, Christian, 1, 2f
Barratt-Boyes, Brian, 11
Base, 189
Basement membrane, 203f
Basic cardiac procedures, 213-257
  CPB, 230-250
  myocardial protection, 250-256
  thoracic incisions, 213-230
Basic sternotomy sets, 77
Basilic veins, 282
Basophils, 480t
Batista, Randas J. V., 272
Batista procedure, 272
Baue, Arthur E., 51
Baumgarten, Gwyn, 8
Beating heart surgery
  concepts/techniques, 268b, 269b
  intraoperative considerations, 148b,
     149b
  myocardial protection, 256
  operative procedure, 289-291
  special considerations, 77b
  structural standards, 73-75
  ventricular assistance, 246-247
Beck, Claude, 4, 12, 13, 258
Beck aorta clamp, 71f
Beck aorta clamp tip, 71f
Belly band, 159
Benign left atrial myxoma, 566f
Bentall-DeBono procedure, 409-410
Bicaval cannulation of right atrium,
     242-243
Bicuspid aortic valve, 344f, 528t
Bigelow, W. G., 6
Bilateral en bloc lung transplantation,
     488
Bilateral lung transplantation, 491-
     492
Bilateral sequential lung
     transplantation, 488
Bilateral submammary incision, 217f

Billowing mitral valve, 313b
Billroth, Theodor, 1
Biologic circulatory assistance. *See* Mechanical/biologic circulatory assistance.
Biologic prostheses, 85
Biologic valve prostheses, 336t
Biologic valves, 86
Biomedicus centrifugal pump, 439, 440f
Bioprosthesis, 90f
Bird baths, 58
Biventricular pacing, 516
Blalock, Alfred, 11
Blanket warmers, 69
Blind aneurysmectomies, 521
Blood banking, 6
Blood cardioplegia solutions, 252
Blood chemistry, 113t
Blood conservation, 160-161
Blood conservation agents, 169
Blood oxygenation, 65-66
Blood preservation, 6
Blood pressure, 123
Blood pressure cuff, 154t
Blood refrigerators, 69
Blood salvaging devices, 161
Blood substitutes, 6
Blood transfusion, 160-161
Blood transfusions, 6
Blood typing, 6
Blower-mister, 75, 76f
Blunt thoracic injuries, 550-551
Body positioning, 155, 158
Bone wax, 167t
Borrowing equipment, 35
Brachial artery, 208f
Brachial plexus nerve injury, 177
Brachiocephalic artery, 208f
Bradydysrhythmias, 508-517, 521
Brain death, 465
Brandt, Lisbeth, 9
Braunwald, Eugene, 187
Bretylium, 157t
Bretylol, 157t
Brevital, 156t
Brock, Lord, 13
Bruits, 123
Bubble method, 65
Bubble oxygenators, 231t, 233
Bulldog clamp, 83f
Bullock, Barbara L., 15, 95
Bundle branches, 200
Bundle of His, 194
Burley, Wanda, 17
Bypass pump, 64
Bypass tubing, 236-237

C

CABG. *See* Surgery for CAD.
Cabrol technique, 412, 414, 415f
Cachexia, 97b
CAD, 258-263. *See also* Surgery for CAD.
Calan, 157t
Calcium chloride, 156t

Cancellation of surgery, 153
Cannon, Alice, 8
Cannon, John, 14
Cannulation of aorta, 240-241
Cannulation of femoral artery, 241
Cannulation of right atrium, 242
Cannulation for venous return, 242-243
Capillaries, 209
Capnography, 154t
Cardiac catheterization, 107-112, 379-380, 532
Cardiac chambers, 191-194
Cardiac cycle, 204-205
Cardiac dysrhythmias, 495-526
   ablation therapy, 508
   AEDs, 521
   AF, 517-521
   AVNRT, 517
   bradydysrhythmias, 508-517, 521
   categorizing dysrhythmias, 501-502
   conduction system, 495-500
   diagnostic evaluation, 503-507
   documentation, 514b
   glossary of terms, 496b
   ICDs, 522-523
   nursing care, 510t, 511t
   pacemakers, 508-517
   patient teaching, 512-513
   pharmacologic therapy, 507-508
   procedural considerations, 502-503
   safety measures, 514b
   signal-averaged ECG, 503-504
   special considerations, 514b
   supplies, 514b
   supraventricular dysrhythmias, 508-521
   tachydysrhythmias, 517-524
   ventricular dysrhythmias, 521-524
   WPW syndrome, 517
Cardiac enzymes, 112, 113t
Cardiac index (CI), 206t
Cardiac myocyte, 202-203
Cardiac nuclear imaging, 104-106
Cardiac output (CO), 205-207
Cardiac rehabilitation, 182-183
Cardiac resynchronization therapy (CRT), 516
Cardiac rhythm, 124
Cardiac structures/coronary supply, 261t
Cardiac suite, 53. *See also* Structural standards.
Cardiac surgery course outline, 28b
Cardiac Surgery and the OR Nurse, 17
Cardiac surgical organizations, 25
Cardiac Surgical Patient, The (Powers/Storlie), 14
Cardiac tamponade, 555-556
Cardiac team members, 32-33
Cardiac trauma. *See* Emergency situations.
Cardiac tumors, 565-568
Cardiac valve prostheses, 86-91. *See also* Valve prostheses.

Cardiac valves, 194-196
Cardiac veins, 199
Cardiac venting catheters, 235-236
Cardiac wall, 189
Cardinal symptoms, 97b
Cardiomyopathy, 434f, 444
Cardiomyoplasty, 457-459
Cardio-omentopexy, 13
Cardioplegia, 252-253
Cardioplegia solutions, 252-253
Cardiopulmonary bypass, 230-250
   advances/discovery, 230t
   adverse effects, 238-239
   bicaval cannulation of right atrium, 242-243
   blood activation, 238t, 239f
   bypass tubing, 236-237
   cannulation of aorta, 240-241
   cannulation of femoral artery, 241
   cannulation of right atrium, 242
   cannulation for venous return, 242-243
   cerebroplegia, 250
   components of bypass system, 231t
   deep hypothermia with circulatory arrest, 248, 250
   discontinuation of CPB, 243-244
   ECLS, 247-248
   effects, 249t
   emergency extracorporal support, 244-245
   endovascular systems, 245-246
   heparin, 231-233
   hypothermia, 230-231
   partial CPB, 233
   percutaneous CPB, 244-246
   postoperative care, 248
   priming solution, 237
   protamine sulfate, 233
   pumps/oxygenators, 233
   removal of cannulas, 244
   RNFA considerations, 238b
   safety considerations, 234t, 237-238
   suction devices, 233-235
   surgical procedures, 239-244
   thoracic aortic disease, 408
   total CPB, 233
   venting devices, 235-236
   ventricular assistance for beating heart surgery, 246-247
Cardiopulmonary bypass circuit, 231, 232f
Cardiopulmonary bypass pump, 64f
Cardiopulmonary technologists, 33
Cardiosurgical Nursing Care (Chow), 18
Cardiotomy suction, 233, 235
Cardiovalvulotome, 12
Cardiovascular anesthesiologists, 32
Cardiovascular draping system, 158-159
Cardiovascular Nursing, 18
Cardiovascular Nursing Care (Chow), 15
Cardiovascular nursing literature, 17-18

Cardiovascular Nursing: Rationale for Theory and Nursing Approach, 15
Cardiovascular risk factors, 263t
Cardiovascular Surgical Nursing (Fordham), 12, 17
CardioWest (CWT) C-70 total artificial heart, 451
Care of the Cardiac Surgical Patient (King), 15, 18
Care plans, 135-144
Carpentier, Alain, 375
Carpentier annuloplasty ring technique, 385, 388f
Carpentier-Edwards Perimount bovine pericardial valve prosthesis, 86f
Carpentier rings, 328, 330f
Carpentier tricuspid rings, 383
Carrel, Alexis, 5, 7, 258, 463
Castenada, Aldo, 12
Castroviejo needle holders, 73, 74f
CCS classification system, 96b
Cefadyl, 157t
Celiac artery, 208f, 270f
Cellular contraction, 204
Central fibrous body, 377f, 499f
Central fibrous skeleton, 194
Central venous pressure (CVP) line, 154t
Centrifugal blood pump, 67f
Centrifugal pumps, 231t, 233, 439-440
Cephalic vein, 282
Cephalosporins, 157t
Cerebroplegia, 250
Certified registered nurse anesthetists (CRNAs), 32
Cervical plexus vein, 210f
Chargoff, Erwin, 6
Chart review, 153
Chemical injury, 177
Chest drainage system, 64f
Chest pain, 97b, 122
Chest radiography, 532
Chest tube insertion, 166-168
Choosing, 126, 134
Chordae tendineae, 192, 194f, 310f
Chordal dysfunction, 314
Chordal replacement, 330
Chordal transfer, 330
Chow, Rita, 15
Chronic aortic insufficiency, 349
Chronic congestive heart failure, 431
Chronotropy, 202
CI, 206t
Circulatory assist devices, 434t, 435-438. *See also* Mechanical/biologic circulatory assistance.
Circulatory system, 207-212
Circumflex artery, 194f
Circumflex branch of left coronary artery, 377f
Circumflex coronary artery, 197
Circus movement, 502, 517
Circus movement tachycardia, 496b
CK-MB, 113

CK-MB1, 113
CK-MB2, 113
Clamp, 71
Clamshell, 214t, 217f
Cleaning/checking instruments, 34
Clinical advances, 3t, 4t
Clinical collaboration, 25
Clinical Disorders of the Heart Beat (Lewis), 2
Clopidogrel, 114t
Closed mitral commissurotomy, 325, 326f
CO, 205-207
Coagulation profile, 113t
Coarctation of the aorta, 542-546
Code of ethics, 35
Codman internal mammary artery kit, 74f
Cold injuries, 178
Cold topical solutions, 58, 59f
Collaboration, 24-26
Collapse, 97b
Collins sternal retractor, 72f
Color flow echocardiography, 379
Colp, Ralph, 5
Commissure, 343
Commissuroplasty, 328
Commissurotomy, 13
Committees, 37
Common carotid artery, 188f, 190f
Common iliac artery, 208f
Common iliac vein, 210f
Communicating, 117, 132
Communication, 37
Competency statements
 abbreviations, 49
 assessment, 43-45
 evaluation, 48-49
 implementation, 45-48
 planning, 45
Competent nurse, 29-30
Completion of procedure, 168
Computed tomography (CT), 106
Computer terminals, 69
Concurrent evaluation, 175
Conduction delay and block, 501
Conduction system, 199-200
Conductivity, 496b
Conduits, 91-92
Congenital aneurysms, 398
Congenital heart disease, 527-546
 ASD, 536-541
 cardiac catheterization, 532
 chest radiography, 532
 coarctation of aorta, 542-546
 congenital malformations, 530-531
 diagnostic evaluation, 531-532
 ECG, 531-532
 echocardiography, 532
 intrauterine circulation, 529
 most frequent malformations, 527b
 PDA, 532-536
 postnatal circulatory changes, 530
 types of lesions/malformations, 528t, 530t

Congenital malformations, 344, 530-531
Constrictive pericarditis, 570
Continuous axial-flow systems, 452
Contractility, 206t, 207
Contrast echocardiography, 104
Conus arteriosus, 190f, 192, 194f
Cooley, Denton A., 1, 7, 8, 18, 396b
Cooley jaws, 71f
Cooley sternal retractors, 72f
Cooper, Joel D., 15, 464
Coronary anastomosis, 287-289
Coronary arteries, 196-199
Coronary arteriography, 110
Coronary artery bypass, 259t. *See also* Surgery for CAD.
Coronary artery bypass conduits, 280-286
Coronary artery bypass instrument extras, 79b
Coronary artery disease (CAD), 258-263. *See also* Surgery for CAD.
Coronary artery fistula, 528t
Coronary Artery Surgery (Ochsner), 18
Coronary balloon angioplasty procedure, 265f
Coronary blood flow, 198
Coronary endarterectomy, 295-296
Coronary sinus, 194f, 198f, 377f, 498f
Coronary sulcus, 190f, 191
Corridor procedure, 518
Cosgrove annuloplasty ring technique, 386-387
Cosgrove-Edwards annuloplasty ring, 384
Cosgrove ring, 328
Cough, 97b
Coumadin, 114t
Coumadin anticoagulation therapy, 318b
CPB. *See* Cardiopulmonary bypass.
Crafoord, Clarence, 11
Creatinine kinase (CK), 112-113
Crile, George, 6
Crista supraventricularis, 192, 193f
Crista terminalis, 191
CRNAs, 32
Crossing the Quality Chasm: a New Health System for the 21st Century, 37
CRT, 516
Crystalloid cardioplegia solution, 253
CT scan, 106
Cultural diversity, 23
Customized suture packs, 82f
Custom packs, 34
Cutler, Elliott, 12
Cutting instruments, 79b, 80b
CVP line, 154t
Cyanosis, 97b
Cyclosporine, 15, 480b, 481
Cystic medial necrosis, 399
Cytoskeleton, 203

D

Dack, Simon, 129
Davis, Ludmilla, 15
Davis, Nancy, 9, 19
DDAVP, 157t, 165
Deairing the heart, 235
Death, 465
DeBakey, Michael, 7, 14
DeBakey jaws, 71f
DeBakey multipurpose vascular clamp, 71f
DeBakey multipurpose vascular clamp tip, 71f
Decision-making exercises, 30, 49-50
Decision-making process, 36-37
Decoupling, 464
Deep femoral artery, 208f
Deep medial circumflex femoral artery, 208f
Defibrillation, 161-163
Defibrillator, 59-62
Defibrillator model, 34-35
Degenerative calcific stenosis of trileaflet aortic valve, 346f
Delayed sternal closure, 217-219
de Leval, Marc R., 22
Demikhov, Vladimir, 463
Denervated heart, 479
Depolarization, 496b
Descending branch artery, 208f
Desflurane, 156t
Desmopressin, 157t, 165
Desmopressin acetate, 169t
De Vega suture annuloplasty technique, 385, 386f
DeVries, William, 1
DeWall, Richard, 7
Diagnosis-related group codes, 53b
Diagnostic procedures
  aortic valve surgery, 350
  blunt thoracic injuries, 550-551
  cardiac catheterization, 107-112
  cardiac nuclear imaging, 104-106
  congenital heart disease, 531-532
  CT scan, 106
  dysrhythmias, 503-507
  ECG, 100
  mitral valve surgery, 315, 317f
  MRI, 107
  penetrating thoracic injuries, 552-554
  pulmonary valve disease, 392
  radiography, 101-102
  stress test, 100-101
  thoracic aortic disease, 401-403
  tricuspid valve surgery, 379-380
  tumors, 565-566
Diastasis, 205
Diazepam, 157t
Dietrich scissors, 74f
Digital artery, 208f
Digital conversion, 104
Digoxin, 157t
Dilated cardiomyopathy, 434
Diller, Doris, 13

Diprivan, 156t
Dipyridamole, 101, 114t, 169t
Direct myocardial revascularization, 13
Direct revascularization techniques, 14
Discard suction, 235
Discharge concerns requiring immediate attention, 182b
Disposable bulldog clamps, 83f
Dissecting aortic aneurysm, 397
Diversity issues, 23
Dobutamine, 101, 156t
Dobutrex, 156t
Dodge, Renee, 272b
Doggett, Willard M., 299b
Dominance, 197
Domino donor procedure, 477
Donor organs, 464-466
Dopamine, 156t
Doppler devices, 69
Doppler echocardiography, 379
Dor procedure, 272-273
Dorsal metatarsal artery, 208f
Dorsal sympathectomy, 13
Dorsal venous arch, 210f
Double valve replacement, 339f, 371
Draping, 158-159
DRGs, 53b
Dual-chamber cardiac pacemaker generator, 512f
Ductus arteriosus, 209
Durable powers of attorney, 151
Duran annuloplasty rings, 92f, 384
Duran annuloplasty ring technique, 386
Duran annuloplasty technique, 331f
Dynamic cardiomyoplasty, 457-459
Dyskinesis, 263b
Dyspnea, 97b
Dysrhythmias. *See* Cardiac dysrhythmias.

E

Early developments. *See* History of cardiac surgery.
Early extubation, 180, 274t
EBCT, 106
Ebstein's anomaly, 376, 379f
ECABG, 259t
ECG, 100, 154t
ECG waveform components, 100f
Echinacea, 116t
Echo Boomers, 24t
Echocardiography, 102-104, 379, 532
ECLS, 247-248
ECMO, 247
Ectopy, 496b
Edema, 97b, 123
Effective refractory period, 496b
Ehlers-Danlos syndrome, 401
Ejection fraction, 206t
Ejection phase, 205
Electrical injuries, 178
Electrical outlets, 34

Electrocardiogram (ECG), 100, 154t, 531
Electroencephalogram, 154t
Electrolyte levels, 112
Electron beam computed tomography (EBCT), 106
Electrophysiologic studies, 504-507
Electrophysiology studies, 112
Electrosurgical unit, 62-63
Elephant trunk technique, 419
Ellison, Dorothy, 17
Ellison, Marie, 17
Elongated arterial cannulas, 66f
Emergency extracorporeal support, 244-245
Emergency situations, 547-564
  blunt thoracic injuries, 550-551
  cardiac tamponade, 555-556
  diagnostic evaluation, 505-551, 552-554
  epidemiology, 547
  iatrogenic injuries, 554
  mechanism of injury, 548-549
  nursing considerations, 549, 557
  nursing intervention classifications, 558t
  open cardiac wounds, 554-555
  pacemaker wire removal, 563
  penetrating thoracic injuries, 552-556
  penetrating wounds to major vessels, 555
  postoperative complications, 561-563
  procedural considerations, 561
  prompt intervention, 547, 557
  pulmonary embolus, 559-561
  questions to ask, 550b
  sternal exploration (ICU), 562
  transected aorta, 551-552
  trauma, 547
Endarterectomy loops, 277f
Endocarditis, 376
Endocardium, 189
Endocrine system, 125-126
Endomyocardial biopsy, 111, 480, 481
Endoscopic coronary artery bypass graft (ECABG), 259t
Endothelin, 434
Endovascular cardiopulmonary bypass, 65f
Endovascular systems, 245-246
Endoventricular circular patch plasty, 272
Enflurane, 156t
Enhanced normal automaticity, 496b
Enlargement of small aortic root, 362-364
Entry into operating room, 151-153
Environmental service employees, 33
Eosinophils, 480t
Ephedra, 116t
Ephedrine, 156t
Epicardium, 189
Epinephrine, 156t, 165, 167t

epsilon-Aminocaproic acid, 169t
EP studies, 504-507
Eptifibatide, 114t
Error, 38
Error detection/prevention, 37-40
Espersen, Christine, 19
Ethical considerations, 35-36
Ethrane, 156t
Ethylene oxide, 177
Etiologic factors, 96b
Eustachian valve, 191, 498f
Evaluation, 173-186
    additional methods, 185
    AF, 181
    anxiety, 176
    bleeding, 180
    cardiac output, 179-180
    competence, 48-49
    early extubation, 180
    evidence-based practice, 174
    of fiscal/material resources, 184-185
    fluid/electrolyte status, 178
    human resource management, 183-
        184
    infection, 182
    injury, 177-178
    intraoperative period, 177-180
    knowledge, 176-177, 181-182
    neurologic outcomes, 181
    of nursing care, 183
    pain, 180
    patient care management, 175-183
    postoperative period, 180-183
    preoperative period, 176-177
    rehabilitation, 182-183
    skin integrity, 179
    STS database, 174-175
    tissue integrity, 179
Evidence-based clinical practice, 174
Exchanging, 120-126, 133-134
Excision technique, 403, 404f
Excitability, 496b
Excitation-contraction of cardiac cell,
    202-204
Exercise ECG, 100-101
Experts, 31-32
Explanted porcine mitral valve
    prosthesis, 314f
External carotid, 208f
External defibrillation pads, 523f
External features of heart, 190
External iliac artery, 208f, 270f
External iliac vein, 210f
External jugular vein, 210f
Extracorporeal circulation, 7
Extracorporeal life support (ECLS),
    247-248
Extracorporeal membrane
    oxygenation (ECMO), 247

F

Facial artery, 208f
Fallot, Etienne-Louis Arthur, 11
False aneurysms, 398, 399f
Families, 177

Family, 152
Fascicles, 200
Fast sodium channel, 204
Fast-track cardiac surgery, 169
Fatigue, 97b, 123
Favaloro, Rene G., 2, 14, 269b
Feeling, 118, 132
Femoral artery, 208f
Femoral vein, 210f
Femoral vein-femoral artery bypass,
    421-422
Fentanyl, 156t
Fetal circulation, 209-212
Fever and chills, 97b
Fibrillar collagen, 203f
Fibrillator, 62
Fibrin glue, 165, 167t, 168f
Fibrinolysis, 115f
First assistant, 32
Fish mouth mitral valve, 312f
Flail mitral valve, 313b
Flap closure of sternum, 223-226
Floppy mitral valve, 313b
Fluothane, 156t
Foramen ovale, 192, 209
Forane, 156t
Fordham, Mary E., 12
Forme fruste, 347
Fossa ovalis, 192f, 193f
Franck, Francois, 258
Frank-Starling mechanism, 433
Frazier, O. H., 444b
Furosemide, 157t
Fusiform aneurysms, 398, 399f

G

Garlic, 116t
Garrett, Edward, 14
Gastroepiploic artery (GEA), 270f,
    286
Gastrointestinal system, 125
Gated SPECT imaging, 105
GEA, 270f, 286
Geha, Alexander S., 51
Gelfilm, 167t
Gelfoam, 167t
Gender differences. *See* Women.
General appearance, 120
Generational differences, 23-24
Generation X, 24t
Generation Y, 24t
Generic care plans, 135-144
Gibbon, John H., Jr., 6, 7, 213
Ginkgo, 116t
Ginseng, 116t
Glover patent ductus clamp, 71f
Glover patent ductus clamp tip, 71f
Glycopyrrolate, 156t
Goal conflicts, 36
Goetz, Robert, 14
Gordon, Marjorie, 129
Gott shunt, 421f, 422
Graft valve conduits, 91-92
Grant, F. C., 161
Great cardiac vein, 198f, 377f

Greater saphenous vein, 210f, 270f,
    283
Green, George, 14
Gross, Robert E., 11, 12, 527
Guide to procedures. *See* Operative
    procedures.
Guthrie, Charles, 5

H

Halothane, 156t
Handbook of Cardiology for Nurses
    (Modell), 13
Hardy, James, 487
Harken, Dwight E., 1, 11, 13, 343
Harkin caged bill valve, 344f
Harmon, Elizabeth, 14
Harmonic imaging, 104
Hartin, Peggy, 15-16
Harvey, William, 1, 187
Hauser, Elizabeth, 187
HCM, 349, 434
Hct, 113t
Headlight, 57
Healthful foods, 33b
Heart failure
    acute/chronic, 431
    causes, 432b
    compensatory mechanisms, 432-433
    defined, 431
    initial medical management,
        433, 435
    sequence of events resulting in,
        431f
Heart-lung machine, 64
Heart-lung transplantation, 464, 483-
    487
HeartMate I system, 449
Heart rate, 206
HeartSaver VAD, 451-452
Heart sounds, 123, 136b
Heart transplantation, 467-483
    autotransplantation, 482-483
    CAD, 482
    contraindications, 467b
    denervation of heart, 479
    discharge planning, 482
    domino donor procedure, 477
    endomyocardial biopsy, 480, 481
    etiology, 467
    heterotopic transplantation, 477
    history, 463
    immunosuppression, 481-482
    infection, 482
    nursing care, 474b-476b
    operating room setup, 469f, 470f
    operative procedure, 473-477
    orthotopic transplantation, 471-477
    patient teaching, 468, 482
    postoperative care, 477-479
    procedural considerations, 468
    rejection, 479-481
    selection criteria, 467-468
Helistat, 167t
Hemaseel, 167t
Hematocrit (Hct), 113t

Hematologic tests, 112
Hemiarch replacement, 419
Hemoglobin (Hgb), 6, 113t
Hemoptysis, 97b
Hemopump, 438
Hemostasis, 115f, 165-166
Heparin, 6, 114t, 157t, 231-233
Heparin-coated CPB circuits, 237
Hepatic vein, 210f
Herbal medicines, 112, 116t
Heterotopic transplantation, 477
Hgb, 6, 113t
Hibernating myocardium, 204t
Higgins, Virginia, 15
High-risk industries, 39
High-sensitivity C-reactive protein
    (hs-CRP), 119
Himmelstein sternal retractor, 72f
His bundle, 499f
History of cardiac surgery, 1-21
    aortic valve surgery, 13
    atrial septal defects, 11-12
    blood transfusions, 6
    blood vessel surgery, 5
    cardiac resuscitation, 3-4
    cardiac valve prostheses, 10-11
    cardiopulmonary bypass, 6-7
    cardiovascular nursing literature,
        17-18
    chest radiographs, 2
    clinical advances, 3t, 4t
    coarctation of the aorta, 11
    congenital heart disease, 11-12
    coronary artery disease, 13-14
    cross-circulation, 7
    defibrillation, 4
    electrocardiography, 2
    extracorporal circulation, 7
    heparin/protamine, 6
    instruments, 7-9
    mitral valve surgery, 12-13
    operating room nursing, 16
    patent ductus arteriosus, 11
    perioperative cardiac nurse, 18-19
    prosthetic implants, 10
    selective coronary arteriography,
        2-3
    supplies/equipment, 9-10
    surgical procedures, 11-12
    suture, 9
    tetralogy of Fallot, 11
    textbooks, 16
    thoracic anesthesia, 5
    transplantation, 14-16
    valvular heart surgery, 12-16
Hoarseness, 97b
Holding instruments, 79b, 80b
Homocysteine, 119
Homografts, 91, 353
Homologous blood transfusion, 160
Hooker, Donald, 4
hs-CRP, 119
Hubbard, John P., 11, 527
Hufnagel, Charles, 13
Hufnagel valve, 344f

Human leukocyte antigen
    sensitization, 457
Human response patterns and
    associated diagnoses,
    132-135
Hymolysis, 455-456
Hyperacute rejection, 480
Hyperkalemia, 116
Hypertension, 123
Hypertrophic cardiomyopathy
    (HCM), 349, 433
Hypokalemia, 116
Hypokinesis, 263b
Hypothermia
    CPB, 230-231
    exchanging, 134
    inadvertent, 557, 559
    myocardial protection, 251-252
Hypothermia/hyperthermia units, 58

I

IABP, 68, 435-438
Iatrogenic injury, 554
Idiopathic hypertrophic subaortic
    stenosis (IHSS), 349
IHSS, 349
Illumination of surgical field, 34
Implantable axial flow systems, 452
Implantable cardioverter
    defibrillators (ICDs), 69, 522-
    523
Implantable VADs, 448-450
Implementation, 146-172
    admission to cardiac ICU, 171b
    admission to cardiac service, 146,
        149b
    advance directives, 151
    cancellation of surgery, 153
    chart review, 153
    chest tube insertion, 166-168
    competency, 145-148
    completion of procedure, 168
    defibrillation, 161-163
    draping, 158-159
    entry into operating room, 151-153
    family, 152
    fast-track cardiac surgery, 169
    hemostasis, 165-166
    infection control measures, 159-160
    intraoperative medications, 155-157
    monitoring, 153-154
    patient transfer report, 171b
    positioning, 155, 158
    postoperative management, 170-172
    preoperative patient teaching, 146-
        151
    room preparations, 151
    skin preparation, 158
    temporary epicardial pacing, 163-
        165
    transfusion therapy/blood conser-
        vation, 160-161
Impulse conduction, 501
Impulse formation, 501
Inadvertent hypothermia, 557-559

Incisions. *See* Thoracic incisions.
Inclusion technique, 403, 404f
Inclusion wrap technique, 413
Increased sympathetic activity, 433
Increasing angina, 261
Infant PDA, 532-536
Infection, 182
Infection control measures, 159-160
Infective endocarditis, 339
Inferior epigastric artery, 270f
Inferior mesenteric artery, 208f, 270f
Inferior mesenteric vein, 210f
Inferior vena cava, 190f, 191, 192f,
    193f, 194f, 210f
Informal meetings, 37
Infundibulum, 192, 193f
Injury, 177-178
Innervation of heart, 200-201
Innominate artery, 188f, 190f
Innominate vein, 190f
Inocor, 156t
Inotropy, 202
Instat, 167t
Instruments, cleaning/checking, 34
Insulin, 157t
Integrilin, 114t
Interleukin-2 receptor antagonists,
    482
Intermediate anginal syndrome, 261
Internal carotid, 208f
Internal defibrillator paddle tips, 61f
Internal iliac artery, 208f, 270f
Internal iliac vein, 210f
Internal jugular vein, 190f, 210f
Internal mammary arteries, 187, 190f
Internal paddles, 35
Interpersonal communication, 37
Interventricular septum, 193f
Interventricular sulcus, 191
Intraaortic balloon pump (IABP), 68,
    435-438
Intraarterial catheter, 154t
Intracardiac fetal circulation, 529f
Intracoronary stenting, 266
Intraluminal prostheses, 423
Intraluminal tube grafts, 85
Intraoperative aortic dissections, 401
Intraoperative electrophysiologic
    studies, 507
Intraoperative medications, 155-157
Intrapulmonary balloon pump
    (IPBP), 438
Intrauterine circulation, 529
Intravascular ultrasonography
    (IVUS), 104
INTrEPID, 449
Intropin, 156t
Ion, Edwinia James, 10, 18
IPBP, 438
Ischemia, 261-263
Ischemic myocardium, 204t
Isoflurane, 156t
Isoproterenol, 156t
Isoptin, 157t
Isovolumic contraction, 205

Isovolumic relaxation, 205
Isuprel, 156t
IVUS, 104

J

James, Edwinia E., 18
Jaw patterns, 71
Jehovah's Witnesses, 161
Johnson, Dudley, 14
Jude, James, 4
Judkins technique, 109f, 110f

K

Kadow, Susan J., 19
Kalke double-leaflet valve, 334f
Kay bicuspidization technique, 385
Keflex, 157t
Keflin, 157t
Keller, Manelva Wylie, 5, 13
Kent bundles, 517
Kernicki, Jeannette, 15, 95
Kidney function tests, 116
King, Ouida M., 15, 18
Kirklin, James, 7
Kirklin, John, 7
Knickerbocker, Guy, 4
Knotted grafts, 84-85
Knowing, 118-120, 132-133
Knowledge, 176-177, 181-182
Knowledge error, 38
Kolessov, Vasily, 14
Konno-Rastan procedure, 364, 366f,
      367f
Kouwenhoven, William, 4
Kussmaul's sign, 570

L

Laboratory tests, 112-117
LA catheter, 154t
LAD coronary artery, 197
Landsteiner, Karl, 6
Langworthy, O. R., 4
Lanoxin, 157t
LAO projection, 110
Lapse, 38
Lasers, 69
Lasix, 157t
LAST, 214t
LATCAB, 259t
Latent failures, 38
Late potentials, 503
Lateral anterior thoracotomy
      coronary artery bypass
      (LATCAB), 259t
Lateral border of ventricle, 190f
Lateral chest x-ray film, 102f
Lateral positioning, 155
Lateral thoracic artery, 208f
Lateral thoracotomy, 214t
Leaflet disorders, 314
Left anteriolateral thoracotomy, 559f
Left anterior descending (LAD)
      coronary artery, 197
Left anterior oblique (LAO)
      projection, 110

Left anterior small thoracotomy
      (LAST), 214t
Left atrial appendage, 193
Left atrial (LA) catheter, 154t
Left atrial-distal aorta bypass, 421, 422
Left atrium, 192-193
Left basilic vein, 210f, 270f
Left brachiocephalic vein, 210f
Left bundle branch, 498f
Left cephalic vein, 210f, 270f
Left common carotid artery, 208f
Left coronary artery, 208f, 377f
Left coronary cusp, 192f
Left coronary ostium, 192f
Left coronary vein, 210f
Left dominant, 197
Left fibrous trigone, 194, 311f, 377f,
      499f
Left free wall, 499f
Left full-lateral position, 155
Left internal jugular vein, 188f
Left internal mammary artery, 270f
Left phrenic nerve, 188f
Left pulmonary artery, 188f, 190f,
      194f, 310f
Left pulmonary veins, 188f, 192f
Left semilateral position, 155
Left-sided heart bypass, 239
Left-sided heart catheterization, 109,
      110f
Left subclavian artery, 208f
Left subclavian vein, 188f, 210f
Left vagus nerve, 188f
Left ventricle, 193-194
Left ventricular aneurysm repair, 296-
      298
Left ventricular apicoabdominal
      aortic conduit, 364, 368f
Left ventricular outflow tract
      (LVOT), 349
Left ventricular trabeculations, 310f
Left ventricular wall, 194f, 310f
Left ventriculography, 111
Lesser saphenous vein, 270f, 283
Levine, Samuel, 12
Levophed, 156t
Lewis, Sir Thomas, 2
Lidocaine, 157t
Lidocaine 1%, 157t
LIFEPAK 9 defibrillator, 61f
LIFEPAK 12, 60f
Ligamentum arteriosum, 212
Lighting, 34
Lillehei, C. Walton, 1, 7
Limbus, 192
Limbus marginalis, 193
Lindbergh, Charles, 7
Lister, Joseph, 16
Litwak, Robert S., 129
Liver function tests, 116
Living wills, 151
Lone atrial fibrillation, 518
Longmire, William, 14
Long thoracic vein, 210f
Lorazepam, 156t

Loupes, 57
Lower, Richard, 15, 463
Low-molecular-weight heparin, 114t
Lung transplantation, 487-492
   advantages of single-lung transplan-
      tation, 488b
   bilateral transplantation, 491-492
   history, 464, 487-488
   operative procedure, 488-491
   postoperative period, 492
   procedural considerations, 488
LVOT obstruction, 349

M

Mack, Michael, 51
Macrophages, 480t
Made-to-order suture packs, 78, 82f
Magnetic resonance imaging (MRI),
      107
Main pulmonary artery, 193f
Major dysrhythmias, 501
Mandol, 157t
Mannitol, 157t
Manouguian procedure, 364, 365f
Manubrium, 187, 188f
Marfan's syndrome, 399-400
Mass spectrometry, 154t
Matas, Rudolph, 395
Matthews, Joan, 15, 95
Mattox, Kenneth L., 547, 559b
Mayo tray, 78
Maze procedure, 518f
Maze II procedure, 519
Maze III procedure, 519-521
McLean, Jay, 6
MCS devices. *See* Mechanical/biologic
      circulatory assistance.
Mechanical/biologic circulatory
      assistance, 430-462
   bleeding, 454
   cardiomyoplasty, 457-459
   circulatory assist devices, 434t, 435-
      438
   complications, 454-457
   device-related complications, 457
   future challenges, 459-460
   hemolysis, 455-456
   hemopump, 438
   human leukocyte antigen sensitiza-
      tion, 457
   IABP, 435-438
   infection, 455
   IPBP, 438
   patient considerations, 453-454
   pericardial devices, 459
   right ventricular failure, 456-457
   skeletal muscle-powered assist
      devices, 459
   special considerations, 456b
   thromboembolism, 454-455
   training, 452-453
   VADs, 438-452. *See also* Ventricular
      assist devices (VADs).
Mechanical prostheses, 86
Mechanical valve prostheses, 335t

Medawar, Peter, 463
Medial degeneration, 399
Medial papillary muscle, 193f, 196
Median basilic vein, 210f
Median sternotomy, 213-226
Medtronic BioMedicus pump, 439, 440f
Medtronic Freestyle aortic root bioprosthesis, 87f
Medtronic Hall tilting disk valve prosthesis, 88f
Medtronic Mosaic aortic porcine bioprosthesis, 87f
Medtronic Mosaic porcine mitral bioprosthesis, 87f
Membrane method, 66
Membrane oxygenators, 66, 67f, 231t, 233
Membranous septum, 192f, 193, 377f, 499f
Mended Hearts, Inc., 119, 176, 185, 565
Merz, William, 8, 71
Methohexital, 156t
Microbubbles, 104
Midazolam, 156t
MIDCAB, 259t, 267
Middle scallop, 311f
Millenialists, 24t
Mills, Noel, 18
Milrinone, 156t
Minimal access surgery, 75-78, 213
Minimally invasive direct coronary artery bypass (MIDCAB), 259t, 267
Minimally invasive Maze III procedure, 520-521
Minimally invasive saphenous vein harvesting, 283
Minimally invasive surgery, 213
Mini-sternotomy, 214t, 215
Minor dysrhythmias, 501
Mirowski, Michel, 5
Mistake, 38
Misuse, 174
Mitochondria, 203
Mitral annuloplasty, 327-328
Mitral apparatus, 196
Mitral commissurotomy, 325-327
Mitral complex, 196
Mitral valve, 192f, 194-196, 377f
Mitral valve annulus, 310f
Mitral valve apparatus, 309, 310f, 311f
Mitral valve exposure, 323f
Mitral valve prolapse, 313-314
Mitral valve repair, 317-331
Mitral valve replacement, 331-339
Mitral valve surgery, 309-342
  abnormalities of mitral apparatus, 312t
  annular dilation, 314
  bacterial endocarditis, 312
  CAD, 339
  chordal dysfunction, 314
  completion of procedure, 339-340

Mitral valve surgery—cont'd
  diagnostic evaluation, 315, 317f
  documentation, 319b
  equipment, 319b
  infective endocarditis, 339
  leaflet disorders, 314
  medical history, 316
  mitral annuloplasty, 327-328
  mitral commissurotomy, 325-327
  mitral regurgitation, 313-315
  mitral stenosis, 311-313
  mitral valve apparatus, 309, 310f, 311f
  mitral valve disease, 310-315
  mitral valve prolapse, 313-314
  mitral valvuloplasty, 329-331
  multiple valve surgery, 339
  nursing care, 320t, 321t
  papillary muscle dysfunction, 314
  patient-related factors, 333b
  patient teaching, 318, 331-332
  postoperative complications, 340-341
  procedural considerations, 318-322, 333-335
  reoperation, 339
  reparative procedures, 317-331
  replacement, 331-339
  RFNA considerations, 317b
  rheumatic fever, 311
  safety measures, 319b
  signs/symptoms of disease, 316t
  skin preparation, 319b
  special considerations, 319b
  valve prostheses, 334-336
  valve-related risks, 333b
  warfarin (commadin) anticoagulation therapy, 318b
Mitral valvuloplasty, 329-331
MMF, 481-482
M-mode echocardiography, 103
Modell, Walter, 13
Moderator band, 192, 193f, 498f
Modified anterolateral position, 155
Modified Bentall-DeBono procedure, 410-414
Modified human hemoglobin, 169t
Monitoring devices, 69
Monoclonal, 15
Monocytes, 480t
Monofilament sutures, 78
Montgomery, Jill Gorman, 12
Morfan's syndrome, 347
Morphine, 156t
Morrow procedure, 368-371
Moving, 120, 133
MRI, 107
MUGA studies, 104
Multifilament polyester sutures, 78
Multiple-uptake gated acquisition (MUGA) studies, 104
Multiple valve surgery, 339
Mural leaflet, 196
Murmurs, 123, 136b
Muscular septum, 193
Muscular ventricular septum, 192f

MVo2, 207
Mycophenolate mofetil (MMF), 481-482
Mycotic aneurysms, 400
Myocardial ischemia, 261-263
Myocardial oxygen consumption (MVo2), 207
Myocardial oxygen deprivation, 260b
Myocardial perfusion imaging, 105
Myocardial protection, 250-256
  antegrade/retrograde blood cardioplegia infusion, 253-256
  beating heart surgery, 256
  cardioplegia, 252-253
  hypothermia, 251-252
  warm heart surgery, 251-252
Myocardial revascularization. *See* Surgery for CAD.
Myocardium, 189

N

National databases (morbidity/mortality), 51
National Patient Safety Foundation, 37
NBHDs, 465
Nebcin, 157t
Necrosis, 204t, 261
Needle holders, 73, 74f
Negative self-talk, 33b
Neo-Synephrine, 156t
Neurologic outcomes, 181
Neurologic status, 125
Neutrophils, 480t
New-onset AF, 518
NH region, 498
Nicks procedure, 362-364
Nifedipine, 157t
Nipride, 1565
Nitric oxide (NO), 157t
Nitroglycerin, 156t
Nitroprusside, 156t
NO, 157t
Nocturia, 97b
Nodal (N) region, 498
Nodal-His (NH) region, 498
Noise levels, 34
Non-beating heart donors (NBHDs), 465
Noncoronary cusp, 343
Nonthoracotomy ICD lead configurations, 524f
Norcuron, 156t
Norepinephrine, 156t
Northern New England Cardiovascular Disease Study Group, 174
Novacor left ventricular assist device, 449f
Novice circulating nurses, 28
Novice nurses, 27
N region, 498
Nuclear cardiology, 104-106
Nursing care
  aortic valve surgery, 355t, 356t
  CABG, 279t, 280t

Nursing care—cont'd
  cardiac dysrhythmias, 510t, 511t
  heart/lung transplantation, 474b-
    476b
  mitral valve surgery, 320t, 321t
  thoracic aortic disease, 405t
  tricuspid valve procedures, 381t
  VADs, 443b, 444b
"Nursing Care of the Open Heart Patient"
    (James/Ion), 18
Nursing Care of the Surgical Patient
    (Harmon), 14
Nursing diagnoses, 129, 130b
Nursing of the Open-Heart Surgery
    Patient (Aspinall), 18
Nursing roles, 26-32
Nutritional status, 125
NYHA classification system, 96b

O

Objective evaluations of outcomes,
    175
Occipital artery, 208f
Octopus, 290
Octopus 3 coronary stabilizer, 75f
O'Kane, Hugh, 51
OKT3, 482
Old/young, physiologic features, 121t
Olson, Kenneth, 6
Omental flap, 223, 225f
Omnibus Reconciliation Act of 1986,
    151
Open cardiac wounds, 554-555
Open mitral commissurotomy, 325,
    327f
Operating room, 34, 54f. *See also*
    Structural standards.
Operating Room Technique
    (Alexander), 17
Operative procedures
  allograft replacement of aortic
    valve, 364-368
  allograft replacement of tricuspid
    valve, 389-390
  antigrade/retrograde blood cardio-
    plegia infusion, 253-256
  aortic arch replacement, 417-419
  aortic valve replacement, 359-362
  ascending thoracic aortic aneurysm,
    409-414
  ASD, 539-541
  atrial myxoma, 567-568
  Bentall-DeBono procedure, 409-410
  bicaval cannulation of right atrium,
    242-243
  CABG, 280-292
  cannulation of aorta, 240-241
  cannulation of femoral artery, 241
  cannulation of right atrium, 242
  cannulation for venous return, 242-
    243
  coarctation of aorta, 544
  coronary endarterectomy, 295-296
  deep hypothermia with circulatory
    arrest, 250

Operative procedures—cont'd
  descending thoracic aortic
    aneurysm, 422-423
  emergency extracorporeal support,
    244-245
  enlargement of small aortic root,
    362-364
  flap closure of sternum, 223-226
  heart-lung transplantation, 484-487
  heart transplantation, 473-477
  IABP insertion, 436
  ICD, insertion of, 523
  implantable VADs, 449-450
  infant PDA, 534-536
  Konno-Rastan procedure, 364, 366f,
    367f
  left ventricular aneurysm patch
    repair, 297
  left ventricular apicoabdominal aor-
    tic conduit, 364, 368f
  lung transplantation, 488-491
  Manouguian procedure, 364, 365f
  Maze III procedure, 519-521
  mitral annuloplasty, 327-328
  mitral commissurotomy, 326-327
  mitral valve repair, 322-324
  mitral valve replacement, 336-339
  mitral valvuloplasty, 329-331
  modified Bentall-DeBono tech-
    nique, 410-414
  Morrow procedure, 368-371
  myomyectomy for hypertrophic
    subaortic stenosis, 368-371
  Nicks procedure, 362-364
  open heart wounds, 554
  pacemakers, 513-576
  patch enlargement of proximal
    ascending aorta, 362, 363f
  pericardial window, 569-570
  pericardiectomy, 571
  pulmonary embolectomy, 561
  pulmonary valve surgery, 393
  removal of aortic cannula, 244
  repeat sternotomy, 219-220
  sternal closure, 217
  sternal exploration (ICU), 562
  sternotomy, 215-217
  thoracoabdominal aortic aneurysm,
    424-425
  transected aorta, 552
  tricuspid valve commissurotomy, 387
  tricuspid valve repair, 384-387
  tricuspid valve replacement, 388
  tricuspid valvulectomy, 390
  VSD repair, 300-303
Organizational learning factors, 23
Organ recovery, 465-466
Orifice of coronary sinus, 192f
Orringer, Mark B., 173
Orthotopic heart transplantation,
    471-477
Oscillating saw, 57f, 58
O'Shaughnessy, Laurence, 13
Ostium primum atrial septal defect,
    528t, 537f

Ostium secundum, 192
Ostium secundum atrial septal defect,
    528t, 537f
Otto, Catherine M., 343
Outcome standards, 131b
Overuse, 174
Oxycel, 167t

P

PACAB, 259t, 292
PA catheter, 154t
Pacemakers, 68, 508-517
Pacemaker wire removal, 563
Paget, Sir Stephen, 1
Palmar arch (deep) artery, 208f
Palmar arch (superficial) artery, 208f
Palpitations, 122-123
Pancuronium, 156t
Panel of reactive antibodies (PRA)
    test, 457
Papaverine, 157t
Papillary muscle of conus, 498f
Papillary muscle dysfunction, 314
Papillary muscle repair, 331
Parasternotomy, 214t
Parasympathetic nervous system,
    202
Parietal band, 192, 193f
Parietal pericardium, 187
Partial CPB, 233
Partial-occluding clamps, 79b
Partial thromboplastin time (PTT),
    113t
Partnerships, 25
Pasteur, Louis, 16, 547
Patch enlargement of proximal
    ascending aorta, 362, 363f
Patent ductus arteriosus (PDA), 532-
    536
Patient interview, 117-127
  cardiovascular status, 122-124
  choosing, 126
  communicating, 117
  ears/eyes/nose/throat, 125
  endocrine system, 125-126
  exchanging, 120-126
  feeling, 118
  gastrointestinal system, 125
  general appearance, 120
  knowing, 118-120
  moving, 120
  neurologic status, 125
  nutritional status, 125
  perceiving, 117-118
  peripheral vascular status, 124-125
  relating, 126
  respiratory status, 122
  skin integrity, 121-122
  urinary/renal status, 125
  valuing, 126
Patient outcome standards, 131b
Patient-provider partnerships, 26
Patient safety, 37-40
Patient satisfaction questionnaires, 185
Patient Self-Determination Act, 151

Patient teaching
  aortic valve surgery, 354
  CABG, 273-274
  heart transplantation, 464, 482
  mitral valve repair, 318
  mitral valve replacement, 331-333
  pacemakers, 512-513
  preoperative, 146-151
  thoracic aortic disease, 404
  tricuspid valve surgery, 381-382
Patient transfer report, 171b
Pavulon, 156t
PBAV, 351
PCI, 264-267
PCTA, 264-266
Pectinate muscles, 191
Pectoralis muscle flap, 223, 224
Pediatric cardiac self-retaining
    retractor, 73f
Pediatric instrumentation, 80b
Penetrating bundle, 498f
Penetrating thoracic injuries, 552-556
Penetrating wounds to major vessels,
    555
Penfield dissector, 277f
Perceiving, 117-118, 132
Percutaneous balloon aortic
    valvuloplasty (PBAV), 351
Percutaneous coronary intervention
    (PCI), 264-267
Percutaneous CPB, 68, 244-246
Percutaneous transluminal coronary
    angioplasty (PCTA), 264-266
Perfluorochemicals, 169t
Perforated aortic valve leaflets, 346f
Perfusionists, 32
Pericak-Vance, Margaret, 187
Pericardial devices, 459
Pericardial disease, 568-572
Pericardial effusion, 568
Pericardial sarcoma, 567b
Pericardial tamponade, 556f
Pericardial window, 568-570
Pericardiectomy, 571
Pericardiocentesis, 568, 569f
Pericardium, 187-189
Perioperative Nursing Data Set, 95,
    129-132
Peripheral vascular status, 124-125
Permanent pacing, 68, 509
Peroneal artery, 208f
Peroneal vein, 210f
PES, 505
PET, 105
Pfister, Albert J., 258
Phagocytes, 480t
Pharmacologic blood conservation
    agents, 169
Phases of cardiac rehabilitation, 182-
    183
Phentolamine, 156t
Phenylpinephrine, 156t
Phrenic nerves, 189, 190f
Physical hazards, 178
Physician anesthesiologists, 32

Physiologic factors, 96b
Physiologic features (very
    young/old), 121t
Physiology. See Anatomy and
    physiology.
Picket fence, 57f
Piggyback transplantation, 477
Pilling, William, 8
Pilling-Wolvek sternal approximator
    and fixation system, 218f
Pipecuronium, 156t
Planning, 45, 135-144
Plavix, 114t
Pledgeted suture, 82f, 166f
Pledgets, 78
Poirier, Victor, 430
Policies and procedures, 52b
Polypropylene, 78
Polytetrafluoroethylene (PTFE), 85
Popliteal artery, 208f
Popliteal vein, 210f
Port-access CAB, 259t, 292
Port-access coronary artery bypass
    (PACAB), 259t, 292
Port-access robotic dissecting
    instrument tips, 277f
Portal vein, 210f
Positioning, 155, 158
Positron emission tomography (PET),
    105
Posterior commissural leaflet, 311f
Posterior descending coronary artery,
    197
Posterior leaflet, 192f, 196
Posterior papillary muscle, 192f, 193f,
    194f
Posterior scallop, 311f
Posterior septal, 499f
Posterior tibial artery, 208f
Posterior tibial vein, 210f
Posterolateral leaflet, 196
Posterolateral thoracotomy, 214t,
    228f, 229f
Posteromedial papillary muscle, 310f
Postinfarction VSD repair, 298-303
Postoperative false aneurysms, 401
Postoperative management, 170-172
Postperfusion syndrome, 238
Potassium, 157t
Potts, Willis, 8
Potts-Smith scissors, 74f
Potts-type scissors, 73, 74f
Powerlessness, 132
Powers, Maryann, 14, 173
PRA test, 457
Preceptor, 27, 29
Predeposit donation, 161
Preexcitation, 496b
Preinfarction angina, 261
Preload, 206-207
Premature atrial depolarization, 502f
Premature ventricular depolarization,
    502f
Preoperative assessment, 95-128
  background information, 95-98

Preoperative assessment—cont'd
  cardiac catheterization, 107-112
  cardiac nuclear imaging, 104-106
  competency, 43-45
  CT scan, 106
  diagnostic procedures, 98-112
  ECG, 100
  echocardiography, 102-104
  electrophysiology studies, 112
  laboratory tests, 112-117
  MRI, 107
  patient interview, 117-127. See also
    Patient interview.
  radiography, 101-102
  resources, 95
  stress test, 100-101
Preoperative patient interview. See
    Patient interview.
Preoperative patient teaching, 146-
    151
Pretest/posttest, 27, 41-42
Primary tumors, 565
Priming solution, 237
Procainamide, 157t
Procardia, 157t
Procedural guide. See Operative
    procedures.
Procedures outside operating room,
    56b
Professional cardiac surgical
    organizations, 25
Proficiency, 27-32
Proficient nurses, 30-31
Programmed electrical stimulation
    (PES), 505
Prolapse of the mitral valve, 313b
Pronestyl, 157t
Propofol, 156t
Prostaglandin E 1, 156t
Prosthetic heart valves, 86-91
Prosthetic implants, 81-93
  annuloplasty rings, 92-93
  aortic graft valve prostheses, 91-92
  aortic/pulmonary allografts, 91
  biologic grafts, 85
  prosthetic heart valves, 85-91
  synthetic grafts, 83-85
Prostin VR, 156t
Protamine, 6
Protamine sulfate, 157t, 233
Prothrombin time (PT), 113t, 115f
Pseudoaneurysms, 401
Pseudomonas aeruginosa, 390
Psychologic reactions, 119
Psychomotor skills, 27
Psychosocial skills, 27
PT, 113t, 115f
PTFE, 85
PTT, 113t
Pulmonary allografts, 91, 354
Pulmonary artery, 190f, 192, 208f
Pulmonary artery (PA) catheter, 154t
Pulmonary autografts, 354
Pulmonary circulation, 209
Pulmonary embolectomy, 561

Pulmonary embolus, 559-561
Pulmonary valve, 192, 193f, 196
Pulmonary valve disease, 391-392
Pulmonary valve procedures, 391-393
Pulmonary valve stenosis, 528t
Pulmonary veins, 192, 210f
Pulmonic valve, 377f
Pulsatile VADs, 441-448
Pulsating hematomas, 398
Pulse oximeter, 154t
Pulse oximetry finger cot., 26f
Pulses, 123
Pump, 64
Pump oxygenator, 64-68
Purkinje fibers, 200
Purkinje system, 500

Q

Qp/Qs, 537
Quantitative coronary analysis, 261f
Quinidine, 157t

R

Raber, Theo, 4, 28
Radial artery, 208f, 270f
Radiant heaters, 58
Radiography, 101-102
Radiopaque coronary graft markers, 83f
RAO projection, 110
Rapid filling phase, 205
RCP, 416
Recombinant human erythropoietin, 169t
Recommended Practices for Safety through Identification of Potential Hazards in the Perioperative Environment, 52
Rectus abdominus flap, 223, 225f
Recurrent paroxysmal AF, 518
Reentry, 496b
Reentry mechanism, 501
Refractory period, 496b
Refrigerators, 69
Regitine, 156t
Rehabilitation, 182-183
Rehn, Ludwig, 1
Reitz, Bruce, 15
Relating, 126, 134
Relative refractory period, 496b
Remifentanil, 156t
Remodeling, 432
Removal of aortic cannula, 244
Removal of femoral artery cannula, 244
Renal artery, 208f
Renal function tests, 116
Renal/urinary status, 125
Renin-angiotensin-aldosterone system, 433-434
ReoPro, 114t
Repeat sternotomy, 219-220
Reperfusion injury, 250, 251b
Reperfusion management, 253
Repolarization, 496b

Respiratory status, 122
Rest angina, 261
Resting membrane potential, 496b
Restrictive cardiomyopathy, 434
Reteplase (r-PA), 114t
Retractors, 72-73, 79b, 80b
Retrograde cardioplegia infusion catheter, 67f
Retrograde cerebral perfusion (RCP), 416
Retrograde infusion, 253-255
Retrospective reviews, 175
Rheumatic fever, 311, 345
Rheumatic trileaflet, 345f
Rhythm disturbances. *See* Cardiac dysrhythmias.
Rhythmicity, 199, 496b
Right anterior mini-thoracotomy, 214t
Right anterior oblique (RAO) projection, 110
Right anterior papillary muscle, 192f
Right atrial appendage, 192
Right atrium, 191-192
Right basilic vein, 270f
Right brachiocephalic vein, 210f
Right bundle branch, 498f
Right cephalic vein, 270f
Right common carotid artery, 208f
Right coronary artery, 208f, 377f
Right coronary cusp, 192f
Right coronary ostium, 192f
Right coronary vein, 210f
Right dominant, 197
Right fibrous trigone, 194, 311f, 499f
Right free wall, 499f
Right internal mammary artery, 270f
Right posterior papillary muscle, 192f
Right pulmonary artery, 194f, 310f
Right-sided heart bypass, 239
Right-sided heart catheterization, 109
Right subclavian vein, 210f
Right ventricle, 190f, 192
Ring annuloplasty, 328, 330f
Rinsing procedure (bioprosthesis), 90f
Risk factors, 119, 263t
RNFA, 19
RNFA novice, 27
RN First Assistant (RNFA), 19
Robinul, 156t
Robotic CAB, 259t
Robotic grasping forcep, 278f
Robotic surgery, CABG, 292-295
Robots, 69-70
Rocuronium, 156t
Roentgen, Wilhelm, 2
Role conflicts, 36
Roller pumps, 231t, 233, 441
Room preparation, 34, 151
Room temperature, 34
Ross, Donald, 11, 358b
Ross procedure, 368
Rothrock, Jane C., 19, 22
r-PA, 114t
Rule-based error, 38

S

S₁, 123, 136b
S₂, 123, 136b
S₃, 123, 136b
S₄, 123, 136b
Saccular aneurysms, 398, 399f
Safe Medical Devices Act, 53
Safety, 38
Saline ice units, 58
SAM, 349
Samways, D. W., 309
SA node, 199-200
Sarcolemma, 202, 203f
Sarcomeres, 203
Sarcoplasmic reticulum, 203
Sauerbruch, Ferdinand, 5
Saying "I'm sorry", 40
SCD, 521, 522
Schwendeman, Mary, 17
Scopolamine, 156t
Scrub nurse, 29
Seifert, Patricia, 19
Senile calcific aortic stenosis, 345
Septal band, 192, 193f
Septal leaflet, 196
Septal tricuspid leaflet, 498f
Sevoflurane, 156t
"Shared Statement of Ethical Principles for Everyone in Health Care", 36
Short saphenous vein, 283
Shumacker, Harris B., 1
Shumway, Norman, 15, 463
Side pockets, 159
Signal-averaged ECG, 503-504
Silastic vessel loop, 76f
Silent ischemia, 261
Silicone vessel loops, 75, 76f
Simulations, 30, 49-50
Single photon emission computed tomography (SPECT), 105
Sinoatrial (SA) node, 199-200, 497, 498f
Sinous venosus ASD, 528t, 537f
Sinus of Valsalva aneurysm, 528t
Sinuses of Valsalva, 196
Sizing obturators, 92f
Skeletal muscle-powered assist devices, 459
Skeletal muscle ventricles (SMV), 459
Skill-based error, 38
Skin integrity, 121-122
Skin preparation, 158
Sliding technique (SAM), 328
Slip, 38
Slow sodium channel, 204
SMV, 459
Society of Thoracic Surgeons (STS), 25
Sodium bicarbonate, 157t
Sones, F. Mason, 3
Sones technique, 109f, 110f
Spinal cord injury, 420-422
Splenic artery, 208f, 270f
Splenic vein, 210f
Stabilizers, 75

Stable angina, 261
Staff dynamics, 36-37
Staffing issues, 23-24
Staffing shortages, 23
Stafford, Edward S., 13
Stages of proficiency, 27-32
Standard aortic cannulas, 66f
Standards of nursing care. *See*
    Nursing care.
Staphylococcus aureus, 345, 390
Starfish left ventricular suction
    device, 75f
Starr, Albert, 8, 9, 11, 18
Starr-Edwards ball-and-cage valve,
    334f
Starr-Edwards ball-and-cage valve
    prosthesis, 87f
Stenotic unicuspid aortic valve, 345f
Stentless aortic porcine bioprosthesis,
    352f
Step-by-step procedure. *See* Operative
    procedures.
Step-up, 537
Sternal body, 187
Sternal exploration (ICU), 562
Sternal incision, 215-219
Sternal infection, 220-222
Sternal retractors, 73
Sternal saw, 57-58
Sternotomy, 213-226, 408
Steroids, 480b
St. John's wort, 116t
St. Jude Medical bileaflet tilting disk
    valve prosthesis, 89f
Stone, John, 495
Stone heart, 250
Storage space, 34
Storlie, Frances, 14, 173
Straight sinus vein, 210f
Streptokinase, 114t
Stress, 33-37
    communication, 37
    decision-making process, 36-37
    equipment/material resources,
        34-35
    ethical considerations, 35-36
    goal conflicts, 36
    patient factors, 35
    role conflicts, 36
    staff dynamics, 36-37
    work environment, 34
Stress echocardiography, 104
Stress test, 100-101
Stroke volume, 206t
Structural standards, 51-94
    autotransfusion system, 63-64
    beating heart surgery, 73-75, 77b
    cardiac suite, 53-55
    circulatory assist devices, 68
    defibrillator, 59-62
    electrosurgical unit, 62-63
    fibrillator, 62
    financial considerations, 52
    furniture, 56
    guidelines, 51

Structural standards—cont'd
    headlight, 57
    hypothermia/hyperthermia
        units, 58
    implantable cardioverter defibrilla-
        tors, 69
    loupes, 57
    minimal access surgery, 75-78
    pacemakers, 68
    positioning equipment, 56-57
    prosthetic implants, 83-93. *See also*
        Prosthetic implants.
    pump oxygenator, 64-68
    radiant heaters, 58
    recommended resources, 54b, 55b
    regulatory considerations, 53
    robots, 69-70
    saline ice units, 58
    sternal saw, 57-58
    supplies, 81
    suture, 78, 81
    ultrasonic scalpel, 63
Strurli, Adriano, 6
STS, 25
STS database, 51, 173-175
Stunned myocardium, 204t
Subclavian artery, 190f
Subclavian vein, 190f
Subjective evaluations, 175
Sublimaze, 156t
Subxiphoid incision, 214t
Suction devices, 233-235
Sudden cardiac death (SCD), 521, 522
Sufenta, 156t
Sufentanil, 156t
Sulcus terminalis, 191
Superior epigastric artery, 270f
Superior mesenteric artery, 208f,
    210f, 270f
Superior sagittal sinus vein, 210f
Superior vena cava, 190f, 193f, 198f,
    210f
Supine position, 155
Supplies, 81
Supply coordinators, 33
Supportive staff, 33
Suprane, 156t
Suprasternal notch, 187, 188f
Supraventricular dysrhythmias, 508-521
Supraventricular tachycardia, 503f
Surgeon, 32
Surgery for CAD, 258-308
    Batista procedure, 272
    beating heart procedures, 289-291
    clinical outcomes, 304
    completion of procedures, 303
    conduits, 269-271, 280-286, 306
    coronary endarterectomy, 295-296
    Dor procedure, 272-273
    early extubation, 274t
    end-stage heart disease, 272
    hybrid procedures, 267
    intracoronary stenting, 266
    left ventricular aneurysm repair,
        296-298

Surgery for CAD—cont'd
    management strategies (reduction
        of morbidity/mortality), 271t
    MIDCAB, 267
    mitral valve surgery, 339
    new techniques, 267
    nursing care, 279t, 280t
    operative procedure, 280-292
    patient teaching, 273-274
    PCI, 246-247
    port access, 292
    postoperative complications, 304,
        305t
    preoperative evaluation, 275
    procedural considerations, 275
    PTCA, 264-266
    quality of life, 304
    reoperation, 304, 306
    RNFA considerations, 282b
    robotic surgery, 292-295
    sequelae of coronary artery disease,
        271
    thrombolytic/antiplatelet therapy,
        263-264
    TMR/TMLR, 272
    types of bypass procedures, 259t
    VSD repair, 298-303
    women, 273
"Surgery of the Heart and Great
    Vessels" (Brandt), 9
Surgery-related errors, 38
Surgical procedures. *See* Operative
    procedures.
Surgical suites. *See* Structural
    standards.
Surgical technologists, 33
Surgical valvuloplasty, 351
Surgicel, 167t
Suture, 78, 81
Sutureless anastomoses, 291
Suture method, 5
Suturing instruments, 79b, 80b
Symbion Jarvik-7 total artificial heart,
    430f
Sympathectomy, 13
Sympathetic nervous system, 202
Syncope, 97b
Syndrome X, 118
Synergy, 263b
Synthetic grafts, 83-85
Syphilis, 400
Syphillitic aortitis, 347
Systemic blood pressures, 123
Systemic circulation, 207-209
Systolic anterior motion (SAM), 349

T

Tachydysrhythmias, 517-524
Tacrolimus, 481, 482
Takayasu's disease, 401
Taussig, Helen, 11
Teaching. *See* Patient teaching.
Team roles, 32-33
TECAB, 259t
Technetium angiography, 104

Technetium imaging, 104
TEE, 103
Telephone follow-up, 143
Temporary epicardial pacing, 163-165
Temporary pacing, 68, 509
Tendon of Todaro, 498f
TET, 451
Tetralogy of Fallot (TOF), 528t
Texas Heart Institute (THI), 19
Textbook of Surgery for Nurses, A
     (Diller), 13
Textbook of Surgical Nursing
     (Colp/Keller), 5
Thabesian valve, 191
Thallium imaging, 104
Thebesian valve, 192f
THI, 19
Thiopental, 156t
Thomas, Vivian, 11
Thoracic aortic disease, 395-429
   anatomy, 396
   aneurysm, 396-401
   annuloaortic ectasia, 400
   aortic arch surgery, 414-419
   aortic dissection, 396-397
   atherosclerosis, 400
   Bentall-DeBono procedure, 409-410
   classification of aneurysms/dissec-
       tions, 397-401
   completion of procedure, 425
   CPB, 408
   diagnostic tests, 401-403
   documentation, 407t
   excision technique, 403, 404f
   inclusion technique, 403, 404f
   initial therapy, 404
   Marfan's syndrome, 399-400
   medial degeneration, 399
   modified Bentall-DeBono proce-
       dure, 410-414
   nursing care, 405t
   patient teaching, 404
   postoperative complications, 426t,
       427t
   prosthesis, 423
   repair of ascending aortic
       aneurysm, 407-414
   repair of descending thoracic aorta,
       419-423
   RNFA considerations, 408b
   safety measures, 407t
   signs/symptoms, 401, 402t
   special considerations, 406t, 407t
   spinal cord injury, 420-422
   sternotomy, 408
   supplies, 406t
   thoracoabdominal aneurysm, 423-425
   trauma, 400
Thoracic diaphragm, 188f
Thoracic incisions, 213-230
   decision tree, 221f
   delayed sternal closure, 217-219
   median sternotomy, 213-226
   repeat sternotomy, 219-220
   RNFA considerations, 216b

Thoracic incisions—cont'd
   sternal infection, 220-222
   tissue flap wound closure, 222-226
   types of incisions, 214, 226, 230
   weak sternums, 217
Thoracoabdominal aneurysm, 423-
       425
Thoracoabdominal incision, 214t
Thoracotomy ICD insertion, 522f
Thoracotomy instrument extras, 80b
Thoratec VAD, 444-445
Three-dimensional echocardiography,
       104
Threshold potential, 496b
Thrombin, 167t
Thrombin time, 113f, 115f
Thromboembolism (TE), 331, 454-455
Thrombogen, 167t
Thrombostat, 167t
Ticlid, 114t
Ticlopidine, 114t
Tissue flap wound closure, 222-226
Tissue-type plasminogen activator (t-
       PA), 114t
TMLR, 272
TMR, 69, 272
TnI, 116
TnT, 116
Tobramycin, 157t
To Err is Human: Building a Safer
     Health System, 37, 135
TOF, 528t
Topical hemostatic agents, 157t
Total artificial heart, 451
Total CPB, 233
Totally endoscopic coronary artery
       bypass (TECAB), 259t
Total-occluding clamps, 79b
t-PA, 114t
Trabeculae carneae, 192, 193f, 194f
Tranexamic acid, 169t
Transcutaneous energy transfer
       (TET), 451
Transected aorta, 551-552
Transesophageal echocardiography
       (TEE), 103, 153, 154t
Transfusion therapy/blood
       conservation, 160-161
Transient ischemia, 204t
Transmyocardial laser
       revascularization (TMLR), 272
Transmyocardial revascularization
       (TMR), 69, 272
Transplantation, 463-494
   bilateral lung, 491-492
   donor organs, 464-466
   emotional aspects, 464-465
   general considerations, 463-464
   heart. *See* Heart transplantation.
   heart-lung, 483-487
   lung. *See* Lung transplantation.
   nursing care, 474b-476b
   organ recovery, 465-466
   recipient preparation, 466
   xenotransplantation, 467

Transposition of the great arteries,
       531f
Transsternal bilateral anterior
       thoracotomy, 214t, 217f
Transthoracic DeBakey vascular
       clamps, 77f
Transthoracic echocardiography
       (TTE), 103
Transvenous endomyocardial biopsy,
       480, 481
Trauma, 547. *See also* Emergency
       situations.
Triangulation, 5f
Tricuspid apparatus, 375
Tricuspid atresia, 531f
Tricuspid insufficiency, 378f
Tricuspid regurgitation, 376-377
Tricuspid stenosis, 377
Tricuspid valve, 192f, 193f, 196, 377f
Tricuspid valve commissurotomy, 387
Tricuspid valve disease, 375-378
Tricuspid valve procedures, 375-391
   CAD, 376
   cardiac catheterization, 379-380
   diagnostic evaluation, 378-380
   documentation, 382b
   Ebstein's anomaly, 376, 379f
   echocardiography, 379
   endocarditis, 376
   equipment, 382b
   Marfan's syndrome, 376
   nursing care, 381t
   patient teaching, 381-382
   physical examination, 378
   postoperative complications, 390-
       391
   procedural considerations, 382-383
   reparative procedures, 384-387
   replacement, 387-390
   rheumatic disease, 376
   RNFA considerations, 383b
   tricuspid apparatus, 375
   tricuspid regurgitation, 376-377
   tricuspid stenosis, 377
   tricuspid valve commissurotomy,
       387
   tricuspid valvulectomy, 390
Tricuspid valve replacement, 387-390
Tricuspid valvulectomy, 390
Tridil, 156t
Triggered activity, 501
Triple-vessel coronary artery disease,
       198
Troponin, 116
Troponin C, 116
Troponin I (TnI), 116
Troponin T (TnT), 116
True aneurysms, 398, 399f
TTE, 103
Tube grafts, 84
Tuffier, Theodore, 13
Tumors, 565-568
Tunica adventitia, 209f, 395
Tunica intima, 209f, 395
Tunica media, 209f, 395

Two-dimensional echocardiograms, 103
Type I neurologic injury, 181
Type II neurologic injury, 181

U

Ulnar artery, 208f, 274
Ultane, 156t
Ultiva, 156t
Ultrasonic energy, 63
Ultrasonic scalpel, 63
Unclassified cardiomyopathy, 434
Underuse, 174
Uniform Anatomical Gift Act, 151
Uniform Determination of Death Act, 465
United Network of Organ Sharing (UNOS), 466
UNOS, 466
Unstable angina, 261
Unstented aortic valve allograft, 353f
Upright tilt-table test, 504
Urinalysis, 113t
Urinary drainage catheter, 154t
Urinary/renal status, 125
Urokinase, 114t

V

VADs. *See* Ventricular assist devices (VADs).
Valium, 157t
Vallari, Rosalind, 17
Valuing, 126, 134
Valve instrument extras, 80b
Valve prostheses
    aortic valve, 343, 344f, 352-353
    mitral valve, 334-336
    thoracic aorta, 423
    tricuspid valve, 388
Vancomycin, 157t
Vascular clamps, 79b, 80b
Vasopressin, 434
VATS, 551
Vecuronium, 156t

Venoarterial bypass, 247, 248f
Venous cannulas, 66f
Venous circulation, 210f
Venovenous bypass, 247, 248f
Venting devices, 235-236
Ventricular assist devices (VADs), 438-452. *See also* Mechanical/biologic circulatory assistance
    Abiomed system, 442-444
    centrifugal pumps, 439-440
    contradictions/considerations, 441b
    HeartSaver VAD, 451-452
    implantable axial flow systems, 452
    implantable systems, 448-450
    implantation, 444b
    nursing care, 443b, 444b
    operative considerations, 445-448
    pulsatile devices, 441-448
    roller pumps, 441
    Thoratec system, 444-445
    total artificial heart, 451
Ventricular asynergy, 263b
Ventricular conduction, 499-500
Ventricular dysrhythmias, 521-524
Ventricular endoaneurysmorrhaphy, 296-298
Ventricular fibrillation (VF), 502f, 521-524
Ventricular hypertrophy, 433
Ventricular septal defect (VSD), 528t
Ventricular septal defect (VSD) repair, 298-303
Ventricular septum, 193, 194f
Ventricular tachycardia (VT), 503f, 521-524
Verapamil, 157t
Versed, 156t
VF, 502f, 521-524
Video-assisted thoracic surgery (VATS), 551
Video monitors, 6f9
Vineberg, Arthur, 14
Virtual Reality (VR) technology, 25

Visceral pericardium, 187
Volar digital vein, 210f
Volume expanders, 169t
von Decastello, Alfred, 6
VR technology, 25
VSD, 528t
VSD repair, 298-303
VT, 521-524

W

Waller, Augustus, 2
Warfarin, 114t
Warfarin (coumadin) anticoagulation therapy, 318b
Warm heart surgery, 251-252
Waters, Daniel James, 95; 430
West, John, 13
What if exercises, 30, 49-50
Wiggers, Carl, 4
Williams, Chizuko, 18
Wolff-Parkinson-White (WPW) syndrome, 517
Women
    CAD, 99t, 273
    hemodynamic responses to exercise, 101t
Work environment, 34
Woven grafts, 83
WPW syndrome, 517

X

Xenotransplantation, 467
X-ers, 24
Xiphoid process, 187, 188f
Xylocaine, 157t

Y

Young/old, physiologic features, 121t

Z

Zemuron, 156t
Zipes, Douglas P., 495